Textbook of Neurology

Textbook of Neurology

Julien Bogousslavsky, M.D.

Professor and Chairman, University Department of Neurology, and Chief of Neurology Service, Centre Hospitalier Universitaire Vaudois, Lausanne, Switzerland

Marc Fisher, M.D.

Professor of Neurology and Radiology, University of Massachusetts Medical School, Worcester

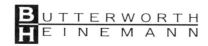

Boston   Oxford   Johannesburg   Melbourne   New Delhi   Singapore

Library of Congress Cataloging-in-Publication Data

Textbook of neurology/ [edited by] Julien Bogousslavsky, Marc Fisher.

     p.   cm.

     Includes bibliographical references and index.

     ISBN 0-7506-9918-3

     1. Nervous system--Diseases.   2. Neurology.   I. Bogousslavsky,

Julien.   II. Fisher, Marc, 1948-

     [DNLM: 1. Nervous System Diseases.   WL 140 T3545 1998]

     RC346.T448   1998

     616.8--dc21

     DNLM/DLC

     for Library of Congress   98-21166

                                          CIP

British Library Cataloguing-in-Publication Data
A catalogue record for this book is available from the British Library.

Contents

Contributing Authors

Alberto Albanese, M.D.
Professor and Chairman of Neurology, University of Lausanne, Lausanne, Switzerland

Ursula E. Anwer, M.D.
Assistant Professor of Neurology, University of Massachusetts Medical School, Worcester

Gil Assal, M.D.
Professor of Neuropsychology, Centre Hospitalier Universitaire Vaudois, Lausanne, Switzerland

Sevin Balkan, M.D.
Professor of Neurology and Anatomy, Department of Neurology, Akdeniz University School of Medicine, Antalya, Turkey

Frederick G. Barker II, M.D.
Instructor in Surgery, Harvard Medical School, Boston; Assistant in Neurosurgery, Massachusetts General Hospital

Kyra J. Becker, M.D.
Assistant Professor of Neurology and Neurological Surgery, University of Washington School of Medicine, Seattle

James P. Bennett, Jr., M.D., Ph.D.
Professor of Neurology and Psychiatric Research and Director, Center for the Study of Neurodegenerative Diseases, University of Virginia School of Medicine, Charlottesville

James L. Bernat, M.D.
Professor of Neurology, Dartmouth Medical School, Hanover, New Hampshire; Senior Neurologist, Dartmouth-Hitchcock Medical Center, Lebanon

Nadir E. Bharucha, M.D., F.A.M.S. (India), F.R.C.P. (Lond), F.R.C.P. Neurology (Canada), Diplomate, American Board of Neurology and Psychiatry (N)
Associate Professor of Neurology and Consultant Neurologist, Bombay Hospital Institute of Medical Sciences, Mumbai, India; Head, Department of Neuroepidemiology, Medical Research Centre, Bombay Hospital Trust, Mumbai

Julien Bogousslavsky, M.D.
Professor and Chairman, University Department of Neurology, and Chief of Neurology Service, Centre Hospitalier Universitaire Vaudois, Lausanne, Switzerland

Thomas Brandt, M.D., F.R.C.P.
Chairman of Neurology, Klinikum Grosshadern, Ludwig-Maximilians-University, Munich, Germany

Louis R. Caplan, M.D.
Professor and Chair of Neurology and Professor of Medicine, Tufts University School of Medicine, Boston; Neurologist-in-Chief, New England Medical Center, Boston

Chantal Ceuterick, Ph.D.
Lecturer, University of Antwerp, Antwerp, Belgium; Head, Laboratory of Electron Microscopy of the Born-Bunge Foundation, University of Antwerp

David A. Chad, M.D.
Professor of Neurology and Pathology, University of Massachusetts Medical School, Worcester

Richard K.T. Chan, M.B., B.S., M.R.C.P. (UK)
Consultant Neurologist, Department of Medicine, National University Hospital, Singapore

Stephanie Clarke, M.D.
Assistant Professor, Division of Neuropsychology, Centre Hospitalier Universitaire Vaudois, Lausanne, Switzerland

Patricia K. Coyle, M.D.
Professor of Neurology, State University of New York at Stony Brook School of Medicine; Attending Neurologist, Stony Brook University Medical Center

Robin I. Davidson, M.D.
Associate Professor of Neurosurgery, University of Massachusetts Medical School, Worcester

Stephen M. Davis, M.B., B.S., M.D., F.R.A.C.P.
Professor of Neurology, University of Melbourne, Parkville, Victoria, Australia; Director of Neurology, Royal Melbourne Hospital, Parkville

Oscar H. Del Brutto, M.D.
Assistant Professor of Clinical Neurology, Neurology Postgraduate School, School of Medicine, Catholic University, Guayaquil, Ecuador; Chief of Neurology, Luis Vernaza Hospital, Guayaquil

Giuseppe De Michele, M.D.
Assistant Professor of Neurology, Federico II University, Naples, Italy

Annelise Dewarrat, M.D.
Department of Neurology, Centre Hospitalier Universitaire Vaudois, Lausanne, Switzerland

Marianne Dieterich, M.D.
Professor, Department of Neurology, Klinikum Grosshadern, Ludwig-Maximilians-University, Munich, Germany

David A. Drachman, M.D.
Professor and Chairman, Department of Neurology, University of Massachusetts Medical School, Worcester

C.M. Ellis, B.Sc., M.R.C.P.
Research Registrar in Neurology, Department of Clinical Neurosciences, Institute of Psychiatry, London

Alessandro Filla, M.D.
Associate Professor of Neurology, Federico II University, Naples, Italy

Marc Fisher, M.D.
Professor of Neurology and Radiology, University of Massachusetts Medical School, Worcester

Hans-Joachim Freund, M.D., F.R.C.P.
Professor and Chairman of Neurology, Heinrich-Heine-Universität Düsseldorf, Düsseldorf, Germany

Bertrand Gaymard, M.D., Ph.D.
Department of Neurophysiology, Hôpital de la Salpêtrière, Paris

Joseph Ghika, M.D.
Department of Neurology, Centre Hospitalier Universitaire Vaudois, Lausanne, Switzerland

Flemming Gjerris, M.D., D.Sc.
Professor and Chairman, University Clinic of Neurosurgery, Rigshospitalet, Copenhagen, Denmark

Francesc Graus, M.D.
Assistant Professor of Medicine, Service of Neurology, Hospital Clinic, Universitat de Barcelona, Catalonia, Spain

Steven M. Greenberg, M.D., Ph.D.
Assistant Professor of Neurology, Harvard Medical School and Massachusetts General Hospital, Boston

Patrice Guex, M.D.
Médecin-Chef, Service de Psychiatrie de Liaison, Centre Hospitalier Universitaire Vaudois, Lausanne, Switzerland

Jean-Marc Guglielmi, M.D.
Chef de Clinique-Assistant, Service de Neurologie Adulte, Centre Hospitalier, Universitaire de Bicêtre, Le Kremlin-Bicêtre, France

David H. Gutmann, M.D., Ph.D.
Assistant Professor of Neurology, Pediatrics, and Genetics and Director, Neurofibromatosis Program, St. Louis Children's Hospital and Washington University School of Medicine, St. Louis

Vladimir Hachinski, M.D., F.R.C.P.(C), M.Sc. (DME), D.Sc. (Med)
Richard and Beryl Ivey Professor and Chair, Department of Clinical Neurosciences, The University of Western Ontario, London, Ontario, Canada; Chairman and Consultant Neurologist, London Health Sciences Centre-University Campus, London

Werner Hacke, M.D., Ph.D.
Professor and Chairman, Department of Neurology, Ruprecht-Karls-University, Medical School, Heidelberg, Germany

Alexander Halim, M.P.H., M.Phil.
Doctoral Candidate, Department of Epidemiology (Public Health), Columbia University Graduate School of Arts and Sciences, New York

Daniel Hanley, M.D.
Professor of Neurology and Director, Division of Neurosciences Critical Care, Johns Hopkins Hospital, Baltimore

Christian W. Hess, M.D.
Professor of Neurology, University of Bern Medical Faculty, Bern, Switzerland; Medical Director (Chairman), University Department of Neurology, Inselspital Bern

Chung Y. Hsu, M.D., Ph.D.
Professor and Head, Cerebrovascular Disease Section, Department of Neurology, Washington University School of Medicine and Barnes-Jewish Hospital, St. Louis

Manabu Ikeda, M.D., Ph.D.
Assistant Professor of Neuropsychiatry, Ehime University School of Medicine, Shigenobu, Onsen-gun, Ehime, Japan

Douglas E. Kargman, M.D., M.S.
Assistant Professor of Neurology, Columbia University College of Physicians and Surgeons, New York; Assistant Attending Neurologist, Presbyterian Hospital of the City of New York

John J. Kelly, Jr., M.D.
Professor and Chair of Neurology, The George Washington University Medical Center and The George Washington University Hospital, Washington, D.C.

Christine J. Kilpatrick, M.B., B.S., M.D., F.R.A.C.P.
Deputy Director of Neurology, Head of Comprehensive Epilepsy Programme, The Melbourne Neuroscience Centre, The Royal Melbourne Hospital, Parkville, Victoria, Australia

Jong Sung Kim, M.D.
Associate Professor of Neurology, University of Ulsan, Asan Medical Center, Seoul, South Korea

Thierry Kuntzer, M.D.
Médecin Adjoint, Department of Neurology, Centre Hospitalier Universitaire Vaudois, Lausanne, Switzerland

Catherine Lamy, M.D.
Neurologist, Hôpital Sainte-Anne, Paris

P. Nigel Leigh, B.Sc., Ph.D., F.R.C.P.
Professor of Clinical Neurology, Institute of Psychiatry and King's College School of Medicine and Dentistry, London

David Leppert, M.D.
Consultant, University Department of Neurology, Katonsspital Basel, Basel, Switzerland

Kerry H. Levin, M.D.
Staff Neurologist, Cleveland Clinic Foundation; Clinical Associate Professor, Department of Neurology, Pennsylvania State University School of Medicine, Hershey

Teng-nan Lin, Ph.D.
Assistant Research Fellow, Division of Neuroscience, Institute of Biomedical Sciences, Academia Sinica, Taipei, Taiwan

N. Scott Litofsky, M.D., F.A.C.S.
Associate Professor, Division of Neurological Surgery; Co-Director, Center for Skull Base Diseases, University of Massachusetts Medical School, Worcester

Randall R. Long, M.D., Ph.D.
Associate Professor and Vice-Chair of Neurology, University of Massachusetts Medical School, Worcester

Jean-Jacques Martin, M.D.
Professor of Neurology, University of Antwerp, Antwerp, Belgium; Head of Neurology, University Hospital of Antwerp

Jean-Louis Mas, M.D.
Professor of Neurology, University René Descartes, Paris; Head of Neurology, Hôpital Sainte-Anne, Paris

Christopher J. Mathias, D.Phil., D.Sc., F.R.C.P.
Professor of Neurovascular Medicine, University of London, Neurovascular Medicine Unit, Division of Neuroscience and Psychological Medicine, Imperial College School of Medicine at St. Mary's; and Autonomic Unit, University Department of Clinical Neurology, Institute of Neurology, University College, London; Consultant Physician, St. Mary Hospital, Western Eye Hospital, and The National Hospital for Neurology and Neurosurgery, London

Aaron Miller, M.D.
Professor of Clinical Neurology, State University of New York Health Sciences Center at Brooklyn; Director, Division of Neurology, Maimonides Medical Center, Brooklyn

Kazuo Minematsu, M.D., Ph.D.
Director, Cerebrovascular Division, National Cardiovascular Center, Osaka, Japan

Patricia M. Moore, M.D.
Associate Professor of Neurology, Wayne State University School of Medicine, Detroit

Bernard Nater, M.D.
Associate Neurologist, Centre Hospitalier Universitaire Vaudois, Lausanne, Switzerland

Christopher S. Ogilvy, M.D.
Associate Professor of Surgery, Harvard Medical School, Boston; Associate Visiting Neurosurgeon and Director, Cerebrovascular Surgery, Massachusetts General Hospital, Boston

Mehmet Zülküf Önal, M.D.
Specialist of Neurology, Akdeniz University School of Medicine, Antalya, Turkey

Charles Pierrot-Deseilligny, M.D.
Professor of Neurology, University Paris VI; Chairman of Neurology, Hôpital de la Salpêtrière, Paris

Pierre Pollak, M.D.
Professor of Neurology, Joseph Fourier Universitaire de Grenoble, Grenoble, France; Chairman of Neurology, Centre Hospitalier Universitaire de Grenoble

Disya Ratanakorn, M.D.
Assistant Professor, Division of Neurology, Department of Medicine, Faculty of Medicine, Ramathibodi Hospital, Mahidol University, Bangkok, Thailand

Roberta H. Raven, B.A. (Sydney), M.B.B.S. (Sydney), D.R.C.O.G. (UK)
Honorary Research Associate, Department of Neuroepidemiology, Medical
Research Centre, Bombay Hospital Trust, Mumbai, India

Lawrence D. Recht, M.D.
Professor of Neurology, University of Massachusetts Medical School, Worcester

Ramón Reñé, M.D.
Staff, Service of Neurology, Ciutat Sanitaria i Universitaria de Bellvitge, Barcelona,
Spain

E. Bernd Ringelstein, M.D.
Professor of Neurology, Klinik und Poliklinik für Neurologie, Westfälische,
Wilhelms-Universität Münster, Münster, Germany

Gustavo C. Román, M.D., F.A.C.P.
Clinical Professor of Neurology, University of Texas Medical School at San Antonio

Kai M. Rösler, M.D.
Lecturer and Consultant of Clinical Neurophysiology, University of Bern, Bern,
Switzerland; Head of Electroneuromyographic Unit, University Department of
Neurology, Inselspital Bern

Ralph L. Sacco, M.D., M.S.
Associate Professor of Neurology and Public Health (Epidemiology) and Associate
Chairman of Neurology, Columbia University College of Physicians and Surgeons,
New York; Associate Attending Neurologist, Presbyterian Hospital of the City of
New York

Gerard Said, M.D.
Chef de Service, Service de Neurologie Adulte, Centre Hospitalier, Universitaire de
Bicêtre, Le Kremlin-Bicêtre, France

Akira Sano, M.D., Ph.D.
Associate Professor of Neuropsychiatry, Ehime University School of Medicine,
Shigenobu, Onsen-gun, Ehime, Japan

Stefan Schwarz, M.D.
Department of Neurology, University of Heidelberg, Heidelberg, Germany

Adolf Pou Serradell, M.D.
Professor of Neurology, Universitat Autonoma de Barcelona, Barcelona, Spain;
Chief of Neurology, Hospital Universitari del Mar, Barcelona

Christian J.M. Sindic, M.D., Ph.D.
Professor of Neurology, Laboratory of Neurochemistry, Université Catholique de
Louvain, Faculté de Médecine, Brussels, Belgium

Andreas J. Steck, M.D.
Professor and Chairman of Neurology, University Hospitals, Basel, Switzerland

Friedrich Stiefel, M.D.
Chef de Clinique, Service de Psychiatrie de Liaison, Centre Hospitalier Universitaire Vaudois, Lausanne, Switzerland

Terri Strassburger, M.D.
Neuromuscular Fellow, The George Washington University Medical Center, Washington, D.C.

Lewis Sudarsky, M.D.
Associate Professor of Clinical Neurology, Harvard Medical School, Boston; Assistant Chief, Neurology Service, Veterans Administration Medical Center, West Roxbury, Massachusetts; Director, Movement Disorders Division, Brigham and Women's Hospital, Boston

Joan M. Swearer, Ph.D.
Assistant Professor of Neurology and Psychiatry, University of Massachusetts Medical School, Worcester

Naoko Tachibana, M.D., Ph.D.
Assistant Professor of Neuropsychiatry, Ehime University School of Medicine, Shigenobu, Onsen-gun, Ehime, Japan

Hirotaka Tanabe, M.D., Ph.D.
Professor and Chairman of Neuropsychiatry, Ehime University School of Medicine, Shigenobu, Onsen-gun, Ehime, Japan

Charles H. Tegeler, M.D.
Associate Professor of Neurology; Head, Section on Stroke and Cerebrovascular Disease; and Director, Neurosonology Laboratory, Bowman Gray School of Medicine of Wake Forest University, Winston-Salem, North Carolina

Philippe Vuadens, M.D.
Associate Doctor, Department of Neurology, Centre Hospitalier Universitaire Vaudois, Lausanne, Switzerland

Patrik Vuilleumier, M.D.
Visiting Research Fellow, Department of Neurology, University of California, Davis, School of Medicine and Veterans Affairs Medical Center, Martinez

Atsushi Yamadori, M.D.
Professor, Section of Neuropsychology, Division of Disability Science, Tohoku University Graduate School of Medicine, Sendai, Japan

Preface

Neurology is undergoing a dramatic change in focus and practice. Disorders of the brain, spinal cord, peripheral nerves, and muscles encompass the traditional discipline of neurology, which has expanded over the years to include electrodiagnosis (e.g., electroencephalography, electromyography), neuroradiology, sonology, and other areas. Neurologic examination and history form the cornerstones of clinical assessment of patients with neurologic disorders, and they must be performed skillfully. Exposure to the basics of imaging, ultrasound, and electrodiagnostic principles; neuropsychology, and epidemiology is also valuable. Neurologic diagnosis can in some cases be made from a thorough understanding of symptoms (such as coma), patterns of weakness, sensory dysfunction, and characteristic abnormalities. Other neurologic diagnoses require a reasonable familiarity with specific disorders that affect the central and peripheral nervous systems. This book is therefore organized into three distinct sections: introductory principles of neurology, commonly encountered symptoms and signs, and specific neurologic disorders.

The intent of this book is to serve as an introduction to the field of neurology for medical students and more advanced trainees who are beginning to explore this fascinating and common medical discipline. It is our hope that this book will also serve as a reliable, easily approachable, and fairly comprehensive resource for practicing physicians who encounter neurologic problems. It is not intended to be an exhaustive, in-depth treatise on neurology; rather, it is a reader-friendly, general reference that will stimulate readers to pursue other, more in-depth neurologic texts and articles.

The contributors to this book represent five continents and 16 countries, providing a unique global perspective. With the current explosion of communication technology, knowledge can be exchanged all over the world instantaneously, weaving a truly international web for information transfers. This volume was specifically designed to reflect the truly global knowledge base currently available about the nervous system and its disorders. We hope that a worldwide audience will take advantage of the information provided by this book's talented, knowledgeable, and dedicated contributing authors. Without their inspired efforts, this work would not have been possible.

As we move into the next millennium, those interested in the nervous system and its disorders can anticipate many exciting and important advances. It is hoped that future editions will reflect the expanding knowledge in this important area and inspire interested readers to participate in the effort to understand how the nervous system functions and to correct its maladies.

J.B
M.F.

Textbook of Neurology

Section I
Basic Principles of Neurology

Chapter 1
The Neurologic Examination

Louis R. Caplan

Chapter Plan

One of the great attractions of clinical neurology is that experienced clinicians, after obtaining a history and performing general and neurologic examinations, can make reasonably accurate predictions of the location of a problem within the nervous system and are able to generate a logical list of causes and probable disease mechanisms. Most other medical specialists must rely on the laboratory to derive such a list. Important lesions within the central and peripheral nervous systems nearly always cause abnormalities evident to the patient (symptoms) and to the alert examining physician (signs). The neurologic examination should consist of part routine and part hypothesis testing. An effective clinician plans and tailors the general and neurologic examinations to hypotheses generated from the history. We see what we look for. During the history, the clinician should make hypotheses about the type of disease process (*What* is the nature of the pathologic condition?) and the location of the disease in the nervous system (*Where* are the abnormalities located?). As the examination proceeds, these hypotheses may need revision if there are unexpected findings.

The most unique feature that separates doctor–patient interactions from those of other professions, businesses, and endeavors is examination of the human body. The examination is often sensitive, occasionally uncomfortable, and often accompanied by anxiety as to what the physician might find. The physician's handling of the examination is very important to patients. The laying on of hands during the examination can be quite therapeutic. A careful, thorough, and thoughtful examination does much to assure patients that they are in good hands. A hurried, cursory, or insensitive examination is not readily forgotten. It is important to perform at least some parts of the examination on all physician visits.

An example will help to illustrate the hypothesis-testing aspect of the initial neurologic examination.

The history reveals that a 55-year-old woman with past hypertension has noted some intermittent numbness and weakness in her right hand during the past month. She has not noted pain and is uncertain of the exact location of the numbness. As she relates the history, the clinician is thinking about the likely nervous system localizations that might explain the symptoms. A lesion in the left sensory-motor cortex adjacent to the central sulcus over the cerebral convexity could yield motor and sensory symptoms. A vascular occlusive process could explain the intermittency of the symptoms. Alternatively, a right cervical spinal root or cord lesion or a lesion of the right ulnar or median nerve in the arm or at the wrist is also plausible. Changes in position or activity in a patient with mechanical compression might explain the variability of symptoms. Considering these possibilities, the physician plans to test left cerebral functions, especially language. Neck mobility and discomfort with motion would also be worth examining, considering the possibility of a localization in the cervical spine. Defining any weakness, atrophy, loss of sensation, and reflex abnormalities in the hand will be essential for localization. The physician plans to test the specific muscles innervated by the median and ulnar nerves, and to test for a Tinel's sign and for the induction of paresthesiae when the wrist is flexed.

In the scenario presented, if the initial testing of the mental state shows a naming, language, or reading and writing abnormality, then other tests of left cerebral function are important for localizing the lesion. Furthermore, when there is one cerebral lesion, there may be others lurking so that cerebral functions will be tested in more detail than if no brain lesion is suspected. Suppose that cortical functions were normal but examination of the right arm revealed hyperreflexia and that the right Babinski's response was extensor. Then careful testing to attempt to localize the lesion along the pyramidal tract pathway would be pursued. Thus, the initial findings influence and dictate further testing. An alert clinician keeps in mind the differential diagnostic possibilities and notes with each examination result whether the finding favors or excludes any of the extant possibilities or raises new diagnostic considerations. The strategy can be likened to a football coach who carefully plans the first plays from prior knowledge of the other team. Subsequent plays depend on the success of the ini-

tial plays and data gleaned from the response of the opponents. Similarly, a clinician must maintain mental flexibility and alertness as the examination proceeds. At the end of the examination, the clinician must be prepared to make preliminary *what* and *where* diagnoses and to plan investigations if necessary to confirm, elaborate, or refute these diagnostic possibilities.

Content and Technique of the Examination

The traditional neurologic examination consists of five parts: mental state testing, cranial nerve testing, motor testing, sensory testing, and reflex testing. Some parts of the examination are specific to brain locations, whereas in other parts of the examination the distribution, nature, and association of different types of abnormalities are necessary to localize the nervous system lesion. Abnormalities of mental (cognitive and behavioral) functions are rather specific to the cerebral hemispheres. Cranial nerve tests assess the functions of the brain stem and its nerves and pathways. In contrast, motor abnormalities could arise from the cerebrum, brain stem, cerebellum, spinal cord, nerve roots, peripheral nerves, or skeletal muscle. Localization of the abnormality depends on the nature of the findings (e.g., atrophy, fasciculations, tenderness); the distribution of the findings (bilateral, proximal, distal, one limb, or one side of the body); and association with sensory, reflex, cranial nerve, and cognitive and behavioral signs. Similarly, sensory abnormalities can arise at many levels, and localization depends mostly on the type of abnormality (e.g., pain and temperature, touch, position sense, all modalities), the distribution (ulnar nerve, radicular, hemicorporeal, etc.), and associated motor, reflex, and other signs. Some reflexes are attributable to local reflex arcs (e.g., knee, ankle, and cutaneous reflexes), although they are also influenced by brain and spinal pathways, whereas others (e.g., Babinski's and Hoffmann's reflexes) reflect pyramidal tract disease rostral to the level of the abnormality.

The neurologic examination should be integrated with the general examination for ease of performance and comfort to the patient. The examination should begin with the mental state while the patient is seated and before he or she undresses. Cranial nerves are tested during the examinations of the facial structures: eyes, ears, nose, and mouth. The motor, sensory, and reflex functions in each limb are tested, and a general examination of the skin, joints, and pulses within the limbs is performed. Ordinarily, the hands and arms are tested, then the lower limbs. Although all neurologic functions are tested concurrently in the limbs, it is always best to record and think of the findings in respect to motor, sensory, and reflex functions.

Probably the most important areas of the examination are testing of mental functions, vision and eye motions, and muscle strength. These areas are almost never tested adequately by non-neurologists and require practice and experience for interpretation. Mental state tests are an integral part of the neurologist's examination and should not be relegated to a neuropsychologist as part of formal neurometric testing. Similarly, visual functions and eye movements cannot be delegated to optometrists and ophthalmologists, and muscle testing cannot be left solely to physical therapists and physiatrists. Space limitations prevent full discussion here of the techniques and distribution of abnormalities. Standard texts on the neurologic examination should be consulted for those details.

Examination of the Mental State

Testing of cerebral functions is critical for most patients with neurologic symptoms or signs, yet this part of the examination is often omitted or poorly performed. Analysis of cognitive and behavioral abilities begins when the patient is greeted in the waiting room or examining room or in the hospital bed. Appearance, facial expression, dress, grooming, social interactions, and vocabulary all give clues to mental state abnormalities. The patient's history also gives great insight into cognitive abilities. The patient should always be allowed to begin the presentation uninterrupted. What they choose to present; the vocabulary, grammar, and syntax used; the organization of the material; and its precision and detail give an alert clinician a very good idea of native intelligence and language functions as well as provide historical details.

Six major categories of mental functions should be assessed: (1) awakeness and alertness; (2) language; (3) memory; (4) visual-spatial abilities; (5) orientation, attention, and distractibility; and (6) quantitative and timing aspects of behavior—the amount of speech and interchange (Are they laconic, loquacious, or average?); spontaneity; the latency and length of replies; the ability to persevere with tasks and answers to queries; the length and depth of replies.

Mental state evaluation can be divided into two broad categories: (1) observation of the patient's intellect and behavior during the interview and examination, which can be thought of as *gestalt* observation, since it is general, unfocused, and informally assessed; and (2) *formal* testing of intellect and behavior. Formal testing should routinely consist of assessment of memory; speech functions; visual-spatial abilities; and tests of orientation, attention, and concentration. These functions are emphasized in formal testing because focal brain lesions can cause isolated dysfunction of one or more of these capabilities and because these functions are difficult to assess and quantitate without specific tests. Neurologists should assess the mental state in each patient they see. When the symptoms suggest possible brain disease, formal testing should be done. In some patients with symptoms that indicate disease of muscle or the peripheral nervous system, testing is often informal, gestalt-type evaluation. The main purpose of examining a patient's mental state is to detect focal brain disease, not to quantitate the patient's intelligence or degree of impairment. Lack of intelligence is quite common in the general population, and most of these persons have no neurologic disease. Moreover, the brief time usually spent on mental state testing does not allow adequate quantification of intellectual ability. In practice, physicians who test general knowledge and try to quantify intelligence make a quick biased judgment of whether a patient is up to his or her usual par. They then gauge the questions by a rough estimate of the patient's education and possible IQ. If the patient is dressed humbly and works as a menial laborer, very simple questions are asked. If the patient is a bright-looking person and possibly a college student, quite different questions are used. In either case, the examiner can find the patient's intelligence wanting by making the questions too difficult or can overlook loss of intelligence by aiming the questions too low. Let's look at the usual general intelligence questions asked: Who is the president? Who are your senators, congressmembers, and the mayor? Name in reverse the last six presidents. What are the capitals of Colorado, Germany, and the Netherlands? Who won the Super Bowl and the World Series last year? Who pitches for the Red Sox? Tell me about Sputnik, Watergate, the Gulf War. What were the dates of the Civil War and World War II? These questions are answered quite variably by "normal" persons encountered on the street or in a physician's office because people's interests, experiences, and backgrounds are quite different. Also, many patients are offended or put off by this type of questioning. When neurologists need to measure and quantify a patient's IQ, it should be done by formal full-length evaluation using standard tests such as the Wechsler Adult Intelligence Scale (WAIS). General gestalt estimates based on dress, hair style, manners, interpersonal behavior, hygiene, mannerisms, gestures, and vocabulary are probably as useful as biased nonstandard brief questioning. Much can be learned about each patient by close scrutiny during the history-taking interview. Ask the patient for specific data: names, address, dates, times. When the patient gives a general answer, press for more specific information. When did that happen? What was the doctor's name? Do you recall the address, phone number, and date of your visit? Note how the patient organizes the history. What vocabulary is used? Are reports consistent?

Let us now turn to the content of formal testing. It is useful to begin by asking the patient to write a paragraph. Evaluating a patient's use of written language is an excellent way to screen language capability. No aphasic patient writes and reads normally. The paragraph can be about a general topic of the patient's choosing or a specific dictated subject. Sample topics include: Write a letter to a relative describing your symptoms. Write a paragraph about the town where you live. Tell a young person why he or she should or should not practice your profession. Alternatively, patients could be asked, while waiting to be called into the office, to write unassisted a paragraph describing their medical symptoms and why they have come to see the physician. Ask patients to identify their paragraphs by writing their name, address, and the date at the top of the paper. This tests orientation without directly calling attention to it. Note the vocabulary, grammar, syntax, and organization of the paragraph and the patient's use of space. If a language abnormality is suspected, ask the patient to write lists of objects,

for example, 10 zoo animals, the 10 largest U.S. cities, 10 articles of clothing, five means of transportation, 10 common hobbies or avocations. This tests naming, spelling, and the ability to persevere with tasks. While the patient still has pencil and paper in hand, test *visual-spatial* capabilities by asking the patient to spontaneously draw an object. Choose a simple common object with some symmetrical features, such as a clock, house, daisy, or bicycle. Next draw an abstract figure and ask the patient to copy it as exactly as possible.

Disorders of drawing and copying can be caused by either left or right cerebral lesions, usually located posteriorly in the hemispheres. Patients with right parietal damage usually copy very poorly. In their spontaneous figures, they often omit features on the left; sizes, angles, and proportions are often misjudged. Copying does not improve performance. In contrast, patients with left parietal damage often draw very simple rudimentary figures but do not omit one side of the drawing and generally estimate sizes, angles, and proportions well. They are able to copy well, greatly improving their spontaneous performance. Their problem is conceptualization of the abstract idea of the object. Patients with right parietal lobe damage have a normal concept of the object, but they cannot construct the visual-spatial components. It is just as important to test constructual abilities in patients suspected of having right cerebral lesions as it is to test language in patients with possible left cerebral disease. Speech abnormalities usually predict dominant hemisphere perisylvian disease, whereas poor copying ability suggests a right inferior parietal lobe abnormality. Still using paper and pencil, the patient can be asked to perform calculations and computations.

After patients have put the pencil and paper aside, ask them to read a paragraph. Choose a suitable paragraph from a packet of materials collected for higher cortical function testing. An Aesop's fable approximately 100 words long copied in large print on white index cards makes excellent testing material. Ask the patient to read the paragraph aloud. Notice especially articulation of the words, listening for the rhythm and ease of speech production and for dysarthria and dysphonia. Listen for omissions, word errors, pauses, and paralexic errors. Does the patient become distracted from the task? Does the loudness or force of speech diminish as the patient reads? Does tone become more nasal, as in some myasthenics? Then,

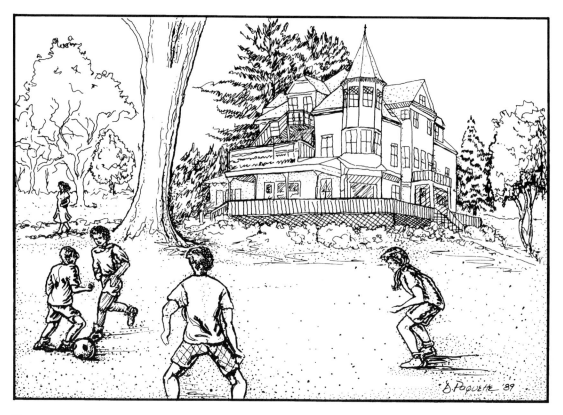

Figure 1-1. Sample picture shown to patients. (Reprinted from LR Caplan. The Effective Clinical Neurologist. Boston: Blackwell Scientific, 1990. With permission.)

ask the patient to describe the meaning of the story. If the patient was reading the story to a child, how would the patient explain the author's message? Has the patient understood what was read? Can the patient explain the message in abstract terms? Use the paragraph later as one memory item to test the patient's recall ability. If no packet of test materials is handy, an appropriate paragraph for reading can be chosen from a newspaper, magazine, or book— ubiquitous objects in doctors' offices and in the patient rooms of hospitals.

Next, show the patient a series of pictures. Some patients seem to resent "school tests" of general information, objecting that the clinician is checking if they have "lost their marbles," but very few patients object to looking at pictures because they think vision is being tested. Choose pictures of scenes cut from magazines such as *National Geographic*. The pictures chosen should have multiple people or objects scattered on the left and right sides. Figure 1-1 is an example of the type of pic-

ture used. Hold the picture in front of the patient for approximately 10 seconds. If the patient has poor visual acuity, give the picture to the patient to examine. After withdrawing the picture, ask the patient what he or she saw. After a general description, ask for specific details. When and where did the scene take place? How old are the individuals? How are they dressed? Much can be learned from the patient's performance. Watch the patient's eyes as they scan the picture. Do they search symmetrically? Have they seen the whole picture? What vocabulary does the patient use to describe the contents? Has the patient grasped the general gestalt of the picture or instead focused on a minor peripheral aspect? Patients with right cerebral hemisphere lesions often neglect figures on the left. Patients with frontal lobe disease often scan poorly and are satisfied with telling about the first feature that catches their eye. They do not extract further information from the scene. Show two or three pictures and use them for memory items later. Pictures from magazines, especially advertisements, can substitute for your own pictures. Next, show the patient pictures of well-known individuals pasted on index cards to test naming and memory. Use pictures of a variety of different individuals—prominent men and women in the fields of politics, art, and sports and comic characters. Select from these five or 10 individuals, chosen with the age, sex, and background of the patient in mind. Ask the patient to name the individuals as they are shown, or if the patient cannot name the persons, ask the patient to describe them. After a patient has named all of the individuals, I review with the patient the pictures that are still laid out on the desk. Encourage grouping, for example, pictures showing two individuals together and pictures of men or women, and figures from different occupations. For example, the clinician might say, "You have been shown three single pictures, all women (Jacqueline Onassis, Barbra Streisand, Hillary Clinton); five men, all political figures—two pairs (Franklin Delano Roosevelt with Winston Churchill, Dwight Eisenhower with Richard Nixon) and one single picture of Ronald Reagan—and one comic character, Mickey Mouse. As the individuals are named, point to the pictures grouped together to facilitate recall. Always tell patients that they will later be asked to remember what pictures they have been shown. A patient's ability to name and describe the individuals tests naming and language functions and recall of past information. After completing the neurologic examination, ask the patient to describe (1) the paragraph he or she read, (2) the scenes he or she saw, and (3) the names of the people in the pictures. This usually includes 14 data items from memory—one paragraph, three scenes, and 10 individuals. Amnesia, the inability to make new memories and to recall recent events and recently learned data, can be caused by focal lesions of the brain. Lesions causing memory loss usually affect structures within the Papez circuit—the mamillary bodies, mamillothalamic tracts, medial thalamic nuclei, fornices, and medial temporal lobes including the hippocampi and amygdala. Bilateral lesions of these structures are usually required to produce permanent amnesia, but unilateral left-sided lesions can cause amnesia lasting up to 6 months. Lesions of the septal nuclei and basal frontal lobes involving the basal nuclei of Meynert can also cause abnormalities of memory function. It is always important to test memory actively by giving patients material and later

checking recall ability. Passive memory testing—that is, asking patients what they had for breakfast or what they did yesterday—is unsatisfactory because answers can be made up or confabulated and checking the accuracy of the answers is difficult. Other active tests can also be used to check memory. Patients can be given three items to recall: for example, a horse, Santa Claus, and 125 Park Avenue. Patients should be told that they will be asked to recall the items later. Ask patients to repeat the items to be sure they have heard and retained them. Alternatively, use a story with a number of data items—for example, "Tom, Bill, and Harry went fishing in the Adirondack Mountains on July 4. They caught three mackerel and two bass, and then each had a roast beef sandwich and a bottle of Budweiser beer." This story contains 10 key facts. At the end of the examination, the degree of recall can be assessed. In aphasic patients who may be unable to reliably recite the names of items, it is usually best to cite objects in the room. The patient later is asked to point to the objects. Money is especially effective. For example, place a $5 bill under the phone, a $1 bill in the desk drawer, and 50 cents under a piece of paper. The patient is told that he or she will be asked to recall the objects and where they are located.

The clinician has now screened the patient for language, visual-spatial, memory dysfunction, and orientation. If abnormalities are found on screening tests, the evaluation of these functions should be tested further. If an abnormality of speech is present, more extensive testing of spoken language production, naming, repetition of spoken language, and comprehension of spoken and written language is necessary. A particularly useful test easily administered at the bedside is the token test of DeRenzi and Vignolo. Tokens of different sizes (small and large), shapes (triangles and squares), and colors (red, yellow, blue, green) are used. These can be made easily from wood, cardboard, or plastic and colored with a child's painting set. The patient is first given directions using a single descriptor, then two adjectives, then three descriptors. If the patient performs correctly, six descriptors are used. Relation words, which are especially difficult for aphasics, can be checked ("hold the blue one above [below, over, instead of, with] the red one"). Gray's standardized reading paragraphs are also useful for quantifying reading difficulty. Visual-spatial abnormalities can be further checked by having the patient copy a Rey figure (Figure 1-2) or construct mosaics using Koh's blocks, which are small cubes with surfaces that are one color (red, blue, and white) or split colors (red and white, blue and white, or red and blue). Diagrams of models of mosaics to be copied are available in Wechsler-Bellevue kits, since testing with Koh's blocks is a standard part of this IQ test. This subtest of the WAIS is easily administered in the office or at the bedside and is very useful in quantifying the severity of constructional visual-spatial deficits. More detailed tests of memory using various items from different sensory modalities for presentation (visual, auditory, tactile) can be given. Usually, patients with left thalamic-temporal lobe disease have difficulty remembering verbal language material, whereas right thalamic-temporal disease causes more visual memory difficulty. The other types of screening procedures that are useful as part of the mental state evaluation test a patient's ability to concentrate on and handle tasks that require persistent effort. Concentration can be tested by asking the patient to repeat series of numbers forward and backward. The numbers are given slowly ("1 . . . 7 . . . 9 . . . 5"), and then the patient repeats them as given or transposes them (5, 9, 7, 1). Normally, patients should be able to retain at least six numbers forward and five in reverse. Some patients perform this task inconsistently, transposing six numbers correctly and then failing to transpose five in the next attempt. Spelling the word "worlds" backwards is a similar task. Addition or subtraction of serial twos or threes is a similar type of concentration task, since the patient must concentrate on and recall the previous number before each addition and subtraction, a phenomenon called *working memory*. Patients with a variety of different lesions have difficulty performing long tasks. Patients with large frontal lesions or extensive bilateral cerebral disease are often abulic. *Abulia* is defined as (1) lack of spontaneity in speech and activity, (2) long latency in beginning tasks or in responding to queries or directions, (3) short, terse replies, and (4) difficulty persevering with tasks. Some tests useful in screening for abulia are counting backward as quickly as possible from 20 to 0, crossing off all the A's in a long paragraph, or instructing the patient to say "up" or "down" each time you move his or her finger. Abulic patients will often wait to begin tasks,

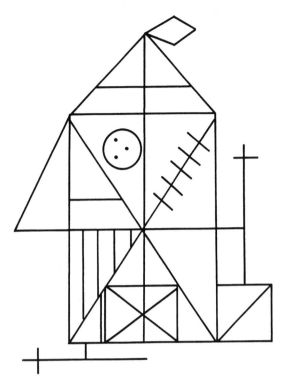

Figure 1-2. A Rey figure for copying.

sometimes requiring repetition of the directions and exhortation. Shortly after starting, they will often slow down, become distracted, or stop. For example, counting backward, they will say "20 . . 19 . . . 18 . . . . 17 . . . . . 16." They will require stimulation from the clinician to continue ("Come along. What's next?"). Some, after beginning to count backward correctly, will start to count forward (20 . . 19 . . . 18 . . . . 17 . . . . . 16 . . . . 15 . . . 16 . . 17 . . 18"). When asked to cross off all the A's on a page, they will correctly find the first few A's and then erratically choose some A's or simply stop the task. When testing position sense, abulic patients may respond correctly for the first few finger movements, then will stop responding. The examiner must prompt them ("What direction was that?" or "Now.") each time the finger is moved to elicit a verbal response.

Patients with frontal lobe lesions often have difficulty switching from one subject or task to another. Luria described a number of tests for perseveration. The patient is asked to write repeatedly a series of two

Table 1-1. Suggested Components of a Kit for Handy Cognitive Function Testing

1. A series of paragraphs (e.g., Aesop's fables)
2. Gray's reading paragraphs
3. Pictures from magazines (e.g., *National Geographic*)
4. Pictures of well-known individuals (e.g., cut from *People* or other magazines)
5. Small pictures of common objects (e.g., telephone, window shade, lamp, chimney)
6. Common objects (e.g., comb, spoon, fork, paper clip, safety pin)
7. Koh's blocks and mosaic patterns
8. Tokens (DeRenzi and Vignolo token test)
9. Identical photographs of faces for matching (e.g., taken from annual "mug shots" of house staff)
10. Colored plastic or fabric swatches for color matching and naming
11. Rey's figure
12. Short, written directions and queries (Stick out your tongue. Close your eyes. Touch your left thumb to your right ear. How old are you? Are you wearing a hat?)

lems. Orally presented computations are variably handled by normal people, and difficulty performing sequential arithmetic manipulations is a very nonspecific finding. Tests of judgment usually involve asking patients how they would behave under certain hypothetical conditions (What would you do if someone in a movie theater yelled fire? What would you do if you found stamped, addressed letters on the street?). These are intellectual tests of gamesmanship. Behavior and "judgment" under the actual circumstances are often quite different than the replies. Throughout this section, various materials useful for cortical function testing have been mentioned. It is useful for neurologists to keep small test kits in their bags or offices for ease of testing. This kit is probably more practically useful than a reflex hammer or sharp pin—objects that most neurologists find indispensable. Table 1-1 is a list of suggested components of such kits. These materials are easily collected and should be maintained and refurbished as times change.

squares, one circle, two squares, one circle, two squares, and one circle; patients with frontal lobe disease may have difficulty in switching from square to circle and will make more than two squares. Frontal lobe disease can also affect the ability to plan tasks. Ask patients to make a floor plan of a one-story house suitable for their needs. This task requires preliminary thinking to decide on the number of bedrooms and baths and the placement of the kitchen, dining area, and living room and their relation to each other and to the entrances and pathways within the house. Patients with frontal lobe dysfunction often begin impulsively without forethought, and the relations, sizes, and proportions are poorly considered.

The entire screening mental state testing should take no longer than 7–10 minutes (less if patients write their paragraphs while waiting to be seen). A number of standard tests suggested by others, for example, tests of general information, proverb interpretation, subtraction of serial 7s from 100, and so-called tests of judgment, have been intentionally omitted herein. These general information tests are biased and not diagnostic. Most individuals have been told proverbs since they were children and associate them with didactic sermons about proper behavior. By adulthood, they are sick of hearing proverbs and cannot interpret them as fresh prob-

Examination of the Cranial Nerves

Olfactory Nerves

Smell need not be routinely tested in each patient, but the neurologist should have olfactory stimuli readily available. The following are indications for testing the sense of smell:

1. Head injury. The olfactory nerves or tracts can be torn or contused. Olfactory nerve injury is especially likely if cerebrospinal fluid rhinorrhea is present.
2. Dementia. Tumors located at the base of the frontal lobe within the anterior cranial fossa such as olfactory groove meningiomas often involve or compress the olfactory nerves on one or both sides. Decreased sense of smell is also common in Alzheimer's disease.
3. Meningoencephalitis. Unilateral or bilateral anosmia may be a clue to the presence of herpes simplex virus encephalitis.
4. Unilateral gradual loss of vision in one or both eyes. Tumors and inflammatory disorders that affect the optic nerves also sometimes involve the more medially placed olfactory nerves.

When testing smell, care should be used to avoid caustic volatile substances that irritate fifth nerve endings in the nares, giving the patient a false sense of smell. Keep five vials or test tubes handy for testing smell and taste, and fill them with coffee, pipe tobacco, water, salt, and sugar. For smell, use water, salt, or sugar as controls. Have the patient occlude one nostril with a finger and then, with eyes closed, smell one of the vials with the open nostril. Patients should be able to differentiate no odor (control vials) from an odor and to tell that two odors—for example, coffee and tobacco—are different. It is not necessary to identify or name odors correctly. Identification of odors requires experience, intelligence, memory, and speech, functions that involve a large portion of the brain. We are now testing just the olfactory nerves.

Optic Nerves

Visual Acuity

Check visual acuity even when there are no visual symptoms. So many neurologic diseases affect vision that the baseline visual acuity measurement may be useful later. Use a hand-held card calibrated for visual acuity. If a chart is not handy, acuity can be estimated by whether the patient can see the head of a small pin or read newspaper print. If visual loss is severe, can the patient count fingers or detect hand movements or light? Corrected vision should be checked with glasses or contact lenses if they are worn. If patients do not have their glasses, a pinhole can be used. When visual loss can be corrected by glasses or a pinhole, it is caused by ocular refractive problems and not neurologic disease.

Visual Fields

Test the visual fields by confrontation, testing each eye individually while the patient holds one hand over the other eye. Watch the patient's eyes to ensure they are fixating on your eye. First use finger movements in the periphery of each visual field; then use a white- or red-topped pin. The key to interpreting the patient's response is the patient's answer when given an instruction ("Tell me when you see something move. Tell me when you know I have a pin. Tell me when you know the color of the pin."). The field for movement is much larger than the field for color. In patients with suspected cerebral lesions, I also test functional use of the visual fields. Walk patients over to a window and ask them what they see outside. Use pictures on the wall, advertisements and pictures in magazines, or pictures in a cortical function testing kit. Neglect of one side of visual space may be much more apparent during functional testing than during formal visual fields testing. Optokinetic nystagmus using a striped tape or rotating striped drum can also help to localize lesions that cause visual field defects.

Ophthalmoscopy

Careful observation of the ocular fundus is one of the most important parts of the physical and neurologic examination. Be sure to take time to view the disk, macula, arteries and veins, and peripheral fundus oculi adequately.

Oculomotor, Trochlear, and Abducens Nerves

Pupils and Their Reactions

Note the size and shape of the pupils and their position within the iris. Check both the direct and consensual reaction of the pupils to a bright flashlight. The latency, magnitude of response, and maintenance of constriction are all important. Note any asymmetry of response. Also check the response of the pupils to near fixation. When looking for a subtle Horner's syndrome, it is often useful to see if the pupil in question dilates in a dark room.

Eyelid Position

Check the position of the eyelids in reference to the corneas and pupils, noting ptosis or asymmetries. In Horner's syndrome, the lower lid is often slightly raised in addition to ptosis of the upper lid.

Eye Position and Movements

First note whether the eyes are focused straight ahead or if one eye is positioned inward or outward or if both eyes are deviated conjugately to one side. Conjugacy can be tested by using a flashlight to see if light hits the same region of the pupil in both eyes. If the ocular axes are not conjugate, use the cover/uncover test to see if the patient fixates alternately with each eye. This indicates strabismus as opposed to an acquired oculomotor disorder. Always begin analysis of eye movements by testing each eye individually, before checking conjugate horizontal and vertical gaze. The sixth nerve innervation of the lateral rectus muscle pulls the eye laterally outward (abduction). With the eye in the abducted position, the superior rectus pulls the eye upward, and the inferior rectus pulls the eye downward. The medial rectus pulls the eye inward (adduction). When the eye is adducted, the inferior oblique pulls the eye upward and the superior oblique (fourth nerve) pulls the eye downward. The third nerve innervates the medial, superior, and inferior recti and the inferior oblique muscles.

Next, examine movements of both eyes together. Check horizontal movements by giving the direction to look left and look right, and then ask the patient to follow your finger to each side. Check rapid fixations (saccades) as well as slow following movements. Note whether the two eyes move fully and together and look for nystagmus. Red glass testing is not used unless the patient reports diplopia.

Trigeminal Nerve

Corneal Reflex

Check the corneal reflex using a wisp of cotton to touch the lateral cornea when symptoms suggest a possible middle or posterior fossa lesion such as an acoustic neuroma. Look for eye closure in both the ipsilateral (direct response) and contralateral eye (consensual response). Ask the patient whether he or she feels the stimulus and whether it is the same in both eyes. In some patients, excessive blinking interferes with testing the corneal reflex. Touching the eyelash in these patients elicits a blink response, which is also a V–VII nerve reflex.

Facial Sensation

Check appreciation of touch and pin or cold sensation on the face when (1) the patient reports face pain, numbness, or paresthesiae; (2) a middle or posterior fossa lesion or multiple sclerosis is suspected; and (3) a cerebral hemispheral lesion involving the sensory cortex or parietal lobe might be present. Especially on the face, warm and cold stimuli are preferable to sharp pins. Patients, especially the very young and very old and those with trigeminal neuralgia, do not like to be jabbed with pins on their faces and cannot maintain objectivity in reporting their pin perception. A cold object (e.g., a tuning fork) is usually tolerated well, and patients can report if one area is cooler than another. In patients with cortical lesions, it is very useful to test localization of touch stimuli and extinction of bilateral stimuli. This is done by having the patient, with the eyes closed, touch the precise place on the face that you touch. Can the patient detect simultaneous touches on both sides of the face?

Jaw Strength and Reflex

Ask the patient to hold the mouth open and then closed against resistance. Feel the masticatory muscles below the temporomandibular joint to see if contractions are symmetrical. The jaw reflex can be tested by tapping a finger placed on the middle or sides of the jaw with a reflex hammer. An exaggerated reflex suggests involvement of the pyramidal tract in the rostral pons or above on one or both sides. Sometimes the reflex is more exaggerated when the jaw is tapped on the left or right side.

Facial Nerve

Facial Muscles and Their Strength

Carefully observe the patient's face while obtaining the history, not only for asymmetries, but also for blinking and facial expression. Are there parkinsonian features? Facial weakness can be elicited by asking patients to show their teeth, close their eyes, wrinkle their forehead, and grimace. Asymmetries are sometimes more evident when patients smile or laugh. A nonsensical query (e.g., "What would you do if you found a hyena in your bathtub?") often elicits a grin. The platysma is an especially useful muscle to test because asymmetries are common in patients with upper motor neuron facial weakness. Ask the patient to jut out the chin and grunt; this maneuver shows the platysma muscles bilaterally. The platysma contraction will be less present on the side opposite the upper motor neuron facial weakness. Facial reflexes can be tested by tapping the corner of the mouth or the glabella with a reflex hammer. When there is an upper motor neuron lesion, the orbicularis oculi will contract.

Taste

Gustatory ability need not be routinely tested. It should be checked if the patient has a lower motor neuron facial paralysis to differentiate a brainstem lesion from a lesion within the fallopian canal and when the patient reports abnormal smell or taste. When taste is tested, use salt and sugar. Hold the tongue out with a pad, moisten a swab, and apply salt or sugar to the side of the anterior part of the tongue where the taste buds are located. Ask the patient to raise one hand if he or she tastes something. Patients with normal taste should be able to tell water from salt and salt from sugar.

Eighth Nerve Auditory and Vestibular Portions

Hearing

It is easy to perform a simple audiogram at the bedside by using stimuli of different frequency. Going from highest to lowest frequency—a watch tick, fingers rubbing, whispered numbers, and 256- and 128-Hz tuning forks—provides a wide spectrum of sound frequencies. Patients with neurologically important hearing loss usually have difficulty hearing voice ranges. Inability to hear a watch tick is often caused by presbyacusis or noise trauma. Patients are usually quite deaf before they lose the ability to hear the tuning forks (low ranges). Test each ear separately, masking the other ear by finger rubbing or other noise. The Weber and Rinne tuning fork tests take time and are unrevealing if the patient has no hearing problem. Perform these tests only when the patient reports or you find a unilateral hearing loss.

Vestibular Testing

Vestibular testing is not routine. When the patient reports episodic or persistent dizziness or light-headed feelings, I do perform positional maneuvers

and simple caloric testing in the office or at the bedside. Most important, if a patient says that he or she develops dizziness in certain positions or circumstances, watch the patient as he or she performs these maneuvers (e.g., stooping, turning, lying with the head to the right, bending to look under a table). Look for the development of nystagmus. Examining for positional nystagmus is very useful. In the office, use two adjoining chairs, asking the patient to sit sideways on one chair with the back not restricted by a chair arm or back. Holding the patient's chin in one hand, gently ease the patient's head and trunk backward, holding your knee under the patient's back for support. The head is turned to one side while looking carefully for nystagmus as the patient is brought into the head-to-the-side position. Then the patient is quickly brought to the upright position, again watching for nystagmus and asking about sensations of dizziness. The same maneuvers are then repeated with the head turned to the other side. At the bedside, the test can be performed by having the patient sit on the side of the bed and then propelling the head and trunk backward, turning the head to the side. Patients with benign positional vertigo (the most common cause of positional dizziness), after a brief delay, have rotatory nystagmus with subjective vertigo when the head is turned to one side.

The minicaloric test of Nelson can also be administered at the bedside. A small quantity of ice water is injected into the external ear canal using a tuberculin-sized syringe. The duration of the nystagmus on the two sides is compared. The positional maneuvers and caloric testing often reproduce the patient's sensation of vertigo. When physicians are able to reproduce the sensation that patients experience spontaneously in their attacks, patients gain confidence that the clinician understands their symptoms and will be able to help. Another useful maneuver in patients with vertigo is to check for past pointing. This term does not mean cerebellar-type overshooting of the target. The patient, with eyes open, touches the nose and then the examiner's finger held outstretched near the midline. Then the patient closes his or her eyes and continues to touch the same finger. Patients with vestibular lesions with eyes closed often point past the finger to the same side no matter which arm is used. Past pointing usually indicates a peripheral vestibular lesion as opposed to a brain lesion.

Glossopharyngeal and Vagus Nerves

*Pharyngeal and Palatal Position
and Movement and Gag Reflex*

Note whether the uvula is in the midline and whether one side of the palate is drooped compared with the other side. Watch the uvula and pharyngeal pillars as the patient says "Ah." Note the extent and symmetry of the movement. Does the uvula pull to one side? Testing of the gag reflex is unpleasant for the patient and is seldom revealing. The gag reflex need not be routinely checked. Although many physicians and nurses are taught that patients with neurologic lesions should not be fed until they have a gag reflex, the relationship of the gag reflex to swallowing is the same as the relation of the biceps reflex to arm flexion. Patients with an absent biceps reflex often have normal biceps muscle strength. Similarly, some patients with absent gag reflexes swallow normally; other patients with active and hyperactive gag reflexes swallow poorly and repeatedly aspirate. The only way to judge the patient's swallowing ability is to watch the patient swallow food or liquid.

Sensation

When the patient describes numbness inside the mouth and when a posterior fossa lesion is suspected, sensation in the mouth and soft and hard palate can be tested using a stick with cotton on the end or a tongue blade.

Spinal Accessory Nerve

Neck flexor weakness is a prominent finding in patients with myopathy and motor neuron disease. Neck muscle strength should be tested in patients who have prominent widespread or diffuse muscle weakness and in patients with abnormalities of adjacent cranial nerves (nerves X and XII). Local lesions in or near the jugular foramen can affect cranial nerves IX, X, and XI together; sometimes the lesion also includes the more medially placed hypoglossal foramen, causing tongue weakness. Test the sternocleidomastoid muscles by palpating the ipsilateral muscle as the patient turns the neck to the opposite side. Shoulder shrug tests the trapezius muscles.

Hypoglossal Nerve

Can the patient protrude the tongue fully and in the midline? Is there tongue atrophy or fasciculations? Tongue strength is best tested by having the patient push the tongue forcefully into the cheek on each side while the clinician tries to resist the force of the movement by pushing the cheek from the outside.

Examination of the Motor System

Tests of strength and muscle function, limb coordination, and analysis of gait are all included during evaluation of motor functions.

Muscle Function and Strength Testing

First, inspect the limbs for loss of muscle bulk (atrophy) and for fasciculations. When the patient can exert enough force to use the limb against gravity, strength of muscles is tested by determining how well the patient can move the limb to exert force against the examiner, and if there is pain, how well the patient can maintain isometric muscle contraction against the examiner's attempt to move the part. Check proximal, middle, and distal muscles in each limb, and muscles in each nerve root and nerve distribution. The suggested muscles to routinely test and their root and nerve innervations are listed in Table 1-2.

Grade the degree of muscle weakness so that later you or other examiners can determine whether weakness is the same, worse, or improved. Use a 10-point scale, which is simply a doubling of the standard 5-point system. In the 5-point system, nearly all patients can exert force against resistance and so are graded between 4 and 5. Decimal differentiators—for example, 4.2 or 4.4—are awkward. In the 10-point system, 6 is resistance against gravity and is equivalent to 3 in the 5-point scale. The muscle strength grading system is noted in Table 1-3.

Patterns of Weakness

Experienced clinicians look for patterns of weakness that can point to various likely locations of disease and pathophysiologic conditions.

Table 1-2. Muscle Strengths to Test Routinely

Muscles	Nerve Roots	Peripheral Nerves
Upper limbs		
Deltoid	C5	Axillary
Supra- and infraspinati	C5	Nerve to the spinati
Biceps	C5–C6	Musculocutaneous
Triceps	C7	Radial
Wrist flexors	C6–C7	Median
Wrist extensors	C6–C8	Radial
Abductor pollicis brevis	C8	Median
Abductor digiti minimi	T1	Ulnar
Lower limbs		
Psoas	L2–L4	Femoral
Thigh adduction	L2–L4	Obturator
Thigh abductors	L4–S1	Superior gluteal
Thigh extensors-glutei	L5–S2	Superior and inferior gluteal
Quadriceps	L3–L4	Femoral
Hamstrings	L4–S1	Sciatic
Tibialis anterior	L4–L5	Peroneal
Foot flexors	L5–S1	Posterior tibial
Foot invertor	L5–S2	Posterior tibial
Foot abductors	L5–S1	Peroneal

Table 1-3. Muscle Strength Grading Scale

Grade	Response
1	No contraction
2	Minimal muscle contraction, no movement
3	Stronger muscle contraction, no movement
4	Slight movement of part with gravity eliminated
5	Moves limb well with gravity eliminated Can resist gravity feebly and temporarily
6	Can lift limb well against gravity but not against resistance
7	Limb easily overcome by resistance
8	Moderate resistance needed to overcome limb
9	Slight but definite weakness
10	Normal

Unilateral Pyramidal Tract Lesions (Cerebral, Brain Stem, Occasionally Spinal)

Weakness involves the limbs or parts of the limbs on one side of the body. Weakness is usually accompanied by hyperreflexia and a Babinski's sign. Weakness is usually most severe in the extensors and abductors of the upper extremity and in the thigh and leg extensors and the foot everters and extensors in the lower extremity. Arm strength on the two sides can be compared by asking the patient to hold and maintain the arms outstretched at the same level. Drift of one arm is the most common finding in patients with unilateral weakness, but in some patients the wrist or hand on the weak side will flex, showing asymmetric weakness. Extension of the metacarpal phalangeal joints and flexion of the proximal and distal interphalangeal joints are early signs of hand weakness. In some patients, when the hands are held outstretched, the little finger on the weak side will become hyperab-

ducted (digiti minimi sign). Patients with bilateral cerebral lesions or lesions of the brain stem or spinal cord that affect both sides have pyramidal distribution weakness on both sides of the body that is often asymmetrical.

Myopathies

Muscle diseases most often affect the proximal muscles in the limbs and the limb girdles bilaterally and roughly symmetrically. Most often the thighs are weaker than the shoulder muscles.

Peripheral Polyneuropathies

Weakness when present is most pronounced in the distal portions of the limbs—the hands and feet. Acute neuropathies can also cause proximal muscle weakness that is almost always accompanied by distal limb weakness, loss of deep tendon reflexes, and a glove-and-stocking type of sensory loss. In patients with postinfectious radiculoneuropathy (Guillain-Barré syndrome), there is usually combined proximal and distal limb weakness along with areflexia and bifacial paresis.

Single Peripheral Nerves (Mononeuropathies) or Nerve Roots

The weakness is in the distribution of a nerve root or peripheral nerve often with a radicular or peripheral nerve distribution sensory loss.

Coordination (Cerebellar Functions)

Coordination in the limbs should be routinely checked using finger-to-nose and toe-to-object testing. Rapid alternating movements of the hand, hand patting, touching each finger with the thumb quickly and successively, tapping quickly the end of the bent index finger on the distal interphalangeal joint of the thumb, drawing a small circle or square with the toe, and tapping the foot in rhythm are other useful tests of cerebellar functions. Abnormalities can be unilateral or bilateral.

When tremor is present, note the relative extent and nature of the tremor at rest and on finger-to-nose testing. Cerebellar-type tremors are often accentuated when patients hold their arms in the wing-beating posture.

Gait

Gait is the single most important motor function to test. Some physicians customarily watch the patient walk before they begin formal neurologic testing. Others watch gait after the rest of the examination. Be sure to notice the posture and movements of the upper limbs in addition to the legs. Note the speed, stability, and coordination of the gait.

Testing of Reflexes

Deep Tendon Reflexes

Check routinely the biceps, triceps, and brachioradialis reflexes in the upper limbs and the knee and ankle jerks in the lower limbs. Reflexes are usually graded on a 0–4 scale, with 0 being absent, 1 being underactive, 2 and 3 being average, and 4 being clearly hyperactive. Testing the jaw, facial, and glabella reflexes is important in patients with brainstem and cerebral lesions. Reflexes can be conveniently noted on a small stick figure. Asymmetry of reflexes and absent reflexes are usually significant.

Some non-neurologists limit their neurologic examination to testing of deep tendon reflexes. Very seldom is one or more abnormal reflexes the only abnormality. More often, abnormal reflexes corroborate other symptoms and signs. When looking for a subtle reflex asymmetry, it is useful to check reflexes that are normally hard to elicit—pectoral, trapezius, wrist extensor, finger flexor, thigh adductor, hamstring, and posterior tibial reflexes. On the side opposite an upper motor neuron lesion, it is often possible to elicit these reflexes, whereas they are absent in the contralateral limbs. It is easier to differentiate a positive reflex from no response than a 2+ from 3+ reflex.

Superficial Cutaneous Reflexes

The abdominal (T7–T9 upper abdominal, T11–T12 lower abdominal) and cremasteric (L1–L2) reflexes are often reduced on the side opposite a pyramidal tract lesion and the toe response (Babinski sign) is extensor. For a variety of reasons, the plantar response may be difficult to interpret. Ticklishness, hypersensitivity, toe grasp, and withdrawal are sometimes present when the Babinski response is elicited in the usual way with a key or sharp object. In these patients, either gentle stimulation with your own thumb or using the patient's thumb to elicit the plantar response avoids withdrawal. The upper or lower abdominal reflexes may be absent on one or both sides in patients with lesions in the lower thoracic spinal cord. Testing the bulbocavernosus and anal wink reflexes is useful in patients with suspected sacral cord or root lesions. Absence of a red axon flare response to scratching of the skin with a pin can indicate an abnormal autonomic nervous system response. Other autonomic function tests examine sweating, piloerection, and vascular responses to a Valsalva's maneuver.

Primitive Reflexes

Grasp, suck, rooting, and palmomental responses can indicate a release of primitive reflexes as a result of loss of cerebral function. These reflexes are seldom useful in practice.

Testing of Sensation

Patients often report subtle sensory symptoms—numbness and paresthesiae before any objective sensory abnormalities can be elicited. Extensive routine

Figure 1-3. A sample sensory chart. A patient with a severe peripheral polyneuropathy.

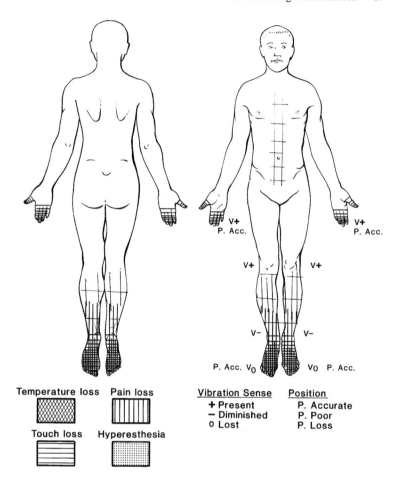

Temperature loss	Pain loss

Touch loss	Hyperesthesia

Vibration Sense	Position
+ Present	P. Accurate
— Diminished	P. Poor
0 Lost	P. Loss

sensory testing is seldom revealing when there are no sensory symptoms. Carefully check regions with sensory symptoms. Also, routinely check the face and distal limbs for touch (cotton), cold (cool tuning fork), and vibration and position sense. Check vibration sense with a l28-Hz tuning fork. Determine how long the patient can continue to feel the vibration; compare the finding with your own ability to continue to feel the vibration. When testing objective sensitivity, ask the patient to close his or her eyes and see if the patient can distinguish one object from another. Use cotton, finger touch, the sharp end of the pin, and the blunt end of the pin. This type of testing is more useful than comparing the patient's estimate of the degree of normality (e.g., if 100 represents normal sensitivity, does this sensation rate 80, 40, 60, etc.?). Thermal testing is preferred over the use of a pin. Cool objects such as a spoon, tuning fork, or metal portion of the reflex

hammer are good stimuli. Some patients, especially youngsters, lose their objectivity when approached with a sharp object. In patients with reduced alertness or those who might not be reliable observers, intersperse controls (e.g., no vibration, dull finger instead of sharp pin) amid the test stimuli to be sure that the patient is paying attention and the responses are consistent.

Record any abnormalities of elementary sensations on a sensory chart. Charts or sketches are much more revealing than verbal descriptions for showing the distribution of sensory changes on a limb or the trunk. On the chart, you can also record the results of vibration sense and position sense testing and severity and gradations of sensory loss. Figure 1-3 shows a sample sensory chart. In patients with suspected cerebral lesions, testing of touch localization in the opposite limbs, recognition of objects in the contralateral hand, and extinction of bilateral, simultaneously presented tactile stimuli are important. Some normal patients have poor graphesthesia, making this test less useful than stereognosis. Two-point discrimination is tedious and requires extensive attention and cooperation. The ability to discriminate two points differs in the proximal, middle, and distal limbs and varies with the stimuli—a compass point, pin, or the sharp end of a pencil. Abnormalities of two-point discrimination are often not reproducible.

As with the interpretation of abnormalities in the motor examination, localization of the lesions that cause sensory abnormalities depends on the nature and distribution of the findings and their association with motor and reflex signs. Certain patterns are common:

1. Cerebral hemisphere and thalamic lesions causing contralateral hemisensory loss, especially of the "cortical type" as described above
2. Brain stem lesions that cause sensory loss in a contralateral tract pattern (medial lemniscus or spinothalamic tract), sometimes with ipsilateral spinal tract of nerve V loss of pain and temperature sensation on the face
3. Spinal lesions that cause bilateral tract or Brown-Séquard–type sensory loss (ipsilateral posterior column and contralateral spinothalamic tract abnormalities)
4. Focal sensory loss in a radicular or peripheral nerve distribution
5. Peripheral polyneuropathy with glove-and-stocking distribution loss of more than one sensory modality

The most important aspect of the examination is that it be directed toward the testing of hypotheses generated from the history. When the examiner does not know what to look for, the odds are high that little of importance will be found. Even during the examination, positive findings should generate new hypotheses, which are then tested as the examination proceeds. The neurologic examination should be thorough and complete. The information gleaned cannot be duplicated by any present or future technology.

Suggested Reading

Bing R, Haymaker W. Compendium of Regional Diagnosis in Lesions of the Brain and Spinal Cord (11th ed). St. Louis: Mosby, 1940.

Brazis PW, Masdeu JC, Biller J. Localization in Clinical Neurology (3rd ed). Boston: Little, Brown, 1996.

Caplan LR. The Effective Clinical Neurologist. Boston: Blackwell Scientific, 1990.

Dawson DM, Hallett M, Millender LH. Entrapment Neuropathies. Boston: Little, Brown, 1983.

Denny-Brown D, Dawson DM, Tyler HR. Handbook of Neurological Examination and Case Recording (3rd ed). Cambridge, MA: Harvard University Press, 1982.

DeRenzi E, Vignolo L. The token test: a sensitive test to detect receptive disturbances in aphasics. Brain 1962;85:665.

Devinsky O, Feldmann E. Examination of the Cranial and Peripheral Nerves. New York: Churchill Livingstone, 1988.

Fisher CM. The neurological examination of the comatose patient. Acta Neurol Scand 1969;45(Suppl 36):1.

Haerer AF. DeJong's The Neurologic Examination (5th ed). Philadelphia: Lippincott, 1992.

Haymaker W, Woodhall B. Peripheral Nerve Injuries: Principles of Diagnosis (2nd ed). Philadelphia: Saunders, 1953.

Hier DB, Gorelick PB, Shindler AG. Topics in Behavioral Neurology and Neuropsychology. Boston: Butterworths, 1987.

Kendall FR, Kendall FP. Muscles: Testing and Function. Baltimore: Williams & Wilkins, 1949.

Luria AR. Higher Cortical Functions in Man. New York: Basic Books, 1966.

Monard-Krohn GH, Refsum S. The Clinical Examination of the Nervous System (12th ed). New York: Hoeber Medical Division of Harper & Row, 1964.

Nelson J. The minimal ice water caloric test. Neurology 1969;19:577.

Strub RL, Black FW. The Mental Status Examination in Neurology. Philadelphia: Davis, 1977.

van Gijn J. The Babinski Sign—A Centenary. Utrecht, The Netherlands: University of Utrecht, 1996.

Wartenberg R. The Examination of Reflexes: A Simplification. Chicago: Yearbook, 1945.

Chapter 2
Clinical and Biochemical Neuroanatomy

Sevin Balkan and Mehmet Zülküf Önal

Chapter Plan

Cerebral cortex
    Motor areas
    Sensory areas
    Association areas
    Cerebral dominance
Diencephalon and limbic systems
    Thalamus
    Hypothalamus
    Epithalamus
    Subthalamus
    Limbic system
Basal ganglia
    Afferents
    Internal circuits
    Efferents
    Functional and clinical considerations
Autonomic nervous system
    Sympathetic system
    Parasympathetic system
Brain stem and reticular formation
    Midbrain
    Pons
    Medulla
    Brain stem lesions
    Reticular formation
Cranial nerves
Cerebellum
Spinal cord with ascending and descending pathways
    Gray matter
    White matter

Neurovascular anatomy
    Arterial supply
    Venous drainage
Meninges, ventricular system, and cerebrospinal fluid
    Meninges
    Ventricles and cerebrospinal fluid
    Blood-brain barrier
Neurochemistry
    Acetylcholine
    Catecholamines
    Dopamine
    Noradrenaline
    Adrenaline
    Serotonin
    Histamine
    Amino acid neurotransmitters
    Excitatory amino acids
    Inhibitory amino acids
    Glycine
    Neuropeptides
    Opioid peptides

The fields of neuroanatomy and neurochemistry are the most rapidly expanding disciplines in neuroscience. The nervous system, which is bilateral and essentially symmetrical, consists of central and peripheral components, which are interconnected and interactive. The central nervous system (CNS) consists of the brain (i.e., the cerebrum, brain stem, and cerebellum) and the spinal cord. The peripheral nervous system consists of ganglia, cranial nerves

(CNs), and peripheral nerves that lie outside the brain and spinal cord. In humans, the cerebrum dominates all of the other parts of the nervous system. This system, with its complex arrangement, enables the organism to respond to internal and external stimuli on the basis of information coming from the peripheral receptors. The human brain, which has a larger memory than any known computer, gives commands for the coordinated movements of muscles, regulates somatic and visceral functions, stores and retrieves information, and regulates emotions and behavior. The malfunctioning of the nervous system lends itself to clinical interpretation better than any other organ. In particular, two modern imaging techniques (i.e., magnetic resonance imaging and positron emission tomography) have engendered a revolution in the noninvasive study of the regional, structural, and functional neuroanatomy in the living human brain.

The functional unit of the nervous system is the neuron, which is highly specialized. The neuron has a cell body, typically many dendrites for reception of information, and a single axon for transmission of this information. The rapid and precise communication between neurons is made possible by two basic mechanisms: axonal conduction and synaptic transmission (electrical or chemical). Electrical transmission is mediated by direct flow of the current through gap junctions, and the predominant chemical transmission involves transmitter release presynaptically and receptor activation postsynaptically, either excitatory or inhibitory. The nature of each neuron is determined by gene expression in the course of the brain's development and subsequently is modified by experience. The information transfer between neurons is supported externally by glial cells (i.e., astrocytes, oligodendrocytes, ependymal cells, and microglia), which support the neurons physically and sustain them metabolically. In the peripheral nervous system, the glia cell (Schwann cell) produces the myelin sheath around axons for facilitating conduction.

Cerebral Cortex

The cerebral cortex, which covers the surface of the brain as a mantle of gray matter, is composed of a complex network of neurons, dendrites, axons, neu-roglia, and blood vessels. The cortex has a corrugated appearance, with the crest of each fold called a *gyrus* and the depression between gyri called a *sulcus*. Because of these foldings, only about one-third of the cortex lies exposed. Its unfolded area is approximately 0.25 m^2, and the estimated number of neurons in the cerebral cortex is approximately 14–16 billion. The thickness of the cortex varies from 1.5 to 4.5 mm. The areas of the cortex have extensive afferent and efferent connections with each other and with parts of the CNS.

Based on histologic and phylogenetic criteria, the cerebral cortex is subdivided into archicortex, paleocortex, and neocortex. The archicortex's hippocampal formation is the oldest region and is associated with emotion and behavior. The paleocortex is principally olfactory in nature and includes the lateral olfactory gyrus, the uncus, and the parahippocampal gyrus. The neocortex, which constitutes 90% of the human cerebral cortex, is phylogenetically recent. There are two main types of neocortex: (1) the homotypical cortex, with a six-layer arrangement (75% of the cortex is of this type), and (2) the heterotypical cortex, in which layers are less distinct.

Clinicopathologic, neurophysiologic, and other diagnostic studies in humans and electrophysiologic and ablation studies in animals have produced evidence that the function of the different areas of the cerebral cortex is specialized. On the basis of cytoarchitectural criteria, the most commonly employed system is Brodmann's classification system (Figure 2-1). In the CNS, some myelinated nerve fibers in the white matter interconnect various cortical regions. These are (1) the association fibers within the same hemisphere, (2) the commissural fibers connecting the corresponding regions of the two hemispheres, and (3) the projection fibers connecting the cortex to lower portions of the brain or spinal cord. The cortex can be functionally divided into motor, sensory, and association areas. The cerebral cortex is not uniform and performs a wide range of sensory, motor, and mnemonic processes associated with cognition besides its organization for affective behavior. The relationship between the cerebral cortex and the thalamus is especially important because thalamic excitation of the cortex is necessary in performing different functions. The loss of cerebral function incurred when the thalamus

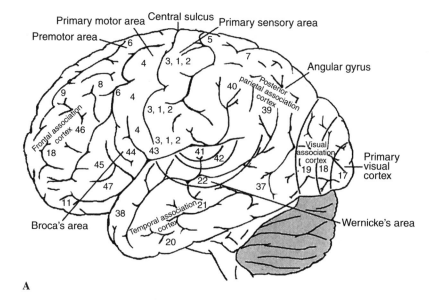

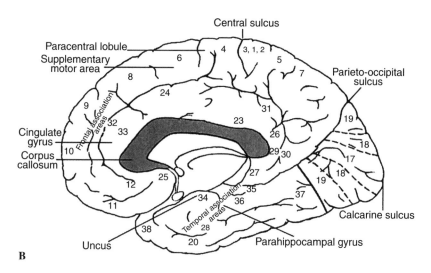

Figure 2-1. Brodmann's areas. (A) Lateral view. (B) Medial view.

is damaged along with the cortex is much more extensive than when only the cortex is damaged.

The cerebral cortex is also divided topographically into five lobes: frontal, parietal, temporal, occipital, and limbic. The frontal lobe is the largest and extends from the rostral pole to the central sulcus. The parietal lobe extends from the central sulcus to the parieto-occipital sulcus and medially to the cingulate gyrus. The temporal lobe is inferior to the lateral fissure and extends posteriorly to the preoccipital notch. The occipital lobe is situated behind the parieto-occipital fissure. The limbic lobe is located in the medial surface of the hemispheres and is composed of the cingulate gyrus and the hippocampal and parahippocampal gyri.

Motor Areas

The motor cortical areas are primary and secondary and have extensive and reciprocal projections. The primary motor cortex (M-I) (see Figure 2-1, area 4) is in the precentral gyrus, which mediates fine control of contralateral voluntary motor activity. M-I participates in the suprasegmental control of movements through its numerous influences on other brain regions involved in motor control. It contributes projections to the spinal cord (via the corticospinal tract), brain stem motor nuclei (via the corticobulbar tract), striatum, thalamus, cerebellum, premotor cortex (PMC), supplementary motor area (SMA), and somatosensory cortex. There is a somatotopic representation of the body within M-I called the *motor homonculus,* with the head, trunk, and upper extremity represented laterally and the lower extremity medially. The neurons of M-I have the lowest threshold, and when stimulated (such as by irritative lesions) produce contralateral stereotypical muscle contraction and relaxation (jacksonian epilepsy). Destructive lesions of M-I produce contralateral flaccid paralysis; spasticity occurs if area 6 is also destroyed.

The secondary motor areas are the PMC, SMA, frontal eye field, and parietal motor areas. The PMC (area 6) is in front of M-I, on the lateral surface. The PMC projects to M-I and the SMA and also contributes to the corticospinal tract. Stimulation of the PMC produces contralateral movements of the limbs, adversive movements such as turning the head and eyes, and twisting movements of the trunk. Lesions of the PMC produce an apraxia condition in which the patient is unable to move the arms simultaneously, and they also produce weakness contralaterally. The SMA is located on the superior and medial aspect of area 6. The SMA contributes to the corticospinal tract besides projecting to M-I, the PMC, and the contralateral SMA. The SMA plays a crucial role in motivating a person to execute motor behavior involving both sides of the body and in the basic drive to produce speech. This area contains a somatotopic representation of the body. Stimulation of the SMA produces symmetric vocalizations, facial expressions, and limb movements. Lesions of the SMA produce deficits in bimanual coordination; the patient has apraxia while performing different movements simultaneously. Thus, the PMC and SMA are concerned with planning and initiation of motor behavior, which in turn stimulates M-I for the final command signal. The frontal eye field (area 8) is anterior to area 6. It coordinates horizontal eye movements. Lesions of this area produce ipsilateral conjugated eye deviation. The somatosensory cortex (areas 3, 1, and 2) also contributes to the corticospinal tract, with an esti-

mated ratio of 30%. Lesions of this area also cause weakness contralaterally. The frontal operculum includes areas 44 and 45. In the dominant hemisphere, this region constitutes Broca's area and is involved in motor aspects of linguistic expression. Lesions of this area result in motor aphasia. In the nondominant hemisphere, these areas mediate motor control of the mouth, tongue, palate, and vocal cords.

Sensory Areas

The sensory areas are divided into primary and secondary sensory areas. The primary sensory areas of the cortex receive afferent projections from specific thalamic relay nuclei, and in general they contain a precise map of the sensory information. These areas are the following:

1. The somatosensory cortex (S-I) (areas 3, 1, and 2). Like M-I, S-I is also organized somatotopically in the same representation. This area together with the posterior parietal areas is responsible for pain localization and integration. Damage to this area produces contralateral loss of two-point discrimination, stereognosis, texture discrimination, and vibratory and position sense. Pain and temperature sensory loss is minimal. In S-I, the fibers conveying information from the lower limbs and perineum terminate on the medial surface in the paracentral lobule. Lesions of this area cause incontinence.

2. The primary visual cortex (area 17). This area receives the optic radiations. Lesions of this area produce contralateral homonymous hemianopsia with macular sparing.

3. The primary auditory cortex (Heschl's gyrus, areas 41 and 42). This area receives projections from the medial geniculate body and is organized tonotopically. Unilateral lesions of this area produce slight hearing loss and are undetectable clinically because this area receives information from both ears (mostly from the opposite ear).

4. The taste cortex (area 43). Gustatory information is relayed in the thalamus (ventral posteromedial nucleus), unlikely in an uncrossed pathway that projects to the operculoinsular area.

The secondary sensory areas are adjacent to the primary sensory areas and receive input mainly from the related primary sensory areas for perception; this is integrated with the information they receive from other systems. The secondary sensory areas are the following:

1. Areas 5 and 7 for S-I. These are important for memory and recall of somatosensory information. Lesions of these areas seldom produce the sensory deficits that are seen with S-I lesions.
2. Areas 18 and 19 for the visual cortex. These are visual association areas and play a role in visual perception. Lesions of these areas produce visual agnosia and color agnosia (achromatopsia).
3. Area 22 for the auditory cortex. This is in the superior temporal gyrus and is involved in the discrimination of auditory frequency and the sequence of sound and retention of auditory information. Destruction results in slight hearing loss contralaterally.

Association Areas

In the cerebral cortex, those areas that are not pure motor or sensory areas are named *association areas*. These areas receive and analyze signals from multiple regions of the cortex and subcortical structures. The association cortices are involved in higher brain functions, including language and communication skills, cognition, personality, emotional behavior, sensory perception, and memory. There are three association areas involved in different higher functions (see Figure 2-1). The prefrontal association cortex includes frontal cortical areas rostral to the motor areas. The dorsolateral prefrontal region (areas 9, 10, and 46) is concerned with various types of high-level intellectual abilities (e.g., mental operations that require retrieval and manipulation of information, especially for a creative production). This region is also concerned with problem solving. The orbitofrontal region (areas 11 and 12) is concerned with judgment, planning, and decision making and is more directly associated with emotional disturbances. The superior mesial region (areas 8, 9, and 32) is concerned with personality characteristics (e.g., introversion, extroversion, and obsessions) and also with maintenance of the optimal state of arousal and alertness. Patients with prefrontal association cortex lesions exhibit socially inappropriate behavior with a labile emotional state. The posterior parietal association cortex includes areas 5, 7, 39, and 40. Areas 5 and 7 project to M-I and to both the SMA

and PMC. These areas are concerned with the tactile and visual aspects of reaching and guiding movements. Lesions of these areas in the nondominant lobe produce principally neglect of the contralateral external space in sensory, motor, cognition, and attentional dimensions. The patient neglects the contralateral parts of his or her body while dressing, has problems in recognizing the objects by touch (astereognosis), draws only the ipsilateral half of an object, and describes a scene he or she sees only ipsilaterally. There is also ataxia as a result of neglect and deficit in initiating the movement of the contralateral limbs. In the dominant hemisphere, damage of the inferior regions produces astereognosis; aphasia; tactile agnosia (the inability to perceive objects); and Gerstmann's syndrome, which is characterized by (1) dysgraphia and dyslexia, (2) dyscalculi, (3) right-left disorientation, and (4) finger agnosia. The temporal association cortex includes all temporal cortical areas except the primary auditory cortex. The superior region, area 22 in the dominant hemisphere, comprises Wernicke's area and is specialized for understanding speech and the perception of written language. Destruction of this area results in receptive (sensorial) aphasia. The inferolateral region (areas 20, 21, 37, and 38) has an important role in higher-order aspects of visual processing. Damage to this area results in difficulty in the performance of visual discrimination. This region is also involved in memory. Lesions of this area in the nondominant and dominant hemispheres result in severe deficits in short-term visual memory and verbal memory, respectively. Bilateral lesions of this region produce prosopagnosia (an inability to recognize familiar faces). The mesial temporal region (areas 27, 28, 35, and 36) includes the parahippocampal system and is specialized for memory; the dominant hippocampal system is dedicated to verbal material and the nondominant system to nonverbal material. This system is important for the acquisition of new information (anterograde memory).

Cerebral Dominance

There is a considerable variation between the degree of lateralization of different cortical functions. Among these, the localization of speech centers is the traditional criterion for determining dominance. Almost all of right-handed and 60–70% of left-handed persons have a dominant left hemisphere. The dominant

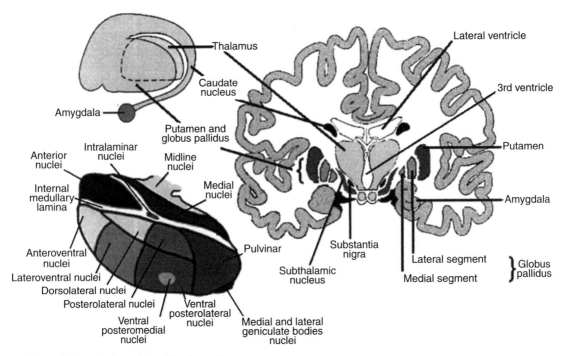

Figure 2-2. Thalamic nuclei and basal ganglia.

hemisphere performs calculations, intellectual functions involving decisions, problem solving, and symbolic thought processes besides speech and language. The nondominant hemisphere is usually responsible for visual and tactile recognition of complex three-dimensional structures, musical ability, nonverbal thought processes, and creative abilities.

Diencephalon and Limbic Systems

The diencephalon is the rostral expansion of the midbrain and lies between the cerebral hemispheres. The two halves of the diencephalon are separated by the third ventricle. The diencephalon includes the thalamus, hypothalamus, epithalamus, and subthalamus.

Thalamus

The thalamus, with its geniculate bodies, is the major component of the diencephalon. It plays an important role in sensory and motor systems integration and also is involved in the maintenance of consciousness and in autonomic reactions. The thalamus is a paired, large, and ovoid gray mass of nuclei located between

the third ventricle and the internal capsule. There are five groups of thalamic nuclei. In the rostrocaudal direction, the thalamus is roughly divided into three nuclear mass groups by the internal medullary lamina, a thin sheet of myelinated fibers (Figure 2-2). These are the anterior nuclei, the medial nuclei (intralaminar nuclei and dorsomedial nucleus), and the lateral nuclei (reticular nucleus, anteroventral nucleus, dorsolateral nucleus, lateroventral nucleus, posterolateral nucleus, ventral posterolateral nucleus, and ventral posteromedial nucleus). Besides these groups, there is a group of midline nuclei in the interthalamic region lining the third ventricle (the most prominent is the centromedian nucleus) and a group of posterior nuclei (pulvinar nucleus, medial and lateral geniculate bodies). These thalamic nuclei relay all ascending subcortical information destined for cortical processing except for the olfactory sensation. Most of the direct input to the cerebral cortex is derived from the thalamus. The aforementioned thalamic nuclei, according to their functional connections, can be divided into specific and nonspecific nuclei.

The specific nuclei are (1) the somatosensory relay nuclei (ventral posteromedial and ventral posterolateral), receiving the sensations of touch, pressure, position, pain, and temperature; (2) the auditory relay nucleus (medial geniculate body), receiving the auditory afferent fibers from the inferior colliculus; (3) the visual relay nucleus (lateral geniculate body), receiving the optic tract; (4) the motor relay nuclei (anteroventral, lateroventral), receiving afferents from the dentate nucleus, globus pallidus, and substantia nigra; (5) the gustatory relay nucleus (ventral posteromedial), receiving taste sensation; (6) the vestibular relay nuclei, receiving projections from the vestibular nuclei; and (7) the limbic relay nuclei (anterior dorsomedial), receiving afferents from the limbic system.

The nonspecific nuclei of the thalamus are the following:

1. The intralaminar nuclei, receiving afferents from the cerebellum, basal ganglia, brain stem, reticular formation, and spinothalamic tract. These nuclei have widespread projections to cortical areas, with the greatest contribution to the motor areas, and play a role in cortical arousal and sensorimotor integration.
2. The midline nuclei, receiving afferents from the locus ceruleus, raphe nuclei, hypothalamus, and epithalamus. These nuclei play a role in integration of visceral activities.

The thalamic reticular nucleus modulates and modifies the level of activity in both the thalamus and cerebral cortex. This nucleus does not project to the cortex; its axons project to all other thalamic nuclei. It has also a major role in the synchronizing effects of the thalamus such as rhythmic brain activity and phasic and tonic movements.

The afferents and efferents of the thalamic nuclei also can be divided into two categories: specific and nonspecific. The specific afferents synapse in a specific relay nuclei and specific efferents project to a restricted cortical area (e.g., optic tract → lateral geniculate body → area 17). The nonspecific afferents synapse in more than one nucleus, and nonspecific efferents project more diffusely (e.g., ascending serotonergic and adrenergic projections). There is a point-to-point reciprocal connection of the thalamus and cortex—that is, all thalamic nuclei receive descending input from the cerebral cortex, principally from the cortical areas to which they project (two-way feedback system). This interconnection may regulate the subsequent information to that cortical area. These thalamocortical and corticothalamic fibers course through the internal cap-

sule and are called the *thalamic radiation*. The thalamus by these aforementioned connections has a significant role in the conscious appreciation of sensation; in addition it relays information about motor behavior to the motor areas of the cortex. In addition, the thalamus is involved in autonomic reactions, which regulate levels of awareness and emotional aspects of sensorial experiences. In the thalamic syndrome, which occurs as a result of thrombosis of posterior choroidal or posterior cerebral arteries, the threshold for pain, temperature, and tactile sensations is raised on the contralateral side of the body, and contralateral hemianalgesia, spontaneous paroxysmal pain without any external stimulus, can be seen.

Hypothalamus

The hypothalamus, the lowermost portion of the diencephalon, lies between the third ventricle and subthalamus and is connected to the hypophysis by the infundibulum. It is an important integrator of autonomic and neuroendocrine activities, maintains the constancy of the internal environment (homeostasis), and establishes behavioral patterns. The hypothalamus can be grossly divided into lateral, medial, and periventricular regions. Among these, the lateral region contains short and long ascending and descending fibers projecting to the cortex, brain stem, and spinal cord. The medial region contains most of the nuclei of the hypothalamus and is divided into three portions along the anterior-posterior axis: (1) the most anterior supraoptic portion, containing the supraoptic, paraventricular, and suprachiasmatic nuclei; (2) the tuberal portion, containing the dorsomedial, ventromedial, and arcuate nuclei; and (3) the most posterior mamillary region, containing the mamillary and posterior nuclei. The periventricular region contains small neurons that secrete the substances that control the release of anterior pituitary hormones. Each of these hypothalamic nuclei subserves a variety of functions.

The hypothalamus has extensive connections with various parts of the CNS. The major inputs are from the hippocampus, cingulate cortex, amygdala, frontal association cortex, basal ganglia, limbic system, thalamus, reticular formation, cerebellum, and retina. The outputs project to the thalamus, reticular

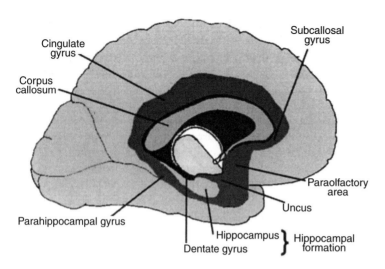

Figure 2-3. Limbic system.

formation, autonomic neurons in the brain stem and spinal cord, hypophysis, hippocampus, and cerebellum. The hypothalamus regulates the endocrine system by controlling the anterior (adenohypophysis) and posterior (neurohypophysis) parts of the pituitary gland. The releasing factors, which are produced by the hypothalamus, travel down the hypothalamo-hypophyseal venous portal system and stimulate formation of certain hormones from the adenohypophysis that regulate adrenal, thyroid, and gonadal function besides growth and lactation. The second part of the pituitary gland, the neurohypophysis, stores and releases two hormones—vasopressin (ADH) and oxytocin—which are produced in the supraoptic and paraventricular nuclei and carried down in the hypothalamo-hypophyseal tract. These hormones regulate water balance, blood pressure, milk ejection, and uterine contractions. The hypothalamus, by these connections, regulates autonomic function, eating, body temperature, water balance, and the endocrine system and also is involved in the control of circadian rhythms, such as sleep (by the suprachiasmatic nucleus), and behavioral processes, such as sexual, ingestive, maternal, and emotional behaviors.

Epithalamus

The epithalamus is the most dorsal division of the diencephalon and consists of the pineal body (epiphysis, pineal gland), habenular trigone, and posterior commissure. The pineal body is a small mass located over the tectum of the midbrain and is continuous with

the habenular and posterior commissures. Its main function is to secrete melatonin. Tumors of this gland causes Parinaud's syndrome with upward gaze paralysis. The habenular trigone contains the habenular nuclei, which receive the afferents from the hypothalamus and the brain stem, including the interpeduncular nucleus and raphe nuclei, and the efferents project to the interpeduncular nuclei (fasciculus retroflexus). The posterior commissure connects the two superior colliculi and is involved in consensual light reflex.

Subthalamus

The subthalamus is located between the midbrain and dorsal thalamus, which contains the zona incerta, Forel's tegmental field H (which may be a rostral extension of reticular nuclei), and the subthalamic nucleus of Luys. The subthalamic nucleus has interconnections with the globus pallidus and striatum. Lesions of this nucleus result in hemiballismus, which affects one side of the body as intermittent flailing of the affected extremities. The subthalamus has sensory, motor, and reticular functions.

Limbic System

The limbic system is a phylogenetically ancient system in the medial aspect of the hemispheres (Figure 2-3). This system has extensive reciprocal connections with many areas of the cortex, the diencephalon, and the brain stem. It includes the limbic lobe (i.e., subcallosal gyrus, cingulate gyrus, and parahippocampal gyrus), the hippocampal formation (i.e., hippocampus and dentate gyrus), the anterior nucleus of the thalamus, and the hypothalamus, which are highly interconnected. The limbic system is involved with emotional and motivational behaviors (e.g., the reactions of fear, rage, aggression, anger, and emotions with sexual behavior), recent memory, learning, autonomic responses associated with emotional changes, and olfaction.

Basal Ganglia

The *basal ganglia* is a descriptive anatomic name for a group of subcortical cellular masses that receive input from wide regions of the cerebral cortex, mostly from the prefrontal association cortex. These nuclei project to both the motor and prefrontal cortex via a relay in the thalamus. The basal ganglia play an integral part in controlling movement as well as the maintenance of posture and cognitive function. The main components of the basal ganglia are the striatum or neostriatum (comprising the putamen, caudate nucleus, and nucleus accumbens), the globus pallidus (or pallidum, paleostriatum), the subthalamic nucleus (or corpus Luys), and the substantia nigra (see Figure 2-2). Together the putamen and the globus pallidus are also termed the *lentiform nucleus* because their form is similar to that of a lens. Among these, the striatum and the substantia nigra are the key structures of this system (see Figure 2-2).

Afferents

Almost all afferent connections of the basal ganglia terminate in the striatum and are received from two major sources: the cerebral cortex and the thalamus. Virtually all areas of the cerebral cortex, including the motor, premotor, somatosensory, association, and limbic areas, project to different parts of neostriatum. Among these, the motor and the somatosensory cortices project predominantly to the putamen; the association cortices project to the caudate; and the limbic cortices (i.e., medial and lateral temporal cortices) and hippocampus project to the nucleus accumbens. The putamen is primarily involved in motor control; the caudate is involved in control of eye movements and certain cognitive functions; and the nucleus

accumbens is involved in the control of limbic functions. The second main source of the afferents is the thalamus, mainly its intralaminar and centromedian nuclei. The intralaminar nuclei project predominantly to the caudate, and the centromedian nucleus projects to the putamen. Besides these sources, the basal nucleus of the amygdala, locus ceruleus, and dorsal raphe nucleus also project to the basal ganglia. All of these afferents are predominantly in an excitatory manner.

Internal Circuits

The intrinsic nuclei have interconnections with the input and output nuclei. There are two major circuits through the basal ganglia. These circuits are in parallel; however, they have opposite effects on the cortex. One is the direct pathway, which projects from the striatum to the medial globus pallidus (striatopallidal pathway) and to the substantia nigra pars reticularis (striatonigral pathway). The direct pathway inhibits inhibitory neurons in the medial globus pallidus and substantia nigra pars reticularis; it then projects and disinhibits the thalamus, which projects to the cortex. This circuit increases cortical activity. The second circuit is the indirect pathway, which is projected from the striatum to the lateral globus pallidus and then to the subthalamic nucleus. This pathway is inhibitory, leading to excitation of the substantia nigra pars reticularis and globus pallidus medialis. The excitation of these nuclei inhibits the thalamic relay nuclei and thus decreases cortical activity. So, the direct and indirect pathways counterbalance one another. Another internal circuit is between the substantia nigra and the striatum. The dopaminergic (DAergic) projection from the substantia nigra pars compacta has several effects on striatal cholinergic interneurons. These are both excitatory and inhibitory. DA excites the direct pathway neurons through D_1 receptors but inhibits the indirect pathway through D_2 receptors.

Efferents

The efferents of the basal ganglia have ascending and descending components. Information leaving the basal ganglia projects to the frontal cortex via a relay in the dorsal thalamus. The major inhibitory ascending output is from the globus medialis and projects first to the thalamus (ventral anterior, ventral lateral, and dorsomedial nuclei) by the pathways of the ansa lenticularis and fasciculus lenticularis and then to motor, premotor, and supplementary cortical areas, which give rise to corticospinal, corticobulbar, and corticocerebellar pathways. Thus, this output is primarily involved with limb movements. The second ascending output projects from the substantia nigra pars reticularis to the thalamus (anteroventral medial and dorsomedial nuclei). These nuclei are connected to the frontal eye field area (area 8) and prefrontal cortical areas and thus are involved with eye, orofacial, head, and neck movements. The descending outputs of the basal ganglia project from the globus pallidus to the midbrain pedunculopontine nucleus of the reticular formation and from the substantia nigra to the colliculus superior (which controls vestibuloocular reflexes and eye movements).

The limbic component of the basal ganglia is mainly through the nucleus accumbens and globus pallidus to the thalamus and hypothalamus, which are connected to orbital, medial, and frontal limbic cortices. This system is implicated in emotional behavior and psychiatric disorders. Thus, this system modulates motor activities through direct and indirect feedback projections between the basal ganglia, associated nuclei, thalamus, and cortex.

Functional and Clinical Considerations

Malfunctioning of the basal ganglia characteristically produces involuntary movements such as decreased movement (i.e., hypokinesia) or excessive movement (i.e., hyperkinesia). It is not possible to precisely state the anatomic locus when disorders associated with these abnormal movements occur because of the aforementioned complex anatomic connections and physiologic associations. Symptoms are usually observed bilaterally; if they are unilaterally observed, the lesion is in the contralateral basal ganglia. Hypokinesias such as bradykinesia (i.e., slowness of movement) or akinesia (i.e., inability to move) are mostly seen unilaterally or bilaterally in Parkinson's disease, which is characterized also by hypertonia (muscle rigidity) and static tremor.

The diseases that are associated with hyperkinetic movements are chorea (rapid, jerky, nonstereotypic movements), athetosis (slow, writhing movements), dystonia (sustained, twisting, repetitive movements), ballism (violent, flail-like movements of the extremities on one side), and tics (sudden, stereotyped movements).

Autonomic Nervous System

The autonomic nervous system is an involuntary system that functions in parallel with the somatic motor system to adjust the body to internal and external environmental changes (homeostasis). This system innervates smooth muscles of the visceral organs, the cardiovascular system, and glands. It includes portions of the central and peripheral nervous systems and has two principal divisions: sympathetic and the parasympathetic. Autonomic reflex activity in the spinal cord and brain stem is modulated by higher centers, such as the cerebral neocortex, the limbic system, the cerebellum, and the hypothalamus. Among these, the hypothalamus is the principal regulator of autonomic function. Figure 2-4 illustrates the autonomic nervous system, both the sympathetic and parasympathetic divisions. The sympathetic and parasympathetic innervations have nearly opposite effects on effector organs as shown in Table 2-1.

Sympathetic System

The sympathetic (thoracolumbar) division of the autonomic nervous system arises from preganglionic cell bodies located in the intermediolateral cell columns of the spinal cord gray matter, which extends from T1 to L3. Axons of these neurons exit the spinal cord in the ventral roots and enter the paravertebral sympathetic chain via the white communicating rami from the thoracic and lumbar levels only. Those from the upper thoracic level ascend to the cervical ganglia and those from lumbar level descend to the sacral ganglia. There are three cervical, 11–12 thoracic, and four to six lumbar ganglia and a variable number of sacral ganglia in the sympathetic chain. Here some of the axons synapse with the ganglia neurons; some pass up or down in the chain to synapse with ganglion cells at higher or lower levels; and some (from the lower seven thoracic and lumbar regions) pass through the trunk

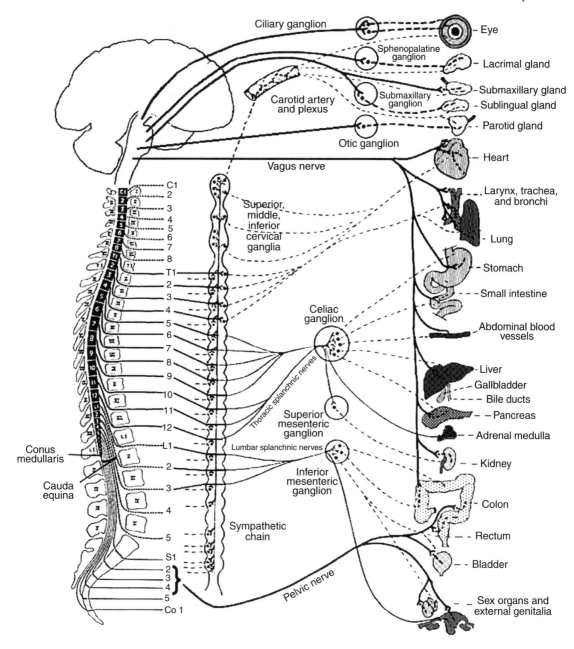

Figure 2-4. Spinal cord and its relationship with the vertebral column. Cervical and lumbar spinal nerves are represented as dashed lines; thoracic and sacrococcygeal spinal nerves as thin lines. Autonomic nervous system: Thick lines represent the preganglionic parasympathetic, thin lines the preganglionic sympathetic, and dashed lines the postganglionic parasympathetic and sympathetic fibers.

without synapsing and route to the prevertebral sympathetic ganglia (i.e., celiac, superior, and inferior mesenteric ganglia) as splanchnic nerves, whose postganglionic axons then reach to the abdominal viscera via the celiac and hypogastric plexuses. At the thoracic and the first two to three lumbar levels, the postganglionic fibers of the sympathetic chain form the gray communicating rami and join the spinal nerves. Neurons of the cervical ganglia (superior, middle, inferior, or stellate ganglia), which form

Table 2-1. Functional Summary of the Autonomic Nervous System

Effector Organ	Sympathetic Stimulation	Parasympathetic Stimulation
Eye	Mydriasis	Miosis
Salivary glands	Mucus secretion	Serous secretion
Lacrimal glands	No effect	Secretion
Nasopharyngeal glands	No effect	Secretion
Heart	Increased heart rate	Decreased heart rate
Systemic blood vessels	Vasoconstriction	Vasodilation
Systemic veins	Vasoconstriction	No effect
Respiratory system		
Bronchioles	Dilation	Constriction
Bronchial glands	Decreased (β_1) and increased (β_2) secretion	Increased secretion
Gastrointestinal tract		
Peristalsis	Inhibition	Stimulation
Sphincters	Contraction	Relaxation
Glands	No effect	Increased secretion
Blood flow	Vasoconstriction	Vasodilation
Liver	Glycogenolysis and gluco-neogenesis	Glycogenesis
Pancreas		
Acinar cells	Decreased secretion	Increased secretion
Islet cells	Decreased secretion	Increased secretion
Urinary bladder		
Detrusor muscle	No effect	Contraction
Sphincter muscle	Contraction	Relaxation
Reproductive organs		
Male	Ejaculation	Erection of penis
Female	Orgasm	Engorgement of clitoris

the cervical part of the sympathetic trunk, receive preganglionic fibers from the first four to five thoracic segments and innervate structures in the head (cranial and peripheral vessels, sweat glands, lacrimal and salivary glands, hair follicles, pupilla), thoracal visceral organs, and upper extremity. The upper abdominal viscera are supplied by the thoracic splanchnic nerves from the spinal levels of T5–T12, and the lower abdominal and pelvic viscera are supplied from the lumbar splanchnic nerves. Horner's syndrome (miosis, ptosis, anhidrosis) results from an injury to the cervical portion of the sympathetic system (primarily the superior cervical ganglion).

Parasympathetic System

The parasympathetic (craniocervical) division of the autonomic nervous system arises from four of the brain stem CN nuclei (CNs III, VII, IX, and X) and the sacral spinal cord (S2–S4). Among these, CNs

III, VII, and IX provide the parasympathetic innervation of the head through the ciliary, pterygopalatine (sphenopalatine), and submandibular ganglia (submaxillary) and CN X provides the innervation of the entire thoracic and most of the abdominal viscera (except the descending colon, sigmoid, rectum, anus, and pelvic viscera, which are innervated by S2–S4 spinal levels through pelvic ganglia). In the parasympathetic system, the terminal peripheral ganglion cells are located close to the viscera or are actually embedded in them, in contrast to the sympathetic ganglia. Therefore, this system has short postganglionic fibers.

Brain Stem and Reticular Formation

The short portion of the CNS between the cerebral hemispheres and the spinal cord is called the *brain stem*. It has three main divisions: the midbrain (mesencephalon), the pons, and the medulla

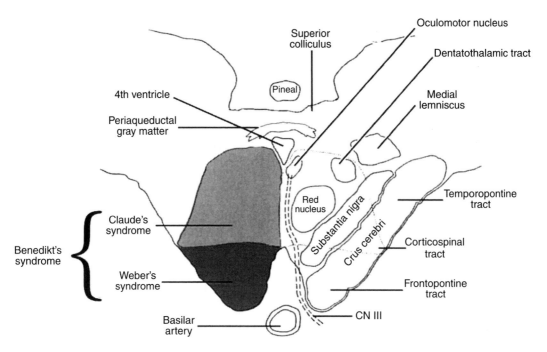

Figure 2-5. The midbrain. (CN = cranial nerve.)

(medulla oblongata, bulbus). Each of these regions contains groupings of cell bodies (nuclei) and bundles of axons (tracts), which are intermingled in contrast to the spinal cord.

Midbrain

The midbrain has three main parts: the basis, the tegmentum, and the tectum (Figure 2-5).

Base

The base of the midbrain on the anterior aspect contains the crus cerebri and the substantia nigra. The crus cerebri is a massive fiber bundle that includes the corticospinal, corticobulbar, and corticopontine pathways. The corticobulbar fibers accompany the corticospinal tract and project to the nuclei of the CNs bilaterally except the lower nucleus of the facial nerve and hypoglossus, which are crossed and unilateral. The substantia nigra, which has two parts (pars compacta, pars reticularis), contains pigmented DAergic neuromelanin cells. It receives afferents from the cortex and striatum and projects back to the striatum. Degeneration of these cells causes parkinsonism.

Tegmentum

The tegmentum lies between the tectum and the base and contains all of the ascending tracts (from the spinal cord and lower brain stem) and most of the descending tracts. This part of the midbrain includes the rich, vascularized red nucleus, trochlear nucleus, oculomotor nucleus (both the motor and parasympathetic Edinger-Westphal nucleus), nucleus of Darkschevich of the reticular formation, the mesencephalic nucleus of CN V, and the interpeduncular nucleus. The superior cerebellar peduncles, which contain efferent fibers from the dentate nucleus of the cerebellum to the opposite red nucleus, enter the tegmentum. The central periaqueductal gray matter, containing the descending autonomic tracts as well as endorphin-producing cells that suppress pain, is continuous posteriorly with the gray substance of the third ventricle.

Tectum

The tectum is the dorsal aspect and roof of the midbrain and contains four hillocks (two superior and two inferior colliculi) called the *corpora quadrigemina*. The superior colliculi are larger and associated with

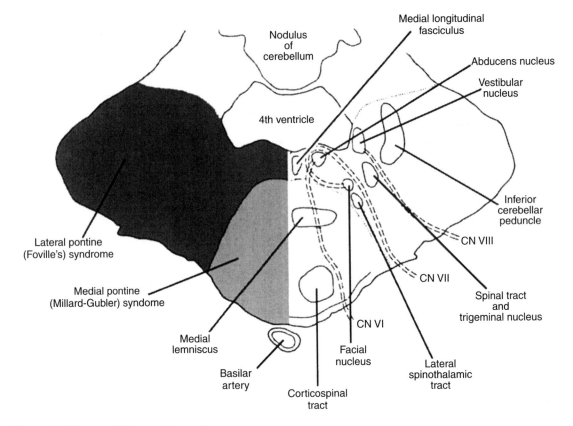

Figure 2-6. The pons. (CN = cranial nerve.)

the optic system and upward gaze. The inferior colli-culi are more prominent and associated with the auditory system. Beneath the tectum extends the rhomboid fossa, which forms the floor of the fourth ventricle. The midbrain is traversed by a narrow channel, the cerebral aqueduct, which connects the third ventricle to the fourth ventricle. The cerebral peduncle includes the tegmentum, the substantia nigra, and the basis pedunculi and excludes the tectum.

Pons

The pons has two main parts, the basis and tegmentum, and is located between the midbrain and the medulla (Figure 2-6).

Base

The base of the pons contains (1) the corticospinal tract, (2) the pontine nuclei, which receive input from the cerebral cortex by the corticopontine path-way, and (3) the pontocerebellar fibers, which connect the pontine nuclei to the neocerebellum by the middle cerebellar peduncle.

Tegmentum

The tegmentum is the most complex part of the pons. It contains the nuclei of CN V (the main sensory nucleus, descending spinal trigeminal nucleus, and motor nucleus), the nucleus of CN VI, CN VII (motor, superior salivatory, and gustatory nuclei), the lateral lemniscus and the trapezoid body of the auditory pathways, the inferior cerebellar peduncle, the reticular formation, and the medial lemniscus.

Medulla

The medulla contains the nuclei of CN VIII (two cochlear and four vestibular nuclei in the pontomedullary junction), CN IX (the nucleus ambiguus, inferior salivatory, and solitary nuclei), CN X (dor-

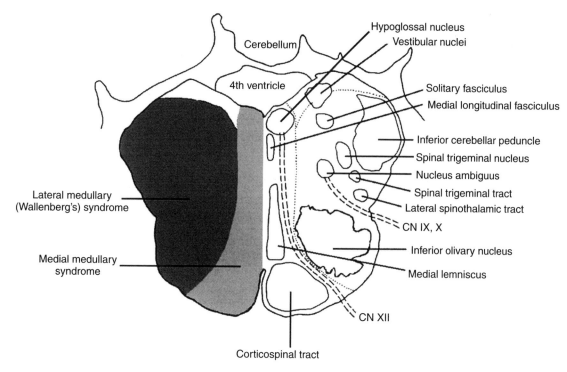

Figure 2-7. The medulla. (CN = cranial nerve.)

sal motor, ambiguus, solitary), CN XI (nucleus ambiguus), and CN XII (hypoglossal nuclei) (Figure 2-7). This part of the brain stem also contains the reticular formation, the relay nuclei of the dorsal column pathway (nucleus gracilis and cuneatus), the medial lemniscus, the spinal trigeminal nucleus, the spinothalamic tract, the spinocerebellar tracts (ventral and dorsal), and the inferior cerebellar peduncle.

The medial longitudinal fasciculus (MLF) interconnects the oculomotor, trochlear, abducens, and vestibular nuclei and also descends to the upper cervical segments. The MLF is in the dorsal tegmentum, in a paramedian location and close to the opposite MLF; thus, an intrinsic brain stem lesion usually causes MLF syndrome (internuclear ophthalmoplegia) with bilateral involvement (see Figures 2-6 and 2-7). The MLF coordinates eye, neck, and head movements in response to visual and vestibular stimuli.

Brain Stem Lesions

Because the brain stem is an anatomically compact structure, several nuclei, tracts, pathways, or reflex centers can be damaged by a small lesion. From an anatomicopathologic point of view, the brain stem provides the best example of close correlation between the clinical signs and symptoms and the damaged anatomic structure. The diseases affecting the brain stem in general involve a combination of CNs and long tracts (motor, sensorial, autonomic) and are divided into extrinsic and intrinsic diseases. The extrinsic diseases such as tumors of the cerebellopontine angle, cerebellum, and pineal gland; developmental bony degenerative diseases; and vascular diseases (hemorrhage, aneurysms) frequently involve multiple CNs and cause increase of intracranial pressure, loss of equilibrium, and truncal ataxia. The intrinsic diseases occur much more frequently and involve unilaterally or bilaterally the nuclei or CNs and the long tracts. These are ischemic-occlusive vascular diseases of the vertebral basilar arteries, intrinsic tumors, demyelinating diseases, and degenerative diseases such as syringobulbia and amyotrophic lateral sclerosis (ALS). Table 2-2 summarizes the most common syndromes of the brain stem.

Table 2-2. Major Brain Stem Syndromes

Syndrome	Structures Involved	Signs
	Mesencephalon	
Weber	CN III, corticospinal tract	Oculomotor palsy, crossed hemiplegia
Claude	CN III, red nucleus, superior cerebellar peduncle	Oculomotor palsy, contralateral tremor and ataxia
Benedikt	Structures involved in Claude and Weber syndromes	Signs as in Claude and Weber syndromes
Parinaud	Colliculus superior	Vertical gaze palsy
	Pons	
Millard-Gubler	CN VI, CN VII, corticospinal tract	Peripheral palsy
Foville	CN VI, CN VII, MLF, PPRF, middle cerebellar peduncle, and spinothalamic tract	Abducens palsy, facial peripheral palsy, internuclear ophthalmoplegia (uni- or bilateral), conjugate gaze palsy, contralateral ataxia, and crossed impaired pain sensation
	Medulla	
Wallenberg (lateral medullary)	CN V (spinal nucleus), CN IX, CN X, inferior cerebellar peduncle, spinothalamic tract, and descending sympathetic pathway	Impaired facial sensation, dysphagia, hoarseness, paralysis of soft palate, cerebellar ataxia, crossed impaired pain sensation, Horner's syndrome
Medial medullary	CN XII, corticospinal tract	Ipsilateral hypoglossal palsy, contralateral hemiplegia

CN = cranial nerve; MLF = medial longitudinal fasciculus; PPRF = paramedian pontine reticular formation.

Reticular Formation

The reticular formation is a complex organization of several interconnected nuclei extending throughout the brain stem. This system integrates motor (tone, reflexes, and body posture), sensory, autonomic, and limbic functions and plays a role in cortical arousal mechanisms, alertness, sleep cycles, pain modulation, and the control of vital functions such as regulation of blood pressure and respiratory rhythms. The nuclei of the reticular formation have extensive afferent and efferent connections with other parts of the CNS. They are divided into three columns based on their anatomic locations: the median, the medial, and the lateral columns. The median column consists of unpaired raphe nuclei, which extend in the midline of the brain stem. Many of these neurons contain serotonin (5-HT). The caudal median column plays a key role in modulation of pain transmission and the rostral median column regulates limbic system functions. The medial column consists of the paired ventral reticular nucleus and the gigantocellular and pontine reticular nuclei (including the paramedian pontine reticular formation). The long ascending and descending tracts of the reticular formation mainly originate from this column. The lateral column includes the paired pedunculopontine, cuneiform, parabrachial, and parvicellular nuclei. This column is the afferent component of the reticular formation. The principal afferent projections to the reticular formation are mainly from all somatic and visceral pathways and the cortex, striatum, hypothalamus, cerebellum, limbic structures, periaqueductal gray matter, CNs, and spinal cord. The efferents project to the thalamus, hypothalamus, hippocampus, cortex, periaqueductal gray matter, CN nuclei, and spinal cord. In the reticular formation, a projection system called the ascending reticular activating system (ARAS) activates the cortical, hypothalamic, and limbic structures and provides the level of consciousness and the emotional and behavioral responses to sensorial stimuli (e.g., response to pain). Lesions that destroy ARAS pathways lead to an altered level of consciousness or coma.

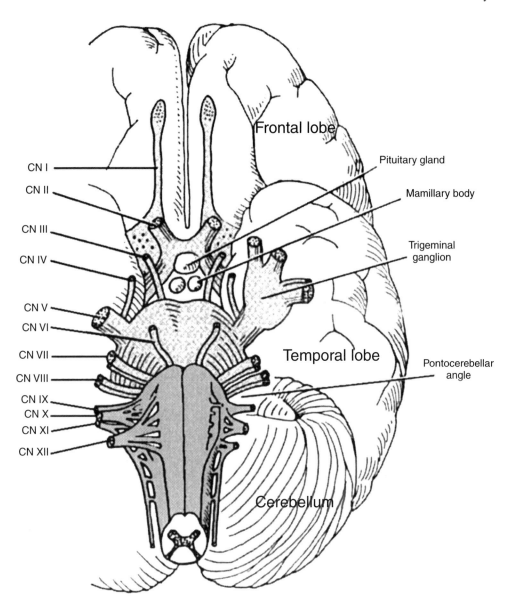

Figure 2-8. The cranial nerves (CNs) (antero-inferior view).

Cranial Nerves

Cranial nerves (CNs) are the peripheral nerves of the brain that transmit input from the special sensors (i.e., smell, vision, hearing, and taste); receive sensory information from the skin, muscles, and joints of the head; control motor output to muscles of the eyes, face, and neck; and control parasympathetic innervation of the structures in the head and visceral organs. There are 12 pairs of CNs, 10 of which have their

nuclei in the brain stem. CN I (the olfactory nerve) and CN II (the optic nerve) are not true peripheral nerves but are actually tracts of the CNS (Figure 2-8). The location of cell bodies, function, lesions, and foramina at the base of the skull related to the CNs are shown in Table 2-3. The CNs are pure motor, pure sensory, or mixed in nature. All of the CNs enter or exit the brain stem ventrally or ventrolaterally, but CN IV (the trochlear nerve) exits from the dorsal surface, and it is the only crossed CN. CNs with motor function

Table 2-3. Cranial Nerves

Cranial Nerve	Origin	Function	Lesion	Foramen
I. Olfactory	Bipolar olfactory neuroepithelial cells	Olfaction	Anosmia	Cribriform plate
II. Optic	Retinal ganglion cells	Vision	Loss of vision	Optic foramen
III. Oculomotor				Superior orbital fissure
Parasympathetic	Edinger-Westphal nucleus-preganglionic to ciliary ganglion	Pupillary constriction and accommodation of lens for near vision	Mydriasis and paralysis of accommodation	
Motor	Oculomotor nucleus	Innervation of the levator palpebrae and eye muscles (except lateral rectus and superior oblique)	Ptosis and deviation of the eye inferiorly and laterally Diplopia	
IV. Trochlear	Trochlear nucleus	Innervation of the superior oblique muscle	Unable to look downward while in adduction Diplopia	Superior orbital fissure
V. Trigeminal				Superior orbital fissure (ophthalmic), foramen rotundum (maxillary), foramen ovale (mandibular)
Motor	Motor nucleus	Innervation of mastication muscles and tensor tympani muscle	Difficulty in mastication, deviation of the jaw ipsilaterally Hypoacusis	
Sensory	Mesencephalic, main sensorial and spinal trigeminal nuclei	Cutaneous and proprioceptive sensations from skin and muscles of the face, nose, mouth, anterior two-thirds of the tongue, temporomandibular joint, and meninges	Ipsilateral diminished tactile sensation in the face, tongue, and mucous membranes	
VI. Abducens	Abducens nucleus	Innervation of the lateral rectus muscle	Medial deviation of the eye Diplopia	Superior orbital fissure
VII. Facial				Internal auditory meatus → facial canal → stylomastoid foramen
Parasympathetic	Superior salivatory nucleus-preganglionic to geniculate, sphenopalatine, and submaxillary ganglions	Secretion of lacrimal, nasal submaxillary, sublingual, and palatal glands	Loss of tearing and reduced salivation	
Motor	Facial motor nucleus	Innervation of the facial expression, platysma, and stapedius muscles	Ipsilateral facial paralysis of peripheral type (e.g., Bell's palsy) Hyperacusis	

Cranial Nerve	**Origin**	**Function**	**Lesion**	**Foramen**
Sensory	Primary geniculate ganglion, secondary spinal trigeminal tract	Tactile sensation from skin of the external auditory meatus	Loss of sensation	
	Primary geniculate ganglion, secondary nucleus solitarius	Taste sensation of the anterior two-thirds of the tongue	Taste loss	
VIII. Vestibulo-cochlear				Internal auditory meatus
	Primary vestibular ganglion, secondary vestibular nuclei	Equilibrium, orientation in space	Vertigo, nystagmus	
	Primary spiral ganglion, secondary cochlear nuclei	Hearing	Hearing loss, tinnitus	
IX. Glossopharyngeal				Foramen jugulare
Parasympathetic	Inferior salivatory nucleus, preganglionic to otic ganglion	Secretion of parotid gland	Reduced salivation	
Motor	Nucleus ambiguus	Swallowing, innervation of the stylopharyngeus muscle	Difficulty in swallowing (dysphagia)	
Sensory	Primary inferior petrosal ganglion, secondary nucleus solitarius	Taste sensation of posterior one-third of the tongue	Taste loss	
		Cutaneous sensation of posterior one-third of the tongue, tonsil, upper pharynx, tympanic cavity, carotid sinus	Loss of gag reflex ipsilaterally, loss of sensation in tongue, and pharyngeal mucous membrane, impairment of carotid reflex	
	Primary superior ganglion, secondary spinal trigeminal tract	Tactile sensation from back of the ear	Loss of sensation	
X. Vagus				Foramen jugulare
Parasympathetic	Dorsal motor nucleus-preganglionic to terminal ganglia	Innervation of smooth muscles and blood vessels in heart and visceral organs in thorax and abdomen (to the left colic flexure of the large intestine)		
Motor	Nucleus ambiguus	Innervation of the muscles of the pharynx, uvula, levator veli palatini, palatoglossus, and pharyngeal muscles of the upper esophagus	Ipsilateral paralysis of the soft palate, dysphonia, dysarthria, contralateral deviation of the uvula, dysphagia, hoarseness	
Sensory	Superior ganglion	Tactile sensation to external ear	Irritation results in nausea, cough, faint	
	Primary inferior nodosal ganglion, secondary to the nucleus and tractus solitarius	Visceral sensation of pharynx, larynx, aortic body, thorax, and abdominal organs (to the left colic flexure of large intestine)		

Table 2-3. *Continued*

Cranial Nerve	Origin	Function	Lesion	Foramen
XI. Accessory motor (cranial)	Nucleus ambiguus	Taste sensation from epiglottic region Innervates larynx muscles	Paralysis of larynx muscles	Foramen jugulare
Motor (spinal)	C1–C6 ventral horn cells	Innervates sternocleido-mastoid and trapezius muscles	Difficulty in turning the head to the opposite side, shoulderdrop, and winging of the scapula	
XII. Hypoglossal	Hypoglossal nucleus	Innervates intrinsic and extrinsic muscles of the tongue	Atrophy and paralysis in the ipsilateral tongue with protruding toward the lesion	Hypoglossal canal

(i.e., CNs III, IV, V, VI, VII, IX, X, XI, and XII) have their motor nuclei (homologous to the anterior horn cells) innervated by the corticobulbar tract, the fibers of which descend in close proximity to the corticospinal tract. In general, this tract projects to the motor nuclei bilaterally, except to the motor neurons supplying the lower half of the face and the genioglossus muscle, which receive contralateral corticobulbar fibers. Lesions involving one motor cortex or its corticobulbar pathways therefore result in central facial paralysis, with the orbicularis oculi and frontalis muscles being unaffected and with deviation of the tongue on protrusion. CNs with sensory function have their origin cells in the ganglia outside of the brain stem (homologous to the dorsal root ganglia). CNs III (the oculomotor nerve), IV, V (ophthalmic and maxillary divisions of the trigeminal nerve), and VI (the abducens nerve) course in close proximity only in the cavernous sinus. A lesion in this sinus therefore causes ophthalmoplegia in addition to sensory loss in the face. The long intracranial course of CN VI makes it vulnerable to pathologic processes in the middle and posterior cranial fossa (especially with increased intracranial pressure). In the auditory system, there is a bilateral cortical representation with the uncrossed and mostly crossed fibers. Therefore, a unilateral central auditory pathway lesion causes a slight hearing loss that is clinically undetectable. In general, examination of CN IX (the glossopharyngeal nerve) is done with CN X (the vagus nerve), because lesions restricted to the nuclei or nerve roots of CN IX are rare. Unilateral lesions of CN X rarely produce autonomic dysfunction, but bilateral involvement of this nerve usually has a fatal result.

CN X is also important in visceral reflexes such as coughing, vomiting, sneezing, hiccuping, and yawning.

Cerebellum

Cerebellum, meaning "little brain," constitutes only approximately 10% of the total weight of the brain but contains more than one-half of all the neurons. It has three main functions: (1) the coordination of skilled voluntary movements by influencing muscle activity and motor learning, (2) the maintenance of muscle tone, and (3) the control of equilibrium. The cerebellum is situated dorsal to the pons and medulla and occupies the posterior cranial fossa. It is separated from the overlying occipital lobes of the cerebrum by the tentorium cerebelli. It consists of two large hemispheres joined by a smaller midline structure called the vermis. The surface of the cerebellum is highly convoluted by many parallel fissures known as folia, so that approximately 85% of its area is hidden. Two of these fissures—the primary fissure and the posterolateral fissure—are significant because they divide the main body of the cerebellum into three lobes: the anterior lobe, the posterior lobe, and the flocculonodular lobe. Of these, the posterior lobe is the largest. These lobes are divided into the lobules, which are further divided into many folia. Traditionally, the lobules are identified by names, but in the vermis they are identified by Roman numerals I–X. These lobules have no known functional significance, so they are of limited use clinically. They are commonly used for descriptive purposes in experimental studies.

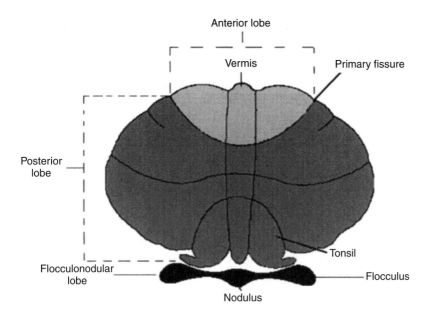

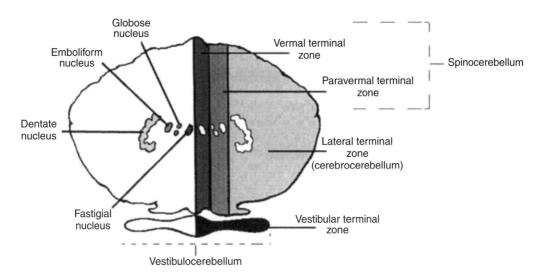

Figure 2-9. Schematic representation of the cerebellar cortex and functional divisions with the cerebellar nuclei.

Functionally and phylogenetically the cerebellum may be divided into three divisions: (1) the paleocerebellum (spinocerebellum), (2) the neocerebellum (pontocerebellum), and (3) the archicerebellum (vestibulocerebellum) (Figure 2-9). The paleocerebellum receives sensory input from the spinal cord for controlling synergy, muscle tone, and posture of stereotyped movements such as walking. The neocerebellum receives projections from the cerebral cortex that relay in the pontine nuclei. This part, which is largest and youngest, coordinates the planning of movements, such as making an operation. The archicerebellum, being the oldest part, has reciprocal connections with the vestibular system for controlling balance and for coordinating eye movements with movements of the head. The internal structure of cerebellum is composed of gray and white matter, like the cerebrum. The gray matter is mainly the cortex of the cerebellum, which covers the entire outer surface and is divided into three layers: (1) the external molecular layer, (2) the middle Purkinje cell layer, and (3) the internal granular layer. These layers contain five basic types of neurons: the stellate and the basket cells in the external layer, the Purkinje cells in the middle layer, the granule and the Golgi cells in the internal layer. There is a somatotopic organization of body parts within the cerebellar cortex. Besides the cortex, there are four masses of gray matter embedded in the white matter of the cerebellum in each hemisphere. From medial to lateral, they are the fastigial nucleus, the globose nucleus, the emboliform nucleus, and, the largest, the dentate nucleus (see Figure 2-9). These nuclei relay the entire output from the cerebellum to other parts of the CNS. The amount of the white matter of the cerebellum is large in the hemispheres but small in the vermis. It is made up of three groups of fibers: (1) intrinsic, (2) afferent, and (3) efferent. Intrinsic fibers connect different parts of the cerebellum on the same side or to the opposite side. These fibers form the inhibitory intracerebellar circuits. The afferent fibers, which are all excitatory, reach the cerebellum mainly through the middle and inferior peduncles and are directed to the cerebellar cortex. There are three axon types in these fibers: (1) the climbing fibers, (2) the mossy fibers, and (3) the aminergic fibers.

Three pairs of fiber bundles, called peduncles, located around the fourth ventricle, attach the cerebellum to the brain stem:

1. The superior cerebellar peduncle (brachium conjunctivum) is composed mostly of efferent fibers, leaving the cerebellum from the globose, emboliform, and dentate nuclei and sending impulses to both the thalamus and spinal cord after a relay in the red nuclei. This peduncle also conveys afferent fibers into the cerebellum from the ventral spinocerebellar tract, the tectocerebellar tract, the rubrocerebellar tract, and from the locus ceruleus.
2. The middle cerebellar peduncle (brachium pontis) is the largest and consists of fibers that originate from the cerebral cortex and project from the contralateral pontine nuclei to the neocerebellum.
3. The inferior cerebellar peduncle (restiform body) allows the entrance of afferent tracts from the spinal cord and lower brain stem to the cerebellum. This peduncle also consists of efferent fibers to the vestibular, olivary, and reticular nuclei.

All of the inputs and outputs of the cerebellum are routed through these peduncles. The inputs of the cerebellum, which have excitatory characteristics, reach its cortex mainly from three major sources: (1) the spinal cord, (2) the vestibular system, and (3) the cerebral cortex. The outputs from the cerebellum are less complex and mostly conveyed by axons of Purkinje cells after relaying in the deep nuclei. These fibers project mainly to the brain stem, thalamus, and cortex. The final output of the cerebellum is inhibitory.

Dysfunction of the cerebellum releases other parts of the nervous system from cerebellar influences (i.e., the loss of the effects of a negative feedback system). Lesions of the cerebellum or its afferents or efferents produce ipsilateral disturbances. From a clinical perspective, cerebellar dysfunction can best be understood according to the four zones of cerebellar organization, which are based on the longitudinal termination of inputs to the cerebellar cortex. These are the vermal, paravermal, lateral, and vestibular zones (see Figure 2-9). The vermal zone consists of the vermis, fastigial nuclei, and related input and output fibers. Functionally this zone is associated with head position, posture, eye movements, and proprioceptive information from the head (particularly from the temporomandibular joint). Cerebellar damage of this localization frequently causes trunk ataxia (loss of equilibrium while standing or walking), nystagmus, tilting of the head, and titubation. The second, the paravermal zone, consists of the paravermal cortex, the globose and emboliform nuclei, and interconnected inputs and outputs. Damage restricted to this zone is found only in experimental animals, and dysfunction of this part causes tonus changes. The third, the lateral zone, consists of the cerebellar hemispheres, the dentate nuclei, and related inputs and outputs. The main input of this zone is from the cerebral cortex, and outputs course to the brain stem and thalamus. Damage to the lateral zone is associated with ataxia, hypotonia, asthenia (an increased propensity for muscle fatigue), intention tremor (kinetic tremor), dysdiadochokinesia (decomposition of movement in tests of alternating repetitive movements), dysmetria (the impaired judgment of distance), nystagmus (with greatest amplitude to the same side as the lesion), dysarthria (slow and labored speech as a result of ataxia of laryngeal muscles), and problems in initiating and terminating motor actions. The vestibular zone is the flocculonodular lobe modulating the descending vestibulospinal and reticulospinal system for maintaining and adjusting body posture. In general, lesions of the deep cerebellar nuclei or superior cerebellar peduncle (i.e., lesions interrupting cerebellar output) produce more severe and lasting (not attenuating) deficits, whereas cerebellar cortex lesions are associated with attenuating deficits with reduction in severity as time passes.

Spinal Cord, with Ascending and Descending Pathways

The spinal cord occupies two-thirds of the adult spinal canal within the vertebral column. It continues rostrally with the brain stem and ends at the lower end of the second lumbar vertebra. The conus medullaris is the conical end of the spinal cord, and the filum terminale attaches the conus medullaris to the first segment of the coccyx. Throughout its length, 31 pairs of spinal nerves (eight cervical, 12 thoracic, five lumbar, five sacral, and one coccygeal) exit the cord through the intervertebral foramina (see Figure 2-4). C1 exits between the atlas and occipital bone; C2–C7 exit above the corresponding vertebrae; C8 exits between C7 and T1; and the rest of the spinal nerves exit below the corresponding vertebrae. Each spinal nerve is composed of dorsal roots, consisting of sensory afferent fibers from the dorsal root ganglion cells, and ventral roots, consisting of motor efferent fibers originating in the ventral and lateral gray columns. The spinal cord has two enlargements—cervical (between C3 and T2) and lumbosacral (between T9 and T12), which correspond with the origins of the peripheral brachial and lumbosacral plexuses, respectively, for motor and sensory innervation of the upper and lower extremities. The lower portion of the dural sac between L2 and S4 contains only nerve roots, which are collectively known as the cauda equina. Clinically, the withdrawal of cerebrospinal fluid is usually done from this segment. In a transverse section, the spinal cord is composed of a butterfly-shaped core of gray matter, consisting of cell bodies and their processes surrounded by white matter, consisting of axons, mostly myelinated. The central canal, extending in the centrum of the gray matter, is filled with cerebrospinal fluid and opens into the fourth ventricle.

Gray Matter

The gray matter is subdivided into dorsal, intermediate, and ventral horns. The dorsal horns contain sensory relay nuclei; the ventral horns contain somatic motor neurons innervating striated muscles; and the intermediate horns contain all visceral motor neurons that innervate neurons in the autonomic ganglia. For the neuronal organization of gray matter, two nomenclatures are used: (1) the columnar and nuclear organization, and (2) Rexed's laminae I–X. The dorsal horn relays sensory information to higher centers after integrating and modulating them. The reflex arcs are also established through the dorsal horn. The nuclei of the dorsal horn are (1) the posterodorsomarginal nucleus, (2) the principal sensory nucleus, (3) the substantia gelatinosa, and (4) the dorsal nucleus of Clarke (in segments C8–L3). The ventral horn contains lower motor neurons for innervation of striated muscles. In the organization of these neurons, the medial motor column for the axial musculature extends the length of the entire cord, but the lateral motor columns are present in the cervical and lumbosacral enlargements for the extremity muscles. The intermediolateral cell column containing preganglionic sympathetic neurons is limited between T1–L3.

White Matter

The white matter is composed of myelinated and unmyelinated fibers and glial cells within the dorsal, ventral, and lateral funiculi. These fibers carry information from the spinal cord to the brain (i.e., the ascending tracts) or information associated with motor function from the brain to the spinal cord (i.e., the descending tracts) (Figure 2-10). There are also extensive connections between the spinal segments, which ascend or descend adjacent to the gray matter; these are called the *fasciculus proprius*.

After the stimulation of peripheral sensory receptors, which are widely distributed over the body, the information is transmitted to the dorsal roots of the spinal cord via fibers in the spinal nerve. The area of skin innervated by a single dorsal root is known as a *dermatome*. The dorsal root fibers all have their cell bodies in the dorsal root ganglia, which lie close to the junction with the ventral root. The major ascending tracts (Table 2-4) are composed of a chain of three neurons, each with a long axon. The first neuron is in the dorsal root ganglia; the second neuron is in the neuraxis

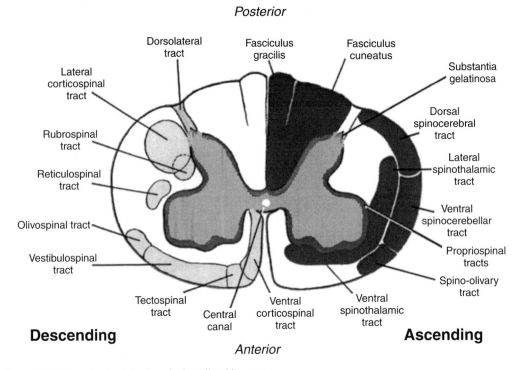

Figure 2-10. The major tracts in the spinal cord's white matter.

(which is different for each as shown in Table 2-4); and the third neuron is in the thalamus, which projects to the sensory cortex for conscious perception or in the brain stem and cerebellum for reflex activity. Sensory information that extends to the spinal cord from one side of the body crosses over the opposite side of the nervous system before being projected to the cerebral cortex. Generally, the axons of the second neuron decussate either within the spinal cord or the brain stem. The net influence of higher centers (i.e., cerebral cortex, basal ganglia, cerebellum, and brain stem) on the spinal cord is projected by the descending tracts (Table 2-5). The descending tracts are located in the lateral and ventral funiculi of the spinal cord white matter. Most of the axons in these tracts terminate on interneurons that project to the motoneurons and a few on the sensory relay neurons for central control of sensory processing. The most prominent descending tract is the lateral corticospinal tract carrying information from the motor cortices and projecting to contralateral motoneurons of the spinal cord (decussation is in the lower medulla). These tracts are concerned

with skilled voluntary movements, posture, and balance. The spinal cord has other descending tracts (the olivospinal and autonomic tracts) and ascending tracts (the spinoreticular, spinotectal, spinocervicothalamic, spinocortical, spinovestibular, spinopontine, and spino-olivary tracts), which are generally inaccessible for clinical evaluation.

Spinal cord diseases and injuries produce signs and symptoms according to the side, level, and extent of the lesion. These can be intrinsic or extrinsic in origin. In these lesions, a motor disability (paresis or paralysis) results when it involves the corticospinal fibers in the lateral column (i.e., upper motor neuron) or the spinomuscular fibers, including the anterior horns or anterior roots (i.e., lower motor neuron). In upper motor neuron lesions, a spastic syndrome consisting of a spasticity in the affected muscles (particularly to the flexors of the arm and extensors of the leg), ipsilateral increased deep tendon reflexes (which is produced by a simple direct connection between sensory and motor neurons) such as hyperreflexia, pathologic reflexes (e.g., Babinski's, clonus), diminished or absent superficial reflexes (i.e.,

Table 2-4. Major Ascending Pathways

Name	Origin	Second Neuron	Termination	Function
Dorsal column	Skin, joints, tendons, and muscles	Nucleus cuneatus (for upper extremity) Nucleus gracilis (for lower extremity)	Areas 3, 1, 2	Contralateral conscious proprioception, pressure, and touch
Lateral spino-thalamic	Skin	Substantia gelatinosa	Areas 3, 1, 2	Contralateral pain and temperature
Ventral spino-thalamic	Skin	Substantia gelatinosa	Areas 3, 1, 2	Contralateral touch and itching
Ventral spino-cerebellar	Skin and muscles	Laminae V, VI, and VII	Paleocerebellum and caudal vermis (via colliculus superior)	Unconscious proprioception (from lower extremities and lower half of the body)
Dorsal spino-cerebellar	Skin and muscles	Clarke's nucleus (C8–L3)	Paleocerebellum and caudal vermis (via colliculus inferior)	Unconscious proprioception from lower extremities and lower half of the body) and tactile impulses

Note: All of the ascending pathways have their first neuron in the dorsal root ganglia, and pathways reaching to the thalamus have (i.e., rows 1–3) a relay nuclei in the thalamus as a third neuron.

Table 2-5. Major Descending Pathways

Name	Origin	Termination	Function
Corticospinal	Areas 4, 6, 3, 1, 2	Anterior horn, α-moto-neuron	Voluntary skilled movement
Tectospinal	Colliculus superior	Anterior horn interneurons	Reflex head and neck movement to visual and auditory stimuli
Vestibulospinal	Lateral vestibular nucleus	Extensor motoneurons and interneurons	Postural reflexes
Reticulospinal	Reticular formation	Anterior horn cells (predominantly flexors)	Posture and balance
Rubrospinal	Nucleus ruber	Anterior horn interneurons	Posture and balance

cutaneous reflexes), and withdrawal responses accompany the motor disability. Isolated lesions of the corticospinal tract usually result in motor disability with normal reflexes and flaccid tone, but because the damage to the lateral column usually involves also the rubrospinal and reticulospinal tracts, the paralysis is spastic. In lower motor neuron lesions, abolition or decreased deep tendon reflexes (i.e., areflexia), muscle atrophy, and muscle fasciculation accompany the flaccid paralysis. In some diseases of the spinal cord (e.g., ALS), there is a combination of upper and lower motor neuron signs and symptoms. The sensorial ascending spinal pathways in general convey tactile, pain, temperature, deep sensibility, and the unconscious proprioceptive impulses. In complete lesions of the dorsal root, all forms of these sensibilities are lost, but if the lesion is incomplete, some are involved. The spinal cord lesions involving the ascending tracts cause sensorial deficit contralaterally below that segment.

Neurovascular Anatomy

The brain constitutes only approximately 2% of total body weight but utilizes approximately 20% of cardiac output. The cerebral blood flow is approximately 50 ml per 100 g brain tissue per minute. The brain tissue must receive a constant flow of oxygen and glu-

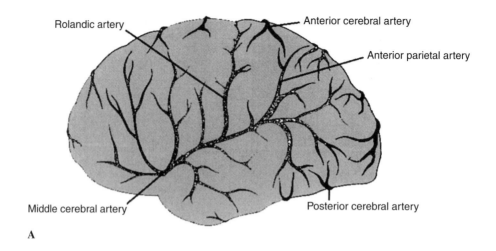

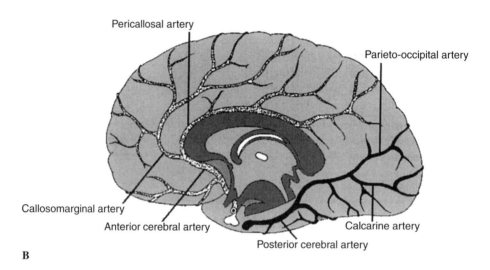

Figure 2-11. The cerebral arteries. (A) Lateral view. (B) Medial view.

cose to survive. Autonomic regulation provides adequate perfusion of the cerebral capillary beds despite variations in systemic blood pressure (cerebral autoregulation) and also provides blood volume shift to one cortical area in case of increased cortical activity. The neurovascular anatomy of the nervous system consists of an arterial and venous system and there is no lymphatic system.

Arterial Supply

The arterial blood supply to the brain is provided by two pairs of arteries: the internal carotid arteries (the

carotid system) and the vertebral arteries (the vertebrobasilar system). These arteries are located at the base of the brain within the subarachnoid space.

The Carotid System

The internal carotid artery (Figure 2-11), a branch of the common carotid artery, ascends the neck and perforates the base of the skull through the foramen lacerum, passes through the carotid canal and the cavernous sinus, and gives off its branches in the region of the anterior perforated substance as follows. The ophthalmic artery supplies the eye, the frontal area of the scalp, and the frontal and ethmoid sinuses. An important branch of this artery is the central retinal artery. The posterior communicating artery joins the posterior cerebral artery, thus forming part of the arterial circle of Willis, and supplies the hypothalamus, ventral thalamus, and cerebral peduncles. The anterior choroidal artery mainly supplies the choroidal plexus of the lateral ventricle. It also gives branches to the optic tract, internal capsule, lateral geniculate body, and crus cerebri. The anterior cerebral artery runs forward on the medial aspect of the hemisphere, where it gives off the branches of the orbital, frontal, pericallosal, and callosomarginal arteries and the penetrating medial striate artery (recurrent artery of Heubner), which supplies the nucleus caudatus, the anterior limb of the internal capsule, the putamen, and the septal nuclei. The cortical branches of the anterior cerebral artery supply all the medial surface of the frontal and parietal cortex. Each of the two anterior cerebral arteries are joined by the anterior communicating artery. The middle cerebral artery is the largest branch of the internal carotid artery. It gives off first the penetrating central branches (lenticulostriate or lateral striate), which enter the anterior perforated substance to supply the globus pallidus, putamen, caudate nucleus, thalamus, genu, and posterior limb of the internal capsule. The middle cerebral artery then runs laterally in the depths of the lateral sulcus and divides into the cortical branches, which supply the entire lateral surface of the hemisphere except the occipital pole and the inferolateral surface.

The Vertebrobasilar System

The posterior portion of the brain is supplied by the two vertebral arteries, which arise from the subclavian arteries. Each enters the vertebral canal at the level of the sixth cervical vertebra and ascends. The two vertebral arteries enter the cranial cavity through the foramen magnum and join at the pontomedullary junction to form the basilar artery. In the intracranial portion before this confluence, each vertebral artery contributes to the formation of the anterior spinal artery supplying the anterior two-thirds of the spinal cord and anteromedial medulla, and to the posterior inferior cerebellar artery, supplying the dorsolateral medulla, inferior cerebellar peduncle, and inferior surface of the cerebellum. The basilar artery gives rise to the anterior inferior cerebellar artery, which supplies the pons, the choroid plexus of the fourth ventricle, and the anterior inferior surface of the cerebellum. The pontine arteries

supply the pons. The labyrinthine artery supplies the cochlea and labyrinth. The superior cerebellar artery supplies the rostral pons, the middle and superior cerebellar peduncles, the superior surface of the cerebellum, and the cerebellar nuclei. The posterior cerebral arteries supply the midbrain, the cerebral peduncles, the inferior medial portion of the temporal cortex, the occipital cortex, and the thalamus. This artery is joined with the internal carotid artery by the posterior communicating artery. The posterior choroidal artery, arising from the posterior cerebral artery, supplies the tectum, the choroid plexus of the third ventricle, and the superior and medial surfaces of the thalamus.

The circle of Willis (circulus arteriosus cerebri) is formed by the junction of the terminal branches of the basilar artery and the two internal carotid arteries, which is achieved by a pair of posterior communicating arteries and an anterior communicating artery (Figure 2-12). There are extensive anastomotic connections in the brain apart from the cerebral arterial circle of Willis between the carotid and vertebral systems. These connections are rich with penetrating arteries, so the occlusion of an artery in the brain can be ineffective or less effective.

Venous Drainage

The venous drainage of the brain is supplied by the brain veins, dural sinuses, meningeal veins, and diploic veins of the skull. Cerebral veins, unlike systemic veins, have no valves. This is also true for the dural sinuses, which are channels located between two layers of dura mater. Although the venous drainage of the cerebellum and brain stem parallels the arterial system, the veins of the brain do not accompany the arteries. The cerebral veins are classified as internal cerebral and cortical veins. The deep or internal cerebral veins (i.e., the thalamostriate and choroidal veins), the basal veins (of Rosenthal), the precentral cerebellar vein, and the upper brain stem veins drain into the great cerebral vein of Galen. This vein drains, respectively, into the straight, lateral, and sigmoid sinuses to the left internal jugular vein. The superficial drainage system—that is, the cortical veins, drain into the nearest vein or sinus. These are divided into two groups:

1. The superior cerebral veins, 6–12 in number, are on the lateral surface of the hemisphere and drain into the superior sagittal sinus.

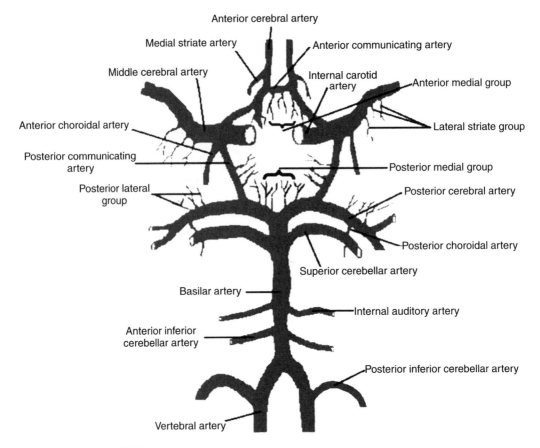

Figure 2-12. The circle of Willis.

2. The inferior cerebral veins drain into the cavernous sinus by the superficial middle cerebral vein or drain into a transverse sinus. This group is connected also to the superior sagittal sinus by the great anastomotic vein of Trolard and by the vein of Labbé. The deep cerebral vein is also in this group and drains into the basal vein, which in turn drains into the straight sinus. The venous drainage of the spinal cord drains into three longitudinal systems, which anastomose extensively: the spinal cord plexus itself and the epidural, internal, and external vertebral plexuses.

Meninges, Ventricular System, and Cerebrospinal Fluid

Meninges

The spinal cord and the brain are covered by three layers of membranes called the *meninges*: the dura mater,

the arachnoid, and the pia mater from the outer surface, respectively (Figure 2-13). The dura mater is a strong, fibrous covering of the CNS and is bounded tightly to the inner surface of the skull but loosely to the vertebral canal. The arachnoid is a delicate structure loosely attached to the dura mater. The pia mater, which is delicate and rich in vascularization, tightly covers the brain and related structures. The meninges are separated from each other by the meningeal spaces. The cranial epidural space contains the meningeal arteries and veins, and the spinal epidural space contains fat tissue, lymphatics, and venous plexuses. The cranial subdural space is traversed by bridging veins, but the spinal subdural space is potentially insignificant. The subarachnoid space ends at the level of the second sacral vertebra and contains the cerebrospinal fluid (CSF). Dural folds—called the *cerebral falx*, the *cerebellar falx*, and the *cerebellar tentorium*—divide the cranial cavity into compartments that are important in the formation of herniation syndromes.

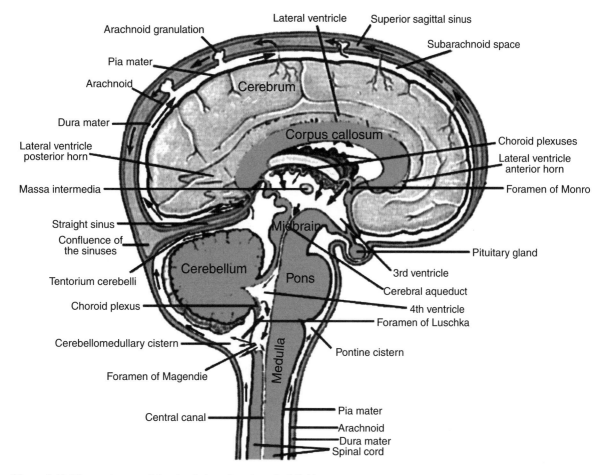

Figure 2-13. The meninges and the circulation of cerebrospinal fluid.

Ventricles and Cerebrospinal Fluid

The brain and spinal cord are extremely soft tissues and therefore require a protective system, which is provided by the bony structures of the cranial cavity and vertebral canal. In this vault, the CNS floats suspended in a pool of CSF. CSF is secreted from the choroidal plexuses at 600–700 ml per day, so that the entire volume of CSF is turned over three to four times a day. The choroid plexus is made of dense capillary networks covered with the pia mater and the modified ependymal cells and is located in the walls of the lateral, the third, and the fourth ventricles. The two lateral ventricles communicate with the third ventricle via the foramen of Monro. The third ventricle, via the cerebral aqueduct (aqueduct of Sylvius), connects with the fourth ventricle. The fourth ventricle communicates with the subarachnoid space via the foramen of Magendie and the two foramina of Luschka. CSF is a clear, colorless, almost acellular (less than 5 mononuclear cells per microliter) fluid with a pressure range of 80–180 mm H_2O. CSF contains glucose (50–75 mg per dl, 66% of blood glucose), protein (15–50 mg per dl), and a small amount of electrolytes. The CSF is absorbed by the arachnoid villi (pacchionian granulation) into the spinal venous plexus and mainly the superior sagittal sinus. CSF protects the CNS against concussive injury, transports hormones and related substances, preserves homeostasis in the nervous system, and removes waste products. Blockage of the flow of CSF results in hydrocephalus. Changes in cellular content (e.g., the existence of red blood cells in the CSF means subarachnoid hemorrhage), glucose, and protein levels are particularly important in the diagnosis of a wide variety of diseases (e.g., meningitis).

Blood-Brain Barrier

Homeostasis in the nervous system occurs because of the specific permeability barriers between blood and the brain, between blood and CSF, and between the brain and CSF. These barriers allow the passage of some molecules from blood into the brain or CSF, or from the brain into the CSF, and also allow the removal waste products. Among these, the blood-brain barrier plays a key role in maintaining intracerebral oxygen, glucose, carbon dioxide, ion, amino acid, protein, and fluid homeostasis. This barrier is located in the specialized endothelial cells of the capillaries. These cells are joined by tight junctions, have a high number of mitochondria providing energy for transport, have few pinocytotic vesicles, and make frequent contact on their brain side with numerous processes of the astrocytes. A continuous basement membrane also surrounds the capillary outside the endothelial cells. The blood-brain barrier penetration can be lipid- or carrier-mediated and can affect both entry and exit of substances. In general, substances that are highly soluble in lipid and small molecules enter the CNS more readily and rapidly. Most larger proteins do not enter at all. The entire CNS parenchyma has a blood-brain barrier, except in the pineal gland, pituitary gland, some areas of the hypothalamus, and the area postrema. In these regions, capillary permeability through the fenestrations of the endothelium resembles that found in non-neural tissues. In pathologic conditions, such as stroke, infections, tumor or trauma, the blood-brain barrier breaks down, and normally excluded substances, such as metabolites and fluid from the blood or CSF, can leak into the CNS. The blood-CSF barrier, which is composed of vascular endothelium, basement membrane and choroid epithelium of the choroid plexus, is an effective one-way entry into the CSF compartment of the brain. The major drainage route of this barrier is the arachnoid villus. The third physiologic barrier is the brain-CSF barrier, between the extracellular compartment of the CNS and the CSF. This is a potential barrier and is composed of ependyma, basement membrane and subependymal glial membrane.

Neurochemistry

CNS neurons receive signals from thousands of synaptic terminals. In this network, rapid and precise communication is made possible by neurotransmitters, neurohormones, and neuromodulators. Neurotransmitters are small organic molecules that carry a chemical message from a neuronal axon or dendrite to another cell or nerve. Neurohormones are chemical messengers that can be released from both neuronal and non-neuronal cells into the circulatory system and alter cellular function at a distance. Neuromodulators are transmitters that alter the endogenous activity of the target cell pre- and postsynaptically, in the face of ongoing synaptic activity. Neuromodulation allows a cell or a nerve to adapt its activity to environmental changes. In the last several years, advances in neurochemistry, neurophysiology, and molecular biology, including autoradiographic and immunocytochemical techniques, have helped to elucidate the structure of the neurotransmitters and to map out the anatomic distribution of neurons containing neurotransmitters. A neurotransmitter must be synthesized in the presynaptic neuron, stored in presynaptic vesicles, released by calcium-dependent mechanisms from the presynaptic neuron, active at selective postsynaptic receptors to change membrane potential, and, finally, removed from the synaptic site or destroyed biochemically. Neurotransmitters function in two distinct ways: (1) neurotransmitters produce fast phasic responses by changing the postsynaptic membrane ion channel state, and (2) neurotransmitters act via G-protein-coupled metabotropic receptors through a long-lasting effect via second messengers in a enzymatic cascade. Neurotransmitters mediate a synaptic transmission in a rapid or slow fashion because of the type of the transmitter and receptor that is used. This transmission rate is also affected by the site of synthesis and the metabolic enzymes of the transmitter. Some neurotransmitters are synthesized in the cell body and require axonal transmission for release (e.g., slow peptide transmitters), but some are synthesized and stored in the axon (e.g., fast acetylcholine [ACh], glutamate neurotransmitters). The chemical synapses have four principal advantages: (1) They are unidirectional, so information is transmitted in one preferred direction; (2) synaptic information can be inhibited or excited; (3) they provide a delay for information transfer, which allows the arrival to be timed appropriately; and (4) chemical synapses can undergo plastic changes—that is, they can alter their efficacy (plasticity). Neurotransmitters are grouped into six categories: acetylcholine, catecholamines, indole amines, histamine, amino acids (inhibitory and excitatory), and neuropeptides. There are probably many more transmitters, but they are currently unknown. In the future, they should be identified to explain how the brain works with more detailed information.

Acetylcholine

ACh is the principal neurotransmitter of the neuromuscular junctions, sympathetic and parasympathetic preganglionic neurons, parasympathetic postganglionic neurons, which innervate the viscera, and sympathetic postganglionic neurons, which innervate major sweat glands of the skin. It also is used at many synapses throughout the brain. In the brain, cholinergic neurons are found in the septal nuclei, the basal nucleus of Meynert, the striatum, and the brain stem motor and parasympathetic nuclei. Major central projections are to the frontal and parietal neocortex, the hypothalamus, the thalamus, and the hippocampus. In the spinal cord, the preganglionic sympathetic and parasympathetic preganglionic neurons and alpha motor neurons contain ACh. There are two kinds of ACh receptors: nicotinic and muscarinic. Nicotinic receptors are found at the neuromuscular junction and autonomic ganglia and also in the brain. Nicotinic and muscarinic receptors have five subunits. ACh generally functions as an excitatory neurotransmitter throughout the nervous system. The cholinergic pathway in the ARAS is necessary for consciousness. ACh neurons play a role in motor control and the cognition process. ACh is partly or completely responsible for a wide spectrum of neurologic diseases, including myasthenia gravis, Lambert-Eaton myasthenic syndrome, familial dysautonomia, Huntington's disease, tardive dyskinesia, and Alzheimer's disease.

Catecholamines

All of the neurotransmitters in the catecholamine group (e.g., DA, noradrenaline [NA], adrenaline) are synthesized from the amino acid tyrosine as follows: tyrosine $\rightarrow$ dihydroxyphenylalanine (DOPA) $\rightarrow$ DA $\rightarrow$ NA $\rightarrow$ adrenaline. Two enzymes—monoamino oxidase and catechol-o-methyl-transferase—degrade the catecholamines.

Dopamine

DA is the major catecholamine neurotransmitter and neuromodulator in the human nervous system. The principal DAergic neurons are located in the substantia nigra pars compacta, and ventral tegmental area of the midbrain. Neurons of the substantia nigra project to striatum (mesostriatal), and neurons in the ventral tegmental area project to the limbic system (mesolimbic) and cerebral neocortex (mesocortical). Besides these localizations, olfactory bulb, retina, and hypothalamus also include DAergic interneurons. The mesostriatal pathway accounts for approximately 80% of the brain DA and is involved in the control of voluntary movement. The mesolimbic and mesocortical pathways are associated with emotion, mood alteration, and cognitive function. DA is also found as an interneuron in the peripheral autonomic ganglia. There are two major types of DA receptors: (1) D_1-like receptors, with two subtypes (D_1, D_5), mainly excitatory postsynaptic; and (2) D_2-like receptors, with three subtypes (D_2, D_3, D_4), inhibitory presynaptic and postsynaptic. DAergic synapses include D_1, D_2, or both. In general, DA is an inhibitory neurotransmitter. Degeneration of the DAergic neurons in the substantia nigra causes Parkinson's disease and hyperactivity in the DAergic synapses causes involuntary movements and psychosis.

Noradrenaline

The NA system is less specific than the DAergic system. In the CNS, the NAergic neurons are located in the locus ceruleus and lateral tegmental nuclei, both of which have ascending and descending projections diffusely throughout the cortex, thalamus, limbic system, hypothalamus, cerebellum, olfactory bulb, medulla, and spinal cord. In the peripheral nervous system, NA is the transmitter of the postganglionic sympathetic neurons. These projections are involved in activation of cognitive function, arousal, motivation, mood, memory, pain, and control of autonomic and endocrine functions. Like DA, the NAergic synapses can be excitatory or inhibitory. Adrenergic receptors are divided into two major subtypes, alpha (α) and beta (β), which are located presynaptically and postsynaptically and have subtypes α_1 and α_2 and β_1, β_2, and β_3. In general, α-adrenergic activation is excitatory and β-adrenergic activation tends to be predominantly inhibitory.

Adrenaline

The adrenergic neurons are located in the lateral and dorsal tegmental nuclei, which project to the hypothalamus, locus ceruleus, and spinal cord intermediolateral cell columns. These projections regulate endocrine and autonomic functions. Adrenaline is also released from the adrenal medulla and postganglionic sympathetic nerve endings with NA. Adrenaline also acts on α and β receptors and has inhibiting functions in the CNS. There is no major neurologic disease related directly to improper adrenergic and NAergic activity.

Serotonin

5-HT is produced from tryptophan and functions as a neurotransmitter and neuromodulator. The concentration of 5-HT is very high in the periphery (platelets, mast cells, and the gastrointestinal system) but low (1–2% of the total amount of serotonin) in the brain. The serotonergic system, however, is the most extensive monoaminergic system in the brain and originates from the raphe nuclei located in the brain stem. These nuclei project to all areas of the cerebral cortex (i.e., neocortex, paleocortex, and archicortex), thalamus, hypothalamus, limbic system, basal ganglia, and cerebellum, whereas caudal raphe nuclei project to the spinal cord. There are seven types of 5-HT receptors. The first three also have subtypes, with each having different pharmacologic properties and biologic responses; as inhibitory and or excitatory. Among these, some 5-HT$_1$ receptors are autoreceptors, with their highest activity rate during wakefulness. As a whole, most serotonergic synapses are inhibitory to the postsynaptic neuron. The ascending projections of the serotonergic system modulate cortical activity and have been implicated in sleep, higher cognitive functions, arousal, vigilance, emotion, mood, sexual behavior, body temperature regulation, blood pressure regulation, pain perception, and neurohumoral regulation of CSF secretion. The descending projections play a key role in the modulation of pain transmission; they inhibit the spinal sensory neurons and excite the motor neuron. The affective disorders, schizophrenia, anxiety states, phobic disorders, obsessive-compulsive disorder, cerebral aging, Alzheimer's disease, carcinoid syndrome, migraine, and sleep disorders are all related to improper 5-HT function.

Histamine

Histamine, which is derived from histidine, acts as a CNS neurotransmitter and neuromodulator. It is found in the mast cells and also the CNS. The histaminergic neurons are located in the ventral posterior portion of the hypothalamus and project to innervate the cerebral cortex diffusely, the thalamus, the striatum, limbic structures, the cerebellum, and the spinal cord. There are three known receptors: H$_1$, H$_2$, and H$_3$. Histamine by these receptors in general regulates autonomic responses, control of appetite, regulation of pituitary hormone secretion, and control of vestibular reactivity. It also regulates vegetative functions, has a role in arousal, and regulates behavioral and mental states. Histamine also stimulates chemosensitive nociceptors after injury or inflammation.

Amino Acid Neurotransmitters

On the basis of neurophysiologic and biochemical studies, amino acids have gained recognition as major, widely distributed, fast transmitters in the mammalian CNS. Amino acids have been separated into two groups: excitatory amino acids (glutamic acid, aspartic acid, cysteic acid and homocysteic acid), which depolarize neurons, and inhibitory amino acids (gamma-aminobutyric acid [GABA], glycine, taurine, and β-alanine), which hyperpolarize neurons in the CNS.

Excitatory Amino Acids

The principal excitatory neurotransmitters are glutamate and aspartate, which depolarize neurons in the CNS. Glutamate, which is formed from glutamine, is the major fast excitatory neurotransmitter of the brain and spinal cord. Glutamate is a product of the Krebs cycle; it excites virtually all central neurons and is found in very high concentrations in the nerve terminals. Essentially all efferent projections of the cortex to the striatum, thalamus, subthalamus, and brain stem and afferents of the cerebellum and efferents of the hippocampal cells use glutamate. Almost all cells in the brain have receptors that respond to glutamate. There are five types of glutamate receptors, each having distinct physiologic characteristics: (1) N-methyl-D-aspartate (NMDA), with R$_1$ and R$_2$ subtypes, including glutamate, glycine, phencyclidine, magnesium, polyamine, and quinolinic acid sites; (2) kainate; (3) quisqualate (α-amino-3-hydroxy-5-methyl-4-isoxazole-propionic acid [AMPA]); and (4) metabotropic (trans-1-aminocyclopentane-1-3-dicarboxylic acid [ACPD]), and (5) 1,2-amino-4-phosphonobutyrate (AP_4) autoreceptor. The activation of non-NMDA receptors produces excitatory postsynaptic potentials (EPSPs). A high-frequency stimulation of certain synapses produces prolonged potentiation of the EPSPs. This long-term potentiation (LTP) depends mainly on NMDA receptor stimulation and is involved in short-term memory and learning. Excessive amounts of glutamate are highly toxic to neurons. This is due to the excessive influx of Ca^{2+} into the neurons through the NMDA receptors, which in turn activate intracellular Ca-dependent enzymes, leading to free radical production, which is highly toxic to neurons. Glutamate neurotoxicity may contribute acute brain injury such as stroke, trauma, status epilepticus, cerebral aging, various neurodegenerative disorders (e.g., Parkinson's disease, dementia, and ALS), and viral disorders (e.g., acquired immunodeficiency disorder). Aspartate is a less potent excitatory neurotransmitter that is not as widely distributed as glutamate. It is also a product of the Krebs cycle and activates the same receptors as glutamate.

Inhibitory Amino Acids

The principal inhibitory CNS neurotransmitters are GABA and glycine. GABA is the inhibitory transmitter involved in the internal circuits of the brain and spinal cord. It is also found in the pancreas and adrenal glands. GABA is synthesized from glutamate. Both neurons and glial cells have a high affinity for GABA. There are two types of GABA receptors that respond rapidly like excitatory ones. GABA-A is a postsynaptic receptor that has binding sites for GABA, barbiturate, and benzodiazepine. This receptor allows the conduction of chloride ions, which decrease the depolarizing effects of the excitatory input and depress excitability. GABA-B is a presynaptic receptor that functions as a modulator of GABA release. GABAergic neurons are found in the cerebral cortex, cerebellum, olfactory bulb, basal ganglia, retina, hippocampus, caudal hypothalamus, and spinal cord. Nearly all neurons of the cerebral cortex are either glutaminergic or GABAergic. Inhibitory

signals, which are generated by GABAergic interneurons, are essential for the processing of information at the level of the cortex. In the basal ganglia, the projections from the striatum to the thalamus via the globus pallidus medialis and substantia nigra in the direct loop and projections from the striatum to the subthalamic nucleus via the globus pallidus lateralis in the indirect loop are all inhibitory (GABAergic). The cholinergic interneurons in the striatum excite these GABA striatal efferents in the indirect loop and thus counterbalance the cortical reinforcing effect of the DAergic neurons. Inhibitory spinal interneurons, mostly in the dorsal horn, are GABAergic. GABA plays a role in the pathogenesis of a group of diseases. In Huntington's disease, striatal GABAergic and cholinergic neurons are destroyed. In epilepsy, there is a reduction in cortical inhibition mediated by GABA. In parkinsonism, schizophrenia, tardive dyskinesia, and dementia, the GABAergic system is also affected. Drugs that increase the amount of GABA cause disturbances of conscioiusnes leading to coma and death.

Glycine

Glycine, which structurally is the simplest amino acid, is a less common inhibitor neurotransmitter. The concentration of glycine in the spinal cord, in the central and ventral location, is much higher than the level in whole brain.

Neuropeptides

More than 50 active neuropeptides have been described; most of these have been defined by the technical advances in molecular biology. Neuropeptides are slow neurotransmitters or neuromodulators and are present in small amounts in the CNS. They are synthesized in the cell body and are axonally transported to the nerve terminal. Neuropeptides generally are classified in at least 10 groups, but for convenience they are grouped as nonopioid peptides and opioid peptides.

Nonopioid Peptides

Many of the peptides in the group of nonopioid peptides are named in relation to the localization of the discovery of the compound, such as hypothalamic neurohormones (e.g., thyrotropin, soma-totropin, and corticotropin-releasing hormones), pituitary peptides (e.g., prolactin and growth hormone), neurohypophyseal hormones (oxytocin and vasopressin), gastrointestinal peptides (e.g., substance P, cholecystokinin, vasoactive intestinal polypeptide), and others (e.g., calcitonin gene–related peptide, sleep peptide, bradykinin, and angiotensin II [vasoactive peptides]). Among these, substance P was the first peptide neurotransmitter discovered in the gastrointestinal system. Substance P is a member of the family of neurokinins and has an excitatory effect in the CNS in mainly two locations: (1) the substantia gelatinosa in the spinal cord gray matter, and (2) the striatum. In the spinal cord, substance P is secreted by the dorsal root ganglion cells conveying pain from the periphery to the posterior horn in the case of painful stimuli. Here, the descending serotonergic pathways simultaneously stimulate the release of opiates in the substantia gelatinosa, which blocks the secretion of substance P. The direct pathway from the striatum to output nuclei is mediated by GABA and substance P.

Opioid Peptides

Opioid peptides are putative transmitters that bind to opiate receptors. These are actually the "morphine" of the brain and are important in analgesia and euphoria. Opioid peptides are particularly found in the striatum, globus pallidus, limbic system, raphe nuclei, hypothalamus, cerebellum, somatosensory pathways, and spinal cord. These neurotransmitters are derived from three genetically distinct precursors: proenkephalin, pro-opiomelanocortin, and pro-dynorphin. Proenkephalin was first identified in the adrenal medulla and it is the precursor of enkephalin and enkephalin-related peptides. Enkephalin is found in high concentrations in the striatum and

globus pallidus; however, it is also distributed throughout the neocortex, diencephalon, brain stem, cerebellum, and spinal cord. Pro-opiomelanocortin is mainly the precursor of alpha, beta, and gamma endorphins, the cell bodies of which are in the pituitary gland, hypothalamus, and nucleus of the solitary tract and projecting mainly to the brain stem reticular nuclei, periaqueductal gray matter, and spinal cord. Prodynorphin is the precursor of dynorphin. Dynorphins are heavily concentrated in the posterior pituitary, hypothalamus, and limbic system and also in the neocortex and cerebellum. The opioid receptors have subtypes, the best known of which are the mu (endorphin), delta (enkephalin), and kappa (dynorphin) receptors.

Suggested Reading

Burt AM. Textbook of Neuroanatomy. Philadelphia: Saunders, 1992.

Conn PM. Neuroscience in Medicine. Philadelphia: Lippincott, 1995.

Cooper JR, Bloom FE, Roth RH. The Biochemical Basis of Neuropharmacology (7th ed). New York: Oxford University Press, 1996.

DeMyer W. Neuroanatomy, The National Medical Series for Independent Study. New York: John Wiley, 1988.

Gilman S, Newman SW. Manter and Gatz's Essentials of Clinical Neuroanatomy and Neurophysiology (9th ed). Philadelphia: Davis, 1996.

Guyton AC. Basic Neuroscience, Anatomy and Physiology (2nd ed). Philadelphia: Saunders, 1992.

Jennes L, Traurig HH, Conn PM. Atlas of the Human Brain. Philadelphia: Lippincott–Raven, 1995.

Joseph R. Neuropsychiatry, Neuropsychology and Clinical Neuroscience. Baltimore: Williams & Wilkins, 1996.

Kandell ER, Schwartz JH, Jessell TM. Principles of Neural Science (3rd ed). New York: Elsevier, 1991.

Noback CR, Demarest RJ. Human Nervous System (4th ed). Columbia: Lea & Febiger, 1991.

Snell RS. Clinical Anatomy for Medical Students (5th ed). Boston: Little, Brown, 1995.

Chapter 3
Neuroimaging

Kazuo Minematsu

Chapter Plan

Observation is the first step of natural science. Attempts to see through the body have led to the current developments in imaging technology. X-ray computed tomography (CT) represented a significant breakthrough in the diagnosis of neurologic disorders in the mid-1970s, when plain radiography, invasive contrast angiography, pneumoencephalography, and myelography were the only available neuroradiologic methods. Since the era of CT began, less invasive and more accurate neuroimaging methods have become available. They include magnetic resonance imaging (MRI), magnetic resonance angiography (MRA), single-photon emission CT (SPECT), and positron emission tomography (PET).

In this chapter, the neuroimaging techniques currently used for clinical neurology and neuroscience are briefly reviewed. The discussion is focused mainly on methodologic issues and major clinical applications.

Structural Imaging

X-Ray Computed Tomography

CT uses differential absorption of thin-section x-ray beams passed through the target organ to construct a map of relative tissue densities. The gray scale of CT images represents the relative values of x-ray attenuation. The computer-generated attenuation number of water is arbitrarily defined to be 0 Hounsfield units (HU). The values are +10 HU for spinal fluid, +30 ~ +40 HU for soft tissues including the white and gray matters, +40 ~ +50 HU for liquid blood, +50 ~ +100 HU for clotted blood, above +100 HU for bone, and −50 ~ −100 HU for fat. The appearance of a CT image can be modified by changing the range of CT numbers selected for a given display, which is termed the *window*. The reference CT number, or the center of the window, is called the *level*. On routine examination where the level is selected to be 40 or 50 HU, spinal fluid appears dark, and clotted blood looks fairly bright. Calcification, fresh hemorrhage,

Table 3-1. Advantages and Disadvantages of Computed Tomography (CT)
and Magnetic Resonance Imaging (MRI)

	CT	MRI
Ionizing radiation	Present	Absent
Spatial resolution	Excellent	Fair
Contrast resolution	Poor	Excellent
Information	Simple	Complex (T1, T2, proton density, flow, diffusion)
Diagnosis of vascular patency	Impossible	Possible (flow void)
Imaging of acute hemorrhage	Excellent	Poor
Multiplanar imaging	Difficult	Easy
Examination time	Short	Relatively long[a]
Artifacts by bone	Often	Absent
Contraindication	Not specific	Uncooperative or very ill patients; claustrophobic patients; patients with ferromagnetic objects[b]
Costs	Less expensive	Expensive

[a]Fast (within seconds) and ultrafast (<1 sec) techniques are currently available.
[b]Includes cardiac pacemakers, cochlear implants, aneurysm clips, prosthetic heart valves, and so forth.

and blood stasis look hyperdense relative to the normal brain parenchyma. In contrast, infarcted and necrotic tissue, brain edema, and demyelinating lesions cause various degrees of hypodensity. When a CT scan is performed with the intravenous administration of iodinated contrast agents, abnormal enhancement is shown in the tissue with breakdown of the blood-brain barrier (BBB) or with increased vascularity. The major disadvantages of CT scanning are the artifacts that arise from adjacent bones, especially in the posterior fossa and spinal canal. To minimize this problem, scans within the posterior fossa are often obtained at 5-mm thickness, whereas 1-cm slices are adequate above the tentorium for routine clinical purposes.

CT scans are now available in most hospitals, and the method has become standard for neurologic diagnosis. Currently available CT techniques allow rapid image acquisition, excellent spatial resolution, and great differentiation between normal and pathologic tissue. Although MRI is quickly replacing CT scanning as the most sensitive method for detecting various types of neurologic disorders, CT remains the quickest, easiest, least expensive, and relatively accurate way for the diagnosis of neurologic emergencies. CT examinations are indicated for patients with intracranial aneurysm clips, for patients with cardiac pacemakers, and for very ill or uncooperative patients who cannot easily be examined with

MRI (Table 3-1). CT is superior to MRI for the diagnosis of acute trauma, suspected acute intracranial hemorrhage, bone fractures, and neoplasms that contain calcification (e.g., granuloma, glioma, meningioma, teratoma).

CT scanning should be performed immediately if acute intracranial hemorrhage is suspected. Acute clotted blood is visualized on a CT scan as a localized parenchymal hyperdensity in brain hemorrhage and as diffuse areas of increased density within the basal cisterns and sylvian fissure in subarachnoid hemorrhage (SAH). In acute brain hemorrhage, the volume and location of an area of hyperdensity on CT images are excellent predictors of a patient's outcome and may help establish the indication for surgical evacuation. In SAH, the thickness of clot in the cisterns is directly related to the likelihood of subsequent vasospasm.

Usually no abnormalities are apparent on a CT scan during the first hours after acute ischemic stroke. It has been emphasized, however, that early examination with a high-resolution CT scanner, even within 3 hours of stroke onset, may provide evidence of major artery occlusion and early parenchymal ischemic damage. The hyperdense middle cerebral artery (MCA) sign is a hyperdensity in the MCA trunk in the basal cistern and supports the presence of thromboembolic occlusion of the MCA (Figure 3-1). The early CT signs include attenuation (or obscuration) of the lentiform nucleus, loss of the insular ribbon, and hemispheric sulcus effacement. Studies have demonstrated that the presence of two or three of these signs is associated with substantial MCA infarction and a poor outcome (Figure 3-2). They also identify patients with an increased risk of hemorrhagic transformation, particularly after thrombolytic therapy.

In the majority of ischemic stroke patients, an area of hypodensity becomes evident after 24–28 hours. The early changes on CT scans tend to be less distinct than the ones obtained several weeks after a stroke. Delineation between the infarcted and normal tissue may be unclear because of surrounding brain edema. Extensive infarction is often accompanied by ventricular compression or the shift of the midline structures during the initial weeks. Hemorrhagic transformation, which is easily detected on CT scans, may occur in thrombotic or embolic infarction (see Figure 3-2). One to 3 weeks after the stroke onset, ischemic lesions often become iso-dense and demonstrate the so-called fogging effect. Old infarcts are quite distinct on CT scans, having sharp margins and lower density.

Hypodensity may also be produced by tumors and old and recent foci of inflammation or of demyelination. A brain tumor is better visualized on CT scans if it contains hemorrhagic or calcified components. A combination of the findings on plain CT scans and scans with contrast enhancement, the location of the lesion, and other CT characteristics is used to distinguish various tumor types.

A contrast-enhanced CT study may help distinguish such entities as subacute infarcts and hemorrhage, primary and metastatic neoplasms, inflammations, granulomas, acute and large plaques of multiple sclerosis (MS) from old infarction, old plaques of MS, and leukoencephalopathy. Ring enhancement on the margin of a lesion, shaped like a ring or an oval, may be seen in gliomas, resolving infarction or hemorrhage, and abscess.

Magnetic Resonance Imaging

MRI is a more recent imaging modality than CT scanning, and it provides the most accurate localization of lesions without invasive radiation. It uses the varying electromagnetic properties of mobile hydrogen protons contained within biolog-

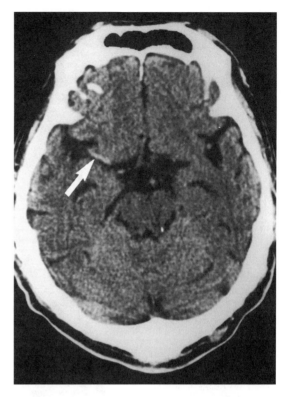

Figure 3-1. Hyperdense middle cerebral artery (MCA) sign (*arrow*) in a patient with cardioembolic infarction. Embolic occlusion of the MCA is confirmed by contrast angiography.

ical tissues. Bone and air give off no signals because they contain very few hydrogen protons. An external magnetic field (B_o) is generated by a magnet located within an MRI scanner. The magnetic field is used to fix the position of protons held within the thermomagnetic lattice structures in the tissue. Radiofrequency (RF) is used to stimulate the protons to a higher energy level. Protons give off relatively intense signals as they decay to the resting state. These signals are detected by receiver coils within the MRI scanner and then used to construct an image of the brain, spinal cord, or other body parts.

MRI offers several advantages over CT scanning in diagnosis of cerebral and spinal pathologic conditions (see Table 3-1). Although the spatial resolution of CT is superior to that of MRI, the contrast resolution is better in the latter than in the former. The contrast in MRI is determined by many tissue variables, including T1 relaxation time, T2 relaxation time, proton density, flow, and molecular diffusion. Among

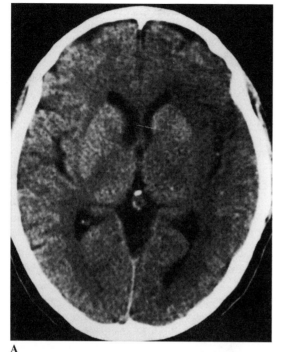

A

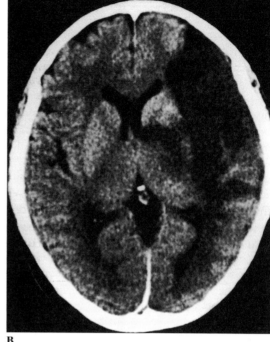

B

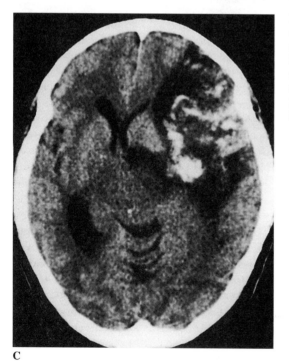

C

Figure 3-2. The early computed tomographic signs and subsequent hemorrhagic transformation. (A) Three hours after the stroke onset. Obscuration of the lentiform nucleus, loss of the insular ribbon, and hemispheric sulcus effacement are evident in the territory of the left middle cerebral artery. (B) Day 2. Hypodensity becomes evident. (C) Day 4. Hyperdense lesions develop within the infarct, indicating hemorrhagic transformation.

them, T1 (longitudinal relaxation) reflects the rate of alignment of protons with the main magnetic field, and T2 (transverse relaxation) reflects the loss of magnetization in the transverse plane. Any one of these variables can be enhanced on an MRI image by modifying the RF pulse sequences. In a T1-weighted image (T1WI), gray and white matter discrimination can easily be achieved, and cerebrospinal fluid (CSF) spaces become black. A T2-weighted image (T2WI) shows high signal intensity in CSF or in areas with high extracellular water content, such as in nonhemorrhagic infarction, vasogenic edema, and demyelinating plaques. Enhancement of the image can be obtained by the use of intravenous gadolinium-diethylenetri-amine penta-acetic acid (Gd-DTPA). Multiplanar imaging is easily achieved with MRI (Figure 3-3). There are, however, several disadvantages in MRI studies. Patients who are confused or agitated by acute brain illness and those who are implanted or surrounded with ferromagnetic materials (pacemakers, clips, respirators, etc.) cannot be examined with MRI.

MRI has become the gold standard for the diagnosis of most neurologic disorders. MRI studies are primarily indicated for a patient with posterior fossa disease, middle fossa disease, disease at the vertex, small paraventricular lesions, demyelinating diseases (e.g., MS), deep white matter infarction, hydrocephalus, small brain tumors, and early infarction and inflammation. Sellar and parasellar masses, pathologic process within the cavernous sinus and cranial canals, or lesions adjacent to the ventricular systems can be visualized easily with MRI in the sagittal or coronal planes. MRI alone can noninvasively and reliably detect myelopathy (e.g., syringomyelia, tumor, infarct, MS, myelitis), disc degeneration, radiculopathy, and metastasis to the spine.

Ischemic lesions may be identified with MRI within 12–24 hours after the onset of symptoms or in even shorter time spans. Compared with CT scanning, MRI can better localize ischemic injury, particularly in the brain stem and cerebellum (Figure 3-4). With conventional MRI sequences (T1WI and T2WI), however, small cortical infarcts can be difficult to detect because of the similarly low or high signal of cortical gray matter and adjacent CSF and the complex convolutional geometry of the surface of the brain. The fluid-attenuated inversion recovery sequence produces a strongly T2WI and suppressed CSF signal, offering advantages in detection of lesions affecting the cortical ribbon.

Conventional MRI is insensitive for detecting acute intracerebral hemorrhage. Strongly susceptibility-weighted MRI such as echo-planar gradient-echo image, however, can detect hemorrhage within 2.5–5.0 hours of onset of clinical symptoms as regions of marked signal loss resulting from susceptibility effects. Signal intensity of hemorrhage changes over weeks in relation to different magnetic properties of hemoglobin metabolites (Table 3-2). The evolving MRI signals make it feasible to image detailed structures of subacute hematoma and to detect old hemorrhage.

Confluent periventricular and punctuate hemispheric foci of abnormaly high signal intensity called *leukoaraiosis* are commonly seen in T2WIs of elderly patients. The majority of these lesions are caused by subtle changes of gliosis and demyelination, presumably from chronic vascular insufficiency.

Gd-enhanced T1WI with a slice thickness of 5 mm is commonly used to detect disease activity in MS. Enhancing lesions correspond to a damaged BBB and perivascular inflammation. The number and extent of Gd-enhancing lesions are well correlated with immunologic markers of disease activity and with short-term outcome in relapsing-remitting and secondary progressive MS. In such patients, the MRI method is currently used for rapid screening of therapies aimed at suppressing new pathologic activity of MS.

New Magnetic Resonance Imaging Techniques: Perfusion and Diffusion Magnetic Resonance Imaging

Conventional MRI studies require several minutes for data acquisition. Recently, fast (within seconds) or ultrafast (less than a second) imaging has become available. The ultrafast technique can prevent motion artifacts in moving organs and provide real-time imaging capability. Echo-planar imaging (EPI) is an important technique for ultrafast imaging that can be used for both diffusion and perfusion imaging and for functional MRI.

EPI is applied to cardiovascular and flow imaging. The method uses intravenously administered paramagnetic contrast agents such as Gd-DTPA, which normally remain within the intravascular space and induce a strong magnetic field gradient in

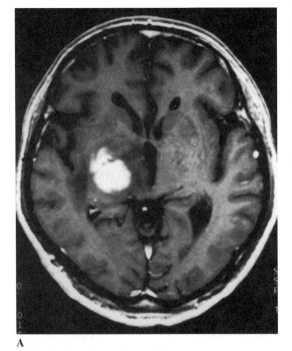

A

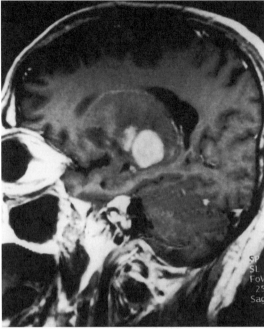

B

Figure 3-3. Multiplanar magnetic resonance imaging studies with Gd-DTPA enhancement in a patient with presumed malignant glioma. (A) Axial image. (B) Sagittal image. (C) Coronal image.

C

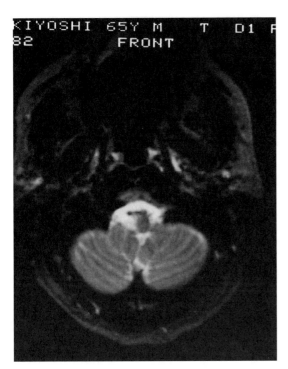

KIYOSHI 65Y M   T   D1
82   FRONT

Figure 3-4. A T2-weighted magnetic resonance imaging study showing a lateral medullary infarction.

Table 3-2. Signal Intensity of Hemoglobin Metabolites in T1- and T2-Weighted Magnetic Resonance Images

Hemoglobin Metabolites	T1-Weighted	T2-Weighted
Oxyhemoglobin in RBCs	Isointense	Isointense
Deoxyhemoglobin in RBCs	Isointense	Hypointense
Methemoglobin in RBCs	Hyperintense	Hypointense
Methemoglobin, extracellular	Hyperintense	Hyperintense
Hemosiderin	Isointense	Hypointense

RBCs = red blood cells.

the capillary space and surrounding tissue. After the bolus injection of a contrast agent, a transient reduction in T2* signal intensity occurs as a function of cerebral blood volume (CBV). Perfusion imaging, or dynamic contrast-enhanced T2*-weighted MRI, is useful in documenting a perfusion failure in patients with acute ischemic stroke. The technique demonstrates lesions early in their clinical course. Perfusion imaging can also be accomplished without injecting contrast agents, and this technique is currently used for functional MRI.

Water diffusion, or translational movement of water molecules, which occurs within all tissues, can be imaged with MRI. By integrating strong, short dephasing and rephasing magnetic field gradients into the standard spin-echo pulse sequence, MRI signals become highly sensitive for the water diffusion. Failure of energy metabolism and associated ionic pumps results in intracellular water accumulation (cytotoxic edema) during pronounced ischemia, making a diffusion-weighted MRI image bright. In animal stroke models, diffusion MRI identified earliest ischemic injury within minutes and hours after arterial

occlusion and could be used for the quantitative assessment of the severity and volume of ischemic injury.

Since diffusion MRI is extremely sensitive to any net translational movement of water molecules, even very slight movement of the head or brain during image acquisition will severely impair the quality of the images. The conventional strategy for MRI is not practical for many patients with acute stroke because it requires 10 minutes or more to perform diffusion MRI. The problem has been solved by the application of EPI. This imaging method has already seen routine clinical use in a few centers (Figure 3-5) and provides important knowledge concerning diagnosis, treatment, and outcome prediction. This method can also differentiate acute from chronic infarcts, which have increased diffusion.

Water diffusion is also affected by directional barriers. Faster or slower diffusion occurs parallel or perpendicular to the long axes of white matter tracts (anisotropic diffusion). This effect is used for the assessment of disease of the white matter. Diffusion imaging is also useful in improving the detection, characterization, and therapeutic management of brain tumors.

Vascular Imaging

Contrast Angiography

Although noninvasive techniques such as ultrasound, MRA, and CT angiography (CTA) are currently avail-

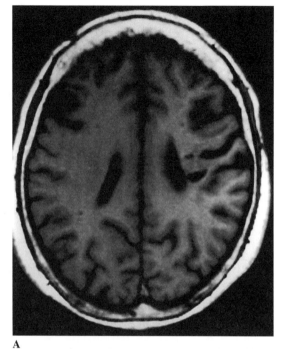

A

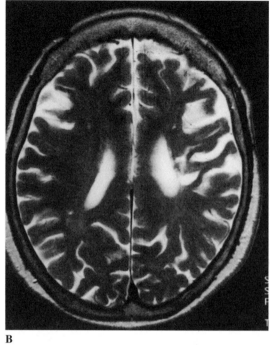

B

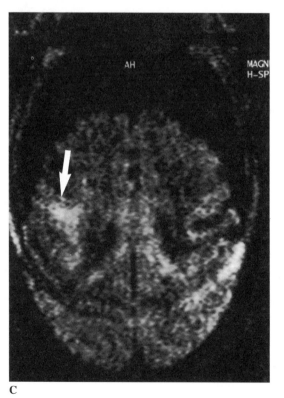

C

Figure 3-5. Diffusion imaging. (A) A T1-weighted image. (B) A T2-weighted image. (C) A diffusion-weighted image. A cortical infarction is visualized only with the diffusion magnetic resonance imaging technique (*arrow*) 120 minutes after the onset of symptoms.

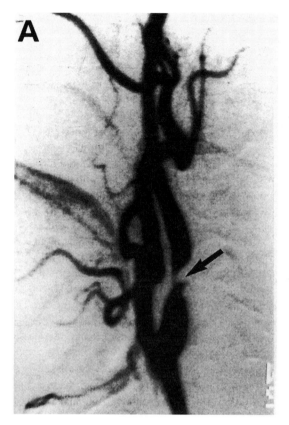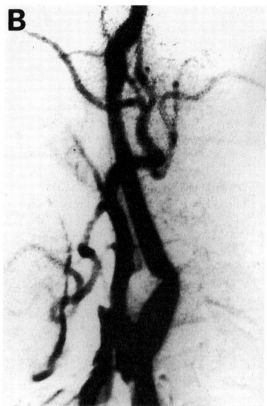

Figure 3-6. Contrast angiography and carotid endarterectomy (CEA). (A) Severe stenosis in the internal carotid artery demonstrated by intra-arterial digital subtraction angiography (*arrow*). (B) A post-CEA angiogram.

able for the evaluation of vascular structures, contrast angiography, including the conventional method and intra-arterial digital subtraction angiography (DSA), remains of value in selected patients. Conventional angiography and intra-arterial DSA require selective catheterization of the extracranial vessels, with subsequent injection of iodinated contrast agents into the target arterial systems. DSA has a number of advantages over the conventional method, which has a 0.5–3.0% risk of stroke, other serious complications, or death. These advantages include a shorter examination time, lower dose of contrast, multiple views, and prompt observation of images; the studies are easier to perform, and there is a lower incidence of complications.

Contrast angiography may be necessary to secure the diagnosis of cerebral arteritis, intracranial aneurysm, arterial dissection, or cortical vein and sinus thrombosis. Angiography is indicated in any patients having a surgical procedure involving the

intra- or extracranial vasculatures: carotid endarterectomy (CEA), clipping of an aneurysm, or resection of an arteriovenous malformation (AVM). After the success of the North American Symptomatic Carotid Endarterectomy Trial (NASCET), European Carotid Surgery Trial (ECST), and Asymptomatic Carotid Atherosclerosis Study (ACAS) in establishing the efficacy of CEA, it is strongly recommended that carotid stenosis be measured with contrast angiography as the gold standard for the indication of surgery (Figure 3-6). Intracranial arterial stenosis or occlusion is identified by noninvasive techniques but requires contrast angiography for confirmation.

Magnetic Resonance Angiography

MRA is a new tool for noninvasive visualization of the intra- and extracranial vasculatures without radi-

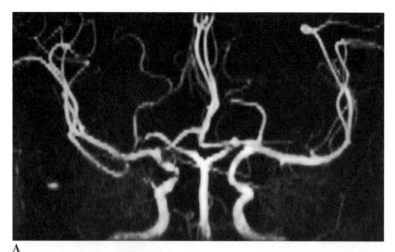

A

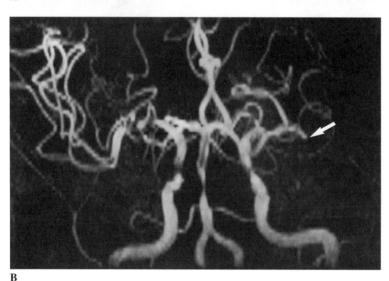

B

Figure 3-7. Magnetic resonance angiography in the circle of Willis. (A) A normal study. (B) The left middle cerebral artery appears completely occluded (*arrow*) and the horizontal portion of the right middle cerebral artery appears partly discontinued, indicating the presence of a severely stenotic lesion.

ation hazard. It does not require injection of a contrast agent and can be performed with routine MRI settings. MRI sequences involve suppression of the signal from stationary background tissue and acquisition of the signal emitted by flowing blood within the volume of interest.

MRA studies are performed most commonly with a three- or two-dimensional time-of-flight technique. MRA has proved to be a valuable, noninvasive screening tool for intracranial aneurysms, AVMs, and major vessel occlusive diseases (Figure 3-7). MRA agrees well with contrast angiography in the extracranial cerebral arteries. With severe stenosis, however, it shows a segment of signal void or discontinuity in the vessel with clearly defined proximal and distal seg-

ments. The signal loss in a stenotic artery occurs because of intravoxel incoherence. Although MRA may overestimate the extent of occlusive disease and miss some ulceration, negative (normal) findings on a study are highly accurate. MRA often fails to demonstrate small arterial pathologic conditions (small-sized aneurysms, distal branch occlusion) mainly because of limited spatial resolution.

Computed Tomographic Angiography

Spiral, or helical, CT is a new technique combining continuous gantry rotation with simultaneous displacement of the examination table throughout acqui-

Figure 3-8. Three-dimensional CT angiography. (A) A large arteriovenous malformation in the left frontal lobe. The nidus and draining veins are clearly visualized. (B) An unruptured aneurysm of the anterior communicating artery (*arrow*).

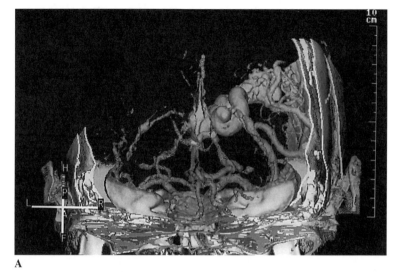

A

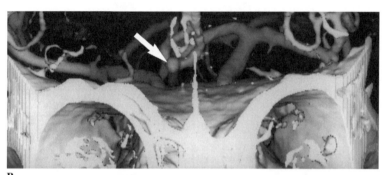

B

sition, allowing data acquisition of a large volume in a short time. When combined with intravenous injection of a contrast agent, thin helical CT images provide excellent visualization of intracranial vasculatures as well as arterial lumens and walls. Three-dimensional reconstruction of intracranial vasculatures on CTA can easily be achieved and used to demonstrate intracranial aneurysms, AVMs, arterial dissection, and occlusive arterial disease (Figure 3-8).

Imaging of Cerebral Blood Flow and Metabolism

Single-Photon Emission Computed Tomography

SPECT is a noninvasive and three-dimensional measurement of cerebral blood flow (CBF) and receptor density. SPECT uses traditional nuclear medicine radioisotopes such as xenon-133 (^{133}Xe), iodine-123 (^{123}I), and technetium-99m (^{99m}Tc). A tracer is tagged with a radionuclide and injected intravenously. A three-dimensional image of the distribution of a radionuclide in the brain then is obtained with a gamma camera and the technique of CT.

Flow tracers combined with lipophilic amines (i.e., ^{123}I-IMP, ^{99m}Tc-HMPAO, and ^{99m}Tc-ECD) cross the BBB easily but leave the brain slowly, and therefore their distribution represents a record of local CBF at the time of injection. Compared with the tracers used for PET, SPECT tracers have a longer half-life and can be prepared in easily usable, commercially available kits and stored for relatively long periods of time before use. The radiation dose per study, however, is larger in SPECT than in PET. Modern SPECT techniques can produce a spatial resolution of 6–9 mm, with data acquisition times of 10–20 minutes.

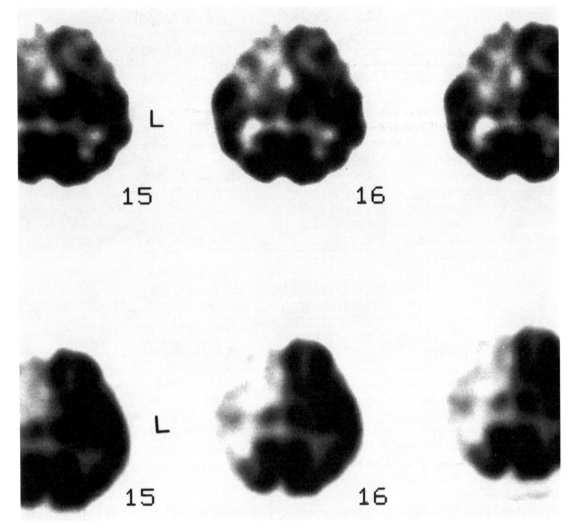

Figure 3-9. Acetazolamide-enhanced single-photon emission computed tomography (SPECT) study in a patient with occlusion of the right internal carotid artery. (Top) A perfusion SPECT image in the resting state. (Bottom) The hemispheric difference in perfusion becomes enhanced after the injection of acetazolamide, suggesting an impairment of the perfusion reserve.

Most routine clinical applications of perfusion SPECT do not quantify CBF values. The result is simply described to be hyper- or hypoperfused or is semiquantified by calculating the relative uptake ratio to that in the contralateral cerebral or ipsilateral cerebellar hemisphere. Unlike PET, SPECT cannot measure local cerebral metabolism. By combining it with the intravenous injection of a strong vasodilating agent (e.g., acetazolamide), perfusion SPECT studies allow the evaluation of cerebral perfusion reserve, which was earlier determined only through PET (Figure 3-9).

SPECT has been applied to the study of stroke, vascular dementia, transient global amnesia, neoplasm, acquired immunodeficiency syndrome encephalopathy, head trauma, seizures, Alzheimer's disease, Huntington's chorea, persistent vegetative state, and brain death. The efficacy of SPECT studies, however, remains unestablished in neurologic disorders except for the detection of acute ischemia and seizure focus and in helping in the clinical diagnosis of Alzheimer's disease. Neuroreceptor SPECT imaging has been done by using the benzodiazepine antagonist ^{123}I-iomazenil in temporal lobe epilepsy or ischemic stroke, and the dopamine D_2-receptor antagonist ^{123}I-iodobenzamide in Parkinson's disease.

Positron Emission Tomography

PET measures various physiologic and biochemical processes using a positron-emitting isotope and a positron camera, which maps the distribution of an injected radiotracer in three-dimensional space. This complex and expensive technique is available only in a few centers equipped with a cyclotron and a team of specialists. The positron-labeled metabolites must be given immediately after they are produced because of their short half-life.

The ^{15}O-gas steady-state inhalation method is popular for the measurement of CBF, cerebral metabolic rate of oxygen ($CMRO_2$), CBV, and oxygen extraction fraction (OEF). This method requires a combined use of oxygen, carbon dioxide, and carbon monoxide, resulting in a long examination time, of at least 60 minutes. Recently the bolus inhalation or injection method has been introduced to shorten the examination time and to increase the reproducibility. [^{18}F]fluoro-deoxyglucose (FDG) is used as a marker for glucose uptake and metabolism. The FDG-PET technique requires an intravenous injection of the tracer, continuous sampling of arterial blood, and a brain scan beginning 40 minutes after injection. Other PET methods for receptor imaging have been developed but are still investigational.

A characteristic disruption of the normal coupling between CBF and metabolism has been demonstrated within areas of brain infarction. In the early infarct, CBF is disproportionately decreased compared with $CMRO_2$ and glucose metabolism, whereas there is a marked increase in OEF. This phenomenon reflects compensation for the reduction of total oxygen supply and is termed *misery perfusion syndrome* (Figure 3-10). Within a week, CBF appears increased, $CMRO_2$ unchanged or depressed, and OEF markedly decreased (*luxury perfusion*).

PET studies can reliably detect derangement of the perfusion reserve in patients with reduced cerebral perfusion pressure (CPP) caused by occlusive arterial diseases, venous thrombosis, or intracranial mass lesions (Table 3-3). When CPP is reduced,

CBV increases as a result of dilation of cerebral vessels with CBF being constant (stage I). When vascular response is maximal and no further vasodilation is possible, CBF begins to decrease, with a subsequent increase in OEF (stage II). Persistent further decline in CPP and CBF results in permanent tissue damage (stage III). The PET examination may quantify the risk of subsequent infarction and predict the hemodynamic efficacy of surgical interventions, although this speculation remains to be confirmed.

FDG-PET is used to detect local metabolic alteration in many neurologic disorders, including Alzheimer's disease and other degenerative diseases, brain tumors, and epilepsy. In these disorders, the pattern of glucose metabolism is rather characteristic and therefore is helpful in making the clinical diagnosis. FDG-PET has allowed us to examine the physiologic effects of a structural lesion in various behavioral disorders.

PET studies in stroke and other neurologic disorders often demonstrate widespread remote metabolic changes in neighboring and distant structures that appear normal on CT or MRI scans. The phenomenon termed *remote effect* or *diaschisis* is often detected in the contralateral cerebellum (*crossed cerebellar diaschisis*), the ipsilateral thalamus and caudate, and other brain structures and is presumably caused by disconnection between the structures. For example, interruption of cerebropontocerebellar pathways is the most likely mechanism of crossed cerebellar diaschisis.

Magnetic Resonance Spectroscopic Imaging

Nuclei with odd numbers of protons or neutrons, such as sodium and phosphorus, can produce MRI signals. The signals from the different metabolites are distinguishable from one another because of the magnetic field strength at the nucleus and hence the resonant frequency varies slightly depending on the electronic environment in chemical bonds surrounding the nucleus (chemical shift). Magnetic resonance spectroscopy (MRS) uses this phenomenon in water nuclei (proton), lactate, phosphate compounds, and some amino acids. In the clinical setting, proton (^{1}H) and phosphorus (^{31}P) MRS imaging is used to map three-dimensional changes in tissue lactate, *N*-acetylaspartate, high-energy

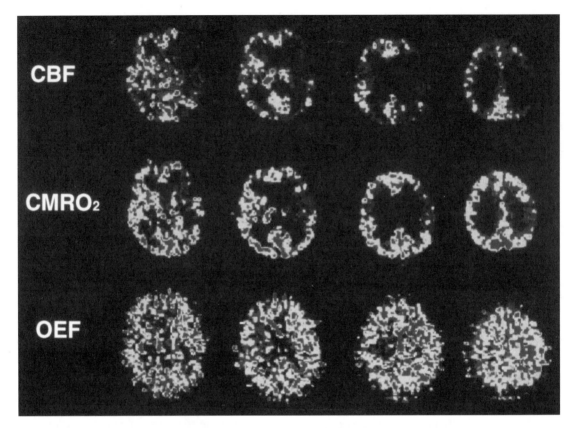

Figure 3-10. A positron emission tomography (PET) study in a patient with acute ischemia of the left middle cerebral artery on day 2. Magnetic resonance imaging lesions were localized within the deep white matter. The PET study demonstrates a diffuse and pronounced increase in the oxygen extraction fraction, indicating acute misery perfusion syndrome. (CBF = cerebral blood flow; $CMRO_2$ = cerebral metabolic rate of oxygen; OEF = oxygen extraction fraction.)

phosphate metabolites, and tissue pH. The sensitivity and resolution of clinical MRS imaging is low, and therefore its clinical utility is still limited.

Functional Imaging

Activation Study with Positron Emission Tomography

The PET method has been increasingly used to study brain areas for specific physiologic and psychological functions in normal volunteers and patients with neurologic disorders. After a bolus injection of ^{15}O, a radioactive atom with a very short half-life of 1.8 minutes, usually in the form of ^{15}O-labeled water, the radioactivity detected in the brain occurs as a linear function of local CBF. When the brain tissue is activated because of increased neuronal function, a local increase in CBF and glucose metabolism is demonstrated within seconds in the normals. Rapid and repetitive measurements of local CBF with the $H_2{}^{15}O$-PET therefore can provide a map of neuronal activation. Anatomic information from MRI can be combined with functional information from the PET study.

Functional Magnetic Resonance Imaging

Functional MRI (FMRI) is a noninvasive tool for mapping human brain function. Changes in local CBF caused by neuronal activation can rapidly be detected by MRI without the injection of a contrast agent or

Table 3-3. Compensatory Response to Reduced Cerebral Perfusion Pressure

Stage	CPP	CBF	CMRO$_2$	CBV	CBF/CBV	OEF	Comment
0	→	→	→	→	→	→	Normal
I	↓	→	→	↑	↓	→	Autoregulation
II	↓↓	↓	→	↑	↓↓	↑	Misery perfusion
III	↓↓↓	↓↓	↓	?	?	?	Ischemic injury

CPP = cerebral perfusion pressure; CBF = cerebral blood flow; CMRO$_2$ = cerebral metabolic rate of oxygen; CBV = cerebral blood volume; OEF = oxygen extraction fraction; → = constant or unchanged; ↑ = increased; ↓ = decreased.

radioactive tracer. A local increase in oxygen delivery beyond metabolic demand and then a decrease in the arteriovenous oxygenation difference occurs in activated brain tissue, where local CBF increases. An increase in oxygenated blood and a decrease in deoxyhemoglobin, which is paramagnetic relative to oxyhemoglobin and surrounding brain tissues, occur within microvasculature of metabolically active brain areas. This phenomenon is accompanied by a local increase in magnetic field homogeneity and an increased MRI signal relative to the resting state, demonstrating functionally activated cortical areas. Because the duration of these signal changes is very short, FMRI studies can be accomplished only with fast or ultrafast image acquisition techniques, such as fast low-angle shot imaging and EPI.

This new MRI approach allows a determination of correlation of brain anatomy with function at a high level of spatial resolution and within a brief temporal interval. FMRI has already been used to determine cerebral dominancy and areas with important brain functions before brain surgery in patients with epilepsy or mass lesions.

Suggested Reading

Baron JC, Frackowiak RSJ, Herholz K, et al. Use of PET for measurement of cerebral energy metabolism and hemodynamics in cerebrovascular disease. J Cereb Blood Flow Metab 1989;9:723.

Binder JR, Rao SM. Human Brain Mapping with Functional Magnetic Resonance Imaging. In A Kertesz (ed), Localization and Neuroimaging in Neuropsychology. San Diego: Academic, 1994;185.

Brant-Zawadzki M, Atkinson D, Detrick M, et al. Fluid-attenuated inversion recovery (FLAIR) for assessment of cerebral infarction. Initial clinical experience in 50 patients. Stroke 1996;27:1187.

Edelman RR, Warach S. Magnetic resonance imaging. Part I and part II. N Engl J Med 1993;328:708, 785.

Fisher M, Sotak CH, Minematsu K, et al. New magnetic resonance techniques for evaluating cerebrovascular disease. Ann Neurol 1992;32:115.

Gomori JM, Grossman RI, Goldberg HI, et al. Intracranial hematomas: imaging by high-field MR. Radiology 1985;157:87.

Hirano T, Minematsu K, Hasegawa Y, et al. Acetazolamide reactivity on ^{123}I-IMP single photon emission computed tomography in patients with major cerebral artery occlusive disease: correlation with positron emission tomography parameters. J Cereb Blood Flow Metab 1994;14:763.

Hugg JW, Duijn JH, Matson GB, et al. Elevated lactate and alkalosis in chronic human brain infarction observed by ^{1}H and ^{31}P MR spectroscopic imaging. J Cereb Blood Flow Metab 1992;12:734.

Miller DH, Albert PS, Barkhof F, et al. Guidelines for the use of magnetic resonance techniques in monitoring the treatment of multiple sclerosis. Ann Neurol 1996;39:6.

Minematsu K, Li L, Fisher M, et al. Diffusion-weighted magnetic resonance imaging: rapid and quantitative detection of focal brain ischemia. Neurology 1992;42:235.

Minematsu K, Yamaguchi T. Management of Intracerebral Hemorrhage. In M Fisher (ed), Stroke Therapy. Boston: Butterworth–Heinemann, 1995;351.

Moulin T, Cattin F, Crepin-Leblond T, et al. Early CT signs in acute middle cerebral artery infarction: predictive value for subsequent infarct locations and outcome. Neurology 1996;47:366.

Okada Y, Yamaguchi T, Minematsu K, et al. Hemorrhagic transformation in cerebral embolism. Stroke 1989;20:598.

Therapeutic and Technology Assessment Subcommittee of the American Academy of Neurology. Assessment of brain SPECT. Neurology 1996;46:278.

Tomura N, Uemura K, Inugami A, et al. Early CT findings in cerebral infarction: obscuration of the lentiform nucleus. Radiology 1988;168:463.

Warach S, Gaa J, Siewert B, et al. Acute human stroke studied by whole brain echo planar diffusion-weighted magnetic resonance imaging. Ann Neurol 1995;37:231.

Chapter 4
Clinical Neurophysiology

Christian W. Hess and Kai M. Rösler

Chapter Plan

In clinical neurology, electrophysiologic testing primarily is used to assess the functional integrity or disruption of the nervous system by measuring the electrical activity of nervous and muscular tissues. In the diagnostic workup of patients, electrophysiologic studies are complementary to the classic imaging methods, such as magnetic resonance imaging (MRI) and computed tomographic (CT) scanning, which basically assess structural changes of the nervous system. For practical purposes it is convenient to discuss the methods used for testing the central nervous (e.g., electroencephalography [EEG]) and the neuromuscular system (e.g., nerve conduction studies) separately, although the two domains tend to converge for methodologic reasons and are now sometimes performed by one laboratory. Also, there are electrodiagnostic procedures, namely evoked potential studies, that are used to assess both the central and the peripheral nervous system. Because the emphasis of evoked potentials clearly lies in assessing the functional integrity of central nervous structures, they will be discussed separately. Conversely, some central nervous system (CNS) investigatory procedures, such as polysomnographic sleep studies or motor evoked potentials (MEPs), imply the measurement of muscle activity.

Electroencephalography

EEG is used primarily for two reasons:

1. To study patients suspected of having epileptic seizures—that is, patients either with a history of tonic-clonic seizures and with loss of consciousness or with attacks of unexplained confusion, reduced responsiveness, falls, or syncope of noncardiac origin. Even when the optimal diagnostic situation of an attack during the recording procedure does not occur, interictal EEG abnormalities often provide important information supporting the diagnosis of epilepsy, and sometimes help to iden-

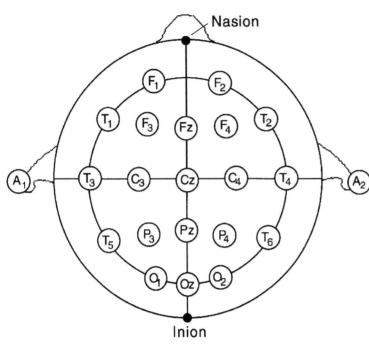

Figure 4-1. Surface electrode positions and designations of the "10-20 system" as commonly used in routine electroencephalography and afferent evoked potential investigations.

tify the type of the epileptic disorder. Conversely, an interictal EEG recording that appears normal does not exclude epilepsy. The workup for epilepsy often requires long-term monitoring.

2. To study patients with confusional states or with lasting disturbances of arousal and consciousness that cannot be explained on the basis of a detectable metabolic disorder or brain lesion (e.g., stroke, hemorrhage, tumor), particularly when encephalitis or nonconvulsive epileptic status must be ruled out. In comatose patients, the EEG (preferably in combination with measurement of somatosensory evoked potentials [SEPs]) can additionally provide important prognostic information. An EEG study performed in the intensive care unit must always take into account possible drug influences, which may hamper its diagnostic and prognostic value.

Methodologic Aspects of Electroencephalographic Recording

The EEG examination measures the spontaneous electrical brain activity from several sites over the scalp through the intact skin and skull (Figure 4-1)

over a given period of time. Since a distant scalp electrode cannot record the activity of a single neuron, only the synchronous activity of an aggregate of horizontally oriented neural elements is measured. The usual EEG session should yield approximately 30–45 minutes of pure recording time, and in situations demanding prolonged recordings, may last several hours or even days (telemetry). The EEG requires high-gain and high-input impedance amplification to make small voltage signals (on the order of a few microvolts) visible and for that reason is relatively prone to pick up "artifactual" electrical activity of different origins, such as neighboring head muscles or external sources (e.g., interference from main currents). The latter particularly may be a problem when recording in an intensive care unit with various electrical machinery working. Detecting and, if possible, eliminating artifacts are therefore chief tasks of the recording and reporting personnel. To minimize artifacts, the electrodes must be placed on carefully prepared skin with an adhesive paste to yield low electric contact resistance, and the patient should be comfortably seated in a relaxed position with the eyes loosely closed during most of the recording. Repeated eye opening for short periods of time is used to check the arousal effect of rest activity (so-called alpha-blocking) on the EEG pattern.

A conventional EEG recorder uses 16–32 separate amplifying units that measure the potential differences between two adjacent electrodes on the scalp (bipolar recording) or the potential difference between each scalp electrode and a common reference electrode (monopolar recording), the reference being, for example, the connected ears or the electronically coupled average of the scalp electrodes. Furthermore, some channels are reserved for the simultaneous recording of the electrocardiogram (ECG) and other optional variables, such as an event marker, certain muscles of interest (myoclonus), an oculogram, oxymetry, and respiratory movements by a strain gauge. The continuous printout of the signals on paper is now increasingly being replaced by digital computer systems, which amplify, display, and process the recorded activity and allow storage on a digital medium (streamer, optical discs). In particular, the montage (how the leads are connected), the gain (usually 70 µV per cm), the time base (usually 10–30 seconds per screen), and the frequency range (usually 0.5–75.0 Hz) can be selected according to the situation off-line—that is, after the actual recording has been terminated.

Because muscles produce much greater electrical activity than the brain, any head, face, jaw, throat, or eye movement will produce artifactual high-amplitude and high-frequency signals that heavily interfere with the genuine EEG activity and sometimes completely obscure it. This is obviously a major handicap when recording during a seizure, when the detection of potential epileptic activity would be most important, but often is not possible. It is all the more crucial to meticulously assess the EEG activity just before and after an attack, and this makes a precise correlation of the EEG recording with the clinical manifestations important. For this reason, the simultaneous videographic recording for behavioral monitoring of the patient has, at least in institutional settings, become a standard procedure in epileptology.

A major limitation of conventional EEG lies in its restricted pickup area, which is confined to the cortex of the brain convexity and misses the deeply situated mesial and basal cortex of the temporal and frontal lobe and also the subcortical nuclei. If necessary, this can be overcome by more invasive procedures to pick up focal epileptic activity, which might be hidden in the depths: foramen ovale electrodes, sphenoidal electrodes, subdural electrodes, or depth electrodes introduced into the brain tissue. These invasive procedures are reserved for patients with refractory seizures for which a surgical treatment is envisioned.

Depending on the clinical situation, a number of activating procedures are carried out:

1. Forced hyperventilation with 3 minutes of vigorous overbreathing provokes epileptic patterns in generalized epilepsies, most reliably in patients with absences.
2. Stroboscopic stimulation with bright flashes at frequencies of 1–25 per second in front of the patient's eyes discloses photosensitivity and activates epileptic discharge patterns in idiopathic epilepsy syndromes, most notably in juvenile myoclonic epilepsy.
3. The patient is allowed to fall asleep to provoke focal epileptic activity, particularly in temporal and frontal lobe epilepsies. Falling asleep is best achieved in the early afternoon after lunch. If seizure activation by sleep is crucial, it might be necessary to use sedative drugs or to keep a patient awake during the previous night. Also, other EEG abnormalities are facilitated by sleep, notably the repetitive complexes in the early stages of Jakob-Creutzfeldt disease or of subacute sclerosing panencephalitis.

Computer-assisted analysis can produce continuous frequency power spectra and has also been used for automatic pattern recognition (e.g., epileptic spikes, apneas, movement signal). It has been of great value in sleep studies and monitoring of consciousness, vigilance, and anesthesia. However, artifacts are readily overlooked or produced in automatically processed EEG studies, which will not be a substitute for a conventional EEG recording. The possibility for inspecting the EEG raw signal at any time is a mandatory feature of automatic EEG processing devices. Electrical brain mapping provides topographically displayed EEG information on a head outline and is an important research tool. However, its general clinical utility has yet to be established.

In unconscious patients, the arousal effect in the EEG is checked by passive eye opening, calling the patient by name, shouting, making loud noises, or perhaps gently applying noxious stimuli to the skin.

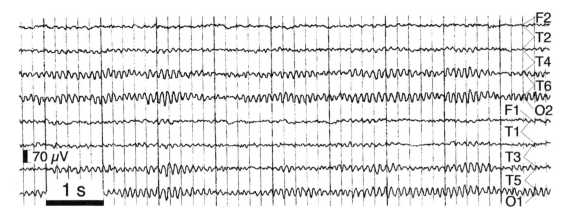

Figure 4-2. Normal resting electroencephalographic activity of an adult in a bipolar montage showing predominant posterior series of waxing and waning alpha waves (10 Hz). The alpha activity is attenuated or blocked when the eyes are opened (not shown).

Long-term EEG studies with simultaneous video monitoring are used to capture seizures. This is done by telemetry equipment, whereby the EEG signal is linked by cable or radio transmission to the recorder while the video camera remains focused on the patient, permitting only limited mobility to the latter. Ambulatory monitoring with a portable cassette in an everyday environment is less reliable because of muscle and movement artifacts and because it lacks videographic recording.

Complete overnight polysomnography includes two or more EEG records, an oculogram, an ECG recording, percutaneous oxymetry readings, measurement of respiratory variables (air flow and thoracoabdominal movements), several EMG records (mental and limb muscles), body position, and infrared videography. Polysomnography has a special role in the investigation of sleep-related breathing disorders, dyssomnias, and parasomnias. Recording, evaluating, and interpreting polysomnographic recordings requires special training and expertise in sleep medicine on the part of both the technician and the academic. The multiple sleep latency test or maintenance of wakefulness test is used for quantifying proneness to fall asleep or the ability to stay awake during the day, respectively. The tests measure the latency to sleep onset by EEG in a standardized fashion four to five times throughout the day, and the subject is each time either allowed to fall asleep in the supine position or instructed to stay awake in the sitting position.

Normal Electroencephalographic Findings

In resting awake adults with eyes closed, the EEG record is dominated by an 8- to 12-Hz, approximately 50-µV amplitude waxing and waning sinusoidal rhythm over both the occipital and parietal regions, the so-called alpha activity (Figure 4-2). This alpha activity is suppressed by eye opening or mental tasks. There are fast- and low-amplitude beta waves (13–30 Hz), predominately over the frontal and central regions, and some slow-amplitude theta waves (4–7 Hz) show over the temporal regions. When a normal subject falls asleep, the alpha rhythm disintegrates, and with deepening of sleep, increasingly slower and higher amplitude waves prevail until the EEG is dominated by high-voltage delta activity (1–3 Hz) during deep "slow wave sleep" (stage 3 and 4 of nonREM sleep according to Rechtschaffen and Kales). Additionally, during light sleep (nonREM stage 2), characteristic single, sharp waves with so-called K complexes and spindles of 12- to 15-Hz waves appear over the vertex.

The EEG is a very sensitive measure for assessing subtle changes in alertness and is also readily influenced by sedative drugs. This is a frequent source of misinterpretation when effects of drowsiness or drugs are not taken into account. Because slowing is a common EEG abnormality and may arise from diverse disorders, it may be difficult to distinguish between the effects of drowsiness and pathologic conditions.

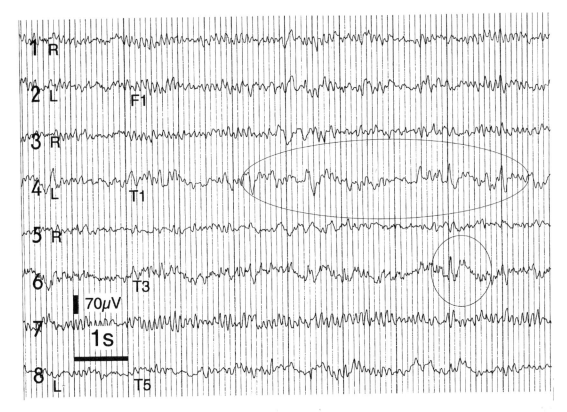

Figure 4-3. Interictal focal slowing and epileptic discharges (sharp and slow waves) on the left temporal side (leads T1 and T3) in a patient with complex partial seizures originating from the left temporal lobe in a monopolar recording. There is also a slowing with delta and theta waves on the contralateral side.

The EEG pattern of children younger than 12 years of age is generally slower, less rhythmic, and more variable, particularly in infants and newborns. Furthermore, specific EEG patterns, such as arousal reaction, hyperventilation-induced changes, or epileptic activity of infants, look quite different from the EEG pattern in adults. Therefore, the interpretation of a pediatric EEG study requires ample and specific experience.

Abnormal Electroencephalographic Patterns

Electroencephalographic Patterns in Epileptic Disorders

Epileptic EEG patterns arise from excessive, hypersynchronous neuronal activity and are characterized by electronegative single or grouped spikes (duration of less than 80 ms) or pointed sharp waves, which must be differentiated from sharp high-frequency muscle artifacts. The epileptic spikes are often associated with a following blunt wave, which then forms the specific epileptic spike-wave or sharp-and-slow wave complexes (Figure 4-3). When a series of such epileptic discharges appears in paroxysmal fashion, it is highly suggestive of epilepsy. However, epileptic EEG patterns are occasionally seen in patients with cerebral disorders without epilepsy. The interpretation of epileptic patterns therefore always depends on the clinical context.

Epileptic discharges may be focal over one or a few adjacent electrodes, as in partial epilepsies, or may be generalized and then appear simultaneously over many leads on both sides symmetrically, as in generalized epilepsies. For instance, in an absence seizure, the epileptic discharges appear suddenly in an otherwise normal EEG pattern in all leads at the same time as a series of regular three-per-second spike-and-waves that persist for several seconds and

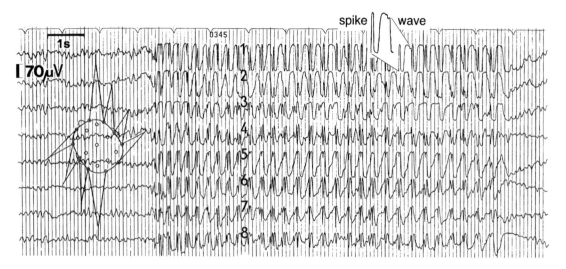

Figure 4-4. Typical brief absence seizure in 15-year-old girl showing high-voltage bilateral, regular, and synchronous 3-Hz spike-wave activity (bipolar recording). Note the abrupt beginning and halt with a normal resting activity prior and after the seizure, which is characteristic of this type of generalized seizure.

disappear all at once (Figure 4-4). If such a generalized discharge is very short, the clinical absence may go unnoticed by an observer or even by the patient (subclinical discharge). Conversely, a clinically manifest generalized seizure is always accompanied by a concurrent EEG discharge, which, however, may not always be absolutely typical. If the spikes are lost or blunted, we are left with more or less rhythmic and synchronous delta wave sequences over both hemispheres.

As opposed to generalized seizures, focal seizures are not invariably accompanied by concurrent discharges in the EEG activity. Partial complex seizures originating from very restricted epileptic activity in deep mesiotemporal or orbitofrontal foci, and oddly also simple partial (focal) seizures originating from primary motor cortex or those with psychic or viscerosensory symptoms, may occasionally remain undetected in the ictal EEG pattern. Also, noncortical myoclonic discharges are not seen with EEG activity. It is therefore important to remember that a normal EEG pattern during a seizure does not always indicate a psychogenic seizure. Moreover, during seizures with ample motor activity, the EEG activity is dominated by muscle and movement artifacts that may obscure possible epileptic discharges. Meticulous analysis of minor EEG changes just before and after the seizure and also of the video-

graphic recording is crucial in these cases and usually allows a firm diagnosis, particularly when several seizures are captured. For instance, an epileptic seizure is sometimes preceded by a short period of attenuated resting EEG activity and followed by postictal slow waves. When several recorded seizures can be compared off-line, the absolutely stereotyped progression of the electroclinical manifestation is the single most important criterion in diagnosing an epileptic as opposed to a psychogenic seizure, and this is occasionally based solely on the videographic analysis.

*Electroencephalographic Patterns
in Disorders of Consciousness*

Diffuse EEG abnormalities reflect general cerebral pathologic conditions and usually are nonspecific. In organic confusional, obtunded, and comatose states, the EEG pattern is abnormal in all conditions and typically shows progressive slowing with increasing clinical deterioration: loss of occipital alpha activity, augmented and widespread theta activity, diffuse or high-amplitude bifrontal delta activity with onset of coma, and, finally, intermittent suppression of any activity, which progresses to total electrical silence in the terminal state. The differential diagnosis of a diffusely abnormal EEG pattern includes toxic-metabolic and infectious encephalopathies and encephalitis. Hepatic encephalopathy, intoxication with barbiturates or other sedative-hypnotic drugs, and effects of diffuse anoxia-ischemia are typical examples in which the CT scan may appear normal. The EEG pattern may also unexpectedly disclose a clinically inapparent continuous epileptic discharge (nonconvulsive status epilepticus). Conversely, the EEG pattern may be absolutely normal, suggesting a psychogenic stupor. Psychotic states, intoxication with hallucinogenic drugs such as lysergic acid diethylamide (LSD), and the majority of cases of mental retardation are associated with no or only minor nonspecific EEG abnormalities. Thus, a normal EEG pattern in a patient who is apathetic, slow, or depressed is a point in favor of the diagnosis of an affective disorder or schizophrenia. Also, delirium tremens and Wernicke-Korsakoff syndrome cause relatively little alteration in the genuine EEG activity apart from abundant movement artifacts.

An important criterion when interpreting the abnormal EEG pattern of a stuporous or comatose patient is the reactivity to passive eye opening, loud noises, or noxious stimuli. Any immediate, clear-cut, and reproducible EEG change in response to the stimulus indicates preserved reactivity of the brain. Other than in the awake state, a comatose patient produces a large slow-wave arousal reaction ("paradoxical arousal response") on application of the stimulus.

Some focal and generalized intermittent or periodic EEG patterns deserve special attention:

1. Periodic lateralized epileptiform discharges (PLEDs) are relatively high-voltage sharp (and slow) waves with a repetition rate of 0.3–0.7 Hz and, when localized over a temporal region in an obtunded patient, are an important diagnostic feature of herpes simplex encephalitis. Bilateral PLEDs in herpes simplex encephalitis typically occur nonsynchronously, indicating independent inflammatory foci in the two temporal lobes.
2. Generalized periodic discharges appear as "triphasic waves" in hepatic and severe posthypoxic encephalopathy, and also occasionally in uremia, electrolyte disorders, and barbiturate overdose. The 0.5- to 1.0-Hz periodic discharges of the fatal Jakob-Creutzfeldt disease are a bit less conspicuous, usually appearing as bisyn-chronous sharp waves, and those of subacute sclerosing panencephalitis of children and adolescents may initially be subtle, repeating at 10- to 20-second intervals.
3. Frontal intermittent rhythmic delta activities are bursts of bilaterally synchronous frontal 2-Hz waves that are attenuated on alerting the patient. It is an unspecific finding that occurs in both toxic-metabolic encephalopathies as well as in lesions of subcortical structures.

The most pathologic finding is that of electrocerebral silence, which means that the surface EEG activity is less than 2 µV or is absent. Acute intoxication with anesthetic levels of drugs such as barbiturates can produce an isoelectric EEG pattern. However, in the absence of nervous system depressants or hypothermia, an isoelectric EEG pattern over the entire scalp is usually the result of global cerebral hypoxia or ischemia and suggests irreversible coma. Intermittent suppression of EEG activity (burst suppression pattern) and isoelectric EEG patterns are both of adverse prognostic import.

Afferent Evoked Potentials Studies

The bright light of a stroboscope induces a small occipital spike that can usually be detected in the EEG background activity. Other, less vigorous sensory stimuli produce more subtle cortical responses, which under normal conditions are too small to be discerned among the much greater waves of EEG resting activity. This obstacle can be overcome when the stimulus is repeated many times and the relevant EEG segments after the stimulus are electronically summed up. With this averaging technique, the aggregated EEG records are precisely timed with respect to the stimulus. As a consequence, all waves occurring at constant intervals after the stimulus will be built up, whereas those that are independent of the stimulus occur at random intervals and will gradually cancel out during the averaging process. Using this averaging technique, stimulus-induced electrical events can be recorded not only from the cortex, but also from the brain stem and peripheral nerves if the active electrode is placed near the target structure. When averaging up to 100 or more sweeps, responses from distant (e.g., subcortical) structures also can be made visible, provided that the indifferent electrode is appropriately located—that is, it is relatively far away from the active one. Because many stimulus variables (stimulus intensity) critically influence not only the amplitude but also the latency of the averaged response, it is crucial to use a standardized method and to compare the normal values of the equipment with published ones by recording the activity of some normal subjects from time to time. Furthermore, it is a general rule of all evoked potential techniques that the reproducibility of the averaged response must be ascertained by repeating each examination at least once.

Afferent evoked potential studies are used to assess the functional integrity over the entire afferent pathway of a specific modality from the excited sense organ or peripheral nerve up to the cortex. Clinical applications include a great variety of issues, ranging from assessing possible deafness in an infant or hysterical blindness in an adult to measuring central conduction delay in multiple sclerosis. With the advent of MRI, evoked potential testing has lost some of its importance in the diagnosis of diseases of the CNS. However, evoked potential testing still is essential in many cases of central disorders in which the MRI study appears normal. Clearly, evoked potential studies remain an indispensable method in the institutional diagnostic workup of neurologic patients.

Visual Evoked Potentials

Visual evoked potential (VEP) studies were the first potential studies introduced into clinical neurology and rightly hold first place within the afferent evoked potential test battery nowadays. Not only are the VEP studies most easily performed and interpreted, but by measuring the conduction of the optic nerves, the sensitivity of VEP testing is not readily exceeded by imaging techniques. Although VEPs are most easily produced by bright stroboscopic lights, flash-induced VEPs have proved unsuitable in assessing the central visual pathways because their responses are generated in many brain regions and can even be recorded in blind patients with an occipital cortex destroyed by ischemia. Conversely, the pattern of evoked visual potentials induced by sudden changes of a viewed checkerboard pattern are generated within the occipital cortex and closely correlate with visual function. These pattern-reversal VEPs are widely adopted as one of the most delicate tests of the visual system. It was found that this technique could demonstrate subclinical conduction delays in the visual pathways of patients with normal visual acuity and no visual field abnormalities who had formerly suffered a demyelinating disease of the visual pathways. Depending on the clinical question, the pattern-reversal stimulus is applied first to one and then to the other eye to detect prechiasmatic lesions (optic nerves), or to the left and right hemifields separately to detect postchiasmatic lesions (optic tract, geniculatum laterale, radiatio optica, and occipital cortex). The pattern-reversal stimulus is presented on a television screen or computer monitor with a checker size of approximately 1 degree of visual angle that shifts once per second in a dark room, and the patient is presented with a point on which to fixate either in the center (or upper border) of the screen when the two eyes are stimulated separately, or at the left or right border of the screen when the two hemifields are stimulated separately. The standardized light intensity of the white and black checkers must be regularly calibrated. One to three active leads are placed in symmetrical fashion over the occipital lobes with a frontal reference electrode (Fz), and 32–128 averaged responses are usually sufficient to generate a sizable triphasic cortical response with negative-positive-negative polarity. The positive deflection with a latency of approximately 100 ms (P100) and an amplitude of 5–20 μV is taken as the most consistent major component. Usually, some reduction in amplitude accompanies the abnormally prolonged latencies. VEP testing also allows a rough estimate of the visual capacity in infants, when the stimulus screen is brought close to the eyes so that the checkerboard cannot be avoided by the look. Alternatively, stroboscopic flashes may be used exceptionally and applied through the closed eyes when even rudimentary visual function of prechiasmatic structures is uncertain.

The VEPs are particularly valuable in proving the existence of active disease or a residual lesion of an optic nerve. The VEPs usually remain abnormally delayed and only rarely normalize completely in patients who have recovered from optic neuritis and whose optic nerves appear normal in MRI studies (Figure 4-5). Also, in multiple sclerosis patients with no history or clinical evidence of

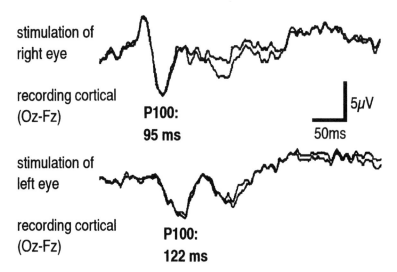

Figure 4-5. Visual evoked potentials in a multiple sclerosis patient, The first major positivity P100 is of normal latency on the right side and clearly delayed on the left side with a latency of 122 ms (upper limit of normal: 113 ms). Two sweeps are superimposed to ascertain reproducibility.

optic nerve involvement, abnormal findings on VEP testing often are found as evidence of a clinically silent lesion. Thus, the finding of an abnormal VEP pattern in a patient with a clinically apparent lesion elsewhere in the CNS provides laboratory-supported evidence of a second lesion, permitting a diagnosis of multiple sclerosis.

Compressive lesions of the optic nerves also will produce delayed and reduced responses, whereas other diseases of the optic nerves, including ischemic optic neuropathy, toxic and nutritional amblyopias, and the Leber-type of hereditary optic neuropathy, primarily show reduced amplitudes or even absent VEP responses. The VEPs are a sensitive means of detecting psychogenic visual disturbances when impaired vision or even blindness is claimed in the presence of a completely normal VEP pattern. In cases of decreased visual acuity, a successively reduced pattern size allows a rough objective measurement of the acuity and comparison with the psychophysical assessment. It must be kept in mind, however, that higher order disturbances such as visual agnosias are compatible with perfectly normal VEP responses. Impaired fixation caused by spontaneous nystagmus produces only an amplitude decrement without latency prolongation. It is also important to consider that some diseases of the eye such as glaucoma may produce increased latencies. On the other hand, impaired visual acuity caused by refractory abnormalities has little effect on VEP latency with the exception of extreme myopia.

Somatosensory Evoked Potentials

Testing of SEPs is performed by applying 3- to 5-Hz painless electrical stimuli, which are approximately two to three times above the motor (mixed nerves) or sensory threshold, over peripheral nerves on both sides separately, typically over the median, ulnar, or tibial nerves. Sometimes, stimulation of purely sensory nerves (e.g., the suralis) or of segmental skin areas (e.g., finger I, III, or V) also is needed to better localize a lesion. Simultaneous recordings must be done over two to three sites: over Erb's point above the clavicle; over the cervical spine; and over the opposite parietal cortex for the upper limbs or over the lumbar (and possibly also the cervical) spine and over the midline parietal cortex for lower limbs. Placement of the reference electrodes influences pickup of far-field potentials of distant generators and must be chosen according to specific requirements. For instance, the parietal signal may be derived relative to a frontal scalp lead to obtain a more or less pure cortical response or, alternatively, to an ear reference to additionally obtain preceding brain stem and subcortical potentials. If enough averagers are available, a signal can be derived using two different references to yield the more easily interpreted near-field signal as well as the combined signal comprising both the near-field and far-field signal components. This may be of great help in pathologic conditions, when small and unequivocal components no longer can be safely discerned. Unlike VEPs, SEPs require averaging of several hundred sweeps to obtain spinal and subcortical signals. The former are crucial in cases of a conduction delay to differentiate between peripheral and central prolongation. For this reason, some laboratories use deeply inserted spinal needle electrodes that bypass the disturbing truncal muscle activity. Also, a comfortable prone position for the patient is an important prerequisite for minimizing muscle artifacts and obtaining good recordings. Sometimes tranquilizers are used to help the patient relax.

The signals recorded depend primarily on large sensory fibers and rapidly conducting afferent pathways of fast proprioceptive and epicritic touch modalities (e.g., the posterior columns of the spinal cord, the medial lemniscal system of the brain stem), neglecting other more slowly conducting afferent routes. Although not invariably correct, the recorded SEP components are assumed to be linked in series, so that interwave abnormalities in latency indicate a conduction defect between the presumed generators of the two peaks involved. The normal waveforms are mostly designated according to the polarity and the mean normal latency by the symbol P (positive) or N (negative) and a number (e.g., N11, N13, N20). In clinical neurophysiology, only the short-latency SEPs, including the primary cortical responses of a latency of less than 50 ms, are used to confirm lesions in the somatic sensory system. SEPs have been most helpful in establishing the existence of lesions in the spinal cord and brain stem when clinical and imaging data are uncertain, such as in some cases of multiple sclerosis and cervical spondylosis. Not surprisingly, the SEPs from the lower limbs and particularly from tibial nerve stimulation have proved most rewarding when looking for spinal afferent conduction failure (Figure 4-6).

Contrary to EEG studies, SEPs are only minimally influenced by sedative drugs, making them a useful tool in the intensive care unit. For instance, SEPs from the upper limbs are used to assess the functional integrity of the cortex in comatose patients and, in particular, may be helpful in defining brain death. The deleterious sign of a bilateral absence of cortical SEPs from the upper limbs must be relied on only when the plexus and cervical responses from medial or ulnar nerve stimulation are normally recordable. Otherwise, a plexus or cord lesion could account for the SEP abnormality

(trauma patients). SEPs from the upper limbs are sometimes used to discern and localize proximal brachial plexus or cervical root lesions.

Auditory Evoked Potentials

Recording auditory evoked potentials (AEPs) requires even more averages than for SEPs: Between 1,024 and 2,048 clicks are delivered by headphones, first to one ear and then to the other while a masking noise is given to the contralateral ear. In routine clinical neurophysiology and audiology, only the short-latency (less than 15 ms) AEPs, which are generated in the brain stem, have attained practical importance. They are recorded by electrodes over both mastoids and over the vertex. Seven waves with positive polarity as viewed from the scalp (or negative polarity as viewed from the mastoid) appear and are usually designated with roman numerals I–VII. Clinical interpretations of AEPs are based mainly on latency measurements of waves I, III, and V. Wave I and perhaps also wave II are generated by the acoustic nerve, wave III on the bulbar level, and wave V on the pontomesencephalic level. The AEPs are a sensitive means of detecting lesions of the eighth cranial nerve (acoustic neuroma and other tumors of the cerebellopontine angle) and of the auditory pathways of the brain stem. They are also useful in assessing hearing in infants, in whom deafness as a cause of behavioral abnormalities should not be missed. In central nervous system (CNS) disorders, AEPs have the least diagnostic impact of all evoked potential studies and are no longer in the first line of diagnostic procedures for these conditions.

Motor Evoked Potentials by Transcranial Brain Stimulation

Unlike the case with afferent evoked potentials, there is no need for averaging with the MEPs. A single pulse of transcranial stimulation of the motor cortex induces a muscle jerk, and therefore a sizable compound muscle action potential (CMAP), which can easily be recorded by surface electrodes taped over the muscle belly. The stimulating coil put over the scalp delivers single magnetic pulses, which by the nature of the rapidly changing mag-

stimulation on right side

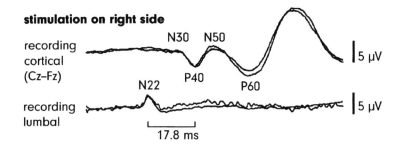

stimulation on left side

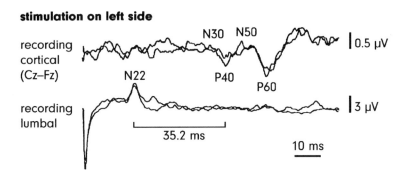

Figure 4-6. Somatosensory evoked potentials from tibial nerve stimulation and parietal recording (two sweeps superimposed). Normal finding on the right side and much delayed and reduced cortical responses on the left side (note the higher gain). The afferent central conduction time between the lumbar potential (recorded at L5 vertebra) and the first major cortical positivity P40 is 17.8 ms on the right and 35.2 ms on the left side.

netic field induce stimulating currents within the brain. Because the magnetic pulse passes unattenuated through scalp and skull directly into the cortex, there is only a trivial skin sensation with each stimulus. The magnetic stimulator triggers an ordinary electromyography (EMG) machine, which suffices to record the responses. The magnetic stimulator excites the rapidly conducting pyramidal system, probably transsynaptically, thereby producing short-latency CMAPs (Figure 4-7).

For diagnostic purposes it is best to use a large circular stimulating coil where the precise coil position is not crucial. For exciting the hand muscles, a large coil may be centered over the vertex, making the lateral coil segment approximately overlay the hand area. For exciting the lower limb muscles, the coil must be shifted to the front and greater stimulus intensities used. Figure-of-eight–shaped twin coils provide a much more focal stimulus and are primarily used for research purposes.

A conspicuous feature of MEPs is their facilitation by a slight voluntary background contraction of the target muscle: The threshold is lowered, the amplitude is increased, and the onset latency is shortened by about 2–3 ms compared with responses from a relaxed muscle. Facilitation is used to periph-

erally "focus" the MEPs to the target muscles because it allows a moderate stimulus intensity to be applied, which excites the contracted muscles but not the relaxed muscles. Facilitation of the recorded target muscles by slight steady precontraction is therefore routinely used when the patient is capable of doing so. If this is not the case, as in plegic limbs or comatose patients, reflexive activation of the target muscle usually achieves the same effect. In cases of severe peripheral nerve lesions, it may be impossible to record MEPs. The small hand muscles (e.g., abductor digiti minimi, first dorsal interosseous), biceps brachii, and the tibialis anterior muscle are particularly suitable target muscles for MEPs. For clinical purposes, it is preferable to assess conduction at least to one upper and one lower limb muscle—for example, to the abductor digiti minimi and tibialis anterior.

The MEP muscle responses vary in latency and amplitude from trial to trial. This inherent variability is in contrast to peripherally evoked motor responses, which are identical when supramaximal nerve stimuli are used. Therefore, at least four responses are usually collected, and the latency is taken from the shortest and the amplitude from the greatest of the four responses. Amplitudes are

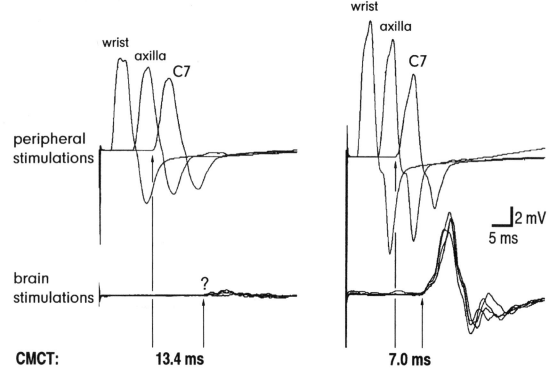

Figure 4-7. Motor evoked potentials recorded from the abductor digiti minimi muscle from peripheral nerve and cortical stimulation (four responses superimposed). An abnormal finding with much reduced and delayed responses in a patient with motor neuron disease is shown on the left part of the figure. With an upper limit of normal of 8.5 ms, the central motor conduction time (CMCT) of approximately 13.4 ms is moderately prolonged. A normal finding is shown on the right part. The CMCT is defined as the difference between the corticomuscular latency and the latency from motor root stimulation over the spine (C7).

preferably expressed as a percentage of response obtained when stimulating the corresponding peripheral nerve. The variability of amplitudes is such that they can be taken as abnormal only if they do not reach 15–20% of the peripherally evoked response. The small amplitudes of normal MEPs are largely caused by the so-called phase cancellation phenomenon of the negative-positive CMAP. It is caused by the relatively great temporal dispersion of the impulses over the entire motor route, including a central and peripheral segment with intercalated synapses.

To calculate a central motor conduction time (CMCT), the peripheral motor conduction time must be subtracted from the total corticomuscular latency. The former may be obtained by F-wave techniques and from cervical or lumbar stimulation by a high-voltage electric or a magnetic stimulator (see "Motor Neurography"). Spinal stimulation is known to excite the motor roots at their exit foramen, allowing the calculated CMCT to include a small peripheral nerve segment.

MEPs are a highly sensitive method for detecting subtle lesions in the pyramidal system in central demyelinating disorders. In multiple sclerosis, MEPs disclose abnormal results more often than VEPs, SEPs, or AEPs. However, the MEPs tend to confirm a clinical abnormality such as hyperreflexia or Babinski's sign, and the detection of a clinically silent lesion clearly occurs less frequently than with VEPs. Therefore, in terms of diagnostic impact in suspected MS, MEPs rank behind VEPs. The MEPs are also of great value in assessing conduction delay in compressive cervical myelopathy, in which they help to judge the clinical relevance of imaging results. Conversely, in axonal disorders such as amyotrophic lateral sclerosis (ALS), the method has a lower sensitivity, particularly in the early stages of the disease. In ALS, the MEPs tend to evoke low-amplitude or absent responses of near normal latency, but occasionally clearly prolonged responses are also encountered. In stroke, the MEPs are often absent or of low amplitude and probably indicate an unfavorable prognosis. But again, CMCT prolongation is also seen in strokes. Therefore, in individual cases, the MEPs do not allow differentiation with certainty between demyelinating and axonal disorders. However, MEPs may help to substantiate the diagnosis of psychogenic weakness: If completely normal MEPs are recorded in a lasting (several days) and complete plegia of a limb, a psychogenic origin is very likely.

High sensitivity, low specificity, and easy performance make the MEPs an ideal screening method. For instance, in a case with doubtful symptoms and equivocal hyperreflexia, clearly abnormal MEPs may prompt further investigations.

Electrodiagnosis of Neuromuscular Disease

Nerve Conduction Studies (Electroneurography)

Since the epochal discovery by von Helmholtz in 1850, who for the first time measured the motor conduction velocity in the sciatic nerve of frogs, it is known that (1) an intact nerve can easily be excited by a brief electrical current and (2) the stimulus-induced muscle twitch is accompanied by an electric CMAP of several millivolts. This is, of course, an artificial situation because the external stimulus excites all nerve fibers simultaneously, producing a synchronous volley of impulses traveling along the nerve. As a consequence, the muscle fibers within a muscle are also activated synchronously, generating the CMAP, which does not occur during natural activation of a muscle. Von Helmholtz measured the nerve conduction velocity by stimulating the nerve at two separate sites, and the distance between the two sites was divided by a time interval between the two motor responses. In today's clinical use, motor nerve conduction studies depend on the same principle, and the technique has been expanded to sensory nerve fibers as well. Because the sensory end organs of the skin do not produce measurable elec-

tricity, they are not accessible to percutaneous recording. For this reason, the conduction of sensory nerve fibers is assessed by percutaneous recording of the compound nerve action potential at different sites over the nerve. A distal sensory nerve segment is stimulated, and a sensory nerve action potential (SNAP) is recorded proximally over the nerve. The electric currents produced by the nerves are much smaller than those of the muscles. When an electric stimulus sets up a synchronous volley of impulses in the entire nerve, a compound SNAP of a few microvolts can nevertheless be recorded through the intact skin. The depolarization of neural membranes produces outside negativity, causing an overlying recording electrode to become negative, which by convention is displayed upward on the screen. When recording from a muscle, the active electrode (i.e., the recording lead) is usually placed over the belly of the muscle, which corresponds approximately to the motor point, where the neuromuscular synapses (i.e., the endplates) are situated. Because the depolarization of the muscle fibers originates at the endplates, the biphasic CMAP measured this way begins with a negative (upward) deflection followed by a positive one. In contrast, recording the electrical activity passing by in a nerve causes a triphasic action potential in which the major negativity of the depolarized zone is preceded and followed by a smaller positivity. When the depolarized zone moves under the recording electrode, it is preceded and followed by positive nondepolarized regions, from which the electrical currents are "sucked off" to the depolarized zone (Figure 4-8).

The duration of a nerve action potential roughly reflects the velocity spectrum of the axons within the nerve, and the potential duration is augmented somewhat with increasing distance from the stimulation site because of the growing dispersion of the impulses that arrive at the recording electrode. When assessing the nerve conduction velocity, the latency is measured from the stimulus artifact to the onset of the negative deflection of a CMAP or to the initial positive peak of a SNAP, respectively, which has proved most reliable. It is important to consider that this assesses the velocity only of the largest and most rapidly conducting nerve fibers. For surface stimulation, a pair of stimulating electrodes is placed over the nerve, with the depolarizing cathode closer to the recording site. On rare occasions

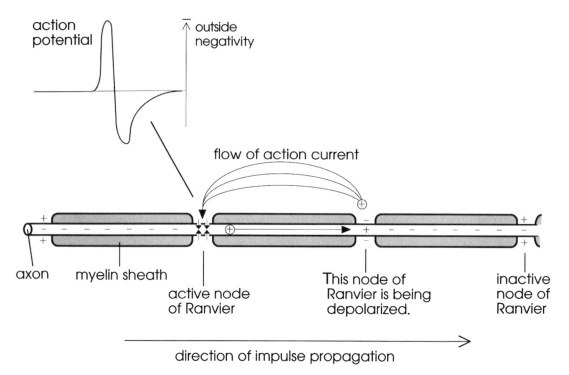

Figure 4-8. Impulse propagation of a myelinated nerve fiber schematically depicted. In reality, the internodal distances are much greater. A negative action potential (displayed upward) is recorded at the outside of a nerve because there is an influx of positive sodium ions into the axons, causing a depolarization at the active nodes of Ranvier. The action currents spread ahead of the impulse and will depolarize the next nodes of Ranvier. The myelin sheaths provide electrical insulation, enabling the action potential to jump from node to node (i.e., saltatory impulse propagation) rather than creep continuously as in unmyelinated fibers.

such as in brachial plexus stimulation, the use of monopolar stimulation, in which a needle electrode is inserted as a cathode close to the nerve, is preferable. A surface electrode on the skin serves as the anode.

Electroneurography is primarily used to diagnose focal or generalized neuropathies in which nerve conduction is in some way deficient. Two basic conduction abnormalities can be distinguished by electrodiagnostic studies: slowing of conduction and loss of conducting nerve fibers (Figure 4-9).

Slowing of Conduction

Slowing of conduction is found in focal and generalized neuropathies. Examples are entrapment or compression neuropathies, in which conduction slowing is confined to the site of impairment, as in carpal tunnel syndrome, or generalized neuropathies with widespread deficiency of the myelin sheaths, as in the inflammatory or the Charcot-Marie-Tooth

neuropathies and related inherited disorders. In these conditions, conduction slowing may typically affect the different axons within a nerve, disparately leading to an abnormally increased dispersion with greatly expanded potential durations.

It is important to notice that conduction slowing as such does not necessarily lead to clinical deficits such as weakness or sensory loss because the number of conducting axons may still be normal. Hence, conduction slowing provides a subclinical measure of nerve disease and therefore adds a new variable to the information collected by clinical examination.

Conduction slowing is usually caused by myelin damage. However, it can also occur in conditions in which previous axonal damage was followed by reinnervation. Reinnervation fibers are of smaller diameter with thinner myelin sheaths and conduct slowly. Moreover, an axonal disease may preferentially injure the fastest-conducting large-diameter fibers, leading to a reduction of the maximum conduction

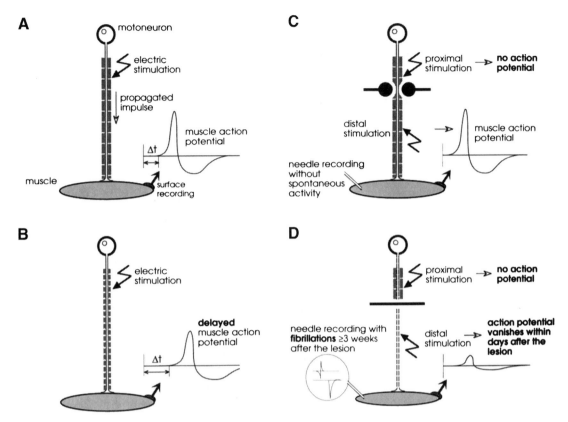

Figure 4-9. The principal motor conduction abnormalities as electrodiagnostically assessed (only one nerve cell and fiber is depicted for simplicity). (A) Normal conduction. (B) Slowed conduction. (C) Conduction block (neurapraxia). (D) Axonal lesion (axonotmesis). Conditions in panels C and D cause clinical weakness. In axonal lesions (D), fibrillation potentials will be recorded by needle myography and the muscle becomes atrophied, whereas in conduction block (C), this is not the case. Note that in clinical reality these distinct conditions virtually never occur purely—that is, homogeneously for all nerve cells and fibers of a nerve, and usually a mixture of several types of abnormality, are encountered, with predominance of one type or the other.

velocity as assessed by neurography, because the remaining small-diameter fibers conduct more slowly. Thus, mild slowing of nerve conduction is also a frequent finding in axonal neuropathies.

Loss of Conducting Nerve Fibers

Loss of conducting axons within a nerve leads to reduced amplitudes or surface areas of the compound action potential (CMAP or SNAP) and may be the result of two entirely different pathogenic mechanisms:

1. It is a characteristic finding of disorders of damaged axons, such as in nerve injuries and toxic neuropathies, or damage of nerve cell somas, such

as in anterior horn diseases. Damage to motor axons additionally leads to signs of denervation or neurogenic transformation in needle myograms (see "Needle Examination of Muscle [Electromyography]").

2. Drop out of conducting axons may also occur in demyelinating diseases, in which nerve fibers sometimes completely fail to propagate impulses in spite of preserved continuity of the axons. This conduction abnormality is called *conduction block* (i.e., neurapraxia). It may also occur in conditions of very little or no structural nerve damage, as in transient compression syndromes (e.g., "Saturday night palsy") or pharmacologic nerve blocks with local anesthetics. Other than with axonal loss, normal amplitude action potentials are obtained if stimulation can be applied beyond the conduction block, and in motor nerve con-

duction block no denervation signs are found in the muscle even if it is a long-standing block. Furthermore, conduction block is associated with a better prognosis than axonal loss. In clinical testing, differentiation between axonal loss and conduction is often difficult, making electrophysiologic study a particularly important diagnostic tool.

In contrast to conduction slowing, loss of conducting axons is invariably accompanied by some clinical deficit. Accordingly, it can be inferred that in a patient with a significant motor or sensory deficit of noncentral origin, there is always a loss of conducting fibers as a result of axonal loss or conduction block.

In clinical reality, the two basic types of abnormality, conduction slowing and drop out of conducting fibers, are often found concurrently: (1) Some disease processes produce both demyelination as well as axonal damage, as in, for example, severe entrapment (focal damage) or in diabetes mellitus (expanded and multifocal damage); (2) a demyelinating disorder may also lead to secondary axonal degeneration, particularly when it is a long-standing disease; (3) in some demyelinating disorders, the combined occurrence of slowed conduction and conduction block is typical, as in inflammatory or postradiation neuropathies.

Conduction studies may appear normal despite widespread axonal degeneration if a critical number of large nerve fibers are unaffected by the disease process because neurography assesses the conduction of the most rapidly conducting, large-diameter fibers and the derived velocities always reflect the status of surviving fibers. For instance, some sensory neuropathies that predominantly or exclusively affect the thinly myelinated and nonmyelinated fibers cannot be detected by conventional neurography because the small diameter sensory fibers do not contribute to the amplitude of SNAP. This is the case in the small-fiber neuropathies, in which conventional nerve conduction studies typically produce normal findings and specific autonomic tests are required to disclose them (see below). Furthermore, after incomplete transection of a nerve, the maximal motor conduction velocity may also be normal in the remaining fibers despite severe weakness in the muscle involved. However, in this case, the CMAP recorded from the muscle is clearly reduced in amplitude and signs of denervation can be recorded by needle myography.

When exploring axonal damage, several methodologic factors must be considered:

1. It is crucial to stimulate the nerve supramaximally to guarantee activation of all nerve axons. It is therefore customary to increase the stimulating intensity until the CMAP or SNAP amplitude is saturated (i.e., maximal stimulation intensity), and then add another 20–30% of stimulating power (supramaximal). In antidromically measured sensory conduction velocity, submaximal stimulation is used, rendering this method unsuitable for assessing axonal damage (see below). For measuring SNAP amplitudes, the orthodromic technique should be used, preferably with surface recording.
2. CMAP or SNAP amplitudes are inherently variable, with a broad range of normal values rendering detection of slight reductions impossible.
3. Signs of acute denervation in needle myography occur only approximately 2–3 weeks after the injury and may be scarce in chronic disease processes or completely absent in predominantly sensory neuropathies. In chronic disease, quantitative motor unit evaluation may nevertheless disclose a neurogenic transformation (see below).
4. It is important to note that in axonal damage, amplitude reduction of the CMAP must also be encountered with the most distal stimulation site. This discriminates from conduction block (neurapraxia), in which the amplitude drop occurs in a stepwise fashion when moving with stimulation proximally.

Any nerve that can be stimulated and recorded through the skin by surface electrodes is accessible to electroneurography. A limitation is encountered when extending neurography to proximal sites, where the nerve trunks are deeply situated and where special techniques are required for stimulation and recording. The accuracy of proximal neurography can be maintained by using needle electrodes to record and sometimes also to stimulate. Furthermore, special techniques are used to assess the cranial nerves or phrenic nerve.

The conduction velocity is determined by dividing the nerve length between two stimulation (motor) or recording (sensory orthodromic) points by the corresponding latency difference. The length of the nerve segment is estimated by measuring the surface distance along the course of the nerve. To maintain a satisfactory accuracy of the assessed conduction velocity, the two stimulation points should be separated by at least 10 cm. However, in the evaluation of a focal lesion, inclusion of the unaffected segments in the calculation dilutes the effect of slowing at the injured site and decreases the sensitivity. Particularly when the clinician is looking for focal slowing or partial conduction block (neurapraxia), stimulation must sometimes be moved across a critical segment in a stepwise fashion to better localize an abnormality that might otherwise escape detection ("inching").

The important influence of limb temperature on nerve conduction velocity must be considered. Nerve impulses propagate slower by 1.5–2.4 meters per second per degree centigrade, and distal latencies increase when the limb is cooled below 37°C. To reduce this type of variability, skin temperature is measured with a plate thermistor on the skin over the measured nerve. If the skin temperature falls below 34°C for motor neurography or below 36°C for orthodromic sensory neurography, it is mandatory that the limbs be warmed with an infrared heat lamp or by immersion in warm water. One should, however, be careful not to heat the limb to above 38°C because of possible hazards (patients with defective thermal and pain sensibility) and the risk of producing false-negative results (Table 4-1).

Motor Neurography

By placing the active muscle recording electrode on the belly of the target muscle (where the motor point is situated) and the indifferent electrode on the tendon, a simple biphasic waveform with initial negativity results. Initial positivity of the CMAP usually suggests inaccurate positioning of the active electrode, which should then be adjusted. The corresponding mixed or motor nerve is stimulated at two or more points along its course with supramaximal strength to excite all nerve fibers and provide a CMAP of full size. The amplitude is usually measured from the baseline to the negative peak, the latency from stimulus to onset of the negative deflection, and the duration from onset to the final return to baseline (Figure 4-10).

Because the latency is the sum of the nerve conduction time and the neuromuscular transmission time, which is not precisely known, a motor conduction velocity cannot be properly derived in the most distal segment. Therefore, the distal motor latency between the most distal stimulus point and

the muscle is left as such and compared with the normal range of the target muscle in question.

Most EMG devices automatically provide the CMAP area under the negative component of the waveform, which reflects the amount of excited muscle fibers more faithfully than the amplitude. This is important when looking for motor conduction block in suspected focal compression, entrapment, or inflammatory neuropathies. Precise localization of a restricted conduction abnormality requires so-called inching by moving the stimulus in short increments along the course of the nerve. An abrupt change in amplitude or area and waveform is found across the site of the conduction abnormality (Figure 4-11). An abrupt prolongation of the CMAP duration, indicating abnormal dispersion or focal conduction slowing, also occurs in focal demyelination. In inflammatory neuropathies such as Guillain-Barré syndrome and its variants, focal conduction abnormalities are sometimes located at proximal and distal extremes of the peripheral nerve, rendering detection difficult and requiring special techniques—for example, the F-wave technique (see below), motor root stimulation over the spine (see below), or even transcranial cortical stimulation. In chronic inflammatory neuropathies, conduction block and focal slowing must be sought at unusual sites—for example, amidst the forearm or upper arm, where entrapment is rare.

Conduction blocks or axonal lesions in the very distal motor nerve terminals are notoriously difficult to localize and sometimes account for very low CMAP amplitudes from stimulation over the entire course of the nerve. Needle myography in a search for denervation signs, motor point stimulation over the muscle to detect very distal conduction block, and assessment of the recruitment pattern of low-threshold motor units are helpful (see "Needle Examination of Muscle [Electromyography]"). Other reasons for very low CMAP amplitudes or even absent motor responses are hypoexcitable or unexcitable nerves in the acute stage of very severe Guillain-Barré syndrome, in long-standing compression neuropathy, or, rarely, in chronic hereditary dysmyelinating neuropathies of the Dejerine-Sottas type. Also, the Eaton-Lambert myasthenic syndrome typically produces low CMAP amplitudes that increase shortly after tonic contraction of the target muscle (postexercise potentiation).

When diagnosing a motor conduction block (neurapraxia), several possible pitfalls must be ruled

Table 4-1. Synopsis of Principal Electrodiagnostic Findings in Neuromuscular Disorders

Abnormal Condition	Duration Type	Pathomechanism	Examples	Neurography		Needle Myography			Special Findings
				CAP Amplitude	Conduction Velocity	Spontaneous Activity	Volitional Activation	MUP Size and Shape	
Abnormal conduction: neurapraxia and/or slowing	Very transient (hours)	Dysfunction of membrane ion channels; ischemia, local edema?	Local anesthetics, "sleeping limb" from local pressure	Conduction block	Normal	None	Reduced IP, fast MUP firing rate	Normal	
	Short duration (days–weeks)	Slight focal (paranodal) myelin damage from acute pressure	Pressure paralysis ("Saturday night palsy")	Conduction block	Sometimes focally reduced	None	Reduced IP, fast MUP firing rate	Normal	Marked motor and sensory deficit
		Widespread or multifocal myelin damage, immune mediated	Acute inflammatory demyelinating polyneuropathy (Guillain-Barré syndrome)	Conduction block frequent	Multifocal (rarely extensive) slowing (often very proximal and/or very distal)	None	Reduced IP, fast MUP firing rate	Normal	Usually predominately motor deficit
	Moderate duration (weeks–months)	Focal myelin damage from chronic compression	Entrapment syndromes (e.g., carpal tunnel syndrome)	Usually normal	Focally reduced	Sparse fibrillations, typical myokymia	Normal	Normal	Only little clinical deficit, secondary axonal degeneration possible
	Long duration (months–years)	Multifocal myelin damage, antibody-induced ion channel dysfunction?	Chronic inflammatory demyelinating polyneuropathy, radiation plexopathy	Conduction block	(Multi-) focal slowing	Often numerous myokymia and fasciculations	Reduced IP, fast MUP firing rate	Normal	Additional axonal damage possible
	Inherited	Myelin formation defective	Charcot-Marie-Tooth disease	Normal	Marked general slowing	None or sparse fibrillations (secondary axonal degeneration)	Normal	Normal	Clinical deficit often trivial

Category								
Axonal and/or neuronal damage	Acute partial nerve injury (axonotmesis)	Axonal disruption with preserved epineural connective tissue	Stretch or crush injury, vasculitic and toxic neuropathy	Reduced	Normal or slightly reduced	Fibrillation and SPW ≥3 weeks after a lesion	Reduced IP, fast MUP firing rate	Large and polyphasic months after a lesion	After reinnervation: axon reflexes, synkinesia due to misrouting after injury possible
	Systemic neuronal degeneration	Nerve cell death	Motorneuron disease, spinal muscular dystrophy	Reduced	Normal or slightly reduced	Fibrillation and SPW, fasciculations	Reduced IP of large amplitude	Large and polyphasic	No axon reflex
	Acute nerve transection (neuronotmesis)	Complete division of all axons and epineural connective tissue	Penetration wound	No response	Not measurable	Fibrillation and SPW after ≥3 weeks	None	Large and polyphasic >6 mos after successful nerve suture	After reinnervation: axon reflexes, synkinesia due to misrouting
Myasthenic syndromes	Chronic disease with exacerbations possible	Defective neuromuscular transmission, immune mediated	Myasthenia gravis; Eaton-Lambert myasthenic syndrome	Progressive decline on repetitive stimulation (3 Hz), Eaton-Lambert myasthenic syndrome: CAP amplitude increases after volitional activation	Normal	None	Progressive decline with prolonged contraction	Sometimes smaller	Single-fiber EMG with increased jitter and blocking
Myopathies	Chronic muscle disease	Degenerative and metabolic muscle fiber damage	Muscular dystrophies	Normal	Normal	None or sparse fibrillations	Full IP of low amplitude, early MUP recruitment	Small and polyphasic	Characteristic myotonic discharges in myotonias
	Myositis subacute-chronic	Inflammatory muscle fiber damage	Polymyositis	Normal	Normal	Fibrillation potentials and SPW	Full IP of low amplitude, early MUP recruitment	Small and polyphasic	

CAP = compound action potential; MUP = motor unit potential; IP = interference pattern; EMG = electromyography; SPW = sharp positive wave.

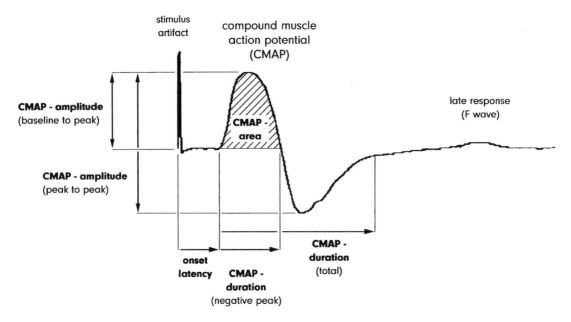

Figure 4-10. Parameters of compound muscle action potentials (CMAP). The onset latency and negative component amplitude measured from baseline to peak are the most important parameters for routine evaluation.

out: (1) Inadequate stimulation at proximal sites that is not supramaximal is a frequent mistake of an inexperienced examiner; (2) innervation anomalies with nerve anastomoses may simulate conduction block because of abrupt amplitude changes; (3) in the first days after an acute lesion before denervation signs occur in the muscle, a conduction block cannot be formally distinguished from an axonal lesion; and (4) local hypoexcitability caused by demyelination producing reduced CMAPs may be mistaken for a conduction block.

Exploring very proximal conduction abnormalities is a challenge to clinical electrophysiologists and calls for experience. It is important in assessing lesions of the brachial plexus and in Guillain-Barré syndrome or chronic inflammatory demyelinating polyneuropathies. Moreover, proximal conduction must be measured in assessing the CMCT from magnetic brain stimulation (see "Motor Evoked Potentials by Transcranial Brain Stimulation"). There are two routinely used techniques: motor root stimulation and F waves.

Motor root stimulation can be achieved using powerful electric or magnetic stimulators. Because with this technique the actual site of stimulation lies relatively distant from the stimulating electrodes or

coils, particular stimulation principles apply. If conduction block at the brachial plexus is sought and therefore supramaximal stimulation is crucial, only special high-voltage low-output impedance electrical stimulators (e.g., D180, DIGITIMER, Electronic Medical Instrumentation Development and Manufacture, Hertfordshire, United Kingdom) are sufficient, and a distance between the stimulating electrodes of approximately 6 cm must be used. The electrodes are preferably placed over the back of the neck in the midline, with the cathode situated just below the spinous process of C7 and the anode above. The stimulating strength must be increased until no further rise in amplitude occurs. It is important to consider that such a vigorous stimulation over the spine must not be used in patients with unstable vertebrae. Furthermore, the stimulus has the tendency of reaching far out into the brachial plexus, rendering latency measurements unreliable. Hence, for latency measurements, just-maximal or submaximal stimulation is additionally used, which has been shown to excite the motor roots at their exit foramen of the spine, and this is the case for both electric and magnetic root stimulation. When using a magnetic stimulator, a large, round coil is put around the C7 spinous process, and with a

Figure 4-11. Motor ulnar nerve neurography in a patient with an immune-mediated multifocal motor neuropathy. Careful movement discloses a partial conduction block along the course of the nerve within the forearm. The compound muscle action potential amplitude shows a sudden drop to approximately half the size without much increase of dispersion (potential duration not much prolonged) when moving with stimulation proximally. Note the unusual site of conduction block typical of these neuropathies. In the ulnar nerve, a conduction block is more commonly found at the elbow from chronic compression.

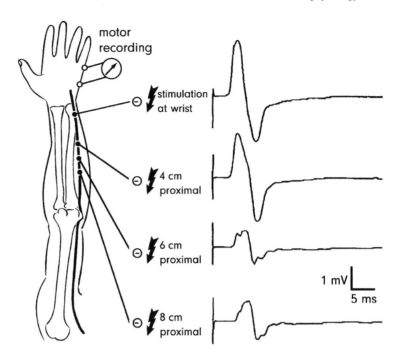

monophasic stimulus, the coil must be turned around to change the direction of the inducing current to stimulate both sides. To fractionate the brachial plexus measurements, supraclavicular electric stimulation over Erb's point is also performed. Corpulent patients sometimes necessitate special techniques for supramaximal Erb's point stimulation—either with a high-voltage stimulator or a unipolar stimulation technique, whereby a large plate over the back of the shoulder serves as the anode. Supramaximal stimulation of the lumbosacral roots is not reliably possible.

Proximal conduction can also be explored using the F-wave technique. The F wave is evoked by a supramaximal stimulus of a mixed or motor nerve and is typically small and variable within a subject. Its latency lies between 28 and 34 ms in the arms and between 36 and 40 ms in the legs. The F wave is produced by antidromically traveling impulses in the motor fibers that activate the anterior horn cells, some of which respond with an orthodromic motor response. The latency of the F waves typically shortens when moving with the stimulus to more proximal sites, and this is also true for other indirect responses (H reflex, axon reflex). An F-wave study requires that at least 10 responses be collected, and 20 or more trials are often required. Absolute latencies or a computed F-wave conduction velocity are compared with normal values established for the distal arm and leg nerves. The most sensitive criterion of abnormality is one-sided absence of F waves or a latency difference between the two sides in a unilateral disorder. F waves must be distinguished from other late responses: (1) H reflexes after submaximal stimulation; and (2) axon reflexes, which, contrary to the F waves, produce responses without latency and amplitude variation but may shorten stepwise with increasing stimulation intensity. The presence of an axon reflex may be a relevant sign as proof of peripheral nerve involvement because it can occur only with a former or recent peripheral lesion.

Sensory Nerve Conduction

Two techniques for testing sensory nerve conduction are routinely used:

1. Antidromic sensory conduction measurement is done by submaximal stimulation of the nerve at different sites along its course and recording of

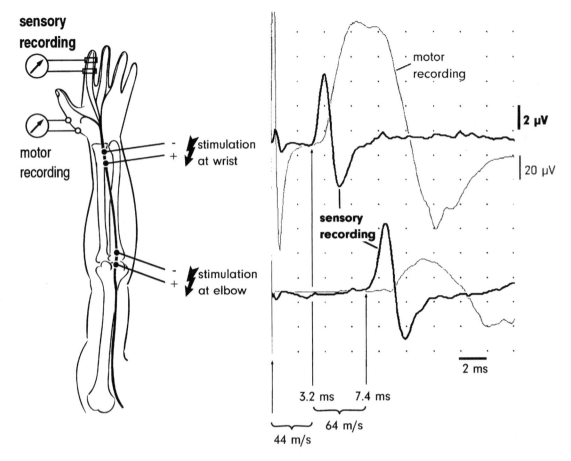

Figure 4-12. Antidromic median sensory conduction study. The nerve is stimulated at different sites along its course and the antidromic sensory action potential is recorded from the index finger using surface ring electrodes. Simultaneous recording of the motor compound muscle action potential is crucial for the antidromic technique. To be taken as genuine, the sensory potential must have a shorter latency than the motor potential (see text).

SNAPs with distal surface electrodes, usually ring electrodes at the fingers for the median and ulnar nerves.

2. Orthodromic sensory conduction measurement is done by supramaximal stimulation of the distal skin area, mostly of digital nerves with ring electrodes, and by recording at different sites over the nerve with surface or needle electrodes insulated except for the tip.

The antidromic technique is easier to perform and perfectly suitable for screening purposes, particularly in assessing sensory conduction of suspected carpal tunnel syndrome. It yields reliable sensory velocities if there is no severe axonal damage involved. It is preferable to average 16–32 responses. The antidromic digital SNAP has an initial negative deflection when recorded with a pair of ring electrodes. Its amplitude is greater than the orthodromic SNAP. However, the antidromic SNAP amplitudes cannot be used as a quantitative estimate of axonal intactness or loss. The antidromic technique does not allow supramaximal nerve stimulation because the antidromic SNAP is easily corrupted by the volume conducted effect from the much larger CMAP. Therefore, the CMAP should be monitored on a second motor channel to ascertain the genuineness of the sensory SNAP. The latter must have an earlier onset than the CMAP (Figure 4-12).

If the antidromic technique yields doubtful results or no proper SNAP, the orthodromic technique is used. Although surface electrodes provide reproducible results and may be preferable for

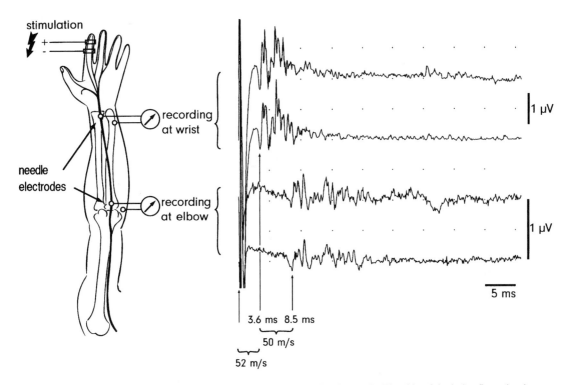

Figure 4-13. Orthodromic needle technique of a median sensory conduction study. The skin of the index finger is stimulated through surface ring electrodes, and the orthodromic sensory nerve potential is recorded by thin needle electrodes that are insulated except for the tip. The active electrode is pushed to the nerve and the reference electrode is inserted approximately 2–3 cm to the side. This technique requires averaging of many sweeps, and two separate potentials are recorded from each site to ascertain reproducibility. The latency to the first positive peak provides the conduction velocity of the fastest fibers. The number of components (i.e., phases) is also evaluated and may be abnormally increased with or without reduction of the conduction velocity.

amplitude measurements (estimation of possible axonal damage), the needle recording is clearly superior and allows the shape and duration of the orthodromic SNAP to be judged as well. The active needle electrode is placed as close as possible to the nerve. To obtain optimal positioning of the electrode in case of mixed nerves, small stimulating currents are sometimes first injected into the active needle electrode, and the precise position is optimized according to the evoked motor response. Averaging of orthodromic responses is essential, and several hundred sweeps must sometimes be collected to obtain a satisfactory SNAP. The patient should be comfortably positioned, with the limb completely relaxed, to avoid volume-conducted contamination of the SNAP from neighboring muscles. In doubtful cases, the averaging procedure must be repeated to ascertain reproducibility.

A needle-recorded orthodromic SNAP with normal onset latency may contain a multitude of components that result from demyelinated, remyelinated, or regenerated fibers. The number of allowable components (≥10% of maximal peak-to-peak amplitude) is defined for each nerve and recording site. The orthodromic SNAP is triphasic, with an initial positive deflection (where the latency is measured) when recorded with the active electrodes near the nerve and the reference electrode 2–3 cm sideways (Figure 4-13). The orthodromic SNAP amplitude is measured between the negative and positive peaks.

Needle Examination of Muscle (Electromyography)

To pick up the low-amplitude asynchronous electrical activity of muscle fibers as it arises from a natu-

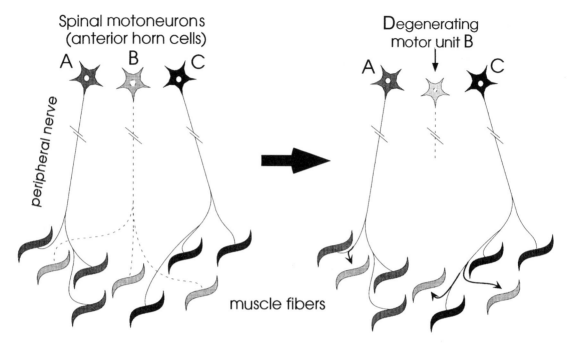

Figure 4-14. The principle of neuromuscular reorganization after a partial axonal lesion leading to enlarged motor units. Three motor units, A–C, are schematically depicted, comprising three muscle fibers each (in reality, there up to several hundred muscle fibers in motor unit). Denervated muscle fibers from the degenerated motoneuron B attract the newly sprouting nerve twigs from the surviving motor units A and C, to which the orphaned fibers are added. As a consequence, motor unit potentials become enlarged (i.e., prolonged duration, greater amplitude, and often also polyphasic), as assessed in needle myography.

rally activated muscle, surface recordings do not suffice, and needle electrodes must be inserted into the muscle. This is done with standardized concentric needle electrodes, where the tip of the wire in the lumen of the needle is the active electrode (the recording lead), which is in proximity to relatively few muscle fibers. The shaft of the needle is in contact over most of its length with the muscle tissue and serves as an indifferent reference electrode. During slight voluntary contraction, the needle recording picks up electrical activity of individual motor units. These motor unit potentials arise each from the simultaneous discharge of the muscle fibers belonging to one motor unit. A single motoneuron in the anterior horn of the spinal cord supplies several muscle fibers in the muscle, constituting a collectively behaving motor unit (Figure 4-14). Thus, the muscle fibers in a normal muscle are always activated as motor units rather than individually.

In pathologic conditions, the motor units show characteristic changes. Chronic partial denervation of a muscle gives rise to enlarged motor units because denervated muscle fibers, as a compensating mechanism, are being linked up by adjacent surviving motor units. The abnormally large motor units lead to enlarged motor unit potentials, and this can be assessed by needle myography. On the other hand, when the muscle itself is diseased, as in myopathy or myositis, in which some muscle fibers of a motor unit may be destroyed or rendered nonfunctional, the population of muscle fibers per motor unit is reduced, and hence the motor unit potentials become abnormally small, splintered, or shortened. It is important to note, however, that very distal neuropathies affecting the terminal branches to the individual muscle fibers may also lead to smaller motor unit potentials, when motor units lose contact with some of their muscle fibers. Furthermore, in relatively recent denervation, abnormal spontaneous discharges in the relaxed state that are produced by isolated muscle fibers may be recorded. The assessment of the motor unit potentials and the search for abnormal spontaneous activity by the intramuscular needle electrodes constitute the bases of needle myography or EMG in the strict sense.

The correct use of recording variables is imperative for needle myography, especially for analysis of motor unit potentials. This is particularly true for the filter setting, which, with the exception of special purposes, must be set at 2 Hz for low filtering and at 10 kHz for high filtering. Raising the low-frequency filtering produces a more stable baseline, but importantly affects the shape and duration of motor units, the normal values of which have commonly been assessed with 2-Hz filtering. Lowering the upper-frequency filtering renders differentiation between proximal and distant muscle activity impossible. A sweep speed of 5–10 ms per cm is best for defining spontaneous and voluntary muscle activity, and the gain is usually set between 100 μV and 1 mV per cm.

No experienced electromyographer would feel comfortable during an examination without acoustic presentation of the EMG signal to complement the screen display. Audio monitoring of the EMG is essential because the ear is more sensitive and quicker than the eye in qualitatively identifying the frequency spectrum of the complex signals and in appraising the rhythmicity of repetitive discharges. For instance, when the needle electrode has not yet penetrated the fascia of a small muscle being explored, the blunt sound of the muscle activity caused by the high-frequency filtering effect of the intercalated tissue immediately indicates to the examiner that he or she must insert the tip of the needle slightly deeper until the sharp sound heard during voluntary activity contraction affirms optimal positioning of the electrode. Also, very low-amplitude, scarce spontaneous activity from a distant site, complete absence of any activity (total silence) from biologic or artificial causes, interference from main currents, and other artifacts are more readily recognized by the ear than by the eye.

Needle myography is performed in three steps by assessing (1) the spontaneous activity in the relaxed muscle, (2) the recruitment and interference pattern during weak and maximal volitional effort, and (3) the motor unit potential (MUP) during minimal contraction. Usually several muscles must be tested because of the varying topography of muscle and peripheral nerve diseases, which may involve some muscles and not others. An adequate EMG study requires exploration in different parts of the limb and sampling of each muscle in several areas.

Spontaneous Activity

Spontaneous activity is assessed by inserting the concentric needle electrode into a completely relaxed muscle and waiting for a few seconds with a high gain of 100 μV per cm using audio monitoring. A minimum of 10 different sites in each muscle should be explored. Normally, a resting muscle is electrically silent. However, inserting or slightly moving the needle regularly causes insertional activity as a result of mechanical excitation of muscle fibers, which normally vanishes within half a second.

Absence of insertional activity suggests fibrotic muscle after ischemic damage or severely atrophied muscle tissue. Another form of normal spontaneous activity that must not be confused with abnormal activity is encountered when the needle is placed near a motor endplate: (1) Very small (approximately 150 μV of amplitude) and brief (0.5–2.0 ms), monophasic, negative, and irregularly firing endplate potentials (endplate spikes); and (2) a conspicuous irregularity in the baseline, so-called endplate noise in the speaker.

Pathologic spontaneous activity and abnormally prolonged insertional activity indicate denervation, myotonic disorders, or myositis, and include the following:

1. Fibrillation potentials and positive sharp waves, which are generated by single muscle fibers and are not accompanied by a visible motion at the skin surface. Sharp positive waves are monophasic, with initial positivity and subsequent slow negativity; the fibrillation potentials are diphasic or triphasic, with initial positivity having a duration of approximately 15 ms and an amplitude of 20–200 μV (Figure 4-15). They typically fire in a regular decelerating pattern of 1–30 Hz. Their presence in at least two different areas of a muscle is considered abnormal. They are frequently but not exclusively encountered in denervation. In acute axonal lesions there is a 2- to 3-week latent period before fibrillations and sharp positive waves appear. They arise very abundantly in

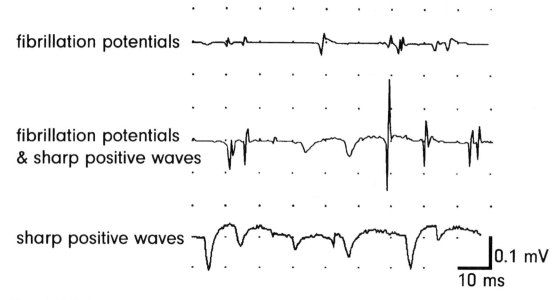

fibrillation potentials

fibrillation potentials
& sharp positive waves

sharp positive waves

0.1 mV

10 ms

Figure 4-15. Fibrillation potentials and sharp positive waves as recorded by needle electrodes. This type of spontaneous activity is typically encountered in partially or totally denervated muscle, and is also found in active myositis. The pathologic significance of fibrillation potentials and sharp positive waves is the same.

severe or near-complete recent axonal lesions, producing a sound similar to "rain on a metal roof." In chronic and partial lesions only scarce fibrillations are found. The distribution of spontaneous potentials is useful for localizing lesions in the spinal cord, root, plexus, or peripheral nerves. Relatively intense fibrillation and sharp positive waves are also typical of active myositis and are, to a lesser extent, found in muscular dystrophies.

2. Fasciculation potentials and myokymic discharges are generated by motor units or otherwise functionally linked groups of muscle fibers and may cause detectable skin movement over a localized area or minute finger jerks (*signe de l'index*). These forms of spontaneous activity are indicative of chronic conditions. Fasciculation potentials basically look like motor unit potentials but fire sporadically and are unaffected by voluntary effort of agonist or antagonist muscles. They are most commonly seen in diseases of anterior horn cells, chronic inflammatory neuropathies, entrapment neuropathies, radiculopathies, and cervical spondylotic myelopathy. They may also normally arise in the gastrocnemius muscle after exertion and occasionally affect individuals without apparent serious disorders ("benign fasciculations"), sometimes

accompanied by myalgia or cramps. Myokymic discharges look like motor unit potentials but fire repetitively in a relaxed muscle. They occur either as grouped discharges of complex bursts with intervals of up to 10 seconds in between or as regularly firing single potentials at a rate of 1–5 Hz. Myokymic discharges originate ectopically in demyelinated nerve fibers and are typical of chronic inflammatory neuropathies (particularly those with conduction block) and in radiation plexopathies. In the facial muscles they suggest multiple sclerosis or brain stem glioma.

3. Complex repetitive, neuromyotonic, and myotonic discharges are relatively high frequency (≥5 Hz) regular discharges that may begin spontaneously or after a needle movement, and they are also confined to chronic conditions. When occurring in abundance in a muscle, they may induce muscle tension or cramp. This is particularly true for the myotonic discharges.

   Complex repetitive discharges are simple (and, strictly speaking, not complex) or serrated potentials (complex), firing with relatively uniform frequency at a rate of 5–30 Hz, occasionally up to 100 Hz. They have an abrupt onset, cessation, or change in configuration, and range from 50 μV to 1 mV in amplitude and last up to 100 ms and sometimes much longer. When of lower frequency, they produce the characteristic sound of a machine gun. Higher-frequency repetitive discharges may resemble myotonic discharges (hence the often-used term *pseudomyotonic discharges*), but they never show waning or waxing amplitudes (see below). They are most commonly found in spinal muscular atrophy, Charcot-Marie-Tooth disease, Duchenne's muscular dystrophy, and other chronic myopathies and neuropathies. High-frequency repetitive discharges are also found in the striated muscle of the urethral sphincter of women with and without urinary retention and rarely in deep muscles of apparently healthy individuals.

Neuromyotonic discharge as an electrodiagnostic term is not universally accepted and describes a very high-frequency (150–300 Hz) firing of motor unit potentials for a few seconds with a waning amplitude. It occurs among other types of spontaneous activity in the rare syndrome of continuous muscle fiber activity with muscle stiffness and cramps, also called *neuromyotonia*. The spontaneous MUP firing does not disappear during sleep or barbiturate anesthesia. Conversely, in the stiff man syndrome, the activity disappears during sleep and while the patient is under anesthesia.

Myotonic discharges are the electrodiagnostic hallmark of myotonic myopathies and consist of the repetitive firing of biphasic spike potentials, usually at a rate of 20–80 Hz (occasionally up to 150 Hz). The amplitude and frequency must both wax and wane, which differentiates myotonic discharges from the complex repetitive discharges and produces a highly characteristic accelerating and decelerating sound like roaring motorcycles (or, for the historically minded, dive-bombers). Myotonic discharges are most frequently found in the dominantly inherited myotonia congenita (Thomsen's disease), in which the discharges are rather short, and in myotonic dystrophy (Curshmann-Batten-Steinert syndrome) and proximal myotonic myopathy, in which they are typically of longer duration and often cause significant muscle cramps. Other less frequent conditions with myotonia are the recessively inherited Becker-type myotonia congenita, the sodium channel myopathies (paramyotonia congenita [i.e., Eulenburg's disease], adynamia episodica hereditaria [i.e., Gamstorp's disease], myotonia

fluctuans, acetazolamide-responsive myotonia congenita), and Pompe's disease.

Recruitment and Interference Pattern

After exploring spontaneous activity with a specific needle position, a slight contraction of the target muscle is performed until some isolated MUPs begin to fire. Constant mild contraction normally causes one to two low-threshold motor units to fire semirhythmically at a rate of approximately 4–5 Hz each. Slowly increasing the contraction induces both recruitment of previously inactive units and more rapid firing of already active units. When, with increasing contraction, a single motor unit enhances its firing frequency to more than 10 Hz without additional units being recruited within the pickup area of the concentric needle electrode, loss of motor units must be assumed because of axonal (and neuronal) damage or conduction block. When two motor units are recruited, the average individual firing frequency must not exceed 20 Hz, and for three recruited motor units, the upper limit is 30 Hz. In very distal conduction block, as sometimes occurs in acute inflammatory neuropathies and which escapes nerve conduction studies (because the most distal stimulating point lies proximal to the block), this abnormal recruitment pattern may be the only abnormality apart from a low CMAP amplitude (see "Motor Neurography").

When enhancing the contraction still further, many motor units begin to fire rapidly, making recognition of individual unit potentials difficult and producing the so-called interference pattern, which is usually assessed with a gain of 1 mV per cm and a sweep speed of 5 cm per second. The interference pattern at maximal volitional effort gives a rough estimate of the number of voluntarily recruitable motor units. Normally, it should be full, with no individual MUPs identifiable, and produce maximal amplitudes of 2–5 mV, with occasional potentials of up to 10 mV, and in very small muscles such as intrinsic hand muscles up to 12 mV. Only in the gastrocnemius muscle is a full interference pattern normally not achieved. The interference pattern can be reduced to a mixed or intermediate pattern, in which some individual MUPs can be identified, but the baseline is still not recognizable. In severe recruitment deficit, individual motor units and the baseline in between can easily be recognized. Obviously, the recruitment of motor units is influenced by a great

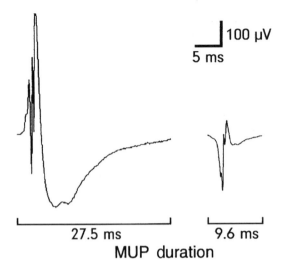

100 μV

5 ms

27.5 ms   9.6 ms

MUP duration

Figure 4-16. Examples of an enlarged and a normal motor unit potential (MUP) as recorded by needle electrodes.

number of factors, and lack of compliance or pain-induced inhibition may significantly rarefy the pattern, apart from loss of motor units. However, only in chronic neurogenic conditions does the maximal amplitude sometimes exceed 10 mV, because of the greatly increased size of the surviving motor units. Conversely, in myopathies and myositis the pattern is typically dense and often diminished in amplitude.

*Quantitative Measurement
of Muscle Unit Potentials*

Only major MUP abnormalities can be assessed with reasonable certainty by visual and acoustic measurement of the size and waveform of the MUP. If spontaneous activity is being assessed, the recruitment and interference patterns fail to reach a conclusion, and quantitative MUP measurement with a standardized and objective method may be necessary.

The MUP is characterized by amplitude, duration, and number of phases. These are the variables influenced by disease processes: Amplitude and duration are enlarged by neurogenic transformation and tend to become smaller and shorter in myopathy, and the number of phases is increased in both situations. In a normal muscle, most MUPs are diphasic or triphasic (Figure 4-16), but up to 12% of potentials in a normal muscle have four or more phases (baseline crossings) and are defined as *polyphasic MUPs*. In the vastus lateralis and tibialis anterior muscles, up to 20% of polyphasic MUPs may be found. Amplitudes and durations vary considerably within a muscle, and only statistical methods yield reliable results. The calculated average of 20–25 distinct MUPs in a muscle as defined by the school of Buchthal is the gold standard of quantitative EMG. Each muscle has its distinct normal values that also depend on the age of the subject. To assess individual MUPs, a minimal contraction is required, which is not always easily achieved, particularly when the patient is anxious or in pain. Only MUPs generated in the proximity of the electrode that produce a sharp sound—that is, with a rise time of less than 500 ms from the initial positive peak to the subsequent negative peak—should be accepted for analysis. Because only two to three MUPs can usually be reliably measured with a given electrode position, the latter must be changed several times by at least 5 mm or inserted at another site. This is important, because a motor unit should not be measured twice and only slight repositioning of the electrode significantly changes the electrical profile of a motor unit, making it look like a different one.

Quantitative MUP analysis can be tedious and depends heavily on the cooperation of the patient. Moreover, the result and value of the study are importantly influenced by the experience and expectations of the examiner, which somewhat hampers its feasibility. Furthermore, analysis only of the lowest threshold MUPs is possible, which is another critical limitation. Consequently, many attempts to get around this problem with computer assistance have been undertaken. They are far too numerous to be mentioned here. Several semiautomatic and interactive MUP decomposition programs are commercially available, validated for numerous muscles, and facilitate the procedure. However, the use of these programs also necessitates much experience. A relatively simple and widely used computer-assisted quantitative EMG analysis was described in 1964 by Willison: an automatic amplitude-turns analysis ("Willison analysis") of the interference pattern, where the amplitudes are related to the number of turns of the composite EMG signal. It will show whether activity of high amplitudes with relatively few potential turns or of low amplitudes with numerous turns are prevailing. The number of turns gives a rough measure of the number of phases, although a turn, strictly speaking, does not equal a phase (zero crossing). The method has been modified and improved and is easy to perform and implemented in many EMG machines. In clinical practice, it yields results comparable to or even superior to the conventional MUP analysis, but normal values are as yet established for only a few muscles.

Testing of the Neuromuscular Junction

There are two principles for assessing deficient neuromuscular transmission in myasthenic syndromes: (1) repetitive stimulation of a motor nerve and measuring the corresponding CMAP, or (2) single fiber recording of volitional activity, in which the temporal stability of interspike intervals within an MUP is measured.

When neuromuscular transmission is impaired in a myasthenic disorder, by botulinum toxin, or by curare, the CMAP shows a typical decrease in amplitude when the motor nerve is repetitively stimulated with intensities well above threshold at a low rate of 3 Hz (1–10 Hz). This decrement is usually most pronounced with the response of the fifth stimulus, where the amplitude is measured and should normally be 90% or more of that of the first response. The incomplete blocking of neuromuscular transmission can be partially reversed with neostigmine, which supplements the diagnostic test. Botulism and the Eaton-Lambert myasthenic syndrome are additionally characterized by a marked post-tetanic facilitation: The CMAPs, which are often very small with the first stimulus, show a dramatic (more than 100%) increase in amplitude immediately after a vigorous volitional effort or during high-frequency stimulation (20–50 Hz) of the nerve, the latter being a rather painful procedure. In myasthenia gravis, this post-tetanic potentiation does not occur, and the amplitude decrement at low frequencies is observed in only clinically or subclinically affected muscles. In contrast to the Eaton-Lambert myasthenic syndrome, in myasthenia gravis the disease process can be restricted to certain parts of the body, and the test muscle must therefore be appropriately chosen. Pure ocular myasthenia may escape this test because the cranial nerves serving ocular movements cannot be stimulated. It is also important to note that the decrement at low frequencies is not specific and can occasionally also be observed in motor neuron diseases.

In the single-fiber EMG technique, the variability of the interpotential interval between two or more single fibers belonging to the same motor unit are measured, and this phenomenon is called *jitter*. The test is performed using a special needle electrode with a small side port on the cannula that serves as the pickup area. The gain is set higher than for conventional EMG, the sweep speed is faster, and the filters are raised to stabilize the baseline and allow very high frequencies. During mild, voluntary contraction, a suitable biphasic potential with a duration of approximately 1 ms is sought by carefully adjusting the needle while a single-fiber spike is triggering the sweep. Increased jitter—that is, an increased interpotential variability of repetitively firing single-fiber spikes or blocking of the second spike—indicates motor endplate instability. This test is highly sensitive for disorders of the neuromuscular junction but quite unspecific because numerous other neuromuscular disorders can also increase the jitter.

Testing of Autonomic Functions

The Sympathetic Skin Response

The sympathetic (galvanic or sudomotor) skin response (SSR) test is an easily performed method for assessing peripheral autonomic nerve conduction. It measures the sympathetic outflow from the spinal cord to the limbs and depends on the distal activity of the eccrine sweat glands. Most of the peripheral sudomotor route uses unmyelinated postganglionic C fibers, with a conduction velocity of approximately 1.3 meters per second. In addition to the thermoregulatory sweat glands are the eccrine sweat glands, which are emotionally activated, and their greatest density is found in the palms and soles. Sudomotor activation induces a slow, initially negative, biphasic or triphasic potential that is most easily recorded with an active surface electrode over the pit of the palm or over the sole just behind the ball of the first toe, and the reference electrode is put over the dorsal surface of the hand or foot, respectively (Figure 4-17). Considering the very slow conduction, recording is done with a sweep length of 5–10 seconds and a low filtering of approximately 0.16 Hz (long time constant).

The sympathetic outflow to the extremities is reflexively activated by a great variety of stimuli,

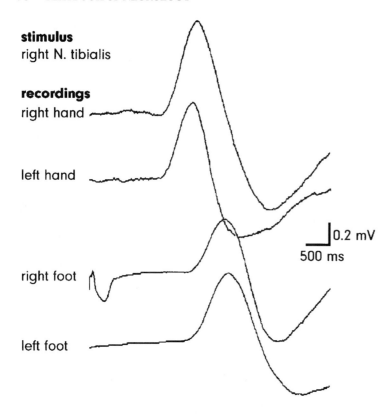

stimulus
right N. tibialis

recordings
right hand

left hand

0.2 mV

500 ms

right foot

left foot

Figure 4-17. Normal sudomotor sympathetic skin response from hands and feet after tibial nerve stimulation. The onset latency is approximately 1.5 seconds for the hands and 2 seconds for the foot (note the long time base). Any nerve may be stimulated to elicit a response, and also a loud click presented by earphones may be used.

such as coughing, taking a deep breath, sudden noises, startles, and the like. Therefore, sudomotor reflex abnormality may also occur in CNS disorders, although its clinical use in CNS disease is limited to a few exceptions (see below). To have a well-defined beginning of the sudomotor reflex, strong (slightly painful) electrical stimulation of a peripheral nerve, which triggers the recording sweep, has proved most useful. Usually, the stimuli are given to the medial or tibial nerve, preferably at a more proximal site (elbow or upper arm) and contralateral to the limb from which the recording is to be made. Alternatively, loud, single clicks delivered to the ears by earphones can be used. Given the slow efferent conduction time of well over 1 second, the rapid afferent conduction over the somatosensory or auditory fibers as well as the relatively rapid central processing can virtually be disregarded, and different afferent conduction times are negligible. The conduction time is measured to the negative onset and is normally found to be 1.5 seconds to the hand and 2 seconds to the foot. The amplitudes are highly variable and usually do not exceed 1 mV on the palm and are on the order of 0.1 mV on the foot. Hence, in terms of sudomotor response size, only the complete

absence of the response can be taken as abnormal. In very old subjects, the SSR normally may be absent. In case of an absent response, it is essential to use alternative stimuli such as a cough, a deep breath, or an unexpected loud noise. This is to rule out an afferent conduction failure as a cause of the absent response—for example, in peripheral neuropathies.

A conspicuous feature of the sudomotor reflex is its rapid habituation with repeated stimulation. As a consequence, the repetition needed to ascertain reproducibility must respect intervals between the stimuli of a minute or so, and the test cannot be done just after a conventional nerve conduction study, with its inevitable electrical stimuli. Furthermore, the patient must be relaxed and comfortably seated or in supine position in a quiet room, with as few external stimuli as possible. Also, local heating of the limb must be strictly avoided because this can cause direct depolarization of the sweat glands.

In clinical diagnosis, the SSR is useful for assessing autonomic function peripheral neuropathies and is frequently found to be abnormal in diabetics, alcoholics, and patients with familial amyloid polyneuropathy. It is also, as a rule, abnormal in axonal neuropathies of various causes. More interestingly, the SSR may also be abnormal in the presence of normal findings on conventional nerve conduction studies. This is occasionally found in diabetes and is a typical feature of the small-fiber neuropathies. Hence, the SSR may be more sensitive in neuropathies primarily affecting the non-myelinated fibers. In Sudeck's reflex sympathetic dystrophy (complex regional pain syndrome) both enhanced and absent SSRs are described, possibly reflecting the variable sympathetic activity at different stages. The SSRs may also be used to monitor the effectiveness of surgical or chemical sympathectomies. Obviously, the SSR may also be abnormal or absent in Sjögren's syndrome.

In acute inflammatory polyneuropathies (i.e., Guillain-Barré syndrome), the SSR is usually obtained, sometimes with a delay. In this condition, an absent SSR may indicate a potentially hazardous autonomic disruption, although the sudomotor involvement or noninvolvement does not necessarily parallel the more significant involvement or non-involvement of autonomic fibers controlling the heart. The latter are clinically relevant because of much-feared cardiac dysrhythmias in Guillain-Barré syndrome. For the specific purpose of assessing autonomic heart control, additional measuring of the beat-to-beat variation of the heart rate is advised (see "Assessing of Heart Rate Variation"). The SSR is usually abnormal or absent in multisystem atrophies (i.e., sporadic olivopontocerebellar atrophy, striatonigral degeneration, Shy-Drager syndrome) because of the degeneration of the preganglionic spinal cell bodies and in idiopathic dysautonomias with orthostatic hypotension caused by postganglionic degeneration. The SSR is usually normal in idiopathic Parkinson's disease, hereditary ataxias, and familial olivoponto-cerebellar atrophy.

Assessing Heart Rate Variation

In normal subjects, the heart rate shows important variations in the beat-to-beat intervals or in frequency, which depend on the autonomic control of the heart—that is, the vagal cardiac innervation. The heart rate is affected by numerous factors, such as respiration, intrathoracic pressure (Valsalva's maneuver), and body position (upright or supine). For instance, in a healthy individual the heart rate increases by more than 15 beats per minute when changing from quiet to forceful breathing. These variations are virtually absent in a transplanted—that is, denervated heart. Likewise, in autonomic neuropathies, the heart rate variation may be diminished or absent. Hence, measuring the beat-to-beat variation, the R-R interval variation (RRIV), is a relatively simple means for assessing autonomic control of the heart. As mentioned above, the autonomic control of the heart is particularly relevant in acute neuropathies such as Guillain-Barré syndrome, but also in some CNS conditions.

The RRIV can be assessed by customary EMG equipment, and common surface electrodes are used to record the electrocardiogram (ECG). The electrodes should be placed over the thorax or upper limbs such as to obtain an ECG with a high-amplitude R spike. The EMG machine is set to make the R spike trigger the sweeps, and several heart beats are then recorded on the screen. At least 20 beat-to-beat intervals should be recorded with the patient in a relaxed supine position during quiet breathing, and this should be repeated several times. Subsequently, the same procedure is done during forceful breathing, ideally with five to six breaths per minute. The variation is expressed either as a percentage or as a ratio. The ratio of the shortest R-R interval during inspiration to the longest R-R interval during expiration (longest divided by the shortest) should be greater than 1.1:1. The RRIV decreases with age and becomes very small in very old people. If the RRIV is virtually absent during this procedure, other trials to alter the heart rate should be undertaken: Valsalva's maneuver, careful carotid massage, immersion of one arm into ice water, a forceful hand grip for several minutes, or changing from a supine to a standing position.

Suggested Reading

Aminoff MJ. Electrodiagnosis in Clinical Neurology (3rd ed). New York: Churchill Livingstone, 1992.

Brown WF, Bolton CE. Clinical Electromyography (2nd ed). Boston: Butterworth–Heinemann, 1993.

Chiappa KH (ed). Evoked Potentials in Clinical Medicine (2nd ed). New York: Raven, 1990.

Daube JR. Clincal Neurophysiology. Philadelphia: Davis, 1996.

Delagi EF, Perotto A, Lazzetti J, Morrison D. Anatomic Guide for the Electromyographer (2nd ed). Springfield, IL: Charles C Thomas, 1980.

Delisa JA, Mackenzie K, Baran EM. Manual of Nerve Conduction Velocity and Somatosensory Evoked Potentials (2nd ed). New York: Raven, 1987.

Gilchrist JM. Single fiber EMG reference values: a collaborative effort. Ad hoc committee of the AAEM special interest group on single fiber EMG. Muscle Nerve 1992;15:151.

Halliday AM. Evoked Potentials in Clinical Testing (2nd ed). Edinburgh: Churchill Livingstone, 1993.

Kiloh LG, McComas AJ, Osselton JW, Upton ARM. Clinical Electroencephalography (4th ed). London: Butterworths, 1981.

Kimura J. Electrodiagnosis in Diseases of Nerve and Muscle: Principles and Practices (2nd ed). Philadelphia: Davis, 1989.

Liveson JA, Ma DM. Laboratory Reference for Clinical Neurophysiology. Philadelphia: Davis, 1992.

Ludin HP. Electromyography in Practice. Stuttgart: Thieme, 1980.

Ludin HP, Tackmann W. Sensory Neurography. Stuttgart: Thieme, 1981.

Niedermeyer E, DaSilva FL. Electroencephalograpy (3rd ed). Baltimore: Williams & Wilkins, 1993.

Petajan JH. AAEM minimonograph #3: motor unit recruitment. Muscle Nerve 1991;14:489.

St Ülberg E, Trontelj JV. Single Fibre Electromyography. Surrey, England: Mirvalle, 1979.

Chapter 5
Neurosonology

Charles H. Tegeler and Disya Ratanakorn

Basic Ultrasound Principles

Sound is a traveling wave of energy, the basic unit of which is a single, complete variation, or cycle. Sound waves are described by the number of cycles per second (frequency), with the unit of measurement being Hertz (Hz). The human ear can detect sound with frequencies between 20 and 20,000 Hz, and the term *ultrasound* implies sound wave frequencies greater than the audible range (>20,000 Hz). When an electrical current is applied to a crystal or ceramic material in an ultrasound transducer, the electrical energy causes this piezoelectric material to rapidly contract and expand, converting the electrical energy into sonic energy—a sound wave. Conversely, when the transducer receives sonic energy, it is converted back to electrical energy as a result of the same piezoelectric properties of the transducer. Diagnostic ultrasound devices usually operate at frequencies of 2–10 MHz (2–10 million cycles per second).

The Doppler Principle

The Doppler effect, described by Christian Andreas Doppler, is the change, or shift, in the frequency or wavelength of a wave that results from the relative movement between a sound source or scatterer and the receiver (Figure 5-1). This change in frequency, called the *Doppler frequency shift* (DFS), equals the difference between the transmitted and the received frequencies. When used to study moving red blood cells, this principle can be used to determine the speed and direction (velocity) of flow and the character of blood flow. If the DFS (in MHz), transmitted frequency (operating frequency of the transducer, *Ft,* in MHz), cosine of the angle of insonation (cos θ), and the sound propagation speed in soft tissue (*C,* in m/s) are known, the speed of the blood flow (*V,* in m/s) can be calculated as follows:

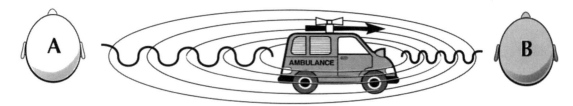

Figure 5-1. A sound source (ambulance siren) is moving toward B and away from A. More sound waves per second hit B (shift to a higher frequency), while fewer waves per second hit A (shift to a lower frequency).

$$V = \frac{DFS \times C}{2 \times \cos \theta}$$

Flow that is moving relatively toward the transducer produces positive DFS values, whereas flow away produces a negative DFS value. Calculation of blood flow velocity depends on the cosine of the angle of insonation (the angle between the direction of the sound beam and the direction of flow). The highest velocity values will occur with a zero angle of insonation (cos 0 = 1), whereas at angles approaching 90 degrees (cos 90 = 0), accurate calculation of velocity becomes difficult or impossible. In clinical practice, Doppler angles between 45 and 60 degrees yield satisfactory results and are usually achievable for extracranial cerebrovascular applications. Standardization of the angle of insonation improves the reproducibility of Doppler results.

There are two main categories of Doppler transducers: those that continuously transmit and receive frequencies (continuous-wave, or cw, Doppler transducers) and those that only intermittently transmit and receive (pulsed-wave, or pw, Doppler transducers). cw Doppler transducers can detect any frequency shifts caused by moving targets anywhere along the sound beam and can accurately detect very high frequency shifts associated with greatly increased flow velocities, but because they are continuously transmitting and receiving, cw Doppler transducers cannot localize the depth at which the signal originated or the source of the signal. Earlier ultrasound testing routinely used cw Doppler instruments.

To be able to separate Doppler signals from different sources—that is, from different vessels along the sound beam—a time factor is used to calculate the depth at which a specific signal arose. By transmitting discrete, brief pulses of sound and then waiting for scattered signals to return before transmitting the next pulse, pw Doppler transducers introduce a time element that allows localization of the depth of origination. The time needed for a pulse to travel to a specific depth and then return can be calculated, and the transducer can be set to only receive signals that return at a specific time or within a time window. This allows selective sampling for any signals that arise from a particular depth or volume of tissue (range gating). Most modern carotid duplex and transcranial Doppler ultrasonography (TCD) instruments use pw Doppler transducers.

Red blood cells move at a variety of speeds and directions within the vessel so that there are a variety of different DFS values (spectrum) from any sample volume within a vessel. This spectrum of DFS values, or velocities, can be evaluated using many variables, including the peak systolic and end-diastolic velocities.

Characteristics of the spectral waveform are determined by flow hemodynamics at the point of sampling, but are also affected by hemodynamic factors proximal and distal to the point of sampling, particularly the distal peripheral vascular resistance. The spectral pattern can infer disease distally or proximally. For example, a spectrum with high pulsatility, low end diastolic velocity (Vd), and a high peak systolic velocity (Vs)/Vd ratio suggests high distal peripheral vascular resistance, as with more distal stenosis or occlusion, whereas low pulsatility, high Vd, a low Vs/Vd ratio, and turbulence are seen within a vessel beyond a tight stenosis, in which the distal peripheral resistance is quite low.

Brightness-Mode Real-Time Imaging

Brightness-mode, or B-mode, imaging provides a two-dimensional gray-scale image of the soft tissue and vessels based on the acoustic properties of the tissue. Tissues with different densities have different values of acoustic impedance, and the greater the difference in acoustic impedance between adjacent tissues, the greater the reflection or scattering that occurs at interfaces or boundaries between the tissues. The returning echoes from along an ultrasound beam are stored in digital memory and assigned a gray-scale value ranging from white (intense signal) to black (no signal). The ultrasound beam can be mechanically or electronically steered across a tissue, creating many scan lines of B-mode information in a single plane. This gray-scale information is used to reconstruct a two-dimensional image in that plane. The appearance depends on the intensity or brightness at each point (more intense signals are assigned whiter gray-scale values). When the two-dimensional B-mode image is updated many times each second (usually 30 times per second), the eye is not able to discern that a series of frozen images is being displayed, and it takes on a dynamic, or real-time, appearance.

Duplex Doppler Ultrasonography

pw Doppler flow velocity sampling is combined with B-mode imaging in duplex ultrasonography to provide both hemodynamic (Doppler) and anatomic (B-mode) information, including image-guided placement of the Doppler sample volume in the region of choice (vessel lumen) as well as the ability to correct for the angle of insonation. This overcomes many pitfalls of using either modality alone, as in years past. The real-time capability allows evaluation of flow hemodynamics, the vessel wall, and the residual lumen throughout the cardiac cycle. Duplex ultrasonography is now used routinely for examination of the carotid, vertebral, and innominate arteries and even the aortic arch.

Color Flow Imaging

Color flow imaging (CFI) superimposes color-coded Doppler data (direction and speed of flow relative to the transducer) on the two-dimensional, gray-scale B-mode display. Most CFI instruments calculate flow velocity using DFS data and display a mean velocity value. Some instruments now calculate velocity using time-domain processing (color velocity imaging

[CVI]), which is based on echo information contained in the B-mode image scan lines. Cross-correlation of echoes from adjacent scan lines identifies differences in the arrival time of the echoes from specific clusters of red blood cells. When the angle of insonation is known, the instrument calculates the distance moved by that cluster of red cells over time, yielding the flow velocity. Velocities are color coded and superimposed on the B-mode image, as with Doppler methods. Potential advantages of such CVI based on time-domain processing include color display of instantaneous peak velocity, high-time and spatial resolution, and lower power requirements.

Potential advantages of all CFI methods over conventional gray-scale duplex ultrasonography include (1) improved visualization of the vessel wall and detection of hypoechoic plaques; (2) differentiation between an ulcerated plaque with craters open to the lumen and intraplaque hemorrhage; (3) rapid recognition of the presence and direction of flow; (4) more accurate placement of the sample volume at the point of highest flow velocity in stenotic lesions or in regions of trickle flow with a nearly occluded lumen; and (5) improved accuracy for determination of the Doppler insonation angle. CFI differentiates between subtotal and total occlusion of the internal carotid artery (ICA) with a sensitivity of 87–100% and a specificity of 84% compared with conventional angiography. Thus, angiography can often be avoided unless the CFI result is equivocal. CFI also allows good visualization of the extracranial vertebral arteries (VAs) and is useful for evaluation of pulsatile neck masses and identification of vascular neck tumors. Because conventional Doppler CFI cannot quantify peak flow velocity, it is used in combination with duplex Doppler flow velocity sampling in order to grade the degree of carotid stenosis.

Power Doppler Ultrasonography

Power Doppler (PD) ultrasonography is a Doppler-based imaging technique that encodes and displays an estimate of the integrated intensity in the Doppler spectrum rather than an estimate of the mean frequency shift or velocity, as with CFI. Although PD is based on the same principles as CFI, once the Doppler shift has been detected, all frequency components are removed so that no velocity information is present. The intensity of the signal is color coded

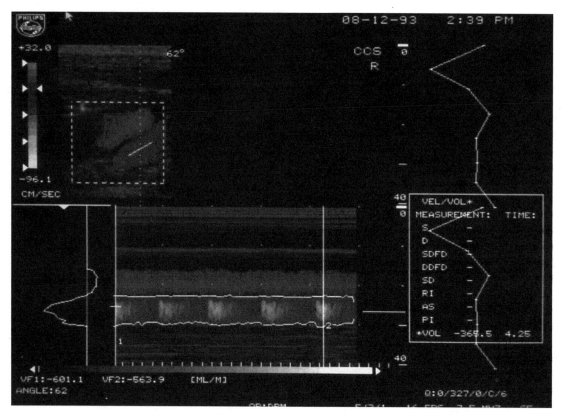

Figure 5-2. Volume flow rate measurement in the common carotid artery with an M-mode scan line through the color velocity imaging (top) and the M-mode color display (bottom) that includes the profile of peak flow velocities across the flow lumen and tracking of the diameter throughout the cardiac cycle. The volume flow rate in this example is 365.5 ml/min.

and superimposed on the gray-scale B-mode image. PD is less angle dependent than CFI, allowing the detection of blood flow even with nearly perpendicular angles of insonation, which is very helpful for evaluating the continuity of tortuous vessels. The excellent sensitivity to flow assists with the detection of very low blood flow. However, PD does not provide the direction or velocity of flow, so it is used in combination with conventional CFI. PD also is reportedly superior to CFI for visualization of orbital vessels, stenosis of the middle cerebral artery (MCA), intracranial aneurysms, significant extracranial ICA stenosis such as string sign in a nearly occluded ICA, and for defining plaque surface morphology.

Volume Flow Rate

Doppler methods can estimate the volume flow rate (VFR) at a specific point in a vessel by multiplying the flow velocity with cross-sectional lumen diameter at that specific point in time. However, Doppler methods lack a profile of instantaneous peak velocities across the entire vessel and cannot adjust for changes in the flow lumen throughout the cardiac cycle. Time-domain processing with CVI (see CFI section) can be combined with an M-mode (motion-mode) color display to provide an instantaneous profile of the peak velocities across the flow lumen as well as a continuous estimate of vessel diameter throughout the cardiac cycle. By assuming a circular vessel and axisymmetric flow, VFR with CVI-quantification (CVI-Q) can be calculated (Figure 5-2).

Applied to normal volunteers, this CVI-Q estimated VFR in the common carotid artery (CCA) at 330 ± 60 ml/min for women and 375 ± 70 ml/min for men. VFR is useful for grading carotid stenosis and evaluating cerebrovascular reserve as well as for identifying feeders, and follow-up studies of intracranial arteriovenous malformations, for quantification of hemodynamic changes in patients with subclavian steal phenomenon, and for assessing vasospasm in patients with subarachnoid hemorrhage. A direct correlation between MCA mean flow velocity, CCA VFR, and end-expiratory carbon dioxide, both before and after breathing carbon dioxide, has been shown in normal subjects. This allows the study of cerebrovascular reactivity in patients with absent or inadequate acoustic temporal windows, which can limit the use of TCD. This method appears helpful in assessing intracranial hemodynamics in a variety of clinical settings.

Carotid Duplex Color Flow Ultrasonography

Clinical Indications

Carotid duplex color flow ultrasonography is considered the initial noninvasive method of choice for evaluating the extracranial carotid system in patients with stroke or cerebrovascular disease. Other common clinical indications include symptomatic and asymptomatic neck bruits, pulsatile neck masses, preoperative evaluation of patients having surgery for other vascular diseases (e.g., coronary artery bypass), postoperative follow-up after carotid endarterectomy, and serial evaluation of patients with known cerebrovascular disease. Carotid duplex color-flow ultrasonography offers a safe, repeatable, portable, and inexpensive way to evaluate the extracranial carotid system, which is quite accurate for identification of significant carotid stenosis. However, these methods are operator dependent, so they must be performed and interpreted by trained, experienced individuals to obtain accurate results. Physical limitations to this method include a high carotid bifurcation, very short neck, extremely deep vessels, and extensive acoustic shadowing, which may prevent adequate visualization/study of the vessels.

Although the exact protocol for carotid duplex color-flow ultrasonography testing varies somewhat among laboratories, certain components are crucial for an adequate examination. This includes examination of both carotid and vertebral arteries with duplex Doppler sampling of the proximal, middle, and distal CCA, proximal and distal ICA, and the external carotid artery (ECA). If disease is detected, then additional sampling should include the vessel proximal to,

at, and distal to the stenosis. The CCA bifurcation (BIF) need not be routinely sampled because of the variability of hemodynamics at that location, but must be studied when any disease is detected. B-mode real-time imaging of the CCA, BIF, ICA, and ECA should include visualization from the anterior, lateral and posterolateral, longitudinal, and transverse views. Many laboratories also obtain lumen measurements in the CCA, BIF, ICA, and ECA, and if any plaque is identified, measurements of plaque thickness and residual lumen are also made. CFI and PD are powerful additions to the interpretation of these studies.

Duplex Doppler Interpretation Parameters

Correct identification of the CCA, BIF, ICA, and ECA is crucial, especially when interpreting carotid stenosis. Many variables are used to distinguish between these vessels, including the size, location in the neck, any branches, the Doppler spectral waveform, and the response to temporal artery tap. Normal duplex Doppler spectral waveforms of the CCA, ICA, and ECA are shown in Figure 5-3.

Intima-Media Thickness

B-mode imaging allows study of the vessel wall to assess thickness, appearance, and any changes caused by atherosclerosis. Although usually used to evaluate advanced atherosclerotic plaque, the earliest measurable changes in vessel walls caused by atherosclerosis are just thickening of the intima-media layers (intima-media thickness, or IMT) of the arterial wall and increased stiffness of the vessels involved. High-resolution B-mode ultrasonography of the carotid artery provides visualization of the vessel wall in detail, as shown in Figure 5-4. This allows very accurate assessment (0.1–0.3 mm changes) of wall thickness. Early phases of atherosclerotic plaque formation may cause thickening of the arterial walls with simultaneous dilatation of the vessel, thereby preserving the residual lumen. Therefore, there is no real hemodynamic effect to cause changes detectable by Doppler techniques, so measurement of IMT is now widely used to study early atherosclerotic change in different clinical research settings as well as to study the regression and progression of atherosclerotic lesions and associations with related risk factors. An increase in IMT at the CCA correlates with increased IMT of

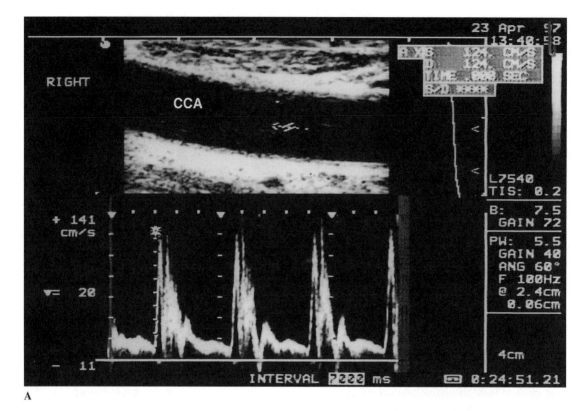

Figure 5-3. Duplex Doppler images of a normal carotid artery. (A) Duplex Doppler image of the common carotid artery (CCA) shows a typical spectral pattern, which usually has a mixture of characteristics of the internal carotid artery (ICA) and external carotid artery (ECA). (B) Duplex Doppler image of the ECA shows a characteristic pattern of a high-resistance vascular bed distally, with a quick upstroke, sharp systolic peak, rapid decrease in velocity after the peak, a dicrotic notch, and little diastolic velocity. (C) Duplex Doppler image of the ICA shows the characteristic pattern of a low-resistance vascular bed distally (brain), with a more gradual upstroke, more rounded peak, gradual fall in velocity after the peak, and persistent diastolic velocity.

the thoracic aorta and also is associated with development of clinically significant atherosclerosis in peripheral arteries. Measurement of carotid IMT has the potential to be useful as a marker for risk of atherosclerosis in other vascular segments or beds and may soon become part of the clinical evaluation.

Plaque Features

A unique strength of B-mode imaging is the ability to assess morphologic characteristics of atherosclerotic plaques in the carotid artery. The acoustic appearance of atherosclerotic plaque on B-mode imaging is described as low-intensity echoes (echolucent, hypoechoic, or anechoic), medium-level echoes (echogenic), and high-level or intense echoes (hyperechoic). Texture describes the uniformity of echoes. The presence of uniform echoes is described as homogeneous, whereas nonuniformity is described as mixed or heterogeneous. Plaques with prominent echolucent or anechoic regions are more likely to have intraplaque hemorrhage on surgical or pathologic examination. Heterogeneous plaques also have more surface abnormalities (irregularity, craters, ulceration). Plaques that are mostly homogeneous and echogenic are primarily fibrous and represent a more stable plaque. The presence of plaque calcification produces a hyperechoic appearance, and because calcium blocks propagation of ultrasound beams, it causes acoustic shadowing (the absence of echoes behind the plaque or calcified structure). Plaques that are heterogeneous, with marked surface abnormalities, or possible intraplaque hemorrhage are often referred to as *complex plaques.*

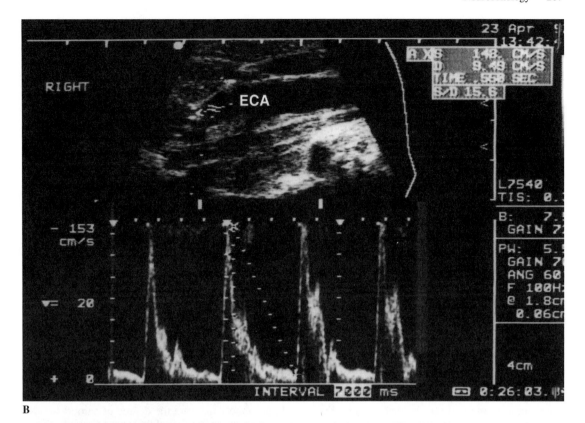

B

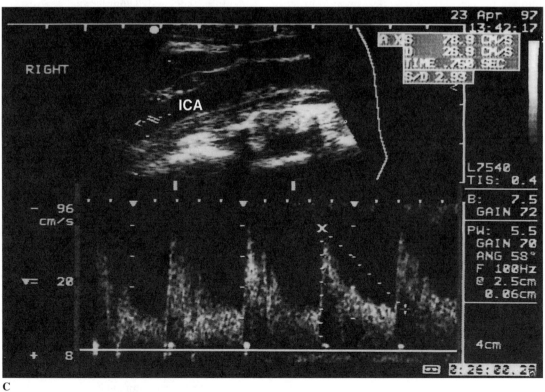

C

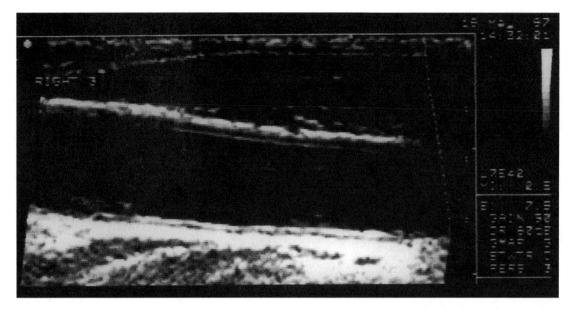

Figure 5-4. Longitudinal B-mode image of a normal common carotid artery, showing typical structures, including the vessel lumen, intima/media complex, adventitia, subcutaneous tissue, and skin surface.

The reporting of plaque features on B-mode ultrasound should include the location and distribution of plaque, surface features (smooth, irregular, crater/ulcer), echodensity (anechoic, hypoechoic, echogenic, hyperechoic, echodense), calcification and shadowing, texture (homogenous, heterogenous/mixed, intraplaque hemorrhage), and the pattern of pulsation throughout the cardiac cycle (radial or longitudinal). Regardless of the severity of any hemodynamic stenosis, a complex plaque is believed to be more unstable and to produce a higher risk for causing cerebral ischemia. An example of an ulcerated plaque is shown in Figure 5-5.

New methods such as video densitometric analysis of B-mode images to evaluate plaque composition and three-dimensional ultrasound reconstructions to evaluate plaque features and volumes may add new insights and allow more precise study of the progression and regression of plaques after specific interventions.

Grading Carotid Stenosis

Since publication of the results of the North American Symptomatic Carotid Endarterectomy Trial (NASCET) and the Asymptomatic Carotid Athero-sclerosis Study (ACAS), there is a clinical mandate to accurately measure the degree of carotid stenosis to identify 70–99% of symptomatic stenosis and 60–99% of asymptomatic stenosis. Carotid duplex color-flow ultrasonography provides a hemodynamic assessment of carotid stenosis rather than merely a linear measurement of stenosis, as with angiographic or B-mode–only approaches. When performed and interpreted by trained personnel, using a standard protocol, with ongoing quality assurance, this technique can reach 90% sensitivity and specificity for detection of significant carotid stenosis.

Progressive worsening of stenosis with decreasing residual lumen diameter causes predictable changes in flow velocity, the characteristics of flow (turbulence and spectral broadening), and the VFR. Peak systolic velocity and end-diastolic velocity remain the key hemodynamic variables for evaluating the degree of carotid stenosis. Other adjunctive variables for interpretation that may be important in specific patients include the ratio of the velocity in the ICA to the velocity in the CCA, the VFR in the CCA, the presence of extensive plaque or the residual lumen diameter on B-mode imaging, a high-resistance Doppler spectral pattern in the CCA, and side-to-side differences. Caution must be used in applying such criteria for inter-

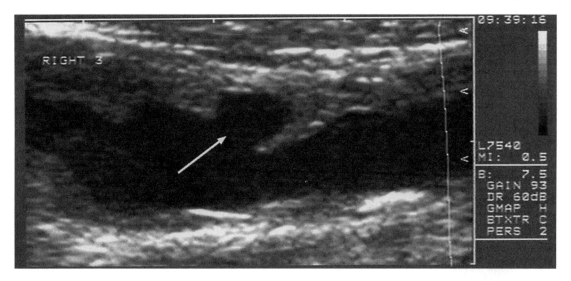

Figure 5-5. Longitudinal B-mode image of a heterogeneous plaque in the internal carotid artery, which has an open crater/ulcer (*arrow*).

preting velocity changes contralateral to severe stenosis or occlusion because collateral flow can increase contralateral velocities, leading to overestimation of stenosis. Measuring VFR in the CCA can help to distinguish between collateral flow and true stenotic flow. Table 5-1 shows the criteria for grading carotid stenosis used in our laboratory. Criteria such as these should not be viewed as rigid or absolute values and cut-points. All variables are considered in each case so that a diagnosis might be made even if absolute velocities do not fit exactly with the criteria values.

With 95–99% stenosis (subtotal occlusion), flow velocity is variable. The use of CFI and PD helps to differentiate between subtotal and total occlusion by demonstrating trickle flow or a string sign and reconstitution of the lumen distally. As mentioned, a residual lumen diameter of less than 2 mm and reduced VFR in the CCA are also helpful as adjunctive data for interpretation. Figure 5-6 shows duplex findings of 95–99% stenosis of the ICA compared with angiographic findings.

Vertebral Doppler Ultrasonography

Ischemic events in the territory of the vertebral or basilar arteries are quite common, and it is important to include a study of the VAs as part of the extracra-

nial cerebrovascular study. There are no widely accepted criteria for grading the degree of stenosis in the VAs, but the presence and direction of flow should be reported. Between C4 and C6, the interosseous VA segments can be identified in nearly 100% of patients, while the origin is seen in 81% on the right and 65% on the left. Evaluation of the VAs is especially helpful for identification of vertebral/subclavian steal syndrome, although the flow direction and spectral waveform at rest depend on the degree of stenosis. When combined with physiologic testing, vertebral duplex ultrasonography allows classification of the stages of subclavian steal and helps determine whether it is a true intracranial steal or a vertebral-to-vertebral overflow phenomenon. Figure 5-7 shows a normal VA duplex study and a subclavian steal.

Transcranial Doppler Ultrasonography

Basic Principles

TCD is a real-time, noninvasive method for evaluating intracranial hemodynamics in the basal cerebral arteries of the circle of Willis. The pw Doppler methods previously described are used for TCD. The thickness of the skull bone limits the penetration of ultrasonic energy from the higher frequency transducers used for other conventional extracranial appli-

Table 5-1. Flow Velocity Criteria Used for Grading Carotid Stenosis in the Neurosonology Laboratory at Wake Forest University Baptist Medical Center

Percentage of Diameter Stenosed	PSV (cm/sec)	EDV (cm/sec)	ICA:CCA Ratio
0–49%	<140	<40	<2
50–74%	>140	<110	>2
75–94%	>>140	>110	>3
95–99%	Variable	Variable	Variable
Occlusion	No flow	No flow	Not applicable

PSV = peak systolic velocity; EDV = end-diastolic velocity; ICA = internal carotid artery; CCA = common carotid artery; >> = much higher.

cations. Low-frequency, 2-MHz pw Doppler ultrasound allows insonation through the skull and study of intracranial blood flow velocities in a variety of cerebrovascular disorders. A number of methods can be used to perform TCD, including hand-held pw Doppler transducers, mapping vessels with the same pw Doppler velocity data, transcranial color-flow duplex ultrasonography (TCCD), transcranial PD ultrasonography, and three-dimensional reconstructions of TCD data. Most widely used is the hand-held TCD, or blind technique, using pw Doppler equipment, in which the data obtained are limited to flow velocity (speed and direction) and characteristics of flow or spectral waveform analysis without imaging of cerebral structures or arteries. This method requires operator and interpreter understanding of cerebrovascular anatomy, hemodynamics, and expected flow velocities and spectral waveforms.

Three standard approaches or acoustic windows are used: (1) the thin portion of the temporal bone anterior to the ear (temporal window) accesses the MCA, the anterior cerebral artery (ACA), and

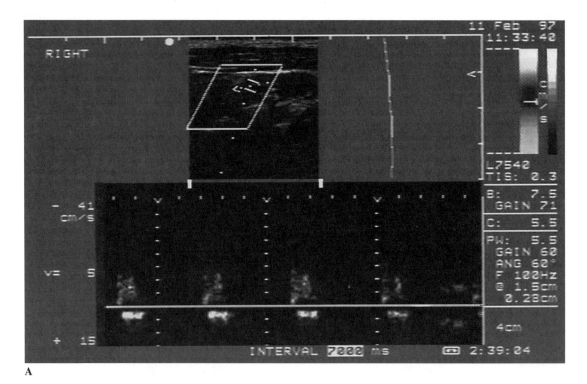

A

Figure 5-6. Color duplex ultrasound findings of 95–99% stenosis of the internal carotid artery (ICA) compared with the angiographic findings. (A) Duplex Doppler signal just proximal to 95–99% stenosis shows a high-resistance, low-velocity signal with some reverberating flow and no diastolic velocity. (B) A color flow image allows easy identification of the 95–99% stenosis with a very narrowed lumen. (C) Cerebral angiography shows the tight ICA stenosis.

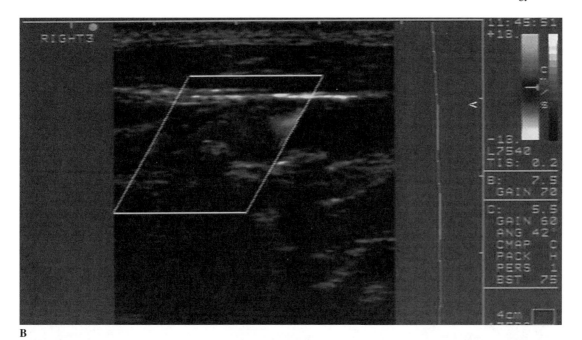

B

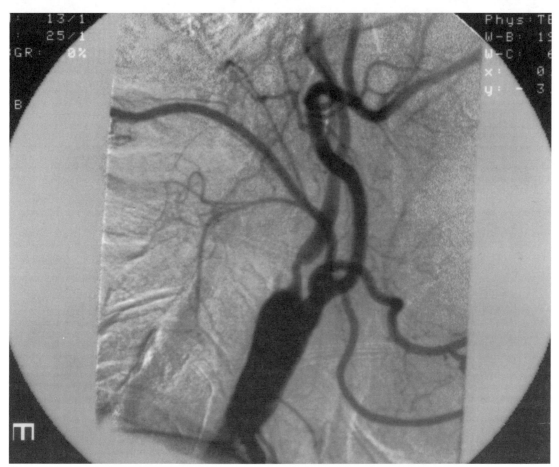

C

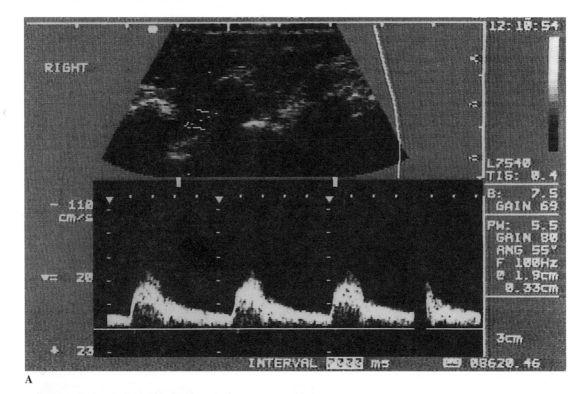

A

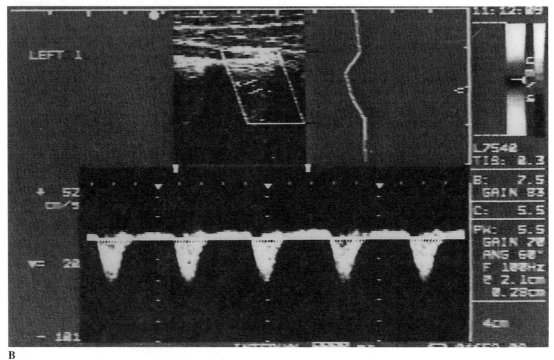

B

Figure 5-7. Vertebral duplex ultrasonography. (A) Duplex Doppler image of a normal vertebral artery. (B) Duplex Doppler image shows reversed flow in systole, suggesting subclavian steal.

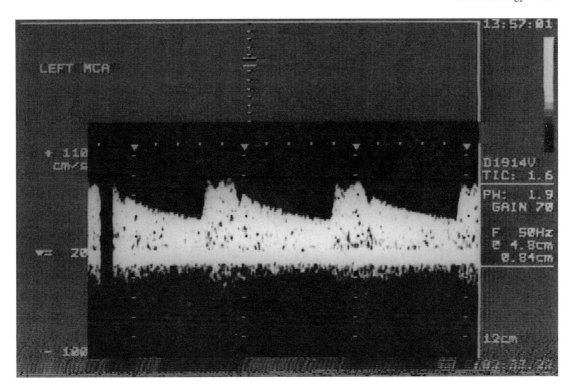

Figure 5-8. Transcranial Doppler spectral waveform of the middle cerebral artery at a depth of 48 mm, with flow toward the transducer.

the posterior cerebral artery (PCA); (2) the suboccipital window with insonation through the foramen magnum accesses the intracranial VA and the basilar artery (BA); and (3) the transorbital window via the orbit or optic foramen accesses the ophthalmic arteries (OAs) and the carotid siphon. A normal MCA spectral waveform is shown in Figure 5-8, and normal values and direction of mean blood flow velocities (Vm) of the basal cerebral arteries as used in our laboratory (time-averaged mean maximum velocity) are shown in Table 5-2.

Inadequacy of either temporal window is the most frequent cause of an insufficient TCD study. Inadequate windows occur in 14.5% of the general population and are especially prevalent in nonwhite women of 60 years of age or older. In addition to inadequacy of the acoustic window, velocities are affected by many factors, including poor angle of insonation, age, heart rate, and hematocrit. TCD data are reproducible, and there are no significant variations between the sides or between studies on different days.

Clinical Indications

Established clinical indications for the use of TCD include detection of severe stenosis or occlusion of the major basal cerebral arteries, assessment of collateral flow in patients with intracranial or extracranial arterial stenosis or occlusion, evaluation of vasospasm (especially after subarachnoid hemorrhage), the identification of arteriovenous malformations and their feeding arteries, and the assessment of potential cerebral circulatory arrest (brain death). The criteria for vasospasm as used in our laboratory (Table 5-3) are slightly different than those used for intracranial stenosis.

TCD can also be used to evaluate cerebrovascular reserve, which is the ability of the cerebral circulation to increase perfusion after vasodilating stimulation to the cerebral resistance vessels, or to maintain perfusion with physiologic challenges that decrease perfusion pressure. Cerebrovascular reserve can be easily evaluated using TCD by monitoring flow velocities during manipulation of arterial carbon dioxide tension with breath-holding, hyperventilation, or inhalation of

Table 5-2. Normal Values for Transcranial Doppler Ultrasonography: Depth, Flow Direction, Velocities

Artery	Depth (mm)	Flow Direction	Mean Velocity (cm/sec)
Middle cerebral artery	50–55	Toward	40–80
Anterior cerebral artery	65–70	Away	35–60
Posterior cerebral artery	60–65	Toward	30–55
Vertebral artery	60–75	Away	25–50
Basilar artery	>75	Away	25–60
Ophthalmic artery	40–55	Toward	15–30
Internal carotid artery siphon	65–75	Variable	40–70

Table 5-3. Transcranial Doppler Ultrasound Criteria for Vasospasm

Severity	Mean Velocity (cm/sec)	Distal x-ICA	MCA/x-ICA
Normal	<85	Normal	<3
Mild	<120	Normal	<3
Moderate	120–150	Normal–↓	3–5
Severe	151–200	↓–↓↓	>6
Critical	>200	↓↓↓	>6

MCA = middle cerebral artery; x-ICA = distal extracranial internal carotid artery by submandibular insonation; Vm = time-averaged mean maximum velocity; MCA/x-ICA = ratio of these velocities; ↓ = decreased.

5% carbon dioxide, or by intravenously administering acetazolamide and evaluating changes in velocity caused by these physiologic stimuli.

Inhalation of 5% carbon dioxide normally induces an increase of about 50% in flow velocity or a change of approximately 5% in velocity for each 1–mm Hg change in end-tidal carbon dioxide tension. In a cooperative patient, even breath-holding causes a 30–50% increase in MCA flow velocity. Flow velocity normally decreases up to 35% with hyperventilation within 15 seconds after optimal hyperventilation is achieved. In response to 1,000 mg acetazolamide intravenously, MCA flow velocity increases within less than 3 minutes before reaching a plateau about 35% higher than baseline values within 10 minutes. This effect persists from 30 minutes to as long as 60–120 minutes, then gradually resolves. These TCD methods for evaluating cerebrovascular reactivity have been widely used in patients with severe stenosis or occlusion of the extracranial carotid arteries to identify those vessels with diminished responses. Such patients are believed to have an increased risk for hemodynamic stroke when faced with any circumstances that would decrease blood flow to the brain. This information may help with decisions regarding the need for treatments such as extracranial-intracranial bypass surgery, carotid endarterectomy, or other revascularization techniques.

Some patients have ischemia only with maneuvers such as head extension or turning, which can affect the VA flow. TCD is used to evaluate changes in velocity over time and in response to mechanical stimuli. For instance, when there is asymmetry of the VA lumen diameter that exceeds 75%, significant reduction of BA flow velocity is observed only after rotating the head to the side of the hypoplastic VA. The correlation of symptoms to hemodynamic findings may help to identify patients with true position-related vertebrobasilar insufficiency.

Embolus Detection

Cerebral microembolism can be reliably detected by TCD in numerous clinical settings, including in those patients with prosthetic cardiac valves, various cardiac conditions, extracranial carotid stenosis, or vertebrobasilar ischemia as well as during carotid endarterectomy, cerebral contrast angiography, carotid angioplasty, and cardiopulmonary bypass. Sequential TCD monitoring for cerebral microembolism may play an important role in the management of patients with acute stroke to assist with classifying the stroke subtype, understanding the prognosis of stroke, and making decisions on the best preventive therapy. "Embolic signals" appear in TCD as a short-duration, frequency-focused, high-intensity signal, predominantly unidirectional and within the Doppler–fast Fourier transform (FFT) spectrum (Figure 5-9) and are accompanied by a characteristic sound (a "pop" or "chirp"). Conversely, Doppler artifacts usually appear as a bidirectional, high-intensity signal with maximum intensity at lower frequencies. Because of their appearance as high-intensity transient signals within the spec-

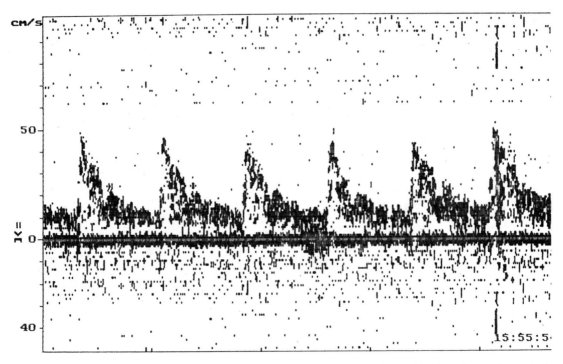

Figure 5-9. Doppler spectral display on transcranial Doppler ultrasonography that shows a high-intensity transient embolic signal in a patient with polycythemia and transient ischemic attacks (TIAs).

tral waveform, this phenomenon has been called "HITS" to describe the signal without invoking a mandate for clinical action. Such signals are more prevalent in patients with cerebral ischemic symptoms, in those with severe carotid stenosis, and on the symptomatic side. They are also present in virtually all cases of cardiopulmonary bypass and in carotid endarterectomy procedures. However, the natural history, the prognostic clinical importance, and the implications for altered treatment in patients with these signals remain to be confirmed.

This same principle can be used to easily identify the presence of a patent foramen ovale with TCD monitoring. The MCA is monitored during the intravenous injection of agitated saline or commercial ultrasound contrast agents. Such bubbles are too large to cross the pulmonary capillary bed, but if there is a patent foramen ovale or a right-to-left intracardiac shunt, the bubbles will quickly cross to the left side of the heart and proceed out the arterial tree, some to the cerebral circulation. Those bubbles that pass through the MCA act as emboli and cause distinct embolic signals. The use of a Valsalva's maneuver increases the diagnostic yield. TCD is

reported to have 77–100% sensitivity and 94–100% specificity for identification of intracardiac shunts compared with contrast transesophageal echocardiography. This easy bedside method may be quite helpful in managing patients with acute stroke.

Transcranial Color-Flow Duplex Ultrasonography

TCCD combines pw Doppler, real-time B-mode imaging, and CFI principles with low-frequency transducers so that intracranial structures can be studied. This allows evaluation of the course of intracranial vessels, the brain parenchyma, and bony structures, as shown in Figure 5-10. Because of the low transducer frequency (2.0–2.5 MHz), the B-mode image is relatively poor, and there are still limitations caused by inadequate acoustic windows. Potential advantages of TCCD compared with conventional TCD include improved vessel identification, the ability to study the course and branches of intracranial vessels, and the ability to image multiple vessels simultaneously. TCCD also allows an oppor-

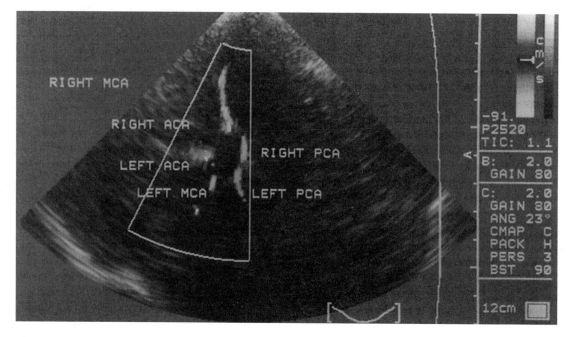

Figure 5-10. Transcranial color duplex image of vessels of the circle of Willis. (MCA = middle cerebral artery; ACA = anterior cerebral artery; PCA = posterior cerebral artery.)

tunity to visualize and detect flow in veins, aneurysms, and arteriovenous malformations, to rapidly and correctly place the Doppler sample volume in a specific segment of the vessel, to obtain angle-corrected flow velocities, and to potentially decrease the examination time. Angle-corrected Doppler flow velocities are approximately 10–15% higher than those recorded with conventional TCD, but the accuracy and clinical utility of angle-corrected flow velocities require further study as well as the definition of "normal values" for angle-corrected peak velocities. Despite this, TCCD may be rapidly performed as a noninvasive bedside procedure to provide prompt and reliable data regarding stroke subtype and mechanism, which may be especially helpful in the setting of acute stroke.

Transcranial duplex sonography with PD, rather than CFI, is equally effective in the detection of the ACA, MCA-M1, and PCA-P1, but is actually better than TCCD with CFI for demonstrating the MCA-M2, PCA-P2, and posterior communicating arteries. Transcranial duplex PD may also have advantages over CFI for study of small-diameter and low-flow arteries and those that have unfavorable Doppler insonation angles.

Integrated Use of Carotid Duplex Color-Flow Ultrasonography and Transcranial Doppler Ultrasonography

As outlined above, ultrasound now offers a safe, noninvasive, accurate, repeatable, and relatively inexpensive way to evaluate patients with stroke or a variety of other cerebrovascular disorders. In deciding what role, if any, ultrasound should have in clinical practice, some basic decisions must be made. First, will any additional diagnostic testing by ultrasound or any other technique help with the diagnosis or management decisions for that specific patient? If not, then additional testing would have little clinical value and should be avoided.

Second, if additional testing is indicated and there are multiple techniques having roughly comparable accuracy from which to choose, then the safe, noninvasive, less expensive method should be used initially, and the more costly, invasive, or risky procedures saved for those who really need them. In this setting, ultrasound is well suited to serve as the initial test of choice for the study of cerebrovascular disease, reserving angiography of all types for those in whom additional data are needed (e.g., patients in

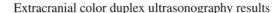

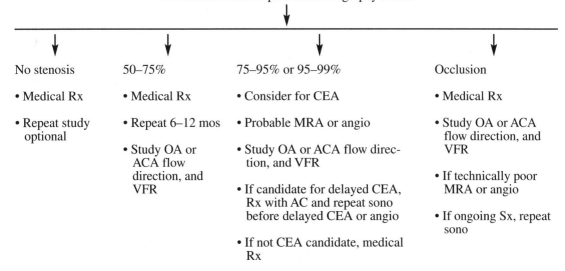

Extracranial color duplex ultrasonography results

No stenosis	50–75%	75–95% or 95–99%	Occlusion
• Medical Rx	• Medical Rx	• Consider for CEA	• Medical Rx
• Repeat study optional	• Repeat 6–12 mos	• Probable MRA or angio	• Study OA or ACA flow direction, and VFR
	• Study OA or ACA flow direction, and VFR	• Study OA or ACA flow direction, and VFR	• If technically poor MRA or angio
		• If candidate for delayed CEA, Rx with AC and repeat sono before delayed CEA or angio	• If ongoing Sx, repeat sono
		• If not CEA candidate, medical Rx	

- If ongoing Sx for any severity of stenosis, consider embolus detection.
- If >75% stenosis, especially if ongoing Sx, consider cerebral vasoreactivity.
- Consider agitated saline study for PFO in any patient with TIA/stroke, especially those with no other identified cause.

A

Figure 5-11. The impact of extracranial carotid color-flow duplex and transcranial Doppler ultrasonography in the diagnosis and management of patients with transient ischemic attacks, stroke, or cerebrovascular disease in clinical practice at Wake Forest University Baptist Medical Center. (A) Extracranial stenosis. (B) Intracranial stenosis. (OA = ophthalmic artery; ACA = anterior cerebral artery; CEA = carotid endarterectomy; MRA = magnetic resonance angiography; VFR = volume flow rate; AC = anticoagulant; PFO = patent foramen ovale; TIA = transient ischemic attack; angio = angiography; sono = ultrasonography.)

whom ultrasound is technically inadequate; those with disease for which ultrasound is not adequate alone, such as cerebral vasculitis; or when additional data are required for making decisions, such as whether carotid surgery should be performed). Using these principles, many physicians now rely on a combination of carotid duplex color-flow ultrasonography and magnetic resonance angiography (MRA), reserving conventional angiography for patients in whom the results of the noninvasive methods disagree or are inadequate. If the surgeon will still require conventional angiograms from which to make the decision on surgery, then multiple preliminary noninvasive tests are not indicated.

Finally, decisions on which tests to use must be individualized for each patient and for the resources and expertise available. Laboratories should have an ongoing program of quality improvement with comparison of results with correlative data such as results of cerebral angiography, MRA, clinical outcome, surgical pathology, or repeat studies. The accuracy data of the laboratories performing all diagnostic procedures should also be available. Another measure of the quality of the ultrasound laboratory is whether it is accredited or whether the sonographers and physicians are certified.

We currently use ultrasound as the initial test of choice for evaluating cerebrovascular disease, usually reserving MRA, computed tomographic angiography, or contrast angiography for those patients with disease or in whom noninvasive results are inadequate, as mentioned above (Figure 5-11). In addition, evaluation with both carotid duplex color-flow ultrasonography and TCD is strongly preferred and recommended because this offers a more complete assessment of the cerebral circulation, and the combination is much more useful clinically for us than one or the other alone.

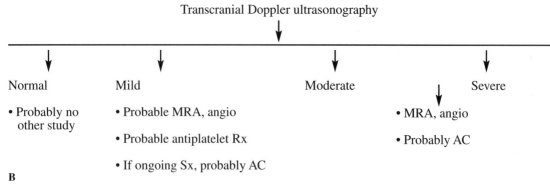

B

Figure 5-11. *Continued.*

Thus, ultrasound now plays an important clinical role in the management of stroke and cerebrovascular disease, and with the new and evolving applications mentioned above, it holds even more promise for the future. Some of the information provided by ultrasound remains unique, and the clinician must learn to effectively integrate ultrasound with other complementary diagnostic techniques to provide the best care for patients, which remains the ultimate goal. The evolution and availability of ultrasound contrast agents and three-dimensional ultrasonography will enhance the diagnostic capability and accuracy of these methods even more.

Suggested Reading

Aaslid R, Markwalder T-M, Nornes H. Noninvasive transcranial Doppler ultrasound recording of flow velocity in basal cerebral arteries. J Neurosurg 1982;57:769.

Alexandrov AV, Brodie DS, Mclean A, et al. Correlation of peak systolic velocity and angiographic measurement of carotid stenosis revisited. Stroke 1997;28:339.

Bartels E, Fuchs H-H, Flugel KA. Duplex ultrasonography of vertebral arteries: examination, technique, normal values, and clinical applications. Angiology 1992;43:169.

Baumgartner RW, Mattle HP, Aaslid R. Transcranial color-coded duplex sonography, magnetic resonance angiography, and computed tomograpy angiography: methods, applications, advantages, and limitations. J Clin Ultrasound 1995;23:89.

Daffertshofer M, Ries S, Schminke U, Hennerici M. High-intensity transient signals in patients with cerebral ischemia. Stroke 1996;27:1844.

Executive Committee for the Asymptomatic Carotid Atherosclerosis Study. Endarterectomy for asymptomatic carotid stenosis. JAMA 1995;273:1421.

Gray-Weale AC, Graham JC, Burnett JR, et al. Carotid artery atheroma: comparison of preoperative B-mode ultrasound appearance with carotid endarterectomy specimen pathology. J Cardiovasc Surg 1988;29:676.

Griewing B, Morgenstern C, Driesner F, et al. Cerebrovascular disease assessed by color-flow and power Doppler ultrasonography. Comparison with digital subtraction angiography in internal carotid artery stenosis. Stroke 1996;27:95.

Howard G, Sharrett AR, Heiss G, et al. Carotid artery intimal-medial thickness distribution in general populations as evaluated by B-mode ultrasound. Stroke 1993;24:1297.

Kremkau FW. Diagnostic Ultrasound: Principles and Instruments. Philadelphia: Saunders, 1993.

North American Symptomatic Carotid Endarterectomy Trial Collaborators. Beneficial effect of carotid endarterectomy in symptomatic patients with high-grade carotid stenosis. JAMA 1991;273:1421.

Ratanakorn D, Greenberg JP, Meads DB, Tegeler CH. Middle cerebral artery flow velocity correlates with common carotid volume flow rate after CO_2 inhalation [abstract]. J Neuroimaging 1997;7:268.

Ratanakorn D, Tegeler CH, Greenberg JP. Risks for inadequate temporal windows in transcranial Doppler sonography [abstract]. Neurology 1997;48:A156.

Ringelstein EB, Sievers C, Ecker S, et al. Noninvasive assessment of CO_2-induced cerebral vasomotor response in normal individuals and patients with internal carotid artery occlusions. Stroke 1988;19:963.

Tegeler CH, Kremkau FW, Hitchings LP. Color velocity imaging: introduction to a new ultrasound technology. J Neuroimaging 1991;1:85.

Chapter 6
Neuroimmunology

David Leppert and Andreas J. Steck

Chapter Plan

The nervous system—not an immunologically
restricted site
Immunity in the nervous system
  Specific immune response and the concept of
  autoimmunity
  Nonspecific immune response
  Role of genetic background for neuroimmunologic
  diseases
  Effector mechanisms of immunity in the nervous
  system
Immunotherapy

This chapter provides an overview of the mechanisms
of immune-mediated neurologic diseases. The interactions between the nervous system and the immune
system are mutual. We briefly discuss how immune
surveillance is exerted by blood-derived immune cells
and resident neural cells in both the peripheral and
central nervous system. On the other hand, the nervous system modifies the functions of the immune
system. We present the current concepts of autoimmunity in the nervous system, discussing specific and
nonspecific immune responses, genetic aspects, and
effector mechanisms. We conclude with an overview
of current and future approaches to immunotherapy.

The Nervous System—Not an
Immunologically Restricted Site

Historically, the nervous system has been considered
an "immune-privileged site," based on the following
observations: (1) the apparent lack of a lymphatic
drainage system, (2) the tightness of the blood-brain
barrier (BBB), which restricts extravasation of
immune cells into the nervous tissue parenchyma,
and (3) the apparent paucity of cells able to present
antigen. The impaired rejection of xenografts
implanted into the brain was considered to be the
functional consequence of the anatomic reclusion of
the nervous system from the vascular system and
hence from immune cells. However, an intact cellular and humoral response caused by an antigenic
challenge can be observed during inflammatory diseases of the nervous system. The BBB is fully pene-
trable by activated immune cells (lymphocytes,
monocytes, granulocytes), which accumulate in the
neural parenchyma during encephalitis or meningitis. The intrathecal production of antibodies (Abs)
during infectious and noninfectious inflammatory
diseases is reflected by the occurrence of oligoclonal
bands in the cerebrospinal fluid (CSF) and an
increased immunoglobulin G (IgG) index.

Recent anatomic studies in several mammalian
species have shown that tracers applied in the brain
interstitium are cleared out by a perivascular
drainage system connected to neck lymph nodes,
where antibody production is modulated. T cells
constantly patrol across the BBB into the brain
parenchyma and are recirculated into the vascular
system. Furthermore, several sites (Table 6-1) have
been identified in the brain where the endothelial
layer does not show the tight junctions typical for
the BBB, but rather fenestrated vessel walls. Across
these anatomic windows to the vascular system,
humoral factors circulating in the blood stream can

Table 6-1. Sites in the Blood-Brain Barrier Where the Vessel Walls Are Fenestrated

1. Area postrema
2. Pineal gland
3. Subfornical organ
4. Organum vasculosum of the lamina terminalis
5. Neurohypophysis
6. Median eminence of the hypothalamus

reach their receptors in the brain without prior disrupture of the BBB. Cytokines such as interleukin (IL)-1, tumor necrosis factor (TNF), and IL-6, which are released at inflammatory sites in the periphery, are able to cross the BBB and modulate the centers that regulate body temperature in the hypothalamus, leading to the phenomenon of fever.

Thus, under physiologic conditions, the nervous system is fully accessible to humoral and cellular components of immune surveillance derived from the vascular system. We discuss later in this chapter how neural cells are also able to exert nonspecific immune functions, and specifically, to present antigens.

Immunity in the Nervous System

The goal of the immune system is to preserve the integrity of the organism. The basic property of the immune system is the ability to distinguish between "foreign" and "self." Its function is to eliminate the former and to exert tolerance toward the latter. Immune-mediated diseases, specifically in the context of the nervous system, cannot be understood solely as a reaction of the organism against "nonself" environmental factors such as infectious agents or toxins. Genetic background and the network of specific and nonspecific immune response mechanisms are additional determinants for immunoregulation, discussed below. The clinical picture of diseases results from the interplay between an antigen and the type of immune response produced. The nervous system is particularly vulnerable to the sequelae of inflammation. The course of inflammatory diseases of the nervous system is therefore determined by the type and extent of the immune response rather than the involved antigen or antigens. The concept of an overactive or autoaggressive immune response is of fundamental importance for

both an understanding of clinical disease and the development of novel therapeutic strategies.

Specific Immune Response and the Concept of Autoimmunity

Specificity of the immune response implies that unique receptors on lymphocytes selectively target single antigenic determinants. Lymphocytes express two categories of antigen-recognizing receptors, which belong to the immunoglobulin superfamily. The T-cell receptor (TCR) is expressed on the surface of T cells. Abs function as membrane-anchored or as secretory products of B cells. A B cell or T cell challenged by an antigen matched to its specific receptor structure responds by proliferation, resulting in clonal expansion of cells with identical antigenic determinants. The multiplication of these cells allows them to target and quantitatively eliminate antigens. The diversity of the immune response (the ability to recognize almost any protein sequence as an antigen) is based on a repertoire of 10^8 different clones of lymphocytes. The repertoire of TCRs is defined during ontogeny and remains finite in later life. On the other hand, the repertoire of Abs undergoes somatic changes, resulting in an adaptive increase in specificity, and hence affinity, toward a given antigen.

With these tools, the immune system can eliminate efficiently most infectious agents and either prevent or overcome clinical disease. Classically, viral and bacterial infections lead to an acute immune response, which manifests clinically as meningitis or encephalitis. In viral encephalitis, Ab- and T-cell–mediated responses occur simultaneously and are equally effective. Bacterial infections in the central nervous system elicit predominantly immune responses related to granulocytes and macrophages recruited from the vascular system after the BBB is opened. They do not lead to strong immune responses that involve active processing of antigens and therefore do not lead to a significant immune memory. In some instances, infectious agents induce a chronic immune response when most or all exogenous antigen is eliminated. The inflammatory response persists or recurs after an interval and targets "self" tissue that is physiologically spared from immune attacks. Thus, exogenous antigens could induce a failure of the state of tolerance toward "self" structures and eventually cause disease.

Table 6-2. Neuroimmune Diseases Triggered by Exogenous Antigens

Disease	Primary Immune Mediator	Target Tissue	Exogenous Antigen
Post–rabies vaccination encephalomyelitis	T cells	White matter	Vaccine
Postrabies neuritis	T cells	White matter	Vaccine
Chorea minor Sydenham	Abs	Caudate and subthalamic neurons	Streptococci
Subacute sclerosing panencephalitis	T cells	White matter	Persistent measles virus
Guillain-Barré syndrome (acute inflammatory demyelinating polyneuropathy)	Abs	Peripheral nerve myelin, Schwann cells, axons	*Campylobacter jejuni,* other antigens
Acute demyelinating encephalomyelitis	T cells and Abs	White matter	Viral antigens
Rasmussen's encephalitis	T cells, antiglutamate receptor-Abs?	Gray matter	Cytomegalovirus?, other viruses?

Abs = antibodies.

Rasmussen's encephalitis has been considered a deleterious autoimmune disorder. Seventy-one percent of patients with Rasmussen's encephalitis (versus 4% in controls) show cytomegalovirus genome in brain biopsy tissue. This, and the successful treatment with ganciclovir in the early stages of the disease, raises the possibility that a latent viral infection accounts for pathogenesis at least during a certain period in the course of the disease. This example highlights the theory that the boundaries between classical inflammatory (caused by exogenous antigens) and autoimmune diseases are not discrete, but represent a continuum. Table 6-2 summarizes other neuroimmunologic disorders that share the same features.

Tolerance is an actively induced condition that leads to the inability of the immune system to react to an antigen. Functionally, this protects the organism from the sequelae of an exaggerated immune response by limiting its extent and duration. Tolerance can be achieved by (1) clonal deletion, (2) ignorance, (3) anergy, and (4) suppression. During ontogeny, the randomly produced repertoire of T-cell clones is actively restricted, as the bulk of self-reactive cells are eliminated in the thymus. This process of clonal deletion excludes most but not all self-reactive T cells. T cells autoreactive against "self" epitopes (e.g., myelin basic protein [MBP]) can be found in peripheral blood cells routinely in healthy donors. In the mature immune system, additional inhibitory mechanisms that prevent the development

of autoimmune reactions are required. Ignorance, which results from diminished traffic of lymphocytes across the BBB, might be only a minor control factor for lymphocytes targeting autoantigens in the nervous system. Anergy occurs when T lymphocytes are exposed to processed antigens—that is, complexed to major histocompatibility complex (MHC) class II proteins, in the absence of additional costimulatory signals (e.g., B7, CD58) on the surface of the antigen-presenting cells (APCs). For B cells, similar mechanisms to induce anergy exist as well. Suppression can be induced by humoral factors (cytokines and Abs [anti-idiotypes]) and specific T cells carrying the CD8 molecule. The earlier concept of CD4 cells as inducer cells and of CD8 cells as suppressor cells is no longer tenable, as cytotoxicity and suppressor functions can be exerted by subtypes of both CD4 and CD8 lineage (see section below on T_{H1} and T_{H2} cells).

The failure of one or several factors to sustain tolerance allows the development or reactivation of autoimmune disease. In the absence of a specific exogenous antigen, this can result from (1) molecular mimicry, (2) activation by superantigens, and (3) bystander activation. Molecular mimicry occurs when peptides of exogenous antigens have amino acid sequences similar to those of endogenous proteins. T cells reactive against the exogenous antigen can therefore cross-react with the endogenous target and eventually cause disease. In the case of

Table 6-3. Autoimmune Neurologic Diseases

Disease	Primary Immune Mediator	Target Structure	Possible Cross-Reactive Immunogen
Multiple sclerosis	T-cells	Myelin	?
Myasthenia gravis	Anti-AChR Abs, anti-striated muscle Abs	Postsynaptic end-plate	Epithelial thymus cells
Eaton-Lambert syndrome	Voltage-gated Ca^{2+} channel Abs	Presynaptic, Ca^{2+} channels	Small lung cancer cells
Chronic inflammatory demyelinating polyneuropathy	Abs >> T cells	Myelin	?
Paraneoplastic cerebellar atrophy	Anti-Yo Abs	Purkinje cells	Tumor cells
Paraneoplastic encephalomyelitis (limbic, brain stem encephalitis)	Anti-Hu, T cells	White matter	Tumor cells
Neuromyotonia (Isaac's syndrome)	Ab	K^+ channels distal motor axon	
Multifocal motor neuropathy	Ab	Ganglioside GM_1	Gram-negative bacteria?
IgM paraproteinemic sensorimotor polyneuropathy	Ab	MAG	?
Stiff-person syndrome	Ab	GAD	Tumor cells?

Ab = antibody; MAG = myelin-associated glycoprotein; GAD = glutamic acid decarboxylase; >> = much higher.

post-measles encephalitis, some patients were found to develop an immune response to MBP. Alternatively, autoreactive T cells can be stimulated by superantigens, proteins that bind to the "outside" (i.e., nonspecifically) of the antigen groove to the TCR. This binding of a superantigen (mostly of bacterial origin) can be sufficient to activate T cells.

Autoimmunity, by definition, implies the absence of an exogenous antigen and the presence of an endogenous antigen. Table 6-3 summarizes the more common neurologic disorders having assumed or proven autoimmune pathogenesis and the corresponding antigenic target. Myasthenia gravis (MG) and paraneoplastic cerebellar atrophy are two diseases in which autoantibodies against structures of the nervous system can be found in most patients and in which titers show a fair correlation with disease activity. For multiple sclerosis (MS) and Guillain-Barré syndrome (GBS), the two major neurologic disorders considered to be of autoimmune nature, no definite endogenous antigen has been found yet, and specific exogenous triggers functioning as superantigens or tar-

gets of molecular mimicry have been implicated at least in some instances. The hypothesis of autoimmune pathogenesis in MS is supported by the fundamental work by Rivers and coworkers. In monkeys, they induced a neuroinflammatory disease, later referred to as experimental autoimmune encephalomyelitis (EAE), which resembles MS. This was achieved by peripheral sensitization with brain homogenates, together with priming of the immune system with noninfectious stimuli, such as Freund's adjuvant. EAE can be induced by different protein components of the white matter, such as MBP and proteolipid protein (PLP). Several specific sequences of these proteins are particularly immunogenic for T cells. However, these observations are not paralleled in MS: (1) MBP-reactive cell clones appear in MS patients as often as in their healthy relatives, and (2) the antigenic determinants of MBP-reactive T cells show a random distribution over the MBP sequence in both groups. Thus, the presence of self-reactive T cells in MS does not allow a conclusion on their possible etiologic role for disease. These findings emphasize the limitations of animal models of specific immune responses for human autoimmune disease.

Nonspecific Immune Response

Whereas antigen recognition is a specific process, other signaling and effector mechanisms are not antigen specific and occur in a stereotypic manner once triggered—that is, show no adaptive property. Nonspecific immune mechanisms encompass (1) antigen presentation, (2) cell recruitment into sites of antigenic challenge, and (3) effector mechanisms of antigen elimination. The combination of specific antigen recognition and nonspecific enhancing/propagation mechanisms explains the efficacy of the immune system in qualitative and quantitative terms. Antigen presentation is based on ingestion and degradation of proteins that are then presented in the form of small oligopeptides (approximately 15 amino acids) on the cell surface. These presenting molecules are encoded by the MHC and belong, as TCRs and Abs, to the immunoglobulin superfamily. Very similar to the recognition by Abs, processed antigens are put into grooves determined by the tertiary and quaternary structure of the heterodimer structure. There are two types of MHC molecules. Class I molecules are encountered genuinely on virtually all cells. Their presence is compulsory for CD8 T cells to kill the cell expressing the antigen; an antigen cannot be targeted in the absence of MHC class I receptors or a xenogeneic receptor that does not correspond to the TCR receptor. For induction of CD4 helper T cells, class II receptors are required. They are expressed genuinely on monocytes and macrophages and are therefore termed "professional" APCs. Blood-derived macrophages are relatively sparse in the neural parenchyma. Astrocytes, microglia, and brain endothelial cells do not express class II receptors under normal conditions. However, astrocytes and microglial cells can be induced for class II expression and can function as facultative APCs. Hence, the nervous system can compensate for its partial lack of professional APCs by induction of class II receptors by glial and other cells of the nervous system. CD4 T cells can be subdivided into at least two different subsets according to their spectrum of secreted cytokines. T_{H1} cells secrete IL-2 and interferon-gamma (IFN-γ), which stimulates T-cell proliferation and activation, and hence promote a cellular immune response. T_{H2} cells produce IL-4, IL-5, and IL-6, cytokines that first were defined to induce B-cell maturation. In addition, they secrete IL-10. The common denominator of T_{H2} cytokines is the induction of a humoral response that goes in hand with a suppression of the cellular, T_{H1}-mediated response. T_{H3} cells, an additional subtype of CD4 cells with suppressive activity, have been defined recently. These cells are found in gut tissue and secrete predominantly transforming growth factor-beta 1 (TGF-β_1). They are believed to play an important role in induction of oral tolerance against exogenous antigens.

Other signaling molecules are eicosanoids, adhesion molecules, and complement factors. An increasing body of evidence has accumulated that cells of the nervous system can express a functional set of molecules of each of these groups. The role of these nonspecific factors of immune mediation is exemplified by their detection in neural tissue and CSF during inflammatory neurologic diseases and the increasing number of novel therapies attempting to block the activity of these molecules (see "Immunotherapy"). The fact that the nervous system can organize its immune surveillance without help from blood-derived immune cells has important therapeutic consequences. In diseases with an elusive etiology, such as MS, new therapeutic approaches will depend on an understanding of the cytokine network and other local immune mediators. The therapeutic progress for immune-mediated neurologic diseases we experienced in the last years resulted almost exclusively from research done on the function of nonspecific responses (summarized in Table 6-4).

Role of Genetic Background for Neuroimmunologic Diseases

A genetic background in the pathogenesis of MS and MG has been sought by studies demonstrating an association of marker genes in a group of affected individuals but not in unaffected controls. The genes coding for the MHC, TCR, and the heavy chains of Abs are likely candidates for determining disease susceptibility in autoimmune disorders. Association studies analyzed the differ-

Table 6-4. Therapies for Neuroimmune Diseases

Therapy	Established Indications	Indications Under Evaluation	Indication Evaluated: Result
Plasma exchange	GBS, CIDP, MG	Neuromyotonia, Rasmussen's encephalitis	MS: no improvement
Intravenous immunoglobulins	GBS, CIDP, Lambert-Eaton syndrome, dermatomyositis	MG, stiff-person syndrome, Rasmussen's encephalitis, paraneoplastic cerebellar atrophy, multifocal motor neuropathy, MS	
Immunosuppressive strategies			
Corticosteroids	MS		
Cytostatic drugs			
Cyclophosphamide			MS: insignificant results
Methotrexate, mitoxanthrone	Chronic progressive MS?		MS: no improvement
Cyclosporin A			
Azathioprine	MS?		
Linomide			MS: unacceptable side effects
Cladribine			MS: no improvement
Effector-mechanism–related strategies			
Cytokines			
Interferon-beta	MS		
Interferon-alpha		CIDP	
Interferon-gamma		Anti-MAG neuropathy	MS: deterioration
TGF beta			MS: unacceptable side effects
Anti-TNF Abs			MS: deterioration
Protease inhibition			
Metalloproteinase inhibitors		MS, GBS?	
Vaccination, tolerization			
Copolymer-1	MS		
Oral myelin			MS: no improvement
Antigen-specific strategies			
Anti-TCR approach		MS	
Anti-TCR Abs		MS	
T-cell vaccination		MS	
TCR peptides forming anti-idiotypes		MS	
Anti-MHC Abs, MCH peptides		MS	
Reconstitutive strategies			
Growth factors (IGF, PDGF, FGF)		MS	
Others			
Thymectomy	MG		
Bone marrow transplantation		MS, POEMS syndrome	

Abs = antibodies; GBS = Guillain-Barré syndrome; CIDP = chronic inflammatory demyelinating polyneuropathy; MG = myasthenia gravis; MS = multiple sclerosis; TGF = tumor growth factor; TNF = tumor necrosis factor; TCR = T-cell receptor; MHC = major histocompatibility complex; IGF = insulin-like growth factor; PDGF = platelet-derived growth factor; POEMS = polyneuropathy, endocrinopathy, M protein, and skin changes syndrome; MAG = myelin-associated glycoprotein; FGF = fibroblast growth factor.

ences in frequencies of marker genes in patients and controls. They yield a relative risk factor for an individual who carries a specific allele compared with a control individual who does not carry the marker. Such associations have been postulated for MHC, TCR, and Abs in MS, and for the MHC in MG. In genetically complex diseases such as MS, association studies also yielded conflicting results and failed to identify a prominent susceptibility gene. Several research groups have tried to elucidate the multigenetic etiology of MS by systematically screening large family cohorts of MS patients by linkage analysis. Here, the co-segregation of a phenotype (patient or healthy) and genes in a certain chromosomal region is analyzed. Other than in association studies, linkage analysis is unbiased toward the known function of genes and allows definition of susceptibility of genes whose pathophysiologic role for disease is not known or not expected to be involved.

The association of an allele coding for an immune-relevant determinant with a disease does not necessarily imply a causal link but could result from a bystander association with the responsible gene or from linkage disequilibrium with other genes. Narcolepsy is such an example, in which the association with the DR2 haplotype of the MHC II is almost 100% in white patients and therefore used as a surrogate marker for diagnosis. On the other hand, there is no evidence that narcolepsy has an immune pathogenesis.

Effector Mechanisms of Immunity in the Nervous System

Cytotoxicity and invasion to sites of antigenic challenge by immune cells are the two effector components of the immune system. Although the signaling mechanisms of the immune response have been studied intensively, the molecular basis of effector mechanisms remains poorly understood. Similar to signaling molecules, it has been recognized that brain cells are able to produce most, if not all, cytotoxic molecules encountered outside the nervous system. Besides the cytokines with effector activity (e.g., TNF-α/β), astrocytes, microglial cells, and endothelial cells produce reactive oxygen molecules and nitric oxide. Matrix metalloproteinases (MMPs) have been implicated as effector molecules in the

process of extravasation of immune cells across the BBB and destruction of white matter. They are also involved in the opening of the BBB during inflammation. In MS and GBS, metalloproteinases are expressed by T cells and macrophages invading into neural tissue. In animal models of these diseases, the drugs suppressing MMP activity ameliorate disease and are likely candidates for treatment of human disease (see later).

Immunotherapy

In parallel with our increasing knowledge of immune-mediated neurologic conditions, we have seen unprecedented advances in the development of new disease-modifying therapies (see Table 6-4). The immunotherapeutic agents that are used today to treat neurologic diseases with an autoimmune pathogenesis are not specific for each disease. Many immunomodulating drugs or procedures are used, often empirically, in different conditions. Although nonspecific immunosuppression still remains the backbone of immunotherapy, the development of new selective or semiselective immunotherapies should allow a more disease-specific manipulation of the immune system and, it is hoped, lead to better therapeutic results.

Plasmapheresis has been shown to be effective as a short-term therapy in MG and other immune-mediated neurologic diseases, such as GBS and chronic inflammatory demyelinating polyneuropathy (CIDP). In recent years, however, high-dose intravenous immunoglobulin is emerging as a major nonspecific immunotherapeutic modality in neurology and is the first choice therapy in GBS and CIDP.

Thymectomy has been used in MG and is considered effective in patients up to the age of 55 years. Its role of action is unclear, but acetylcholine receptors are present in the epithelial cells of the thymus, and they are believed to be a source of autoantigen.

Immunosuppressive drugs are the most widely used for nonspecific immunosuppressive therapy. Corticosteroids exert multiple effects by inhibiting or suppressing the function of T cells and B cells, acting on macrophage differentiation, suppressing numerous cytokines, and having an effect on vascular permeability. The cytostatic drugs include the main drugs in clinical use, such as azathioprine, cyclophosphamide, and chlorambucil. Cyclosporine causes a profound inhibition of T-cell–mediated immunity.

Bone marrow transplantation is a new option in the therapy of autoimmune diseases, because new developments in autologous stem cell transplantation have reduced the risks of this procedure.

In the effector mechanisms related strategy therapy group, the beta-interferons are now widely prescribed for treatment of relapsing forms of MS, reducing annual exacerbation rates by approximately 30% and possibly also reducing the rate of progression in secondary progressive disease. Because TNF-α may be a specific mediator of tissue damage in several autoimmune-mediated disorders, treatment with TNF antagonists is under evaluation. Copolymer 1 (cop-1 glatinamer acetate) reduces exacerbation rates in MS and is now also available for treatment. Another cytokine, IFN-α, has been reported to improve the neuropathy associated with anti–myelin-associated glycoprotein (anti-MAG) Abs.

Metalloproteinase inhibitors act by blocking the cleavage of membrane-bound TNF-α to soluble TNF-α and proteolysis of extracellular matrix. A number of drugs aimed at reducing T-lymphocyte trafficking across vascular endothelial cells are under investigation. Abs to adhesion molecules VLA-4, ICAM-1, and L-selectine have been shown to decrease the expression of adhesion molecules on T lymphocytes and vascular endothelial cells in experimental models. Among the new disease-modifying procedures, immunotherapy directed at antigen-specific alteration has considerable potential. The difficulty with any antigen-specific therapy is the assumption that one knows which antigen is causing the disease. The prototype autoimmune neurologic disease in which the antigen is well defined is MG. In the immune-mediated neuropathies, MAG is the responsible autoantigen target in IgM-associated demyelinating neuropathy and the GQ1b ganglioside is the antigen in the Miller-Fisher variant of GBS. In MS, the identity of the autoantigen is unclear, but myelin peptides are the strongest candidates. On this basis, several antigen-specific strategies involving the injection of peptides that compete with the autoantigen or blockade of TCRs have been proposed. T-cell vaccination and oral tolerance by feeding an autoantigen (acetylcholine receptor or myelin) are procedures under evaluation. Growth factors, such as insulin-like growth factor-1 (IGF-1), that enhance oligodendrocyte survival in vitro may promote maturation of oligodendrocytes and remyelination in demyelinating disorders.

Suggested Reading

Antel J, Birnbaum G, Hartung HP (eds). Clinical Neuroimmunology. Boston: Blackwell Science, 1998.

Bartfai T, Ottoson D (eds). Neuro-Immunology of Fever. Oxford: Pergamon, 1992.

Chen Y, Kuchroo VK, Inobe J, et al. Regulatory T cell clones induced by oral tolerance: suppression of autoimmune encephalomyelitis. Science 1994;265:1237.

Hohlfeld R (ed). Immunology of Neuromuscular Disease. Immunology and Medicine Series (Vol 24). Boston: Kluwer, 1994.

McLachlan MS, Levin S, Blume WT. Treatment of Rasmussen's encephalitis with ganciclovir. Neurology 1996;47:925.

Oksenberg JR, Seboun E, Hauser SL. Genetics of demyelinating diseases. Brain Pathol 1996;6:289.

Rivers TM, Sprunt DH, Berry GP. Observations on attempts to produce acute disseminated encephalomyelitis in monkeys. J Exp Med 1933;58:39.

Roitt I, Brostoff J, Male D. Immunology (4th ed). St. Louis: Mosby, 1994.

Rolak LA, Harati Y (eds). Neuro-Immunology for the Clinician. Boston: Butterworth–Heinemann, 1997.

Tyndall A, Gratwohl A. Bone marrow transplantation in the treatment of autoimmune diseases [editorial]. Br J Rheumatol 1997;36:1.

Chapter 7
Molecular Biology and Genetics in Neurologic Disorders

Chung Y. Hsu, Teng-nan Lin, and David H. Gutmann

Chapter Plan

Application of molecular biology in the study of mechanisms of neurologic disorders
  Detection of gene expression after cerebral ischemia
  Functional significance of gene expression
  Alteration of postischemic gene expression
  Transgenic technology
Identification of neurogenetic disease genes

More advances in the diagnosis and treatment of neurologic diseases have been made in the 1990s, the "decade of the brain," than in any previous decade. To a large extent, this can be attributed to the progress made in molecular biology and genetics, which has enabled neuroscientists to link genetic abnormalities with molecular mechanisms and clinical presentations of neurologic diseases. Development of new molecular biology techniques and genetic tools has revolutionized the thinking about mechanisms of neurologic dysfunction in diseases and has changed our diagnostic approach to neurologic disorders, especially those, old or newly discovered, with the phenotypic presentation of "disease genes." The introduction of gene therapy during this decade also raises the hope that an understanding of the molecular and genetic mechanisms of diseases will lead to the development of more effective therapeutic strategies.

It is not possible in this chapter to even briefly review the current status of molecular biology and genetics in neurologic diseases. We will draw on a few examples of animal stroke models to introduce the application of molecular biology techniques in studies of molecular mechanisms of brain injury and recovery. We will also use a prototype neurogenetic disorder, neurofibromatosis 1 (NF1), to illustrate the approaches to identification of a gene responsible for the clinical presentation of a hereditary neurologic disorder. The discovery of the *NF1* gene has led to the development of more reliable diagnostic tests and brightened the prospect that effective remedies for this disease may be within reach in the coming years.

Application of Molecular Biology in the Study of Mechanisms of Neurologic Disorders

Molecular biology is now widely applied in studying the mechanisms of diseases and developing novel therapeutic applications. We will use animal stroke models to illustrate the utility of molecular biology in basic research. An ischemic insult to the brain triggers a multitude of biochemical and physiologic changes in the ischemic region and its surroundings. New molecular biology techniques have greatly advanced our understanding of the molecular events that may underlie the mechanisms of ischemic brain injury and the scientific basis of functional recovery after stroke.

Table 7-1. Representative Immediate Early Genes Induced By Cerebral Ischemia

Gene	Structural Feature	Function
c-*fos*	Leucine zipper	Transcription factor (AP-1)
fos-B	Leucine zipper	Transcription factor (AP-1)
c-*jun*	Leucine zipper	Transcription factor (AP-1)
jun-B	Leucine zipper	Transcription factor (AP-1)
jun-D	Leucine zipper	Transcription factor (AP-1)
zif/268 (egr-1, TIS-8, Krox 24, NGFI-A)	Zinc finger	Transcription factor
Krox 20 (egr-2)	Zinc finger	Transcription factor
nur/77 (NGFI-B, TIS-1)	Zinc finger	Steroid receptor superfamily

Detection of Gene Expression After Cerebral Ischemia

It has now been extensively documented that transient or permanent cerebral ischemia causes the expression of a large number of genes that serve diverse biologic functions. Immediate early genes are those that express minutes after stimuli and return to baseline levels within hours. Table 7-1 lists selected immediate early genes that have been detected in the ischemic brain and the major function of each gene product. Gene expression can be detected at mRNA or protein levels. For the former, the commonly used techniques are Northern blot analysis or RNase protection assay, which determine semiquantitatively the mRNA content of a specific gene in the brain tissue. The development of the polymerase chain reaction (PCR) added a quick means for screening the increase in the expression of a large number of genes by first reverse transcribing the endogenous mRNA in the brain tissue to cDNA. PCR amplification using the cDNA as the templates can generate a sufficient quantity of cDNA for semiquantitative analysis of the amount of each endogenous mRNA. This procedure, RT-PCR, is being used with increasing frequency to detect gene expression at mRNA levels. RT-PCR is not as reliable as Northern blot analysis or RNase protection assay and frequently requires confirmation with either of the latter two methods. Figures 7-1 and 7-2 show the expression of c-*fos* and c-*jun*, genes that are expressed early after focal cerebral ischemia, by Northern blot analysis. Northern blot analysis, RNase protection assay, or RT-PCR assess the relative content of mRNA of selected genes in the sampled region of the brain. In situ hybridization is applied if information on the regional distribution of mRNA is needed. Figure 7-2 shows the regional expression of c-*fos* mRNA after transient focal cerebral ischemia in a portion of the cortex irrigated by the right middle cerebral artery.

A gene may be expressed at the mRNA level but not the protein level. To determine that the targeted gene is not only transcribed (mRNA synthesis) but also translated (protein synthesis), Western blot analysis or immunoprecipitation methods are used to detect the quantitative increase in gene product. For studying regional distribution, immunohistochemistry is needed.

Functional Significance of Gene Expression

An increase in the amount of a gene product does not necessarily imply that the specific gene function will be fully executed after its expression. Additional studies are needed to detect the gene function. For certain immediate early genes that serve as transcription factors, the resultant increase in gene function can be estimated by studying the binding activity of the transcription factors. For instance, AP-1 is a transcription factor that is a heterodimer formed by gene products of two immediate early genes, c-*fos* and c-*jun*. An increase in AP-1 binding activity after cerebral ischemia as shown in Figure 7-3 is indicative of enhanced gene function mediated by c-*fos* and c-*jun*.

Although numerous genes have been noted to increase their expression after focal cerebral ischemia, the roles of these genes remain poorly

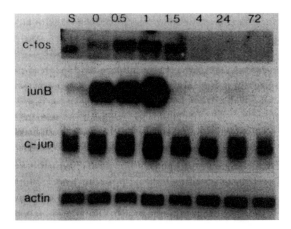

Figure 7-1. Expression of immediate early genes after focal cerebral ischemia-reperfusion. Rats were subjected to transient ischemia for 30 minutes. Severe ischemia is confined to the cerebral cortex in the territory of the right middle cerebral artery (MCA). At variable time intervals after the onset of ischemia, the right MCA cortex was removed to isolate total RNA for Northern blot analysis. The time at which the ischemic cortex was removed is indicated by the number in hours at the top of each sample. Note low baseline mRNA signals in sham-operated animals (S). A transient increase in the expression of immediate early genes, including c-*fos*, *jun*-B, and c-*jun*, was noted within a period of 2 hours after reperfusion. Actin, a housekeeping gene, showed no change in signal after ischemia-reperfusion, indicating only selected genes are activated after an ischemic insult.

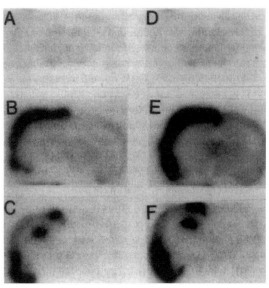

Figure 7-2. Regional distribution of c-*fos* and *jun*-B mRNA after focal cerebral ischemia-reperfusion. The brain slices from animals subjected to focal cerebral ischemia for 30 minutes and reperfusion for 60 minutes were prepared for in situ hybridization. Panels A–C are studies based on a radioactive c-*fos* cDNA probe to identify c-*fos* mRNA signal. Panels D–F are from those using a *jun*-B cDNA probe for *jun*-B mRNA signals. Panels A and D are brain slices from sham-operated animals; panels B and E are from animals subjected to 30 minutes of ischemia and 60 minutes of reperfusion; and panels C and F are from animals with 90 minutes of ischemia and 60 minutes of reperfusion. Note the intense c-*fos* and *jun*-B mRNA signals in the right middle cerebral artery (MCA) cortex, where severe ischemia developed after 30 minutes of ischemia (B, E). Ischemia for 90 minutes resulted in attenuated c-*fos* and *jun*-B mRNA signals in the MCA cortex destined to develop infarction. However, intense expression of c-*fos* and *jun*-B was still noted in the region adjacent to the infarcted cortex and in the ipsilateral hippocampus (C, E).

understood. Products of immediate early genes may function as transcription factors (see Table 7-1), which in turn regulate the expression of other genes. For instance, AP-1 has been found in the promoter regions of a neurotrophin gene, nerve growth factor (NGF). After the postischemic expression of immediate early genes, a number of other genes are expressed in a delayed fashion. Many of these genes, including *NGF* and other neurotrophin genes, may exert trophic actions in the ischemic brain. The possible regulation of these so-called late effector genes by immediate early genes remains to be fully elucidated.

Alteration of Postischemic Gene Expression

The sequential expression of immediate early genes and late effector genes raises the possibility that the expression of the former leads ultimately to the enhanced neurotrophic actions by the late effector genes. If this is indeed the case, the expression of immediate early genes should constitute an early step of a molecular cascade that protects the brain from ischemic insult. Alteration of the postischemic expression of immediate early genes is then expected to alter the outcome after an ischemic insult. The molecular biology techniques described above allow the study of alteration of gene expression after focal cerebral ischemia. Hyperglycemia was found to suppress c-*fos* expression and also

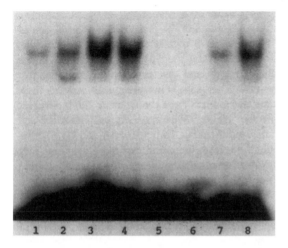

Figure 7-3. Increase in AP-1 binding activity after focal cerebral ischemia-reperfusion. Gel mobility shift assay was used to determine the nuclear content of AP-1 transcription factor, which is a heterodimer formed by Fos and Jun family proteins. The cortex in the territory of the right middle cerebral artery (MCA) was dissected after ischemia-reperfusion and nuclear proteins isolated for determination of the extent of AP-1 binding to a radioactive AP-1 DNA binding sequence (AP-1 motif). (Lane 1) Sham-operated animal. (Lane 2) Thirty minutes after 30 minutes of ischemia. (Lane 3) Four hours after ischemia. (Lane 4) Twenty-four hours after ischemia. (Lane 5) Displacement of AP-1 binding by an unlabeled AP-1 motif. Inhibition of AP-1 binding activity by anti-Fos and anti-Jun B but not by anti-glial fibrillary acidic protein antibodies is shown in lanes 6, 7, and 8, respectively. This figure shows an increase in AP-1 transcription factor after ischemia-reperfusion with a peak level noted 4 hours after ischemia. The specificity of AP-1 binding activity is demonstrated by the ability of the unlabeled AP-1 motif to compete with the radioactive one and inhibition by antibodies to Fos and Jun-B, which constitute the AP-1 transcription factor and lack of effect of a nonspecific antibody against GFAP, a glial protein.

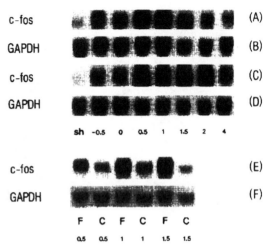

Figure 7-4. Time course of c-*fos* mRNA expression in ischemic cortex in the territory of the right middle cerebral artery (MCA) after ischemia-reperfusion. Northern blot analysis shows that ischemia induced a transient expression of c-*fos* mRNA in rats fed until ischemia (row A). Rats that fasted for 24 hours sustained more intense expression of c-*fos* mRNA for a longer period (row C). The fasted rats had smaller infarct volumes in the right MCA cortex (row C). *GAPDH*, a housekeeping gene that does not change its expression during ischemia-reperfusion, served as the control to normalize the mRNA content of each sample (rows B and D). The lower panel shows quantitative analysis of the relative extent of c-*fos* mRNA signals in fed control and fasted groups.

exaggerated the ischemic brain injury. Figure 7-4 shows that lowering plasma glucose levels was accompanied by an enhanced and prolonged expression of c-*fos* after focal cerebral ischemia and reduced infarct sizes. These findings are consistent with the contention that an increase in c-*fos* expression may be beneficial in the setting of transient focal cerebral ischemia. These results are, however, only correlative and do not prove a causal role of c-*fos* in limiting ischemic brain injury. It should be noted that some of the immediate early genes such as c-*jun* have also been implicated in the pathogen-

esis of apoptosis, which is one of the mechanisms of neuronal death after focal cerebral ischemia.

To further investigate the role of a specific gene in ischemic brain injury, experimental strategies are needed for selectively blocking the gene under investigation. Antisense technology has been used to block expression of targeted genes and has been under development for reducing tumor growth by suppressing the expression of selected oncogenes. Figure 7-5 shows the application of antisense strategy in successfully blocking c-*fos* expression and its function after focal cerebral ischemia. However, there are a number of technical problems to be overcome before antisense strategies can be more reliably applied in the study of gene function and in therapeutic usage. A more definite means for blocking the function of a specific gene is to delete it from genomic DNA by applying transgenic technology.

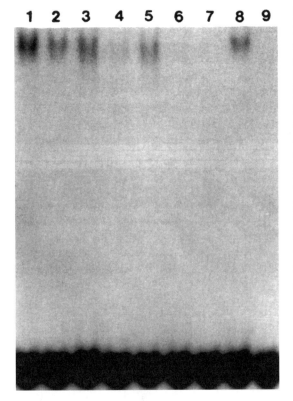

Figure 7-5. Reduction of AP-1 binding activity by an antisense oligonucleotide (ODN) directed at the translation initiation site. Animals were treated with sense ODN, which served as the control (lanes 1, 3, 5) or antisense ODN by intracerebroventricular injection (lanes 2, 4, 6). Sixteen hours later, the animals were subjected to ischemia-reperfusion. Nuclear proteins from ischemic cortex in the territory of the right middle cerebral artery (MCA) were then isolated for gel mobility shift assay as described in Figure 7-3. Note reduced AP-1 binding activity in antisense ODN-treated animals (lanes 2, 4, 6). Lane 7 is a sham-operated control, lane 8 is from an animal subjected to ischemia without injection of ODN, and lane 9 is radioactive AP-1 alone in the absence of nuclear proteins.

Transgenic Technology

The ability to alter gene expression through transgenic technology in selected animal species has greatly enhanced the ability to deduce more precise roles of specific genes in neurologic disorders. Transgenic technology is illustrated by studies on transgenic mice that alter the expression of an endogenous free radical scavenger, superoxide dismutase. Free radicals have been speculated to mediate ischemic brain injury after transient cerebral ischemia-reperfusion. The brain is endowed with an endogenous antioxidant defense mechanism with a high cellular content of antioxidants, including glutathione, ascorbate, and vitamin E, and antioxidant enzymes, including superoxide dismutase, catalase, and glutathione peroxidase. The creation of transgenic mice that overexpress superoxide dismutase led to a series of studies that support the role of superoxide dismutase as a neuroprotective enzyme in the setting of cerebral ischemia-reperfusion and reaffirm the contention that free radicals are generated in and detrimental to the ischemic brain after reperfusion. Figure 7-6 shows the infarct size in a transgenic mouse overexpressing superoxide dismutase in comparison with that of a wild-type mouse. The role of superoxide dismutase is further strengthened by the recent establishment of transgenic mice in which the superoxide dismutase gene is deleted. In these animals, the extent of ischemic brain injury was substantially greater than in the wild-type mice. Figure 7-7 shows the infarct size in a transgenic mouse with superoxide dismutase gene knockout compared with that in a wild-type animal. These findings together support a neuroprotective role of superoxide dismutase and nicely demonstrate that transgenic techniques are powerful tools for studying the molecular mechanisms of neurologic disorders. New methods are available for directing knockout or overexpression to specific tissues or cells.

Identification of Neurogenetic Disease Genes

Inherited neurologic disorders may result from mutations in a single gene or multiple genes. For those disorders resulting from mutations in a single gene, powerful genetic approaches are now available for identifying the gene in question. In most situations, no a priori information is available on the structure or function of the disease gene. Therefore, the only feasible approach available to identify the gene is through positional cloning. The identification of the gene responsible for causing a hereditary disorder, von Recklinghausen's disease, or NF1, is an example of the successful application of molecular genetics. The isolation of the *NF1* gene began with an international collaboration that assembled genetic information from many families with NF1. This

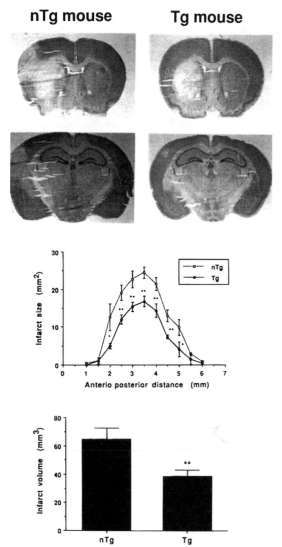

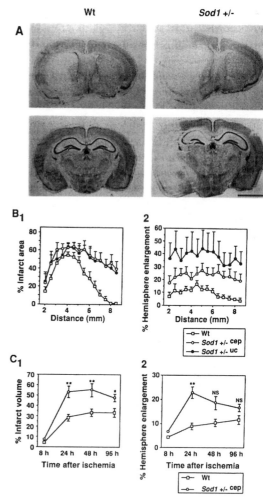

Figure 7-6. Comparison of infarct volume between transgenic mice overexpressing superoxide dismutase (Tg) and wild-type (nontransgenic; nTG) mice after focal cerebral ischemia-reperfusion. The infarction was less apparent (upper panel) and the infarct volumes significantly smaller (lower panel) in Tg compared with nTg mice. (Courtesy of Dr. Pak H. Chan, Stanford University Medical Center, Palo Alto, CA.)

Figure 7-7. Comparison of infarct volume between transgenic mice with heterogeneous deletion of superoxide dismutase (Sod +/–) and wild-type (Wt) mice. The infarction was more extensive (upper panel) and the infarct volumes significantly larger (lower panel) in the Sod +/– mice compared with the Wt mice. (Courtesy of Dr. Pak H. Chan, Stanford University Medical Center, Palo Alto, CA.)

worldwide effort culminated in the construction of a genetic map that narrowed the candidate chromosomes to a handful. Using selected DNA markers, the *NF1* gene was linked to a small region on chromosome 17. The use of additional DNA markers further narrowed the interval on chromosome 17 where the *NF1* gene resided. This high-density genetic linkage map was used to identify candidate genes within a small interval of genomic DNA on chromosome 17. Fortuitously, two patients with NF1 had chromosomal translocations involving the long arm of chromosome 17. These two NF1 patients further narrowed the region on chromosome 17 where the *NF1* gene was located. Using a combination of genetic techniques, candidate genes were identified. Of the first four genes analyzed, only one gene demonstrated mutations in patients affected with NF1. This fourth gene proved to be the *NF1* gene based on two criteria. First, this gene was disrupted in both patients with the chromosomal translocations. Second, more subtle mutations were identified in patients with NF1 that altered the coding potential of this candidate gene. With the identification of the *NF1* gene, it became possible to determine the role of this gene and its protein product in the molecular pathogenesis of NF1. In addition, more reliable genetic tests could be developed.

Our ability to identify neurogenetic disease genes has been greatly enhanced by the progress made in the Human Genome Project. First, an improved set of DNA markers are available to more precisely localize potential disease genes to specific chromosomes. Second, extensive libraries exist that contain most genes expressed in the brain. Third, many potential disease-related genes have now been placed on a genetic map, enabling researchers to rapidly move from family linkage studies to the identification of the gene. This new technique, dubbed "positional-candidate cloning," has greatly condensed the time required for positional cloning efforts. Last, several new exciting approaches to dis-

ease gene identification may result from analyzing complex gene expression patterns in tissues affected by a specific disease. These methodologies will enable researchers to begin to dissect the complex genetic programs associated with neurogenetic diseases.

Suggested Reading

Akins P, Liu PK, Hsu CY. Immediate early gene expression in response to ischemia: friend or foe. Stroke 1996;27:1682.

Chan PH. Role of antioxidants in ischemic brain damage. Stroke 1996;27:1124.

Collins FS. Positional cloning: let's not call it reverse anymore. Nat Genet 1992;1:3.

Green ED, Cox DR, Myers RM. The Human Genome Project and Its Impact on the Study of Human Disease. In CR Scriver, AL Beaudet, WS Sly, D Valle (eds), The Metabolic Basis of Inherited Disease (7th ed). New York: McGraw Hill, 1996;401–436.

Gutmann DH, Collins FS. The neurofibromatosis type 1 gene and its protein product, neurofibromin. Neuron 1993; 10:335.

King MC. Leaving Kansas ... finding genes in 1997. Nat Genet 1997;15:8.

Velculescu V, Zhang L, Vogelstein B, Kinzler KW. Serial analysis of gene expression. Science 1995;270:484.

Chapter 8
Neuropharmacology

James P. Bennett, Jr.

Chapter Plan

Principles of chemical synaptic transmission
    Overview of synaptic transmission
    Neurotransmitter synthesis
    Neurotransmitter catabolism
    Neuropeptides and neuromodulators
    Neurotransmitter storage and release
    Neurotransmitter receptor interactions: principles
        of receptor function
    Secondary actions of neurotransmitters
    Receptor desensitization
Nitric oxide: a novel gaseous free radical neuro-
    transmitter
Long-term molecular effects of neurotransmitters
Conclusion

Although *neuropharmacology* has no precise single definition, operationally it may be considered the study of how drugs affect functioning of the peripheral and central nervous systems. This occurs on several levels. At the molecular level, which is where the greatest advances have been made in the last decade, primary, secondary, and tertiary structures of drug and neurotransmitter receptors and transport proteins have been deduced. At the cellular level, detailed mechanisms are now known of how receptors control ion passage through specific channels and thus modulate neuronal firing, activate second messenger systems, control transcription of multiple genes, and ultimately affect multiple cellular functions, including survival. At the systems

level, the effects of the dynamic actions of multiple converging neurotransmitters on neuronal populations within a given brain region are integrated to affect the output from that region. Finally, at the behavioral level, the combined effects of interacting neuronal systems yield the complex final product known as behavior. Although each of these four major levels of organization is important in its own right and advances in each area complement the others, clinical neurology is ultimately most concerned with the behavioral consequences of brain disease and drugs used to treat those diseases. Thus, the emphasis in this chapter is on correlating the rapidly increasing knowledge of molecular and cellular mechanisms of drug action in the central nervous system (CNS) with brain diseases for which those drugs are used. However, readers should consult individual chapters on specific diseases for details of treatment.

Principles of Chemical Synaptic Transmission

The Nobel laureate neuropharmacologist Julius Axelrod once described the brain as "Nature's finest chemical factory." This is a convenient starting point in a discussion of neuropharmacology and emphasizes an underlying principle: Neurons communicate by releasing chemical neurotransmitters, and all CNS-active drugs act by influencing directly or indirectly the normal process of *synap-*

tic transmission. Drug influences on synaptic transmission may be general, such as the ability of general anesthetics to perturb multiple ion channels, but usually are more specific and involve interactions with one or more receptor molecules. These drug-receptor interactions ultimately mediate both the desired therapeutic actions and frequently troublesome side effects.

Overview of Synaptic Transmission

Effective synaptic transmission requires that the neuron synthesize, store, and release physiologically the neurotransmitter chemical. In many cases, the presynaptic terminal is also responsible for terminating the action of the neurotransmitter, usually by reuptake through specific transport molecules (Figure 8-1).

Neurotransmitter Synthesis

In general, neurotransmitters are specialized molecules that serve few if any other purposes. In some cases, specifically certain amino acid transmitters, such as glutamate or glycine, or the purine transmitter adenosine, the neurotransmitter compartment can be either drawn from the general metabolic pool or provided by specific synthetic pathways. Examples of the latter include conversion of serine to glycine by the enzyme serine transhydroxymethylase or synthesis of glutamic acid from glutamine. Glutamate-utilizing neurons possess the enzyme glutaminase, which makes use of glutamine manufactured in glia (from glutamate by glutamine synthetase). Thus, a circular pathway is established whereby glia surrounding the glutamate synapse assist in removing glutamate, convert it to glutamine, and recycle it back to the glutamate neuron. In other cases, such as for gamma-aminobutyric acid (GABA) or acetylcholine, the neurotransmitter substance is synthesized in a single step from substances in the general metabolic pool (glutamate for GABA, choline and acetyl-CoA for acetylcholine). Biogenic amine transmitters, such as dopamine, norepinephrine, and serotonin, are formed in multiple-step reactions from dietary amino acids. In all cases, at least one enzyme responsible for neurotransmitter synthesis is localized specifically to neu-

rons and nerve endings that utilize that transmitter substance (Table 8-1).

For neuropeptides, the typical scenario is that a precursor peptide is manufactured in the soma and moved by axonal transport to distal endings. There it is cleaved by specific or shared enzymes to the final product. Many precursor peptides are designated by the prefix "prepro-"; examples include preprotachykinin (for substance P and related neurokinins), preproenkephalin (for the delta-opiate peptides leucine-enkephalin and methionine-enkephalin), and preprodynorphin (for the opiate peptide dynorphin).

A general principle in synaptic transmission is that the synthesis and release of neurotransmitters are highly regulated processes. For neurotransmitter synthesis, two basic types of control mechanisms are utilized: regulation of activity of synthetic enzyme or control of availability of substrate. Dopamine terminals are an excellent example of the first type of synthetic control. The rate-limiting step in dopamine synthesis is the enzyme tyrosine hydroxylase, which produces L-dopa, the immediate precursor of dopamine. L-Dopa is rapidly converted to dopamine by an excess activity of dopa-decarboxylase (L-aromatic amino acid decarboxylase). Tyrosine hydroxylase is normally saturated with substrate (tyrosine), and its activity level is controlled by the phosphorylation state of the enzyme and availability of and affinity for its tetrahydrobiopterin cofactor. Activation of tyrosine hydroxylase is associated with an increase in affinity for cofactor. A major regulatory component in enzyme phosphorylation is the dopamine receptors located on the presynaptic nerve ending (autoreceptors), which sense synaptic dopamine levels and increase or decrease tyrosine hydroxylase activity as needed.

Synthesis of serotonin and acetylcholine is an example of the second type of regulation of synthesis. Tryptophan hydroxylase is rate-limiting for serotonin synthesis but is normally not saturated with substrate (L-tryptophan). Thus, tryptophan availability to serotonin neurons determines their serotonin levels. Increased dietary tryptophan intake (and resultant increased blood tryptophan levels) increases serotonin levels and synaptic activity at serotonin synapses. Acetylcholine synthesis depends on availability of choline, which in turn is controlled by activity of the presynaptic choline transporter. Increased activity of cholinergic

Figure 8-1. A typical presynaptic terminal. Axon microtubules transport neurotransmitter synthetic enzymes and neuropeptide precursors to terminals. In some cases (e.g., acetylcholine), a specific presynaptic transporter accumulates the neurotransmitter precursor (choline). Synthesized neurotransmitter is packaged into vesicles, which fuse with the synaptic membrane and release neurotransmitter when a depolarizing wave reaches the terminal and calcium ion enters through voltage-dependent channels. For many neurotransmitters, specific transporters reaccumulate the transmitter and terminate its synaptic action. (NT = neurotransmitter.)

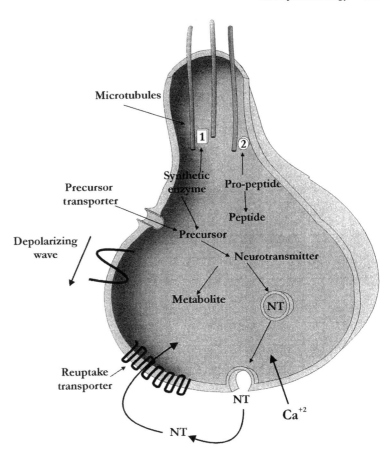

pathways (the septo-hippocampal and habenular-interpeduncular pathways are two of the best studied) yields increased activity of the choline transporter by increasing the apparent affinity of the transporter for choline. This leads to increased presynaptic choline levels and stimulates acetylcholine synthesis.

Neurotransmitter Catabolism

Degradation of neurotransmitters is accomplished by enzymes that are either utilized by a class of transmitters or appear to be neurotransmitter specific. An example of a degrading enzyme used by a neurotransmitter class is monoamine oxidase (MAO) for the biogenic amines (i.e., norepinephrine, dopamine, and serotonin). Two major isoforms of MAO have been identified (type A and B), and they share extensive conservation of their primary sequences. Type

A preferentially oxidatively deaminates serotonin to 5-hydroxyindoleacetic acid, and type B preferentially degrades dopamine to homovanillic acid. Both isoforms of MAO are localized to the outer mitochondrial membrane.

Examples of neurotransmitter-specific degrading enzymes include GABA-transaminase (GABA-T), which is a mitochondrially localized enzyme that converts GABA to succinic acid semialdehyde, which is then oxidized to succinic acid. GABA-T thus allows GABA to be utilized as a metabolic substrate. Another example is acetylcholinesterase, which degrades acetylcholine back to choline and acetate.

From Molecules to Bedside: Inhibition of Neurotransmitter Catabolism and Treatment of Epilepsy
Advances in epilepsy therapeutics have involved drugs that manipulate GABA synaptic function. One class of such agents are those that inhibit GABA breakdown, specifically the "suicide sub-

Table 8-1. Representative Small Molecule Neurotransmitters

Transmitter	Source	Action	Localization
Glutamic acid	Synthesized from glutamine, amino acid pool	Excitatory	Throughout gray matter
Glycine	Synthesized from serine, amino acid pool	Inhibitory	Spinal cord, brain stem, mainly interneurons
GABA	Decarboxylation of glutamate	Inhibitory	Throughout gray matter, both projection neurons and interneurons
Acetylcholine	Choline and acetyl-CoA	Generally excitatory	Throughout gray matter, projection neurons from septum and nucleus basalis, interneurons in striatum
Dopamine	Hydroxylation of tyrosine, followed by decarboxylation of dopa	Excitatory or inhibitory	Projection neurons with cell bodies in midbrain, paracrine neurons in hypothalamus (regulate prolactin secretion)
Histamine	Decarboxylation of histidine		Projection neurons in posterobasal hypothalamus and reticular formation
Norepinephrine	Hydroxylation of dopamine	Inhibitory	Projection neurons with cell bodies in medulla (locus ceruleus)
Serotonin	Hydroxylation of tryptophan followed by decarboxylation of 5-hydroxytryptophan	Inhibitory	Projection neurons in pons/midbrain (raphe nuclei groups)

GABA = gamma-aminobutyric acid.

strate" inhibitors of GABA-T. GABA-T is a mitochondrial enzyme that enables GABA to be used as a metabolic substrate for energy production. In this reaction gamma-acetylenic GABA is utilized as a substrate for GABA-T, and in the course of being acted on by the enzyme, is converted to a reactive intermediate that covalently attacks the enzyme active site and irreversibly inactivates it (Figure 8-2). A related compound, gamma-vinyl GABA (GVG) has been developed for use in humans with epilepsy. GVG treatment of animals can elevate brain GABA levels many-fold, and GVG administration to humans leads to elevated GABA levels in the cerebrospinal fluid. The efficacy of GVG as an anticonvulsant derives from its elevation of synaptic levels of GABA, the major inhibitory transmitter in the forebrain.

Neuropeptides and Neuromodulators

Evolving concepts of neurotransmitter action include both classic neurotransmitters, typically small molecules that alter neuronal firing by interacting with specific postsynaptic receptors, and neuromodulators, which can be either small molecules (e.g., prostaglandins) or peptides that act by altering the actions of classical transmitters. The term *neuropep-*

tide refers to small oligopeptides, usually less than 30 amino acids long, that are found in specific central neurons. Many neuropeptides are also commonly found in enteric neurons. Within the CNS, some neuropeptides are found in neuronal populations that utilize classic transmitters such as dopamine or GABA (Table 8-2). Although much is known about the anatomic localization of neuropeptides and molecular machinery for their synthesis, much less is known about their physiologic functions. Exceptions include the enkephalins, small 5-amino-acid peptides that can stimulate mu and delta opiate receptors and produce analgesia. For other neuropeptides, their predominant actions appear to be to modify the effects of classical neurotransmitters. Examples of this type of action include the enhancement by somatostatin of excitatory actions of acetylcholine and inhibition of dopamine actions by cholecystokinin.

Neurotransmitter Storage and Release

From a purely functional perspective, the brain needs only one excitatory and one inhibitory transmitter to control neuronal firing. The fact that a number of excitatory and inhibitory substances exist, with differing potencies and subtle variations in both mecha-

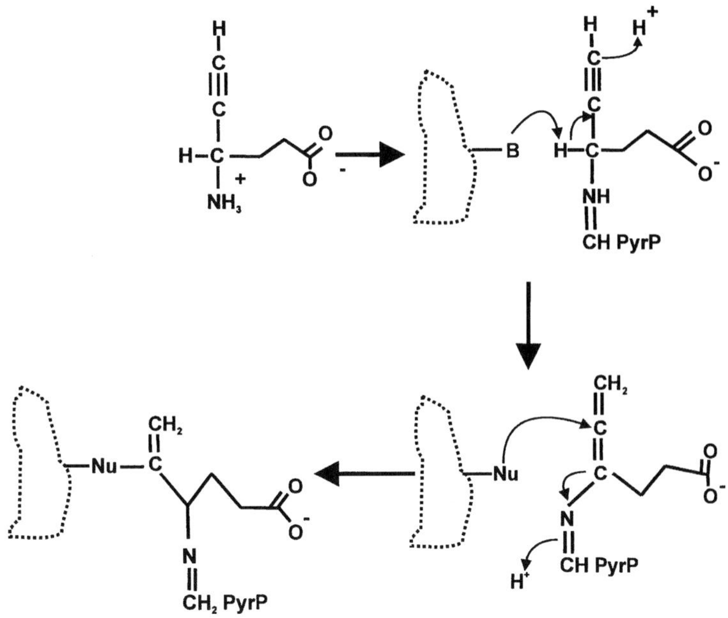

Figure 8-2. Presumed mechanism of irreversible gamma-aminobutyric acid (GABA)-transaminase (GABA-T) inhibition by gamma-acetylenic GABA (GAG), a "suicide substrate." The enzyme active site ("B") extracts a proton to the Schiff base formed with pyridoxal phosphate cofactor (PyrP). A nucleophilic residue on the enzyme is then covalently added to the allene group, leading to enzyme inactivation. Acute GABA-T inhibition has revealed that GABA is rapidly turned over. Brain GABA levels can rise up to sixfold in a few hours after experimental animals are treated with the related compound gamma-vinyl GABA. (Adapted from BW Metcalf, P Casara. Regiospecific 1,4 addition of a propargylic anion. A general synthon for 2-substituted propargylamines as potential catalytic irreversible enzyme inhibitors. Tetrahedron Letters 1975;38:3337–3340).

Table 8-2. Examples of Neuropeptide Colocalization with Classic Neurotransmitters and Other Neuropeptides

Neuropeptide	Colocalized with	Location
Substance P	GABA	Striatonigral neurons
	Calcitonin gene–related peptide	Spinal afferents
Enkephalins	GABA	Striatopallidal neurons
Dynorphin	GABA	Striatonigral neurons
Cholecystokinin	Dopamine	Nigrostriatal and mesolimbic neurons
Somatostatin	Neuropeptide Y, nitric oxide	Striatal interneurons, cortical and limbic neurons

GABA = gamma-aminobutyric acid.

nisms of action and effects on neuronal firing, attests to the extensive degree of chemical "fine-tuning" that has evolved. Because most neurotransmitter substances require at least one specialized chemical step (and therefore a specialized enzyme), neurotransmitters are relatively precious molecules to the cell and must be stored to protect them from intracellular degradation, released only under appropriate circumstances, and conserved. Known intracellular neuro-

transmitter storage mechanisms typically utilize storage vesicles, which are membrane-bound organelles typically found at synaptic endings. In the case of biogenic amines, genes for specific vesicle transport proteins have been cloned and sequenced. It is likely that similar mechanisms also exist for amino acid neurotransmitters and acetylcholine.

Neurotransmitter release occurs when a depolarizing wave invades the nerve terminal and allows calcium influx into the terminal through voltage-sensitive calcium channels. Thus, most neurotransmitter release is a calcium ion–dependent process. Once released, neurotransmitters are subject to competing forces. A molecule can diffuse across the synapse and bind to one or more specific transmitter receptors or be reaccumulated back into the synapse by specific presynaptic reuptake systems. These reuptake sites typically function by sodium ion gradient–driven, carrier-mediated diffusion but are capable of concentrating neurotransmitters several-fold into the presynaptic ending. They serve both to terminate the action of the transmitter substance and to conserve the neurotransmitter. In some cases, specifically that of acetylcholine, synaptic actions are terminated by hydrolysis to its precursors—choline and acetate. Choline is then reaccumulated into the presynaptic ending by a specific transport system so that acetylcholine synthesis can continue.

Presynaptic receptors, including autoreceptors in some cases, participate in regulation of neurotransmitter release. In the case of dopamine terminals, presynaptic receptors of the D_2 and in some areas the D_3 subtypes control the coupling between depolarization and neurotransmitter release. The presynaptic D_2 receptors increase K^+ current, hyperpolarizing the terminal and making it directly resistant to depolarization. Thus, an excess of synaptic dopamine will decrease both its synthesis (by decreasing tyrosine hydroxylase activity) and release (by hyperpolarizing the terminal).

Other neurotransmitter receptors participate in control of release of different transmitters by alternative mechanisms. One of the most widely utilized transmitter receptors for this purpose is the GABA-B subtype. Presynaptic GABA-B receptors block calcium influx, which is necessary for neurotransmitter release. In this manner, they regulate release of multiple substances, including excitatory glutamic acid and nociceptive substance P neuropeptide.

From Molecules to Bedside: Inhibition of Neurotransmitter Release and the Relief of Spasticity
Spasticity arises when spinal cord– and brain stem–mediated muscle stretch reflexes are removed from upper motor neuron suppression and operate under unopposed cerebellar facilitation. One mode of treatment of spasticity involves treatment with baclofen, an agonist at GABA-B receptors. A major site of baclofen action is the presynaptic GABA-B receptor, which is now known to function through-

out the CNS, not just at the spinal cord and brain stem. As shown in Figure 8-3, presynaptic GABA-B receptors block calcium entry through several subtypes of voltage-regulated calcium channels and thus inhibit release of neurotransmitter after nerve terminal depolarization. Inhibition of release of glutamate from spinal cord afferents likely accounts for a substantial portion of baclofen's actions in relieving spasticity. Activation of postsynaptic GABA-B receptors may also play a role. Postsynaptic GABA-B receptors hyperpolarize by increasing K^+ current.

From Molecules to Bedside: Antidepressants and the Therapeutic Effects of Inhibiting Neurotransmitter Uptake
Effective treatment of biological depression is very important to clinical neurology because of the high risk of depression associated with neurodegenerative diseases, poststroke syndromes, and the debilitation associated with chronic neurologic illnesses. Previously used tricyclic antidepressants possessed a multitude of effects on synaptic function, obscuring their potential underlying mechanisms of action. The development of highly selective inhibitors of neurotransmitter uptake transporters has lent additional support to the biogenic amine hypothesis of depression. The most extensively developed are the selective serotonin reuptake inhibitors, which act as antagonists of the serotonin transporter. The serotonin transporter is structurally similar to other transporter molecules that have been cloned and analyzed, including the norepinephrine and dopamine transporters (Figure 8-4). These transporters have 12 potential transmembrane segments. The observation that three clinically useful antidepressants (fluoxetine, paroxetine [Paxil], and sertraline [Zoloft]) all have selective interactions with the 5-hydroxytryptophan transporter and little interaction with other known transporters or neurotransmitter receptors suggests that augmentation of synaptic activity of serotonin alone can be effective treatment of depression.

Neurotransmitter Receptor Interactions: Principles of Receptor Function

Neurotransmitter- and drug-receptor interactions are best conceptualized and modeled by reversible, steady-state kinetic models. There are three underlying assumptions for this commonly used model of drug and neurotransmitter action. First, drug/neurotransmitter binding is reversible. This has been shown to be the case for all classic neurotransmitters studied

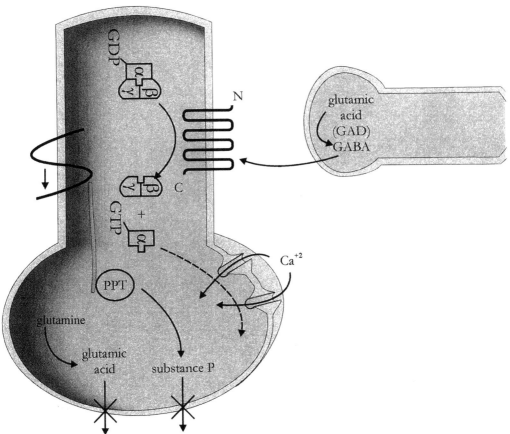

Figure 8-3. Presynaptic inhibition by gamma-aminobutyric acid (GABA) acting at GABA-B receptors. Shown on the left is a nerve ending that releases glutamic acid and substance P. This type of ending can be found in the dorsal gray matter of the spinal cord. Shown to the right is a GABA-releasing ending that exerts presynaptic inhibitory activity on the glutamate synapse. Released GABA (formed from glutamic acid by glutamate decarboxylase [GAD]) interacts with the metabotropic GABA-B receptor, shown with its seven transmembrane segments and extracellular amino (N) and intracellular carboxy (C) ends. Activation of the GABA-B receptor, as is the case for all G protein–coupled receptors, leads to exchange of guanosine triphosphate (GTP) for the guanosine diphosphate (GDP) normally bound to the a subunit and dissociation of the α GTP subunit. This leads to blockade of calcium ion entry into the presynaptic ending when a depolarizing wave enters (shown on left). Substance P, the nociceptive transmitter of dorsal gray pain fibers, and glutamic acid (formed from glutamine) cannot be released because presynaptic calcium entry is blocked. (PPT = preprotachykinin.)

directly. Second, a finite number of specific receptor sites per unit of tissue exists. Third, the biological action or actions associated with drug/neurotransmitter binding to these specific receptor sites are related to the degree of receptor occupancy. These assumptions allow use of binding equations such as the following:

$$[drug] + [receptor] \underset{k_{+1}}{\overset{k_{-1}}{\rightleftarrows}} [drug\text{-}receptor]$$

where k_{+1} and k_{-1} refer to the rate constants for the forward (association) and reverse (dissociation) reac-

tions, respectively, and [drug-receptor] refers to the concentration of drug-receptor complex. At a steady state, the rate of the forward reaction equals the rate of the reverse reaction:

$$k_{+1}[drug][receptor] = k_{-1}[drug\text{-}receptor]$$

The *equilibrium dissociation binding constant*, K_D, is the ratio of k_{-1}/k_{+1} and equals the following:

$$K_D = [drug][receptor]/[drug\text{-}receptor]$$

Thus, drugs or neurotransmitters that bind to their receptors with very high affinity have K_Ds that are

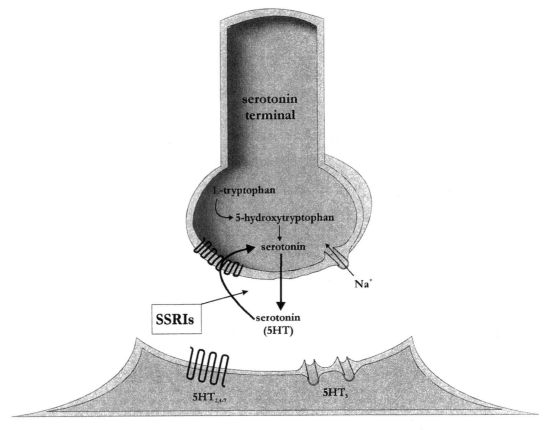

Figure 8-4. Blockade of serotonin reuptake by selective serotonin reuptake inhibitor (SSRI) antidepressants. Shown is a representative serotonin terminal. Serotonin is formed by decarboxylation of 5-hydroxytryptophan (5HT) by the action of the enzyme tryptophan hydroxylase. Tryptophan hydroxylase is normally not saturated with its substrate L-tryptophan, and increasing terminal L-tryptophan levels will increase serotonin synthesis. Released serotonin can interact with either metabotropic ($5HT_{2,4-7}$) or inotropic ($5HT_3$) postsynaptic receptors and is reaccumulated back into the terminal by the serotonin transporter. It shares structural characteristics with other biogenic amine transporters by having 12 transmembrane segments and being operated by the sodium ion gradient.

small in absolute magnitude and vice versa. The potencies of drugs in their interactions with a given neurotransmitter receptor site are commonly defined experimentally in terms of their K_D, which defines the binding affinity of that substance to the receptor. A hypothetical neurotransmitter-receptor binding interaction is presented in Figure 8-5.

Drugs generally act at neurotransmitter receptors either as agonists, mimicking the molecular effects of the endogenous substance, or as antagonists, blocking the actions of the neurotransmitter. In practice, many agonist drugs do not possess the full intrinsic activity of the natural substance and are more properly considered partial agonists. Relevant examples of clinically used partial agonists are the ergot-derived drugs bromocriptine and pergolide, used as dopamine agonists in treating Parkinson's disease or pituitary prolactin-secreting tumors. Drugs that are either precursors of a neurotransmitter (e.g., L-dopa for dopamine), release the transmitter (e.g., amphetamine for dopamine or norepinephrine), or block degradation of the neurotransmitter (e.g., GVG for GABA) are referred to as *indirect agonists.*

Clinically used antagonists are generally full antagonists and possess no agonist activity. For members of the benzodiazepine (BZ) family, a special situation exists with regard to antagonists. Pure antagonists, such as the clinically useful drug flumazenil, serve only to block the actions of exogenous BZ agonists (e.g., diazepam, lorazepam). A special class of BZs

Figure 8-5. Hypothetical binding curve for a neurotransmitter binding to a single homogeneous receptor population. The curve demonstrates the property of saturability. B_{max} refers to the maximum number of specific receptor sites available for neurotransmitter binding. Shown in the inset is a Scatchard plot, which is a linear transformation of binding data used to estimate the equilibrium dissociation binding constant (K_D). (B/F = [bound ligand]/[free ligand]; B = [bound ligand].)

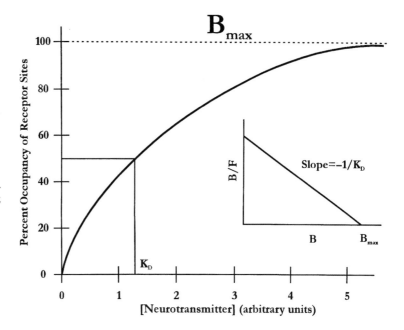

known as *inverse agonists* cause effects opposite to agonists; in other words, they produce seizures. These interactions are diagrammed in Figure 8-6.

Secondary Actions of Neurotransmitters

Known neurotransmitters bring about one of two general actions on neurons or other receptive cells. First, agonist binding can be directly linked to opening a particular ion channel. Receptors that operate in this manner are called *inotropic*. Representatives of inotropic receptors include several amino acids such as glutamate, GABA-A, and glycine (Table 8-3). Other receptors are *metabotropic* and couple through guanine nucleotide–binding proteins to stimulate second messenger systems, such as those responsible for production of cyclic adenosine monophosphate (cAMP) or diacylglycerol/inositol triphosphate. All of the known biogenic amine receptors (i.e., dopamine, norepinephrine, serotonin, muscarinic acetylcholine), a subclass of glutamate receptors, and GABA-B receptors are metabotropic (see Table 8-3).

Modern molecular biology cloning techniques have allowed isolation of the genes for and determination of the primary amino acid sequences of many inotropic and metabotropic receptors, and there are substantial differences between the two families that

have relevance to drug action in the CNS. Inotropic receptors are formed of multiple subunits that associate in heterogeneous formulas to produce functioning receptors. An excellent example is the GABA-A receptor family (Figure 8-7). GABA-A receptors account for the majority of GABA receptors, are coupled to opening an ion channel that passes chloride ion, and generally hyperpolarize the neuron. GABA-A receptors are composed of pentamers of four separate subunits, referred to as α, β, γ, and δ. In the retina is found a fifth subunit, known as r, which combines to form a separate class of GABA receptors known as GABA-C. There are 13 different genes for these subunits: six for α, three for β, three for γ, and one for δ. If these subunits combined randomly, there would be more than 100,000 different combinations of GABA-A receptors. However, there appears to be a preferred combination formula (2 α + 1 β + 2 γ), with 1 δ being able to substitute for 1 γ. With these restrictions, there are approximately 137 combinations. This is potential receptor heterogeneity at its finest, and undoubtedly accounts for the subtle variations in actions of a given GABA agonist in different brain regions. Different combinations of the six a subunits confers varying specificities to BZ agonists, allowing for the presence of type 1 (zolpidem-preferring) or type 2 BZ receptors. One of the challenges of modern mol-

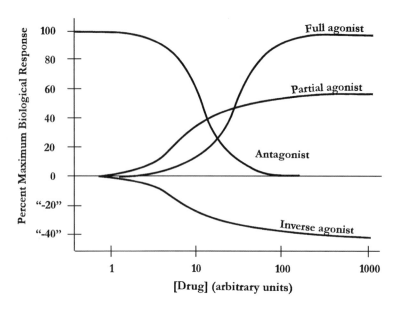

Figure 8-6. Actions of agonists and antagonists at neurotransmitter receptors. A full agonist brings approximately 100% of the maximum biological response but may not need to occupy 100% of receptor sites to do this (i.e., there may be "spare receptors"). A partial agonist cannot bring about a complete response, and an inverse agonist brings about an "opposite" response to that of the neurotransmitter. A pure antagonist only blocks agonist actions.

Table 8-3. Inotropic and Metabotropic Neurotransmitter Receptors

Transmitter	Receptor Subtype	Inotropic (I) or Metabotropic (M)	Second Messenger(s)	Ion Channel(s)
Glutamate	NMDA	I	(–)	Cations, including Ca^{+2}
	AMPA	I	(–)	Na^+
	Kainate	I	(–)	Na^+
	Metabotropic	M	cAMP, IP_3/DAG	
GABA	A	I	(–)	Cl^-
	B	M	cAMP	
Dopamine	D_1, D_5	M	cAMP	
	D_2, D_3, D_4	M	cAMP	K^+, Ca^{+2}
Norepinephrine	Alpha	M	cAMP, IP_3/DAG	
	Beta	M	cAMP	
Serotonin	$5HT_2$	M	IP_3/DAG	
	$5HT_3$	I	(–)	Nonselective cation
	$5HT_{1, 4-7}$	M	cAMP	
Acetylcholine	Muscarinic	M	IP_3/DAG	
	Nicotinic	I	(–)	Na^+, Ca^{+2}
Histamine	H_1	M	IP_3/DAG	
	H_2	M	cAMP	
	H_3	M(?)	?	
Adenosine	A_1	M	cAMP	
	A_2	M	cAMP	

NMDA = N-methyl-D-aspartate; GABA = gamma-aminobutyric acid; cAMP = cyclic adenosine monophosphate; IP_3/DAG = inositol triphosphate/diacylglycerol; 5HT = 5-hydroxytryptophan.

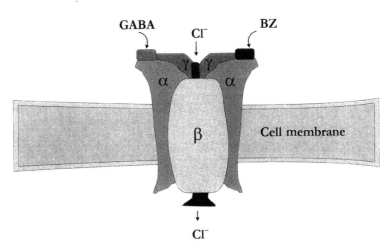

Figure 8-7. The gamma-aminobutyric acid (GABA)-A receptor complex. Shown is a hypothetical pentameric GABA-A receptor complex composed of two alpha subunits, two gamma subunits, and one beta subunit. Separate GABA and benzodiazepine (BZ) binding sites are shown. Cl⁻ and corresponding arrows designate the chloride channel opened by the GABA receptor.

ecular neurobiology is to understand both the anatomic and neurophysiologic variations in receptor subunit heterogeneity and to determine the cellular regulation in health and disease of receptor subunit expression and assembly. For instance, it is unclear exactly how many and in what regions different combinations of pentamers for GABA-A receptors are expressed, and how these combinations vary in disease states such as epilepsy.

From Molecules to Bedside: Benzodiazepines and Modulation of GABA-A Receptor Function
The wide varieties of BZ action, including sedation and antianxiety effects, muscle relaxation, and relief of seizures, appear to derive from specific interactions of BZs with GABA-A receptors. The degree to which a given BZ binds to a regulatory site on the GABA-A receptor depends on the subunit composition (see text for details). Once BZ binding occurs, receptor affinity for GABA increases, which potentiates the capacity of available GABA to open chloride channels and increase neuronal hyperpolarization (Figure 8-8).

Metabotropic receptors follow a more stereotyped structure (Figure 8-9). They are composed of lipophilic stretches of amino acids that are believed to lie within the membrane, with connecting hydrophilic loops that lie in either the extracellular or intracellular spaces. Attached are hydrophilic amino terminals, which are extracellular, and carboxy terminals, which are intracellular. These receptors have highly conserved primary structures for the seven lipophilic transmembrane segments and differ from each other primarily in the structures of their amino and carboxy tails and the primary structure of the intracellular cytoplasmic "loops."

Mutation studies have shown that the third cytoplasmic loop appears to be important for determining with which family of guanine nucleotide binding protein (G protein) the receptor interacts. This is important for determining the ultimate actions of an agonist acting at a given receptor in terms of how the second messenger system is regulated. As an example, if the receptor couples to the G_s, or stimulatory G protein, then activation of the receptor will lead to stimulation of the second messenger system, such as adenylate cyclase. In contrast, coupling to G_i, or inhibitory G protein, will have the opposite effect on second messenger synthesis.

Receptor Desensitization

It has been known for decades that for most receptor-mediated processes, continuous exposure to agonist shifts the dose-response curve to the right (desensitizes). Recent knowledge of primary receptor structure and the ability to express specific receptor subunits in cultured cells have produced insight into how desensitization occurs. For inotropic receptors, desensitization can be rapid, may derive from the phosphorylation state of one or more subunits (e.g., *N*-methyl-D-aspartate [NMDA] glutamate or GABA-A receptors), and can lead to disruption of coupling of receptor subunits to ion channels, increased receptor internalization, and decreased receptor synthesis.

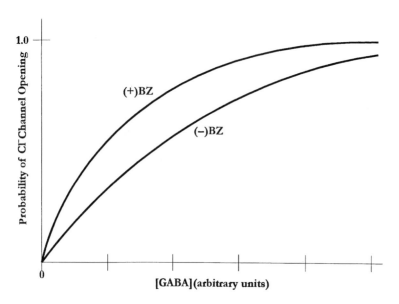

Figure 8-8. Potentiation of gamma-aminobutyric acid (GABA)-A receptor activity by benzodiazepines (BZs). Shown is a hypothetical curve relating the concentration of GABA and the probability of opening the chloride channel operated by the GABA-A receptor complex. The addition of BZ shifts the dose-response curve for GABA to the left and makes it more likely that a given synaptic GABA level will open chloride channels.

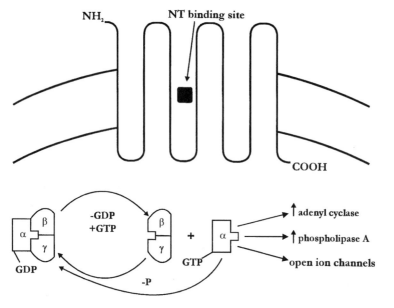

Figure 8-9. A typical metabotropic neurotransmitter receptor. This type of receptor is used by many different neurotransmitters throughout the central nervous system. Shown are the extracellular amino and intracellular carboxy tails, separated by seven transmembrane segments, which form three intracellular and three extracellular loops. The neurotransmitter binding sites are believed to lie deep within the transmembrane segments. Neurotransmitter binding leads to dissociation of guanosine diphosphate (GDP) from the heterotrimeric G protein complex and binding of guanosine triphosphate (GTP) to the alpha subunit. The α-GTP complex then can activate (or in some cases inhibit) second messenger systems or open ion channels. The alpha subunit possesses GTPase activity, so the GTP is eventually hydrolyzed to GDP and the heterotrimeric complex can reform. The α-GTP complex formation lowers affinity for agonist binding by the receptor, and the GDP-bound heterotrimeric complex restores high-affinity agonist binding. (NT = neurotransmitter.)

Figure 8-10. Hypothetical concentration-response curves for changes in receptor affinity. Continuous agonist exposure typically desensitizes receptors and shifts response curves to the right (*arrow A*). Neurotransmitter deficiency or continuous antagonist exposure can make receptors supersensitive and shift the response curve to the left (*arrow B*). As discussed in the text, changes in receptor sensitivity may occur by several mechanisms. If biological response correlates linearly with receptor occupancy (and it may not for a variety of reasons) and if there are no "spare" receptors, then the curves for neurotransmitter receptor binding, and biological responses will be superimposable.

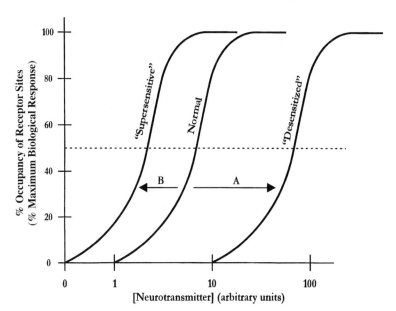

For metabotropic receptors, the molecular mechanisms of receptor desensitization are more completely known. Very short-term regulation of receptor agonist affinity appears to be controlled by the relative amount of completely assembled G protein heterotrimer (α, β, and γ subunits), which binds guanosine diphosphate and keeps the receptor in a high-affinity state for agonist compared with the amount of dissociated G protein, in which the α subunit binds guanosine triphosphate and switches receptors to low affinity for agonist (see Figure 8-9).

A major pathway for longer-term metabotropic receptor desensitization is G protein-coupled receptor kinases, which, when activated, phosphorylate the receptor. The phosphorylated receptor then binds to a family of cytoplasmic proteins called *arrestins,* which serve to uncouple the receptor from interacting with G proteins. Prolonged receptor occupancy by agonists can lead to increased receptor internalization and loss of receptor density on the membrane surface. Hypothetical dose-response curves for supersensitive and desensitized receptors are shown in Figure 8-10.

Nitric Oxide: A Novel Gaseous Free Radical Neurotransmitter

Traditional concepts of neurotransmitter identity and action have had to be modified to accommo-

date evolving knowledge about the function of nitric oxide (NO) in the nervous system. NO appears to be used throughout the body, serving both common and unique functions in different tissues. NO is a gaseous free radical that is synthesized by several isoforms of NO synthase (NOS), with the general reaction involving conversion of L-arginine to L-citrulline. NOS is expressed either constitutively as in the neuronal isoform, or is inducible, which is the isoform typically found in microglia and other inflammatory cells. The constitutive isoform has an absolute requirement for the calcium-calmodulin complex, whereas the inducible isoform has very high affinity for and is normally saturated with calcium-calmodulin. Thus, the constitutive NOS isoform in NOS-producing neurons is always available for NO production, and its activity is determined by intracellular levels of calcium-calmodulin. Inducible NOS is made on demand, typically as a result of the stimulation of inflammatory cells by chemical messengers such as cytokines (Figure 8-11).

The physiologic actions of NO in the brain are still being defined. NO appears to function as a "second messenger," which stimulates guanylate cyclase activity, increasing production of the "third messenger," cyclic guanosine monophosphate (cGMP). cGMP in turn can activate a variety of protein kinase enzymes, whose functions

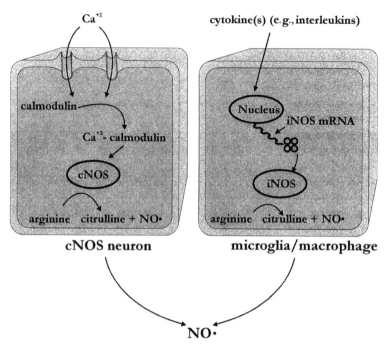

Figure 8-11. Production of nitric oxide (NO) by constitutive and inducible mechanisms. In neurons containing constitutively expressed nitric oxide synthase (cNOS), calcium ion entry appears to exert major control over NOS activity through formation of calcium-calmodulin complexes. Phosphorylation of cNOS also regulates its activity. In cells with inducible NOS capacity, appropriate extracellular stimuli activate transcription of the *iNOS* gene, leading to rapid increases in intracellular iNOS protein. (iNOS = inducible nitric oxide synthase.)

are to phosphorylate other proteins. Drugs that block NOS activity interfere with the acquisition of long-term potentiation, which is a type of synaptic memory. Much more is known about the apparent involvement of NO in models of neurotoxicity. Neuronal NOS activity is increased when NMDA glutamate receptors are activated, probably as a result of increased intracellular calcium levels. NO appears to be involved in and may mediate excitotoxicity caused by a variety of stimuli, such as status epilepticus, hypoxia-ischemia, and hypoglycemia. In addition, mice made neuronal NOS-deficient by gene knockout or treated with NOS inhibitors resist damage to dopamine nerve endings in experimental MPTP parkinsonism, suggesting that NOS may play a role in chronic neurodegenerative diseases such as Parkinson's disease.

NO can have several damaging actions, but by itself it appears to have limited toxicity. Rather, interaction of NO with superoxide anion, commonly formed from the mitochondrial electron transport chain during normal metabolic activity, can lead to the production of a more damaging species, peroxynitrite ion (Figure 8-12). Peroxynitrite appears capable of nitrosylating proteins and

degrading nonenzymatically to hydroxyl radical, which is a highly reactive oxygen free radical that can also attack DNA (see Figure 8-12).

From Molecules to Bedside: Nitric Oxide and Potential Protection from Neurotoxicity

Although not yet in use in humans, agents that modify NO actions in the nervous system will likely enter the clinical trial arena shortly for neural protection after stroke or status epilepticus. NO is a gaseous, diffusible free radical formed by the actions of one or more isoforms of NO synthase on arginine. The major neuronal isoform of NOS is dependent on calcium-calmodulin and can be stimulated by calcium influx into cells after activation of NMDA glutamate receptors (see Figure 8-11). Many acute neurodegenerative models for hypoxia-ischemia, status epilepticus, and hypoglycemia have shown that blockade of NMDA receptors or NOS activity increases neuronal survival. NO appears to function normally as a stimulator of guanylate cyclase, leading to an increase in cGMP production. In states of pathologic overproduction of NO, more reactive free radical species such as peroxynitrite may be formed (see Figure 8-12). Peroxynitrite can damage intracellular proteins and DNA and is an inhibitor of the mitochondrial electron transport chain. Thus, NOS

Figure 8-12. Nitric oxide (NO) as a neurotoxic substance. Situations leading to increased NO production (e.g., high activity at N-methyl-D-aspartate [NMDA] glutamate receptors) or to oxidative stress and increased superoxide ($O_2 \cdot$) production from the mitochondrial electron transport chain can increase intracellular levels of toxic peroxynitrite anion. Peroxynitrite can nitrosylate tyrosine residues in proteins and nonenzymatically decay to the reactive hydroxyl free radical (OH·). This in turn can hydroxylate nucleotide residues in DNA.

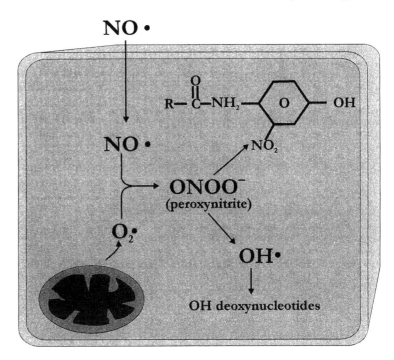

inhibition in the short term can ameliorate excessive NO production, which appears to be a major mediator of neuronal damage.

Long-Term Molecular Effects of Neurotransmitters

In addition to acute effects on neuronal firing, many different classes of neurotransmitters appear to have the potential to alter neuronal function in a more chronic manner. This concept is based on observations that expression of several different immediate early genes, also known as transcription factors, is increased in vitro and in vivo in response to neurotransmitter receptor activation. Immediate early genes code for proteins that appear to serve functions restricted to activating or inhibiting expression of other genes.

The two neurotransmitters studied most extensively are the NMDA glutamate and dopamine systems. In the case of dopamine, the cAMP-mediated intracellular signaling cascades responsible for increased expression of some immediate early genes is known (Figure 8-13). Although these pathways have been defined in several systems, what is not known are the downstream effects of the immediate early genes that are activated. In other words, what further genes are activated and what are the net effects on neuronal functions? At the moment, immediate early gene activation by neurotransmitters provides only potential pathways for additional molecular control of neuronal function.

Conclusion

The human CNS can be viewed as a rich mixture of chemical synapses that utilize multiple molecules of varying complexity and sources. These synapses are regulated at all levels of neurotransmitter synthesis, release, reuptake, and interactions with presynaptic and postsynaptic receptors. Specificity of neurotransmitter action depends mainly on receptors, and the same transmitter chemical can have a multiplicity of actions, depending on the receptor with which it interacts. Neurotransmitter receptors have both short-term (opening of ion channels, stimulation of

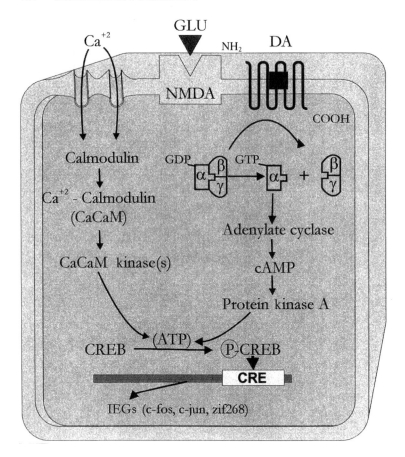

Figure 8-13. Potential mechanisms for long-term molecular effects of neurotransmitters. Increased activity at either *N*-methyl-D-aspartate (NMDA) glutamate or dopamine receptors has been shown to lead to activation by phosphorylation at serine 133 of cyclic AMP-responsive element binding protein (CREB). Activated CREB then can bind to the cyclic AMP-responsive element (CRE) sequences of many genes, leading to increased transcription. There is minimal knowledge about what these "downstream genes" are, but several transcription factors, or "immediate early genes" (IEGs), are activated by CREB-dependent pathways. These IEGs are believed to regulate transcription of additional genes, which ultimately provide long-term molecular changes in neuronal function. (GLU = glutamic acid; DA = dopamine; GDP = guanosine diphosphate; GTP = guanosine triphosphate; cAMP = cyclic adenosine monophosphate; ATP = adenosine triphosphate.)

second messengers) and long-term (activation of immediate early gene cascades) effects on neurons. Novel substances such as NO have pointed out the delicate balance that exists between normal, beneficial actions of transmitters and the destructive, neurotoxic effects of transmitter excess.

There are multiple points at which these basic principles of neuropharmacology can be and are manipulated for therapeutic benefits. As knowledge of the molecular identities and peculiarities of neurotransmitter receptors and transporters are elucidated, more specific and focused therapies will evolve with improved efficacy-to–side effect ratios. Fortunately, the distance between molecules and the bedside is

shortening, to the benefit of our patients afflicted with many previously poorly treated neurologic illnesses.

Suggested Reading

Copper JR, Bloom FE, Roth RH. The Biochemical Basis of Neuropharmacology (7th ed). Oxford: Oxford University Press, 1996.

Bloom FE. Neurotransmission and the Central Nervous System. In JG Hardman, LE Limbird, PB Molinoff, et al. (eds), The Pharmacological Basis of Therapeutics (9th ed). New York: McGraw-Hill, 1996;267–294.

Purves D, Augustine GJ, Fitzpatrick D, et al. (eds). Neuroscience. Sunderland, MA: Sinauer, 1997.

Chapter 9
Neuro-Ophthalmology

Bertrand Gaymard and Charles Pierrot-Deseilligny

Chapter Plan

Visual fields
    Anatomy of the visual pathways
    Visual field examination
    Visual field defects
Eye movements
    Anatomy of the ocular motor pathways
    Eye movement examination
    Eye movement abnormalities

Visual Fields

The visual field examination is essential in clinical neurology. It has great semiologic value because the discovery of a visual field defect generally leads to a precise topographic diagnosis. The accuracy of the diagnosis depends on a firm knowledge of the anatomy of the visual pathways.

Anatomy of the Visual Pathways

The Retina and the Optic Nerve

The visual signal is generated in the receptor cells of the retina by transduction of photic energy into an electric signal. These receptor cells are composed of the cones, responsible for color vision and visual discrimination, and the rods, absent in the foveal region and involved in light perception. The signal is then transmitted to the ganglion cells, whose axons form the optic nerve, and reach the chiasm. At this level, the fibers of the optic nerve connected with the nasal sector of the retina (including the nasal half of the macula) cross the midline, whereas those connected with the temporal sector of the retina remain uncrossed. After the chiasm, these fibers synapse with the cells of the lateral geniculate body, whose fibers, called the *optic radiations*, project to the posterior pole of the occipital lobe, the calcarine area. The optic radiations connected with the upper half of the retina travel in the parietal lobe, and those connected with the lower half of the retina travel in the temporal lobe.

Representation of the Visual Environment

The visual system allows a point-to-point representation of the visual world from the retina to the striate cortex. The part of the visual field that is seen by a visual neuron in the striate cortex is called its visual receptive field. These occipital visual receptive fields are of various sizes, being very large for those connected to the peripheral part of the retina and very small for those connected with the macula. Ninety percent of the visual neurons of the striate cortex are connected with the macula, thus resulting in a magnification of the macular region, where the visual acuity is the best.

Visual Field Examination

Visual field examination should first be done eye by eye and should always be preceded by an examination of visual acuity.

Bedside Examination

Visual field examination can easily be performed on a cooperative patient at the bedside. The patient is asked to maintain fixation on the examiner, one eye being covered. A small object or the examiner's finger is placed laterally, initially in the periphery, then displaced toward the center of the visual field. The patient is asked to mention each time the target is visible. Each eye and each visual field are tested sequentially.

Goldmann's Perimetry

A more precise examination can be performed by using Goldmann's perimetry. The subject fixates the center of a hemisphere placed in front of him or her and must signal each time he or she sees a lateral luminous target. The use of targets of various sizes and luminances allows isopters (i.e., regions of the visual fields in which targets of the same size and luminance are perceived) to be determined. The region of the optic nerve corresponds to the blind spot.

Visual Field Defects

Visual field examination may allow a lesion to be localized on the visual pathways. The defect may be either a scotoma—that is, a blind area surrounded by a normal visual field—or a hemianopia—that is, a blind hemivisual field.

Lesions of the Retina or the Optic Nerve

The major characteristic of a lesion involving the retina or the optic nerve is that it is purely monocular. According to the size of the lesion, it may correspond to a small scotoma or to complete monocular blindness. A lesion of the optic nerve may also lead to an ipsilateral pupillary areflexia.

Lesions of the Chiasm

A lesion of the chiasm mainly involves the decussating fibers—that is, fibers coming from the nasal hemifields of the retina. The typical visual field abnormality resulting from such a lesion is therefore a bitemporal hemianopia—that is, a blindness in each temporal visual field.

Retrochiasmatic Lesions

A unilateral retrochiasmatic lesion involves fibers coming from the ipsilateral temporal retinal hemifield (uncrossed fibers) and from the contralateral nasal retinal hemifield, resulting in a homonymous hemianopia. In a case of congruous homonymous hemianopia—that is, when the visual field defect is identical in both eyes—the lesion is more often located in the striate cortex. Conversely, incongruous homonymous hemianopia more often is caused by a lesion of the optic tract or a lesion in the parietal or temporal lobes. A partial damage of the optic radiations may result in a quadrantic visual field defect: a parietal and a temporal lesion result, respectively, in a superior and an inferior quadrantic defect. Because of the magnification of the macula in the occipital lobe, a lesion in the cortical region often leads to a hemianopia sparing the macula.

Eye Movements

Apart from spontaneous eye movements (e.g., during sleep or mental activity), eye movements have two main goals: either to orientate the gaze toward a center of interest located in the visual field or to maintain the gaze on a stable or moving target. Fast orientating eye movements are called *saccades*. Slow stabilizing eye movements consist of smooth pursuit, which enables the eyes to focus on a small moving target; optokinetic nystagmus, which enables the eyes to observe a moving background; and vestibulo-ocular reflex (VOR), which allows the eyes to be stabilized during head movements. The anatomic structures involved in each type of eye movement are now well known. A precise analysis of eye movements may thus allow an accurate anatomic localization.

Figure 9-1. Sagittal view of the human brain stem. (iC = interstitial nucleus of Cajal; IO = inferior olive; MLF = medial longitudinal fasciculus; Mn = motoneuron; N = nucleus; PC = posterior commissure; PPRF = pontine paramedian reticular formation; Ri MLF = rostral nucleus of the medial longitudinal fasciculus; RN = red nucleus.)

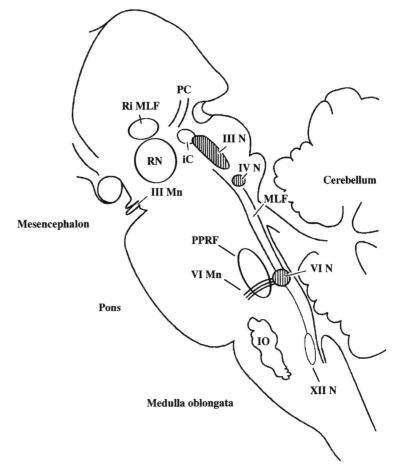

Anatomy of the Ocular Motor Pathways

Two main parts may be distinguished in the ocular motor pathways: the final common pathway, and the premotor structures.

The final common pathway consists of the ocular motor nerves (III, IV, and VI) and their nuclei and is used for all types of eye movements (Figure 9-1). The premotor structures are located upstream to the final common pathway. They are different for each type of eye movement (saccades, smooth pursuit, VOR). The immediate premotor relay for saccades is the pontine paramedian reticular formation (PPRF) for horizontal saccades and the mesencephalic reticular formation (MRF) for vertical saccades (see Figure 9-1). The immediate premotor structure for smooth pursuit and vestibulo-ocular movements is located in the medial vestibular nucleus. These premotor structures project directly to the ocular motor nuclei.

Premotor structures controlling saccades and smooth pursuit are connected with the cortical ocular motor areas. These areas are, in the parietal lobe, the posterior parietal cortex (Brodmann's areas 19 and 37) for smooth pursuit, the parietal eye field (PEF) in the intraparietal sulcus for saccades, and in the frontal lobe, the frontal eye field (FEF) (posterior part of the midfrontal gyrus) and the supplementary eye field (rostral to the supplementary motor area) for both types of eye movements (Figure 9-2).

The frontal lobe is more involved in triggering voluntary eye movements, whereas the parietal lobe is involved chiefly in reflexive-like eye movements (e.g., saccades toward a suddenly appearing visual target). The dorsolateral prefrontal cortex (Brod-

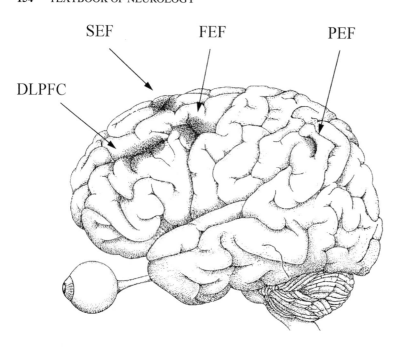

SEF   FEF   PEF

DLPFC

Figure 9-2. Location of the cortical ocular motor areas in the human brain. (DLPFC = dorsolateral prefrontal cortex; FEF = frontal eye field; PEF = parietal eye field; SEF = supplementary eye field.)

mann's area 46) is not an ocular motor area per se, because it does not trigger eye movements, but allows reflexive eye movements (triggered by the parietal lobe) to be inhibited, if necessary, and allows the location of a visual target to be memorized for a short period. Cortical and brain stem premotor structures are connected either by direct pathways or by indirect pathways passing through the basal ganglia or the cerebellum (vermis and flocculus).

Eye Movement Examination

An eye movement examination may be performed either at the bedside or, more accurately, with an eye movement recording.

Bedside Examination of Eye Movements

The visual field should always be tested before an eye movement examination. The examination will also search for strabismus or an eyelid or a pupillary abnormality. During the examination, subjects are asked not to move their head while moving their eyes.

- *Fixation* is studied by asking the subject to fixate a target located successively straight ahead, up, down, right, and left, with the examiner looking for any abnormal eye movements (e.g., nystagmus).
- *Conjugacy* is tested by asking the subject to displace the eyes laterally and up and down, while the examiner checks that both eyes move with the same velocity and amplitude.
- *Saccades* are tested by asking the subject to look successively at the examiner's face and one finger placed laterally, right or left. Vertical saccades are similarly tested, with a finger placed above or below the subject's eyes. Special attention is given to saccade velocity and amplitude. Saccades of normal velocity cannot be "followed" by the examiner's eyes, and saccades of normal amplitude enable the subject to reach the target either directly or with a small corrective saccade.
- *Smooth pursuit* is tested by asking the subject to follow the examiner's finger moving slowly laterally or vertically in front of the subject. Smooth pursuit normally enables a slowly moving target to be followed without the need for catch-up saccades.
- *Vestibulo-ocular* movements may be tested by rapidly rotating the subject's head from a lateral to a central position. A normal VOR enables the

eyes to remain fixed in space, without the need for corrective saccades. The subject may also be asked to read while rotating the head horizontally from side to side. A normal VOR should be able to fully compensate this head movement and thus avoid blurred vision.

Bedside examination of eye movements is reliable and allows a precise anatomic localization of brain stem focal lesions. However, eye movement abnormalities resulting from cortical lesions are subtle and require an eye movement recording.

Eye Movement Recording

Two methods may be easily used for eye movement recordings: electro-oculography, with cutaneous electrodes placed on each side of the eyes, or an infrared device, using the reflection of an infrared light on the cornea.

In either case, the subject is seated in complete darkness, the head immobilized. Visual targets are presented in front of the subject. Eye movements and target displacements are transmitted to and visualized on a computer for off-line analysis.

Saccade latency—that is, the time between the appearance of a target and the beginning of the saccade—is usually approximately 200 ms. Saccade peak velocity is approximately 300 degrees per second for a 25-degree amplitude. Saccade accuracy, measured by the gain—that is, the ratio of saccade amplitude to target eccentricity—is normally between 0.9 and 1.0.

The smooth pursuit and VOR gains—that is, the ratio of peak eye velocity to peak target velocity and peak head velocity, respectively, are measured. In normal subjects, smooth pursuit gain is close to one for slowly moving targets (velocity of less than 40 degrees per second).

Eye Movement Abnormalities

Lesions of the ocular motor nerves or of the immediate brain stem premotor structures can easily be recognized and diagnosed by bedside examination.

Lesions of the Final Common Pathway

Lesions of the final common pathway affect all types of eye movements.

Lesions of the Oculomotor Nerve (Cranial Nerve III). In the most severe cases, the eye is deviated toward the side of the lesion, with a complete ptosis and a nonreactive mydriasis. All vertical and adduction movements are absent in the ipsilateral eye. A more selective lesion, involving partially only several fascicles of the nerve, may occur either after intraorbital lesions or after mesencephalic lesions. However, in the latter, neurologic signs such as a contralateral hemiparesis (Weber's syndrome) or a cerebellar syndrome (Claude's syndrome) are usually associated. An isolated mydriasis may result from an extrinsic compression of the oculomotor nerve by an expansive lesion.

Lesions of the Oculomotor Nuclear Complex. A lesion of the oculomotor nuclear complex is rare. In its complete form, it consists of bilateral ptosis, a complete ipsilateral oculomotor nerve lesion, and a contralateral superior rectus paralysis (with therefore a downward eye deviation). The contralateral superior rectus paralysis is explained by the crossed innervation of this muscle.

Lesions of the Trochlear Nerve (Cranial Nerve IV). A lesion of the trochlear nerve consists of a slight upward drift of the ipsilateral eye. This vertical dysconjugacy increases on downgaze. A contralateral head tilt is often associated.

Lesions of the Abducens Nerve (Cranial Nerve VI). A complete lesion of the abducens nerve consists of an esotropia, the ipsilateral eye being deviated toward abduction. Because of the close vicinity of the facial nerve, a facial palsy is often associated.

Lesions of the Medial Longitudinal Fasciculus. A lesion of the medial longitudinal fasciculus (MLF) produces an internuclear ophthalmoplegia (INO) consisting of an adduction paralysis of the ipsilateral eye, a nystagmus of the contralateral eye during abduction, and a varying degree of impairment of convergence. If the lesion only partially damages the MLF, adduction of the ipsilateral eye is possible but slowed.

Lesions of the Nucleus of the Abducens Nerve. A lesion of the abducens nerve is a very rare condition that consists of a complete ipsilateral gaze paralysis, because this nucleus contains the cell bod-

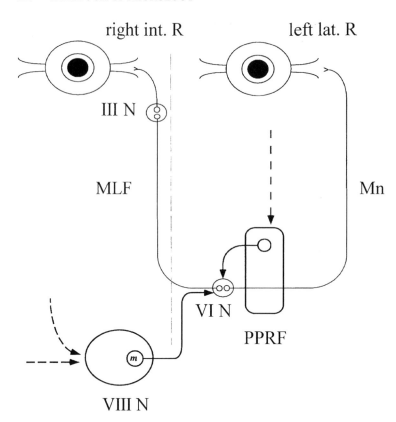

right int. R   left lat. R

III N

MLF   Mn

VI N

PPRF

VIII N

Figure 9-3. Circuitry of horizontal saccades in the pons. (left lat. R = left lateral rectus; MLF = medial longitudinal fasciculus; Mn = abducens motoneuron; PPRF = pontine paramedian reticular formation; right int. R = right internal rectus; III N = oculomotor nucleus; VI N = abducens nucleus; VIII N = vestibular nucleus. The abducens nucleus contains the motoneurons projecting on the ipsilateral lateral rectus muscle and the interneuron projecting on the contralateral subnucleus of the internal rectus muscle [in the oculomotor nucleus].)

ies of both the abducens motoneurons and the internuclear neurons that link the abducens nucleus to the contralateral oculomotor nucleus (Figure 9-3). The association of an INO with a lesion of the abducens nucleus realizes a one-and-a-half syndrome: The only possible horizontal eye movement is nystagmus of the abducting eye. Convergence and vertical eye movements are preserved.

Lesions of the Brain Stem Premotor Structures

Lesions of the brain stem premotor structures may selectively impair one type of eye movement. It is therefore necessary to test saccades, smooth pursuit, and oculovestibular movements separately.

Lesions of the Pontine Paramedian Reticular Formation. A lesion of the PPRF results in a paralysis of all ipsilateral saccades. When the PPRF is only partially damaged, ipsilateral saccades are possible but slowed. If the lesion is restricted to the PPRF, smooth pursuit and vestibulo-ocular move-

ments are preserved because the vestibular nucleus projects directly on the abducens nucleus (see Figure 9-3). However, an abducens nerve lesion is often associated, because the fascicles of this nerve pass through the lower part of the PPRF. The association of an INO and a lesion of the PPRF realizes another form of one-and-a-half syndrome.

Lesions of the Vestibular Nuclear Complex. A lesion limited to the vestibular nuclear complex is extremely rare. It results in a paralysis of ipsilateral vestibulo-ocular and smooth pursuit eye movements.

Lesions of the Mesencephalic Reticular Formation. A lesion of the MRF results in a paralysis of vertical saccades with preservation of the vertical VOR (Parinaud's syndrome). The paralysis may involve more selectively upward or downward saccades.

Lesions of the Cerebellum

Lesions of the Vermis. A lesion of the posterior vermis (lobules VI, VII, and VIII) results in saccade inaccuracy. Saccades are either too large (hypermetria) or too small (hypometria), thus requiring one or more corrective saccades to reach the target. Typically, a lateralized vermal lesion induces ipsilateral hypometria and contralateral hypermetria, but any pattern of dysmetria may be seen. Saccade latency and velocity are normal.

Lesion of the Fastigial Nucleus.   The fastigial nucleus is the main efferent of the vermis. Because the fastigial nucleus is under vermal inhibition, a fastigial lesion typically induces ipsilateral hypermetria and contralateral hypometria.

Lesions of the Cortical Ocular Motor Areas

Posterior Parietal Lesions.   A lesion of the angular gyrus (Brodmann's area 39) induces an increase in reflexive saccade latency and a decreased saccade amplitude. A slightly lower lesion, involving the parietotemporal junction, induces a decrease in ipsilateral smooth pursuit velocity.

Frontal Cortical Lesion.   A lesion in the FEF induces an increase in voluntary saccade latency and reduced ipsilateral smooth pursuit velocity. A slightly more anterior lesion, involving the dorsolateral prefrontal cortex (Brodmann's area 46), results in an inability to suppress reflexive saccades, tested by the antisaccade task. In this paradigm, the subject is asked to make a saccade in the opposite direction to a suddenly appearing visual target. Normal subjects are able to perform this task with an error rate of less than 15% (i.e., saccades directed toward the visual target), whereas the percentage of errors in frontal patients may reach 100%. A clinical antisaccadic test, described by Currie and colleagues, gives analogous results.

Clinical Applications of Eye Movement Recordings

Brain Stem Lesions.   Eye movement examination in a patient with a brain stem lesion enables a diagnosis of great anatomic precision. Its interest, however, has decreased with the introduction of new imaging techniques (magnetic resonance imaging).

Cortical Lesions.   The major interest of recording eye movements in patients with a cortical dysfunction is not topographic but diagnostic. Indeed, this examination may help to differentiate patients with various degenerative disorders, such as parkinsonian syndromes: Parkinson's disease, progressive supranuclear palsy (PSP), corticobasal degeneration (CBD), multisystem atrophy (MSA), and olivopontocerebellar atrophy (OPCA). Such pathologic conditions may initially consist of similar clinical symptoms. An eye movement recording, consisting of several simple tasks such as reflexive saccades, smooth pursuit, and an antisaccade task, often enables the clinician to reveal patterns of abnormalities that allow the diagnosis to be oriented, such as a frontal lobe impairment associated with slow saccades (PSP), an increase in reflexive saccade latency with asymmetric smooth pursuit and saccades of normal velocity (CBD), or dysmetric saccades with an impaired smooth pursuit (MSA or OPCA with a cerebellar syndrome). Usually, idiopathic Parkinson's disease does not result in any marked ocular motor abnormalities, except in later stages of the illness.

Suggested Reading

Büttner U, Brandt T (eds). Clinical Neurology: Ocular Motor Disorders of the Brain Stem. London: Baillière Tindall, 1992.

Leigh RJ, Zee DS. The Neurology of Eye Movements (2nd ed). Philadelphia: Davis, 1991.

Pierrot-Deseilligny C, Rivaud S, Gaymard B, et al. Cortical control of saccades. Ann Neurol 1995;37:557.

Walsh FB, Hoyt WF. Clinical Neuro-Ophthalmology (4th ed). Baltimore: Williams & Wilkins, 1991.

Chapter 10
Neuroepidemiology

Alexander Halim, Douglas E. Kargman,
and Ralph L. Sacco

Chapter Plan

Epidemiology has been described as the study of the *occurrence* of human disease. Neuroepidemiology, then, is simply the study of the occurrence of neurologic diseases. In the clinical setting, epidemiology is a means of organizing all existing information relating to a disease of interest into distinct categories (e.g., patient demographics, risk factors, clinical symptoms, prognosis, recurrence) that can be easily referred to and applied to each subsequent individual patient. This allows the specific presentation of each new patient to be compared with those of prior patients to facilitate diagnosis and decide on the most efficient plan of management. In the research setting, information on exposures or diseases from individual patients are aggregated into rates and proportions in the investigation of etiologic agents, disease characteristics, or morbidity and mortality trends. Observations and inferences based on these epidemiologic data are ultimately used in the public health field to design both prevention and intervention strategies.

Studying the Occurrence of Disease

Disease Mortality

Disease mortality statistics are readily available from routinely collected data sources such as death certificates. Commonly reported mortality data include overall mortality rate, cause-specific mortality rate, and age-specific mortality rate. The cause-specific mortality rate provides the approximate risk of death from a specific cause. The precise risk cannot be obtained because of competing causes of death. For

159

Table 10-1. Crude Prevalences
of Selected Neurologic Diseases

Neurologic Disease	Crude Prevalence per 100,000
Alzheimer's disease (age 65+)	2,000–10,000
Ischemic stroke	500–600
Epilepsy	400–800
Parkinson's disease	18–328
Meningioma (age >55, at autopsy)	100

specific causes, its relative impact in relation to all causes is measured by the proportionate mortality ratio. Age-specific rates account for varying age distributions and allow mortality trends in specific age groups to be studied.

Mortality rates do not accurately reflect disease morbidity rates because many diseases are not immediately fatal, and fatal diseases may be excluded as underlying or contributing causes of death on a death certificate or medical report. Elderly persons in particular often die with several diseases, and the true cause may be omitted. Such surveillance problems are especially germane to neurology. For example, diseases such as Alzheimer's disease, Parkinson's disease, and essential tremor are not always distinguished from the normal aging process and may elude medical attention. Changes in mortality rates should be interpreted with caution, because they can be influenced by changing age distributions as well as changing disease risks. Mortality trends over time are also affected by evolving diagnostic technology, as improved disease ascertainment may be misinterpreted as increased mortality.

Disease Prevalence

The number of cases of disease that *presently exist* in a population represents its burden of the disease and consequently governs the allocation of health services and medical resources. This burden of disease is measured by the prevalence of disease:

$$\text{Prevalence} = \frac{\text{Number of existing cases of disease in a population}}{\text{Number of people at risk for disease in the population}}$$

Prevalences can be obtained from routinely collected data sources (e.g., hospital discharge lists, disease registries) or directly measured through population-based health surveys. Prevalence counts favor disease survivors because patients who are cured, have died, or have moved away from the survey population are excluded. Crude prevalences for some neurologic diseases are reported in Table 10-1. Age- and sex-specific prevalence rates for these diseases are reported elsewhere.

Rate of New Disease Occurrence in a Population: Incidence Density

The risk of acquiring disease is derived through measures of incidence density or cumulative risk. The first method involves a *dynamic* population, which, in contrast to a static population, has continual entry and exit of members (through births, deaths, and migration) during the observation period. Persons within the population are observed for unequal lengths of time. New cases of disease are therefore more appropriately assessed with regard to the sum total of the individual observation periods of each person in the population rather than simply the population size at the beginning of the observation period. This precise measure of incidence, the *incidence density* of disease, measures the *rate* of new disease within the population:

$$\text{Incidence density} = \frac{\text{Number of new cases of disease}}{\text{Sum of total person-time at risk}}$$

The contribution of each individual toward the calculation of risk for the entire population should reflect the actual length of time that individual spends being part of the at-risk population. This difference in time at risk for disease can be adjusted for by measuring the sum of the *person-time* at risk for each individual. The denominator of the incidence density accurately reflects each individual's relative contribution toward the overall measure of risk.

The relative incidence (or relative risk [RR]) of disease compares persons with a putative risk factor (the exposed) with persons without the same putative risk factor (the unexposed). If the risk factor is associated with the disease, then the risk of disease in the exposed is expected to be significantly greater than the risk of disease in the unexposed. When the incidence density is used to derive the measure of risk, then the RR is termed the *incidence density ratio* (IDR). The calculation of the RR is discussed below.

Average Risk of Disease: Cumulative Incidence

The second method of measuring the risk of acquiring disease involves following a *static* population for a specific length of time and determining the number of new cases of disease that occur in the population in that time period. This method gives a less realistic measure of risk, because most populations are dynamic in nature. The *proportion* represents the *average* risk of acquiring disease in that population and is termed the *cumulative incidence.*

$$\text{Cumulative incidence} = \frac{\substack{\text{Number of new cases in a} \\ \text{specified time interval}}}{\substack{\text{The population at the start} \\ \text{of the time interval}}}$$

Cumulative incidence represents a theoretical risk, since it operates under the assumption of no other competing diseases. In practical terms, when comparing the average risk of a disease between people with a risk factor (the putative exposure) and people without, the risks of competing causes are often assumed to be comparable in both groups. The denominator should ideally include only people at risk for the disease in the population. This at-risk population excludes persons who have zero probability of acquiring the disease of interest and persons who have already developed the disease. However, for many incidence rates, individuals who are not at risk are too few in number and their exclusion from the denominator will not significantly alter the true incidence counts.

The measure of RR using cumulative incidence is the cumulative incidence ratio (CIR), which compares the cumulative incidence of disease in those exposed with those unexposed to the putative risk factor.

The following example illustrates the erroneous conclusions that can arise when cumulative incidence is measured instead of incidence density in a dynamic population.

Persons with coronary artery disease (CAD) have double the risk for ischemic stroke compared with persons without CAD. Based on this

statistic, a hypothetical study following 10,000 people with CAD and 10,000 without CAD for 1 year may expect, for example, 20 and 10 new cases of ischemic stroke over the course of the year, respectively. If hypothetically all 10,000 people with CAD die of a myocardial infarction at the end of the sixth month (the midpoint of the study interval), and up to this point in time, there were only 10 cases of stroke, at the end of the year, there will be 10 new cases of ischemic stroke among the 10,000 people who began the year in each of the CAD and non-CAD groups, leading to the erroneous CIR of [(10/10,000)/(10/10,000)] = 1.00. An IDR would derive an incidence density rate of 10 cases among 5,000 person-years for persons with CAD (10,000 people each followed for 0.5 years) and 10 cases among 10,000 person-years for persons without CAD (10,000 people each followed for 1 year). The incidence density of (10/5,000) in the CAD group and (10/10,000) in the non-CAD group thus yields an IDR of 2.0. This latter measure is an accurate reflection of the twofold risk attributed to the presence of CAD.

Effect of Individual Causes: Etiologic Fraction (Attributable Risk Percent)

The impact of a single risk factor on the risk of disease is measured by the proportion of all new cases of disease within a population that are caused by the specific risk factor. It may also be thought of as the proportion of new cases that are potentially eliminated if that risk factor were removed or prevented. For deleterious exposures, the etiologic fraction (EF), or attributable risk percent, is calculated by the following ratio:

$$\text{EF} = \frac{\substack{\text{Number of new cases due to risk} \\ \text{factor in time period}}}{\substack{\text{Total number of new cases} \\ \text{in same time period}}}$$

The numerator is derived by subtracting the number of new cases expected in the absence of exposure (i.e., the number of new cases in the unexposed population) from the total number of new cases occurring within the same time period. It is alternatively interpreted as the probability that a randomly selected patient develops disease as a result of the

Table 10-2. Calculation of Sensitivity and Specificity in Screening

	Persons with Disease (D)	Persons without Disease ($\bar{D}$)	
Positive screen result	True-positives (TP)	False-positives (FP)	High-risk group
Negative screen result	False-negatives (FN)	True-negatives (TN)	Low-risk group

Sensitivity = [(TP)/(TP + FN)]; positive predictive value = [(TP)/(TP + FP)]; specificity = [(TN)/(TN + FP)]; negative predictive value = [(TN)/(TN + FN)].

exposure. The corresponding measure for protective exposures, the prevented fraction (PF), is the proportion of cases expected in the absence of the exposure that has been eliminated because of the presence of the exposure.

$$PF = \frac{\text{Number of new cases prevented by the exposure}}{\text{Sum of prevented and occurred cases}}$$

The numerator for the PF is the number of new cases expected in the absence of exposure minus the number of new cases that actually occurred.

Identifying Presymptomatic Disease: Screening

People are defined as diseased only when they develop symptoms and are subsequently diagnosed as cases. The advantages of detecting presymptomatic disease are a more accurate measure of disease incidence as well as the opportunity to initiate early intervention to prevent the progression toward symptomatic (clinical) disease. The detection of such presymptomatic cases in a presymptomatic population is known as *screening*. The function of screening is to separate people into high-risk and low-risk groups, in which high-risk persons are identified as potential cases of disease and therefore candidates for early intervention. The ultimate goal is to prolong the patient's life by administering the intervention early during the preclinical stage. For example, a stroke screening program would involve measuring blood pressure and blood glucose and also inquiring about cardiac disease and smoking history. The presence of any of these stroke risk factors places an individual at an increased risk for stroke. Interventions may include antihypertensive or diabetes mellitus medication, modification of dietary habits, and reduction or cessation of smoking. It is hoped that these interventions would ulti-

mately prevent the occurrence of stroke by essentially reducing as many modifiable risk factors as possible.

Although screening need not be a diagnostic procedure, the effectiveness of any screening program is measured by how accurately the screening test results agree with results obtained from a "gold standard," which is either a diagnostic test or an established biologic marker. The gold standard results represent the true disease status. The total number of subjects categorized as diseased represents the true disease prevalence in the population being screened.

The *sensitivity* (Table 10-2) of a screening test is the probability that a true case of disease is correctly identified by the screening test. It is measured as the proportion of true positives among all persons with disease, as determined by the gold standard. The *specificity* is the probability that a disease-free individual is correctly identified as such by the screening test and is measured as the proportion of true negatives among all persons without disease. The *positive predictive value* (PPV) indicates the probability that a positive screening result actually detected true disease. The PPV is the proportion of true positives among all positive screening test results (this includes both true positives and false positives). Conversely, the *negative predictive value* (NPV) is the proportion of true negatives among all negative test results and represents the probability that a negative result detected a true absence of disease.

The sensitivity and specificity of a single screening are inversely related. By adjusting the cut-off score of the screening test variable, which distinguishes positive and negative screen results, the screening test itself can be recalibrated to increase either sensitivity or specificity. The decision on which measure to maximize depends on the particular disease being screened. If the priority is to detect all persons who may truly be diseased (perhaps because an effective treatment can be implemented in the preclinical stage and the consequences of a missed diagnosis are life-threatening), then the sensitivity should be maximized at the expense of specificity. Both the positive and NPVs of a screening test (with a fixed sensitivity and specificity) will vary depending on the prevalence of disease in the population screened. The same screening test, holding sensitivity and specificity constant, will yield a higher PPV (and lower NPV) in a population of higher disease prevalence than one of lower disease prevalence.

Studying the Causes of Disease

Causation

If a change in the frequency of an exposure is accompanied by a change in the frequency of a disease, we can say that there is an *association* between exposure and disease. However, to infer *causation* between the exposure and disease, we must first establish that the exposure occurred before the disease—that is, the change in exposure frequency preceded and thus provoked the change in disease frequency. The temporal order between both variables establishes the directionality of the association and is required to establish a causal relationship. Other criteria that support causality include consistency in the findings across different studies, the biologic plausibility of the hypothesized exposure–disease relationship, the strength of association between exposure and disease, a dose-response trend, and the specificity of the exposure. Although these additional criteria support causality, their violation may not necessarily refute it. The inconsistency of results across studies may be caused by different study methodologies. Evidence of biologic plausibility depends on the availability of an appropriate animal model or other experimental data. Some exposures may have an inherently weak yet significant association with the disease. The dose-response criteria disregards threshold or ceiling effects. Finally, the specificity rule, which states that the removal of an exposure will lead to a reduction in disease under the assumption of a one exposure–one disease relationship, is inapplicable to diseases with multiple causes.

An association or causation between an exposure and a disease is numerically represented by a measure of effect greater or less than unity. Measures of effect greater than one indicate that the exposure is deleterious, whereas those less than one suggest a protective effect with respect to the disease. A measure of effect of one denotes an absence of an association between exposure and disease.

Study Designs and Measures of Effect

The study of any exposure-disease relationship generally progresses from the initial generation of a hypothesis based on observed rates and trends for both exposure and disease variables, to the testing of that hypothesis with any of the various observational study designs. Results from these observational studies may lead to the development of potential treatments or intervention programs, whose effectiveness can be tested using experimental studies such as randomized clinical trials (RCTs).

Epidemiologic studies are classified as *experimental*, *quasi-experimental*, or *observational* in design. In an experimental design, the investigator assigns the exposure or exposures under study through randomization. In a quasi-experimental design, the exposure is assigned without randomization. In an observational study, none of the study variables are under the manipulation of the investigator, nor can randomization be utilized.

Ecologic Study

Characteristics.   Different *populations* are compared with regard to the distribution of a specific exposure as well as a specific disease. All derived measures are based on populations and are inherently uninformative with regard to the individuals in each population.

Measure of Effect.   Each population is plotted on a two-dimensional graph, with exposure and disease plotted on each axis. A correlation coefficient is calculated to test for the linear relationship between both variables. A score indicative of a linear trend suggests that an association between exposure and disease may exist and therefore should be studied at the level of the individual person.

Table 10-3. Prevalence Ratio*

	D	$\bar{D}$	
E	a	b	a + b
$\bar{E}$	c	d	c + d
	a + c	b + d	N

E = exposed; $\bar{E}$ = unexposed; D = diseased; $\bar{D}$ = nondiseased; a = persons who have exposure and disease; b = persons who have exposure but are free from disease; c = persons who have disease but are unexposed; d = persons without exposure or disease; N = total number of persons (or total study sample).
*Prevalence ratio = (Prevalence of disease among exposed)/(prevalence of disease among unexposed) = [a/(a + b)]/[c/(c + d)].

Strengths.   Ecologic studies provide a quick, easy, and inexpensive means of generating a hypothesis between an exposure and a disease. Data acquisition relies on available records and is therefore relatively easier compared with other designs.

Weaknesses.   An observed relationship between exposure and disease at the population level does not necessarily imply a relationship at the individual level because individuals with or without the exposure are not necessarily the same individuals with or without disease. An erroneous extrapolation in this manner is known as the ecologic fallacy in which individual risk is inferred from population-based data. It is also impossible to measure confounders at the individual level.

Indication.   Ecologic studies are used to generate hypotheses that are subsequently tested using more appropriate designs based on individual data.

Cross-Sectional Study

Characteristics.   A cross-section of the population is surveyed with respect to the current existence of disease (i.e., prevalent cases) and the concurrent existence of the exposure variable (current exposure).

Measure of Effect.   A comparison can be made in two ways: The prevalence of disease (D) among the exposed (E) is compared with that among the unexposed ($\bar{E}$), or the prevalence of exposure among the diseased (D) is compared with that among those free of disease ($\bar{D}$). In either case, the relative prevalence of one variable is compared with the preva-

lence of the second factor to generate a *prevalence ratio* (Table 10-3). Other measures include prevalence odds ratio and odds ratio (OR).

Strengths.   A cross-sectional survey offers a quick, easy, and relatively cheaper means of hypothesis testing. It offers an instantaneous description of the distributions of both variables within the population surveyed.

Weaknesses.   The information is derived from prevalent exposure and prevalent disease. This usually precludes the determination of the onset of exposure or disease, which in turn can obscure the true temporal order of exposure and disease. Current exposure status may not reflect true exposure status, e.g., nonsmokers may in fact be ex-smokers. In addition, individuals with disease are disease survivors who represent either milder (less fatal) forms of the disease or diseases of longer duration.

Indication.   Cross-sectional studies may be used to either generate or test a hypothesis. In terms of hypothesis testing, it is best suited for exposures (or traits) that are inherited and life-long. One can determine the onset of such exposures and thus establish the temporal relationship.

Case-Control Study

Characteristics.   Individuals with the disease of interest (D) and disease-free controls ($\bar{D}$) are compared with regard to the presence (E) or absence ($\bar{E}$) of the exposure or exposures of interest in the past. The timing of the exposure is set to precede the onset of disease. Ideally, controls should be comparable with cases in all characteristics except for the exposure of interest. Exposure information is obtained through in-person interviews, medical records review, or even biologic measurements, if applicable.

Measure of Effect.   The measure of effect for case-control studies is the *OR*, which compares the odds of exposure in cases to that in controls (Table 10-4).

Strengths.   Compared with cohort studies and clinical trials, case-control studies take less time and are often cheaper. They are also ideal for studying rare diseases and multiple exposures. Case-control studies are not subject to attrition of study subjects because

Table 10-4. Calculation of Odds Ratio*

	D	D̄
E	a	b
Ē	c	d
	Cases	Controls

E = exposed; Ē = unexposed; D = diseased; D̄ = nondiseased;
a = persons who have exposure and disease; b = persons who have
exposure but are free from disease; c = persons who have disease
but are unexposed; d = persons without exposure or disease.
*Odds ratio = (Odds of exposure among cases)/(odds of expo-
sure among controls) = (a/c)/(b/d) = (ad)/(bc).

Table 10-5. Calculation of Relative Risk*

	D	D̄	
E	a	b	a + b
Ē	c	d	c + d

E = exposed; Ē = unexposed; D = diseased; D̄ = nondiseased;
a = persons who have exposure and disease; b = persons who have
exposure but are free from disease; c = persons who have disease
but are unexposed; d = persons without exposure or disease.
*Relative risk = (Proportion developing disease among
exposed)/(proportion developing disease among unexposed) =
[a/(a + b)]/[c/(c + d)].

there is no follow-up, nor are they influenced by the Hawthorne effect (see the section on cohort studies).

Weaknesses.   The temporal order between exposure and disease may be difficult to establish, especially if the disease onset is insidious and the timing
of the exposure is obscure. Recall bias is an inherent limitation of this design because the exposure
measurement is largely, if not entirely, dependent
on the subject's recall.

Indication.   Case-control studies, by improving
the establishment of temporality and using incident
cases of disease, provide a better means of studying
causation compared with cross-sectional studies.
However, when both disease onset and timing of
exposure are unclear, a cohort study design would
be better suited to clarify temporality.

Cohort Studies

Characteristics.   Study subjects free of the disease
of interest are identified and placed into exposed or
unexposed groups (cohorts). Both cohorts are then
followed over time. At the end of the follow-up
period, the proportion of cohort members who have
developed the disease are compared between
cohorts. If the cohorts are highly dynamic, with
members spending significantly different lengths of
time under follow-up (either because of death from
another cause or being lost to follow-up), then the
denominator used in the calculation of risk should
represent the actual length of time each member
contributed during the follow-up period (i.e., person-
time) rather than simply the number of subjects.

Cohort studies may be retrospective or prospective
depending on when disease occurs among cohort

members relative to the beginning of observation. For
diseases in which the exposure of interest may occur
far in advance of disease onset (e.g., invasive head
trauma in early adulthood and subsequent Parkinson's
disease after age 65 years), following cohort members
throughout the lengthy disease process is logistically
difficult, not to mention excessively costly. A retrospective cohort design would be more suitable in such
situations. This design (not to be confused with *retrospective studies*, which is a synonym for case-control
studies) involves obtaining information on past exposures, often through reviewing past medical records to
identify individuals with and without the exposure and
tracking them to the present to determine which cohort
members have been diagnosed with the disease of
interest. In a prospective cohort design, exposure is
measured at the start of the study and cohort members
are followed over actual time until a predetermined
end-point, at which time disease occurrence is measured. Furthermore, because of the potential threat of
attrition of study subjects, greater numbers of subjects
are required to ensure that a study sample with sufficient statistical power (discussed later) will remain at
the end of the study period.

Measure of Effect.   The proportion who developed
disease (D) in each exposure group is represented by
the cumulative incidence, derived at the end of the
follow-up period. Exposed (E) and unexposed (Ē)
cohorts are then compared in terms of the RR or risk
ratio of disease (Table 10-5). If the risk of disease is
derived from incidence density, the *relative rate* (or
rate ratio) is a more appropriate measure of effect
than RR (or risk ratio) (Table 10-6).

Strengths.   Because disease-free individuals are
followed until the disease process occurs, the tem-

Table 10-6. Calculation of Relative Rate*

	D	Person-Time (PT)
E	D/E	Total person-years PT(E)
Ē	D/Ē	Total person-years PT(Ē)

E = persons with exposure; Ē = persons with no exposure; D = persons with disease; D/E = "D given E,"—that is, persons who have disease among all persons with exposure; D/E = "D given Ē " —that is, persons who have disease among all persons without exposure.

*Relative rate = (Incidence density in exposed)/(incidence density in unexposed) =
$$\frac{(D/E)\ /\ [PT(E)]}{(D/\bar{E})\ /\ [PT(\bar{E})]}$$

poral relation between exposure and disease is well established. Measurement of exposure does not depend on the subjects' recollection, thereby eliminating recall bias. Cohort studies are ideal for studying rare exposures and multiple outcomes. Retrospective cohort studies, where applicable, offer a cheaper and less time-consuming alternative to prospective cohort designs.

Weaknesses.   A lengthy follow-up period and increased study cost may offer a severe disadvantage to prospective cohort studies, more so than to retrospective cohort study, when compared with case-control studies. Attrition of study subjects is a major problem. This threat is minimized in retrospective cohort studies because of the reduced participation time by subjects. If the determination of disease is made without blinding the investigators to exposure status, then case ascertainment potentially may be biased. In prospective cohort designs, participants may change their behavior (and ultimately their risk of disease) by virtue of participating in the study. This phenomenon, known as the Hawthorne effect, may under- or overestimate the true risk of disease in either or both cohorts.

Indication.   Cohort studies are superior for establishing temporality because the exposure variable is defined and measured in a nondiseased study population, and subsequent cases of disease are monitored through follow-up.

Randomized Clinical Trial

Characteristics.   In an RCT, study subjects are randomized into groups known as *treatment arms*,

each of which is assigned a different exposure. In drug trials, a placebo is assigned to one group, and the drug or drugs being studied are each assigned to the remaining group or groups. In contrast to other observational study designs, the exposure of interest in RCTs confers protection against adverse outcomes. Because the exposures are not meant to prevent the initial occurrence of disease, these adverse outcomes are usually disease sequelae. Both the study subjects and the investigators are blinded to the actual assignment of the exposures. This is known as *double-blinding*. Being experimental in design, the applicability of RCTs is governed by ethical considerations involving human subjects.

Measure of Effect.   Members of each treatment arm are assessed in terms of the risk of reaching an outcome at the end of the trial period. Outcomes assessed include physiologic changes (e.g., cholesterol reduction) and recurrence of disease (e.g., recurrent ischemic stroke). The measure of effect is the RR (see Table 10-5).

Strengths.   The ability of the investigator to manipulate the exposure variable strengthens the measure and definition of exposure. Randomization distributes known and unknown confounding variables equally across all treatment arms. The greater the size of the study sample, the more equal this distribution will be. The success of randomization can be assessed by comparing the distribution of known confounders among the various arms. The temporal order can be established in RCTs, as exposure is allotted before the occurrence of the outcome. Double-blinding reduces the potential for bias among both subjects and investigators. Blinded subjects are less likely to influence their outcome or switch treatment groups, whereas blinded investigators are prevented from probing for an anticipated outcome.

Weaknesses.   RCTs are often expensive and always susceptible to attrition by trial participants. They also commonly focus on patients with specific characteristics, undermining the extrapolation of study results to the general population. The longitudinal design renders RCTs unsuitable for the study of rare outcomes. Another limitation that threatens the validity of the study is the failure of study subjects to adhere to their assigned treatment regimen.

Indication. RCTs are used to compare the relative success of different interventions, such as drugs, surgical procedures, or educational programs for a disease of interest.

Genetic Epidemiology Study Designs

Hypotheses involving genetic etiologies can be studied using observational study designs, in which the exposure is defined as either the presence of a genetic marker or having a relative with the same disease. The *outcome* is defined as disease in the proband or disease in a relative. There are, however, other observational study designs that are specific for the investigation of genetic etiologies and that have the advantage of an improved measure of exposure and disease. In addition, these designs have the ability to isolate the independent contribution of the genetic factor toward disease risk. These designs include familial aggregation studies, twin studies, sibling studies, adoption studies, segregation analysis, and linkage analysis. Discussions on these genetic approaches and study designs can be found in more advanced genetic epidemiology textbooks.

Bias in Study Design

Bias in epidemiologic studies represents a systematic (nonrandom) error within the research design itself that may obscure the true exposure-disease relationship. There are essentially three types of bias: selection bias, information bias, and confounding.

Selection bias occurs when subjects included in a study are systematically different from the source population targeted for the study in terms of the exposure-disease relationship. In case-control studies, selecting hospitalized cases for a disease that does not always require hospitalization may result in more severe cases of disease in the case group while excluding milder cases (Berkson's bias). With regard to control selection, healthy individuals may volunteer to participate in studies, leading to a self-selection bias, as they may overestimate the "healthiness" of the general disease-free population. The group will potentially provide an underestimation of the true frequency of deleterious exposures in the population. Selection bias is minimized by enrolling cases that are *representative* of all cases in the population and recruiting a *random* sample of disease-free participants.

Information bias is a systematic error in the acquisition of study data that leads to the misclassification of study subjects. Misclassification can occur in either the exposure or the disease variable. If misclassification of one variable occurs independently of the other, it is termed *nondifferential* and will result in the true association being biased toward the null (i.e., no association). Alternatively, if the misclassification is dependent on the other variable, it is *differential*, and the bias can be away or toward the null. Case-control studies are particularly susceptible to recall bias (a form of differential misclassification), as cases may "blame" their disease on the exposure under study or search their memories to a greater degree than controls. This would lead to an overestimation of the odds of exposure among cases. Recall bias may be minimized if the exposure information is obtained from physical measures or historical records rather than based on the recall of study subjects or if the questions on the exposure under study are "buried" among questions on other exposures of lesser interest. Cohort studies may also be affected by information bias. For example, if investigators expect exposed subjects to have a greater disease frequency than unexposed subjects, they may probe exposed subjects more rigorously or misclassify borderline cases of disease among exposed subjects as being fully diseased. This form of information bias is commonly referred to as *interviewer bias* and can be minimized by simply blinding interviewers to the exposure status of the subjects.

Confounding is defined as the obscuring of the estimate of the measure of effect of an exposure (on the disease of interest) because of another variable whose effect is mixed with that of the exposure. In simple terms, it is thought of as a mixing of effects that consequently leads to an overestimation or underestimation of the true effect of the exposure. It may also create an apparent association when none exists, or it may nullify a true association. A *confounding variable* (confounder) is defined as being (1) a risk factor for the disease, (2) associated with the study exposure, and (3) excluded from the causal pathway between exposure and disease. All three criteria must be satisfied for a variable to be considered a confounder. Confounding presents a potential threat to all study designs. Its potential effect can be eliminated at the design phase through restriction, matching, or randomization. With restriction, study subjects with the confounding variable or those who have specific levels of the confounding variable are excluded. This reduces the variability of that confounding variable within the study population. In matching, confounding is prevented by making the distribution of confounding variables similar in both study groups. In case-control studies, cases are often matched to controls with respect to variables such as age, sex, race-ethnicity, and other characteristics. Similarly, exposed and unexposed groups may be matched in cohort designs. Randomization, which is intrinsic to clinical trials, reduces the effect of confounding by creating treatment groups with similar distributions of all potentially confounding variables. It has the added advantage of being able to address unknown confounders, while restriction and matching can only address confounders that are known and measurable. Ideally, all three methods should create study groups that are similar with respect to all characteristics except the ones of interest. Confounding may also be controlled in the analytic phase of a study by other methods discussed below.

Analytic Issues

Statistical Issues

When an exposure-disease hypothesis is tested, there are two critical errors that can lead to a distortion of causal inference. The first involves concluding that an association exists when there is none (type I error); the second involves missing a true association (type II error).

A type I error is mathematically represented by alpha (α), which is the probability that an observed association is due to chance and which represents the statistical significance of the measured effect estimate. Alpha is traditionally set at 0.05, with the corresponding ($1 - \alpha$), or 95%, confidence interval (CI). A 95% CI implies that 95% of the time, the point estimate of the measure of effect will lie within that interval—for example, RR = 2.3 (95% CI, 1.6–3.0). Studies with numerous variables or that employ multiple statistical tests may be inappropriate for an α level of 0.05. For example, if a study analyzes 100 ORs, then five of those ORs will yield an apparent association simply because of chance—the 5% error rate set by α. This problem can be addressed with statistical adjustments such as Bonferroni correction, which are designed to reduce type I error by setting α at a more stringent level—for example, 0.01.

A type II error involves the statistical power of the study. The power ($1 - \beta$) indicates the probability of detecting a true association, while β is the probability of not observing a true association. Most studies set the statistical power at 80%, which indicates a 20% probability of missing a true association when one actually exists. This error can be minimized by increasing the sample size of the study, which raises the statistical power. The sample size of a study is determined by setting the study at specific levels of α and β, specifying the disease prevalence in the population at risk for disease, and accounting for the ratio of the number of study subjects in the two comparison groups (e.g., cases and controls).

Reliability and Validity

The concepts of reliability and validity involve an appreciation of measurement error in either exposure or disease. Random measurement error refers to all unavoidable chance errors inherent in everyday action. Nonrandom error exists as a result of a functional or systematic distortion of the actual measurement process.

Reliability is defined simply as the lack of random error. In epidemiologic studies, it refers to the reproducibility of results obtained using repeated measures by the same instrument. The results are not expected to be perfectly consistent since random error can never be completely eliminated. The concept of reliability also applies to the agreement of results across several instruments. For example, the degree to which several neurologists agree on a diagnosis of tremor on physical examination is a measure of the reliability between the neurologists.

Validity is a measure of "truthfulness." In epidemiology, validity is used to describe the extent to which a measuring instrument actually measures what it is designed to. The validity of a specific measuring instrument is evaluated by comparing its results with those obtained from a more conclusive instrument, often referred to as the "gold standard." This gold standard is not necessarily the reflection of truth, but rather the best available indicator of truth whose own validity is assumed to be maximal. The validity of all other measuring instruments will then be evaluated relative to this standard. A departure from validity is caused by a systematic error that distorts the truth and is not random in nature. These errors may exist either in the form of a bias in the study design or in the form of an inappropriate measuring instrument. Therefore, validity may alternatively be thought of as an absence of systematic (nonrandom) error. Although the lack of reliability undermines validity, reliability itself does not guarantee validity. The concepts of reliability and validity are illustrated in the following example:

We are interested in measuring obesity in a sample of individuals. The various instruments used to measure obesity available include (1) a personal interview during which each subject is asked if he or she was obese; (2) a personal interview during which each subject is asked if he or she was ever diagnosed with obesity by a physician; (3) a visual assessment by one of the investigators of all subjects to determine obesity; (4) measuring each subject's weight on a simple scale; or (5) measuring each subject's height and weight and calculating a body mass index (BMI). If we consider the BMI to be the best available measure of true obesity, then the BMI will be our gold standard. The reliability of each of the five measuring instruments is determined by performing repeated interviews for instruments (1) and (2), and repeated measurements for (3), (4), and (5). Instruments that consistently produce the same result for each subject are deemed reliable. The validity of instruments (1), (2), (3), and (4) is determined by comparing their results with that provided by the BMI for all subjects. The greater the agreement between the results of a particular instrument and the results of the BMI, the greater the validity of that instrument.

Controlling Confounding

In addition to the methods of preventing confounding in the design phase, confounding may also be controlled for in the analytic phase through either stratification or multivariate analysis. In stratified analysis, the exposure-disease relationship is investigated within different levels (strata) of the confounder. In each stratum, the groups being compared have little or no variability with regard to the confounder and will therefore provide an unconfounded estimate. For example, if the association between cigarette smoking and subarachnoid hemorrhage is

suspected to vary across the sexes, then separate analyses performed on the male and on the female strata will respectively yield valid effect estimates for men and for women, and control for any confounding due to sex. If the stratum-specific estimates are *equal* to each other (i.e., the estimate for men equals that for women) but are different from the crude estimate (i.e., the overall unstratified), then confounding exists. If, however, the stratum-specific estimates are *unequal* as well as different from the crude estimate, then effect modification is present. Alternatively, multivariate analysis uses mathematical modeling to assess the independent effect of a putative exposure while simultaneously controlling for other covariates as well as to describe any confounding or effect modification that may be present.

Effect Modification

Effect modification, or interaction, as it is more commonly known, refers to the variation in the exposure-disease relationship according to different levels of a third variable. This combination of effects between the exposure and effect modifier has also been described as synergism, in which the combined effect is greater than the individual effects, or antagonism, in which the combined effect is less. Mathematical models are used to determine if the effect modification operates in a multiplicative or additive manner. Effect modification models have also been applied to elucidating the combined effects of genetic factors and environmental exposures.

Methodologic Issues in Epidemiologic Studies of Neurologic Diseases

Defining and Measuring Exposure

The true measurement of any exposure variable requires a clear and consistent definition of the exposure, a valid and reliable means of measuring it, and an understanding of the disease process to determine the actual timing of the exposure. The definition of the exposure is critical to the comparison of results across studies. For example, when comparing studies investigating the role of hypertension, one has to know the precise systolic and diastolic cut-off points used and also whether the patient has to be currently taking blood pressure lowering medication to be defined as hypertensive. Similarly, studies investigating cigarette smoking or alcohol consumption should clearly define and quantify the exposure. The exposure quantification is especially critical if the exposure is subject to a threshold effect involving lifelong exposure or involves repeated insults. Some exposures may simply elude definition. For example, although an association between rural living and Parkinson's disease has been established, it is unclear if the exposure is a marker for rural living per se, an environmental toxin, or some other undefined exposure or risk factor.

Many exposures that are defined may nonetheless suffer from the absence of a suitable measuring instrument. For example, although the presence of a family history for any disease is easily defined, the degree to which it can be reliably reported depends on the proband's recall and familiarity with family members' medical history. Living relatives may serve as more valid sources of information provided they are aware of and can recall their own medical history. This problem is further complicated if the disease process adversely affects the mental state of the patient. Information on past illnesses may also be limited by the diagnostic procedures available then. Even when the exposure can be detected by physical symptoms or laboratory tests, its measure is still dependent on the reliability of the detection instruments used.

Neurologic diseases that occur late in life, such as Alzheimer's disease, may be induced by exposures that occurred decades earlier. Knowledge of the latency period and the time of disease onset provides an approximation of the time the exposure occurred. This leads to the identification of the critical exposure (the true cause of disease), and allows all unrelated exposures to be disregarded. However, such a determination may be difficult, if not impossible, if the exposure is nebulous or if the disease onset is insidious.

Ascertaining Cases

Neurologic diseases have acute, subacute, or insidious onsets. Diagnosing diseases with an acute onset is relatively straightforward if the appropriate diagnostic tools are available. Case ascertainment then depends on the availability and sensitivity of diagnostic instruments, the consistency of the clinical presentations, and agreement between clinicians making the diagnosis. Diseases with subacute onset are often subjected to delayed diagnosis because the early symptoms do not distinguish them from other diseases with similar presentations. For example, meningitis in its early stages may be misdiagnosed as influenza because of similar presentations. For such diseases, case ascertainment may require prolonged observation but should nevertheless be as definitive as for diseases with acute onset. In diseases with insidious onset, the problem of underascertainment is exacerbated as a result of the extended duration in which cases exhibit vague symptoms that preclude a definitive diagnosis. Consequently, there is a greater likelihood of underdiagnosis.

Other factors that may potentially complicate case ascertainment include age, mental state, and autopsy-dependent diagnosis. The advanced ages at which many neurologic disorders manifest themselves allow for competing morbidities or mortality from other diseases. This situation will obscure the onset and therefore the detection of the distinct neurologic symptoms of the disease of interest and lead to an underestimation of the true incidence. Persons with diminished mental capacity (e.g., dementia, aphasia, anosognosia) may have difficulty complaining of symptoms of other diseases depending on the extent of their cognitive disability. In such a situation, any information necessary for a definitive diagnosis is obtained solely from a clinical examination, laboratory tests, or a proxy. The absence of an antemortem diagnostic test for Parkinson's disease and Alzheimer's disease forces the diagnosis of these diseases to rely on clinical examinations. Case ascertainment therefore depends on the reliability of the clinical examination. In the event that there is significant variation is the diagnostic accuracy of different investigators, the reliability of the diagnostic procedure will be less than optimal, and case ascertainment will be greatly undermined.

Conclusion

Neuroepidemiology studies the characteristics and determinants of neurologic diseases. Traditional epidemiologic measures describe the distributions and trends of neurologic diseases and their putative exposures (i.e., risk factors). Both observational and experimental study designs are used to investigate hypothesized exposure-disease relationships. There are potential methodologic problems that are unique to neuroepidemiology. These problems are influenced by difficulties with measuring past exposures, the insidious nature of many neurologic diseases, the advanced ages at which they manifest themselves, and the performance of available diagnostic instruments. Despite these problems, neuroepidemiologic studies have led to significant advancements in the understanding of the causes and consequences of many neurologic disorders.

Suggested Reading

Anderson DW (ed). Neuroepidemiology: A Tribute to Bruce Schoenberg. Boca Raton, FL: CRC Press, 1991.

Daniel WW. Biostatistics: A Foundation for Analysis in the Health Sciences. New York: John Wiley, 1991.

Fleiss JL. Statistical Methods for Rates and Proportions. New York: John Wiley, 1981.

Gorelick PB, Alter M (eds). Handbook of Neuroepidemiology. New York: Marcel Dekker, 1994.

Kelsey JL, Thompson WD, Evans AS. Methods in Observational Epidemiology. New York: Oxford University Press, 1986.

Khoury MJ, Beaty TH, Cohen BH. Fundamentals of Genetic Epidemiology. New York: Oxford University Press, 1993.

Kleinbaum DG, Kupper LL, Morgenstern H. Epidemiologic Research. New York: Van Nostrand Reinhold, 1982.

Longstreth WT Jr, Kopsell TD, van Belle G. Clinical neuroepidemiology. I. Diagnosis [review]. Arch Neurol 1987; 44:1091.

Macmahon B, Pugh TF. Epidemiology: Principles and Methods. Boston: Little, Brown, 1970.

Miettinen OS. Proportion of disease caused or prevented by a given exposure trait or intervention. Am J Epidemiol 1974;99:325.

Ottman R. An epidemiologic approach to gene-environment interaction. Genet Epidemiol 1990;7:177.

Rothman KJ. Modern Epidemiology. Boston: Little, Brown, 1986.

Sackett DL. Clinical Epidemiology: A Basic Science for Clinical Medicine. Boston: Little, Brown, 1991.

Chapter 11

Cerebrospinal Fluid, Cerebrospinal Fluid Dynamics, and Lumbar Puncture

Christian J.M. Sindic

Chapter Plan

Cerebrospinal Fluid

History

Galen, a Greek physician of the second century, described the cerebrospinal fluid (CSF) as a vaporous humor produced in the cerebral ventricles that provided energy to the entire body. In 1825, Magendie showed the continuity between the subarachnoid spaces and the ventricles and described the anatomic localization of CSF. The study of CSF in neurologic disorders started in 1891, when Quincke did the first lumbar puncture (LP); this had previously only been tried on cadavers. The first comprehensive study on CSF proteins was made by Mestrezat in 1912. This author offered pathophysiologic explanations, which are still valid, of the changes in CSF composition; these were either a result of defective spinal circulation with impaired CSF production and resorption, or plasma transudation through capillaries with abnormal permeability. Currently, four principal roles are attributed to CSF: (1) mechanical protection and support, (2) intracerebral transport, (3) internal milieu, and (4) lymphatic circulation.

Anatomy and Physiology

The CSF is a clear, colorless liquid that fills the ventricles (approximately 35 ml), the subarachnoid spaces surrounding the brain (approximately 25 ml), and the spinal cord (approximately 80 ml) (Figure 11-1). Its total volume is approximately 140 ml, and its mean rate of formation is calculated at 0.4 ml per minute, or 500 ml per day. The entire volume is renewed every 7 hours, a little more than three times daily. The bulk of CSF (approximately 70%) is produced in the choroid plexus; the remainder is derived from the capillary

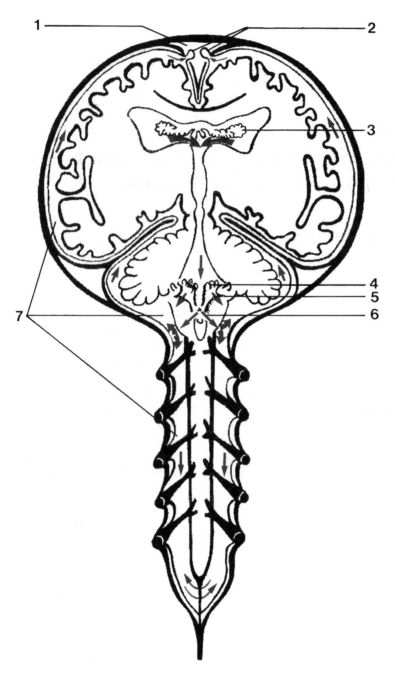

Figure 11-1. Schematic diagram of the CSF circulation. 1. Longitudinal superior sinus. 2. Arachnoid villi. 3. Superior choroid plexus. 4. Inferior choroid plexus. 5. Lateral foramina of Luschka. 6. Foramen of Magendie. 7. Subarachnoid space.

bed of brain and spinal nerve roots, from the vessels traversing the subarachnoid space, and from metabolic water production. The choroid plexus, which regulates the CSF composition, produces CSF by secretion, not by passive diffusion. Sodium and potassium are transported by an energy-dependent sodium-potassium ATPase pump, and water flow is secondary to the gradient produced by this pump. The Cl^- and HCO_3^- anions move passively into CSF.

The internal CSF has a net flow from its primary source, the choroid plexus in the ventricles, and connects with the fluid of the subarachnoid space via the two lateral foramina of Luschka and the foramen of Magendie, located in the lateral recesses and in the midline of the caudal roof of the fourth ventricle, respectively. The external CSF flows both cranially toward the arachnoid villi associated with the superior sagittal sinus, and caudally to the spinal subarachnoid space. Within the spinal subarachnoid space, the CSF flows predominantly caudally in the posterior portion and rostrally in the anterior portion. The arachnoid villi are the main sites of absorption of the CSF into the dural sinuses. It is the hydrostatic pressure difference between the CSF and the sagittal sinus that drives the CSF across the arachnoid villi. An equilibrium between the formation and absorption rates occurs at approximately 11 cm H_2O. Lymphatics of the spinal and cranial nerves could be minor sites of CSF absorption.

The CSF has an important cushioning effect, providing buoyancy and thereby "reducing" the weight of a 1,500-g brain to approximately 50 g. It acts as an important protective device against trauma, stretching, and compressive forces. It is also an important factor in the diffusion of metabolites in and out of the brain. Alterations in its composition markedly influence functions of the central nervous system (CNS). Changes of calcium, potassium, and magnesium concentrations are known to alter blood pressure, heart rate, and other autonomic functions. The CSF has an excretory role whereby unwanted drugs and metabolic products that enter the extracellular fluid of the brain are rapidly diluted by its "sink action."

Content

The chemical composition of CSF compared with that of plasma reveals higher concentrations of sodium, chloride, and magnesium but lower concentrations of potassium, bicarbonate, calcium, phosphate, and glucose. However, the most dramatic difference between plasma and CSF is the protein content, which is on the average approximately 250 times lower in CSF (Table 11-1). This difference is the result of the presence of a blood-brain barrier and a blood-CSF barrier to proteins, first suggested by the early experiments of Goldman with trypan blue. When such a dye was injected into the systemic circulation, it stained most organs but not the brain. As this dye is bound to plasma proteins, the barrier to injected dye was actually to dye-protein

Table 11-1. Overall Composition of Cerebrospinal Fluid Versus Blood

	Cerebrospinal Fluid	Blood
Sodium (mmol/liter)	147.0 ± 2.6	139.7 ± 2.7
Chloride (mmol/liter)	123.3 ± 2.5	103.1 ± 3.3
Magnesium (mmol/liter)	1.12 ± 0.07	0.83 ± 0.04
Potassium (mmol/liter)	2.84 ± 0.17	3.93 ± 0.33
Calcium (mmol/liter)	1.32 ± 0.12	2.36 ± 0.13
HCO_3 (mmol/liter)	21.5	24.7
Glucose (mg/dl)	65.3 ± 8.0	83.2 ± 16.0
Protein (g/liter)	0.29 ± 0.13	74.3 ± 11.9
Leukocytes (per μl)	1–5	4,000–10,000

complexes. In contrast, there is no impediment to protein exchange between the brain-pial surface and the ependymal surface on one hand and the CSF on the other (Figure 11-2).

The cellular composition of CSF also is dramatically different from that of blood, as the CSF contains no more than 5 cells per milliliter, with a cell ratio of two-thirds lymphocytes and one-third monocytes. In normal CSF, there are neither granulocytes nor plasma cells.

"Barrier" Concept

The blood-brain barrier, the blood-CSF barrier, and the blood–spinal root barrier are different barriers and should no longer be considered a single entity. The blood-brain barrier consists primarily of the capillary-glial barrier, and its morphologic basis relies on (1) the presence of tight junctions between the capillary endothelial cells; (2) the glial foot processes surrounding the capillaries; (3) the near absence of pinocytosis and vesicular transport of blood-borne material into and across endothelial cells; and (4) the absence of transendothelial channels. Tight junctions also link adjacent epithelial cells of the choroid plexus; they restrict but do not completely impede the movement of macromolecules and polar (non–lipid-soluble) substances from the fenestrated choroid capillaries to the ventricular CSF. The same tight junctions are also present between cells of the outer arachnoid layer. However, peripheral nerves must pierce the dura mater and traverse the subarachnoid space to reach the

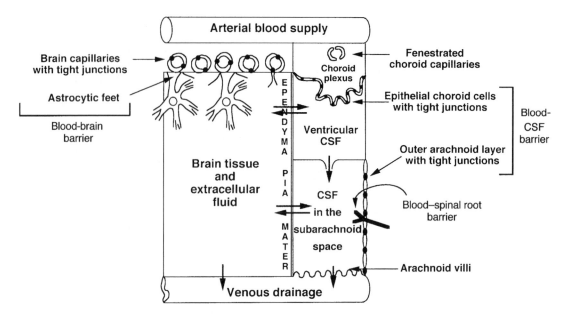

Figure 11-2. Schematic diagram of the blood-brain, blood-CSF, and blood–spinal root barriers. Black dots represent tight junctions between endothelial cells of brain capillaries, epithelial choroid cells, and cells of the outer arachnoid layer. (CSF = cerebrospinal fluid.)

surface of the brain or spinal cord. Where the nerve penetrates the meninges, the more superficial layers of the perineurium diverge from its surface and join the dura and arachnoid layers, whereas the inner layers persist as the deeper part of the root sheath. These inner layers apparently terminate as an open-ended tube near the junction of the peripheral nervous system and CNS. There is therefore continuity between the interstitial space of the endoneurium and the subarachnoid space through gaps or fenestrations between pial cells. The blood–spinal root barrier is thus the most permeable one, also at the level of the vasculature within the dorsal root ganglia, and this explains why the protein content of lumbar CSF, although 250 times lower than in the plasma, is about twice the one of ventricular CSF.

Roster of Cerebrospinal Fluid Proteins

The restricted movement of plasma proteins across the above-described "barriers" accounts for the low protein content of the CSF and for the relative exclusion of proteins of high molecular weight. In healthy people, the absolute CSF levels of plasma-derived proteins depend on many factors, such as their hydrodynamic radii, their serum concentrations, the age-dependent function of the blood-CSF barrier, the CSF flow, and the volume of CSF extracted.

Albumin is the major CSF protein and represents approximately 55% of the total protein content, a proportion similar to that observed in serum. Albumin is synthesized only by hepatocytes and is not catabolized within the CNS. Dynamic studies using intravenously injected radiolabeled albumin have demonstrated that serum albumin is the precursor of CSF albumin and strongly support the use of CSF/serum albumin quotient (Q Alb) to assess the blood-CSF barrier function. The Q Alb is age dependent. The upper reference limit for the first 10 ml of lumbar fluid is 5.0×10^{-3} for patients younger than 15 years; 6.5×10^{-3} for patients younger than 40 years; 8×10^{-3} for patients younger than 60 years, and below 9×10^{-3} for older patients; it may be as high as 28×10^{-3} in newborns.

The same dynamic studies using radiolabeled immunoglobulin G (IgG) have also shown that serum IgG is the precursor of CSF IgG: In normal conditions, CSF IgG originates from the blood and there is no antibody production within the CNS.

Proteins of high molecular weight, such as alpha and beta lipoproteins, fibrinogen, alpha$_2$-macroglobulin, and IgM, are present in CSF only as a minute fraction of their plasma concentration. In addition, up to 20% of CSF proteins are synthesized within the brain or the choroid plexus and released into the relatively small (140 ml) CSF pool. These proteins are mainly the prostaglandin D synthase (formerly called *beta-trace protein*), transthyretin (formerly called *prealbumin*), and cystatin C (formerly called *gamma-trace*). Therefore, the rank order of the major CSF proteins is completely different from that of plasma (Table 11-2).

Prostaglandin D synthase constitutes approximately 8% of the total protein content of normal human CSF, at a concentration approximately seven times higher than that of serum. It is synthesized by glial and choroid cells but also in genital organs. Its biologic significance in CSF remains obscure: Its product, prostaglandin D$_2$, is not detected in significant amounts in normal CSF, and other known prostaglandin synthases are generally located intracellularly. Transthyretin is synthesized in choroid epithelial cells and secreted into the CSF; it mediates the transport of thyroxine from the bloodstream to the brain. Cystatin C is a basic low-molecular-weight protein that has a concentration approximately 5.5 times higher in CSF than in serum. mRNA for this protein is present in the choroid plexus as well as in the brain. Cystatin C is a potent protease inhibitor. Transferrin is also in part synthesized within the brain; the locally produced protein is devoid of sialic acid residues and displays a slower electrophoretic mobility (beta-2 transferrin). The detection of beta-2 transferrin in rhinorrhea is a marker for CSF leakage.

Table 11-2. Roster of the Major Cerebrospinal Fluid Proteins Versus Plasma

Cerebrospinal Fluid	Plasma
1. Albumin	1. Albumin
2. Prostaglandin D synthase (7-fold less)	2. IgG (3-fold less)
3. IgG	3. Beta lipoprotein
4. Transthyretin	4. Alpha lipoprotein
5. Transferrin	5. Fibrinogen
6. Alpha$_1$-antitrypsin	6. Transferrin
7. Apo A-lipoprotein	7. Alpha$_1$-antitrypsin
8. Cystatin C	8. Alpha$_2$-macroglobulin

Source: Adapted from EJ Thompson. The CSF Proteins: A Biochemical Approach. Amsterdam: Elsevier, 1988.

that a meningeal syndrome may be absent, minimal, or delayed in patients with immunodeficiency states, using immunosuppressive drugs, or with alcoholism as well as in patients with chronic CNS infections, meningeal carcinomatosis, and subarachnoid hemorrhage. In the latter case, LP is a more sensitive diagnostic procedure than brain computed tomographic (CT) scanning and is indicated when the CT scan appears normal but clinical suspicion remains high. Analysis of CSF is very specific for meningeal malignancy and must be performed in any patient at risk of developing a chronic meningitis because of an underlying debilitating disease. Bacterial meningitis may present as a febrile coma with acute onset. LP is a valuable adjunct to CT scanning or magnetic resonance imaging (MRI), and to electrodiagnostic tests in the diagnosis of multiple sclerosis, Guillain-Barré syndrome, chronic inflammatory polyneuropathies, and idiopathic intracranial hypertension.

Lumbar Puncture

Indications

An LP is indicated (1) in the presence of a meningeal syndrome; (2) in case of stupor or coma with normal findings on brain imaging, especially if fever is present; and (3) for the diagnosis of a great number of specific diseases of the nervous system.

Currently, the major indication for LP is in the diagnosis of meningitis, encephalitis, myelitis, and meningoradiculitis. One must keep in mind, however,

Contraindications

There are few absolute and some relative contraindications to LP, and one must carefully considered the risk/benefit ratio in each case. Absolute contraindications are

- A local infection and suppuration of the skin and deeper tissues in the lumbar area.
- Evidence of increased intracranial pressure with focal neurologic signs, because transtentorial and foramen magnum herniation may be fatal.

The ideal way is to obtain a CT scan before LP, as a CT scan may show indirect signs of unequal pressures between intracranial compartments. The following CT abnormalities should be considered contraindications to LP:

- The lateral shift of the midline structures (septum pellucidum, third ventricle).
- The loss of the suprachiasmatic and circummesencephalic cisterns (basilar cisterns), indicating high supratentorial pressure pushing structures into the posterior fossa.
- The obliteration of the fourth ventricle or the obliteration of the superior cerebellar and quadrigeminal plate cisterns, with sparing of the ambient cisterns, indicating high infratentorial pressure pushing structures upward as well as through the foramen magnum. Indeed the strongest contraindication to LP is a posterior fossa mass.

Relative contraindications are

- Papilledema. LP is dangerous if the papilledema is related to an intracranial mass but is safe in relation with idiopathic intracranial hypertension.
- Bacteremia. Few patients developing meningitis after LP in the presence of bacteremia have been reported, and this occurrence is probably uncommon. In contrast, bacteremia may often be considered an important indication for LP to rule out concomitant meningitis.
- Presence of a bleeding disorder, with a low platelet count (less than 50,000 per μl), or the use of anticoagulants. In such conditions, the risk of subarachnoid hemorrhage and epidural spinal hematomas is clearly increased. Discontinuation of anticoagulants or administration of protamine, vitamin K, or platelet transfusion should be done before LP. In the same way, administration of anticoagulants should be strictly avoided within the hour after LP.

Complications

The most common complication of the LP is the well-known post-LP syndrome (PLPS), which occurs in approximately 30% of cases and is characterized by headache, back pain, dizziness, nausea, vomiting, increased sweating, and a tendency to orthostatic hypotension. It usually has a delayed onset of 24–48 hours and lasts for 3–4 days, but may occasionally persist for weeks or even for months. In such cases, it could predispose to subdural hematomas. The symptoms are exacerbated by standing and rapidly improved by lying flat. Bed rest and increased fluid intake have shown no satisfactory prophylactic effect on PLPS. The use of thinner needles or of "atraumatic" needles is the only way to reduce the incidence of this syndrome. The application of an epidural blood patch is a very effective treatment for severe PLPS.

The so-called puncture-hole theory is the most accepted explanation for the PLPS. It postulates that there is a persistent seepage of CSF through the LP hole that causes low CSF pressure and painful traction on the meninges and intracranial blood vessels. This seepage has indeed been documented using various imaging techniques. However, this theory does not explain why the PLPS is twice as common in women as in men and occurs less frequently in children and in the elderly.

Technique of Lumbar Puncture

For performing a diagnostic LP in a cooperative patient, the sitting position is generally used. If not, the patient is positioned lying on his or her side, with the knees drawn up to the chest and the head slightly flexed. The imaginary transverse line between the tops of the patient's iliac crests indicate the approximate level of the L3–L4 interspace, the proper site for puncture. Puncture above this level may risk damage to the spinal cord, which ends as low as the L2–L3 level in up to 6% of patients. Alternatively, the L4–L5 interspace may also be used. After meticulous disinfection with iodine and local anesthesia with 5 ml lidocaine, the LP is carried out with a 20- or a 22-gauge cannula with a Quincke bevel or, preferably, with an atraumatic cannula of similar size. The atraumatic cannula is a needle with a tip shaped like a closed circular cone with a rounded profile and is usually used with an outer cannula (introducer). Its lateral opening is larger than the inside diameter. The use of such atraumatic needles has reduced the frequency of PLPS from 30% to 5% of patients.

If the patient complains of pain radiating down the lower extremity, a nerve root of the cauda equina has been struck. The procedure can continue, however, because the nerve roots floating within the CSF will be pushed aside and not damaged by the advancing needle. Once the needle is believed to be resting in the subarachnoid space, the stylet is withdrawn, and as soon as CSF appears, the cannula is connected to the manometer. Normal CSF pressure measured with a patient in the lateral recumbent position ranges 50–200 mm H_2O. Unequivocal elevated CSF pressures are those greater than 250 mm H_2O. CSF pressure levels are less reliable when measured with a patient in the sitting position. After a CSF sample is collected, the stylet must be replaced to prevent aspiration of arachnoid or nerve roots when the needle is withdrawn. Once the cannula is removed, a pressure is applied with sterile gauze on the puncture site. The patient is then advised to lie flat in bed for 3 hours, the first 30 minutes in the abdominal position if possible.

Cerebrospinal Fluid in Neurologic Diseases

Appearance

The normal clear and colorless appearance of CSF can be altered in various disorders to become cloudy, bloody, or xanthochromic. By visual inspection, a CSF sample containing as few as 50 cells per µl may be "snowy" and cloudy at counts of more than 200 per µl. A bloody sample caused by a traumatic LP must be differentiated from one that is bloody from subarachnoid hemorrhage. In the former, tubes that are collected earlier are bloodier than those filled later, the blot may clot, and after centrifugation, the supernatant will not be xanthochromic. In subarachnoid hemorrhage, the CSF will have a uniform appearance from one tube to another, and pigment changes after centrifugation will remain out of proportion to the protein level. Thus, in the absence of severe systemic jaundice, xanthochromic CSF that has either a normal or a slightly increased (less than 150 mg per dl) protein content indicates a previous subarachnoid or intracerebral hemorrhage with bilirubin formation. For values of more than 150 mg per dl, the degree of xanthochromia is related to the total protein content.

Cells

After LP, cells should be counted as soon as possible (preferably within 30–60 minutes), as differential cell loss occurs during CSF storage, neutrophils being the most fragile cells. A count of more than 5 per µl is consistent with disease of the CNS or meninges. As a rule, the presence of any cells in the CSF other than lymphocytes and monocytes is abnormal. The use of the cytospin centrifuge allows cells contained in 300 µl CSF to be concentrated onto a single area of a few square millimeters.

A predominance of polymorphonuclear cells (PMNs) indicates an acute infection by pyogenic bacteria involving the meninges or in close proximity to the meninges (e.g., empyema, brain abscess, mastoiditis). CSF lymphocytosis occurs in viral, fungal, tuberculous, and parasitic meningoencephalitis, postinfectious encephalitis, carcinomatous meningitis, and many other CNS inflammatory diseases. However, only 1% of patients with multiple sclerosis have lymphocyte counts of more than 35 per µl, and a count of more than 50 per µl makes this diagnosis unlikely. The presence of plasma cells in the CSF is always abnormal and may be detected in any disease characterized by the occurrence of CSF-restricted oligoclonal IgG bands (see "Detection of Cerebrospinal Fluid Oligoclonal IgG Bands and Antibodies"). In some cases, these cells are present despite unequivocally normal CSF cell counts.

It should be kept in mind that a PMN predominance is sometimes observed within the first hours of an echovirus meningitis, during a chronic fungal meningitis, and in neuro-Behçet's disease. CSF lymphocytosis is observed in the late phase of a treated pyogenic meningitis and of a subarachnoid hemorrhage, and in some toxic (drug-induced) meningitis. Eosinophils are present in cases of parasitic infections. The definite diagnosis of carcinomatous or lymphomatous meningitis relies on the detection of the corresponding neoplastic cells in the CSF, and this may require special immunocytochemical techniques.

Infectious Agents

In cases of either acute or chronic meningitis, the bacteria will be identified and their sensitivities to antibiotics tested by standard culture techniques. It is essential to prepare a Gram's stain to distinguish between gram-positive cocci and gram-negative rods. In suspected tuberculous meningitis, smears are positive for acid fast bacilli in only 15–25% of cases. Culturing of *Mycobacterium tuberculosis* can take 4–8 weeks and may remain sterile even in cases later proven at necropsy. India ink smear may be helpful for the detection of *Cryptococcus neoformans*. However, the latex agglutination test detecting cryptococcal antigen is the most useful test and may produce positive results in more than 90% of cases, even when the results of cultures and India ink preparations remain negative.

The polymerase chain reaction (PCR) of CSF for the detection of herpes simplex virus (HSV) type 1 or type 2 DNA provides a reliable method for determining an etiologic diagnosis of herpetic encephalitis. The viral DNA can be detected in the first 7–10 days before anti-HSV antibodies are locally produced. Later in the disease, serologic results will be positive and PCR results negative. Therefore, CSF has to be systematically screened for herpes DNA and for anti-HSV antibodies in any case of acute or subacute encephalitis. PCR is also promising for the rapid diagnosis of tuberculous meningitis.

Glucose

The concentration of glucose within the CSF is normally 50–80 mg per dl, which is approximately 60% of its plasma concentration. In case of changing plasma levels, the equilibrium between both compartments is reached in approximately 4 hours. Low CSF glucose levels are observed in pyogenic, tuberculous, parasitic, and fungal meningitis, but also in carcinomatous meningitis and in subarachnoid hemorrhage. In the absence of hypoglycemia, a CSF level of less than 40 mg per dl or a CSF-to-plasma ratio of less than 0.3 is always abnormal. It should be noted that a slightly reduced glucose level may also be observed in some viral infections (i.e., mumps and herpes simplex meningitis, cytomegalovirus polyradiculitis in patients with acquired immunodeficiency syndrome) and in some cases of neuroborreliosis and neurosyphilis. A low CSF glucose level is secondary to an increased glucose utilization rate caused by an increased anaerobic glycolysis by the adjacent brain and spinal cord and to a lesser extent (depending on their number) by polymorphonuclear leukocytes. This explains the increase in CSF lactate levels that is found characteristically with a low glucose level.

An increased CSF glucose level is the result of a hyperglycemia and has no clinical significance.

Lactate

Levels of both CSF lactate and its enzyme (lactate dehydrogenase) are elevated in bacterial meningitis, and they have been suggested to be sensitive aids in its early diagnosis. A CSF lactate level of more than 3.5 mmol per liter in combination with a white cell count more than 800 per µl is indeed a good indicator of bacterial meningitis. Increased CSF lactate levels have also been found in seizures, traumatic brain injury, ischemia, subarachnoid hemorrhage, and comas of toxic or metabolic origin.

Proteins

The protein content of the CSF may be altered by four different but not mutually exclusive mechanisms:

1. An increased passage of plasma proteins into the CSF caused by an abnormal permeability of the blood-brain, blood-CSF, and blood–spinal root barriers
2. A reduced lumbar CSF flow caused by a spinal block, leading to an increased exchange time at the level of a normal blood–spinal root and blood-CSF barrier below the block
3. The synthesis within the CNS of proteins that are normally not synthesized therein (e.g., the immunoglobulins)
4. The increased release into the CSF of proteins normally synthesized by brain cells (e.g., myelin basic protein, S-100 protein, glial fibrillary acidic protein, neuron-specific enolase, ferritin).

Total Protein Content

By analyzing the total protein content and especially the albumin level of the lumbar CSF, one can assess the integrity of the functionally defined blood-CSF and blood–spinal root barriers but not always of the isolated blood-brain barrier. For example, large hemispheric infarcts with a completely broken blood-brain barrier may have no effect on the composition of the lumbar CSF. The same is also observed in multiple sclerosis, in which frequent impairment of the blood-brain barrier, as demonstrated by contrast-enhanced MRI scans, is not detected at the lumbar CSF level. Anatomic constraints (e.g., distance to the ventricles, too small lesions) and the direction of the physiologic CSF flow explain the lack of sensitivity of lumbar CSF analysis to the detection of an impairment restricted to the blood-brain barrier.

Because albumin is the major protein of both plasma and CSF and is synthesized only by hepatocytes, any increase of the CSF albumin level results from an increased transudation from the blood and will lead to an increase in the total CSF protein content. In adults, the upper reference values are 55 mg per dl for the total protein content, 28 mg per dl for albumin, and 8×10^{-3} for Q Alb. As already stated, these limits are age dependent. In contrast to absolute concentrations, quotient values are independent from methods and standards, and this allows direct comparisons between different laboratories. An increased CSF protein content caused by a pathologic transudation process or a reduced lumbar CSF flow is observed unspecifically in a great number of neurologic disorders (Table 11-3).

Quantification of the Humoral Immune Response within the Central Nervous System

The detection of a humoral immune response in the CNS requires an expression of results that will discriminate between blood-derived and brain-derived immunoglobulin fractions in CSF. Such quantitative expressions are based on calculations of the CSF/serum quotients of the various immunoglobulin isotypes (i.e., IgG, IgA, IgM) for comparison with the Q Alb. Mathematical analysis of the immunoglobulin quotients observed in disorders characterized by an impairment of the blood-CSF barrier clearly shows that transudated CSF immunoglobulins are not linearly related to the Q Alb. Linear formulas, such as the IgG index or the formula of Tourtellotte, lead to an important loss of specificity with a high rate of false-

Table 11-3. Neurologic Disorders Regularly Associated with a High Cerebrospinal Fluid Protein Content

Without concomitant increase of CSF cells (albuminocytologic dissociation)
  Guillain-Barré syndrome
  Chronic inflammatory polyradiculoneuropathies
  Other polyneuropathies (diabetic, rarely toxic)
  Leukodystrophies
  Hereditary hypertrophic neuropathies
  Myxedema
  Amyotrophic lateral sclerosis
  Disc herniation
  Ischemic stroke
  Tumor of the central nervous system, either benign or malignant, especially in case of spinal block caused by cord tumor, arachnoiditis, epidural abscess, large midline disc herniation: Froin's syndrome (CSF coagulation)
With concomitant increase of CSF cells
  Meningitis, meningoradiculitis, encephalitis, myelitis
  Carcinomatous or lymphomatous meningitis
  Subarachnoid and brain hemorrhages

CSF = cerebrospinal fluid.

positivity when the blood-CSF barrier is severely disrupted, especially for large molecules such as IgA or IgM.

The graphic representation of the immunoglobulin quotients as a nonlinear hyperbolic function of the Q Alb has been developed by Reiber and Felgenhauer for each isotype and has several advantages for the clinician (Figure 11-3). This graph gives simultaneous information about any local humoral immune response or any barrier dysfunction. In cases in which the immunoglobulin quotient falls above the upper reference line, the excess of CSF immunoglobulins has to be attributed to an intrathecal synthesis. There are four possibilities for this (see Figure 11-3): (1) normal albumin and immunoglobulin quotients; (2) normal Q Alb associated with an increased immunoglobulin quotient—that is, an intrathecal synthesis of immunoglobulins without blood-CSF barrier damage; (3) an increase of both quotients, the immunoglobulin quotient remaining under the upper reference line, in case of a pure transudation process through an impaired blood-CSF barrier; and (4) a disproportionate increase of the immunoglobulin quotient compared with the

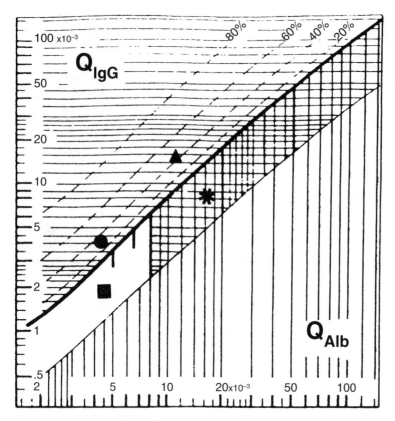

Figure 11-3. The Reiber graph as applied to the detection of an IgG intrathecal production. Q Alb and Q IgG are the cerebrospinal fluid (CSF)/serum ratio × 10⁻³ for albumin and IgG, respectively. Values from normal CSF samples are located in the white area (*black square*). The filled circle represents samples with a normal blood-CSF barrier but a local synthesis of IgG, as observed in approximately 75% of patients with multiple sclerosis. The asterisk represents samples with only abnormal transudation of both albumin and IgG through an impaired blood-CSF barrier. The black triangle represents samples with both an intrathecal IgG synthesis and an impairment of the blood-CSF barrier. (Adapted from H Reiber. External quality assessment in clinical chemistry: survey of analysis for cerebrospinal fluid proteins based on CSF/serum quotients. Clin Chem 1995;41:256.)

increase of the Q Alb, in case of impairment of the blood-CSF barrier associated with an intrathecal synthesis of immunoglobulins.

In clinical practice, the detection of an intrathecal IgG synthesis is the most relevant and is observed, although with less sensitivity, in the same disorders in which CSF-restricted oligoclonal IgG bands are present (Table 11-4). Local IgA synthesis occurs in pyogenic and tuberculous meningitis and in herpetic encephalitis but is quite rare in multiple sclerosis. A strong IgM production is present in neurosyphilis, neuroborreliosis, and CNS trypanosomiasis and decreases in response to specific treatments.

The detection of a specific antibody synthesis may be performed similarly in calculating the ratio between the CSF/serum quotients for specific antibodies (Qspec) and total IgG (Q IgG). This antibody index (AI = Qspec/Q IgG) discriminates between a blood-derived and a pathologic brain-derived specific antibody fraction in the CSF; a value of more than 1.5 indicates a local specific antibody synthesis. Sensitivity and precision are greater if the virus-specific antibodies in the CSF and serum are determined simultaneously with an enzyme immunoassay in continuous concentrations (arbitrary units) instead of titer steps.

Detection of Cerebrospinal Fluid Oligoclonal IgG Bands and Antibodies

It is now widely accepted that the detection of oligoclonal IgG bands specific to the CSF is a more sensitive test for demonstrating an intrathecal immune response than any quantification of the humoral response by any mathematical formulation. However, the detection of such oligoclonal bands requires the following:

- A high electrophoretic resolution, which can be obtained only by isoelectric focusing
- A high sensitivity, which permits the use of unconcentrated CSF

- The possibility of a direct comparison between CSF and serum samples for the detection of "a mirror pattern"
- An immune-enzymatic characterization of the bands by an IgG-specific antibody staining

With such highly sensitive techniques, it is possible to detect five main IgG patterns (Figure 11-4):

1. The *normal pattern* is characterized by a diffuse polyclonal IgG background in both CSF and serum, without detectable oligoclonal banding.
2. The *mirror pattern* is characterized by the presence of identical IgG bands located at the same isoelectric points and similarly immunostained in both CSF and serum. This indicates a systemic immune activation without intrathecal synthesis. The mirror pattern results from the passive transudation of oligoclonal IgG from blood to CSF through a normal *or* an impaired blood-CSF barrier.
3. A particular case of a mirror pattern is the *"paraprotein pattern."* In such cases, the IgG bands are regularly spaced within a short range of pH gradient in both CSF and serum.
4. The pattern characteristic for a *local synthesis* of IgG reveals the presence of at least two oligoclonal IgG bands restricted to the CSF and absent in the corresponding serum.
5. A *mixed pattern* is characterized by the simultaneous presence of a mirror pattern and a local synthesis of some IgG bands. This pattern is mainly observed in systemic inflammation or in infections with CNS involvement, but also in some cases of multiple sclerosis.

Approximately 95% of patients with clinically definite multiple sclerosis display oligoclonal IgG bands restricted to the CSF. However, they are not specific to multiple sclerosis and are also present in various inflammatory disorders as well as in chronic infections of the CNS (see Table 11-4). In contrast, it should be noted that these CSF-restricted bands are *not* observed in acute disseminated encephalomyelitis (parainfectious perivenous encephalitis); in Guillain-Barré syndrome; in vascular, toxic, metabolic, traumatic, or psychiatric disorders; in neurodegenerative diseases, in radicular syndromes; and in most peripheral neuropathies.

Table 11-4. Neurologic Disorders Regularly Associated with the Occurrence of Cerebrospinal Fluid–Restricted Oligoclonal IgG Bands

Inflammatory diseases of the central nervous system
  Multiple sclerosis
  Neurosarcoidosis
  Behçet's disease
  Granulomatous angiitis
  Whipple's disease of the central nervous system
  Neurolupus
  Paraneoplastic disorders (limbic encephalitis, cerebellar degeneration)
Infectious diseases of the central nervous system
  Subacute sclerosing panencephalitis
  Viral encephalitis (herpes, HIV) and myelitis (HTLV 1)
  Viral meningitis (herpesviruses, mumps, HIV, but not picornaviruses)
  Late phase of pyogenic meningitis
  Neurobrucellosis
  Neurosyphilis
  Tuberculous meningitis
  Fungal meningitis (*Candida, Cryptococcus, Aspergillus* organisms)
  Parasitic infections of the central nervous system (toxoplasmosis, neurocysticercosis, schistosomiasis)
  In utero infections with central nervous system involvement (cytomegalovirus, rubella, toxoplasmosis)
Tumors
  Carcinomatous and lymphomatous meningitis
  Primary lymphoma of the central nervous system

HIV = human immunodeficiency virus; HTLV = human T-cell lymphotropic virus.

In some cases of multiple sclerosis, free light chains bands (either kappa or lambda) are present in CSF samples devoid of detectable oligoclonal IgG bands. These bands also represent a sensitive marker of an intrathecal immune response in multiple sclerosis as well as in other inflammatory and infectious disorders of the CNS.

The analysis of the antigen specificity of oligoclonal IgG bands is made possible by an antigen-driven immunoblotting: In this technique, CSF and serum IgG at an identical concentration are first submitted to isoelectric focusing and then transferred by capillary blotting onto a membrane coated with the antigen under study. The presence of oligoclonal antibodies only in the CSF, or more strongly immunostained in the CSF than in the serum, indicates an intrathecal synthesis of these antibodies (Figure 11-5).

THE 5 IgG PATTERNS IN CSF versus SERUM

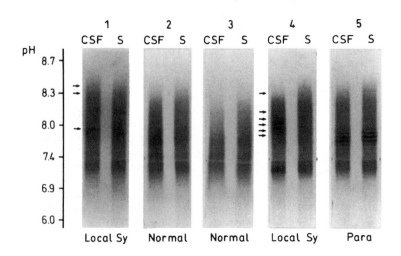

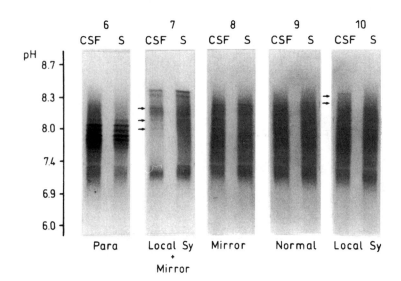

Figure 11-4. Immunoblotting of IgG in cerebrospinal fluid (CSF) and serum tested at the same IgG concentration (50 ng in 10 ml submitted to focusing) from patients with various neurologic disorders. Five IgG patterns have to be discriminated: normal (lanes 2, 3, 9), mirror (lane 8), paraprotein (lanes 5 and 6), local synthesis (Sy, *arrows;* lanes 1, 4, 10: two cases of multiple sclerosis and one case of neurosyphilis), and mixed (i.e., a local synthesis and a mirror pattern; lane 7, a case of subacute sclerosing panencephalitis).

Other Proteins Synthesized Within the Central Nervous System

Various relatively brain-specific proteins may be abnormally released into the CSF during brain trauma, a stroke, or in the course of a postanoxic coma. The most frequently studied proteins have been the neuron-specific enolase, the S-100 protein, the glial fibrillary acidic protein, and the myelin basic protein. As a rule, the higher the CSF concentrations or the more persistent the increases of these proteins, the worse is the outcome of the neurologic disorder. High concentrations of the same proteins are also found in the CSF in Creutzfeldt-Jakob disease because of the massive spongiform destruction of the CNS observed in this disease. Although it was suggested that elevations in myelin basic protein might be a specific marker for demyelination, it has limited diagnostic usefulness because the CSF level is increased by many other causes of myelin breakdown.

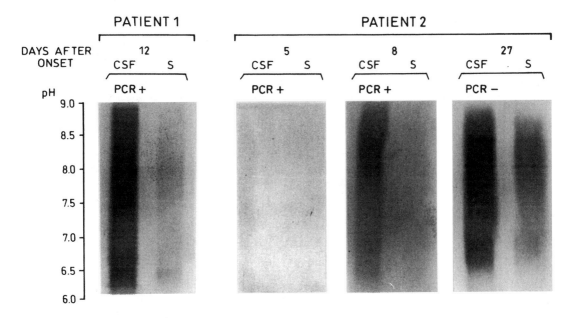

Figure 11-5. Antigen-driven immunoblots of anti–herpes simplex IgG antibodies in two cases of herpetic encephalitis at various days after clinical onset. For the first patient, the cerebrospinal fluid (CSF) contained simultaneously herpes DNA, as detected by polymerase chain reaction (PCR +) and numerous oligoclonal IgG antibodies reacting against herpetic antigens insolubilized onto a polyrinylidene diffluoride (PVDF) membrane. The corresponding serum was devoid of such antibodies. For the second patient, the PCR was positive at days 5 and 8, and a local production of anti-herpes antibodies was present at day 8 and amplified at day 27. (HSV = herpes simplex virus.)

Local synthesis of ferritin by brain cells, especially microglia, occurs even under normal circumstances. Its CSF level is much higher than could be explained by passive transfer across the blood-CSF barrier. An increase in CSF ferritin is found in pathologic processes characterized by either necrosis or hemorrhage involving the brain. After subarachnoid hemorrhage or in the course of herpetic encephalitis, the CSF level may be higher than that of homologous serum. Its determination is more sensitive than the traditional technique of testing for xanthochromia.

ter is far less available than a blood sample, it is necessary to "extract" as much information as possible from individual samples. A basic analysis consists of a bacteriologic culture, cell count, determination of the total protein and the glucose content, calculation of the CSF/serum quotients for albumin and IgG, and, finally, a search for oligoclonal IgG bands by isoelectric focusing and immunoblotting. In suspected infectious diseases of the CNS, lactate determination, detection of an IgM intrathecal synthesis, calculation of specific antibody indices, and, in some cases, specific PCR techniques should be performed as well.

Conclusion

Analysis of the CSF remains a cornerstone in the diagnosis of many neurologic diseases and must often be done in emergency conditions. LP is a safe technique if some precautions are taken. For a comprehensive CSF study, a serum sample must always be collected simultaneously with the CSF sample. Because the lat-

Suggested Reading

Andersson M, Alvarez-Cermano J, Bernardi G, et al. Cerebrospinal fluid in the diagnosis of multiple sclerosis: a consensus report. J Neurol Neurosurg Psychiatry 1994;57:897.

Carson D, Derpell M. Choosing the best needle for diagnostic lumbar puncture. Neurology 1996;47:33.

Cinque P, Cleator GM, Weber T, et al. The role of laboratory investigation in the diagnosis and management of patients with suspected herpes encephalitis: a consensus report. J Neurol Neurosurg Psychiatry 1996;61:339.

Fishman RA. Cerebrospinal Fluid in Diseases of the Nervous System (2nd ed). Philadelphia: Saunders, 1992;183–252.

McConnell H, Bianchine J. Cerebrospinal Fluid in Neurology and Psychiatry. London: Chapman & Hall, 1994;5–33.

Reiber H, Felgenhauer K. Protein transfer at the blood–cerebrospinal fluid barrier and the quantitation of the humoral immune response within the central nervous system. Clin Chim Acta 1987;163:319.

Reiber H, Lange P. Quantification of virus-specific antibodies in cerebrospinal fluid and serum: sensitive and specific detection of antibody synthesis in brain. Clin Chem 1991;37:1153.

Reiber H. External quality assessment in clinical chemistry: survey of analysis for cerebrospinal fluid proteins based on CSF/serum quotients. Clin Chem 1995;41:256.

Sindic CJM, Laterre EC. Oligoclonal free kappa and lambda bands in the cerebrospinal fluid of patients with multiple sclerosis and other neurological diseases. An immunoaffinity-mediated capillary blot study. J Neuroimmunol 1991;33:63.

Sindic CJM, Monteyne Ph, Laterre EC. The intrathecal synthesis of virus-specific oligoclonal IgG in multiple sclerosis. J Neuroimmunol 1994;54:75.

Thompson EJ. The CSF Proteins: A Biochemical Approach. Amsterdam: Elsevier, 1988.

Thompson EJ. Cerebrospinal fluid. J Neurol Neurosurg Psychiatry 1995;59:349.

Chapter 12
Behavioral Neurology

Stephanie Clarke and Gil Assal

Chapter Plan

Delimiting the field
Historical aspects
Diagnosis in behavioral neurology
    Patient history
    Psychological examination
    Anatomic and functional analysis of brain structures
Patient care in behavioral neurology
    Specific rehabilitation
    Accompanying measures

Delimiting the Field

Behavioral neurology is the study of the etiology, diagnosis, and treatment of organic diseases of the brain that affect mental functions and behavior. As a discipline, behavioral neurology has many areas of overlap with neuropsychiatry and neuropsychology, but also some differences from them. *Neuropsychiatry* is intended to be the link between neurologic and psychiatric approaches to disturbances of mood and behavior. Within psychiatry, it emphasizes the neurologic basis of diagnosis and treatment of psychiatric disorders, and within neurology the occurrence and care of psychiatric symptomatology in neurologic diseases. In the newly created journal *Neuropsychologia, neuropsychology* has been defined as an "area of neurology of common interest to neurologists, psychiatrists, psychologists and neurophysiologists." It aims at understanding cognition, emotion, and more generally behavior in terms of brain organization. It contributes to the diagnosis of neurologic diseases and to the monitoring of their evolution. Rehabilitation of behavioral and cognitive deficits after brain lesions is often not conceived as part of neuropsychology, but is often referred to as *neuropsychological rehabilitation.*

Despite its name, behavioral neurology is not an application of behaviorism to neurology. The central tenet of behaviorism, namely that our behavior is the product of conditioning and not determined by thoughts, feeling, and intentions (see, for example, the corresponding entries in *The Oxford Companion to the Mind*), is only of peripheral relevance to the practice of behavioral neurology. Similarly, *behavior therapy*, a term coined in the 1950s to denote a method of treatment of neurotic disorders based on pavlovian or on operant conditioning, is rarely used for treatment of brain-damaged patients. The central focus of contemporary behavioral neurology lies in the multidisciplinary approach to cognitive and behavioral disturbances and in its interactions with basic neurosciences. In particular, it stresses the link between behavior and the functional organization of cortical and subcortical structures. This link is bidirectional; behavioral neurology provides clinical observations that give important indications as to the functional specialization of the different structures, and the understanding of the functional organization of brain structures provides behavioral neurology with useful insights for neurorehabilitation.

Historical Aspects

Although the relationship between the brain and mental functions was firmly established in the eighteenth century, the ascent of behavioral neurology and of neuropsychiatry took place only in the second half of the nineteenth century. Covering the entire history of behavioral neurology is beyond the scope of this chapter, but three movements that influenced deeply today's view of neuropsychiatry, behavioral neurology, and neuropsychological rehabilitation should be mentioned: (1) the humanistic and scientific approach to psychiatry in the early nineteenth century, (2) the clinical-anatomical correlations in the second half of the nineteenth century, and (3) large-scale efforts for rehabilitation of brain-damaged soldiers after World War I.

Neuropsychiatry has its modern origins in the rapidly expanding field of mental illness in the beginning of the nineteenth century. The conditions of mental patients had radically improved at this time, following the reforms introduced by Philippe Pinel in French hospitals. The more humane approach to psychiatric patients was accompanied by brain research. An outstanding example of his time is Jules-Gabriel-François Baillarger, who contributed decisively to both clinical and basic neuroscience. In clinical psychiatry, his favorite subjects were *folie à double forme*, today's manic-depressive disorder; hallucinations, which he believed to be an involuntary replay of memory or imagination; and general paralysis. At the same time, he was keenly interested in the neuropathologic basis of the diseases he observed and he published approximately 20 books on this subject. Because his own studies and those of his contemporaries indicated that the cerebral cortex was greatly involved in psychiatric and neurologic diseases, he became interested in its organization. His name remains attached to the notion that the cerebral cortex is a layered structure, and the outer and inner cortical striae still bear his name.

Behavioral neurology and neuropsychology have their roots in the second half of the nineteenth century. The publication by Paul Pierre Broca (1861) of a case report of speech disorder associated with left frontal damage marked the new era of localizationism. The relationship between different types of aphasia and different localizations of lesions was further explored and described in 1874 by Carl Wernicke. His model of aphasia is still highly relevant for clinical practice; it postulates an anterior speech area (Broca's area) involved in speech production, a posterior speech area (Wernicke's area) involved in speech comprehension, and a connection from the posterior to the anterior area (arcuate fasciculus) critical for repetition of heard information. In the second half of the twentieth century, the neuroanatomy of behavior was reintroduced to clinical neurology by Norman Geschwind. He brought to new life observations by Wernicke and his contemporaries, and he confronted them with new data from neuroanatomic studies in nonhuman primates. His classic papers on disconnection syndromes, hemispheric asymmetries, and cerebral lateralization explained how behavioral disorders such as apraxias could be understood in terms of hemispheric specialization and cortical connectivity.

The term *neuropsychology* is a child of the second half of the twentieth century; it was defined in the editorial of the first number of *Neuropsychologia* in 1963. However, as a discipline, neuropsychology is rooted in the work of Broca, Wernicke, Goldstein, Klüver, and Teuber. In that, its history is not different from behavioral neurology.

Neuropsychological rehabilitation developed in parallel to the work that established neuropsychology (and behavioral neurology) as a distinct discipline. Paul Broca (1865) described his efforts to retrain the reading capacities of an aphasic patient; he noted that in his patient, reading could not be faultlessly acquired again, and that his patient relied on strategies that were different from those used by children. During and after World War I, military hospitals for the rehabilitation of head-injured soldiers were founded in Germany. Walter Poppelreuter clearly recognized the scientific interest in the study of brain-damaged soldiers, but also the need for their treatment and social support. He advocated an interdisciplinary approach integrating psychology, neurology, and psychiatry. Kurt Goldstein introduced the distinction between restorative therapy—that is, trying to restore a patient's earlier capacities—and compensatory therapy—that is, development of substitutive strategies for lost or impaired functions. For Goldstein the decision between the two therapies depended on the size of the lesion. He did not believe in assigning individual functions to strictly defined areas of the brain, which would then be irretrievably lost in the case of

Table 12-1. Domains in which Objective Information Should Be Sought During the Interview with the Patient and Family

1. General information on the patient
   Handedness
   Mother tongue (mono-, bi-, multilingual)
   Educational level
   Profession
   Hobbies, interest, particular expertise
   Premorbid personality
   Premorbid intelligence
   Previous illnesses (somatic or psychiatric)
2. General information on patient's family
   List of family members who interact often with the patient
   Family relationship, structure
   Occurrence of neurologic or psychiatric diseases within the family
3. Current disease
   Time-course of the onset
   Context of the onset
   Nature of cognitive and behavioral disturbances
   Occurrence of deficits in memory, word finding, understanding of other people, reading, writing, numerical skills, dressing, spatial orientation, route finding, recognition and identification of people or objects, thinking and problem solving, professional skills and expertise

Table 12-2. Domains in which a Subjective Account from the Patient Should Be Sought

1. Prior to current disease
   Particular beliefs (religious, philosophical)
   Relationship with family members, friends, colleagues
2. Current disease
   Degree of awareness of the impairment
   Emotional reaction to the impairment
   Emotions and mood generally
   Relationship with family members, friends, colleagues
   Changes in personality and social conduct
   Occurrence of obsessional phenomena, hallucinations, delirious ideations
   Changes in preferences, tastes, and appreciations
   Changes in eating habits
   Changes in sexual behavior
   Interpretation by the patients (and his or her family) of the cognitive and behavioral disturbances

damage. He assumed cooperation between different brain structures underlying one function. If only part of this structure was damaged, restorative therapy would be successful, but if all parts were damaged, compensatory therapy should be used.

Diagnosis in Behavioral Neurology

Diagnosis in behavioral neurology is based on three pillars: the patient's interview, preferably complemented by an interview of the patient's family; the psychological examination; and the anatomic and functional evaluation of damage to brain structures.

Patient History

The aim of interviewing the patient and the patient's family is to obtain an accurate and detailed account of the patient's problems and of their evolution as well as of the patient's experience of these problems. Objective information on the patient's socio-

professional and medical background and the time-course and symptomatology of the present disease (Table 12-1) can be obtained in a structured interview with the patient. Nevertheless, this information should be checked by interviewing other members of the patient's family or witnesses in the case of an accident or epileptic disorder. In many instances, it is difficult to distinguish a true statement from confabulation, to detect gaps in a biography, or to reconstruct the course of an accident from the patient's account alone. If a patient with a frontal tumor confabulates in a structured and reasonably convincing way, the account of his or her professional life may sound true and the interviewer may tend to believe it. Conversely, if an alcoholic patient with a head injury states correctly but in a somewhat exaggerated way that he or she is related to a public figure, we may tend to disbelieve this. Checking of objective information with the family is of great importance in memory disorders because it allows the degree of impairment of episodic memory and possibly its temporal gradient to be determined.

The patient's subjective account of his or her disease is not only of great value to those interested in consciousness and its mechanisms but also contributes to the diagnosis and therapy (Table 12-2). Particular beliefs may influence the patient's attitude to his or her disease. We have examined a patient with disseminated posterior hemispheric lesions caused by meningo-encephalitis that occurred during adolescence. In his early 50s, he was investigated for complex partial epilepsy. He described visual hallucinations of a complex nature that occurred as an overlay of the real world. He saw unreal moving objects and small "scenes" playing within these objects. After he gained confidence in the interviewer, he explained that his visions were sent by extraterrestrial beings who thus revealed to the patient and to the fellow members of his sect (Raelian) how the world had been created. Thus, the patient interpreted the complex visual hallucinations in terms of his beliefs. The sad aftermath of this story is that he gained great standing within his sect because of his visions and refused antiepileptic treatment; 6 months after the first interview we examined him again, only to find an advanced deterioration.

When specifically questioned, some patients deny their disabilities, which may be hemiplegia, paraplegia, loss of a limb, involuntary movements, amputation of the visual field, aphasia, alexia, memory deficits, various cognitive deficits, depression, or inappropriate social behavior. This type of denial is referred to as *anosognosia*. This term, literally lack of knowledge of disease, was introduced in 1914 by Joseph François Félix Babinski to describe the lack of knowledge of left hemiplegia in two patients with right hemispheric lesions. Some patients show awareness but not an appropriate emotional reaction to their disability. This condition is called *anosodiaphoria,* a term also coined by Babinski. Anosognosia and anosodiaphoria are not absolute or lasting phenomena. Many patients deny their disabilities in one context but not in another and may have implicit knowledge of them. The evaluation of anosognosia is of great value to diagnosis and to planning therapy; indeed, the patient has to be aware of his or her disabilities to participate effectively in the treatment.

In some instances, patients may deliberately hide their deficits. This can happen because the deficits appear utterly unbelievable (e.g., a prosopagnosic patient who was examined by us and who, as a farmer, found it unbelievable that he could no longer recognize his cows) or hurt the patient's self-esteem.

The interview should search actively for obsessional phenomena, hallucinations, delirious ideations, paramnesic reduplications, and signs of depression. The best approach is to use open-ended questions on possible changes in visual, auditory, tactile, olfactory, and gustatory experiences and in daily routines.

Psychological Examination

Assessing the patient's mental status can rely on a predominantly clinical appreciation or can include specialized psychological tests. We propose here a short clinical evaluation (Table 12-3), but give also a selection of psychological tests (Tables 12-4 to 12-6). The neurologist should know the classic psychological tests; if a neurologist is trained as a behavioral neurologist, he or she is able to administer them.

Clinical Assessment

A well-trained clinician should be able to arrive at a preliminary diagnosis by carrying out a short survey of the patient's cognitive functions and behavior. Several prototypes of clinical assessment have been published by others. The survey that we propose in Table 12-3 should take 10–20 minutes to carry out and does not need any special materials except a pencil; a sheet of paper; and a small booklet containing the examiner's photograph (passport type), a photograph of a person known by the public at large, a text written across the page, a list of words and pseudowords, a picture of a scene, overlapping figures as proposed by Walther Poppelreuter, a chimeric image (e.g., comb-ruler), and a map without names (Figure 12-1). If the examiner does not wear spectacles, he or she can use for the naming task a watch and its parts (e.g., strap, face, hands). The order of the assessment is the one that we found easiest to administer; the first points are usually well accepted by the patient and help to orient the following explorations. The numbers used below are the same as in Table 12-3, where test items are listed; for pictorial representations, see Figure 12-1.

1. Speech production can be tested with an open-ended question, such as "Why are you in the hospital?" The patient's understanding of this question has to be taken with caution, however, because this type of question is often expected at the beginning of a patient interview. The complexity and clarity of the reply give gen-

Table 12-3. Bedside Assessment for the Clinician

1. Speech production
   "Why are you in the hospital?"
   "What do you see in this picture?" (see Figure 12-1)
2. Automatic series
   Counting
   Days of the week
3. Auditory-verbal understanding
   "The lion was devoured by the tiger. Who is dead?"
   "The dog was bitten by the doctor, there is blood on the
      floor. Who is bleeding?"
   "If there is no blue bird in the room, take off your
      glasses/open your mouth!"
   "If I am wearing glasses, clap your hands!"
4. Repetition
   Auditory-verbal span of five to six digits
   "Methodist Episcopal"
5. Trying to elicit echolalia
   "That's fine!"
   "Beautiful weather!"
   "He is a nice person."
6. Completion of sentences
   "When you are ill, you go to see the . . ."
   "To buy bread, you go to the . . ."
7. Naming
   On visual confrontation
      Objects, parts of objects (e.g., on spectacles: lens,
         frame, sidepiece)
      Picture in Figure 12-1
      Body parts
      Clothing
   On auditory confrontation
      Melodies hummed by the examiner
      Noises produced by the examiner: cough, clap hands
   On tactile presentation
      The examiner's thumb in the patient's left hand
8. Singing of well-known melodies
9. Reading
   Text (presenting it first upside-down; irregular spatial
      disposition)
   Words or pseudowords
10. Writing
    On dictation
    Name and address
    Copy
11. Spelling
    Three words ("animal, rider, household") forward and
       backward
12. Mental arithmetic
    $3 \times 17 =$
    $29 + 34 =$
    $72 - 16 =$
13. Left/right discrimination
    Hand presented at the back of the examiner
14. Ideomotor praxias
    Imitating postures: "butterfly"; touching index finger of
    one hand with the middle finger of the other; miming the
    use of objects: to hammer in a nail; to brush one's teeth;
    to saw with a saw
15. Motor sequences
    Reproduction of hand sequences (fist—external side—
       flat hand), or mouth sequences (open the mouth—
       grimace—protrude the tongue)
16. Constructional praxias
    Completion of Necker cubes
17. Visual recognition
    Overlapping figures (see Figure 12-1): "What do you see
       in this picture?"
    Chimeric image
    Recognition of objects (see point 7) or drawings of objects
       (see Figure 12-1)
    Photograph of the examiner, photograph of person known
       to the patient (see Figure 12-1): "Do you recognize this
       person?" "Is this a man or woman? What is his/her age?"
    Topographic orientation (see Figure 12-1)
18. Search for hemineglect
    Double stimulation: visual, tactile, auditory
    Visuomotor pointing within hemispace ipsilateral or
       contralateral to the pointing arm
    Line bisection
    Recognition of chimeric images, in particular faces
    Description of locations (geographic map, known region)
19. Memory
    Verbal span ("Hebb")
    Visuospatial span ("Corsi")
    Recall of the testing session
    Recall of the three words that were spelled and the three
       calculations
    In case of doubt, learning of a series of 10 words (see also
       Table 12-4)
20. Attention
    Reaction to a letter or a randomly arranged string of letters
21. Executive functions
    Verbal fluency: to name as many animals as possible in
       1 minute
    Antisaccades
    Eliciting utilization behavior: the examiner puts in front
       of the patient several objects of everyday use asking him
       or her not to touch them
    Eliciting imitation behavior: the examiner asks the patient
       to stay still, then holds out his or her hand
    Finding strategies or adaptations to modifications of a
       strategy
22. Reasoning
    "John covers the distance between [Geneva] and
       [Lausanne] at 15 km/h. How old is he?"
    "He buys 1 kg of apples at 15 francs per kg, and 2 kg of
       apples at 10 francs. How much money remains in
       his wallet?"
    "Because of accidents, the last railway carriage was
       removed. Was it a good idea?"

Table 12-4. Selection of Classic Psychological Tests Used in the Assessment of Brain-Damaged Patients

Name of the Test	Authors	Brief Description
Language tests		
Boston Naming	Kaplan et al. 1978; Kaplan et al. 1983	Naming of pictured objects. Original version contains 85 items, revised version 60 items; both are American. For use outside the United States, cultural and linguistic adaptation may be necessary.
Token Test	De Renzi and Vignolo 1962; De Renzi and Faglioni 1978	Understanding of auditory-verbal commands of increasing complexity using tokens of different colors, shapes, and sizes. The original version contains 61 commands, but different short versions have been published. This test can be adapted for understanding of written commands.
Dichotic Listening	Broadbent 1958; Kimura 1961	Repetition of two words presented simultaneously one to each ear. The extinction of stimuli administered in dichotic condition to one ear indicates damage to the contralateral hemisphere.
Nonverbal auditory tests		
Seashore Test of Musical Talent	Seashore et al. 1960	Musical perception.
Visual and visuospatial tests		
Complex Geometrical Figure	Rey 1941; Osterrieth 1945	Visuospatial constructional ability and visuospatial memory.
Judgment of Line Orientation	Benton et al. 1983	Estimation of angular relationships between line segments.
Overlapping Figures	Poppelreuter 1917; Ghent 1956	Discrimination of the shapes of four overlapping line drawings.
Street Completion Test	Street 1931	Completion of pictures for testing of perceptual closure capacities. Not discriminative of brain damage in older subjects.
Gollin Figures	Gollin 1960	Recognition of incomplete drawings.
Bell Test	Gauthier et al. 1985, 1989	Visual detections of 35 bell silhouettes scattered between 280 other objects. A sensitive test of visual inattention without ceiling effect.
Indented Paragraph Reading Test	Caplan 1987	Reading of a text in which line beginnings are not aligned; very effective in eliciting attention errors as well as tendencies to misreading.
Hooper Visual Organization	Hooper 1958	Conceptual rearrangement of pictures that have been cut and disassembled.
Trail Making Test	Army Individual Test Battery 1944	Visual search, attention, mental flexibility, and motor function.
Farnsworth 15 Hues Test	Farnsworth 1957	Color perception: arrangement of colored chips according to hue gradient.
Benton Facial Recognition Test	Benton and Van Allen 1968; Benton 1983; Levin et al. 1975	Matching of unknown faces: photographs from which clothing and hair are shaded out; front views have to be matched with front views, three-quarter views in the same or different lighting conditions.
Memory		
Verbal short-term memory span (Hebb)	Milner 1970, 1971	Short-term retention of digits. The span corresponds to the number of digits correctly repeated.
Visuospatial short-term memory span (Corsi)	Milner 1971	Short-term retention of spatial locations. The span corresponds to the number of locations correctly repeated.
Auditory-Verbal Learning Test (15 words)	Rey 1964; Taylor 1959	Memorizing of 15 words in five repetitions; assesses learning, recognition, and recall.
Visual-Nonverbal Learning Test (15 signs)	Rey 1968; Lanarès et al. 1987	Memorizing of 15 nonfigurative line drawings in five repetitions; assesses learning, recognition, and recall.

Selective Reminding Test	Bushke 1973	Verbal learning and memory during a multiple-trial list-learning task. Distinguishes between short-term and long-term retention.
Consonant Trigrams	Peterson and Peterson 1959	Short-term retention of consonants with intercalated distractor task.
Wechsler Memory Scale-Revised	Wechsler 1945, 1989	Measure of different aspects of memory functions.
Mirror Reading Mirror Drawing	Cohen and Squire 1980	Learning of new visuospatial or motor skills.
Executive functions		
Word Fluency Tests	Benton and Hamsher 1976	Oral production of words beginning with a designated letter.
Design Fluency Test	Jones-Gotman and Milner 1977	Invention of nonfigurative drawings.
Five-Point Test	Regard et al. 1982	Nonverbal fluency in a structured background.
Stroop Test	Stroop 1935	Measure of cognitive flexibility and suppression of habitual responses in favor of an unusual one.
Wisconsin Card Sorting Test	Berg 1948	Ability to form abstract concepts and to adapt to changes of classification criteria.
Raven's Progressive Matrices	Raven 1938, 1947, 1965	Reasoning in the visual modality in Standard version (60 items), Colored version (36 items), and Advanced version (48 items).
Tower of London Test	Shallice 1982	Planning of action to reach a goal. Other versions exist (Tower of Hanoi, Toronto).
Emotion		
Beck Depression Inventory	Beck and Beck 1972	Screening of depression in self-report.

For detailed descriptions of these tests, see Suggested Reading at the end of this chapter.

eral information about cognitive capacities. If the patient's reply is poor, he or she can be asked to describe a picture (see Figure 12-1).

2. If speech elicited under point 1 is nonfluent or shows arthric problems, automatic series should be obtained from the patient. They will point the diagnosis toward anarthria if they are better than nonautomatic speech, or dysarthria if as bad as spontaneous speech.

3. Auditory-verbal understanding can be assessed further by using complex sentences with a question or by giving commands preceded by an "if" clause. The former are also useful for assessing cognitive judgment by asking the patient whether or not these occurrences are frequent. If no replies are obtained in points 1 and 3, simple commands (e.g., "open your mouth," "close your eyes") should be used to ascertain the level of understanding.

4. The repetition task is essential for the evaluation of aphasia. Furthermore, the repetition of a span of five to six digits provides an evaluation of auditory-verbal short-term memory (see point 19) and the repetition of "Methodist Episcopal" a finer evaluation of articulatory capacities.

5. Trying to elicit echolalia is indicated in cases in which transcortical motor or sensory aphasia

or severe executive dysfunction is suspected. Unlike for point 4, the patient should be told not to repeat, but just to listen.

6. The completion of sentences allows testing of word-finding capacities and pragmatic attitudes.

7. The naming of objects should be tested for visual, auditory, and tactile stimuli.

8. Having the patient sing well-known melodies gives an appreciation of musical capacities and possible dissociation between speaking and singing.

9. For a rapid assessment of reading capacity, the patient should be presented with a page on which the text is upside-down. If writing is recognized as such, the patient will turn the page around. If a reading disorder is suspected, reading of words and pseudowords should be tested.

10. Writing can be assessed on dictation or by asking the patient to write his or her name and address or to copy a text.

11. Oral forward and backward spelling should be tested when writing disorders or general deterioration are suspected. Furthermore, the three words used for spelling can be asked for in the memory assessment (point 19).

photograph of the examiner	*photograph of a "famous" person known by the public*

Paris, 5th September
A fire has destroyed large parts of the city yesterday evening. Several houses were completely destroyed. Due to an explosion in one of the buildings one of the fire engines caught fire. The driver was burned severely.

PIPE   NEG
ISLAND   GLEM
CANARY   GORTH
TULIP
AND
THOROUGH

Figure 12-1. Items used for a short clinical assessment of cognitive functions (see Table 12-1 and text). Photographs of the examiner and of a famous person should be limited to the face and should be of the opposite sex and of different age groups. The text as well as words and nonwords should be arranged across the page. Instead of Bobertag's picture, other scenes can be used. Reproduced here is the original version of Poppelreuter's superimposed figures (1917); more modern versions can be used. A chimeric image with different left and right halves is useful for the assessment of visual recognition and of putative hemineglect. The map used should contain outlines of borders, shores, and rivers but no towns and no names; it should be adapted to the country of the patient (Switzerland is used here).

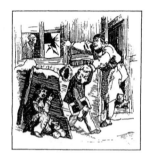

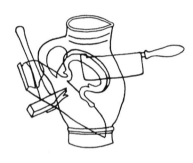

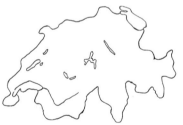

12. The interpretation of results in mental arithmetics depends on the educational level and occupation of the patient. As in the spelling task, these three items can be used for the memory assessment (point 19).

13. Left/right discrimination can be tested by asking the patient to indicate left or right body parts on himself or herself, on the examiner, or on pictures.

14. Ideomotor praxias can be tested either by imitation of hand postures or by miming the use of objects. The imitation of hand posture is more difficult to perform when the examiner and the patient are face-to-face and easier when they are side-to-side. Miming the use of objects should be elicited by verbal command, and if not successful, by imitation. The use of "body-part-as-object" should be looked for. If callosal disconnection is suspected, miming the use of objects should be investigated separately for the left and right hands.

15. The patient can perform motor sequences with either the hand or with the mouth.

16. Constructional praxias can be assessed by asking the patient either to draw a Necker cube or to complete such drawings. In our experience with more than 100 normal subjects, older people with limited education are unable to draw or to copy a Necker cube, but they are able to complete an unfinished drawing.

17. In visual recognition, both apperceptive and semantic aspects should be briefly tested. If object naming, and hence recognition of real objects, was satisfactory, recognition of pictorial representations should be tested (see Figure 12-1). Degraded representations, such as overlapping images, may reveal moderate recognition deficits. In a brief assessment, we recommend testing facial recognition using photographs of the examiner and of a "famous" person known to the general public. Chimeric images can be used for object recognition testing, but also give information about possible hemineglect (see point 18). Topographic orientation can be assessed rapidly by presenting the patient with a map that gives the outlines of borders, shores, and rivers but no towns and no names. The sheet with the map can be handed to the patient upside-down to test nonverbal recognition of the map. The patient is then asked to locate geographic landmarks on the map.

18. Hemineglect should be sought in the visual, auditory, and tactile modality. Useful information on the existence of a visual hemineglect can be readily collected in previous points (reading of a text, description of a picture, recognition of chimeric images, orientation on a geographic map; see Figure 12-1).

19. Short-term memory can be briefly assessed by testing the verbal span that is correctly repeated by most normal subjects of the corresponding age. General recall of the testing session and the recall of specific features (the three words that were spelled, the calculations) gives a rough estimate of anterograde memory.

20. Attention can be grossly assessed by asking the patient to react to a given letter while the examiner recites a list of letters in an arbitrary order.

21. The testing of executive functions will differ between patients who do or do not show overt signs of frontal dysfunction. In a patient displaying few deficits, the testing should concentrate on verbal fluency and capacities for determining strategies. In a patient with overt signs of frontal dysfunction, the severity of the deficits should be determined by trying to elicit imitation or utilization behavior.

22. Reasoning can be assessed roughly by presenting propositions and unrelated questions.

Psychological Tests

The assessment of cognitive functions and behavior can be broadened by the use of specific psychological tests. We give here a selection of classic psychological tests (see Table 12-4) and test batteries (see Table 12-5), as well as a few examples of tests developed for the assessment of specific domains (see Table 12-6). For readers particularly interested in testing procedures, we recommend manuals and compendia listed at the end of this chapter. Most tests listed in Tables 12-4 and 12-5 have been published in ready-to-use forms, including precise descriptions of the administration procedure, scoring sheets, and normative data. The latter represent statistical descriptions of performance of normal subjects and thus allow one to judge whether the performance of a brain-damaged patient is within normal limits. The normative data should, however, be used with caution. Knowing how they were obtained may help to avoid several pitfalls:

1. Normative data are representative of the population that was effectively tested. Thus, if normative data were obtained from psychology undergraduates ages 18–22 years, they are not useful for brain-damaged patients aged 50 years or more unless an additional study has shown that the performance in this particular test does not change with age.

2. A similar observation can be made concerning the socioprofessional level or sex of the control and patient population.

3. The cultural context within which the normative data were obtained may play a role. Thus, testing visual recognition or naming capacities of items related to baseball is a standard procedure in the United States but is not adapted for most European countries.

4. The limit of normal performance is an arbitrary decision. Often, a performance below that of the

Table 12-5. Standard Batteries of Psychological Tests Recommended for Use in Brain-Damaged Patients

Name of the Test	Authors	Brief Description
Language		
Neurosensory Center Comprehensive Examination for Aphasia (NCCEA)	Spreen and Strauss 1977, 1991	Examination of receptive, expressive, and immediate memory components of speech; includes Token Test.
Multilingual Aphasia Examination	Benton and Hamsher 1989	Examination of receptive, expressive, and immediate memory components of speech; includes Token Test. Developed from NCCEA.
Boston Diagnostic Aphasia Examination (BDAE)	Goodglass and Kaplan 1983	Assessment of "components of language" as in the Wernicke-Geschwind model; 34 subtests.
Western Aphasia Battery	Kertesz 1979, 1982	Adapted from BDAE for treatment and research purposes.
Visual and visuospatial functions		
Birmingham Object Recognition Battery	Riddoch and Humphreys 1993	Assessment of apperceptive and associative visual processing.
Memory		
Wechsler Memory Scale	Wechsler 1945, 1987	Measures of different aspects of memory.
Intelligence		
Wechsler Intelligence Tests	Wechsler 1981	Most frequently used measures of overall level of intelligence.
Global assessment		
Mini-Mental State	Folstein et al. 1975	Brief screening of cognitive functions.
Consortium to Establish a Registry for Alzheimer's Disease (CERAD)	Morris et al. 1989	Battery used for assessment of dementia. Includes Mini-Mental State.

poorest control subject or below 95% of the control subjects is considered as the limit between normal and abnormal performance.

Language Functions. There are a very large number of tests assessing different aspects of language; we list only a small selection that we found useful in our daily practice. Working in a non-English environment, we have elaborated French, German, and Italian versions of most of these tests and have elaborated normative data for the Swiss French-speaking population. The choice of testing procedure for language in brain-damaged patients is oriented by the cognitive model adopted by the clinician or researcher. Most clinically oriented tests rely on the Wernicke-Geschwind model and several testing batteries are inspired by the Boston Diagnostic Aphasia Examination.

Nonverbal Auditory Capacities. Compared with language, there are relatively few commercially available tests for recognition of musical items, environmental sounds, or emotional intonations of voices. The Seashore Test of Musical Talent is a useful tool for assessing musical capacities, and several tests of recognition of environmental sounds have been described in the literature. The nonverbal auditory domain remains relatively unexplored, however, and new tests are needed for exploring theoretical models. For example, we have assessed the effect of brain damage on different aspects of nonverbal auditory recognition to investigate the role of parallel and serial processing; the tests that we introduced in this study are listed in Table 12-6.

Visuocognitive and Visuospatial Capacities. There is a large choice of published tests for visual cognitive and visual spatial capacity. The selection given in Tables 12-4 and 12-5 is limited to what we find useful in everyday practice. It allows exploration of visuospatial and apperceptive functions. For the assessment of associative functions, one can rely on visual recognition of items in the Boston Naming Test, on recognition of photographs of famous people (to be adapted to the specific knowledge of the patient), or on specifically developed

Table 12-6. Three Examples of Recent Tests for Visual and Auditory Recognition

Domain	Authors	Brief Description
Recognition of known faces	Sergent and Poncet 1990	Testing procedure for overt and covert recognition of famous faces.
Visual recognition of items from specific categories	Clarke et al. 1997	Visual recognition by prosopagnosic patients with premorbid expertise within tested categories.
Recognition of plants and flowers		Recognition of plants from color photographs or drawings; naming or multiple choice. Patient: learned florist. Control subjects: florists age-matched to the patient.
Recognition of mountains		Recognition of views of Swiss mountains from color photographs. Patient: nurse, keen and active mountaineer. Control subjects: members of the Swiss Alpine Club, age-matched to the patient.
Nonverbal auditory recognition	Clarke et al. 1996	Battery of tests for exploration of the respective roles of parallel and serial processing in nonverbal auditory recognition.
Semantic identification of environmental sounds		Semantic identification of sounds of real objects as judged by means of a multiple choice response test.
Asemantic recognition of environmental sounds		Asemantic recognition of sounds of real objects by judging whether two different sound samples belong to the same object.
Segregation of sound objects		Capacity to segregate sound objects on different cues (intensity steps, coherent temporal modulations, signal onset synchrony).

Note: To investigate domains not covered by classic tests, new approaches have been developed: (1) for overt and covert recognition of famous faces; (2) for visual intracategorical recognition within specialized fields of knowledge; and (3) for nonverbal auditory recognition, introducing the notion of sound object segregation to lesion studies.

tests. Among the latter, we mention overt/covert facial recognition tests developed by Justine Sergent and Michel Poncet in 1990 and tests of within-category recognition for patients with specialized knowledge (see Table 12-6). In patients with well-defined deficits, it may prove interesting to investigate their compensatory strategies.

Memory. Again, there is a wealth of published tests of memory functions and our selection in Tables 12-4 and 12-5 is limited. It allows, however, assessment of short-term and long-term aspects of verbal and nonverbal memory, recognition versus recall capacities, role of interference, as well as procedural memory. An example of dissociation in verbal and nonverbal memory occurring after left anterior thalamic infarction is shown in Figure 12-2. The choice of additional tests is mostly dictated by the field being explored. The recognition aspect of memory is rarely investigated in classic batteries; to fill this gap our division has developed a test of visual recognition of 30 recurring items in a series of 100 for verbal and nonverbal material.

Executive Functions. Our selection is limited to well-established fluency tests (Thurstone's Word Fluency Test, Design Fluency Test, Five-Point Test), a reactive flexibility test (Stroop test), and tests of concept formation and reasoning (Wisconsin Card Sorting Test, Raven's Progressive Matrices, Tower of London Test). While testing patients, it should be kept in mind that their performance in a particular task may depend on the context. We have examined an athymhormic patient for verbal production in the standard testing setting—that is, facing the examiner. Her verbal production was very poor, similar to that in other situations when she was facing the person to whom she was speaking. When alone and speaking on the telephone or into a recorder, her verbal production became relatively rich.

Emotion. Emotional disturbances can influence cognitive task performance in normal and in brain-damaged subjects. Conversely, emotional disturbances can be caused by brain damage. Primarily psychiatric scales, such as the Beck Depression Inventory, can be used with brain-damaged patients.

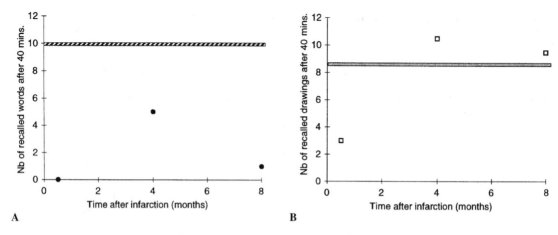

Figure 12-2. Performance in verbal (A) and nonverbal (B) memory at different times after left anterior thalamic infarction. The test consisted of memorizing 15 items—words or drawings—in five repetitions; the scores indicated on the *y*-axis correspond to recalled items 45 minutes after the last repetition from our own data. Bars indicate the lower limit of normal performance in a population matched for age and socioprofessional level to the patient. Note that in the acute stage the patient was deficient in both verbal and nonverbal memory, but later a dissociation between the performance in verbal and nonverbal memory appeared.

Anatomic and Functional Analysis of Brain Structures

Behavioral neurology is intimately linked to brain imaging. Whereas early observations were based on autopsy, modern anatomic analysis makes use of computed tomographic (CT) and magnetic resonance imaging (MRI) technology. New data on the functional organization of the normal and injured brain come from activation studies using positron emission tomography, functional MRI, evoked potentials, or magnetoencephalography.

Relationship Between Behavioral Profiles and Damage to Identified Anatomic Structures

There is a long-standing tradition of anatomoclinical correlations in behavioral neurology. Broca in 1861 and Wernicke in 1874 established a correlation between a circumscribed brain lesion and certain types of language deficits. Their initial observations led to the elaboration of the connectionist model for speech. Today, anatomoclinical correlations are appreciated for several reasons. First, the presence of certain deficits established by a purely psychological assessment can lead to valid predictions concerning the localization of the lesion, even in the absence of imaging data. Such a prediction is based on functional models derived from previous lesion studies (e.g., the above example of speech). Second, the relationship between the severity of a deficit and the anatomically demonstrated localization and extent of the lesion often has a predictive value for the prognosis. Third, the comparison of lesions of patients with or without a given deficit may lead to the identification of functionally relevant regions. Fourth, in the presence of a preexisting model, analysis of new cases of anatomoclinical correlations or the use of new techniques puts the validity of the model to the test. Therefore, the advent of new imaging techniques refined and somewhat complicated the connectionist model for speech. Several studies demonstrated that lesions associated with either Broca's, Wernicke's, or global aphasia were variable and not always limited to or including the corresponding speech areas.

Brain Mapping of the Normal Human Brain

Different brain mapping techniques applied to the human and nonhuman brain have profoundly changed our understanding of brain organization. One of the most striking examples is the human extrastriate visual cortex. Classically, the human extrastriate occipital cortex is often referred to as the visual association cortex and is classically subdivided into three cytoarchitectonic areas. A similar subdivision was proposed for macaque extrastriate cortex, but the work of the last 25 years has shown that it contains more than 30 functionally and anatomically defined visual areas. Early electro-physiologic work of Semir Zeki has shown that certain visual areas are highly specialized, such as area V4 for color and MT-V5 for motion perception. We have applied similar approaches to the human cortex and have shown that visual areas can be anatomically identified in humans. Although only six to eight extrastriate visual areas have so far been identified in humans, the concept of functionally specialized cortical areas becomes a critical issue in neurology and neurorehabilitation.

Another great contribution of imaging techniques to our understanding of brain organization is the visualization of brain activity related to mental functions. Although we cannot summarize most of the outstanding work in this field, we would like to draw attention to some aspects concerning language. The connectionist model postulated the existence of specialized centers within the left hemisphere: Broca's area, mainly involved in speech production, and Wernicke's area, mainly involved in speech reception. Activation studies have presented results that are not compatible with a simple version of this model. In particular, they have shown that in normal subjects both hemispheres are involved in speech, that both Wernicke's and Broca's areas are activated in speech reception, and that both are activated in speech production.

Confrontation of Activation and Lesion Studies

The notion that specific cortical areas are selectively involved in specific functions in normal subjects and that a lesion of these areas is responsible for the deficit in the corresponding function is one of the tenets of behavioral neurology. In rough terms, there is a consensus between activation and lesion studies. For example, prosopagnosia is mostly associated with bilateral posteroinferior lesions, and analysis of facial information has been shown to activate selectively the inferior parts of the temporal and occipital lobes in normal subjects. However, a more detailed comparison between activation and lesion studies shows contradictions that cannot be explained by current models. Activation studies indicate that this large "face area" on the inferior part of the temporo-occipital cortex can be subdi-

vided into a posterior part, involved in apperceptive aspects of face perception, and an anterior part, involved in associative aspects. We had the opportunity to examine two prosopagnosic patients, both with bilateral symmetrical lesions that were limited either to the posterior or the anterior part of the "face area" (Figure 12-3). The type of prosopagnosia observed in either patient could not be deduced from the results of activation studies. The patient with the posterior lesions—involving regions shown to be activated in apperceptive tasks in normal subjects—had a purely associative prosopagnosia and was excellent in several apperceptive tests. The patient with the anterior lesions—sparing regions shown to be activated in apperceptive tasks—had a combined associative and apperceptive prosopagnosia.

Problems Linked to Interindividual Comparisons

Advances in neuropsychology, neuroimaging, and basic human neuroscience make between-case comparisons highly desirable. Individual brains vary greatly, however, in size and shape. Furthermore, the variability of most sulci is such that, with the exception of the lateral, central, calcarine, and parieto-occipital fissures, the identification of individual sulci is hazardous. This represents a serious problem for comparison of data collected in different subjects. Several solutions have been proposed.

1. Use of standard templates for CT and MRI studies has been promoted by Hanna and Antonio Damasio. This methods helps to find roughly corresponding locations on CT or MRI scans and allows a comparison with a standardized map of Brodmann's areas.*
2. Use of a proportional grid and of a coordinate system corrected for size and shape discrepancies has been introduced by Jean Talairach and Pierre Tournoux. This method determines corresponding brain regions by applying a coordinate system anchored in the forebrain commissures and by subdividing the hemispheres into 11 coronal, 12 horizontal, and 8 sagittal slices. The coordinate

---

*The definition of Brodmann's areas outside of cytoarchitectonic applications is renowned to be difficult; within cytoarchitectonic applications it is still difficult to use (because of the lack of precise descriptions and photographic representations), and their subdivisions, such as in the classification by Constantin, are preferred.

right   left

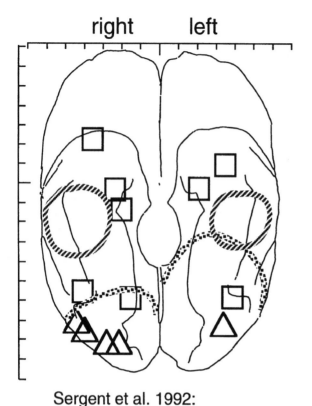

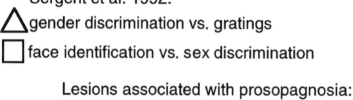

Sergent et al. 1992:
△ gender discrimination vs. gratings
☐ face identification vs. sex discrimination

Lesions associated with prosopagnosia:
(Clarke et al. 1997):
▨ apperceptive and associative
⬚ associative

Figure 12-3. Face recognition: comparison between activation sites in normal subjects and sites of lesions associated with prosopagnosia. Note that bilateral lesion of foci involved in apperceptive aspects of face recognition is not accompanied by an apperceptive deficit in face recognition. Conversely, bilateral lesions outside these foci here are accompanied with both associative and apperceptive prosopagnosia. For details see text. (Reprinted with permission from S Clarke, A Lindemann, P Maeder, et al. Face recognition and postero-inferior hemispheric lesions. Neuropsychologia 1997;35:1555; data from Sergent J, Ohta S, MacDonald B. Functional neuroanatomy of face and object processing. A positron emission tomography study. Brain 1992;115:15.)

system derived from this method is widely used for publication of data from activation studies. We use it currently in our neuropsychological studies.

3. Use of computerized brain atlases has been introduced by several centers (e.g., Computerized Brain Atlas, Karolinska Institute, Stockholm, Sweden; The National Neural Circuitry Database, United States). Similar to the Talairach system, many of the computerized atlases apply a coordinate system to the brain and then use different mapping procedures for superposing what are believed to be corresponding regions in different brains.

Patient Care in Behavioral Neurology

The care of brain-damaged patients with cognitive and behavioral deficits is an enterprise with many facets. Major efforts are directed toward neuropsychological rehabilitation—that is, retraining of lost capacities or adjustment to permanent disabilities. However, measures that accompany neuropsychological rehabilitation should not be underestimated; pharmacotherapy, psychotherapy, ergotherapy, and physiotherapy have specific indications in both the acute and chronic stages of brain damage. A behavioral neurologist is most often directly responsible for neuropsychological rehabilitation and the related pharmacotherapy, but he or she should be able to coordinate psychotherapy, ergotherapy, and physiotherapy when needed. One of the very important tasks is to communicate with the patient and his or her family.

Specific Rehabilitation

Patients who participate in rehabilitation programs often have a spectrum of deficits, although some may predominate. For example, the main problem of a patient with an infarction in the territory of the left middle cerebral artery may be aphasia, with the patient having only minor deficits in praxias and executive functions. A patient with a brain injury after a car crash may have multiple severe deficits, including a dysexecutive syndrome, attention and memory deficits, and aphasia. Before the onset of neuropsychological rehabilitation, detailed information should be obtained about the patient's cognitive status, as well as his or her behavior and personality characteristics. This initial examination should help to set priorities for the treatment. In clinical practice, priorities are often defined by deficits that prevent reaching a set goal (e.g., return to work for a patient with minor brain injuries, independent life at home, relative independence in an institution for patients with more severe injuries).

Specific rehabilitation programs have been designed for aphasia, neglect, memory disorders, and dysexecutive functions. It is beyond the scope of this chapter to enter into details of these programs, but we recommend the selected readings at the end of this chapter.

Accompanying Measures

Specific rehabilitation of cognitive and behavioral deficits is mostly accompanied by other therapies. In the acute stage, pharmacotherapy plays a major role in preventing further brain damage; in the chronic stage it plays a role in treating epilepsy or psychiatric symptoms such as depression. Psychotherapy may prove very useful in helping a patient to adapt to his or her disabilities. These different approaches are usually combined in programs developed by specialized centers for post-acute brain-damaged patients.

Personal contact with the patient and with his or her family is crucial for any rehabilitation. It is extremely important to explain to the patient and to his or her family, as far as they can understand, the nature of the deficits (e.g., aphasia, alexia, amnesia, neglect, dysexecutive syndrome) and the ways in which these deficits have a negative impact on personal and professional life. When compensatory strategies are developed, the collaboration of the patient and his or her family is again very important to ensure effective use of the strategies. Most patients and their families profit from participation in patients' associations. Our practice has more than 20 years of experience with support groups for aphasic patients. These groups are an important step in speech therapy, but they also provide the patient with a social network and very often with emotional support.

Acknowledgments

This work was supported by Swiss National Science Foundation Grant 3231-041607.94 (SCORE A Fellowship to S.C.). We are most grateful to Doctors J. Buttet Sovilla and P.G.H. Clarke, as well as to Ms. A. Bellmann and C. Bindschaedler for comments on the manuscript.

Suggested Reading

Benton AL, Sivan AB, Hamsher KS, Varney NR, Spreen O. Contributions to Neuropsychological Assessment. A Clinical Manual. New York: Oxford University Press, 1994.

Christensen AL, Uzzell BP (eds). Brain Injury and Neuropsychological Rehabilitation. International Perspectives. Hillsdale: LEA, 1994.

Clarke S, Bellmann A, de Ribaupierre F, et al. Non-verbal auditory recognition in normal subjects and brain-damaged patients: evidence for parallel processing. Neuropsychologia 1996;34:587.

Clarke S, Lindemann A, Maeder P, et al. Face recognition and postero-inferior hemispheric lesions. Neuropsychologia 1997;35:1555.

Crawford JR, Parker DM, McKinley WW (eds). A Handbook of Neuropsychological Assessment. Hove, UK: Lawrence Erlbaum Associates, 1992.

Damasio H, Damasio AR. Lesion Analysis in Neuropsychology. New York: Oxford University Press, 1989.

Gregory RL (ed). The Oxford Companion to the Mind. Oxford, UK: Oxford University Press, 1987.

Hodges JR. Cognitive Assessment for Clinicians. Oxford, UK: Oxford University Press, 1994.

Holland AL, Forbes MM (eds). Aphasia Treatment. World Perspectives. London: Chapman and Hall, 1993.

Howard D, Hatfield FM. Aphasia Therapy. Historical and Contemporary Issues. London: Lawrence Erlbaum Associates, 1987.

Lezak MD. Neuropsychological Assessment. New York: Oxford University Press, 1995.

Lishman WA. What is neuropsychiatry? J Neurol Neurosurg Psychiatry 1992;55:983.

Mesulam MM (ed). Principles of Behavioral Neurology. Philadelphia: Davis, 1985.

Poser U, Kohler JA, Schonle PW. A historical review of neuropsychological rehabilitation in Germany. Neuropsych Rehab 1996;6:257.

Prigatano GP, Schacter DL (eds). Awareness of Deficit After Brain Injury. Clinical and Theoretical Issues. New York: Oxford University Press, 1991.

Richardson JTE. Clinical and Neuropsychological Aspects of Closed Head Injury. London: Taylor & Francis, 1990.

Roland P. Brain Activation. New York: Wiley-Liss, 1993.

Rose FD, Johnson DA (eds). Brain Injury and After. Towards Improved Outcome. Chichester, UK: Wiley, 1996.

Spreen O, Strauss E. A Compendium of Neuropsychological Tests. Administration, Norms and Commentary. New York: Oxford University Press, 1991.

Zilles K, Clarke S. Architecture, Connectivity and Transmitter Receptors of Human Extrastriate Cortex: Comparison with Non-Human Primates. In K Rockland, J Kaas, A Peters, et al. (eds), Cerebral Cortex (Vol 12). Extrastriate Cortex. New York: Plenum, 1997;673–742.

Section II
Neurologic Symptoms

Chapter 13
Coma

Kyra J. Becker, Stefan Schwarz, Werner Hacke, and Daniel Hanley

Chapter Plan

In clinical practice, the analysis and management of coma are frequently performed. Approximately 3% of all admissions to the emergency room of large tertiary care centers are the result of coma. Coma is an emergency situation that needs quick and efficient evaluation and immediate treatment to prevent further, and sometimes irreversible, brain damage. This chapter describes coma and other altered states of consciousness and gives a practical approach to evaluating and treating coma.

Definitions

Coma is a state of unresponsiveness or unconsciousness characterized by lack of self- and environmental awareness. For practical purposes, we will use the term *coma* in this chapter to refer to the clinically recognizable state of unresponsiveness. From a clinical perspective, understanding the location and mechanisms of unconsciousness allows for diagnosis and initial therapeutic intervention. The term *consciousness* can be used to refer to a continuum of states ranging from that of awake and alert to that of completely unresponsive (comatose). It is nearly impossible to clearly define the various terms that describe consciousness, and states of altered consciousness such as *stupor*, *coma*, *delirium*, *unresponsiveness*, *lethargy*, *unconsciousness*, *somnolence*, *confusion*, or *obtundation*, since these terms are not strictly medical terms, but also have philosophical, psychological, and literary meanings.

Although it may not be satisfactory from a philosophical point of view to divide the overall cognitive function of the human brain into single aspects, on a physiologic and anatomic basis it is useful to distinguish between two main dimensions of consciousness: wakefulness and awareness.

Table 13-1. The Glasgow Coma Scale

Feature	Score
Best motor response	
Obeys	M6
Localizes	M5
Withdraws	M4
Abnormal flexion	M3
Extensor response	M2
Nil	M1
Verbal response	
Oriented	V5
Confused	V4
Inappropriate words	V3
Incomprehensible sounds	V2
Nil	V1
Eye opening	
Spontaneous	E4
To speech	E3
To pain	E2
Nil	E1

Alterations in Wakefulness

Wakefulness, or arousal, is the quantitative aspect of consciousness and is described with "levels of consciousness."

Alterations of arousal are recognized as relative unresponsiveness to external stimuli. Alterations of arousal do not localize to discrete levels of dysfunction. The various summary terms used to categorize the continuum of behavioral states ranging from *full alertness* to *total unresponsiveness* have no clear anatomic or physiologic basis. Because these terms are seldom used unambiguously, a narrative description of the response to external stimuli is often the best way to describe the clinical situation of a patient. However, four categories along the continuum of arousal are frequently employed to characterize the wakefulness of a patient: alert, somnolent, stuporous, and comatose.

- Alert: The patient is fully awake and responds adequately to stimuli.
- Somnolent: The patient is in a drowsy, sleep-like state, with the eyes closed, but can be easily aroused by calling or touching him or her. Although the patient may not become fully alert, he or she opens the eyes and is able to follow simple commands and to give adequate

verbal answers. If the arousal is not continued, the patient quickly falls asleep and has to be aroused again.
- Stuporous: The patient can be aroused only by repeated and painful stimuli. Aroused, the patient opens his or her eyes. A verbal response cannot be evoked or is unintelligible. Commands are followed only inconsistently, but the patient makes at least some purposeful movements to avoid noxious stimuli.
- Comatose: The patient is not arousable even by vigorous painful stimulation. Purposeful movements or attempts to avoid noxious stimuli are not made. The eyes are constantly closed. In light coma, the patient is still able to react to painful stimuli with primitive and disorganized motor responses. The majority of the brain stem reflexes are present, and the patient breathes sufficiently. In deep coma, only stereotyped responses such as flexor/extensor posturing or no motor reaction at all can be noted. The brain stem reflexes become absent. The patient still breathes spontaneously, but the breathing pattern is frequently abnormal and breathing is insufficient.

Several attempts have been made to standardize clinical findings in comatose patients. One widely used coma scale is the Glasgow Coma Scale (GCS), which was originally established for patients with head trauma but is often applied to any patient with an altered state of consciousness (Table 13-1). It is a responsiveness scale; the score is obtained by assigning points to the categories of eye opening, best motor response, and best verbal response. Other essential neurologic variables such as brain stem reflexes are not included. Its use is further limited in aphasic or sedated patients. Because of its simplicity and reproducibility, the GCS is generally used by emergency and ambulance teams for the initial evaluation of a comatose patient.

Alterations in Awareness

Awareness is the qualitative dimension of consciousness, epitomized as the "content" of consciousness—that is, the sum of all cognitive and affective mental functions and memories. Although wakefulness without awareness can be present, awareness without wakefulness is not possible.

In patients with altered awareness, their perception, orientation, emotions, mnestic functions, or initiative are disturbed to various extents. Patients with this type of alteration of consciousness are awake or easily arousable, but with an inadequate behavior, which occurs either spontaneously or in their reaction to external stimuli. If any, only the simplest commands can be followed. The term *confusion* describes an acute or chronic condition with a disturbed orientation to time, place, pertinent personal data, and an impaired ability to comprehend the immediate situation. Mnestic functions and emotions are typically abnormal in these patients. Subacute or chronic states of confusion are often difficult to differentiate from dementia. The term *delirium* denotes a subgroup of confusional states in which psychomotor hyperactivity is the prominent sign. The patient is in a state of constant physical activity and agitation. Anxiety, illusions, or vivid hallucinations are frequently present. Elevated blood pressure, tachycardia, fever, and excess sweating indicate the overactivity of the autonomic nervous system. Delirium may occur after fever, shock, or exhaustion, but the most frequent causes of delirium are alcohol or drug overdose.

Functional Basis of Consciousness

The basic neuroscience of consciousness is a subject of active investigation. Understanding consciousness is a complex task. Being familiar with the historical development of our knowledge of conscious behavior is helpful to the clinical application of basic physiologic principles in the diagnosis of coma.

Evaluation of the sleep-wake cycle in the 1930s and 1940s led to the concept of a reticular activating system (RAS). This is a network of neurons that acquire multiple sensory inputs, allow for the neural interconnection of these inputs as a diffuse system, and have projections to the cognitive areas of the nervous system, particularly the hemispheres. This system was demonstrated to be necessary and sufficient for arousal from the sleeping state. Specifically, it was observed that lesions in the region of the RAS were associated with the loss of arousal. Furthermore, stimulation of the midbrain tegmental region produced arousal in sleeping cats. The location of lesions that produce an unarousable state, or "coma," was cataloged and described in the 1950s and 1960s.

The basic observations remain valid today—that destruction of the tegmental tissue extending from the pons to the thalamus leads to impaired or absent arousal. Conversely, the destruction of all cerebral cortex tissue leads to the situation of arousal without behavioral events of so-called human content. Thus, the clinical definition of *coma* fits either state. It is clear that coma results from (1) injury to the RAS and adjacent structures, (2) from bilateral hemispheric injury, or (3) from dysfunction of neural tissue at both sites. Understanding how the RAS and other neural systems produce the full effects of human conscious behavior has yet to be accomplished. A preliminary definition of neural transmitter systems that project diffusely to the thalamus and cortex has been accomplished.

These brain stem systems include a noradrenergic system, a cholinergic system, a serotonergic system, and a GABAergic system. Each is composed of neurons that are located predominantly within the region of the RAS as defined by sleep and clinical-pathologic correlates derived from coma patients. The adrenergic nuclei extend from the medullary A1 sites to the locus ceruleus and hypothalamic sites caudal to the thalamus and cortex. The serotonergic nuclei extend from the raphe nuclei and the cholinergic nuclei from the pons and basal forebrain. GABAergic cells can be found in the thalamus and subthalamus. All project rostrally and caudally. The importance and relative function of each neurotransmitter system in producing consciousness remain unclear; however, their existence correlates with the ability of specific receptor blocking drugs to impair the arousal mechanism of humans and other animals. Because of the absence of specific data regarding each neurotransmitter system, the concept of a RAS as a diffuse arousal system continues to dominate clinical thought. Because the oculomotor, oculofacial, and oculovestibular reflex systems are in close anatomic association with the midbrain and pontine RAS, the evaluations of the midbrain and pontine cranial nerve nuclei are accepted as surrogates that correlate with the activity of the RAS.

Clinical Approach to a Comatose Patient

The importance of an accurate description of the patient's level of arousal has been already stressed.

Table 13-2. Approach to an Unconscious Patient

Start intravenous line, draw blood for
1. Glucose
2. ABG, pH
3. Na^+, K^+, Ca^{++}, PO_4
4. Toxicology screen
5. BUN, creatinine
6. ALT, AST, NH_4^+

Administer the following:
1. Oxygen
2. D50, 1 ampule IV; thiamine, 100 mg IV
3. Naloxone, 0.4–2.0 mg IV (and potentially flumazenil, approximately 0.2 mg IV)*

Examine patient/initiate treatment
1. Focal or localizing signs versus no localizing signs
2. External evidence of trauma or signs of increased ICP
3. Consider treating mass effect:
   Hyperventilate to PCO_2 of 25–30 mm Hg
   Mannitol, 0.5–1.0 g/kg IV
   Lasix, 20 mg IV
4. Emergent head CT scan

ABG = arterial blood gas; BUN = blood urea nitrogen; ALT = alanine aminotransferase; AST = aspartate aminotransferase; ICP = intracranial pressure; CT = computed tomography.
*Use of flumazenil should not be considered routine as it can precipitate seizures in certain subsets of patients.

It is important to differentiate those patients with disordered levels of consciousness from those with disordered contents of consciousness, or delirium, because the diagnostic and therapeutic strategies differ. A change in the level of consciousness can be symptomatic of many different diseases and does not represent a unique illness in itself. Adequate management of the comatose patient depends on identification of the underlying disease process and initiation of disease-appropriate treatment. There are, however, certain common principles of therapy that are applicable to all comatose patients irrespective of the mechanism of injury.

Because many forms of coma are fully reversible, two major goals should guide the clinician rendering therapy. First, prompt institution of basic critical care can prevent ongoing neurologic injury. Second, rapid recognition and treatment of remediable causes of coma can restore neurologic function. Acute coma of nonmetabolic causes is often associated with rostrocaudal deterioration or the so-called herniation syndrome. Thus, the presence of an altered level of consciousness associated with focal hemispheric signs progressing to midbrain signs over a short period of time strongly suggests a localized mass and secondary brain stem compression. For this reason, the emergent treatment of a presumed mass is often an early therapeutic consideration in the management of a comatose patient.

Emergent Initial Therapy

On first encounter with an unresponsive patient, the immediate concern should be that the ABCs (airway, breathing, circulation) of cerebral resuscitation are initiated. The airway must be secured and adequate ventilation, oxygenation, and perfusion established. Failure to do so rapidly may result in hypoxic ischemic injury in addition to the injury produced by the underlying disease process. A secure airway implies that the airway is free of obstruction and that the patient is not at risk for aspiration. Thus, depending on the patient's condition, the airway can be secured with placement of an oral obturator, a nasal trumpet, or an endotracheal tube. The need to assist ventilation generally requires endotracheal intubation. The neck needs to be immobilized in any unconscious patient with a potential acute spinal injury to decrease the risk of cervical cord damage and quadriplegia. This should be done before attempts at intubation. Oxygenation can be readily assessed with the use of pulse oximetry (Table 13-2). For traumatic coma, an initial assessment to determine the GCS score is very helpful. This scale is divided into three parts: eye opening, verbal response, and motor response. It can be performed rapidly and reproducibly by physicians and nurses. This is a universally accepted, reliable method of rapidly assessing head injuries. It has been applied to other types of brain injury with varying degrees of acceptance.

Because hypoglycemia can produce coma and cause permanent neurologic dysfunction, unless a glucose oxidase test for serum glucose can be performed immediately, all unresponsive patients should be given intravenous glucose; an ampule of D50 intravenously; and thiamine, 100 mg intravenously, to prevent Wernicke's encephalopathy. The risks of prolonged hypoglycemia far outweigh the risks of transient hyperglycemia, but there is now mounting evidence that hyperglycemia can be detrimental to the injured brain. If the cause of the coma is not readily apparent, initial evaluation must include a blood electrolyte and chemistry profile as well as blood and urine toxicology screens. Blood specimens should be obtained at the time intravenous access is established for glucose administration. Despite noninvasive pulse oximetry and capnography, arterial blood gas determination is important not only for documentation of adequate ventilation and oxygenation, but also because the arterial pH may yield clues to the cause of the unresponsiveness. All of the major causes of anion gap acidoses, lactic acidosis, ketoacidosis, and poisonings (salicylates, ethanol, methanol, and ethylene glycol) can cause coma. Naloxone (Narcan), 0.4–2.0 mg intravenously, should be given to any patient in whom narcotic use is suspected. The drug should be administered in increments of 40–80 μg to avoid the side effects of acute narcotic withdrawal. Flumazenil (Romazicon) should be administered with the same precautions because it can precipitate seizures in normal subjects as well as in patients with benzodiazepine overdose.

Subsequent Diagnostic Evaluation and Examination

Once the patient is rendered stable, diagnostic evaluation should ensue. The history is particularly helpful in defining the role of metabolic impairment in the cause of the patient's presentation. Unfortunately, many patients with drug overdoses and intoxications present without an accompanying person to provide a history. In this situation, the laboratory screen for drugs and metabolic disorders must be performed and the history deferred until the patient awakens or family members are identified. Thus, the clinician must be able to perform a rapid and goal-directed examination that focuses on the diagnostic aspects of the most plausible of the possible treatable causes of coma (Table 13-3). A fundamental knowledge of the neuroanatomic correlates of consciousness allows one to develop a diagnostic approach that significantly abridges the examination and evaluation of the comatose patient.

The requisite for consciousness includes function of the RAS and at least one functional cerebral hemisphere. Coma therefore results from bihemispheric dysfunction, brain stem dysfunction, or both. The dysfunction can be caused by toxic meta-

Table 13-3. Common Differential Diagnoses of Coma

Bihemispheric dysfunction
  Metabolic
    Hypoxia, hypoglycemia, hyperammonemia, uremia, hyponatremia, hypernatremia, hyperglycemic hyperosmolar nonketotic coma, hypothyroidism (myxedema coma)
  Toxic
    Drug overdose, drugs of abuse (e.g., narcotics, barbiturates, benzodiazepines), therapeutic drugs (e.g., anticholinergics, tricyclics)
  Infectious
    Meningitis/meningoencephalitis, encephalitis
  Nonconvulsive status epilepticus
Structural lesions
  Infarction
    Bilateral hemispheric infarcts, basilar artery infarct
  Mass lesions
    Unilateral, bilateral hemispheric with elevated intracranial pressure or local mass effect with brainstem dysfunction
Disorders that can mimic coma
  Bilateral pontine infarcts (locked-in syndrome)
  Neuromuscular weakness
  Acute inflammatory demyelinating polyneuropathy
  Myasthenia gravis
  Botulism
  Drug-induced neuromuscular blockade
  Psychiatric
  Malignant catatonia
  Psychogenic unresponsiveness

bolic insults or by structural lesions. Structural lesions are those masses that can be visualized to produce compartmental shifts on neuroimaging studies such as computed tomographic (CT) scanning or magnetic resonance imaging (MRI). These include infarcts and space-occupying lesions such as hemorrhages, tumors, and abscesses. Strategically placed lesions within the brain stem or cerebral cortices, if bilateral, can produce coma in the absence of a significant mass effect. More commonly, however, lesions in noneloquent cortex or brain stem produce coma by virtue of associated cerebral edema and brain stem compression or midline shift. If midline shift is substantial, dysfunction of the contralateral hemisphere can result. By contrast, toxic or metabolic insults generally result in global cortical dysfunction with preservation of the brain stem examination, although some toxic substances (such as barbiturates) will eventually paralyze all brain stem reflexes if present at high enough levels. Focal neurologic deficits are characteristically absent with metabolic intoxication. The presence of a focal neurologic deficit should alert one to the existence of a structural lesion and dictates emergent neuroimaging. While waiting for laboratory results, the patient should be examined in detail for important clues to the cause of coma.

Responsiveness

The various states of consciousness have been defined in detail previously. An exact narrative description of the patient's responses is preferable to summary terms. A sequence of progressively intensive stimuli is applied with a description of the maximal state of arousal and the response of the patient. The patient is first observed without stimulation. Then, verbal stimuli are used in increasing loudness—for example, calling the patient's name or giving simple commands such as to open the eyes or to press the examiner's hand. Finally, painful pressure to the trunk and limbs should be attempted to arouse the patient or to evoke a motor response. A careful neurologic examination for focal hemispheric and brain stem signs is essential, as it will help to differentiate between cerebral dysfunction resulting from structural lesions and cerebral dysfunction mediated by drug or metabolic intoxications. The most important part of the hemispheric examination is a systematic evaluation of the head and each limb with respect to response to pain. Asymmetry in motor response, muscle tone, or reflexes suggests localizing hemispheric dysfunction. The most important aspects of the brain stem examination are the pupillary responses and extraocular movements.

Posture

The spontaneous posture of the patient gives important diagnostic clues. Patients who move spontaneously or who are swallowing and yawning are closest to being awake. In most patients with stupor or light coma, the eyes and mouth are closed. An open mouth with weak masseter muscular tone and open, immobile eyes indicate deep coma. Absence of spontaneous movements can be seen in hemiparetic, quadriparetic, and comatose patients. Signs of hemispheric lesions are unilateral absent movements, flaccid extremities on the affected side, external rotation of one leg, and conjugate deviation of the eyes and head. In unilateral hemispheric lesions, the plantar reflex (Babinski's sign) is frequently present, indicating lesions within the pyramidal tract. Rhythmic movements of one extremity, the extremities of one side, or of the entire body indicates persistent epileptic seizures. Ominous signs are decerebrate or decorticate posturing. These terms have been adapted from animal experiments in which the brain stem has been transected at various levels. Posturing may occur spontaneously or be elicited by external stimuli. Posturing can be mistaken for spontaneous movement. Decerebrate posturing is an extensor response with extension of the legs and adduction, internal rotation, and extension of the upper extremities. Although the anatomic correlation is not constant, decerebrate posturing is a relatively frequent sign in patients with bilateral lesions of the midbrain or pons or in patients with impending transtentorial herniation. Decorticate posturing results from various lesions, mostly above the brain stem. It is characterized as extension of the lower extremities and flexion at the elbows and wrists with shoulder adduction. Unilateral flexor or extensor postures are relatively frequent signs in unilateral hemispheric lesions and lack the prognostic significance of bilateral decorticate or decerebrate postures.

Brain Stem Reflexes

Normal pupillary size, shape, and reaction to light reflect the function of the upper midbrain, the optic nerve, and the parasympathetic fibers of the third nerve. Unilateral pupillary enlargement and unresponsiveness to light are signs either of an intrinsic midbrain lesion, a peripheral third nerve palsy, or a warning sign of secondary brain stem involvement in large space-occupying supratentorial lesions via distension of the third nerve or compression of the midbrain in transtentorial herniation. Bilateral fixed and dilated pupils are a sign of severe midbrain damage, and are most frequently observed late in patients with transtentorial herniation. Unilateral pupillary enlargement should be differentiated from miosis of the other pupil, as in Horner's syndrome or (seldom) in large ipsilateral supratentorial lesions. Small and reactive pupils are present in thalamic and pontine lesions, as well as opiate intoxications. Supratentorial lesions above the thalamus have no direct influence on pupillary reactivity; one exception is focal frontal lobe seizures, which can produce transient unilateral dilation. The absence of brain stem reflexes (e.g., oculocephalics, calorics, corneals) in the presence of reactive pupils suggests a toxic metabolic insult.

The corneal reflex (afferent limb: trigeminal nerve; efferent limb: bilateral facial nerves) is bilaterally absent in deep coma. Its unilateral absence denotes a pontine lesion or damage to the fifth or seventh nerves.

The resting position and spontaneous movements of the eyes are first noticed after elevating the lids. Horizontal divergence of the eyes occurs frequently in stupor. An adducted eye at rest is a sign of sixth nerve palsy; an abducted eye may indicate third nerve palsy. Skew deviation means vertical divergence of the ocular axes and is the result of cerebellar or pontine lesions. Conjugate deviation of the eyes is present in hemispheric (deviation toward the affected side) or pontine lesions (deviation away from the affected side). Nystagmus in a comatose patient is suggestive of epileptic seizures and should be further evaluated with an electroencephalogram (EEG).

The oculocephalic reflex, or doll's eye maneuver, is tested by sudden passive movement of the head from side to side or vertically. The normal reflex consists of a conjugate eye movement in the opposite direction of the passive head movement and requires the function of the labyrinths, vestibular nuclei, and cervical proprioceptors. Thus, the oculocephalic reflex tests the integrity of a large segment of the brain stem from the cervical spine to the midbrain (where the third nerve originates). In awake patients, this reflex is suppressed by visual fixation. No movement in either eye indicates a brain stem or vestibular lesion. If the eyes move appropriately only when the head is rotated in one direction, a unilateral lesion of the pontine reticular formation is suspected. In the presence of third or fourth nerve palsy, only one eye moves.

If oculocephalic testing reveals no response or if testing is impossible because of cervical spine insta-bility, cold water calorics must be done. Caloric testing of the oculovestibular reflex is usually done with application of 10 ml of ice-cold water into one ear canal, with the patient's head held 30 degrees above the supine position (defects of the tympanic membrane must be excluded before the test). The normal response is a tonic conjugate deviation of both eyes toward the stimulated ear with rapid nystagmus-like movements of the eyes toward the midline (fast phase). Both canals should be tested. The clinical significance is similar to the oculocephalic reflexes. Spontaneous "ocular bobbing" is a rhythmic rapid conjugate downward movement followed by slow upward phases. It appears if spontaneous and reflex horizontal eye movements are absent and is (in their typical, bilateral appearance) a pathognomonic sign of severe bilateral pontine lesions.

Abnormal Breathing Patterns

Abnormal patterns of respiration are a frequent finding in comatose patients. Normal, regular breathing is the function of a complex system of respiratory centers in the medulla and brain stem. Cheyne-Stokes respiration is a breathing pattern characterized by a period of apnea (lasting 10–60 seconds) followed by gradually increasing and later decreasing depth and frequency of respiration. Cheyne-Stokes respiration is associated with diffuse widespread hemispheric or diencephalic damage. Other pathologic breathing patterns are correlated with various lesions within the brain stem. Neurogenic hyperventilation means rapid breathing with up to 60 breaths per minute. It occurs seldom and should be differentiated from reactive tachypnea resulting from cardiac or pulmonary causes. The apneustic breathing pattern refers to sustained inspiratory effort with a pause of breathing at inspiration. Ataxic breathing is a pattern characterized by irregular rate, rhythm, and depth of breathing. It is frequently a late clinical symptom of brain stem compression in transtentorial herniation.

Altered Vegetative Functions

In most comatose patients, there is evidence of disturbed vegetative functions. Central hyperthermia originates from lesions within the temperature-regulating hypothalamic centers. Hyperthermia is a common symptom in patients with hydrocephalus or transtentorial herniation. With progression of the depth of coma, the temperature may abruptly decrease. In critically ill patients, it is often not possible to differentiate central hyperthermia from fever caused by systemic infection. Therefore, the diagnosis of central hyperthermia should only be established after the exclusion of an infectious origin. In patients with increased intracranial pressures (ICPs), pressor centers within the medulla oblongata activate the sympathetic system. The classic Cushing's response consists of arterial hypertension combined with tachycardia. Neurogenic arrhythmia caused by sympathetic overactivity is also a frequent finding in patients with elevated ICP, although the incidence of neurogenic pulmonary edema remains still unclear.

Increased Intracranial Pressure

The neurologic examination is often sensitive but is not specific for diagnosing increased intracranial pressure. The examiner must be aware of the pitfalls of diagnosis. Although bilaterally fixed and dilated pupils may result from drug intoxications (e.g., atropine, phencyclidine) and brain death, they can also be manifestations of increased ICP. The presence of papilledema, although not always seen acutely, can be helpful. The presence of unilateral mydriasis in a comatose patient, however, is indicative of early herniation and requires institution of ICP-reducing therapy without delay. This includes intubation and hyperventilation to a P_{CO_2} of 25–30 mm Hg and osmotherapy, usually with intravenous mannitol, 0.5–1.0 g per kg.

Patients with signs of increased ICP must undergo CT scanning as soon as it is feasible, since the identification of a surgically remediable lesion (e.g., epidural, subdural, or lobar hematoma), subarachnoid hemorrhage, or hydrocephalus may be lifesaving. The presence of asymmetric findings on neurologic examination in the absence of signs of increased ICP also dictates urgent neuroimaging, as early detection and treatment of a mass lesion may avert impending herniation. Evidence of external trauma implies intracranial injury as the cause of the coma, and again, surgically remediable lesions should be identified as quickly as possible.

General Appearance

The general physical examination is also important in determining the cause of coma and is particularly useful in a patient with bilateral cerebral dysfunction. The presence of an arteriovenous fistula or a peritoneal dialysis catheter should suggest renal disease and uremia. Jaundice, ascites, or gastrointestinal bleeding suggests the presence of hepatic disease and hyperammonemia. Knowledge of the core body temperature is extremely important because severely hypothermic patients can appear brain dead and yet recover completely with appropriate therapy. Fever and nuchal rigidity suggest meningitis or meningoencephalitis. Broad-spectrum antibiotic therapy should be started immediately if meningitis is suspected. Delay of antibiotics until the lumbar puncture is performed is not necessary because cerebrospinal fluid cultures will remain positive up to 4 hours after the institution of antibiotics and the Gram's stain and counterimmunoelectrophoreses will reveal diagnostic information despite antibiotic therapy. CT scanning is necessary before lumbar puncture if there are focal neurologic signs. The possibility of nonconvulsive status epilepticus must also be considered in comatose patients. The diagnosis is easy to make if it is suspected but difficult to make if it is not. Whereas in a young patient with a history of seizures the index of suspicion is usually high, the frequency of nonconvulsive status among elderly patients admitted to the hospital with a change in the level of consciousness is usually underestimated. An urgent EEG can confirm the clinical diagnosis. If the suspicion is great enough, a therapeutic trial of lorazepam (Ativan), 0.5–2.0 mg intravenously, in an adult can be given while awaiting the EEG if the airway is secured and ventilation is adequate. In patients in whom the diagnosis is less clear, administration of benzodiazepines should be avoided until there is EEG confirmation of seizures, as they will only serve to further depress the patient's level of consciousness.

Technical Studies in Coma

Electrocardiography, routine laboratory studies, and pulse oximetry have been already mentioned as essential tools in the emergency evaluation of comatose patients. In all patients in whom a metabolic cause of coma is not evident from the immediate clinical evaluation, a cranial CT scan is the next diagnostic step of choice to detect or exclude major structural damage of the brain and to demonstrate signs of secondary brain stem damage from space-occupying supratentorial lesions. Although MRI has a greater sensitivity for detecting subtle intraparenchymal lesions, it is generally not appropriate for most critically ill patients because of its longer examination times. Moreover, the CT scan has a greater sensitivity for detecting skull fractures and intracranial blood. However, a CT scan may fail to detect infarcts in the very acute phase, meningitis, encephalitis, and fresh isodense subdural blood. If occlusion of large arterial vessels or a venous sinus is suspected, a CT angiogram with intravenous contrast medium can be obtained.

Doppler ultrasound is the method of choice for the rapid detection of large artery occlusion, although this technique is strongly dependent on the expertise of the examiner. For the emergency evaluation of a comatose patient, the use of the EEG is mainly confined to the diagnosis of suspected epileptic seizures. Once the patient is in a stable condition, the EEG can be helpful in the diagnosis of metabolic coma. In hepatic encephalopathy, bilateral, broad, high-amplitude triphasic waves are present. Herpes simplex encephalitis may be suggested with the finding of a sharp wave focus over the temporal lobe. In most patients with altered states of consciousness, the EEG reveals a nonspecific decrease of the background rhythm to an irregular theta activity.

The prognostic significance of evoked potential studies has been repeatedly demonstrated. In addition to the CT scan, which provides information about brain structure, evoked potentials give information about the functional integrity of the tested sensory systems and may indicate the location of brain stem lesions, whereas CT scanning often fails to detect small lesions.

Special States Related to Coma

Important disease entities that mimic coma must be eliminated from the differential diagnosis. These include those states in which the patient is awake and alert but is unable to respond to the environment.

Locked-In Syndrome

The classic example of a disease entity that mimics coma is a patient with bilateral pontine infarcts, or the "locked-in" patient. The locked-in syndrome is a state in which both awareness and wakefulness are retained but movements and communication are nearly impossible because of the disruption of the voluntary motor system. The anatomic basis is a lesion in the corticospinal and corticobulbar at or below the pons. Breathing is possible in some patients. Patients with locked-in syndrome are usually able to communicate with vertical eye and lid movements because these movements are generated from the midbrain, which is spared by the pontine lesion. Neuroradiologic imaging reveals the extent of the lesion. The EEG appears normal. The most frequent cause of the locked-in syndrome is basilar artery thrombosis with infarction of the ventral pons.

Neuromuscular Diseases

Other examples of disease states that mimic coma are conditions of profound neuromuscular weakness such as acute inflammatory demyelinating polyneuropathy (AIDP) (Guillain-Barré syndrome), severe myasthenia gravis, and drug- or toxin-induced (such as botulism) neuromuscular blockade. The pupils are spared in AIDP and myasthenia gravis, and administration of acetylcholinesterase inhibitors such as neostigmine (1–2 mg intravenously) will reverse the effects of nondepolarizing muscle blockade and may improve the examination of a myasthenic patient.

Psychiatric Diseases

Some psychiatric conditions may mimic coma, such as psychogenic unresponsiveness and malignant catatonia. Clues to the psychiatric nature of unresponsiveness include forced eye closure and the presence of visual tracking responses. The latter is best tested by attempting to get the patient to track the reflection of his or her own eyes in a moving mirror; this is a reflex that cannot be suppressed by a conscious patient.

Persistent Vegetative State

The persistent vegetative state (PVS) is a condition in which the patient is fully awake but lacks awareness of self and the surroundings. It is defined as a state of unconsciousness with the "inability to experience the environment." The term *vegetative state* emphasizes the discrepancy between the integrity of vegetative functions and the loss of mental abilities. Typically, patients in PVS emerge from coma. The feature that distinguishes PVS from coma is the presence of intermittent wakefulness and the stabilization of sleep-wake cycles. The phases of wakefulness are not accompanied by any sign of detectable self-awareness, attention, language comprehension, or purposeful reactions to external stimuli. Patients in PVS randomly move their trunk and extremities, which can be easily mistaken as purposeful movements. Although yawning may be sometimes observed, nutrition is possible only via a gastric tube. Fecal and urinary incontinence are consistent symptoms. Patients in PVS do not fixate on a visual target but often show primitive orienting reflexes in turning their head or eyes toward auditory stimuli or environmental movements. As a consequence of sufficiently preserved brain stem and hypothalamic functions, survival is possible for years with adequate nursing care. The EEG reveals a theta or slow alpha rhythm. The vegetative state is defined as persistent if the syndrome lasts longer than 6 months. Recovery from a PVS lasting longer than 3 months is rare and at best associated with moderate or severe disability. Recovery appears to be age-dependent, with a higher percentage and delayed recoveries occurring in pediatric patients. See Chapter 14 for a more extensive discussion of PVS.

Brain Death

Brain death is defined as the complete and irreversible loss of all brain functions and is synonymous with global cerebral infarction. Brain death without preceding circulatory arrest is a consequence of modern intensive care medicine. Without artificial ventilation, lesions of the brain stem respiratory centers induce central respiratory arrest and subsequent circulatory failure before global brain death occurs. With the possibility of artificial venti-

lation, it has become possible to preserve the functions of the human organism for a limited period of time despite the loss of all brain functions.

Although the exact criteria for determining brain death are subject to legislation and there are some slight national differences, the following are a commonly accepted standard among physicians:

1. Coma. The patient is completely unresponsive and not arousable, even to noxious external stimuli. A proximate cause of coma should be identifiable.
2. Absence of potentially reversible causes such as hypothermia, intoxication (especially barbiturates), and severe metabolic disturbance.
3. Complete loss of all brain stem reflexes. The absence of spinal reflexes is not required because the spinal cord remains intact in most cases.
4. Apnea. To check safely the absence of spontaneous respirations in the intubated and ventilated patient, the patient is ventilated with pure oxygen over a period of time for hyperoxygenated eucapnia. Then the patient is disconnected from the respirator for an appropriate interval (10 minutes) while oxygen is administered via a thin tracheal catheter. Apnea is proven if there is a further rise of the carbon dioxide level over this time period without an observed respiratory effort.
5. Electrophysiologic silence. An isoelectrical EEG and the loss of central latencies of evoked potentials demonstrate the absence of detectable electrical activity (not mandatory in all countries).
6. Absence of cerebral blood flow. The absence of cerebral circulation may be demonstrated with angiography, nuclear scans, or ultrasound (not mandatory in most countries).

See Chapter 14 for a more extensive discussion of brain death.

Prognosis in Specific Disease States Producing Coma

Some of the most important questions regarding the comatose state are "Will the patient awaken?" and, if so, "When will this awakening occur, and will return to consciousness occur with full neurologic capabilities?" Starting in the late 1970s the evaluation of prognosis in comatose patients was undertaken in an organized manner. The results of several prospective studies and many case series are now available, and they suggest some general rules about predicting the clinical outcome of a comatose patient. The first studies were those of Levy and Plum, who investigated medical coma, and Jennett and Teasdale, who investigated traumatic coma. Both demonstrated that coma was a high mortality event. In the case of acute medical coma defined as unresponsiveness on serial neurologic examinations over a 6-hour period (excluding all drug overdoses), the survival rate was approximately 10–20%. For acute head injury and coma (defined as a GCS score of 8 or less), the survival rate is much higher, on the order of 70–80%. Predicting the level of recovery after coma has proved substantially more difficult. Factors associated with full recovery, as defined by a return to the premorbid state of daily independence, seem to be related to the specific illness, the severity of the illness, the role of specific treatments in modifying the illness, and the age of the individual patient. The examination of the nervous system at the time of coma can produce information about the cause and the extent of injury; thus, the neurologic state of a patient may help define the likelihood of the victim achieving a poor outcome. However, the neurologic examination is less likely to provide specific prognostic information about the level of good outcome that can be achieved. As a general rule, good recovery seems to be predicted by the length of time it takes to return to consciousness and the prognosis of the underlying disease that produced the coma.

Data for specific diseases exist. For herpes simplex encephalitis, a post hoc analysis has suggested that the age of the patient and the level of consciousness as defined by the GCS were both prognostic factors associated with a higher likelihood of recovery. Cutoff points in this analysis were age younger than 30 years and the initial GCS score of more than 6 at the time of first treatment with the antiviral acyclovir. For basilar artery occlusion, multiple retrospective cohorts suggest that quadriplegia or coma of more than 6 hours' duration is associated with a fatal outcome, whereas recanalization has a better prognosis (mortality falling from approximately 90% to approximately 45%). Anterior circulation stroke can lead to coma when the entire ICA territory is included. The patient usually deteriorates gradually over a 2- to 4-day period, with increasing unresponsiveness. Predictive factors for death are not clear. In one series of

patients, intervention with craniotomy was associated with a higher incidence of good outcomes. Predicting the outcome of coma in head trauma is more complex. Good outcome is related to age, initial GCS score, absence of initial hypoxia, and intensive care unit management without impaired cerebral perfusion pressure (i.e., mean arterial pressure of more than 70 mm Hg and ICP of less than 30 mm Hg).

Recommendations

Detailing specific therapy for each of the diseases that can produce coma is beyond the scope of this chapter. When the patient has been stabilized and (1) immediately remediable forms of coma have been treated (e.g., hypoglycemia, hypoxia, and drug overdose); (2) elevated ICP, if present, has been treated; and (3) surgical intervention, when appropriate, has been obtained, the clinician has some time to embark on further diagnostic evaluation and therapy of the medically remediable causes of coma. If one adheres to the basic principles of critical care, a comatose patient can be prevented from experiencing further neurologic injury. If the cause of the coma is determined through an accurate history review and neuroanatomic diagnosis, then delivery of the appropriate therapy can frequently restore consciousness.

Suggested Reading

Becker KJ, Purcell LL, Hacke W, Hanley DF. Vertebrobasilar thrombosis: diagnosis, management and the use of intraarterial thrombolytics. Crit Care Med 1996;10:1729.

Brandt T, von Kummer R, Muller-Kuppers M, Hacke W. Thrombolytic therapy of acute basilar artery occlusion. Stroke 1996;27:875.

Foulkes MA, Eisenberg HM, Jane J, et al. and the Traumatic Coma Data Bank. Design methods and baseline characteristics. J Neurosurgery 1991;75:S8.

Hacke W, Schwab S, Horn M, et al. Malignant middle cerebral artery territory infarction: clinical course and prognostic signs. Arch Neurol 1996;53:309.

Hanley DF. Neurocritical care for coma, intracranial pressure, head injury, and neoplasia. Curr Opin Neurol 1993;6:829.

Jennett B. Epidemiology of head injury. J Neurol Neurosurg Psychiatry 1996;60:362.

Kandel E. Principles of Neural Science (3rd ed). New York: Elsevier, 1991;792–822.

Levy DE, Bates D, Caronna JJ, et al. Prognosis in nontraumatic coma. Ann Intern Med 1981;94:293.

Plum F, Posner JB. The Diagnosis of Stupor and Coma (3rd ed). Philadelphia: Davis, 1980.

Rieke K, Schwab S, Kreiger D, et al. Decompressive surgery in space-occupying hemispheric infarction: results of an open prospective trial. Crit Care Med 1995; 23:1576.

Teasdale G, Jennett B. Assessment of coma and impaired consciousness: a practical scale. Lancet 1974;2:81.

The Multisociety Task Force on PVS. Medical aspects of the persistent vegetative state. N Engl J Med 1994;330:1499.

Whitley RJ, Alford CA, Hirsch MS, et al. Factors indicative of outcome in a comparative trial of acyclovir and vidarabine for biopsy-proven herpes simplex encephalitis. Infection 1987;15(Suppl 1):S3.

Chapter 14
Brain Death and the Persistent Vegetative State

James L. Bernat

Chapter Plan

Diffuse global damage to the brain may result in the tragic states of brain death and the persistent vegetative state. Neurologists need to understand the diagnostic criteria and the examination findings of both these conditions to be able to diagnose them accurately and confidently. To manage such patients optimally, neurologists also need to understand the profound ethical and legal issues that may arise in the course of their care.

Brain Death

Brain death is the colloquial term for human death determined by specific tests showing the irreversible absence of all clinical functions of the brain. Alternative terms such as "cerebral death" or "neocortical death," despite their sophisticated ring, should not be used in place of "brain death" because they wrongly imply that patients are dead when they have lost only cortical functions. In the United Kingdom, the term "brain stem death" has been used synonymously to acknowledge that the primary functions tested in the determination of brain death originate in the brain stem or pass through it. A determination of brain death requires that the clinician demonstrate that all clinical functions of the brain are absent and that their absence is irreversible.

Pathogenesis

Brain death can be caused by any profound, diffuse insult to the brain. The most common causes are acute traumatic brain injury; hypoxic-ischemic neuronal damage during cardiorespiratory arrest, drowning, or other causes of asphyxiation; massive brain hemorrhage or infarction; Reye's syndrome; and herniation resulting from the expansion of an intracranial mass lesion, such as from neoplasm, abscess, meningitis, or encephalitis.

During the course of the process leading to brain death, intracranial pressure rises until it exceeds mean arterial blood pressure. At this point, intracranial circulation ceases, and essentially all neurons that were not killed by the initial pathologic process then die of secondary ischemia. Intracranial pressure subsequently falls and blood flow to the necrotic brain is re-established. The so-called respirator brain is an utterly autolyzed brain resulting from total infarction.

Examination

The three cardinal features of the examination of a brain dead patient are unresponsiveness, brain stem areflexia, and apnea. The cause of the brain injury should be known, and its extent and severity should be sufficient to cause the irreversible loss of all brain clinical functions. All potentially reversible significant metabolic and toxic contributions to the patient's coma, brain stem areflexia, and apnea must be excluded.

Brain death should be suspected when any patient is rendered comatose and apneic from a severe, diffuse insult. A brain dead patient exhibits the most profound possible coma and unresponsiveness. With the ventilator disconnected, the patient makes no spontaneous movements whatsoever. The application of noxious stimuli, bright lights, and loud noises are utterly without response. The unprecedented depth of the coma seen in brain death led French neurologists in the 1950s to coin the term *coma dépassé,* meaning "a state beyond coma."

One rare and transient exception to the patients' unresponsiveness is the presence of the so-called Lazarus sign. Occasionally, when a brain dead patient is undergoing an apnea test, the patient will be observed to spontaneously elevate one or both arms and flex the arms across the chest or even to flex the neck or sit up. This bizarre and unusual response is believed to represent the spontaneous firing of hypoxic cervical and thoracic spinal cord motoneurons. Despite appearances, it is not indicative of brain functioning.

Brain stem areflexia is determined by showing the absence of all cranial nerve reflexes integrated through the brain stem. Pupillary diameters in brain dead patients either are midposition or large. Pupillary reflexes to light and dark must be absent; there should be no pupilloconstriction to a bright light shone into the pupil or dilatation in response to darkness. Corneal reflexes to touch must be absent. Vestibulo-ocular reflexes to large-volume ice water caloric irrigation of the external auditory canal must be absent, with no eye movement or other response to this test. Similarly, gag and cough reflexes, such as those occurring normally by suctioning of the endotracheal tube, must be absent. Limb deep tendon reflexes integrated at a spinal cord level may be present—their presence or absence is not directly indicative of brain activity.

Apnea must be present for brain death to be determined, but it must be tested properly. The goal in apnea testing is to safely permit the arterial carbon dioxide tension ($Paco_2$) to exceed the threshold necessary to stimulate the brain stem respiratory centers maximally. Because most intensive care unit patients are maintained with $Paco_2$ values of less than 30 mm Hg and because the brain stem respiratory centers respond most strongly to a hypercapnic stimulus, briefly disconnecting the patient from the ventilator to see if there is spontaneous breathing is not an adequate test for apnea.

To test for apnea properly, the patient's $Paco_2$ first should be restored to the normal value of 40 mm Hg by adjusting the ventilator settings. The arterial oxygen tension (Pao_2) should be maximized by increasing the partial pressure of inspired air to 100% oxygen and ventilating the patient for 20–30 minutes. In the absence of intrinsic pulmonary disease, such as neurogenic pulmonary edema, this maneuver should elevate the Pao_2 to more than 400 mm Hg. At this point, the ventilator can be discontinued and a catheter passively infusing high-flow 100% oxygen advanced down the endotracheal tube to the carina. Such passive "apneic oxygenation" usually can maintain a safe level of Pao_2 through the duration of the apnea test.

The ventilator should be disconnected to permit the $Paco_2$ to passively climb to at least 50 mm Hg, although some experts recommend 60 mm Hg for this purpose. In most adults, the $Paco_2$ climbs at a rate of 3.0–3.5 mm Hg per minute. Thus, if the $Paco_2$ was 40 mm Hg when the test began, the ventilator would have to be disconnected for approximately 6–7 minutes to permit the $Paco_2$ to exceed 60 mm Hg. In most patients, the Pao_2 drops only to the range of 100–200 mm Hg during that time. The arterial blood pressure usually climbs slowly during apnea. If it falls or if there is acidosis or ventricular ectopy, the apnea test should be stopped immediately because these signs suggest hypoxemia. If the initial Pao_2 cannot be raised to more than 300 mm Hg, the apnea test should be performed cautiously because of fear of inducing hypoxemia. During the time the patient is disconnected from the ventilator, the patient should be watched carefully for any signs of breathing, sighing, or hiccuping, which, if present, mean that the patient does not have apnea.

The presence of unresponsiveness, brain stem areflexia, and apnea suggests the diagnosis of brain death. To prove that these signs are indicative of an irreversible pathologic process, the clinician must know that the lesion is structural and is sufficient to cause the syndrome. In the setting of acute traumatic brain injury and intracerebral hemorrhage, brain imaging by computed tomography (CT) or magnetic resonance imaging (MRI) can show the extent and severity of the structural lesion. However, in hypoxic-ischemic encephalopathy, early CT or MRI scanning may appear normal or may reveal nonspecific abnormalities. In such cases, a clear history of cardiopulmonary arrest with a documented long duration of inadequate ventilation and circulation should be demonstrated in order to support the presence of a sufficiently severe structural lesion.

The clinician must exclude the presence of reversible metabolic and toxic factors because these factors are potentially reversible and could mislead the clinician into thinking that the structural lesion was more severe than it was. Depressant drugs, such as barbiturates and benzodiazepines, should not be present in sufficient concentrations to interfere with the determination. The exact concentrations of depressant drugs allowable is unclear, but the presence of toxic serum levels should preclude brain death determination unless confirmed by a test revealing absent intracranial blood flow. Similarly, drugs producing neuromuscular blockade should not be present in therapeutic or toxic concentrations. Hypothermia (of less than 32.2°C) should not be present, nor should severe electrolyte or acid-base disorders because each can produce a potentially reversible encephalopathy that may mimic brain death or may contribute to depressed brain functioning.

Confirmatory Tests

The diagnosis of brain death is a clinical diagnosis made at the bedside. Several laboratory tests are available to confirm the clinical diagnosis. These tests may be of value in three circumstances. First, they may be useful in cases in which the clinical examination cannot be performed. For example, in some cases of massive head trauma with damage to the eyes and ears, tests for brain stem areflexia cannot be performed. Similarly, in a patient with carbon dioxide–retaining chronic obstructive pulmonary disease, the apnea test cannot be performed because the patient may be breathing more from a hypoxic drive than from a hypercapnic drive. Second, confirmatory tests may be useful to shorten the mandated interval between examinations to permit more rapid organ donation. Third, they may be useful in some medicolegal cases in which the clinician believes that adjunctive objective data would be useful in court to supplement the clinician's examination.

Confirmatory tests comprise two classes: electrophysiologic and cerebral blood flow determinations. The first group includes the electroencephalogram (EEG), brain stem auditory evoked responses (BAERs), and somatosensory evoked responses (SSERs). The EEG is the oldest confirmatory test for brain death, but alone it is an inadequate test. It measures only hemispheric neuronal function, so it is insensitive to the presence of brain stem disease. It is of value only when used in conjunction with a test measuring brain stem neuronal function. Thus, the EEG plus BAERs or the EEG plus BAERs and SSERs represent a reasonable confirmatory test battery for brain death. To confirm brain death, the EEG must reveal electrocerebral silence, and the BAERs must show an absence of all waves except the cochlear microphonic potential.

Tests measuring intracranial blood flow have become attractive confirmatory tests because they can demonstrate the cessation of intracranial blood flow, the sine qua non of brain death. Contrast angiography of the carotid and vertebral arteries is the oldest test but is cumbersome and invasive. More recent and less invasive tests include radionuclide angiography, intracranial scintigraphy with [99mTc]-HMPAO, xenon-inhalation CT scanning, and transcranial Doppler (TCD) ultrasound. In radionuclide angiography and scintigraphy, the radioisotope must be shown not to enter the intradural extent of the carotid and vertebral arteries. The easiest test to perform and interpret is TCD ultrasound. In this test, the presence of reverberating flow is detected in the carotid and vertebral arteries and their branches in the circle of Willis. During systole, TCD reveals the presence of a small forward blood flow, but during diastole, the flow reverses to return to the starting point. This pattern is relatively easy to detect and is a reliable indicator of absent intracranial circulation in brain death.

Determination

Brain death can be determined when the patient has satisfied two consecutive sets of brain death tests and when reversible disorders have been excluded. The interval separating consecutive tests varies as a function of the patient's age and the nature of the brain injury. Children from 1 week of age to 2 months should have a 48-hour interval and a confirmatory test. Children from 2 months of age to 1 year should have a 24-hour interval plus a confirmatory test. Children older than age 1 year are treated the same as adults as follows.

An interexamination interval of 6 hours from the injury is sufficient in cases of massive brain trauma or intracerebral hemorrhage, in which the causative lesion can be seen easily on imaging studies and judged confidently to be irreversible. Clinicians should allow a 24-hour interval between examinations in cases of hypoxic-ischemic encephalopathy because the severity and extent of the lesion cannot usually be proved by an imaging study. However, if a confirmatory test also is performed, the latter interval can be reduced to 6 hours.

Patients are declared brain dead after they satisfy the second clinical test or the confirmatory test after the second test. Patients who are not going to serve as organ donors should be extubated immediately after brain death is declared. Patients serving as organ donors should be reattached to the ventilator and taken to the organ procurement suite as soon as it is ready.

Differential Diagnosis

Patients satisfying all the tests and prerequisites for brain death should be declared dead and extubated.

The only "differential diagnosis" to consider is that some of the signs of brain death may be false-positive findings. Clinicians must be wary of these and exert the utmost care to interpret the findings correctly. True apnea may not be present if the presence of breathing is tested incorrectly. Survey studies have shown that apnea frequently is tested incorrectly in clinical practice. Absent pupillary reflexes and vestibulo-ocular reflexes may have been a preexisting finding and not from the new brain insult. For example, some diabetics have no pupillary light reflexes, and some patients given toxic doses of aminoglycoside antibiotics may have absent vestibulo-ocular reflexes. Barbiturate intoxication and severe hypothermia may mimic the clinical findings of brain death, yet each is totally reversible. Even electrocerebral silence on the EEG may be produced by barbiturate overdose. The BAERs and SSERs, however, are much more resistant to metabolic and toxic suppression and do not usually produce false-positive readings.

Prognosis

There has never been a case recorded of a patient properly declared brain dead who has recovered or survived. Most patients declared brain dead will experience asystole within a few days or weeks of the determination, regardless of treatment, because medullary damage produces widespread vasodilatation and high-output congestive heart failure. Continued somatic treatment despite brain death is technically difficult. Brain dead patients usually become severely hypotensive and require vasopressors for blood pressure support. They also become septic, develop renal failure, and disseminated intravascular coagulation. They lose the capacity for temperature regulation, and most develop diabetes insipidus. Nevertheless, there have been a few recorded cases in which aggressive and highly sophisticated somatic support was continued on young brain dead patients in whom asystole was delayed for as long as a few months, despite the absence of any sign of neurologic improvement.

Ethical Issues

Ethical issues in brain death include the response of the clinician to cases in which patients' families refuse to accept the concept of brain death for religious or other reasons, and the physician's duty to continue somatic support on a brain dead pregnant woman to try to permit her infant's live birth. Brain death has been accepted by the religions and cultures of the majority of the Western world, but there remain a few exceptions. Some ultra-orthodox Jews and Roman Catholics reject the concept of brain death on religious grounds. Faced with such a bona fide religious refusal, the compassionate physician should acquiesce and not insist on extubation. However, there is no ethical duty to continue to treat such a patient aggressively given the hopelessness of the prognosis.

More commonly, families may urge physicians to maintain ventilation and other treatment despite brain death because of their emotional inability to accept the tragic death of their loved one. In this circumstance, the compassionate physician needs to explain carefully the nature of the injury and that the patient is dead. If such explanations fail, continuing somatic treatment of the brain dead patient for a day or two may allow the family to gradually accept the hopelessness of the situation and to accept the inevitable death. Also, the offer of organ donation helps produce some good out of an otherwise senseless death and helps many grieving families to cope better.

Several cases have been reported of brain dead pregnant women who have undergone aggressive somatic support until their children could be born alive. In one case, such treatment continued for more than 100 days. The vexing decision to proceed with such a course of treatment probably should be made by the prospective father. The ethical duty for physicians to urge the prospective father to permit continued treatment increases with increasing fetal age and viability.

Legal Issues

Brain death has been accepted as legal death throughout the United States, Canada, Australia, and Western Europe, with the exception of Denmark. Although Japan has not yet accepted the concept of brain death, a pitched battle currently is taking place there between some physicians and scientists who wish the culture to embrace the concept and some traditionalists who do not. Many South American,

Asian, and African countries also have accepted the concept, although some have not.

In general, the societal acceptance of multiorgan transplantation accompanies the societal acceptance of brain death. Multiorgan transplantation and brain death are related in that the former cannot occur until the latter is declared. It is critical, however, that no member of the transplantation team participate in the brain death determination to prevent a conflict of interest or objectivity.

In the United States, public laws have been enacted requiring physicians caring for brain dead patients to inquire from their families if they wish the patients to serve as multiorgan donors. There remains a great shortage of transplantable organs, and this law was intended to encourage greater organ donation by patients and families. To date it has had only a modest effect. A few countries have experimented with an implied consent law under which a brain dead patient's organs can be donated without specific consent unless the patient had previously stipulated otherwise.

Some physicians, philosophers, and lawyers, principally in the United States, have advocated changing the criterion of death from "whole brain death," as it is practiced currently, to "neocortical death." They want to dissociate the determination of death from the presence of brain stem functioning and consider patients in persistent vegetative states (see below) as dead. To date, there has been relatively little public support for this radical redefinition of death, and it is unlikely to succeed as public policy in the foreseeable future.

Persistent Vegetative State

Many patients suffering diffuse brain injuries of less severity than those producing brain death suffer damage to their cortical neurons and thalamus to an extent far greater than to their brain stem neurons. Such patients may develop a chronic form of unconsciousness called the *vegetative state*, in which sleep-wake cycles and wakefulness return but awareness of themselves and their environment remains absent. If such a vegetative state lasts longer than 1 month, by convention it is termed the *persistent vegetative state* (PVS). Because PVS patients are unequivocally alive and because they may persist in this state for years, the ethical issues in managing PVS patients generally are more troubling than those encountered in brain dead patients.

Consciousness has two dimensions: wakefulness and awareness. Patients in coma clearly are unconscious because they lack both wakefulness and awareness. Patients in PVS are wakeful but unaware. Should PVS patients therefore be classified as unconscious? In practice, PVS patients are ordinarily classified as unconscious because awareness is a more relevant component of consciousness than is wakefulness. After all, what is the point of an organism being wakeful if it cannot also be aware? Despite the important technical distinction between coma and PVS, for all practical purposes both should be classified as states of unconsciousness.

It is important to distinguish PVS from other states of impaired consciousness or responsiveness. The locked-in syndrome is a state of pseudocoma in which the patient is fully awake and aware but is so severely paralyzed that responses to verbal and other stimuli cannot be made, with the exception of vertical eye movements, which remain under voluntary control. Akinetic mutism is a severe form of dementia in which awareness is retained but verbal and motor responses to stimuli are poor. The *apallic syndrome* is an anachronistic synonym for *PVS* but one that should be avoided because of its imprecise definition.

Pathogenesis

Three major pathogenetic mechanisms produce PVS. The most well-known group of mechanisms consists of acute brain injuries similar to those causing brain death, such as brain trauma; hypoxic-ischemic neuronal injury during cardiopulmonary arrest; intracerebral hemorrhage and infarction; asphyxia; and structural lesions of the cerebral hemispheres (e.g., neoplasms, meningoencephalitis). The second group of mechanisms consists of end-stage chronic, progressive, degenerative brain disorders, such as Alzheimer's disease and other types of dementia, Parkinson's disease, Huntington's disease, and childhood neurodegenerative diseases. The final group consists of developmental disorders presenting in neonates, such as anencephaly, hydranencephaly, and severe microcephaly.

PVS has become a relatively common disorder in the United States and other developed parts of the world because of the success of physicians in saving the lives of patients with devastating brain injuries and illnesses who in the past would have died. It was estimated that in the United States in 1993, there were between 10,000 and 25,000 adults and between 4,000 and 10,000 children in PVS.

PVS occurs because of selective vulnerability of cortical neurons to injury. Cortical neurons are phylogenetically newer than the neurons of the brain stem. They are more vulnerable to traumatic, metabolic, and ischemic injury than are the neurons of the brain stem. A PVS is produced when a diffuse brain insult damages a critical number of cortical neurons but a sufficient number of brain stem neurons survive to maintain brain stem functioning.

Two distinct neuropathologic patterns are seen in the majority of patients in acute PVS. In PVS caused by an acute diffuse hypoxic-ischemic injury, the brain reveals diffuse laminar cortical necrosis and thalamic necrosis. In PVS caused by an acute brain injury, the brain reveals diffuse axonal injury. Obviously, in cases of PVS resulting from stroke, tumor, or encephalitis, the specific neuropathologic findings of these entities also are present.

Because wakefulness and alertness are subserved by the brain stem ascending reticular activating system and its connections, these arousal functions return to normal, usually within several weeks of the brain insult. However, because awareness, sentience, memory, and the capacity to experience reside in the cortex and its connections to the thalamus and other structures, these higher integrative functions are lost. The PVS patient has the tragic and ironic combination of alertness and wakefulness but unawareness of self or environment.

Examination

In 1994, the Multi-Society Task Force on PVS identified the seven criteria for the diagnosis of PVS based on examination findings. The PVS patient has

(1) no evidence of awareness of self or environment and an inability to interact with others; (2) no evidence of sustained, reproducible, purposeful, or voluntary behavioral responses to visual, auditory, tactile, or noxious stimuli; (3) no evidence of language comprehension or expression; (4) intermittent wakefulness manifested by

the presence of sleep-wake cycles; (5) sufficiently preserved hypothalamic and brain stem autonomic functions to permit survival with medical and nursing care; (6) bowel and bladder incontinence; and (7) variably preserved cranial nerve reflexes (pupillary, oculocephalic, corneal, vestibulo-ocular, and gag) and spinal reflexes.

Examining a PVS patient is challenging. It is critical for the clinician to examine the patient during a period of wakefulness to be able to distinguish PVS from coma. During wakefulness, the patient's eyes are open and moving, there is regular, spontaneous breathing, the patient is usually mute but there may be some vocalizations, and the patient often does react to noxious stimuli by grimace or withdrawal or by motor posturing. Many PVS patients make spontaneous movements, but usually movements seem to serve no clear purpose. They exhibit no sustained visual pursuit. A small degree of visual pursuit may be present despite PVS, however, because the brain stem subserves this visuospatial orienting function even in the absence of conscious awareness.

How can examiners know for certain that PVS patients are utterly unaware and nonsentient? Could they not simply be imprisoned in a mind that remains aware but unable to respond and communicate? The answer to this question cannot be known for certain because our only method of knowing the quality of other persons' conscious experiences is to interact with them and, on the basis of their responses to our stimuli, make an informed judgment about their level of awareness and sentience.

Despite this limitation, there are three lines of evidence that suggest that PVS patients are, in fact, unaware and nonsentient. First, they make neither purposeful movements nor respond to the examiner in any way that is recognizably aware or purposeful. Second, their responses to pain resemble reflex responses that do not require awareness and experience. Finally, studies of regional cortical glucose metabolism (described in "Laboratory Tests") in PVS patients reveal levels that are depressed to the equivalent of those of normal patients when in the deepest planes of general anesthesia, whom all would agree are insensate. Most authorities therefore accept that a PVS patient is incapable of experience, awareness, and suffering.

Laboratory Tests

PVS is a clinical diagnosis, and the majority of laboratory tests intended to confirm PVS are diagnostically nonspecific. Imaging of the brain by CT or MRI scanning may reveal few or no findings acutely in a diffuse hypoxic-ischemic injury. Within several days, MRI may reveal loss of distinction between the gray and white matter. Later, diffuse cortical and thalamic atrophy can be imaged. EEG and evoked potential studies also show nonspecific findings. The EEG is usually diffusely slow and occasionally may show electrocerebral silence in the most severe cases. BAERs usually are normal, but SSERs may show prolongation of central conduction.

The only laboratory test that provides a high positive predictive value for PVS is positron emission tomography (PET) scanning, which measures the regional cortical metabolic rate of glucose consumption ($rCMR_{glu}$). In the few PVS patients studied, the $rCMR_{glu}$ was found to be depressed to levels between one-third and one-half of normal values. This range is almost never seen in any other disease and is seen only during the deepest planes of general anesthesia when the cortical neurons have been rendered iatrogenically hypometabolic. The lack of availability of this test severely limits its clinical usefulness, however.

Differential Diagnosis

The other major condition in the differential diagnosis for PVS is severe dementia with preserved awareness. In traumatic and acute nontraumatic injuries as well as in the late stages of neurodegenerative disorders, it may not be easy for the clinician to discern with confidence if the severely impaired patient has retained some slight degree of awareness. There is a reasonably good but not high concordance of opinion among examiners whether such patients are in a PVS. Some neurologists believe that some patients diagnosed clinically as in a PVS do retain some rudimentary level of awareness. Complicating this disagreement is the fact that some patients may alternate between PVS and severe dementia, depending on changing metabolic factors such as the presence of fever and dehydration.

It should be relatively easy for an experienced neurologist to distinguish between the locked-in syndrome and PVS. In the locked-in syndrome, the patient is awake and aware but simply cannot communicate his or her awareness to the examiner because of severe paralysis. In the typical case of locked-in syndrome caused by an infarction or hemorrhage in the base and tegmentum of the pons, the patient is quadriplegic and has a severe pseudobulbar palsy. The only retained voluntary movements are vertical eye movements, because the neural pathways for these movements all are located rostral to the lesion. Patients with brain stem infarctions or hemorrhages who have pinpoint pupils suggesting a pontine location should be asked to look up and look down to test for the presence of locked-in syndrome. A similar degree of severe de-efferentation on a peripheral nervous system basis can be seen in very advanced cases of amyotrophic lateral sclerosis, Guillain-Barré syndrome, and myasthenia gravis.

Prognosis

Defining the prognosis is often the most important issue facing a neurologist caring for an acute PVS patient. Although the terms *persistent* and *permanent* may sound similar, an important distinction separates them. *Persistent vegetative state* is a diagnosis, whereas *permanent vegetative state* is a prognosis. Some patients in PVS do later recover awareness. The probability that a persistent vegetative state will become a permanent vegetative state has been the subject of several studies.

The Multi-Society Task Force on PVS reviewed these prognostic data. They distinguished two groups of acute PVS patients who had different natural histories based on pathogenesis. In this study, PVS resulting from traumatic brain injury generally had a better prognosis than PVS resulting from hypoxic-ischemic neuronal damage. PVS from stroke and other nontraumatic causes had an intermediate prognosis but was closer to that of the hypoxic-ischemic group. Age also was a minor factor, with young patients faring somewhat better than older patients.

The Task Force generated the following prognostic rules for defining the probability of recovering awareness after acute PVS. In adults and children with PVS resulting from traumatic brain injury, if the PVS lasts longer than 12 months, recovery of awareness is highly unlikely. In adults and children with PVS resulting from nontraumatic brain injuries, if the PVS lasts longer than 3 months, recovery of awareness is highly unlikely. The probability of a patient making a late recovery of awareness outside these limits has been estimated to be 0.001.

Survival in PVS was also measured by the Task Force. Their mean survival is approximately 2 years. Approximately 70% of PVS patients will have died by 3 years and 84% by 5 years. An important caveat in these estimates is that the patient illness data from which they were obtained did not necessarily examine the true natural history of treated PVS. In these studies, many PVS patients who died were allowed to die by purposeful nontreatment of intercurrent illnesses, such as pneumonia and urosepsis. Thus, these natural history data are most valid for a PVS patient who has a do-not-resuscitate order and for whom serious infections will not be treated.

Treatment

Specific treatment of PVS patients aimed at restoring cortical functioning and accelerating recovery of awareness generally has been unsuccessful. So-called coma stimulation programs remain controversial, and there are only anecdotal, uncontrolled reports of benefit. Nevertheless, several active coma stimulation hospitals and programs remain in existence and treat patients mostly with brain trauma.

Patients in PVS develop a series of medical complications resulting from their severe debility, including pulmonary, urinary tract, and skin infections; contractures; and decubitus ulcers. PVS patients require skilled nursing care, including careful skin care, bowel and bladder care, pulmonary toilet, and daily range-of-motion exercises. They require gastrostomy feeding tubes, careful nutritional management, and, usually, tracheostomies. Despite optimal nursing care, they usually develop severe limb contractures that further complicate their daily care. They often require repeated courses of antibiotics to treat infectious complications.

Ethical Issues

The principal ethical issue in the management of a PVS patient is to identify and carry out the appropriate level of treatment. In this regard, any previous directive that had been executed by the patient, while competent, should instruct the physician about the level of treatment the patient should receive. Following the terms of an advance directive allows a patient's autonomy to be respected even after the patient has become incompetent. In the absence of a written directive, a proxy decision maker should choose the level of treatment for the PVS patient based on the proxy's understanding of the wishes of the patient in this situation.

The proxy decision maker should first attempt to fulfill the standard of "substituted judgment" by attempting to reproduce the exact decision the patient would have made in this situation based on an understanding of the patient's values and preferences. In the absence of knowledge of the patient's values and preferences, the proxy should employ a "best interest" standard and weigh the benefits and burdens of continued therapy, thereby choosing the level of treatment that the proxy believes represents the patient's best interest.

Clinicians should outline the available treatment modalities and explain that it is acceptable medical practice to withhold any or all of these modalities, depending on the proxy's consent or refusal, except for dignified and respectful treatment of the patient. Clinicians should explain to proxies that artificial hydration and nutrition can be discontinued, along with other therapies if the proxy so chooses, based on a substituted judgment or best interest decision. Medical societies in the United States, Canada, and the United Kingdom have stated that artificial hydration and nutrition in PVS patients should be considered as a form of medical therapy that can be refused by the proxies of PVS patients.

Survey studies of both healthy subjects and ill patients have shown that the overwhelming majority of people would not wish to receive continued treatment if they were in a hopeless PVS with no reasonable chance of recovery. It is reasonable medical practice for clinicians to share these data with families and proxies who are uncertain about whether to authorize continued long-term treatment of a PVS patient.

Legal Issues

Unlike a brain-dead patient, a PVS patient is regarded as alive in every jurisdiction in the world. Despite the arguable loss of "personhood" in PVS patients, and because they are considered alive, most societies grant them the full panoply of rights as a citizen. PVS patients may be permitted to die by purposeful nontreatment, as described above, but such an act should be regarded as permitting a living person to die. Some scholars wish to extend the brain death concept to PVS patients and to permit organ transplantation from them, but this idea has not generated consensus in any jurisdiction.

There is considerable case law in the United States, Canada, the United Kingdom, and Australia supporting the validity of a decision to permit PVS patients to die by purposeful nontreatment if that is the clearly considered wish of the proxy decision maker. The U.S. Supreme Court ruled in *Cruzan* in 1990 that artificial hydration and nutrition can be withheld from PVS patients and other incompetent patients because artificial hydration and nutrition count as a form of medical treatment that can be refused by proxy decision makers.

Suggested Reading

Bernat JL. Ethical Issues in Neurology. Boston: Butterworth–Heinemann, 1994;113–174.

Bernat JL. How much of the brain must die in brain death? J Clin Ethics 1992;3:21.

Bernat JL. The boundaries of the persistent vegetative state. J Clin Ethics 1992;3:176.

Jeret JS, Benjamin JL. Risk of hypotension during apnea testing. Arch Neurol 1994;51:595.

Kantor JE, Hoskins IA. Brain death in pregnant women. J Clin Ethics 1993;4:308.

Machado C. Death on neurological grounds. J Neurol Sci 1994;38:209.

Multi-Society Task Force on PVS. Medical aspects of the persistent vegetative state: statement of a multi-society task force. Parts I and II. N Engl J Med 1994;330:1499; 1572.

Pallis C. ABC of Brainstem Death. London: British Medical Journal Publishers, 1983.

Payne K, Taylor RM, Stocking C, Sachs GA. Physicians' attitudes about the care of patients in the persistent vegetative state: a national survey. Ann Intern Med 1996; 125:104.

President's Commission for the Study of Ethical Problems in Medicine and Biomedical and Behavioral Research.

Defining Death: Medical, Ethical, and Legal Issues in the Determination of Death. Washington, DC: US Government Printing Office, 1981.

Quality Standards Subcommittee of the American Academy of Neurology. Practice parameters for determining brain death in adults (summary statement). Neurology 1995;45:1012.

Task Force for the Determination of Brain Death in Children. Guidelines for the determination of brain death in children. Arch Neurol 1987;44:587.

Walker AE. Cerebral Death (3rd ed). Baltimore: Urban & Schwarzenberg, 1985.

Wijdicks EFM. Determining brain death in adults. Neurology 1995;45:1003.

Wilson K, Gordon L, Selby JB Jr. The diagnosis of brain death with Tc-99m HMPAO. Clin Nucl Med 1993;18:428.

Chapter 15

Headache and Facial Pain

Bernard Nater and Julien Bogousslavsky

Chapter Plan

Headache is one of the most common symptoms that both general physicians and neurologists have to face. Lifetime prevalence varies from 69% to 93% among men and from 94% to 99% among women in the United States and Western Europe. Causes of headaches are numerous, but only a small part are secondary to an underlying life-threatening disease. However, the first role of the physician is to recognize secondary headaches, which can sometimes constitute an emergency. Whereas headache generally is a benign condition, an accurate diagnosis must be achieved in order to allow an appropriate management.

Clinical Diagnosis

In the great majority of cases, diagnosis is performed by history rather than by physical examination or paraclinical investigations. The history must be detailed (Table 15-1), including a description of the evolution of the headache. Sudden or progressive headache requires prompt investigations. For example, a sudden and explosive headache, sometimes provoked by exertion, cough, defecation, or sexual activity, suggests subarachnoid hemorrhage. On the other hand, recurrent or chronic nonprogressive headache is more often benign.

The quality of the pain often helps to identify various types of headaches: throbbing for migraine, pressing for tension-type headache, intense and boring for cluster headache, shocklike stab or series of stabs for trigeminal neuralgia. Provocative factors also must be considered. Postural headaches, occurring or worsening after sitting or standing and disappearing or improving when lying down, suggest low cerebrospinal fluid pressure. Factors triggering facial pain such as talking, chewing, swallowing, or touching the face are typical for trigeminal neuralgia. Associated symptoms can help with the diagnosis. Vomiting may be associated with intracranial hypertension, but it may also be a symptom of migraine. Progressive neuropsychological impairment, neurologic deficits, and seizures are common features of brain tumor. Transient visual or sensory

Table 15-1. Headache History

Age of onset
Frequency and duration
Time of onset
Early warning symptoms: fatigue, hunger, thirst, yawn, mood disorder
Quality: stabbing, throbbing, tightening, pressing, explosive, lancinating
Associated symptoms: nausea, vomiting, photophobia, phonophobia, visual disturbance, hemisensory symptoms, hemiparesis, dysphasia, conjunctival injection, lacrimation, nasal congestion, rhinorrhea, miosis, ptosis, eyelid edema
Precipitating factors: exercise, sexual activity, cough, menstruation, pregnancy, alcohol, drugs, food, movement of the face
Aggravating and relieving factors: Valsalva's maneuver, neck movements, exercise, upright position, rest, emotional state
Family history
Evaluation of previous treatments
Effect on the patient and his or her life patterns

Table 15-2. International Headache Society Classification of Headache Disorders, Cranial Neuralgias, and Facial Pain

1. Migraine
2. Tension-type headache
3. Cluster headache and chronic paroxysmal hemicrania
4. Miscellaneous headaches unassociated with structural lesions
5. Headache associated with head trauma
6. Headache associated with vascular disorders
7. Headache associated with nonvascular intracranial disorder
8. Headache associated with substances or their withdrawal
9. Headache associated with noncephalic infection
10. Headache associated with metabolic disorder
11. Headache or facial pain associated with disorders of cranium, neck, eyes, ears, nose, sinuses, teeth, mouth, or other facial or cranial structures
12. Cranial neuralgias, nerve trunk pain, and deafferentation pain
13. Headache not classifiable

symptoms suggest migrainous aura or transient ischemic attack (TIA). Fever may be the expression of noncephalic infection or less often of intracranial infection such as meningitis, encephalitis, brain abscess, or subdural empyema. The history must include an exhaustive list of the drugs that can provoke or worsen headaches.

Neurologic examination should rule out papilledema, meningismus, and a focal deficit. For example, an isolated and persistent Horner's sign is commonly associated with a carotid dissection. In elderly patients, physical examination also includes the palpation of temporal arteries. When necessary, examination of the eyes, ears, sinuses, teeth, and mouth should be performed. Laboratory investigations (e.g., brain computed tomographic scan or magnetic resonance imaging, lumbar puncture, electroencephalogram, blood tests) are indicated only if the clinical evaluation suggests a secondary headache or occasionally when the patient is obsessed with the fear of having a brain tumor.

Classification

In 1988, the International Headache Society (IHS) published a classification with diagnostic criteria for headache disorders, cranial neuralgias, and facial pain. Headaches are divided into 13 groups (Table 15-2). Groups 1–4 concern primary headaches and groups 5–11 secondary headaches. The twelfth group includes cranial neuralgias, nerve trunk pain, and deafferentation pain, and the last group is unclassifiable headaches.

The criteria for each type of headache are strictly defined. They are helpful for the clinician, but they do not replace clinical judgment. This chapter focuses on primary headaches and on special problems frequently encountered by the physician. Neurologic diseases such as stroke, in which headache is not the main feature, and non-neurologic disorders are not described here.

Primary Headaches

Migraine

Migraine is an episodic headache with accompanying symptoms, including nausea, vomiting, phonophobia, and photophobia (Table 15-3). The prevalence of migraine is approximately 6% among men and 15–17% among women. The highest prevalence occurs between 25 and 55 years of age, then a decline is observed in both men and women.

Migraine is classified into migraine without aura (previously termed common migraine) and migraine with aura (previously termed *classic migraine, migraine accompagnée*), depending on the absence or presence of neurologic symptoms. The aura is defined as the clinical manifestation of a focal cerebral cortical or brain stem dysfunction that develops gradually over a period of more than 4 minutes. Aura symptoms normally do not last more than 60 minutes. The duration of the aura can be prolonged proportionally if there is more than one symptom that develops sequentially. The aura may occur before the headache, with a free interval of up to 60 minutes, but sometimes also just before or even during the headache.

Visual and sensory symptoms are the most frequent manifestations. Visual symptoms affect both eyes in most cases. They include flickering spots and zig-zag sensations with blurred vision, which may lead to a scintillating fortification with scotoma. Hemianopia is less frequent. Sensory symptoms usually follow visual manifestations. They generally have a cheiro-oral distribution. Other neurologic symptoms are infrequent in adults. The description of a progression of the neurologic symptoms as well as their features and duration is very suggestive of a migrainous aura, allowing a TIA or a seizure to be excluded.

The pathophysiology of migraine is unclear. It appears that, because of an altered migrainous threshold, under certain conditions migraineurs may develop a transient perturbation of neuronal activity that particularly affects the serotonin system and secondarily the cranial circulation and the nociceptive trigeminal vascular system. Although no external factor can be identified in many people, precipitating factors are often found, such as menstruation, oral contraceptives, alcohol, foods, odors, exertion, psychological factors, sleep disturbance, weather, and caffeine withdrawal.

From the medical point of view migraine is a benign disorder, although economic and social implications are important. The main complication is migrainous infarction, an exceptional and probably overdiagnosed disease, which is strictly defined as a cerebral infarction occurring during the course of a typical migraine attack and in the absence of other causes of infarction.

Medical treatments include avoiding triggering factors and abortive and prophylactic treatments.

Table 15-3. Migraine Without Aura—International Headache Society Diagnostic Criteria

---

A. At least five attacks fulfilling B–D
B. Headache attacks lasting 4–72 hours (untreated or unsuccessfully treated)
C. Headache has at least two of the following characteristics
  1. Unilateral location
  2. Pulsating quality
  3. Moderate or severe intensity
  4. Aggravation by walking stairs or similar routine physical activity
D. During headache at least one of the following
  1. Nausea and/or vomiting
  2. Photophobia and phonophobia
E. No evidence of related organic disease

Paracetamol and nonsteroidal anti-inflammatory drugs are the first choice of treatment for patients with mild to moderate migraine attacks. Antiemetic drugs such as metoclopramide and domperidone enhance the effectiveness of analgesic drugs through removal of normal gastrointestinal activity. Dihydroergotamine and 5-HT$_1$ receptor selective agonists are recommended for severe migraine attacks. Ergotamine preparations should be avoided in case of frequent attacks because of the risk of ergotamine-induced headache. Prophylactic treatment is indicated if attacks occur more than two to three times a month, if attacks are severe or of long duration, or if attacks are associated with prolonged aura. Preventive treatment has to be continued for at least 6 months. Short-term prevention should be limited to special periods, such as menstruation or weekends. Drugs for long-term therapy include beta-blockers with lack of partial agonist activity (e.g., metoprolol, propranolol, atenolol, timolol), calcium channel blockers (e.g., flunarizine, verapamil), serotonin antagonists, valproate, and tricyclic antidepressants.

Tension-Type Headache

Tension-type headache is one of the most commonly diagnosed type of headaches. Differentiation between migraine and tension-type headache is not always easy. In tension-type headache, pain is less severe, there is no or only mild phonophobia and photophobia, and pain is not or only mildly aggravated by

Table 15-4. Differential Features Between Cluster Headache and Trigeminal Neuralgia

Differential Feature	Cluster Headache	Trigeminal Neuralgia
Age of onset (years)	20–40	50–70
Sex	Male predominance	Female predominance
Localization	Ocular, supraorbital, temporal	Territory of the maxillary and/or mandibular nerve
Duration of attacks	15–180 minutes	Seconds
Frequency of attacks	Up to 8 per day	Several
Autonomic features	Present	Absent
Quality of pain	Excruciating, boring, pressing, burning	Excruciating, electric-like, stabbing
Provocative factors	Alcohol	Stimulation of trigger zone, movements of the face
Remission periods	Months to years	Variable

physical activity in comparison with migraine. The headache is often bilateral and affects the occipital areas, the neck, vertex, base of the nose, or the whole head. The IHS classification distinguishes episodic (less than 180 days per year) and chronic (more than 180 days per year) tension-type headache depending on the number of days with headache per year, with subdivisions relating to the presence of increased tenderness of pericranial muscles.

The cause and pathophysiology of this disorder is unclear and controversial. Vascular factors, muscular contraction, and mainly psychological factors are the most frequently proposed mechanisms.

Episodic tension-type headache is very frequent but is more rarely a cause of medical consultation because of its mild severity. On the other hand, chronic tension-type headache sufferers are current medical advice seekers. Treatment includes psychological management, relaxation exercises, and, if necessary, tricyclic antidepressants such as amitriptyline and doxepin.

Cluster Headache

Clinical features of cluster headache are very characteristic, with periods of recurrent unilateral pain attacks of 15–180 minutes and ipsilateral vegetative disturbances (e.g., conjunctival injection, lacrimation, nasal congestion, rhinorrhea, forehead and facial sweating, miosis, ptosis, or eyelid edema). Attacks often recur at a particular time of the day or night. These criteria are very helpful in distinguishing among cluster headache, migraine, and trigeminal neuralgia (Table 15-4).

Cluster headache predominantly affects men. Its prevalence in the entire population is at least 0.1%. Its pathogenesis remains unclear. Hypotheses include an inflammatory process of unknown origin within the cavernous system and central factors affecting biologic clock mechanisms located in the hypothalamus.

Symptomatic forms of cluster headache, such as those associated with pituitary adenoma, vascular malformation, and nasopharyngeal carcinoma, are infrequent but should be suspected if the neurologic examination results are abnormal, if pain is more chronic and nonepisodic, or if therapy is ineffective.

Chronic paroxysmal hemicrania is a rare variety of cluster headache affecting predominantly women. Attacks are more frequent (7–22 per day) but shorter (5–45 minutes) than in cluster headache. Indomethacin is characteristically effective.

Inhalation of 100% oxygen at 7 liters per minute via a facial mask for 15 minutes or subcutaneous sumatriptan, at most twice daily, are the recommended drugs for the acute treatment of cluster headache. Verapamil is the drug of choice for prophylactic treatment. Methysergide, lithium carbonate, and prednisone for a short time are also recommended in prevention of cluster attacks.

Miscellaneous Headaches Unassociated with Structural Lesions

Idiopathic Stabbing Headache

Idiopathic stabbing headache (previously termed "ice-pick pains") is located mostly in the first division of the trigeminal nerve and occurs as a single stab during a fraction of a second or as a series of stabs. Such pain affects particularly migraineurs.

External Compression Headache

The application of a pressure on the head (tight hat, band, swim goggles) may lead to an external compression headache.

Cold Stimulus Headache

External application of a cold stimulus or ingestion of cold food or drink may induce a cold stimulus headache.

Benign Cough, Exertional, and Sexual Headache

Benign cough headache is defined as a bilateral headache with sudden onset, lasting less than 1 minute and precipitated by cough. Benign exertional headache is a bilateral, throbbing headache lasting from 5 minutes to 24 hours that is provoked by any kind of exercise. Headache associated with sexual activity is subdivided in three types: a dull type that intensifies as sexual excitement increases, an explosive type that occurs during orgasm, and a postural type that develops after coitus. The term *benign* signifies that a symptomatic disorder such as a Chiari malformation or an aneurysmal subarachnoid hemorrhage has been ruled out.

Special Headaches

Thunderclap Headache

Thunderclap headache is often seen in emergency departments. Pain is very severe and has an abrupt onset. The symptomatic causes include subarachnoid hemorrhage, dissection of the carotid or vertebral artery, migraine, and cerebral venous sinus thrombosis. These conditions should always be ruled out by appropriate investigations (i.e., neurologic examination, brain computed tomography scan, lumbar puncture and, if necessary brain magnetic resonance imaging and angiography). A benign idiopathic form has been reported, which is frequently associated with vasospasm. Benign thunderclap headache has a spontaneous resolution over 1 week.

Post-Traumatic Headache

Headaches occurring soon after a head trauma are frequent. In the acute phase, intracranial bleeding or contusion of the scalp should be excluded. The chronic form of post-traumatic headache is often part of the post-traumatic syndrome, and the headache is then often associated with dizziness, inability to concentrate, disturbed sleep, and fatigue. The features of this headache are very similar to migraine or tension-type headache. The diagnosis is mainly based on the temporal relationship between the traumatic event and the appearance of the headache (less than 14 days after the injury or regaining consciousness according to IHS criteria). The absence of correlation between the severity of the head trauma and the transformation of chronic post-traumatic headache suggests that psychological dysfunction associated with trauma may play an important role in the persistence of the headache.

Trigeminal Neuralgia

Trigeminal neuralgia is a relatively rare facial pain with specific features (see Table 15-4). Pain is severe, nearly always unilateral, in one or more divisions of the trigeminal nerve, but only rarely in the first division. Pain is sudden, intense, such as lightning or an electric shock. Attacks last from a few seconds to less than 2 minutes. Light touch or movement of the face can precipitate an attack. Trigeminal neuralgia is a paroxysmal condition with periods of remission. Neurologic examination results are normal in the idiopathic form. There is no specific investigation, and the diagnosis is purely clinical. However, investigations are useful to detect symptomatic trigeminal neuralgia, which may occur with multiple sclerosis, tumors, basilar impression, vascular compression, or pontomedullary infarction.

Anticonvulsants, typically carbamazepine, are the first-line of treatment for idiopathic trigeminal neuralgia. If medical treatment is not successful, microvascular decompression at the root-entry zone may be proposed. This technique has a low mortality and morbidity. Neurologic complications are cranial nerve damage (cranial nerves V, VII, VIII), meningitis, intracranial hemorrhage or infarction, cerebellar edema, and cerebrospinal fluid leakage. These good results suggest that a vascular compression of the fifth nerve root could be a cause of trigeminal neuralgia in some patients. An alternative treatment, percutaneous thermocoagulation of the gasserian ganglion or percutaneous retrogasserian glycerol rhizotomy can be proposed to elderly patients or patients with an anesthetic risk. However, these percutaneous procedures produce sensory loss in the affected area and have a higher recurrence rate (up to 72% for retrogasserian glycerol injections).

Headache in the Elderly

The prevalence of primary headache declines in the elderly. A recent headache in an elderly person should always be considered as a symptom of an underlying disease, including metastatic or primary tumor and subdural hematoma.

Headache caused by giant cell arteritis (temporal arteritis) is a headache of advancing age; its prevalence in people in their 50s is 6.8 per 100,000, versus 73 per 100,000 in people in their 80s. Pain is temporal, unilateral or diffuse, moderate to severe, throbbing or not, persistent throughout the day, and particularly severe at night. Headache is often associated with weight loss, swollen and tender superficial temporal artery, polymyalgia rheumatica, painful tongue, and claudication of the jaw. This disorder must be recognized in order to prevent blindness and stroke, which are the most important complications of this type of arteritis. The sedimentation rate is most frequently elevated (more than 40 mm/hour), but 5–15% of patients have a normal sedimentation rate. Temporal artery biopsy and response to prednisone allow the diagnosis to be confirmed.

Ophthalmic zoster is also mainly a disease of the elderly. Pain is burning, constant, sometimes associated with electric shock-like pain, and located in the ophthalmic division of the trigeminal nerve. Touching the affected area can be painful. Treatment includes tricyclic antidepressants, anticonvulsants, and topic application of capsaicin or lidocaine.

Many drugs can produce mild to moderate, diffuse headaches in the elderly. An attempt to stop the suspected drugs may be warranted. It must be emphasized that, contrary to the common view, mild or moderate arterial hypertension does not cause headache.

The implication of cervical spine dysfunction as a cause of headache is controversial. However, spondylosis on radiologic examination is not sufficient to explain a headache.

Chronic Daily Headache

Chronic daily headache is a descriptive term for headaches recurring daily or almost daily for months to years. Chronic daily headaches include several types of headaches except those in relation to an underlying structural lesion. Chronic daily headaches are often a transformation of episodic migraine (transformed migraine), but in some cases with a long evolution, the distinction between migraine and tension-type headache remains difficult. The main causes of transformation of primary headaches are the overuse of drugs (ergotamine, analgesics) and psychological factors. This complex chronic headache often requires a special management in headache centers. Treatment commonly involves withdrawal of analgesics or ergotamine, prophylactic pharmacotherapy of primary headaches, and psychological and behavior techniques.

Suggested Reading

Edmeads J, Takahashi A. Headache in the Elderly. In J Olesen, P Tfelt-Hansen, KMA Welch (eds), The Headaches. New York: Raven, 1993;809–813.

Haas DC. Chronic post-traumatic headaches classified and compared with natural headaches. Cephalalgia 1996; 16:486.

Headache Classification Committee of the International Headache Society. Classification and diagnostic criteria for headache disorders, cranial neuralgias and facial pain. Cephalalgia 1988;8(Suppl 7):1.

Lance JW. Current concepts of migraine pathogenesis. Neurology 1993;43(Suppl 3):S11.

Lance JW. Mechanism and Management of Headache (5th ed). Oxford, UK: Butterworth–Heinemann, 1993;31–45.

Mathew NT. Chronic refractory headache. Neurology 1993;43(Suppl 3):S26.

Pascual J, Iglesias F, Oterino A, et al. Cough, exertional, and sexual headaches: an analysis of 72 benign and symptomatic cases. Neurology 1996;46:1520.

Slivka A, Philbrook B. Clinical and angiographic features of thunderclap headache. Headache 1995;35:1.

Stewart WF, Shechter A, Rasmussen BK. Migraine prevalence. A review of population-based studies. Neurology 1994;44(Suppl 4):S17.

Zakrzewska JM. Trigeminal Neuralgia. London: Saunders, 1995;5–20.

Chapter 16
Neck and Low Back Pain

Marc Fisher

Chapter Plan

Pain in the neck or lower back is a very frequent complaint of patients seeking medical attention. Involvement of nervous system structures such as the nerve roots and spinal cord occurs regularly in patients with cervical or lumbosacral pain, especially if the pain radiates into an extremity and is associated with numbness or weakness in that limb. This chapter discusses a practical approach to patients with neck and lower back pain, emphasizing neurologically related disorders.

Neck Pain

Anatomic Description

The cervical spine consists of seven vertebrae and their interconnections. Each cervical vertebra contains two major parts: the cylindrical vertebral body and the vertebral arch structures (Figure 16-1). The pedicles and lamina unite these two vertebral components and form the vertebral foramen, enclosing the spinal cord in a protective bony canal. The superior and inferior articular processes contain true joint capsules and interconnect each individual vertebra to its rostral and caudal neighbors. The articular processes are important contributors to the range of motions subserved by the cervical spine. Intervertebral discs lie between each vertebral body and are composed of an eccentrically lying viscous nucleus pulposus and the fibrous annulus fibrosus. Several major ligaments serve to interconnect and anchor the osseous components of the cervical spine, with the anterior longitudinal ligament, the ligamentum flavum, and the posterior longitudinal ligament being the most important ones. The spinal nerves formed by dorsal and ventral nerve roots exit the spinal column through the intervertebral foramina, and the cervical nerve root exiting each foramen has the same numerical designation as the

233

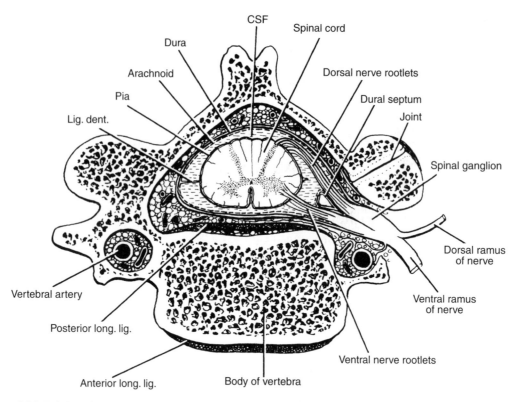

Figure 16-1. Relation of dura to bone and nerve roots shown in an oblique transverse section. (CSF = cerebrospinal fluid; Long. lig. = longitudinal ligament; Lig. dent. = dentate ligament.) (Reprinted with permission from M Wilkinson. Cervical Spondylosis: Its Early Diagnosis and Treatment. Philadelphia: Saunders, 1971.)

inferior disc forming the intervertebral foramen—that is, at the C4–5 level the C5 nerve root exits. The first two cervical vertebrae are unique and form the atlantoaxial complex, which interconnects the spine with the skull and allows for complex head and neck movements. The seventh cervical vertebra is also somewhat unique, serving as a transitional structure between the cervical and thoracic spine.

Differential Diagnosis

In the vast majority of patients with neck pain, the discomfort is secondary to musculoskeletal abnormalities unrelated to neural structures in the region. The most common cause of localized, nonradiating neck pain is muscle spasm. Other relatively common causes of localized neck pain are rheumatoid arthritis and osteoarthritis, whiplash injury, and meningeal irritation. These disorders are beyond the scope of this discussion; the focus here is on neck and associated arm pain that is related to spinal cord, nerve root, and peripheral nervous system structures and that can be confused with radiculopathies. Spinal cord abnormalities that cause neck pain include cervical myelopathy related to osseous overgrowth, intramedullary and extramedullary tumors, syringomyelia, dural cysts, and vascular malformations. Cervical radiculopathy is most commonly caused by a herniated intervertebral disc, but it can also be secondary to cervical spondylosis, traumatic nerve root injury, tumors (either intrinsic to the nerve or metastasis), abscess formation, or herpes zoster. Disorders of the brachial plexus typically cause pain at the base of the neck, the shoulder, and into the arm, leading to diagnostic confusion with cervical radiculopathies. A range of upper extremity mononeuropathies and multiple mononeuropathies can cause radiating arm pain, sensory loss, and weakness, sometimes leading to consideration of and confusion with a cervical radiculopathy. The clinical features of brachial plexus and upper extremity mononeuropathies usually allow the clinician to readily distinguish between these disorders and a cervical radiculopathy.

Cervical Radiculopathy

The cervical nerve roots can be injured by a number of pathologic processes, as outlined in Table 16-1. In younger patients, intervertebral disc herniations are the most common cause, whereas in the elderly, cervical spondylosis is most likely and may be associated with a myelopathy. Cervical disc herniations have been documented to occur at a frequency of 6 per 100,000 per year, involving both sexes equally. The most common cervical nerve root involved in radiculopathies is C7, followed in frequency by C6 and C5. C8 involvement is relatively less common, and the more proximal cervical nerve roots are rarely involved. The symptoms and signs of typical cervical radiculopathies usually allow for relatively accurate localization, and Table 16-2 outlines the usual sensory and pain patterns, motor deficits, and reflex findings. Neck pain and numbness radiating into the arm are common, but occasionally radiating numbness occurs without pain. Knowledge of the cervical sensory dermatomes is helpful for interpreting a patient's history and sensory testing results. The sensory dermatomal map presented in Figure 16-2 can be used to help localize to a particular cervical nerve root distribution. The patient should be asked to trace the distribution of radiating pain and numbness with one finger. This information can then be overlaid on this dermatomal map to ascertain the involved nerve root territory in many cases. Sensory and pain symptoms can be

Table 16-1. Common Causes of Cervical Radiculopathy

Herniated intervertebral disc
Osteoarthritis
Trauma
Tumors, primary and metastatic
Herpes zoster
Diabetes mellitus
Meningeal carcinomatosis
Lyme disease

elicited by abducting the shoulder and raising the hand above the head to induce a radiating pattern.

Diagnostic testing can be useful for confirming the cause of a cervical radiculopathy. Figure 16-3 outlines a suggested approach to the use of diagnostic testing and treatment for patients with suspected cervical radiculopathy. Acute neck pain without radiating pain does not require any initial radiographic investigations unless there is an associated fever, history of trauma, or underlying neoplasm. With persistent, localized neck pain of 3–4 weeks' duration or with pain radiating to an arm, the initial study is a cervical spine series of routine radiographs. Plain x-ray films will identify an obvious bony deformity or metastatic deposit in bones. If the patient continues to have radiating neck pain or neurologic deficits, an imaging study should be considered. Currently, a cervical magnetic resonance imaging (MRI) scan is the imaging study of choice because MRI very accurately depicts the anatomy of the cervical spine and does not require the injection of intrathecal contrast agents. Cervical MRI usually demonstrates nerve root impingement by herniated discs or osseous abnormalities, but it is not infallible (Figure 16-4). Computed tomographic (CT)-myelography with the injection of intrathecal contrast is perhaps more accurate than MRI and should be considered in patients strongly suspected

Table 16-2. Clinical Features of Cervical Radiculopathy

Nerve Root (reflex loss)	Pain and Numbness and Localization	Weakness
C5 (biceps)	Neck, lateral arm, forearm	Deltoid, biceps
C6 (brachioradialis)	Neck, lateral forearm, thumb, index finger	Brachioradialis, pronator teres, wrist flexors
C7 (triceps)	Neck to back of forearm, middle finger	Triceps, wrist, finger extensors
C8 (?triceps)	Neck to medial forearm, small finger, half of ring finger	Intrinsic hand, muscles, finger extensors

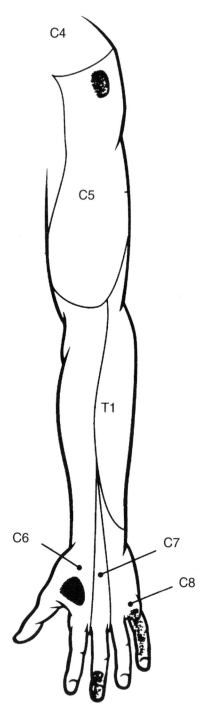

Figure 16-2. A depiction of the cervical dermatomes on the dorsum of the arm, with the hatched areas representing sites most likely to have diminished sensation with the more common radiculopathies. (Reprinted with permission from RB Rosenbaum, SM Campbell, JT Rosenbaum. Clinical Neurology of Rheumatic Disease. Boston: Butterworth–Heinemann, 1996.)

of having a nerve root impingement who have negative findings on MRI. Either MRI or CT-myelography should be considered for patients who have failed conservative management and who are candidates for surgical therapy, if not previously performed. Electromyographic (EMG) investigation is another diagnostic procedure than can be helpful in documenting and localizing cervical nerve root compression, although this procedure will not identify the cause. The needle examination is the most helpful part of EMG testing for cervical radiculopathy and can demonstrate both acute and chronic denervative changes. EMG testing should not be done routinely, but reserved for more difficult diagnostic situations. EMG testing should also be used before surgery to confirm that there is physiologic evidence of denervation in the nerve root to be operated on.

The initial management of patients with neck pain, be it localized or radiating, should be conservative except in those patients with a rapidly progressive myelopathy. Conservative measures include avoiding heavy straining or lifting, local heat or cold, a soft cervical collar, analgesics, anti-inflammatory medications, and muscle relaxants. Not all modalities are needed in each case, but some combination of these interventions is useful in many patients. If the symptoms persist, referral for physical therapy and cervical traction for patients with evidence of a radiculopathy should be considered. Cervical manipulation is also useful for patients with localized neck pain in whom a radiculopathy or myelopathy is not present. The great majority of patients with localized neck pain and cervical radiculopathies respond to conservative management and do not require surgery. Surgery should be considered for patients with intractable pain or weakness that has not responded to conservative treatment after 4–6 weeks. Obviously, an imaging study will have to demonstrate an abnormality appropriate for surgical intervention, such as a herniated disc or bony overgrowth. For disc surgery, both anterior and posterior approaches can be used and both types of surgery afford substantial improvement in most but not all patients.

Cervical Myelopathy

Narrowing of the sagittal diameter of the cervical canal is the most important predisposing factor for

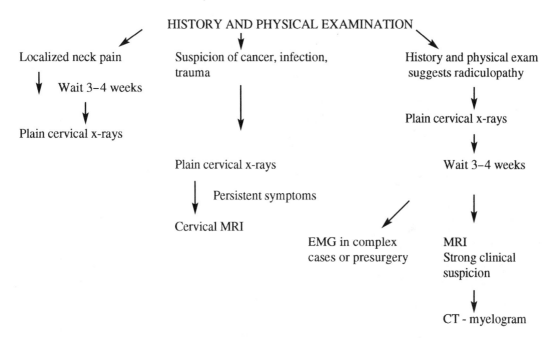

Figure 16-3. A flow diagram suggesting an approach to the diagnosis and management of patients with suspected cervical radiculopathy. (MRI = magnetic resonance imaging; EMG = electromyography; CT = computed tomography.)

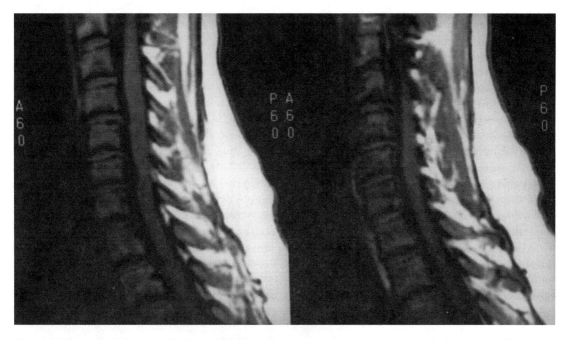

Figure 16-4. A sagittal view on magnetic resonance imaging demonstrating a lateral cervical disc herniation at C6–C7 that caused nerve root impingement.

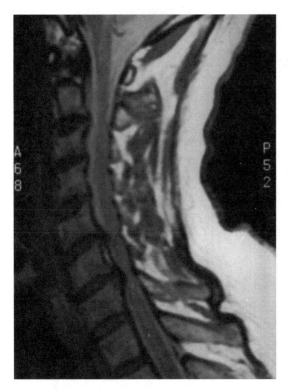

Figure 16-5. A magnetic resonance imaging of the cervical spine showing multiple cervical herniations and narrowing of the anterior-posterior diameter of the spinal canal, consistent with spinal stenosis.

the development of spinal cord compromise and a myelopathy (Figure 16-5). Narrowing can be congenital, induced by bony overgrowth with osteoarthritis, or by upper cervical instability, as occurs in rheumatoid arthritis. Cervical disc herniation centrally or ligamentum flavum degeneration can be the precipitating event in inducing the clinical syndrome of cervical myelopathy. There may also be a role for spinal cord ischemia because of vascular compromise by osseous elements in the development of cervical myelopathy, but this component remains controversial.

The clinical syndrome of cervical myelopathy typically causes spasticity and weakness in the legs, with numbness and clumsiness in the hands. Leg involvement is usually more prominent, and patients may present primarily with a gait abnormality. One leg may be more spastic than the other, and there may be an asymmetry of leg reflexes and an extensor plantar response only on one side. Vibration and joint position sensory loss is typically more prominent in the legs and loss of pain sensation more prominent in the hands, although a discrete sensory level for pain sensation loss is unusual. Wasting and weakness of intrinsic hand muscles may occur. Occasionally, patients with a cervical myelopathy have a concurrent cervical radiculopathy. Urinary urgency and frequency may develop as the syndrome progresses. Neck pain may not be a major complaint in some patients, and a cervical myelopathy must be considered in patients without neck pain who manifest the previously outlined symptoms and signs.

Imaging of the cervical spine is required for demonstrating compromise of the cervical spinal cord. Plain x-ray films can identify osseous abnormalities that might lead to cervical spinal cord compromise. MRI should be the initial, comprehensive imaging study used because it is noninvasive and accurately demonstrates the anatomy of the cervical vertebrae and the spinal cord. Both T1- and T2-weighted MRI sequences should be obtained. T2-weighted MRI may in some cases demonstrate hyperintensity within the spinal cord, perhaps secondary to inflammation or edema of the spinal cord. CT-myelography is also useful for depicting osseous and disc abnormalities that might be the cause of cervical myelopathy, but this investigation is invasive and not routinely done. EMG testing is not typically useful for patients with a clinical myelopathy. Somatosensory evoked responses can document posterior column sensory loss.

The clinical course of patients with cervical myelopathy can be slowly progressive or occasionally a rapid deterioration. In elderly patients with mild deficits and an indolent course, conservative management with pain control, a cervical collar, and physical therapy for gait training is appropriate. Surgical intervention should be considered if deterioration is rapid and neurologic deficits are worsening. Before surgery is considered, it is imperative that other disorders such as amyotrophic lateral sclerosis, multiple sclerosis, and metabolic myelopathies be excluded, especially in patients without much neck pain. Decompressive surgery by an anterior or posterior approach is used. Surgery may only be effective in 60–80% of patients with cervical myelopathy, and the value of surgery has been questioned.

Brachial Plexus and Upper Extremity Mononeuropathies

Brachial plexus disorders are sometimes confused with cervical radiculopathy because the patient typically has pain in the shoulder and the base of the neck that radiates into the arm. The pain syndrome is usually associated with weakness and numbness in the arm, again suggesting the possibility of a cervical radiculopathy. Distinguishing features that suggest a brachial plexopathy and not a cervical radiculopathy are outlined in Table 16-3. The most important indicators of brachial plexus involvement are numbness or weakness that involves the distribution of more than one nerve root. This clinical feature is not infallible, because some patients with cervical root disease can have a polyradiculopathy, as might occur with a large lateral cervical disc herniation. The most common causes of brachial plexopathy are trauma, radiation, invasion by cancer (lung and breast most commonly), idiopathic brachial plexopathy (which may be postinfectious or postvaccination), or related to the thoracic outlet syndrome. With the thoracic outlet syndrome, a cervical rib attached to the C7 vertebra is typically present, and vascular as well as neuropathic symptoms occur. A droopy or low-hanging shoulder is present in some patients with thoracic outlet syndrome; typically, these are women who also have long necks and prominent horizontal or downsloping clavicles.

Mononeuropathies in the arm are occasionally confused with cervical radiculopathies, especially when pain or numbness extends proximally. Carpal tunnel syndrome is the most common upper extremity mononeuropathy. The associated pain and numbness is usually restricted to below the wrist, but occasionally it does radiate up the arm to the shoulder. Carpal tunnel syndrome is usually easily differentiated from a C6 or C7 radiculopathy, and the presence of Phalen's sign on prolonged wrist flexion is particularly helpful for localizing the nerve impingement to the wrist. Some patients have coexistent carpal tunnel syndrome and a cervical radiculopathy (a "double-crush syndrome"), likely because these disorders are both relatively common and can occur independently by chance. Ulnar neuropathy at the level of the ulnar groove is the second most common upper extremity mononeuropathy and can be confused with a C8 radiculopathy. Patients with an

Table 16-3. Clinical Features Suggestive of a Brachial Plexus Abnormality

1. Diffuse weakness in more than one nerve root or peripheral nerve
2. Widespread sensory loss to pain stimulation
3. Suppression of more than one reflex
4. Pain primarily in the shoulder and upper arm; electromyographic evidence of widespread denervation

ulnar neuropathy typically have pain that radiates from the elbow down the medial aspect of the forearm to the fifth finger and the medial half of the ring finger. They do not have neck pain or radiating symptoms in the upper arm. At times, the distribution of sensory and motor abnormalities with ulnar neuropathy can be confused with a C8 radiculopathy without radiating pain. Radial, axillary, and musculocutaneous neuropathies are much less common and not usually confused with cervical radiculopathy.

Low Back Pain

Anatomic Description

Low back pain can be related to the lumbar, sacral, and coccygeal portions of the spine, although the latter structure is not discussed in this chapter. The lumbar spine consists of five vertebrae that are thicker and squatter than those in the cervical spine. The sacral spine consists of six segments. The spinal cord usually ends between the first and second lumbar vertebrae, giving rise to the cauda equina, which contains all of the lumbar, sacral, and coccygeal nerve roots. The nerve roots exit through the intervertebral foramina and the nerve root involved with a lumbar disc herniation is typically the same as the superior vertebral body—that is, an L5–S1 herniation will involve the L5 nerve root. The spinal nerves, after exiting the intervertebral foramina, form the lumbosacral plexus, which can be divided into an upper lumbar plexus and a lower lumbosacral plexus (Figure 16-6). The lumbar plexus gives rise to the femoral, lateral femoral cutaneous, and obturator nerves, whereas the lumbosacral plexus forms the sciatic, peroneal, posterior tibial, and gluteal nerves. The pelvis, specifically the sacroiliac portion, is another important anatomic consideration, because

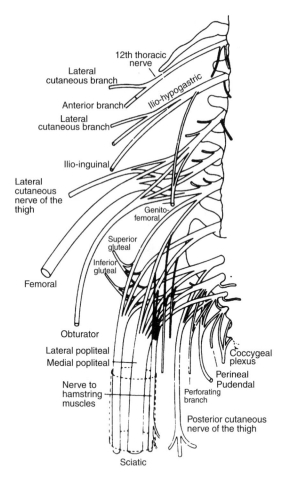

12th thoracic nerve

Lateral cutaneous branch

Anterior branch

Lateral cutaneous branch

Ilio-hypogastric

Ilio-inguinal

Lateral cutaneous nerve of the thigh

Genito-femoral

Superior gluteal

Inferior gluteal

Femoral

Obturator

Lateral popliteal

Medial popliteal

Nerve to hamstring muscles

Coccygeal plexus

Perineal

Pudendal

Perforating branch

Posterior cutaneous nerve of the thigh

Sciatic

Figure 16-6. A diagrammatic representation of the lumbo-sacral plexus. (Reprinted with permission from WG Bradley. Disorders of Peripheral Nerves. Oxford, UK: Blackwell, 1974;29.)

pain in the sacroiliac joint from inflammation or arthritis may be confused with more proximal lower back discomfort.

Differential Diagnosis of Lower Back Pain

Pain in the lower back is a common and debilitating problem that has a plethora of causes. The prevalence of lower back pain at a particular point in time approaches 20% of the population. Low back pain is more common with advancing age, multiparity, and certain occupations, especially those requiring heavy lifting and repetitive pushing and pulling. The prevalence of radiating pain into a

leg, sciatica, is much lower, and this distinction between localized low back pain and radiating pain is important when trying to distinguish nerve root involvement from non-neurologic causes for the pain syndrome. The most common causes of localized, acute low back pain are muscular or ligamentous in origin, and these patients usually respond to conservative measures such as rest, local heat or cold, analgesics, manipulation, and physical therapy. An infection, malignancy, fracture, or intra-abdominal catastrophe should be considered if the pain is severe and unrelenting. More chronic localized low back pain is usually related to osseous degeneration with associated muscle spasm, spondyloarthropathies (e.g., Reiter's syndrome, ankylosing spondylitis), or fibromyalgia. Acute low back pain with radiation to one or even occasionally both legs suggests nerve root impingement. In younger patients, a disc herniation is an important consideration, but epidural abscess or malignancy is a possibility in the appropriate clinical setting. With bladder or bowel compromise and bilateral leg symptoms, impingement of the cauda equina is suggested, and urgent diagnosis and treatment are necessary. Subacute or chronic radiating low back pain can be related to a disc herniation, but osseous degeneration such as spondylolisthesis, facet enlargement, or lumbar spinal stenosis are other important considerations.

Lumbosacral Radiculopathy

Disc herniations and osseous degeneration are the two most common causes of lumbosacral radiculopathy. Involvement of the L5 nerve root is most common, followed by S1 and L4. Involvement of more proximal lumbar nerve roots is relatively rare. Knowledge of the lumbar and sacral (Figure 16-7) dermatomes and myotomes can help the clinician localize which nerve root is most likely involved in a lumbosacral radiculopathy. The patient should be asked to trace the radiation of the pain with one finger from the lower back down the leg. Neurologic examination should include careful testing of motor power, pain sensation, and reflexes to determine the presence of any abnormalities. In addition to the routine elicitation of the knee and ankle reflexes, a hamstring reflex should be performed, as this reflex tests the L5 root not otherwise examined. Using the results of this preliminary examination and relating them to Table 16-4, the clinician may be able to localize which nerve root is compromised. Pain can be elicited by the straight-leg raising test, performed by flexing the hip while keeping the knee straight. This test stretches the sciatic nerve. Pain that occurs in the lower back or along the course of the nerve is considered a positive result. Pain elicited at 10–20 degrees of hip flexion is not related to sciatic nerve stretching. A variation of the straight-leg raising test is to dorsiflex the ankle at a level of hip flexion just before straight-leg raising induces discomfort. A femoral nerve stretch test should also be performed if injury to an upper lumbar nerve root or the lumbar plexus is considered. This test is performed by having the patient in a prone position and extending the hip to determine if this maneuver induces pain.

Diagnostic testing (Figure 16-8) of patients with radiating low back pain includes plain radiographs of the lumbosacral spine, imaging with MRI or CT scanning (including CT-myelography), and EMG testing. Many patients with acute radiating low back pain require no studies initially. If the patient has a fever, recent major trauma, or a malignancy by history, early diagnostic evaluation with plain films and MRI should be considered. In patients without these "red flags," persistent localized pain for 3–4 weeks is an indication for plain x-ray films of the lumbosacral spine with extension-flexion views. Patients with radiating low back pain for several weeks should have an imaging study and MRI as the initial consideration (Figure 16-9). MRI provides extensive coverage of the lumbosacral spine with excellent anatomic detail. The presence of a central disc bulge is of no significance. Even a disc herniation may be present in a minority of asymptomatic individuals, so this finding must be correlated with the clinical picture. Plain CT scanning must be directed by the clinician to the suspected level of nerve root involvement and is not as sensitive as MRI. CT-myelography with the injection of contrast increases the sensitivity, but is invasive. CT-myelography should be considered when the clinical suggestion of a lumbosacral radiculopathy is strong and the MRI findings are negative. EMG studies can provide electrical confirmation of a lumbosacral radiculopathy and should be considered in more complex cases and before surgery.

Patients with radiating low back pain should initially be managed conservatively. In patients with a

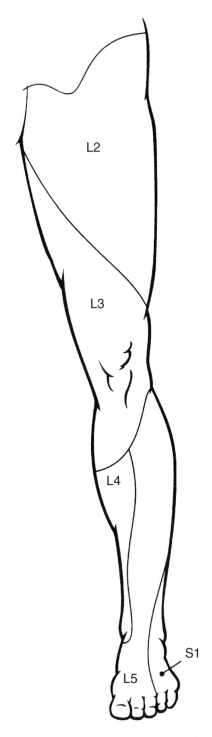

Figure 16-7. A dermatomal map of the leg. (Reprinted with permission from RB Rosenbaum, SM Campbell, JT Rosenbaum. Clinical Neurology of Rheumatic Disease. Boston: Butterworth–Heinemann, 1996.)

Table 16-4. Clinical Features of Common Lumbosacral Radiculopathies

Nerve Root (Reflex Loss)	Pain and Numbness Localization	Weakness
L4 (quadriceps)	Back and buttocks to medial foreleg	Quadriceps and tibialis
L5 (hamstring)	Back and buttocks to foreleg, medial malleolus, and foot	Extensor hallucis, peroneus longus, anterior tibialis
S1 (Achilles)	Back and buttocks to posterior foreleg, lateral malleolus, and foot	Gastrocnemius (rarely)

likely uncomplicated lumbosacral radiculopathy, the initial management should be similar to patients with nonradiating low back pain. Conservative therapy includes bed rest, analgesics, anti-inflammatory medication, treatment of muscle spasm, manipulation, and physical therapy. Recently, the utility of prolonged bed rest was questioned, and it may be prudent to limit the bed rest to a few days. In patients with persistent, radiating low back pain for 3–4 weeks despite conservative measures, an imaging study with MRI should be performed. If there is evidence of a disc herniation or osseous nerve root compression with unrelenting, persistent pain or weakness, the patient should be considered for surgical intervention. Microsurgery is available and effective for patients with uncomplicated disc herniations. With microsurgery, patients can be discharged from the hospital more quickly than with a traditional

laminectomy. Unfortunately, not all patients will have successful results from surgery, and some who initially benefit will suffer a relapse. Surgical failure may occur because of subsequent arachnoiditis, surgically induced nerve root injury, or progression of osseous degeneration. The management of patients with persistent radiating low back pain in whom surgery fails is a vexing problem.

Cauda Equina Syndrome

Lesions of the cauda equina and the conus medullaris cause pain in the lower back that may radiate to one or both legs. Weakness may also occur in both legs and involve muscles supplied by several nerve roots. Loss of pain sensation over the buttocks occurs, and both the knee and ankle reflexes may be lost in one

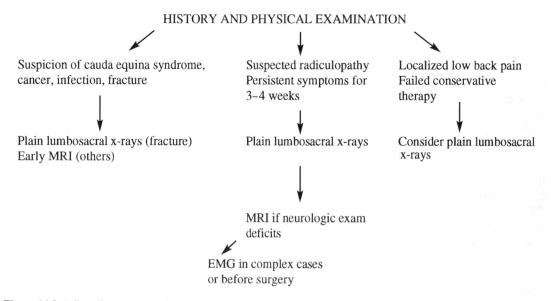

HISTORY AND PHYSICAL EXAMINATION

Suspicion of cauda equina syndrome, cancer, infection, fracture

Plain lumbosacral x-rays (fracture)
Early MRI (others)

Suspected radiculopathy
Persistent symptoms for
3–4 weeks

Plain lumbosacral x-rays

Localized low back pain
Failed conservative
therapy

Consider plain lumbosacral
x-rays

MRI if neurologic exam
deficits

EMG in complex cases
or before surgery

Figure 16-8. A flow diagram suggesting an approach to the diagnosis and management of patients with suspected lumbosacral radiculopathy. (MRI = magnetic resonance imaging; EMG = electromyography.)

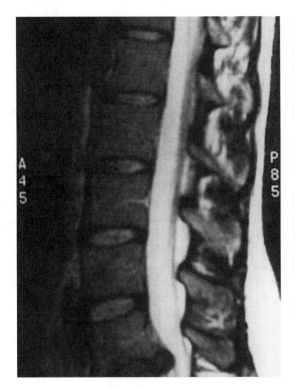

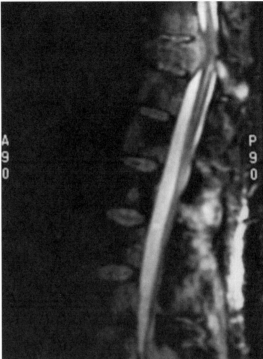

Figure 16-9. A sagittal magnetic resonance image of the lumbar spine demonstrating a disc herniation.

Figure 16-10. A tumor extending from the lower thoracic vertebral bodies to compress the cauda equina is shown on this sagittal magnetic resonance imaging view.

or both legs. Sphincter disturbances may occur. With conus medullaris syndrome, which is a similar syndrome in presentation and differential diagnosis, pain is less severe and marked sphincter disturbance occurs sooner. The most common cause of cauda equina compromise is a central disc herniation; other causes include primary or metastatic tumors (Figure 16-10), hematoma, abscess, lumbosacral fractures, and surgical complications. If a cauda equina or conus medullaris syndrome is suspected, urgent imaging should be performed. MRI is the imaging procedure of choice, although some clinicians rely on CT-myelography. The demonstration of a compressive lesion will lead to early surgery.

Lumbar Spinal Stenosis

Spinal stenosis—that is, narrowing of the anterior-posterior diameter of the lumbar spinal canal—can cause low back pain and compromise of the lumbosacral nerve roots. Narrowing can be caused by several potential mechanisms, including facet joint hypertrophy, degeneration of lumbar discs, osteophyte formation, and ligamentous hypertrophy. Discomfort in the lower back with radiation to the buttocks and legs is common and is typically more troublesome with an erect posture such as with walking or prolonged standing. The elicitation of radiating pain with walking is called *neurogenic pseudoclaudication* and should be distinguished from vascular claudication. A history of weakness or numbness with an erect posture is very helpful when considering the diagnosis of pseudoclaudication induced by lumbar spinal stenosis, as are findings such as an absent knee or ankle reflex, muscle weakness, and positive results on the straight-leg raising test. The symptoms and signs of lumbar spinal stenosis usually develop insidiously, and the patients are typically older than patients with straightforward disc herniations. Congenital narrowing of the lumbar spinal canal occurs infre-

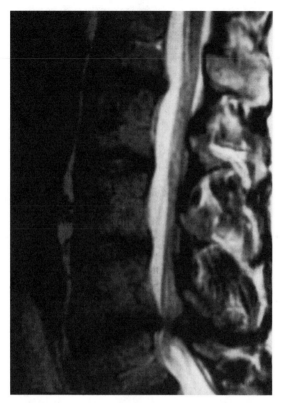

Figure 16-11. A sagittal magnetic resonance image demonstrating multiple-level disc herniations with obvious narrowing of the anterior-posterior diameter of the spinal canal, consistent with lumbar spinal stenosis.

an MRI scan is the imaging study of choice, because it will provide an accurate depiction of the sagittal anatomy (Figure 16-11). CT-myelography is an alternative procedure with a similar degree of diagnostic accuracy, although it will require the injection of contrast material into the subarachnoid space. With both MRI and CT-myelography, there may be false-positive findings. EMG testing can provide evidence of denervation in one or more lumbosacral nerve roots, but results may be negative in some patients with symptomatic lumbar spinal stenosis.

Conservative management with analgesics, anti-inflammatory medication, muscle relaxants, and physical therapy should be used for symptomatic relief. Surgery is indicated if the pain is not tolerable or if the patient develops neurologic deficits. Foraminotomies and multiple laminectomies may be required in some patients, whereas in others surgery at a single level is all that is necessary. The majority of patients with lumbar spinal stenosis who are treated surgically will have some improvement in their symptoms, but a substantial minority will have no benefit. Because medical therapy is usually only palliative, patients for whom surgery fails may not receive adequate relief of their symptoms.

Lumbosacral Plexopathies and Lower Extremity Mononeuropathies

Disorders of the lumbosacral plexus and peripheral nerves in the legs may at times be confused with radiculopathies or lumbar spinal stenosis. Involvement of the lumbar portion of the lumbosacral plexus causes pain, weakness, and sensory loss in the proximal part of the leg, whereas involvement of the sacral portion causes more distal abnormalities. A disorder of the lumbosacral plexus should be considered when the neurologic signs and symptoms in a leg involve more than one nerve root or one peripheral nerve. EMG testing can be helpful in documenting widespread denervation. Specifically, if the EMG study shows paraspinal denervation, then a plexopathy or more distal nerve injury can be excluded. The differential diagnosis of lumbosacral plexopathy includes hematoma, tumor infiltration, trauma, surgical injury, vasculitis, radiation plexopathy, and idiopathic plexopathy. Dia-

quently. In some patients, the slow development of symptoms is punctuated by a rapid escalation, and this should suggest the possibility of a lumbar disc herniation superimposed on a narrowed lumbar spinal canal. The pathogenesis of neurogenic pseudoclaudication remains uncertain. Vascular compromise of lumbosacral nerve roots is one proposed mechanism; the other leading hypothesis is mechanical irritation of the nerve roots by osseous deformities or herniated disc material.

Imaging of the spine is essential for the diagnosis of lumbar spinal stenosis. Plain x-ray films of the lumbar spine are of limited utility, but the lateral projection can provide clues to a narrowing of the spinal canal by osteoarthritic changes. Plain x-ray films should be performed in patients with mild symptoms and no neurologic deficits. In patients with more severe symptoms or neurologic findings, betic proximal neuropathy has a presentation similar to that of lumbosacral plexopathies but may involve both legs in an asymmetric fashion. The typical features include proximal leg weakness, severe upper leg and buttock pain, proximal sensory loss, and an absent or reduced knee reflex. The pain usually resolves spontaneously over 3–4 weeks, but the weakness takes much longer to resolve. Femoral neuropathies, also typical in diabetics, present with pain radiating from the hip or buttock to the upper leg anteriorly. Weakness of the iliopsoas and quadriceps with loss of the knee reflex is common, and this condition can be easily confused with an upper lumbar radiculopathy or diabetic proximal neuropathy. A lateral femoral cutaneous neuropathy causes pain and sensory loss discretely over the lateral thigh and should not be confused with a radiculopathy in most cases. A peroneal neuropathy at the fibular head causes anterior compartment weakness, varying sensory loss, and some discomfort distally in the leg and foot. Peroneal neuropathies are occasionally confused with L5 radiculopathies that do not have radiating pain. Isolated sciatic neuropathies are uncommon, but can occur after pelvic trauma, hematomas in the posterior thigh, after hip replacement surgery, or with endometriosis at the sciatic notch. The pain with sciatic neuropathies should not involve the lower back, and the amount of weakness and sensory loss is greater than with a monoradiculopathy. MRI studies of the pelvis and EMG testing should be performed if there is a strong suspicion of sciatic neuropathy.

Suggested Reading

Braakman R. Management of cervical spondylytic myelopathy and neuropathy. J Neurol Neurosurg Psychiatry 1994;57:257.

Carey TS, Garrett J, Jackman A, et al. The outcomes and costs of care for acute low back pain among patients seen by primary care practitioners, chiropractors, and orthopedic surgeons. N Engl J Med 1995;333:913.

Connell MD, Wiesel SW. Natural history and pathogenesis of cervical disc disease. Orthop Clin North Am 1992; 23:369.

Deyo RA, Rainville J, Kent DL. What can history and physical examination tell us about back pain? JAMA 1992; 286:760.

Frymoyer JW. Back pain and sciatica. N Engl J Med 1988;318:291.

Frymoyer JW, Cats-Baril WL. An overview of the incidences and costs of low back pain. Orthop Clin North Am 1991;22:263.

Gaskill MF, Lukin R, Wiot JG. Lumbar disc disease and stenosis. Radiol Clin North Am 1991;29:751.

Jensen MC, Brandt-Zawadski MN, Obuchowski N, et al. Magnetic resonance imaging of the lumbar spine in people without back pain. N Engl J Med 1994;332:69.

Krauss WE, McCormick PC. Cervical spondylytic myelopathy. Semin Neurol 1993;13:343.

Lestini WF, Wiesel SW. The pathogenesis of cervical spondylosis. Clin Orthop 1989;239:69.

Rowland LP. Surgical treatment of cervical spondylytic myelopathy: time for a controlled trial. Neurology 1992;42:5.

Swift TR, Sethi KD. Arm and Neck Pain. In WG Bradley, RB Daroff, GM Fenichel, CD Marsden (eds), Neurology in Clinical Practice (2nd ed). Boston: Butterworth–Heinemann, 1996;421–432.

Chapter 17
Dyskinesias

Joseph Ghika and Alberto Albanese

Chapter Plan

Tremor
Tics
Dystonia
Chorea, athetosis, ballism
Myoclonus
Other dyskinesias
   Akathisia
   Restless legs syndrome
   Syndrome of painful legs and moving toes
   Abnormal startle
   Tardive dyskinesias
   Psychogenic dyskinesias

Dyskinesia is a generic term encompassing all involuntary movements (e.g., tremor, tic, dystonia). This term is currently used more commonly than the synonym *hyperkinesia*, which has a longer historical tradition. Other motor abnormalities, such as akinesia, ataxia, or paralysis, are not considered dyskinesias.

As a neurologic sign, dyskinesias can be transient, permanent, or paroxysmal (which means that they have an abrupt onset, usually in relation to a voluntary movement). Based on topography, dyskinesias may be focal (just one body part), segmental (two contiguous body parts), multifocal (two noncontiguous body parts), or generalized. As a nosologic entity, dyskinesias are clinical syndromes characterized by a number of clinical signs and symptoms in which dyskinesias are a prominent clinical feature. Usually, just the same dyskinesia term (e.g., chorea, dystonia) is used at times with reference to the occurrence of a clinical sign or, alternatively, to indicate a nosologic entity characterized by a prominent occurrence of the homonymous clinical sign.

The student or resident who tries to address the clinical issues related to dyskinesias will find this task quite difficult. At first sight, involuntary movements very much resemble each other; they may appear funny, bizarre, or frightening to the inexperienced. This explains why, historically, dyskinesias have been defined quite late in the neurologic literature. The chronology of the first official recognition of the main dyskinesias is reported in Table 17-1. It is remarkable to note that students and residents usually learn to recognize dyskinesias with a similar sequence. The chronology of clinical observations therefore parallels the common chronology of the learning curve of an inexperienced clinician.

In a synthetic chapter such as this, it is not possible to describe dyskinesias in full, nor is it possible to teach the inexperienced. Learning in this field requires a good degree of careful observation.

Tremor

Tremor consists of an involuntary, rhythmic, oscillatory movement around a joint. Resting tremor occurs when muscles are entirely relaxed; postural tremor is present on maintaining active postures

Table 17-1. Learning of Diagnostic Skills in the Field of Dyskinesia Reflects the Chronology of First Identification

Date	Dyskinesia	First Usage
Ancient Greece	Tremor	τρεμω (to tremble, to fear)
Fourteenth century	Chorea	Choreomania (ritual dance)
Seventeenth century	Tic	Horse breeders
1871	Athetosis	Hammond
1881	Myoclonus	Friedreich
1885	Ballism	Kussmaul
1911	Dystonia	Oppenheim

Table 17-3. Tremor Classification by Frequency

Frequency	Tremor Type
1–4 Hz	Cerebellar
1–5 Hz	Parkinsonian
5–8 Hz	Essential
7–8 Hz	Shivering, fear
8–12 Hz	Physiologic
8–16 Hz	Orthostatic
10–16 Hz	Thyrotoxic

Table 17-2. Tremor Classification by Relation with Voluntary Movement

Feature	Disorder
Rest*	Parkinson's disease, "midbrain" tremor
Postural	Thyrotoxic, alcoholic, hepatic, essential, orthostatic, paleocerebellar syndrome, Parkinson's disease, "midbrain" tremor, peripheral neuropathies
Action	Neocerebellar syndrome, "midbrain" tremor

*Also called *parkinsonian tremor.*

(e.g., holding the arms against gravity); action tremor (i.e., kinetic tremor) occurs during voluntary motion. *Intention tremor* is a term encompassing postural and action tremor (Tables 17-2 and 17-3). The motion of a tremor can be graphically represented by a sine curve, the amplitude of which reflects the amplitude of the joint displacement produced by the tremor. Tremors of very low amplitude are difficult to detect, as in the case of physiologic tremor, which is usually not seen because of its very low amplitude. Rather, it becomes evident in some physiologic conditions (i.e., stress, fear, cold, hypoglycemia), after administration or deprivation of drugs, or after endocrinologic changes. The expression "enhanced physiologic tremor" is used to indicate such paraphysiologic conditions.

Tremor is thought to be produced by a closed feedback neural loop that comes into a state of oscillation after increased gain, reduced conduction along the loop, or both. Different motor loops (central or peripheral) are responsible for different forms of tremor.

Physiologic tremor is a normal postural and action tremor with a frequency between 5 and 15 Hz (mean, 8–12 Hz, decreasing with age to about 6 Hz) resulting from peripheral mechanical properties of the musculoskeletal system. Parkinsonian tremor occurs at rest. It is usually asymmetric and has a frequency of 4–6 Hz. As a rule, parkinsonian tremor decreases in amplitude or disappears when an active movement is performed. Some parkinsonian patients also have a postural tremor that generally has a slightly higher frequency. Parkinsonian tremor classically affects the hands, with flexion-extension or abduction-adduction of the fingers ("pill-rolling"), but it can be observed in the legs, the chin, or the head in patients with tremor-dominant forms of Parkinson's disease. A postural tremor similar to essential action tremor can also be observed. Antiparkinsonian medications have a moderate effect on parkinsonian tremor, which instead responds to lesions or to high-frequency stimulation of the ventrointermedio-median (Vim) thalamic nucleus or of the subthalamic nucleus.

Essential tremor is a sporadic or familial disorder characterized by the occurrence of postural tremor with a frequency of 5–8 Hz, which is similar to physiologic tremor but has a higher amplitude. A number of patients affected by essential tremor report benefit with consumption of alcohol, and in more than 60% of them there is a family history. Beta-blockers and primidone are the most effective drugs; benzodiazepines are also of some value. Approximately 30% of essential tremor patients do not have benefit from any drug therapy and can be effectively treated by implanting a high-frequency stimulator in the Vim thalamic nucleus.

Cerebellar tremor is an action tremor of low frequency (1–4 Hz) that appears during fine voluntary movements. It is well demonstrated by the finger-to-nose or heel-to-knee maneuver. Cerebellar tremor is associated with other cerebellar features. Its treatment has been disappointing.

A combination of resting and postural tremors can be seen after lesions of the midbrain. Such tremors are capable of interrupting at one time the nigrostriatal pathway and the cerebellar pathway. This is the so-called rubral or mesencephalic tremor, which has, in fact, been shown not to be related to a lesion of the red nucleus.

Primary writing tremor is a rare condition that resembles essential tremor but occurs only during handwriting. Holding the arms outstretched does not produce tremor. This condition is considered to be a mild form of upper limb focal dystonia. Orthostatic tremor is also a rare form of high-frequency (14–18 Hz) tremor that occurs while standing.

Tics

Tics may be motor, vocal, or mixed. They may be simple or complex and are usually preceded by an uncomfortable sensation or by a compulsive thought (mental tic). Tics are repetitive, unpredictable, stereotyped, and generally brief. Examples of simple motor tics are blinking, tongue protrusion, eyebrow elevation, eye rotation, brisk motions of the neck, and shoulder shrugging. Examples of complex motor tics are rubbing, touching, jumping, hopping, stamping, and squatting. Patients with tics may also have peculiar features, such as copropraxia (obscene gestures) or echopraxia (imitating someone's gestures). Examples of simple vocal tics are barking, humming, sniffing, coughing, grunting, or the emission of high-pitched or loud sounds. Examples of complex tics are coprolalia (obscene expressions or sentences) and palilalia (repetition of the last syllables of a word). The pathophysiology of tics is still obscure; some degree of dysfunction of dopaminergic neurotransmission has been advocated.

Tics are often preceded by a sensory sensation ("sensory tics"); these recurrent, involuntary somatic perceptions in joints, muscles, throat, or other parts of the body often precede the motor tic of the same body part. A feeling of relief from the sensory perception is usually associated with the motor tic.

Obsessive-compulsive disorder is usually associated with tics. Obsessions are the fixation of the mind on a word, a sentence, or an idea thought or heard. Compulsions consist of a repetition of a simple or complex movement or gesture.

Gilles de la Tourette's syndrome is a familial disease with incomplete autosomal dominant transmission that is characterized by the association of tics and obsessive-compulsive features. Attention deficit and hyperactivity disorder is often seen in children who carry the Gilles de la Tourette's gene. The *Diagnostic and Statistical Manual for Mental Disorders* (DSM) has set some artificial guidelines that have been repeatedly changed for the classification of tic disorders and Gilles de la Tourette's syndrome. Tics, which are not associated with the other features of Gilles de la Tourette's syndrome, are also usually familiar and occur more frequently in families carrying the Gilles de la Tourette's gene. The physiopathology of this condition is still unknown. An abnormality in dopaminergic neurotransmission is generally believed to be a possible cause; abnormalities in the size of the basal ganglia have also been reported. The symptomatic treatment of tics is with neuroleptics (e.g., tiapride, haloperidol, lithium). Antidepressants are usually associated with other drugs in Gilles de la Tourette's syndrome.

Dystonia

Dystonia is characterized by sustained muscle contractions, which cause twisting or repetitive movements or gestures. Dystonia usually presents as a focal, segmental, or generalized disorder. Some forms of focal dystonias have specific names that are commonly used in clinical practice: Dystonia of the eyelids is called *blepharospasm*, dystonia of the vocal folds is called *spasmodic dysphonia*, cervical dystonia is called *torticollis*, and upper limb dystonia is often called *writer's cramp* (other names, such as "musician's cramp" or "professional cramp" are used for other task-specific dystonias of the upper limbs).

Dystonia is characterized by a typical combination of dystonic postures and dystonic movements. Dystonic postures are generally associated with a feeling of rigidity, traction, pain, or a cramp in relation to flexion, extension, or abnormal rotation of a body part along its major axis (torsion). Dystonic movements may be fast or slow and are superimposed on dystonic postures; in some cases, the jerky movement is very similar to tremor (although irregular at times). Dystonia is typically associated with some peculiar voluntary movements that the patient performs in order to overcome abnormal postures; these are called "sensory tricks" or "gestes antagonistes." Their observation is very useful in confirming the diagnosis.

The severity of dystonia is variable. In milder forms, dystonia occurs when a specific voluntary movement is performed; in more severe forms, dystonia occurs in association with more than one kind of voluntary movement of the affected body part; in very severe forms, dystonia occurs when any body part is voluntarily moved or even at rest. These differences in relation to voluntary movement are seen either in focal or in generalized forms of dystonia with increasing severity.

The pathophysiology of dystonia is still unclear. Lesions at all levels of the basal ganglia, from the caudate nucleus to the thalamus, have been associated with dystonia, but peripheral nerve and spinal cord lesions have also been described in association with focal dystonia.

Focal dystonias generally appear in adults and are usually sporadic. In the majority of cases, focal dystonia is idiopathic, as no obvious cause or lesion is observed. A significant number of these cases occur with familial aggregation and are of genetic origin. Post-traumatic or symptomatic focal dystonia has also been described. In a number of cases, and particularly in familial cases, focal dystonia tends to spread to contiguous body parts, giving rise to segmental or generalized forms. Blepharospasm is a spasmodic contraction of the orbicularis oculi that is usually bilateral and is often triggered by exposure to light (hence, dark glasses worn by the patients). Talking often decreases the spasm. Patients can be functionally blind. A peculiar form of blepharospasm, called *pretarsal blepharospasm*, or apraxia of lid opening, causes an intermittent inability to open the eyelids. Spasmodic torticollis is the most common focal adult dystonia. An abnormal posture of the neck is generally observed at rest, producing a rotation (torticollis), inclination (laterocollis), anteflexion (antecollis), or retroflexion (retrocollis). In addition, mixed forms, in which different involuntary forms of movements and postures are superimposed, are quite frequent. A compensatory scoliosis, the elevation of the shoulder, as well as a postural tremor are frequently associated. Spasmodic dysphonia is caused by an abnormal contraction of the vocal muscles typically presenting with adduction ("strangled" or high-pitched voice) or abduction ("aphonic voice") of the vocal cords. Meige's syndrome is characterized by a variable combination of blepharospasm and oromandibular dystonia. Writer's cramp is a focal involuntary contraction of the forearm muscles that usually worsens with handwriting, while other motor tasks are well preserved. When a task-specific dystonia occurs during the use of a musical instrument or another professional tool, the professional or occupational dystonia bears a different name (e.g., pianist's cramp, typist's cramp).

Hemidystonia is generally symptomatic of a lesion in the contralateral hemisphere. Generalized dystonia occurs more commonly in childhood and generally is of familial origin.

Autosomal dominant, recessive, and X-linked forms of dystonia have been described. Clinical-genetic correlates of dystonia are currently one of the more lively areas of research in movement disorders. The gene *DYT-1* for generalized dystonia has been found in Ashkenazic Jews; other genes for focal dystonias have been localized or are being sought. The pathogenesis of dystonia is not understood. Dopa-responsive dystonia responds to low doses of levodopa. Other forms are treated with systemic medications or with local injections of botulinum toxin.

Chorea, Athetosis, and Ballism

Chorea is an irregular, unpredictable, involuntary movement with variable sequences, usually composed of very brisk and short-lasting jerks. Sometimes, choreic movements are slower and more complex, mimicking dystonia. Rapid flexion-extension, rotation, or crossing of the upper or lower limbs are frequent, together with some grimacing, tongue protrusion, vocalization, or respiratory noises. Two clinical features are specific for chorea and allow this dyskinesia to be distinguished from other movement disorders. First, choreic movements are fluent, meaning that they involve contiguous body parts in sequence and almost invariably affect the face; second, chorea is associated with hypotonia and with motor impersistence, meaning that a patient is unable to hold a posture (e.g., sustained tongue protrusion, fist closure, or lateral rotation of the eyes) for 20 seconds or more. These features are so specific for chorea that they occur not only in Huntington's disease, but also in Sydenham's chorea and in other choreic disorders. Will can control chorea for only a few seconds. Choreic motor patterns are often combined with voluntary executed movements, which explains in part why many patients are often unaware of their chorea (Figure 17-1).

Athetosis is an old term that groups together two quite different dyskinesias. In some instances, athetosis is used to name a slower form of chorea, essentially distal and of low amplitude, irregular, and more stereotyped with snakelike motions. In other instances, the term refers to dystonia. Extension of the neck, flexion or torsion of the limbs or of the axial segments, or slow grimacing and dysphonic voice are characteristic features of dystonic "double athetosis," which is a common aftermath of cerebral palsy.

A proximal and axial form of chorea with large throwing movements of amplitude is called *ballism*. Ballism is increased by stress and emotions and can be confused with action myoclonus. Unilateral ballism (hemiballism) is by far the most frequent presentation. Ballism is characteristically associated with lesions of the subthalamic nucleus, but examples of different anatomic lesions have been reported.

Chorea, athetosis, and ballism can be symptomatic of a focal lesion in the basal ganglia or the thalamus. In such cases, the presentation is usually unilateral (hemichorea-hemiballism). In many instances, chorea is the result of hereditary causes (e.g., Huntington's disease, acanthocytosis, benign familial chorea, paroxysmal choreoathetosis, Hallervorden-Spatz disease, Wilson's disease). Inflammatory diseases (e.g., Sydenham's chorea, lupoid chorea, subacute sclerosing panencephalitis, Henoch-Schönlein purpura, vaccines), and drugs (e.g., levodopa, dopamine agonists, anticonvulsants, oral contraceptives, amphetamines, isoniazid, lithium) are also other important causes of chorea. Choreoathetosis and ballism can be treated symptomatically with neuroleptics.

Myoclonus

Myoclonus is a brisk and brief involuntary muscle contraction, that is usually intermittent and arrhythmic but occasionally rhythmic or repetitive. Myoclonus never produces abnormal postures or torsion of a limb. Positive myoclonus is a muscle contraction associated with a synchronous short EMG burst lasting 50–300 ms; negative myoclonus (asterixis) (Figure 17-2) is a sudden muscle decontraction associated with a brief loss of muscle activity that produces a sudden drop when maintaining postures. As with other dyskinesias, myoclonus can be focal, segmental, generalized, or multifocal. The amplitude may be variable with partial or global involvement of just a segment of a limb or the entire limb or the entire body.

Myoclonus is a reflex phenomenon that is usually trigged by a stimulus (a somatic sensation or an active or a passive movement) that may also occur without any apparent triggering phenomenon. Spontaneous myoclonus is thought to be a reflex response to common stimuli of low intensity that are not perceived as triggering factors. Reflex myoclonus is usually evoked by external stimuli (e.g., a noise, light, a sensory stimulus). Being a reflex phenomenon, myoclonus may be integrated at the level of the cerebral cortex (cortical myoclonus) or the brain stem (reticular myoclonus). Cortical reflex myoclonus is usually a focal or multifocal action myoclonus; reticular myoclonus is usually axial or proximal, whereas spinal myoclonus is usually focal.

Physiologic myoclonus occurs in the first stages of sleep or as a familial condition denominated essential benign myoclonus. In addition, myoclonus is a pathologic phenomenon that can be seen in many brain diseases (e.g., after anoxic injury) and in intoxications. Anticonvulsant medications are generally effective in the treatment of myoclonus.

Other Dyskinesias

Akathisia

Akathisia is the inability to stay put. Akathisia is associated with a state of physical and mental unease and the urge to move with an aimless, poorly organized motor hyperactivity. Akathisia has

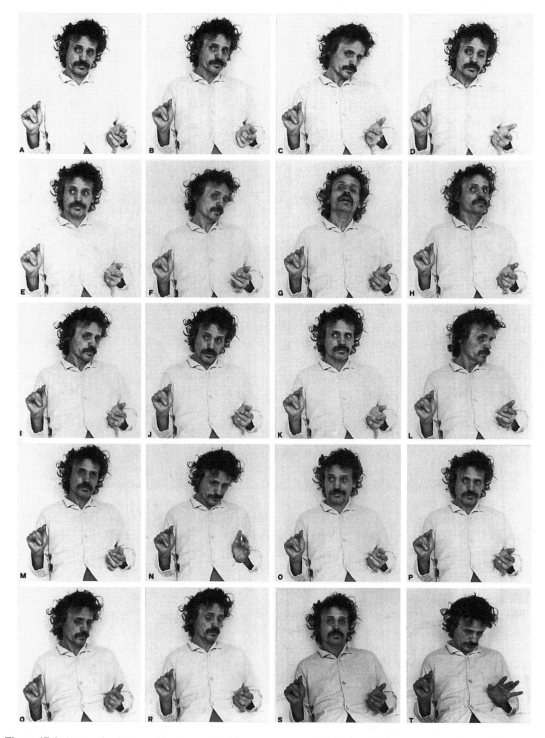

Figure 17-1. Automatic photographic sequence (1.5 frames per second) of the involuntary movements observed in a patient with Huntington's disease. The time lapse between two consecutive images is approximately 600 ms. It can be observed that choreic movements are fast and fluent. Chorea is stereotyped (e.g., compare C and N). The high speed of choreic movements is demonstrated by the observation of a change in posture in two consecutive frames. (Reprinted with permission from A Albanese. I Gangli Motori e i Disturbi del Movimento. Padua: Piccin, 1991.)

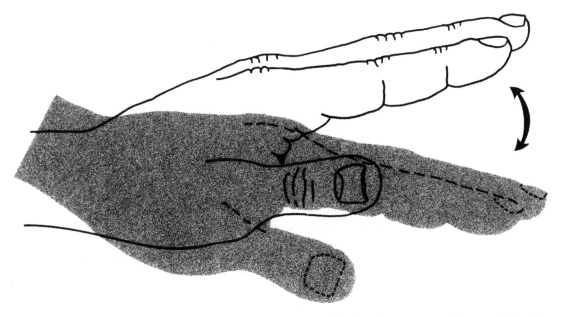

Figure 17-2. Asterixis is a negative myoclonus that can be elicited by asking the patient to outstretch the arms. Under this condition, the hand flexes abruptly and soon afterward regains the original position. (Reprinted with permission from A Albanese. I Gangli Motori e i Disturbi del Movimento. Padua: Piccin, 1991.)

no specific clinical features; it appears as an odd movement disorder that is described as an inner restlessness, a feeling of tension, an urge to move, or a distressing sensation in the limbs or trunk, usually associated with anxiety.

Akathisia is typically secondary to the use of neuroleptics and can occur within hours to years after the start of medication. Discontinuance of neuroleptics is the best treatment. In addition, akathisia is frequently seen in Parkinson's disease.

Restless Legs Syndrome

Restless legs syndrome is characterized by sensory and motor features. The sensory syndrome is an uncomfortable sensation frequently reported in the legs, sometimes in the trunk, arms, or face, rarely asymmetric or alternating, which is usually ill-described by the patients. Adjectives such as creeping, stretching, itching, and burning are used. Characteristically, the symptoms occur only when the limbs are at rest, lying or sitting, especially in the evening and at night. Some mild discomfort can be described during the day. The motor features are

an irresistible urge to move the limbs followed by some relief in the symptoms. The patients may rub the skin, stretch, kick, swing the legs or walk, or press one foot against the other or against the calf. The pathophysiology is unknown. Familial restless legs syndrome can be associated with a polyneuropathy. Symptomatic forms can be associated with the use of various drugs, particularly with their withdrawal. The treatment mainly consists of dopaminergic drugs (levodopa or dopamine agonists).

Syndrome of Painful Legs and Moving Toes

Painful legs and moving toes is a dysesthetic dyskinesia characterized by pain in the legs or feet (rarely the hands) that is described as aching, burning, a feeling of pressure, or pulling with variable degrees in intensity. It is often decreased by immersion in water and it is associated with movements of the toes (e.g., wiggling, fanning, clawing), the feet, or the legs. These movements are stereotyped, are continuous or intermittent, and can be suppressed for a few seconds voluntarily. The syndrome is generally bilateral; it starts usually after

40 years of age and may present in two forms: with or without polyneuropathy. The other main condition in the differential diagnosis is restless legs, which occur only at rest.

Abnormal Startle

Startle is a normal physiologic reaction of a newborn to unexpected stimuli. It is elicited as a reflex phenomenon by pediatricians (reflex of Moro) and disappears with normal development. In some people, based on their genetic makeup, startle is maintained into adult life. People with such features suffer from a disease called *hyperexplexia*. The milder form is expressed as an increased startle reaction to unexpected stimuli, whereas in the severe form, startle is accompanied by a muscular rigidity of short duration with hyperextension of the arms. Families with hyperexplexias have been described in the United States ("Jumping Frenchmen of Maine") and elsewhere. In these cases, everyday life becomes very much impaired because of a series of startle reactions and of violent jumping after normal stimuli. Automatic obedience, echolalia, and echopraxia are also features observed in these forms. The treatment of choice is benzodiazepines.

Tardive Dyskinesias

Tardive dyskinesias are the movement disorders produced by a chronic administration of neuroleptic drugs. They usually present the features of a focal or segmental dystonia, which is often combined with some facial chorea, akathisia, and parkinsonian features. Tardive dyskinesias are most commonly involved and often have the aspect of art movement disorders. A history of neuroleptic administration may be concealed or may not be immediately recognized, particularly in those individuals who take neuroleptics for circulatory disorders (e.g., flunarizine, cinnarizine) or for gastrointestinal disturbances (e.g., tiapride).

Psychogenic Dyskinesias

Psychogenic dyskinesias are not a rare occurrence and can resemble any movement disorder (e.g., chorea, dystonia, tremor). Psychogenic dyskinesias are sometimes difficult to differentiate from organic dyskinesias, as the emotional impact of the doctor–patient relationship sometimes does not allow for an objective evaluation of the clinical features. These movement disorders must also be differentiated from tardive dyskinesia, which also occurs in patients who have psychopathologic traits and usually have complex or bizarre clinical presentations. According to DSM criteria, psychogenic dyskinesia should be classified as somatoform disorders or malingering.

Suggested Reading

Albanese A. I Gangli Motori e i Disturbi del Movimento. Padua: Piccin, 1991.

Findley LJ, Koller WC. Handbook of Tremor Disorders. New York: Marcel Dekker, 1995.

Ghika J, Bogousslavsky J. Movement Disorders. In J Bogousslavsky, L Caplan (eds), Stroke Syndromes. Cambridge, UK: Cambridge University Press, 1995;91–101.

Marsden CD, Fahn S. Movement Disorders 1, 2, 3. Boston: Butterworth–Heinnemann, 1992, 1994, 1996.

Sachdev P. Akathisia and Restless Legs. Cambridge, UK: Cambridge University Press, 1995.

Shapiro AK, Shapiro ES, Young JG, Feinberg TE. Gilles de la Tourette Syndrome. New York: Raven, 1988.

Shulman LM, Weiner WJ. Paroxysmal movement disorders. Semin Neurol 1995;15:188.

Young J. Movement Disorders in Neurology and Neuropsychology. Oxford, UK: Blackwell, 1995.

Chapter 18
Dizziness and Vertigo

Marianne Dieterich and Thomas Brandt

Chapter Plan

Vertigo is an erroneous perception of self-motion or object motion or an unpleasant distortion of static gravitational orientation that is caused by a mismatch between the three sensory systems: the vestibular, the visual, and the somatosensory. These systems are mutually interactive and redundant in that orientation and balance are guided by simultaneous reafferent cues (Figure 18-1). The functional ranges of the three systems overlap so that they are able to compensate in part for each other's deficiencies. Thus, vertigo is not a well-defined disease entity, but rather a multisensory syndrome induced either by stimulation of the intact sensorimotor system by motion (as in motion sickness or height vertigo) or by pathologic dysfunction of any of the stabilizing sensory systems (as in vestibular neuritis).

The reflexes that provide postural and ocular motor responses to head motion are mediated from the semicircular canals and otoliths via the vestibular nuclei in the medullary brain stem to the ocular motor nuclei in the mesencephalic brain stem—that is, the vestibulo-ocular reflex (VOR), which allows compensatory eye movements during head movements. The VOR has three major planes of action: (1) the *yaw plane,* with *horizontal* eye and head movements about the *vertical Z axis*; (2) the *pitch plane,* with *vertical* eye and head movements about the *horizontal Y axis*; and (3) the *roll plane,* with *torsional* eye and head movements about the line of sight, the *horizontal X axis*.

These planes represent the three-dimensional space in the vestibular and oculomotor system. The paired vestibular nuclei receive neural input from all three sensory systems and transmit this information to the spinal cord (for postural stabilization), the vestibular nuclei thalamus and cortex (for motion perception and spatial orientation), and the upper brain stem and cerebellum (for the VOR) (Figure 18-2). Lesions along these pathways can induce vertigo, which manifests in a combination of phenomena that are dependent on the site within these vestibular pathways. Clinical phenomena—characteristic for both physiologic as well as clinical vertigo syndromes—therefore include postural, perceptual, oculomotor, and veg-

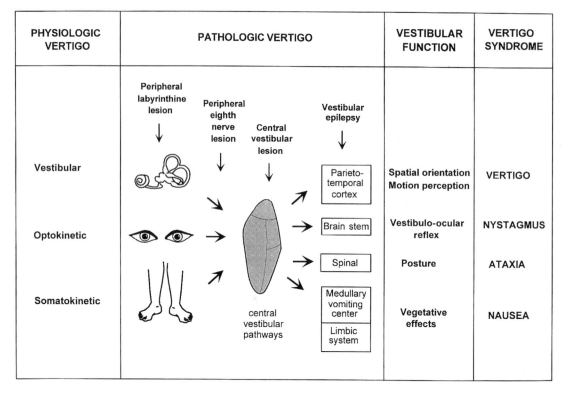

Figure 18-1. Origin and classification of the different types of vertigo. These are not clinical entities but different multisensory syndromes arising from unusual stimulation or lesional dysfunction.

etative syndromes, which manifest with ataxia, nystagmus, vertigo, and nausea. These four manifestations correlate with different aspects of vestibular function: Postural imbalance and vestibular ataxia are caused by an abnormal activation or dysfunction of the vestibulospinal pathways; nystagmus is caused by a direction-specific imbalance in the VOR activating brain stem neuronal circuitry; vertigo itself is caused by a disturbance of cortical spatial orientation; and the unpleasant vegetative effects—nausea and vomiting—are caused by an activation of the reticular formation, the vomiting center, in the medullary brain stem.

The differential diagnosis of peripheral labyrinthine and central vestibular vertigo syndromes is guided by the duration and frequency of vertigo, manifestations of ear signs (e.g., Ménière's disease, perilymphatic fistula, neurovascular cross-compression) or brain stem signs (e.g., central positional vertigo, vertebrobasilar ischemia, basilar artery migraine, paroxysmal ataxia/dysarthria), certain provoking factors such

as head motion (e.g., benign paroxysmal positioning vertigo [BPPV], central positional vertigo, neurovascular cross-compression, bilateral vestibulopathy), or family history (e.g., congenital vertigo). Four typical vertigo patterns are helpful in the differential diagnosis: (1) attacks of rotational vertigo, (2) sustained rotational vertigo, (3) positional vertigo, and (4) dizziness with postural imbalance. Careful history taking makes it possible to diagnose 70% of the patients with vertigo. The most common vertigo syndromes are listed in Table 18-1.

General Treatment

Because the central nervous system has a strong impulse to compensate for, or habituate to, a persisting sensory mismatch, all therapy for vertigo should avoid disturbing these naturally compensatory mechanisms, centered within the vestibular nuclei. It must be stressed that the central nervous

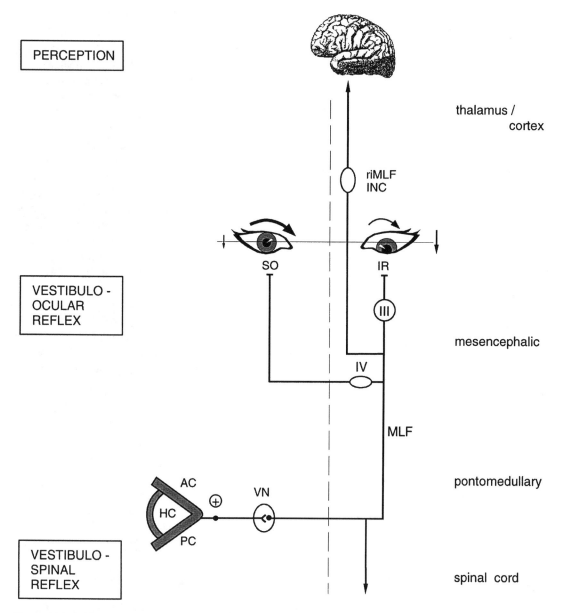

PERCEPTION

thalamus /
cortex

riMLF
INC

SO   IR

VESTIBULO -
OCULAR
REFLEX

III

mesencephalic

IV

MLF

AC

VN

HC

pontomedullary

PC

VESTIBULO -
SPINAL
REFLEX

spinal cord

Figure 18-2. Schematic representations of the vestibulo-ocular reflex (VOR); elements that contribute to the overall senso-rimotor vestibular response. Inputs from the horizontal (HC), anterior (AC), and posterior (PC) semicircular canals converge with otolithic, visual, and somatosensory afferents in the vestibular nuclear complex (VN). The outputs from the neural network in the VN contact the extraocular muscles; here, the principal three-neuron arc connections of the PC are shown passing to the trochlear (IV) and oculomotor nuclei (III), which contact the superior oblique (SO) and inferior rectus (IR) muscles. In addition, connections from the AC and PC contact the interstitial nucleus of Cajal (INC), which is important for eye-head coordination in roll and in vertical gaze-holding and the rostral interstitial nucleus of the medial longitudinal fasciculus (riMLF), which is important for generating quick phases of vestibular nystagmus in the vertical and torsional planes. The VN output also projects to the spinal cord to generate vestibulospinal reflexes, and to the thalamus and cortex to provide inputs for perception of movements. Thus, VOR pathways also mediate posture and perception.

Table 18-1. Frequency of Different Vertigo Syndromes in 406 Patients Seen in a Dizziness Unit in 1996

Diagnosis	Frequency	
	Number	Percent
1. Benign paroxysmal positioning vertigo	74	18.2
2. Central-vestibular vertigo	63	15.5
3. Phobic postural vertigo	59	14.5
4. Basilar migraine	35	8.6
5. Peripheral vestibulopathy	31	7.6
6. Ménière's disease	26	6.4
7. Bilateral vestibulopathy	14	3.4
8. Vestibular paroxysmia	8	2.0
9. Psychogenic vertigo (without 3)	4	1.0
10. Perilymph fistula	2	0.5
Unknown cause	19	4.8
Other (central vestibular syndromes without vertigo)	71	17.5

system needs the stimulus of the sensory mismatch for habituation and compensation. Adequate therapy for vertigo (Table 18-2) must consider that antivertiginous drugs will suppress such mechanisms, because most of these drugs are vestibular sedatives. Therefore, vestibular suppressants should be applied only when vertigo is accompanied by distressing nausea and vomiting—that is, in acute peripheral vestibulopathy and in acute brain stem and cerebellar lesions (near the vestibular nuclei)—or to prevent motion sickness. These drugs are not indicated in patients suffering from chronic dizziness or positioning vertigo. If possible, specific therapies directed at the underlying cause should be chosen. In some cases, it is best to recommend rehabilitation because the central nervous system compensates by itself over time for the lesioned function. Vestibular rehabilitation is often needed to speed recovery and central compensation.

If nausea is a prominent symptom of a vestibular vertigo syndrome, vestibular sedatives should be administered for symptomatic relief despite the major side effect of general sedation. The most commonly used antivertiginous drugs are the antihistamines, anticholinergic drugs, phenothiazines,

Table 18-2. Pharmacologic, Physical, and Surgical Therapies for Vertigo

Therapy	Vertigo Syndrome
Pharmacologic	
Antiepileptic drugs	Vestibular epilepsy, vestibular paroxysmia (disabling positional vertigo), paroxysmal dysarthria and ataxia in multiple sclerosis, other central vestibular syndromes, superior oblique myokymia
Vestibular suppressants	Symptomatic relief of nausea (in acute peripheral and vestibular nuclear lesions), prevention of motion sickness
Beta-receptor blockers	Basilar artery migraine (benign recurrent vertigo)
Betahistine	Ménière's disease
Ototoxic antibiotics	Ménière's disease (vestibular drop attacks in Ménière's disease)
Baclofen	Downbeat or upbeat nystagmus syndrome
Acetazolamide	Familial periodic ataxia or vertigo
Physical	
Deliberate maneuvers	Benign paroxysmal positioning vertigo (BPPV)
Vestibular exercises	Central compensation of acute vestibular loss, habituation for prevention of motion sickness, improvement of balance skills
Physical therapy (neck collar)	Cervical vertigo (?)
Surgical	
Surgical decompression	Tumors (acoustic neurinoma)
Ampullary nerve section or canal plugging	BPPV
Vestibular nerve section or labyrinthectomy	Ménière's disease
Neurovascular decompression?	Vestibular paroxysmia (disabling positional vertigo)
Surgical patching	Perilymph fistula

benzodiazepines, and butyrophenones. Anticholinergic drugs (e.g., scopolamine) have been given in combination with noradrenergic substances (e.g., ephedrine), but double-blind, placebo-controlled studies have reported no significant difference when scopolamine was given alone or in combination with ephedrine. The only known similarity among the drugs used to counter labyrinthine vertigo and motion sickness is their capacity to act as acetylcholine antagonists by competitive inhibition. The most probable sites of their primary action are the synapses of the vestibular nuclei, which exhibit reduced discharges and diminished neuronal responses to body rotation (see Table 18-2).

Peripheral Labyrinthine Vertigo Syndromes

Benign Paroxysmal Positioning Vertigo

BPPV is a mechanical disorder of the inner ear in which precipitating positioning of the head causes an abnormal stimulation, usually of the posterior semicircular canal of the undermost ear. Patients with this most common form of vertigo develop brief attacks of rotational vertigo and concomitant rotatory nystagmus precipitated by rapid head tilt toward the affected ear or by head extension, typically when turning over in bed, extending the neck to look up, or lifting the head after bending over. The clinician can induce the symptoms by rapid position changes from the sitting to the head-hanging-to-the-right or -left positions (Hallpike maneuver). Rotatory nystagmus starts after a few seconds' latency and beats with a crescendo-decrescendo rate, reaching a maximum within a few seconds and lasting 10–60 seconds. When the patient returns to the sitting position, nystagmus is in the opposite direction. The typical nystagmus pattern and the characteristics of short latency, limited duration, reversal on returning to the upright position, and fatigability on repeated provocation are sufficient to establish the diagnosis. This strong correlation between vertigo and rotatory nystagmus makes the diagnosis unlikely if a patient reports intense vertigo but no nystagmus. The most common causes are idiopathic (50%), head injury (17%), viral neurolabyrinthitis (15%), and long bed confinement. Although a striking preponderance of females (female-to-male ratio of 2:1) was found in the idiopathic group, the two

sexes were equally distributed among post-traumatic and postviral groups. In general, it is a disease of elderly people, with a peak of occurrence between the ages of 50 and 70 years.

In 1969, Schuknecht hypothesized that heavy debris settles on the cupula (cupulolithiasis) of the canal, transforming it from a transducer of angular acceleration into a transducer of linear acceleration. It is now generally accepted that in most cases the debris floats freely within the endolymph of the canal (canalolithiasis). The debris (possibly particles detached from the otoliths) gravitates to the most dependent part of the semicircular canal during head-position changes (Figure 18-3).

In 1980, the first effective physical therapy, the positional exercises after Brandt and Daroff, was proposed. These exercises consist of a sequence of rapid lateral head-trunk tilts repeated serially. Meanwhile, single liberatory maneuvers were introduced by Semont and co-workers (1988) as well as by Epley (1992). If performed properly, all forms of physical therapy—the Brandt-Daroff exercises and the Semont and Epley liberatory maneuvers—are effective in BPPV patients. Because the liberatory maneuvers often require only a single session (see Figure 18-3), they should be preferred in cases of canalolithiasis of the posterior semicircular canal.

In case of the rare anterior canal BPPV, spontaneous symptoms occur when the affected ear is uppermost. The Brandt-Daroff exercises, with repeated lateral head-trunk tilts to both sides from a sitting position, seem to be more effective than liberatory maneuvers in patients with the equally rare horizontal canal BPPV. All maneuvers should be performed serially until vertigo and rotatory nystagmus have completely disappeared.

Surgical transection of the posterior ampullar nerve via a middle ear approach can be considered in the very few patients with intense BPPV over many years who do not respond completely to physical therapy. However, sensorineural hearing loss is a possible complication, and it is difficult to locate surgically the particular semicircular canal nerve.

Acute Peripheral Vestibulopathy

An acute onset of prolonged severe rotational vertigo, which is associated with horizontal-rotatory

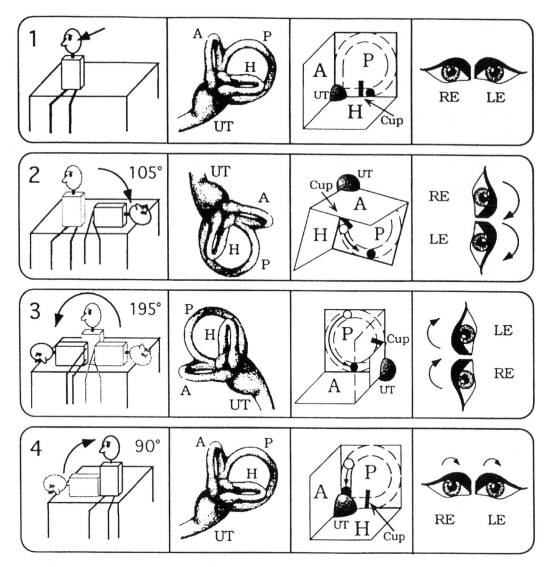

Figure 18-3. Schematic drawing of the Semont liberatory maneuver in a patient with typical benign paroxysmal positioning vertigo (BPPV) of the left ear. Boxes from left to right: position of head and body, position of the labyrinth in space, position and movement of the clot in the posterior canal and resulting cupula deflection, and direction of the rotatory nystagmus. The clot is depicted as an open circle within the canal; a black circle represents the final resting position of the clot. (1) In the sitting position, the head is turned horizontally 45 degrees to the unaffected ear. The clot, which is heavier than endolymph, settles at the base of left posterior semicircular canal. (2) The patient is tilted approximately 105 degrees toward the left (affected) ear. The change in head position, relative to gravity, causes the clot to gravitate to the lowermost part of the canal and the cupula to deflect downward, inducing BPPV with rotatory nystagmus beating toward the undermost ear. The patient maintains this position for 3 minutes. (3) The patient is turned approximately 195 degrees, with the nose down, causing the clot to move toward the exit of the canal. The endolymphatic flow again deflects the cupula such that a nystagmus beats toward the left ear, now uppermost. The patient remains in this position for 3 minutes. (4) The patient is slowly moved to the sitting position; this causes the clot to enter the utricular cavity. (A, P, H = anterior, posterior, horizontal semicircular canals; Cup = cupula; UT = utricular cavity; RE = right eye; LE = left eye.) (Reprinted with permission from T Brandt, S Steddin, RB Danoff. Therapy of benign paroxysmal positioning vertigo, revisited. Neurology 1994;44:796.)

spontaneous nystagmus toward the affected side, a falling tendency to the normal side, and severe nausea and vomiting that gradually resolves over days to weeks, results from an acute unilateral peripheral vestibulopathy, the third most common cause of peripheral vestibular vertigo. It accounts for approximately 5% of patients referred to a neurologic dizziness unit (see Table 18-1). The cause may be bacterial labyrinthitis (otitis media), stroke, or trauma, but in most cases viral involvement of parts of the vestibular nerve is the common cause (*vestibular neuritis* is its idiopathic form). Concomitant auditory dysfunction is absent in vestibular neuritis, which is characterized by a partial rather than a complete vestibular paresis with predominant involvement of the horizontal and anterior semicircular canal fibers, sparing the posterior semicircular canal fibers. This condition mainly affects patients 30–60 years old. Caloric testing invariably shows ipsilateral hyporesponsiveness (33%) or nonresponsiveness (66%) of the horizontal semicircular canal function, which resolves in 50–70% of the patients over months. Diagnosis is based on an acute unilateral peripheral vestibular loss (demonstrated by caloric testing, bedside testing of high-frequency VOR) after clinical exclusion of a neurologic disorder. Relief of the symptoms over 2–3 weeks (rarely up to 6 weeks) is the result of the central compensation of the lesional vestibular tone imbalance. Later on a restoration of peripheral function takes place, which may lead to a mild spontaneous nystagmus beating in the opposite direction. In the few cases of no or only minor peripheral restoration of labyrinthine function, oscillopsia may persist *during* rapid head movements. This is caused by a persisting deficit of the VOR in the higher frequency range, which cannot be compensated for centrally.

Vestibular sedatives should be administered parenterally on days 1–3, when nausea and vomiting are severe, for symptomatic relief while the patient rests in bed and avoids head movements. These drugs should be given only as long as nausea lasts, because antivertiginous drugs suppress the mechanisms of central compensation. Treatment with steroids (methylprednisolone sodium succinate) should be considered in cases of viral vestibular neuritis, because steroids may accelerate the process of central compensation as well as peripheral restoration. Further management includes physical ther-

apy, with the first exercises being done in bed (days 3–5) to suppress nystagmus by visual fixation: Voluntary saccades and eccentric gaze-holding should be performed in addition to sitting freely. During days 5–7 (approximately), when the spontaneous nystagmus is suppressed by fixation but there is continued gaze nystagmus in the direction of fast phase, upright stance and then head oscillations during free stance should be trained. Afterward, during weeks 2–3 and later on, balance exercises should become more complex, gradually increasing in difficulty (e.g., during active head oscillations with increasing frequencies) to reach a level above the demands for postural control under daily life conditions. All these exercises are used to recalibrate the VOR in its three major planes of action, the yaw, pitch, and roll planes, for perfect eye-head coordination.

Ménière's Disease

Ménière's disease is characterized by an episodic triad of rotational vertigo, tinnitus, and fluctuating low-tone sensorineural hearing loss (often accompanied by hyperacusis) and aural pressure or fullness in the affected ear. Spontaneous nystagmus is always present during the attack; the intensity of the nystagmus and vertigo is influenced by head position. One-third of the patients report an increase of tinnitus and hearing loss as well as a subjective feeling of fullness of the ear, which precedes the vertigo attack as a kind of aura. The attacks slowly subside after a few hours, but some dizziness and unsteadiness usually remain for a few days after the attack. In the early stages, patients are symptom free in the vertigo-free interval, but the majority subsequently develop slowly progressive tinnitus, hearing loss, and reduction in vestibular function, as measured by caloric testing. The usual age of onset lies in the fourth to sixth decades; there is an equal distribution between males and females. The longer one follows patients with Ménière's disease, the greater the percentage of patients who develop bilateral disease (15% in the first 2 years, 30% after one decade, up to 60% after two decades).

The underlying pathologic condition is endolymphatic hydrops, which can be classified as embryopathic, acquired, or idiopathic. It is caused by distention and temporary rupture of the membranous labyrinth secondary to increased endolymphatic pressure, altered endolymphatic sac function, relative overproduction of endolymph, defects in endolymph absorption, or a combination of these factors. Membranous labyrinth rupture results in a disruption of endolymph-perilymph sodium and potassium barriers, leading to paralysis of the surrounding vestibular or cochlear hair cells and neural structures.

The acute attack is self-limiting and subsides within a few hours (rarely less than 1 hour or more than a day). If nausea is prominent, vestibular sedatives should be administered parenterally. Treatment in the remission phase is aimed at reducing the frequency of the attacks and preserving hearing. The histamine derivative betahistine is the only drug that has proved to be effective in a prospective double-blind study. Its action is attributed to the improvement of the microcirculation of the stria vascularis and to inhibitory effects on polysynaptic vestibular nucleus neurons. Intratympanic treatment with ototoxic antibiotics (e.g., gentamicin sulfate) instilled via a transmeatal approach is able to selectively damage the secretory epithelium before significantly affecting vestibular and cochlear function. Some authors prefer intramuscular streptomycin injections rather than intratympanic injections. For patients in whom conservative procedures have failed, selective destructive surgical techniques (vestibular nerve section) have been proposed with the intention of preserving serviceable hearing function.

Vestibular Paroxysmia (Neurovascular Cross-Compression of the Eighth Nerve)

Analogous to trigeminal neuralgia, the diagnosis of vestibular paroxysmia (also termed disabling positional vertigo) is based on a few characteristic features. As a result of neurovascular cross-compression of the eighth cranial nerve close to the brain stem, short attacks of vertigo are characterized by (1) rotational or to-and-fro vertigo lasting from seconds to minutes; (2) frequently a dependency on the particular head position and a duration that can be modified by changing head position; (3) hypacusis or tinnitus (permanently or during the attack); (4) auditory or vestibular deficits measurable by

neurophysiologic methods; and (5) response to carbamazepine therapy.

Because this disorder has not yet been well-defined and surgery entails a craniotomy of the posterior fossa for microvascular decompression of the eighth nerve at its root-entry zone (mortality of up to 1%, neurologic complications of up to 10%), carbamazepine is recommended as the therapy of first choice of suspected vestibular paroxysmia before an operation is contemplated. Carbamazepine (Tegretol), the drug of first choice in trigeminal neuralgia, phenytoin, and pimozide have been effective in several patients with vestibular paroxysmia.

Perilymphatic Fistula

Perilymphatic fistulas may lead to episodic vertigo and sensorineural hearing loss. The clinical picture ranges from no symptoms to pure vestibular symptoms, pure hearing loss, or combinations of both. Vestibular dysfunction is more frequent than hearing loss and often begins after barotrauma, heavy lifting, or surgery. The symptoms are caused by a pathologic elasticity of the otic capsule, usually at the oval and round windows, which permits abnormal transfer of pressure changes to the receptors of the maculae and cupulae. Thus, symptoms are exacerbated by sneezing, pressing, and lifting heavy weights. Despite the availability of clinical fistula tests (i.e., pressure fistula test, vascular fistula test), a definite diagnosis can only be made by exploratory tympanotomy with inspection of the round and oval windows.

Because most fistulas heal spontaneously, conservative therapy is recommended as the first choice in the acute phase. Conservative therapy consists of bedrest with the head elevated for 2–3 weeks, and avoidance of sneezing, coughing, pressing, and head-hanging positions. Mild tranquilizers and stool softeners may be helpful. Physical activity should be limited, and heavy lifting or straining should be avoided for several weeks. When symptoms persist for more than 4 weeks or when hearing loss worsens, surgical exploration via a posterior tympanotomy should be considered, even though the results of the surgical intervention are not encouraging (improvement rate for the hearing deficit, 25–50%; for the vestibular symptoms, 50–70%). The recurrence rate of symptoms exceeds 10%.

Central Vestibular Disorders

Vestibular Syndromes in Yaw, Pitch, and Roll Planes

Vestibular syndromes can be classified clinically according to the three major planes of action of the VOR: yaw, pitch, and roll. The plane-specific vestibular syndromes are characterized by ocular motor, postural, and perceptual signs, which allow for a precise topographic diagnosis of brain stem lesions as to their level and side (Figure 18-4).

Yaw plane signs are horizontal nystagmus, past-pointing, rotational and lateral body falls, and deviation of perceived straight-ahead. Pure syndromes in yaw are rare because the small causative area covering the vestibular nucleus is not only adjacent to but is overlapped by the structures that also subserve the roll and pitch functions. The lesional sites of yaw syndromes are restricted to the pontomedullary level because of the short distance between the vestibular nuclei and the integration center for horizontal eye movements in the paramedian pontine reticular formation.

Pitch plane signs include upbeat and downbeat nystagmus, forward/backward tilts and falls, and deviations of the perceived horizontal. A tone imbalance in pitch indicates bilateral paramedian lesions or bilateral dysfunction of the flocculus. In patients with downbeat nystagmus, structural or functional lesions involve either the pontine brain stem between the vestibular nuclei at the floor of the fourth ventricle or the flocculus bilaterally. The two most common causes of downbeat nystagmus are cerebellar ectopia (25%) and cerebellar degeneration (25%), including alcoholic cerebellar degeneration; other conditions causing downbeat nystagmus are multiple sclerosis, intoxication, ischemia, hematoma, vitamin B_{12} deficiency, and magnesium depletion. Upbeat nystagmus presents with lesions of the pontomesencephalic or pontomedullary brain stem, which may be due to brain stem infarctions, hematomas, tumors, cavernomas, plaques in multiple sclerosis, abscess, alcoholic degeneration, or drug intoxication. In contrast to downbeat nystagmus, upbeat nystagmus generally has a dramatic onset with nausea, vomiting, and severe oscillopsia, but ceases spontaneously over a few weeks.

Roll plane signs include torsional nystagmus, skew deviation, ocular torsion, tilts of the head and body, and perceived visual vertical (Figure 18-5). A tone imbalance in roll indicates unilateral lesions along a pathway that runs from the ipsilateral vestibular nucleus via the contralateral medial longitudinal fasciculus (MLF) to the contralateral ocular motor nuclei and the contralateral integration center for vertical and torsional eye movements, the nucleus of Cajal (INC). Because these pathways, which transduce input from the vertical semicircular canals and otoliths, cross the midline at the pontine level, unilateral pontomedullary lesions cause ipsiversive tilts, whereas unilateral pontomesencephalic lesions cause contraversive tilts. A unilateral lesion or stimulation of these "graviceptive" pathways affects function in roll; bilateral lesions or stimulation affect function in pitch. Thus, the vestibular system is able to change its functional plane of action from roll to pitch by switching from a unilateral to a bilateral mode of operation.

The treatment depends on the cause. At first, elimination of the underlying cause should be attempted—for example, remove the drugs in intoxications, substitute vitamins, remove the tumor, treat the multiple sclerosis with corticoids. In patients with Arnold-Chiari malformation, a surgical suboccipital decompression may be discussed to improve the compression of the herniating cerebellum against the caudal brain stem. This can gradually reduce nystagmus. In patients with persistent syndromes caused by brain defects or degeneration, medical treatment with baclofen, clonazepam, gabapentin, and scopolamine in upbeat/downbeat nystagmus may be helpful. The GABAergic drug baclofen, given at a dose of 5–15 mg three times a day, suppresses nystagmus and oscillopsia in approximately 50% of patients.

Vertebrobasilar Ischemia

Most of the central vestibular syndromes and some of the peripheral vestibular syndromes can have vascular causes. Ischemia will sometimes produce a combination of central and peripheral symptoms, as in anterior inferior cerebellar artery infarctions, the territory of which encompasses the labyrinth and pontine and cerebellar structures. In migraine and in vertebrobasilar ischemia, it may not be pos-

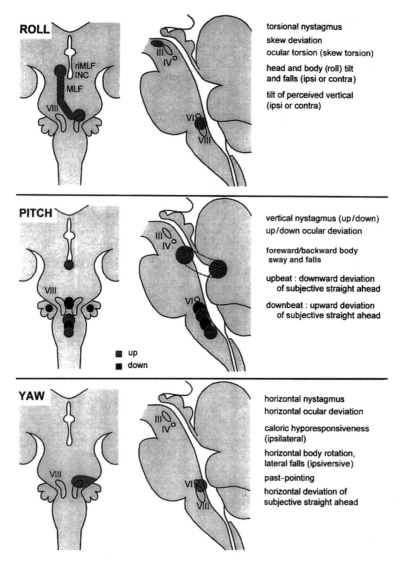

Figure 18-4. Topographic diagnosis of vestibular syndromes in the roll, pitch, and yaw planes. Schematic presentation of the distinct areas within the brain stem and vestibulo-cerebellum (frontal and sagittal views) in which a lesion induces a vestibulo-ocular tone imbalance in the roll, pitch, or yaw plane. Typical ocular motor, postural, and perceptual signs are listed (right). A tone imbalance in roll indicates unilateral "graviceptive" pathway lesions from the medial or superior vestibular nuclei (i.e., inducing ipsiversive signs), crossing the midline to the contralateral medial longitudinal fasciculus (MLF) and the rostral integration center for vertical and torsional eye movements, the interstitial nucleus of Cajal (INC) (i.e., inducing contraversive signs). A tone imbalance in pitch indicates paramedian bilateral brain stem lesions at the pontomesencephalic or pontomedullary level, the brachium conjunctivum, or the flocculi. It is striking that pontomedullary lesions may induce either upbeat or downbeat nystagmus or transitions between the two, whereas binocular flocculus lesions result only in downbeat nystagmus and a pontomesencephalic lesion only in upbeat nystagmus. A tone imbalance in yaw indicates a unilateral pontomedullary lesion involving the medial and superior vestibular nucleus. This area overlaps with the roll and pitch functions of the vestibulo-ocular reflex (VOR), which explains the frequency of mixed vestibular syndromes in more than one plane. (III = oculomotor nucleus; IV = trochlear nucleus; VI = abducens nucleus; VIII = vestibular nucleus.) (Reprinted with permission from T Brandt, M Dieterich. Central vestibular syndromes in roll, pitch, and yaw planes. Neuro-Ophthalmology 1995;15:291.)

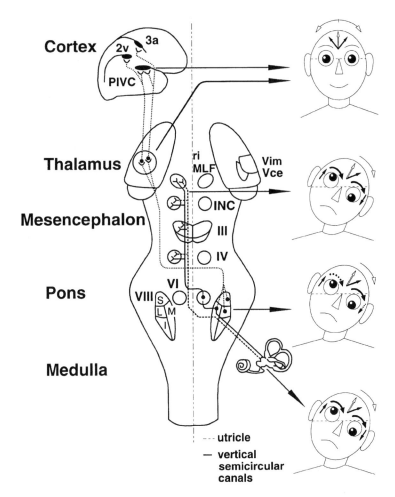

Figure 18-5. "Graviceptive" pathways from otoliths and vertical semicircular canals mediating vestibular function in the roll plane. The projections from the otoliths and the vertical semicircular canals to the ocular motor nuclei (IV = trochlear nucleus; III = oculomotor nucleus; VI = abducens nucleus) and the supranuclear centers of the interstitial nucleus of Cajal (INC), and the rostral interstitial nucleus of the medial longitudinal fasciculus (riMLF) are shown. They subserve the vestibulo-ocular reflex (VOR) in three planes. The VOR is part of a more complex vestibular reaction that also involves vestibulospinal connections via the medial and lateral vestibulospinal tracts for head and body posture control. Furthermore, connections to the assumed vestibular cortex (areas 2v and 3a and the parietoinsular vestibular cortex [PIVC]) via the vestibular nuclei of the thalamus (Vim, Vce) are depicted. "Graviceptive" vestibular pathways for the roll plane cross at the pontine level. Eye and head tilt reactions are depicted schematically on the right in relation to the level of the lesion—that is, ipsiversive tilts with peripheral and pontomedullary lesions, contraversive tilts with pontomesencephalic lesions. In vestibular thalamus lesions, the tilts of subjective visual vertical may be contraversive or ipsiversive; in vestibular cortex lesions they are preferably contraversive. Head tilt, ocular torsion, and vertical divergence of the eyes are not induced by supratentorial lesions above the level of the INC. (Reprinted with permission from T Brandt, M Dieterich. Vestibules syndromes in the roll plane. Ann Neurol 1994;36:337.)

sible to determine whether the vertigo is a symptom of a peripheral or a central vestibular syndrome. The vertigo itself, which is usually abrupt in onset and frequently transient in ischemic attacks, must be differentiated from the episodic vertigo com-monly seen in other conditions, such as Ménière's disease, basilar migraine, and vestibular epilepsy. Basilar insufficiency, resulting from vertebrobasilar ischemia, is a disease of the elderly and most often presents with transient attacks of rotational or to-

and-fro vertigo as an early symptom. Over time, additional brain stem symptoms (e.g., dysarthria, double vision, numbness, drop attacks) may occur in varying combinations and to varying extents. The syndrome is based on the steep pressure gradient from the aorta to the long circumferential terminal pontine arteries, which provide a highly vulnerable blood supply for the vestibular nuclei in the pontomedullary brain stem. In addition to the arteriosclerosis of the small arteries, a functional compression of the vertebral artery secondary to atheromas or cervical spondylosis or osteophytes, which narrow the transverse foramina, can often be found. In these cases, vertigo, postural imbalance, and nystagmus are induced when the head is maximally rotated or extended while standing. Because the blood supply of the inner ear (labyrinthine artery) originates from the anterior inferior cerebellar artery, it is also possible that a transient ischemia of a labyrinth can cause these transient attacks of vertigo. For therapy, antiplatelet agents or anticoagulants may be effective.

Basilar Artery Migraine

Basilar artery migraine is characterized by transient attacks of variable combinations of vertigo, nausea, vomiting, ataxia, visual disturbances, and other brain stem signs, followed by headache, which is more commonly occipital than hemicranial. Impairment or loss of consciousness is a rare facultative symptom. The acute onset of the syndrome, the sequence of events, the occurrence of other more common migraine attacks at other times, the short duration of the single attack (minutes to hours), and a family history of migraine confirm the diagnosis. In some cases, the syndrome is monosymptomatic, presenting only with rotational vertigo and not accompanied by headache, so that the diagnosis is difficult to differentiate from transient ischemic brain stem attacks. Diagnosis is then supported by a longer sequence of identical attacks, the complete recovery of the symptoms, and mild central-vestibular oculomotor signs even during the symptom-free interval. Basilar artery migraine typically starts in childhood or early adolescence, affecting predominantly girls (female-to-male ratio of 3:1), especially for the more violent form with various symptoms. The monosymptomatic form,

presenting with rotational vertigo as the main symptom, has a more continuous disease onset between the tenth and seventeenth year of age, with a broad-based plateau of occurrence between the ages of 35 and 55 years. The attacks occur irregularly and infrequently, sometimes in clusters and most often show a spontaneous improvement with age.

The *benign paroxysmal vertigo of childhood* (BPV) with onset within the first 4 years of life is probably related to migraine. These sudden attacks last seconds to minutes and do not require drug therapy. The natural history is spontaneous relief within months or years. *Benign recurrent vertigo* might be a migraine equivalent in adults, and is also characterized by short rotational vertigo attacks without headache.

Pharmacologic management of the acute migraine attack is identical to that for other migraine attacks. They can be suppressed by ergotamines, sumatriptan, acetylsalicylic acid, or paracetamol. In most cases it is not possible to abort acute basilar migraine attack because of the sudden onset and the spontaneous recovery within a short duration. In these cases and when the attacks occur at least twice a month or present with significant brain stem deficits, a preventive medication with a beta-blocker (e.g., metoprolol, propranolol) should be tried for a period of 9–12 months. Other preventive medications are flunarizine and serotonin antagonists.

Paroxysmal Central Vertigo

Nonepileptic paroxysmal attacks of vertigo, ataxia, and dysarthria are well known—perhaps as the initial symptom—in multiple sclerosis. The attacks, lasting from a few seconds to a few minutes, occur with a varying frequency from a few to 200 per day, sometimes provoked by hyperventilation or when rising. The character of the vertigo is sometimes rotatory but more often to-and-fro or a kind of lack of postural coordination with ataxia and broad-based gait and associated with nystagmus and other central ocular motor signs. The suggested mechanism of the attacks is a transversally spreading ephaptic activation of adjacent axons within a partially demyelinated lesion in fiber tracts of the pontine tegmentum with an involvement of the brachium conjunctivum. Carbamazepine is a most effective treatment, with complete disappearance of the attacks, which otherwise may persist for months if untreated.

Psychogenic Vertigo

The sensation of vertigo, a subjective complaint, is a frequent symptom of psychiatric illness, in particular in anxiety, depression, and personality disorders and less frequently in psychosis. The two most frequent episodic forms are acrophobia and phobic postural vertigo.

Acrophobia

Neurotic acrophobia results when physiologic height vertigo induces a conditioned phobic reaction that is characterized by a dissociation between the objective and subjective risk of falling. Although acrophobic patients are normally aware of this dissociation, they cannot overcome their avoidance behavior. The long-term course of untreated anxiety neurosis indicates that, during a 5- to 6-year interval, most children's phobias and 40–60% of adults' phobias either recover or improve substantially.

Psychotherapy is dominated by behavioral approaches, which can be classified as either systematic or in vivo desensitization procedures. Drugs used for symptomatic relief from panic attacks are either tranquilizers or antidepressants such as imipramine.

Phobic Postural Vertigo

The syndrome of phobic postural vertigo attacks, the third most common cause of vertigo and distinguishable from agoraphobia and acrophobia, is characterized by the combination of a dizziness and subjective disturbance of balance in an upright static position and during motion in the form of postural vertigo attacks. The diagnosis is based on the following seven characteristic features:

1. Dizziness and subjective disturbance in upright posture and during gait despite normal findings on clinical balance tests.
2. Postural vertigo, which is described as fluctuating unsteadiness, often in the form of attacks (seconds to minutes), or sometimes the perception of illusionary body perturbations for a mere fraction of a second.
3. These attacks occur spontaneously as well as with particular constellations of perceptual stimuli (e.g., bridges, staircases, empty rooms, streets, driving a car) or social situations (e.g., store, restaurant, cinema, concert, meeting, reception) from which the patient has difficulty in withdrawing and which are recognized as provoking factors. There is a tendency for rapid conditioning, generalization, and avoidance behavior to develop.
4. Anxiety and distressing vegetative symptoms often (57%), but not always, accompany the vertigo attack, the symptoms of which have to be elicited by direct questioning.
5. Most patients experience vertigo attacks both with and without excess anxiety.
6. Typically, an obsessive-compulsive type personality is often found to have affective liability and mild reactive (to the subjective vertigo) depression.
7. The onset of the condition is frequently after the patient has experienced an illness (37%), usually a vestibular disorder (21%), or after important psychosocial stress and psychodynamic conflicts.

In a neurologic and psychiatric follow-up study of 42 patients with phobic postural vertigo, it was found that, although an association with anxiety disorders was evident, not all patients presented with symptoms of anxiety or panic during attacks of vertigo; rather they (42%) developed a disabling phobic-avoidance pattern with recurrent vertigo attacks without anxiety disorder. The course of the illness varies depending on the neurologic syndrome of vertigo on one hand, and the concomitant psychopathologic syndromes on the other. Despite a considerable rate of improvement (79%) in the vertigo complaints, the group of patients with phobic postural vertigo as a whole presented with significant psychopathologic problems at follow-up term (74%), requiring specific psychiatric and psychotherapeutic interventions. Dependent or avoidant personality traits, a pronounced somatic concept of illness, and hypochondria were prognostic of a more negative course of illness.

The therapeutic regimen consists mainly of relieving the patients of their fear of an occult organic disease and of giving a detailed explanation of the mechanism that causes and the factors that provoke the phobic reactions. Then a controlled self-desensitization (by repeated exposure to situations that evoke the condition) within the context of behavioral therapy is recommended.

Suggested Reading

Baloh RW, Halmagyi GM. Disorders of the Vestibular System. New York: Oxford University Press, 1996.

Baloh RW, Honrubia V. Clinical Neurophysiology of the Vestibular System (2nd ed). Philadelphia: Davis, 1990.

Brandt T, Dieterich M. Central vestibular syndromes in roll, pitch, and yaw planes. Neuro-Ophthalmology 1995; 15:291.

Brandt T, Dieterich M. Vascular compression of the eighth nerve: vestibular paroxysmia. Lancet 1994;343:798.

Brandt T, Dieterich M. Vestibular syndromes in the roll plane: topographic diagnosis from brainstem to cortex. Ann Neurol 1994;36:337.

Brandt T, Huppert D, Dieterich M. Phobic postural vertigo, a first follow-up. J Neurol 1994;241:191.

Brandt T, Steddin S, Daroff RB. Therapy of benign paroxysmal positioning vertigo, revisited. Neurology 1994; 44:796.

Brandt T. Vertigo. Its Multisensory Syndromes (2nd ed). London: Springer, 1991.

De La Cruz A, Robertson DD. Ménière's Disease. In C Conn (ed), Conn's Current Therapy. Philadelphia: Saunders, 1997;928–931.

Dieterich M. Episodic Vertigo. In C Conn (ed), Conn's Current Therapy. Philadelphia: Saunders 1997;921–928.

Epley JM. The canalith repositioning procedure for treatment of benign paroxysmal positioning vertigo. Otolaryngol Head Neck Surg 1992;107:399.

Jannetta PJ, Moller MB, Moller AR. Disabling positional vertigo. N Engl J Med 1984;310:1700.

Kapfhammer HP, Mayer C, Hock U, et al. Course of illness in phobic postural vertigo. Acta Neurol Scand 1997; 95:23.

Schuknecht HF. Cupulolithiasis. Arch Otolaryngol 1969; 90:765.

Semont A, Freyss E, Vitte P. Curing the BPPV with a liberatory maneuver. Adv Otorhinolaryngol 1988;42:290.

Chapter 19
Neurologic Disorders of Gait

Lewis Sudarsky

Chapter Plan

Normal gait: anatomy and physiology
Gait disorders: prevalence and morbidity
Common patterns of gait disorders and their causes
    Spastic gait
    Extrapyramidal disorder
    Frontal gait disorder (gait apraxia)
    Cerebellar gait
    Sensory ataxia and disequilibrium
    Neuromuscular disease
    Toxic and metabolic disorders
    Psychogenic gait disorder
    Other identifiable cause
Diagnostic evaluation
Treatment

Gait is an important and fundamental motor performance. The skill is acquired by the nervous system in the first year or two of life. Thereafter, locomotor control is maintained at an unconscious level, so that we can direct our attention to other matters. Disturbances of walking are common. The performance is affected by minor degrees of orthopedic abnormality and is highly sensitive to diseases of the nervous system. A gait disorder is often the presenting feature of a neurologic illness, and examination of the nervous system is not complete until the gait has been observed.

Normal Gait: Anatomy and Physiology

The events of the gait cycle are reviewed in Figure 19-1. The cycle begins as the right heel makes contact with the floor, which marks the beginning of the stance phase for the right leg. Roughly 60% of the cycle time is spent with the right leg in contact with the support surface (in stance); the leg advances during the remaining 40% (the swing phase). The stance phase for the two limbs overlaps, such that both feet are in simultaneous contact with the floor for 20% of the cycle (double-limb stance), although the center of mass continues its forward progression. Electromyographic (EMG) study reveals an orderly, cyclic pattern of activation of leg muscles: Flexor muscles are active during the swing phase and extensor muscles during stance.

There are two tasks the nervous system must address in order to produce a stable gait: (1) generation of the motor sequence for locomotion, and (2) maintenance of dynamic balance. Spinal pattern generators linked through the propriospinal system produce locomotor movements in animals but are not sufficient to support independent spinal walking in primates and humans. A network of brain stem and cerebellar circuits orchestrates locomotion, the most significant of which is the mesencephalic locomotor region (MLR). The MLR, located in the vicinity of the nucleus

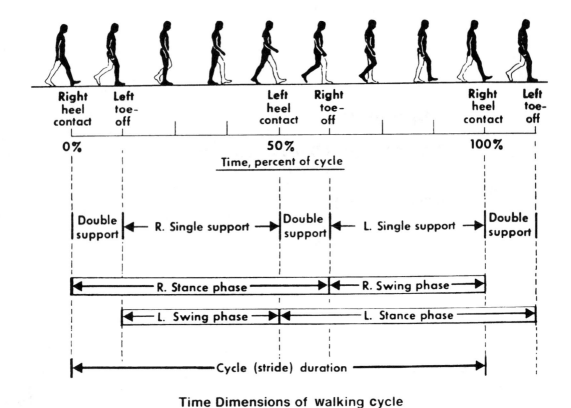

Right   Left   Left   Right   Right   Left
heel   toe-   heel   toe-   heel   toe-
contact   off   contact   off   contact   off

0%   50%   100%
Time, percent of cycle

Double |←—— R. Single support ——→| Double |←—— L. Single support ——→| Double
support | support | support

|←————————— R. Stance phase —————————→|←—— R. Swing phase ——→|

|←—— L. Swing phase ——→|←————————— L. Stance phase —————————→|

|←——————————— Cycle (stride) duration ———————————→|

Time Dimensions of walking cycle

Figure 19-1. Events of the gait cycle are depicted with respect to time. There is a cyclic pattern of activation of the leg muscles: flexor muscles during the swing phase, extensor muscles during stance. (Reprinted with permission from VT Inman, HJ Ralston, F Todd. Human Walking. Baltimore: Williams & Wilkins, 1981.)

cuneiformis and cholinergic pedunculopontine nucleus, projects to nucleus reticularis gigantocellularis, which has descending projections via the reticulospinal tract. The basal ganglia contribute to initiation and maintenance of brain stem locomotor drive. Frontal cortical regions oversee the direction of the performance, adapting locomotor synergies to fit our needs and purposes.

Dynamic balance is maintained during locomotion through the action of postural supporting responses, known in the older physiology literature as righting reflexes. Activity in the anterior compartment muscles can be recorded beginning 110 msec after a toe-up perturbation. These responses are presumed to originate at or above the level of the lateral vestibular nucleus (Deiter's nucleus), although the anatomy has not been well-characterized. Control of balance is dependent on good quality sensory information from the vestibular system,

vision, and proprioceptive input from the lower limbs. Some studies suggest that muscle spindle afferents also contribute to kinesthetic sense and balance.

Gait Disorders: Prevalence and Morbidity

As there is a large range of normal variations, it is helpful to define an abnormality of gait for clinical purposes. We consider that a patient has a gait disorder if there is a substantial reduction in velocity, instability, or a pattern of walking with reduced ergonomic efficiency and increased effort. A healthy older person normally walks at a speed of 0.8–1.2 meters per second. Some older patients with gait impairment are able to cruise at this velocity but are unable to increase the pace of their walking when it might be appropriate to do so.

Table 19-1. Classification of Gait Disorders in 120 Patients According to Cause

Cause	1980–1982	1990–1994	Total	Percent
Myelopathy	8	12	20	16.7
Parkinsonism	5	9	14	11.7
Hydrocephalus	2	6	8	6.7
Multiple infarcts	8	10	18	15.0
Cerebellar degeneration	4	4	8	6.7
Sensory deficits	9	13	22	18.3
Toxic/metabolic	3	0	3	2.5
Psychogenic	1	3	4	3.3
Other	3	3	6	5.0
Unknown cause	7	10	17	14.2

Source: Reprinted from J Masdeu, L Sudarsky, LI Wolfson. Gait Disorders of Aging: Falls and Therapeutic Strategies. New York: Lippincott–Raven, 1997.

The population so defined is heterogeneous, and it is difficult to obtain adequate data about the prevalence of gait disorders. In a survey study in Durham, North Carolina, the prevalence was estimated at 15% of those older than 60 years of age. By age 80, one person in four will use mechanical aids to assist in ambulation. In a recent study in East Boston, more than 40% of those age 85 and older exhibited shuffling or abnormality in turning, features suggestive of a neurologic disturbance of gait.

Gait disorder in the elderly is an established risk factor for falls and fall-related injuries. Accidental injury is the sixth leading cause of death in the elderly, and falls are the principal cause. Many older people develop an inordinate fear of falling and voluntarily restrict their activity. Disturbances of mobility in the elderly (gait disorder and falls) limit independence and are a factor in nursing home admission. Nonambulatory nursing home patients have accelerated morbidity and mortality.

Common Patterns of Gait Disorders and Their Causes

The diversity of gait disorders seen clinically reflects the large network of anatomy involved in the production of gait. Many different failures are possible involving locomotion, balance, and their integrative control. Gait disorders are consequently a heterogeneous group. They are sometimes multifactorial. Musculoskeletal disorders must be distinguished from those that are primarily neurologic.

One approach to the classification of gait disorders is to look at causes. Our survey study in 1983 examined a group of patients older than 65 years of age referred to a neurologist for abnormal gait. An etiologic diagnosis was ultimately made in 86%. Table 19-1 reviews the common causes, updated to include patients examined in 1990–1993 with the aid of magnetic resonance imaging (MRI).

Gait disorders can also be classified descriptively based on classical principles of neuroanatomy and physiology. Nutt, Thompson, and Marsden published such a classification in 1993. One pitfall of this approach is the range of phenomenologic overlap. Many failing gaits appear fundamentally similar; frontal ataxia can resemble cerebellar gait. *The gait disorder observed clinically is the product of a physiologic abnormality and an adaptive response.* In many gait disorders, the biomechanical adaptations overwhelm the distinctive characteristics. Information from gait observation must always be combined with that derived from the history and physical examination. Certain patterns of gait abnormality can be distinguished by a trained clinical eye. We review these patterns and for each consider some of the common causes.

Spastic Gait

Spastic gait is characterized by stiffness and "bounce" in the legs and a tendency to circumduct and scuff the feet. In extreme instances, there is excess adduction, or "scissoring," of the legs because of increased tone. Shoes often reflect an uneven pattern of wear across the outside front of the soles. Spasticity is a component of the upper motor neuron syndrome and can be spinal or cerebral in origin. Myelopathy from cervical spondylosis is the common cause of spastic or spastic-ataxic gait in the elderly. Spondylitic bars and ligamentous hypertrophy narrow the canal, causing mechanical compression and vascular compromise. Some degree of standing imbalance and bladder dysfunction (urgency, incontinence) accompanies a mild spastic weakness of the legs. MRI studies have improved the ease of diagnosis, although MRI sometimes demonstrates advanced pathologic conditions in the cervical spine in minimally symptomatic patients. Other causes of myelopathy in the elderly include vitamin B_{12} deficiency and degenerative disease (e.g., primary lateral sclerosis, hereditary spastic paraplegia).

Demyelinating disease and trauma are the common causes of myelopathy in younger patients. In chronic progressive myelopathy of unknown cause, cerebrospinal fluid studies and MRI will sometimes establishes a diagnosis of multiple sclerosis. It is important to rule out a structural lesion, such as a tumor or dural or spinal vascular malformation. Tropical spastic paraparesis related to human T-cell lymphotrophic virus (HTLV)-1 is endemic in parts of the Caribbean and South America.

With cerebral spasticity, some involvement of the upper extremities is often observed, and dysarthria is usually present. Common causes in adult patients include vascular disease (stroke) and multiple sclerosis. With perinatal injury to the nervous system (cerebral palsy), a mild spastic diplegia is the most frequently observed syndrome.

Extrapyramidal Disorder

Parkinson's disease is common, affecting 1.5% of the population older than 65 years of age. The flexed attitude in posture and shuffling gait are highly characteristic and distinctive. There may be difficulty with initiation and a tendency to turn en bloc. Patients sometimes accelerate (festinate) with progression or display retropulsion. Of patients presenting with axial stiffness, postural instability, and a shuffling gait, some will have a related neurodegenerative disorder, such as progressive supranuclear palsy. Drug-induced parkinsonism is increasingly recognized as a cause of impaired gait and balance. The disorder is caused by the effect of major tranquilizers on D2 dopamine receptors. It is particularly common in psychiatric hospitals and nursing homes.

Hyperkinetic movement disorders also produce distinctive and recognizable disturbances in gait. The gait in Huntington's disease is characterized by the unpredictable occurrence of choreic movements, which give a dancing quality. In generalized dystonia, muscular spasms produce a dysfunctional posture of the legs: typically adduction and inversion, sometimes with torsion of the trunk. Many of the odd, stereotypic gait disorders seen in chronic psychiatric patients are manifestations of tardive dyskinesia.

Frontal Gait Disorder (Gait Apraxia)

Frontal gait disorder, sometimes known as *gait apraxia*, is more common in the elderly and has a variety of causes. Typical clinical features include a wide base of support, a short stride, a tendency to shuffle along the floor, and start and turn hesitation. Many exhibit freezing and difficulty with gait initiation, descriptively characterized as the "slipping clutch" syndrome or gait ignition failure. There is difficulty getting out of a chair, and invariably a degree of imbalance. In studies seeking clinicopathologic correlation, lesions are usually found in the deep frontal white matter.

Communicating hydrocephalus in an adult often presents with this type of gait. Other features of the diagnostic triad (mental change, incontinence) may be absent in the initial stages. MRI demonstrates ventricular enlargement, an enlarged flow void about the aqueduct, and a variable degree of periventricular white matter changes. Hydrocephalus cannot easily be distinguished from brain atrophy using imaging criteria, and a dynamic test is necessary to confirm the diagnosis.

The frontal gait disorder is often caused by the effects of cerebrovascular disease: strokes and small vessel disease. Gait is usually abnormal in hypertensive patients with ischemic lesions of the deep hemisphere white matter (Binswanger's disease). The clinical syndrome includes mental changes (variable in degree), dysarthria, pseudobulbar affect, increased tone, and hyperreflexia in the lower limbs.

Cerebellar Gait

Cerebellar ataxia of gait is one of the most recognizable and distinctive locomotor disorders. The gait is typically slow and halting, with a widened base of support. Truncal instability is more evident when the patient attempts to stand or walk on a narrow base. Patients cannot walk tandem, heel to toe, and have difficulty maintaining their balance when they turn rapidly or change direction. Nonetheless, postural compensation is usually preserved to some degree, and patients are often able to avoid falls in everyday life. Foot placement is irregular, which results in a lurching quality as the upper body segments struggle to maintain alignment.

Slowly progressive ataxia in adult patients presents a diagnostic challenge. Demyelinating disease and posterior fossa tumors must be considered. A variety of hereditary and sporadic cerebellar degenerations have been described. Several forms of autosomal dominant cerebellar ataxia have been characterized genetically. A primarily truncal ataxia with degeneration of the midline vermis occurs among chronic alcoholics. Other causes of cerebellar atrophy include toxins and paraneoplastic cerebellar degeneration.

Sensory Ataxia and Disequilibrium

Sensory ataxia can be distinguished from cerebellar ataxia by a more narrow base, a regular stride, and dependence of locomotion on visual control. Patients with sensory ataxia often suffer recurrent falls. Balance depends on high-quality information from the visual system, the vestibular system, and proprioceptive afferents. When this information is degraded, balance is compromised, and instability results. Patients with impaired proprioception cannot stand steady on a narrow base with the eyes closed (Romberg's sign).

The classic example of sensory ataxia occurs in patients with tabetic neurosyphilis. The disorder is well described in the writings of Romberg and Gowers from the nineteenth century. The contemporary equivalent is the patient with neuropathy affecting large fiber afferents. Patients with bilateral vestibular deficits also have a form of sensory ataxia. Older people seem more vulnerable to imbalance with a loss of afferents from a single modality. Some older patients exhibit a syndrome of dizziness and standing imbalance from the combined effects of multiple sensory deficits.

Neuromuscular Disease

Patients with neuromuscular disease often have an abnormal gait, although it is not typically a presenting feature. With distal weakness (e.g., peripheral neuropathy), the step height is increased to compensate for footdrop, and the sole of the foot may slap on the floor during weight acceptance. Neuropathy may be associated with a degree of sensory ataxia, as described above. Patients with myopathy or muscular dystrophy have primarily proximal weakness. They often have difficulty getting up from a chair. Weakness of the hip girdle may produce a degree of excess pelvic rotation (waddle) during gait.

Toxic and Metabolic Disorders

Unquestionably the most common cause of difficulty walking on any given Saturday night is alcohol intoxication. Chronic toxicity from medications and metabolic disturbances can likewise impair motor function and gait, although the results are more subtle. Static equilibrium is disturbed, and such patients are easily displaced back. This is particularly dramatic in patients with chronic renal disease and those with hepatic failure, in whom asterixis may impair postural support. Sedative drugs, especially neuroleptics and long-acting benzodiazepines, affect postural control and increase the risk for falls. These disorders are important to recognize because they are treatable.

Psychogenic Gait Disorder

Psychogenic disturbances of gait are among the most spectacular disorders encountered in neurology. Odd gyrations of posture (astasia-abasia) and dramatic fluctuations over time may be observed in hysterical patients. Dramatic cures are often possible. Patients with anxiety disorders who are phobic about falling walk with exaggerated caution, as if walking on a slippery surface, and cling to the walls for support. Depressed patients exhibit primarily slowness, a manifestation of psychomotor retardation, and lack of purpose in their stride.

Other Identifiable Causes

A few patients with gait disorders have a mass lesion: primary central nervous system tumor or metastatic cancer. Lumbar spinal stenosis can severely limit ambulation and sometimes produces a tendency toward flexion in posture. Subdural hematoma should be ruled out in a patient with subacute evolution and a history of falls.

Diagnostic Evaluation

In taking a history, it is important to inquire about the pace of the illness. Most patients present with a slowly progressive decline in their walking over months to a year or more. Acute inability to ambulate is a neurologic emergency and a problem of a different character. Stepwise evolution or sudden progression suggests vascular disease. First awareness of a balance problem often follows a fall. Back pain or headache may be clues to a structural pathologic condition, particularly in patients whose illness evolves more rapidly (over weeks). Gait disorder may be associated with urinary urgency and incontinence in patients with subcortical frontal disease or spinal disease. It is always important to discuss the use of alcohol and medications known to affect gait and balance (including anticonvulsants).

Because the list of possible diagnoses is lengthy, information on localization derived from the neurologic examination can be used to narrow the search. The standard neurologic examination is often informative, despite its emphasis on corticospinal systems and distal limb movements. Gait relies primarily on phylogenetically older descending pathways, and the corticospinal tract plays a minor role in locomotor control.

Gait observation provides an immediate sense of the patient's degree of disability. Cadence (steps per minute), velocity, and stride length can be recorded by timing a patient over a fixed distance. Watching the patient get out of a chair provides a good functional assessment of balance. Characteristic patterns of abnormality are sometimes observed, as reviewed above.

Brain imaging studies (computed tomographic or MRI scans) are often informative in patients with an undiagnosed disorder of gait. MRI is sensitive for cerebral lesions of vascular or demyelinating disease and a good screening test for occult hydrocephalus. Many elderly patients with gait and balance difficulty have small strokes or lesions in the periventricular region and centrum semiovale. Sometimes a neurodegenerative disease such as progressive supranuclear palsy or striatonigral degeneration can be recognized by its pattern of atrophy on MRI scans.

Treatment

Of older patients with a chronic and slowly progressive disturbance of gait, 20–25% will have a treatable disorder, such as Parkinson's disease, hydrocephalus, frontal tumor, or abscess. Psychogenic gait disorders are also treatable in an overwhelming majority of cases. Even when no treatable disease is found, a variety of rehabilitation strategies are available to improve the effectiveness and stability of ambulation. Muscle strength training with resistance exercise machines and free weights can improve muscle mass and strength even for people in their 80s and 90s, and modest improvements in habitual gait velocity are achieved. Sensory balance retraining is particularly effective in patients with a cautious fearful gait and those with vestibular or sensory ataxia.

A number of practical measures are helpful to reduce the risk for falls. Patients should have appropriate footwear to reduce the risk for slipping and tripping falls. Assistive devices such as a tripod cane or walker may be appropriate when there is substantial instability. The visiting nurse association (or its equivalent) may be able to arrange a home visit to look for environmental hazards.

Suggested Reading

Alexander NB. Postural control in older adults. J Am Geriatr Soc 1994;42:93.

Armstrong DM. The supraspinal control of mammalian locomotion. J Physiol 1988;405:1.

Fife TD, Baloh RW. Disequilibrium of unknown cause in older people. Ann Neurol 1993;34:694.

Fisher CM. Hydrocephalus as a cause of disturbances of gait in the elderly. Neurology 1982;32:1358.

Masdeu J, Sudarsky L, Wolfson LI. Gait Disorders of Aging: Falls and Therapeutic Strategies. New York: Lippincott–Raven, 1997.

Nutt JG, Marsden CD, Thompson PD. Human walking and higher level gait disorders, particularly in the elderly. Neurology 1993;43:268.

Odenheimer G, Funkenstein HH, Beckett L, et al. Comparison of neurologic changes in successfully aging persons vs the total aging population. Arch Neurol 1994;51:573.

Sudarsky L. Gait disorders in the elderly. N Engl J Med 1990;322:1441.

Tinetti ME, Speechley M, Ginter S. Risk factors for falls among elderly persons living in the community. N Engl J Med 1988;319:1701.

Chapter 20

Neuro-Urogenital and Anal Sphincter Dysfunction

Thierry Kuntzer

Chapter Plan

Various disorders of bladder function, urinary and fecal incontinence, and disorders of orgasm, erection, and ejaculation should be regarded as potentially neurologic symptoms and investigated and managed appropriately. This chapter presents the field of these disorders by integrating the neuroanatomic findings, derived from the history and neurologic examination findings, with the results of neuro-urologic tests. Symptoms of sphincter disturbance are an unpleasant and troublesome burden for the patient but should be considered among the potentially treatable neurologic deficits in the view of the development of a number of successful methods of treatment.

Normal Regulation

Most observations of the physiology, pharmacology, and innervation of the urinary bladder, sexual function, and gastrointestinal motility have been made in experimental animals, and there is a paucity of human data. Newer diagnostic methods, such as neurophysiologic testing and cystometric monitoring, in conjunction with magnetic resonance imaging (MRI) of the central nervous system (CNS) might reveal information on human pelvic organ function.

The urogenital organs and distal bowel exhibit a number of common functional characteristics, most notably an intermittent pattern of activation consisting of long periods of quiescence interspersed with short periods of maximal activity or elimination. These properties are dependent on the coordination of visceral and somatic effector organs and are mediated by reflex pathways in the lumbosacral spinal cord. The functions of these organs are also under voluntary control or are influenced by involuntary inputs from supraspinal centers. Thus, the regulation of the pelvic viscera is complex, involving neurons at various levels of the neuraxis, ranging from the cerebral cortex to the sacral spinal cord and peripheral autonomic ganglia (Figure 20-1). From a pharmacologic point of view, the urinary bladder is predominantly under parasympathetic control, and efferent limbs of voiding reflexes include parasym-

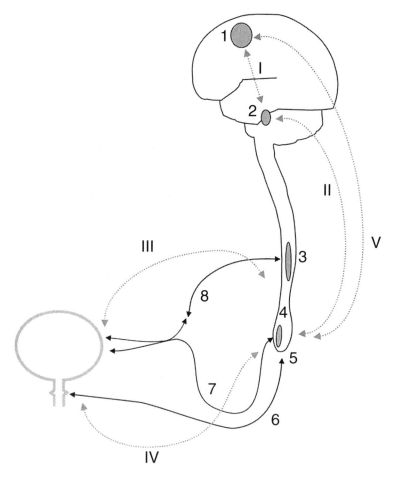

Figure 20-1. The pathways involved in the control of micturition. 1 = Frontal micturition regulating center; 2 = pontine micturition center; 3 = sympathetic motor neurons of the intermediolateral cell column (T10–L1); 4 = parasympathetic motor neurons in the intermediolateral sacral cell column innervating the detrusor via S2–S4 and the pelvic ganglia and nerves; 5 = pudendal somatic motor cells in Onuf's nucleus; 6 = pudendal axons originating from the sacral plexus and innervating the external urinary sphincter and penis or clitoris; 7 = the pelvic nerves formed from the S2–S4 ventral roots combine with the hypogastric nerves to form the pelvic plexus and more distally the vesical plexus and local autonomic ganglia; axons from the vesical plexus innervate the bladder and urethra; 8 = most sympathetic axons synapse in the hypogastric plexus, whereas the preganglionic parasympathetic axons synapse in ganglia located in the pelvic plexus and intramural ganglia to give the principal motor supply of the detrusor. The three sets of peripheral nerves (thoracolumbar sympathetic, sacral parasympathetic, and pudendal) all contain afferent nerve fibers. The afferent fibers that pass in the pelvic nerve carry the sensation of bladder distention. The role of the hypogastric afferents is uncertain, but they may transmit some sensation of bladder distention and pain. The pudendal somatic afferents transmit sensations of flow of urine, pain, and temperature from the urethra. The principal location of areas in the central nervous system concerned with bladder innervation include the frontal cortex, the rostral lateral portion of the pontine tegmentum, and portions of the gray matter of the conus medullaris. The crucial event in the initiation of normal voiding is a coordinated detrusor reflex contraction, with a resultant smooth, sustained rise in intravesical pressure and concurrent relaxation of the external urinary sphincter. Five reflex pathways concur with the control of the urinary bladder. The first represents the mechanism underlying volitional control of bladder function, with relays between the frontal cortex and the pontine detrusor nucleus. The second coordinates and sustains detrusor and sphincter contraction and relaxation from the pontine center and conus medullaris. The third promotes sphincter relaxation when the detrusor is active via detrusor afferents and pudendal motoneurons. The fourth maintains sphincter tone when the detrusor is active through urethral afferents and pudendal motoneurons. The fifth promotes voluntary control of the sphincters.

Table 20-1. Male Sexual Reflexes

Response	Afferent Source	Efferent Source	Central Pathway	Effector Organ
Penile erection				
Reflexogenic	Pudendal nerve	Sacral parasympathetic	Sacral spinal reflex	Dilatation of arterial supply to
Psychogenic	Auditory, olfactory, visual, imaginative	Lumbar sympathetic	Supraspinal origin	corpus cavernosum and spongiosum
Glandular secretion	Pudendal nerve	Lumbosacral sympathetic and parasympathetic	Sacral spinal reflex	Seminal vesicles and prostate
Seminal emission	Pudendal nerve	Lumbar sympathetic	Intersegmental spinal reflex	Contraction of vas deferens, ampulla, prostate, and bladder neck closure
Ejaculation	Pudendal nerve	Somatic efferents in pudendal nerves	Sacral spinal reflex	Rhythmic contractions of bulbo- and ischio-cavernous muscles

Source: Reprinted with permission from WC de Groat. Urol Clin North Am 1993;20:383.

pathetic (cholinergic and purinergic) contraction of the detrusor, and parasympathetic (nitrergic) relaxation of the proximal urethra. In contrast, the predominant neural control of the male accessory sexual organs is sympathetic (adrenergic and purinergic), with efferent reflex limbs being responsible for the motor activity of the vas deferens, prostate gland, and seminal vesicles that leads to emission. There is also sympathetic (adrenergic) control over the proximal urethra, which leads to its constriction during emission and ejaculation, thus preventing retrograde ejaculation into the bladder. Penile erection seems to be under parasympathetic control for tumescence and maintenance of erection (cholinergic, peptidergic, and nitrergic), and sympathetic control for detumescence (adrenergic). Thus, the activity of the parasympathetic and sympathetic nervous systems are not only antagonistic, but also complementary; additionally, sensory and somatomotor pathways contribute to the control of urine storage, micturition, emission, ejaculation, and maintenance of penile rigidity. There is a considerable degree of anatomic overlap in all the neural pathways, and there are many interactions occurring at the level of the spinal cord, peripheral ganglia, and neuromuscular junction.

The reflex mechanisms controlling sexual function in males are described in Table 20-1 and have recently been reviewed. There are both components, the psychogenic and reflexogenic pathways, but it is not known whether psychogenic impulses selectively facilitate the lumbar sympathetic pathway, the sacral parasympathetic pathway, or both. Nocturnal erections occurring during rapid eye movement sleep are evidently brain-initiated and may use different descending pathways. There is a center for erection in the conus medullaris, with a parasympathetic erectile outflow at the S2–S3 level. There are sympathetic erectile and antierectile outflows at approximately the T12 level. There are descending erectile and antierectile pathways in the lateral columns. Several mechanisms are present for the neural control of the arterial and venous resistance in the penis: Alpha-adrenergic blockers, depleters of adrenergic nerve terminals (guanethidine), and direct smooth-muscle relaxant drugs (papaverine, thymoxamine) will all induce intracavernosal arterial opening and venous closure and hence full cavernosal erection when injected intracavernosally. Intracavernosal metaraminol will quickly abolish such erections. Strong stimulation of S2 ventral roots causes erection by way of fine myelinated fibers in the parasympathetic outflow. Strong electrical stimulation of the hypogastric plexus in men induces erection, indicating a sympathetic erectile pathway at the T11–T12 level. Lesions of the superior hypogastric plexus may occur (e.g., after para-aortic lymph node dissection). Such lesions, if complete, cause failure of seminal emission and, in a minority of men, also cause erectile failure. The sympathetic and parasympathetic erectile pathways probably link in the inferior hypogastric plexus and may share some of the same postganglionic axons.

Table 20-2. Typical Neuro-Urologic and Urodynamic Findings in Lesions at Different Levels of the Neuraxis

Disorder	Typical Clinical Findings	Typical Urodynamics
I. Brain disease		
Cerebral diffuse	Unembarrassed enuresis	Reflex detrusor contractions
Cerebral localized	Embarrassed enuresis	Reflex detrusor contractions
Brain stem	Enuresis or retention	Variable
II. Spinal cord disease		
Complete	Dyssynergic voiding, initiated by reflexes	Detrusor-sphincter dyssynergia, unstable urethra, reflex detrusor contractions, low compliance bladder
Incomplete	Dyssynergic voiding, initiated voluntarily or by reflexes	As above
III. Peripheral disease		
Cauda equina lesions and peripheral neuropathy	Stress incontinence, fecal incontinence, impotence, poor voiding	Atonic bladder, voiding by strain, sphincter denervation
Autonomic failure	As above, plus postural features	As above

Source: Reprinted with permission from DN Rushton. Handbook of Neuro-Urology. New York: Marcel Dekker, 1994;123.

Although the distal bowel has the same storage and excretory functions as those of the lower urinary tract and the neurochemistry and central projections are similar, the organization of the reflex pathways controlling the bowel is different. The inhibitory sympathetic outflow to the colon is not mediated by supraspinal mechanisms or spinal afferent input, but is generated by endogenous oscillator circuits in the lumbar cord. The parasympathetic defecation reflex is mediated by a long latency, polysynaptic spinal pathway. This reflex is depressed transiently in acute spinal transection preparations, but is essentially unchanged in animals with chronic spinal transection. Moreover, the micturition and defecation reflex pathways have prominent inhibitory interactions and may partly account for the beneficial effects of vaginal and anal stimulation for the treatment of bladder hyperactivity and incontinence.

Sphincter Disturbance in Neurologic Disease

Disorders of Bladder Function

The symptoms and findings in neurologic impairment of urinary bladder function depend more on the site of the lesion than on the specific disease (Table 20-2). Cerebral disorders can affect bladder function by causing loss of control over the transition between filling and voiding states. This leads to loss of inhibition and facilitation of the detrusor reflex, resulting in urgency, incontinence, hesitancy, or more rarely, retention because of a failure of voluntary initiation of the voiding reflex. After studying patients with cerebral lesions, it was deduced that the cortical loci controlling micturition are in the superior-medial part of the frontal lobes in the region of the anterior cingulate and superior frontal gyri. Also important are white matter tracts that run to and from the genu of the corpus callosum. The cerebral lesions can be diffuse (e.g., as in Alzheimer's, Pick's, Creutzfeldt-Jakob, Huntington's, and Parkinson's diseases; myxedema; or hydrocephalus) or localized (e.g., as in head injury, multiple sclerosis, cerebrovascular disease, or frontal tumor). In stroke syndromes, incontinence is said to be common but transient in approximately one-half of the patients. Incontinence can be a continuing problem for approximately 15% of the patients at 1 year poststroke and is associated with a poor outcome with severe functional loss. Incontinence with incomplete emptying of the bladder is also related to other factors than directly to the brain damage, such as inability to walk, speech disorders, and mental changes.

The pontine micturition center lies in the dorsal tegmentum of the pons, and abnormalities affecting this area give rise to disorders of voiding, usually with other neurologic deficits; however, occasionally a lesion can be sufficiently dorsal and discrete to produce predominantly a defect of bladder function. An internuclear ophthalmoplegia is a

Table 20-3. Symptoms and Signs Differentiating Between Lesions of the Conus Medullaris and Cauda Equina

	Conus Medullaris	**Cauda Equina**
Onset	Sudden and bilateral	Gradual and unilateral
Spontaneous pain	Not common or severe, bilateral and symmetric, in perineum or thighs	May be most prominent symptom. Severe, radicular in type, unilateral or asymmetric, in distribution of sacral nerves
Sensory deficit	Saddle distribution, dissociation of sensation	Saddle distribution, may be unilateral, no dissociation of sensation
Motor loss	Symmetric	Asymmetric
Reflex loss	Only Achilles reflex absent	Patellar and Achilles reflexes may be absent
Bladder and rectal symptoms	Early and marked	Late and less marked
Trophic changes	Decubiti common	Decubiti less marked
Sexual functions	Erection and ejaculation impaired	Less marked impairment

Source: Adapted from AF Haerer. The Neurologic Examination. Philadelphia: Lippincott, 1992.

frequent additional sign because of the proximity of the median longitudinal fasciculus.

Any spinal cord lesion involving the lateral columns bilaterally, such as trauma, multiple sclerosis, transverse myelitis, vitamin B_{12} deficiency, cervical spondylotic myelopathy, or tethered cord syndrome, will also result in urinary disturbance. In spinal cord lesions, the bladder is isolated from the pontine micturition center. The coordination of the voiding act itself, as well as its inhibition, initiation, and completion, is impaired, and the normal coordinated relaxation of the sphincter that precedes and accompanies a detrusor contraction is lost, so that "detrusor-sphincter dyssynergia" occurs. Retention alone is uncommon, except in the early phase of spinal shock. Thus, in a chronic spinal lesion, abnormal voiding is common, accompanied by detrusor hyperreflexia, with urgency and frequency, difficulty of voluntary initiation or interrupted stream, and incomplete emptying. Because of the relative levels at which the innervation of the lower limbs and the bladder arise, it is unusual to have a lesion between the pons and the sacral part of the cord giving rise to a neurogenic bladder that does not also produce other neurologic signs in the lower limbs. A possible exception might be expected from a conus or cauda equina lesion affecting only S2–S4 (Table 20-3).

The peripheral efferent and afferent innervation of the bladder arises largely from the S2–S4 roots. Damage to the preganglionic parasympathetic efferents causes detrusor areflexia; damage to the innervation of the sphincter leads to sphincter weakness; loss of afferent innervation results in loss of bladder sensation as well as sacral anesthesia. This combination of abnormalities is commonly seen after injury to the conus and cauda equina and damage to the pelvic nerve plexus in extensive pelvic surgery, such as abdominoperineal hysterectomy. Central protrusion of a lumbar disc is a common cause of damage to the cauda equina, occurring most commonly at the L4 or L5 level. Poor bladder emptying can occur as part of the progressive cauda equina disorder that may complicate long-standing ankylosing spondylitis. The cauda equina and conus medullaris may be involved by tumors or tabes dorsalis. Urinary retention owing to a sacral myeloradiculopathy has been well described, associated with herpes simplex, cytomegalovirus, Epstein-Barr, or *Borrelia burgdorferi* infections with or without acquired immunodeficiency syndrome. Because a cerebrospinal fluid lymphocytosis is essential to diagnosing a myeloradiculopathy, a lumbar puncture should be performed in patients after the onset of acute urinary retention.

Bladder and sexual dysfunction are prominent features of system degenerations, of which there are varying degrees of autonomic failure with cerebellar, ocular, extrapyramidal, and pyramidal signs. In system degenerations, there may be degeneration of the intermediolateral cell columns in the thoracic spinal cord and of Onuf's nucleus in the sacral cord, with incontinence resulting from sphincter failure as well as retention resulting from atonic bladder.

Many forms of neuropathy are length dependent, the maximum deficit being evident in the longest fibers, whereas the nerve fibers to the bladder are comparatively short. For the innervation of the bladder to have been affected as part of a generalized neuropathy, there should be clinical evidence of extensive disease, with loss of both knee and ankle jerks and sensory impairment in small fibers to a level well above the ankles. However, some neuropathies purportedly affect the parasympathetic before sympathetic system or distal peripheral nerve function, such as those seen in diabetes mellitus and Chagas' disease.

Disorders of Sexual Function in Men

Disorders of sexual function in men have been recently reviewed (see Table 20-1). Vascular and endocrine disorders are outside the scope of this chapter. Very many drugs are suspected of causing erectile impotence; in searching for publications on the effects of particular drugs, it is useful to know that they are indexed by MEDLINE under "impotence/cy" (impotence: chemically induced). Cerebral lesions are generally followed by some important alterations in sexual life concerning both behavior and patients' feelings about sexuality. Associated neurologic features as well as the side of the hemispheric lesion do not seem to play a crucial role. Aberrant sexual behavior, together with psychic blindness, hypermetamorphosis, aphasia, and visual agnosia, is seen in Klüver-Bucy syndrome, a well-known consequence of lesions of the temporal lobe. Sexually aggressive and inappropriate behaviors may respond to treatment with leuprolide.

In paraplegic men with a cord lesion above T12 and evidence of an intact conus, there is a great variation in reflex erections. In some, they can be elicited by handling the penis, catheterization, or spontaneously; in others, they are unobtainable. Obviously, the psychogenic pathway has been interrupted. The majority of men with sacral anterior root stimulator implants with stimulation of the sacral parasympathetic erectomotor pathway show an erectile response. Whether the sympathetic erectomotor pathway in men is constantly present is not known. In many but not all men with a complete cord or cauda equina lesion with its upper level below T12, psychogenic erections may occur via the sympathetic outflow pathway, reflex erections being absent. Patients with thoracic cordotomies aimed at bilateral section of the spinothalamic tracts may report loss of erection and ejaculation or loss only of erotic and orgasmic sensations, with preserved ejaculation. Patients with pure posterior column lesions rarely report such changes.

Many men with complete or incomplete spinal cord lesions above T12 have reflex erections but fail to ejaculate during intercourse or masturbation; however, reflex ejaculation via strong vibration of the glans is present. Facilitated reflex ejaculation via cholinergic mechanisms is not obtainable if the lesion is at T12–L2, suggesting that the reflex center is at that level. Retrograde ejaculation is present if urine that passes after ejaculation failure contains semen; it is often associated with early autonomic lesion, because of the preprostatic sphincter weakness. Retrograde ejaculation may be an early symptom of diabetic autonomic neuropathy (may sometimes be reversed with an adrenergic reuptake blocker such as desipramine) and follows bladder neck surgery or prostatectomy.

Autonomic neuropathy is a common cause of erectile failure, and psychogenic and reflexogenic erections are usually equally affected. Diabetes mellitus is the most common cause of symptomatic autonomic neuropathy, including neuropathic impotence. Erectile failure may be correlated with a loss of cavernosal neurotransmitters. Similarly, erectile failure may be an early symptom of progressive autonomic system failure or multiple system atrophy.

Anal Sphincter Failure

Denervation or surgical division of the anal sphincters causes loss of control of flatus and loose stool, while denervation or loss of the puborectalis muscle causes fecal incontinence. On the sensory side, loss of anal sensation in pudendal neuropathy or cauda equina lesions may also be associated with fecal incontinence. Anal incontinence may therefore occur in disorders of the sensory roots, conus, motor roots (S3–S4), or peripheral nerves (pelvic or pudendal neuropathy). In addition to the reduction in tone of the sphincters, the loss of parasympathetic input leads to a loss of effective propulsion of stool, causing constipation and fecal impaction. Such patients usually have good abdominal musculature to assist in defecation by raising intra-abdominal pressure and are primarily troubled by fecal leakage. Two nontraumatic disorders are of clinical importance: stress and fecal incontinence caused by selective degeneration of Onuf's nucleus seen in multiple systemic atrophies. Another, more frequent disorder, is the pelvic floor neuropathy, which is characterized by abnormal descent of the pelvic floor with urinary and anal incontinence, clinical and electromyographic evidence of pelvic floor and sphincter denervation, and partial or complete rupture of the anal sphincters demonstrated ultrasonographically. Treatment is surgical. Obviously, control of defecation or continence is lost in the presence of diffuse lesions of the brain, especially those associated with frontal or bifrontal dysfunction. The loss of voluntary control and the preservation of the spinal activity center may produce a situation analogous to detrusor-sphincter dyssynergia, with difficulty in emptying and chronic constipation.

Sphincter Disturbance History and Examination

Three groups of patients with pelvic dysfunction can be recognized. The first group comprises those patients who present with a neurologic problem requiring diagnosis. The first aim is to establish a unifying diagnosis that will account for all the symptoms and signs. The second group consists of patients with urologic symptoms that may have a neurologic cause. These patients will usually be seen by a urologist or gynecologist. This often happens after a process of exclusion by examination and investigation. The third group comprises those patients with established neurologic diseases who have as part of their illness a disorder of pelvic visceral function that requires treatment.

In patient group 1, the presenting complaint may be nonurologic, and it will be necessary to run through precise questioning about urinary habits and bowel and sexual function. If there are urologic features, the examination must be sufficient to exclude a local cause (e.g., prostatic hypertrophy or uterine prolapse) before accepting the urologic features of the history as part of the neurologic picture. The presence of pelvic visceral symptoms should

also prompt a more detailed neurologic examination of the sacral segments.

Patients in group 2 are likely to have predominantly urologic symptoms and might not appreciate the relevance of other neuro-urologic disturbances (e.g., impotence, orthostatic hypotension, difficulties in walking). The other problem for the physician is to distinguish these patients from the many patients with similar symptoms of non-neurologic causes and to decide which patients require a detailed neurologic examination.

In patient group 3, what the physician is seeking is not an overall diagnosis, because that has already been made, but clarification of the pathophysiology sufficient to point to the possible best methods of treatment. It is important to focus on the presenting symptoms, but these must be taken in context of the overall clinical picture (e.g., mental state, mobility, hand function). A detailed local neurologic examination is usually needed, with particular attention given to the sacral segments (Table 20-4).

The neuro-urologic history guides the examination and investigation process. It may indicate the cause of a problem, its severity, and its duration. Besides the local symptoms relating to the specific complaint, a broader picture must be sought. It is important not to miss a history of substance abuse and to note every drug being taken, a history of sexually transmitted diseases, a history of previous recurrent urinary tract infections or pelvic surgery that may indicate an anatomic anomaly, and a history of relevant general disorders (such as diabetes, back pain, or epilepsy) or congenital conditions (such as spina bifida occulta).

The pelvic musculature should be examined in detail. Digital assessment of the ability to perform voluntary and cough-induced contractions of the anal sphincter and pelvic floor, of anal sphincter and puborectalis tone, and of the anal skin and bulbocavernous reflex is indicated (see Table 20-4). However, urethral sphincter tone and function cannot be assessed clinically (but see the section on planning investigations that follows). In patients with anorectal incontinence, clinical examination with straining can demonstrate excessive pelvic floor descent, and the clinical impression can be supplemented by neurophysiologic testing and tests of rectal capacity (see the section on planning investigations that follows). Rectal examination is

Table 20-4. Neurologic Clinical Examination in Urogenital and Distal Bowel Disorders

Examination	Relevance of Information
Mental status	Diffuse cerebral disease with signs of dementia causes enuresis. Severe depression may also cause incontinence.
Cranial nerves	Anosmia (frontal meningioma?), visual loss (multiple sclerosis, cerebral tumor, hydrocephalus, diabetes?), abnormal pupils (atropinelike drugs, syphilis?), oculomotor signs (diabetes, multiple sclerosis, multiple system atrophy, other lesions of the pons?).
Motor system	Resting tremor, acinesia, rigidity, loss of postural responses (Parkinson's disease and multiple system atrophy?), spastic limb weakness (spinal cord lesion?), myoclonus (Creutzfeldt-Jakob disease, subacute sclerosing panencephalitis?), cerebellar ataxia (multiple system atrophy, multiple sclerosis, and many others?).
Sensory system	Sensory level suggests spinal cord lesion; suspended spinothalamic loss suggests intrinsic cord pathology. Peripheral sensory loss suggests peripheral neuropathy, which may be associated with autonomic involvement.
Neuro-urologic system	Patulous anus is seen when there is loss of both striated and smooth sphincter tone. Perineal sensory loss suggests a cauda equina, individual root, and pudendal nerve lesions.
	Superficial anal reflex consists of a contraction of the external sphincter in response to stroking or pricking the skin or mucous membrane in the perianal region. This reflex is innervated by the inferior hemorrhoidal nerve (S2–S4).
	The bulbocavernous reflex. Stroking, pricking, or pinching the dorsum of the glans penis is followed by contraction of the bulbocavernous muscle and the urethral constrictor, which may be palpated when a finger is placed on the perineum behind the scrotum with pressure on the urethra. This reflex is supplied by S3 and S4.
	The internal anal sphincter reflex. Contraction of the internal sphincter of the anus may be observed on introduction of the gloved finger into the anus. This reflex is supplied by postganglionic fibers of the sympathetic division through the hypogastric plexus (presacral nerves).

essential to look for prostatic enlargement, carcinoma, hemorrhoids, fissure-in-ano, or fistula-in-ano. Vaginal examination is needed to look for pelvic weakness or prolapse.

Planning Investigations

Disorders of Bladder Function

In patient groups 1 and 3 (see Sphincter Disturbance History and Examination), investigations of bladder symptoms are carried out to understand the pathophysiologic basis for the patient's symptoms and to obtain information on which to base recommendations for managing incontinence. In this instance, investigations are based on recording bladder pressures (urodynamic recordings) after excluding structural abnormalities by a pelvic examination and cystoscopy. In patient group 2, investigations are carried out, with the clinician seeking a neurologic cause (neurogenic bladder): In this instance investigations are of a neurologic and neurophysiologic nature.

Poor bladder control is a common feature of many types of neurologic diseases, especially of the spinal cord. The most common complaints are urgency, frequency, and urge incontinence, reflecting a combination of detrusor hyperreflexia and a disorder of emptying caused by detrusor sphincter dyssynergia and poorly sustained detrusor contractions. If the bladder does not empty completely, the persistent postmicturition residual volume acts as a stimulus for repeated detrusor contractions, so that efforts to treat detrusor hyperreflexia are unlikely to succeed until effective emptying is achieved. The most effective treatment for detrusor hyperreflexia is an anticholinergic drug (e.g., oxybutynin), but there is no oral medication that improves neurogenic voiding disorders, and the best management is intermittent catheterization performed by the patient or caregiver. The single most important investigation in patients with neurogenic bladder is therefore measurement of the postmicturition residual volume. This can either be done by ultrasound or by "in-out" catheterization. A further point about treatment with anticholinergic drugs is that although they may be effective in lessening detrusor hyperreflexia, they can affect bladder emptying. If a patient takes these drugs and fails to respond, it is advisable to repeat the assessment of the postmicturition residual volume. If this volume exceeds 100 ml, it will be necessary to teach the patient how to perform intermittent self-catheterization.

However, assessment of urodynamics is essential for the effective long-term management of neurologic patients. Urodynamic investigations allow not only for the diagnosis of complex lower urinary tract dysfunction, but also the prospective identification of patients at risk of progressive upper tract disease. Often a filling cystometrogram together with uroflowmetry and postvoid residual measurement are sufficient. In unknown lower urinary tract disorders or if the patient fails to respond to a simple treatment regimen, complex urodynamic investigations are needed, with cystometry, videocystourethrography, urethral pressure profilometry, and other urodynamic assessment methods.

The role of urodynamics in trying to decide if a patient has a neurogenic bladder is limited. In most patients referred by urologists or gynecologists to neurologists, filling cystometry has disclosed bladder overactivity. In this instance, the neurologist must confirm or refute that there is a neurologic basis for the problem based on the findings of clinical examination.

From the preceding section emphasizing the value of clinical examination, it is apparent that nervous system imaging is particularly indicated to exclude a suprapontine abnormality or a subsacral cauda equina lesion. Magnetic resonance imaging of the spinal cord and cauda equina is now the investigational method of first choice.

Pelvic floor neurophysiologic investigations can disclose two conditions that might not otherwise be evident:

1. In young women with bladder dysfunction and usually retention but no other neurologic deficit, electromyography (EMG) study of the urethral sphincter may show an abnormal complex repetitive discharge activity. It may be associated with evidence of sphincter denervation and reinnervation and with polycystic ovaries.
2. If there are neurologic features of parkinsonism, cerebellar ataxia, postural instability or hypotension, or symptoms suggesting laryngeal stridor, a diagnosis of multiple system atrophy should be considered. EMG studies of the sphincter have proved a valuable test in detecting these disorders by showing pronounced changes of denervation and reinnervation in the striated muscles of the urethral and anal sphincters. In expert hands, neurophysiologic investigations may also be useful for investigating the pathophysiologic basis of urinary incontinence in conjunction with urodynamic and ultrasonographic tests.

Anal Investigation

Manometry is useful in investigating the anal region because it enables the examiner to collect reproducible data concerning resting and contraction pressures in the anal sphincter region and to assess the separate contribution of the internal and external sphincter muscles in this system. Neurophysiologic investigations are also needed in the syndrome of pelvic floor neuropathy to analyze the striated anal sphincter musculature and to assess the distribution of neurogenic change in the pelvic floor musculature. Needle EMG study, especially single-fiber recording, is useful for this purpose because its results can be quantified. Studies of the innervation of the striated muscles of the pelvic floor can also be achieved by measuring the pudendal or perineal nerve terminal motor latencies using the method pioneered at St. Mark's Hospital in London. The integrity of the more proximal innervation of these muscles can even be assessed by direct stimulation of the motor nerve roots in the cauda equina by using the electrical or magnetic stimulator designed for cortical stimulation in humans.

Treatments

Disorders of Bladder Function

The main goals of management are the preservation of renal function and the avoidance of renal and bladder infection. In addition, it is important to contribute to social independence by achieving continence. The different ways of management cannot be discussed in this chapter and have recently been reviewed. The mainstays of therapy are essentially conservative and involve, as already mentioned (see the section on planning investigations), the use of pharmacologic agents, physical activities, and intermittent catheterization. In selected cases, when other methods have failed, carefully planned and meticulously performed surgical procedures may dramatically enhance a patient's quality of life. Electrical stimulation and sacral deafferentation are effective methods of managing the bladder in some patients, and artificial sphincters are now used.

Disorders of Sexual Function

Treatment of disorders of sexual function have been recently reviewed and is based on many different methods: drugs taken by mouth, intracavernosal injection of smooth-muscle relaxants, psychological treatments, penile prostheses, electroejaculation methods, and hypogastric plexus stimulator devices.

Bowel and Anal Dysfunction

Treatment regimens and procedures have been recently discussed and are different according to the acute or chronic stage of the lesion. In the chronic stage, the primary aims of management are to achieve adequate movement of large bowel contents into the rectum and controlled defecation at chosen times without incontinence. This can be accomplished by simple to complex treatment procedures: diet, laxatives, suppositories, digital stimulation, manual evacuation, and electrical stimulation by the development of implantable electrical stimulators.

Suggested Reading

Althof SE, Levine SB. Clinical approach to the sexuality of patients with spinal cord injury. Urol Clin North Am 1993;20:527.

Betts CD, D'Mellow MT, Fowler CJ. Urinary symptoms and the neurological features of bladder dysfunction in multiple sclerosis. J Neurol Neurosurg Psychiatry 1993; 56:245.

Brindley GS. Neuroprostheses used to restore male sexual or reproductive function. Baillieres Clin Neurol 1995;4:15.

Cheong DM, Vaccaro CA, Salanga VD, et al. Electrodiagnostic evaluation of fecal incontinence. Muscle Nerve 1995;18:612.

Chia YW, Gill KP, Jameson JS, et al. Paradoxical puborectalis contraction is a feature of constipation in patients with multiple sclerosis. J Neurol Neurosurg Psychiatry 1996;60:31.

de Groat WC. Anatomy and physiology of the lower urinary tract. Urol Clin North Am 1993;20:383.

Fowler CJ. Investigation of the neurogenic bladder. J Neurol Neurosurg Psychiatry 1996;60:6.

Fowler CJ. Pelvic Floor Neurophysiology. In CD Binnie, R Cooper, CJ Fowler, et al. (eds), Clinical Neurophysiology. Boston: Butterworth–Heinemann, 1995;232–250.

Ghika-Schmid F, Assal G, De Tribolet N, et al. Kluver-Bucy syndrome after left anterior temporal resection. Neuropsychologia 1995;33:101.

Ghoniem GM. Pharmacologic therapy for urinary incontinence. Urol Nursing 1996;16:55.

Jorge JMN, Wexner SD. Fecal incontinence: etiology, evaluation, and management. Dis Colon Rectum 1993;26:77.

Kirby RS. Impotence: diagnosis and management of male erectile dysfunction. BMJ 1994;308:957.

Low PA. Clinical Autonomic Disorders. Boston: Little, Brown, 1993.

Ott BR. Leuprolide treatment of sexual aggression in a patient with dementia and the Kluver-Bucy syndrome. Clin Neuropharmacol 1995;18:443.

Rushton DN. Handbook of Neuro-Urology. New York: Marcel Dekker, 1994.

Swash M. Faecal incontinence. BMJ 1993;307:636.

Chapter 21
Cortical Motor Dysfunction

Hans-Joachim Freund

Chapter Plan

The modular organization of sensorimotor functions
Factors determining the effects of lesions on function
Functional organization of cortical motor areas
    The agranular frontal cortical motor fields
    Parietal lobe
    Apraxia and the left hemisphere
Other higher-order motor disturbances
Recovery of motor function

The Modular Organization of Sensorimotor Functions

This chapter is organized such that the neurologic symptoms and signs of cortical motor dysfunctions are discussed in relation to lesion site. This approach allows an understanding of the clinical picture and the underlying pathophysiology on the basis of the functional organization of the sensorimotor system as it emerged from experimental and human lesion, stimulation, and activation studies. These data have provided evidence that the body parts to be moved are determined by the recruitment of topographically organized motor representations in the primary motor cortex (MI), whereas different types of movements are encoded by the interaction of distinct functional modules in parietal and premotor association areas in conjunction with the MI. The concept of such a modular organization of the sensorimotor cortex does

not revive the old center doctrine, but considers modules as nodal points in distributed, highly dynamically organized functional networks. This type of organization allows a high degree of functional specialization combined with an astonishing plasticity, even in the adult nervous system. The fine grain of the functional architecture can be experimentally demonstrated by transient focal deactivations achieved by neurotransmitter agonists/antagonists. Muscimol injections in the anterior part of the intraparietal sulcus in monkeys selectively interfere with the act of grasping, whereas more dorsolateral deactivation is followed by reaching deficits. Although such microlesions are rarely seen in patients, some lesions are small enough to disturb particular motor acts selectively. Whereas focal damage to the primary motor cortex is reflected by the somatotropic distribution of paresis, lesions in the parietal or frontal sensorimotor association cortex are associated with specific higher-order motor dysfunctions. They typically affect more complex or specific aspects of motor function characteristic for processing areas upstream of the primary motor cortex. A complementary approach to reveal this functional architecture is the use of positron emission tomography (PET) or functional magnetic resonance imaging (fMRI) activation studies. In a mirrorlike fashion they show task-specific activations at those cortical sites where lesions produce deficits. The advantage of functional imaging is its ability to visualize not only prominent nodal points, but also

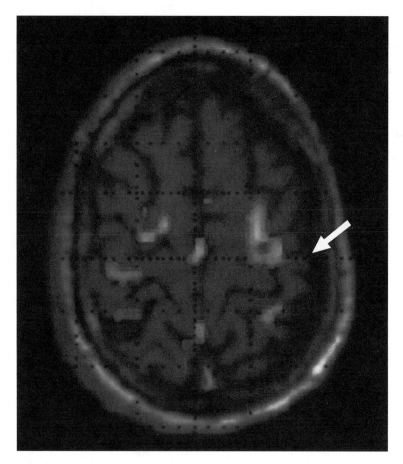

Figure 21-1. Functional magnetic resonance imaging study during tactile exploration of an object that has to be identified with closed eyes by the left hand. The left hemisphere is on the right side. Activations occur in the supplementary motor area, the dorsolateral premotor cortex, the anterior intraparietal sulcus on both sides, and in the left primary motor cortex. The arrow points to the central sulcus.

the involved network. This is illustrated by Figure 21-1, which shows the prominent bilateral activation of the supplementary motor area (SMA) along with dorsolateral premotor and parietal activations in a normal subject during active touch. The primary sensorimotor cortex is activated only contralateral to the moving hand.

Factors Determining the Effects of Lesions on Function

It is important for the clinician to understand that the regional specificity of the various sensorimotor areas can be recognized only when the lesions are restricted to particular areas, as in the case of carefully mapped surgical excisions or in small well-defined lesions as shown by high-resolution MRI studies. MRI allows purely cortical lesions to be distinguished from the more common combined cortical-subcortical lesion.

Only on the basis of this distinction is it possible to disentangle the effects of damage to local cortical circuitry from disconnection syndromes caused by the interruption of long transcortical fiber systems.

Another major factor influencing functional impairment is what Jackson called "lesion momentum." Acute brain damage has functional implications that are quite different from those of chronically developing brain damage. Whereas acute lesions cause deficits that are maximal initially and recover to some extent in most cases, slowly developing tumors are frequently not associated with any deficit at all, except after the onset of focal seizures.

Not only lesion site and momentum, but also the functional organization of the system that is damaged play a major role in its liability to functional impairment. The term *eloquent brain areas* designates those regions where acute acquired lesions cause major and persisting loss of function. Conversely, damage to noneloquent brain areas usually shows

Figure 21-2. Lateral view of the left hemisphere and upper part of the medial aspect of the right hemisphere of the human brain. The latter shows the medial wall motor areas, where the primary motor cortex (MI) (see text) = area 4, SMA = area 6aα, and Pre-SMA = area 6aβ. For the lateral aspect, the cytoarchitectonic areas are given. Area 4 = MI, area 6aα is the likely homolog of the PMv in monkeys, and area 6aβ of PMd. The postcentral gyrus with somatosensory projection cortex (areas 1, 2, and 3) is shown in black. Sensory association cortex of the posterior parietal lobule comprises areas 5, 7, 39, and 40. (CMAc = caudal cingulate motor area; CMAr = rostral cingulate motor area.) (Modified from H-J Freund. Die Organisation der Sensomotorik. Neuroforum 1997;2:42.)

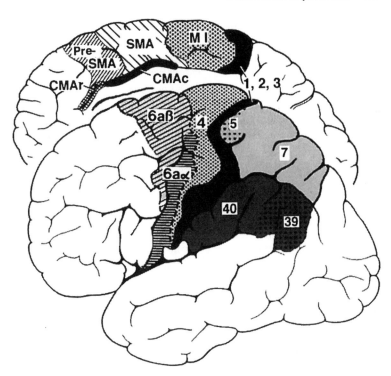

rapid and nearly complete recovery. This liability depends on several factors. One is the complexity of the level of organization of the damaged part. Acute damage to primary sensory or motor cortex usually causes severe, persisting deficits of the elementary aspects of sensation or motor control, whereas compensation is better for impairment of more complex, widely distributed "network" functions. Bilateral versus unilateral organization is another factor determining functional outcome. In the case of the sensorimotor cortex, the eloquent areas either have preferentially unilateral projection systems (primary motor and somatosensory cortex) or represent lateralized functions (Broca's area; inferior posterior parietal cortex). Damage to bilaterally organized systems such as the premotor cortex and supplementary motor area usually produces minor and transient clinical deficits.

Functional Organization of Cortical Motor Areas

The Agranular Frontal Cortical Motor Fields

In humans, approximately eight frontal motor fields are presently distinguished on the basis of probable homologies with monkeys and from lesion, stimulation, and activation studies (Figure 21-2): the MI, the ventral and dorsal premotor cortex (PMv and PMd), the supplementary motor area (SMA), the rostral and caudal cingulate motor areas (CMAr and CMAc), the frontal eye field, and Broca's area. A pre-SMA and a supplementary eye field have also been delineated. In addition to these frontal areas, the parietal cortex plays an important role in motor control. Accordingly, parietal lobe damage causes distinct disturbances of motor behavior. The clinical deficits typically seen after acute damage of the respective functional zones are described first for the frontal cortex and then for the parietal cortex.

Primary Motor Cortex and the Pyramidal Syndrome

Homologous to monkeys, the MI is regarded as coextensive with Brodmann's area 4. Area 4 is mainly restricted to the anterior bank of the central sulcus and the dorsal part of the precentral gyrus (see Figure 21-1). In spite of its small cortical representation (60% of the cortex is buried in the sulci), most pyramidal output fibers originate in the MI.

Damage to the MI or its descending pyramidal fibers causes the pyramidal or upper motor neuron syndrome: weakness, loss of dexterity, spasticity with increased tendon reflexes and muscle tone, and release of flexor reflexes. The nature of the disturbance is purely executional. The relative contribution of each of these features to the actual functional deficit varies considerably. This is particularly true for lesions of the pyramidal tract at different levels along its route. Whereas pyramidal damage above the brain stem level is usually associated with spasticity, lesions at the level of the medulla oblongata often produce hypotonic paresis. This is because of the different compositions of the fiber bundle at the various levels. Cortical surgical resections restricted to the precentral gyrus may produce no spasticity at all. Although the distribution of paresis after small cortical lesions reflects the somatotopic pattern of the motor homunculus, distal fine motor control is often most severely affected. Focal seizures or electrical stimulation of the motor cortex mirror the somatotopic pattern, as does functional activation.

Restoration of function after pyramidal damage is characterized by the reappearance of complex movement synergies, eventually followed by the capacity to perform single movements. The most frequent residual deficit is a disturbance of the fractionated finger movements so that the hand remains clumsy with permanent disturbance of motor skills.

Lesions of the Medial Wall Motor Areas:
The Supplementary Motor Area
and Cingulate Motor Areas

The medial wall motor areas in monkeys include the SMA and CMAs located caudally on the ventral and dorsal banks of the cingulate sulcus. They all have direct corticospinal projections. In humans, a likely homologue of the CMA can be identified anatomically. The SMA was first defined as a separate area by Penfield and Welch on the basis of intraoperative stimulation studies. The major difficulty is that many reports on SMA damage describe the effects of lesions that are not confined to the SMA but in most cases comprise the cingulate gyrus and more prefrontal medial cortex, mostly including the underlying white matter. This is typically seen after infarcts in the territory of the anterior cerebral artery or in cases of surgical excisions of epileptic foci in the medial frontal cortex. There are very few selective lesions of the SMA or CMA that allow their respective clinical deficits to be distinguished.

The typical deficit resulting from damage to the medial wall motor areas is a severe reduction of spontaneous motor activity that is most pronounced contralaterally and often accompanied by a reduction of speech and an emotional facial palsy. Disturbances of bimanual coordination and motor copying have also been reported. These deficits recede during the first weeks. The only persistent deficit is sometimes a slowing of alternating serial movements of both hands. This reciprocal coordination disorder may persist, whereas serial unimanual performances are unaffected.

The transient nature of the initial disturbances is contrasted by the severe and persisting deficits seen after bilateral SMA damage. These are characterized by complete akinesia and mutism, which may improve poorly. This dramatic difference between the cases of unilateral and bilateral damage is typical for the functional impairment that follows damage to bilaterally organized systems. These deficits reveal the significance of the medial wall motor areas for the initiation and preparation of self-generated movements, which is also demonstrated by their strong activation during internally generated movements or their imagination.

Dorsolateral Premotor Cortex

The issue of homologies between the premotor cortex of monkeys and humans is still debated. Fulton originally designated the human premotor area as the frontal agranular cortex rostral to the precentral sulcus corresponding to Vogts' area 6aβ (dorsal part of Brodmann's area 6). This area shows particular enlargement in humans, where it is five times larger than area 4, compared with a 1:1 relationship in macaques. As shown in Figure 21-2, a smaller ventral part of Brodmann's area 6 (Vogts' area 6aα) lies on the precentral gyrus. If the inferior part of the precentral sulcus in humans represents the homologue of the postarcuate sulcus in monkeys, area 6aα, which covers the anterior part of the precentral gyrus, is likely to correspond to the monkey's ventral premotor area (PMv). The large part of the PM in front of the precentral sulcus (area 6aβ) then corresponds to its dorsal compartment (PMd), as outlined for monkeys.

The PET or fMRI studies conducted so far show frequent activations of the cortex lining the precentral sulcus (see Figure 21-1). This is compatible with the view that the PMv represents some sort of a skill strip anterior to the motor representation in the MI. The PMv in monkeys has direct projections to the spinal cord, as has the SMA and CMA. Correspondingly, even the smallest precentral lesions so far do not produce any differential deficits between area 4 and area 6aα other than causing the pyramidal syndrome irrespective of their more anterior or posterior location on the gyrus.

Regarding damage to area 6aβ (PMd), Foerster described more than 40 patients in whom he had excised that area. The observed initial transient weakness was associated with a slowing and poverty of movements on the contralateral side, which was proximally accentuated. Loss of the kinetic melody, disintegration of complex skilled movements, and a disturbance of the kinetic structure of the motor acts have also been described. A special form of limb-kinetic apraxia is characterized by incoordination between the two arms or legs during such tasks as making a windmill movement with the arms or a pedaling movement with the legs. In contrast, distal bilateral movements such as rotating the thumbs or performing a repertoire of bimanual coordination tasks are normal. On testing, complex dysfunctions in sensory conditional motor learning can be observed, so that the patients are severely disturbed in their ability to learn the association between different arm postures and particular sensory cues. Another deficit is a severe disturbance in rhythm reproduction from memory in the absence of difficulties in producing the rhythms under auditory pacing and without problems in rhythm discrimination.

Electrical stimulation of the human PMd elicits mainly proximal movements similar to those observed after SMA stimulation with a consistent pattern of arm movements involving abduction and elevation of the arm, thus resembling a gesture of reaching. Turning movements of the trunk, head, and eyes toward the elevated arm are usually associated. This movement pattern is reproduced by focal seizures generated in that area.

Bilateral damage to the premotor cortex has dramatic and persistent neurologic sequelae, with gait and stance disturbances so severe that patients may be unable to walk and stand. It is not clear whether the dysbasia seen in cases with hydrocephalus is related to premotor circuitry dysfunction. Foerster's classic ablation and stimulation studies arrived at the conclusion that part of the premotor cortex is involved in the cortical control of posture. This notion would be compatible with a predominant projection of the anterior agranular premotor cortex to the brain stem. Whereas in monkeys the descending projection from the SMA and of the postarcuate premotor cortex is part of the pyramidal system, a major projection of the dorsal premotor cortex (Vogts' area 6aβ) is directed toward the magnocellular nucleus of the reticular formation. The reticular formation in turn sends off a bilateral reticulospinal projection to the spinal cord. This reticulospinal projection, including vestibulospinal, tectospinal, and interstitiospinal fiber systems, constitutes the major descending motor projection in addition to the pyramidal tract. The rubrospinal tract, which plays an important role in nonhuman primates and other mammals, is nonexistent or exists in a rudimentary fashion in humans.

The premotor–brain stem–spinal projection system thus represents the basic motor system by which the brain controls automatic movement, the maintenance of posture, the integration of body and limb movements, and the adjustment of the periaxial muscles between the two sides. The pyramidal system amplifies the brain stem control systems and in addition provides the capacity for fractionated distal movements. It is amazing how little we know about the cortical control of posture and locomotion—an issue of such paramount clinical importance. This is because of the difficulty of conducting activation or recording studies during stance and locomotion.

Broca's area also represents agranular and dysgranular frontal cortex specialized for the fine fractionated movement repertoire, with its complex coordination between breathing and the orolaryngeal muscles. Remarkably, this is the frontal motor area with a strongly lateralized function so that only damage to the language dominant hemisphere produces motor aphasia.

The frontal eye fields are discussed in Chapter 9.

Parietal Lobe

Lesions of the Anterior Parietal Lobe

Surgical excisions of the postcentral gyrus lead initially to a complete anesthesia, areflexia, and hypotonia of the contralateral side and to a disturbance of motility with slightly diminished force and slowing of movement. The execution of accurate movements or the selective muscle activation required for fractionated finger movements is impossible. During regression of the mild initial weakness, ataxia becomes prominent and closely resembles that seen after dorsal root section. Movements during prehension and object manipulation are impaired.

Lesions of the Superior Posterior Parietal Lobule

Tactuomotor Dysfunctions. Damage to the posterior parietal lobe, as with damage to the premotor cortex, is characterized by higher-order motor disturbances. In contrast to the disturbances of elementary sensation with their secondary effects on movement precision, damage to the superior posterior parietal lobule leads to the impairment of complex somatosensory functions, such as object recognition, identification of surface textures, and spatial information, without deficits of elementary sensation. On the motor side, hand function is severely compromised, so that active touch, object exploration, and manipulation become impossible. The hand and finger movements show a derangement of the dynamics of the digital palpation of objects, along with a breakdown of the finely tuned scanning process of the fingers, which prevents the sequential sampling of mechanoreceptive information. The essence of this disturbance lies in the impairment of the conception and generation of the spatial-temporal movement patterns required to bring those receptor sheets into action that would normally provide the information required for the identification and manipulation of objects. This

deficit is strictly unimodal, and, in part, visual guidance provides compensation. Because the dysfunction is characterized by misconceived and deranged movements that are functionally useless, the nature of the disturbance resembles an apraxia more than an ataxia. Because of this, the term *tactile apraxia* or *manipulative apraxia* is more adequate for characterizing the pathophysiology of the dysfunction. It shows that the extraction of sensory features relies on the adequacy of the purposive motor act and that the somatosensory association cortex is not only involved in the processing of somatosensory information, but also in the elaboration of the movement concepts. The unimodal nature of this dysfunction is the result of lesions of unimodal somatosensory association cortex—that is, the human homolog of areas 5 and 7b in monkeys.

Visuomotor Dysfunctions. Correspondingly, lesions of a visual association area (7a) produce another unimodal higher-order motor disturbance, optic ataxia. This condition is the inability to direct the arm, head, and eyes adequately toward a target. It is usually seen after bilateral parieto-occipital lesions. The movement disturbance affects only visually guided motor acts. Again, there are perceptive, cognitive, and motor aspects of the dysfunction: the imperfect perception of distances and spatial relationships paralleled by inadequate target-directed adjustment of the arm and eyes and by a grossly deranged movement pattern. This makes the condition different from purely ataxic disturbances and from motor behavior observed in acutely blind patients, who can easily perform smooth and accurate movements to remembered targets. In contrast, these patients show grossly abnormal trajectories of reaching, aiming, grasping, and hand preshaping. Their ability to learn to reach for targets with known locations cued by proprioceptive or acoustic input is poor. Because of this, the dysfunction represents another unimodal apraxia. Whereas tactile apraxia affects solely the contralateral side of the body, visuomotor apraxia may affect not only the opposite hemifield and arm, but also the ipsilateral side. Bilateral parieto-pontine-cerebellar-thalamo-frontal cortical projections play an important part in visuomotor processing. By this route, the basic brain stem–cerebellar system for eye-hand-body coordination is incorporated in the cortical processing streams.

Lesions of the Inferior Posterior Parietal Lobule

Damage to the posterior part of the inferior parietal lobule (IPL) affects motor behavior differently depending on the side of the lesion. Lesions of this area on the side of the language-dominant hemisphere lead to the classic forms of ideational or ideomotor apraxia. According to Liepmann's definition, ideational apraxia is characterized by a deficit of the conception of the movement so that the patient does not know what to do or how to organize movement sequences. Clinically, patients with ideational apraxia are often severely compromised in their daily activities. In contrast, ideokinetic (ideomotor) apraxia is examination bound. The patient does not know how to imitate particular motor act–like gestures. The disturbance affects both sides of the body and is often associated with aphasia. On the basis of the apraxias, Liepmann postulated that the left hemisphere is not only dominant for language but also for praxis. The apraxias seen after IPL damage are supramodal in nature. This is compatible with the presumed supramodal organization of the human IPL.

The frequent association of apraxia and aphasia raises the possibility that the two disorders are the expression of a common underlying deficit of communication affecting linguistic and gestural behavior in a general sense. There has been a long-standing discussion regarding the nature of the speech deficit seen in the Wernicke type of sensory aphasia, in which comprehension is preferentially affected but where speech production is grossly deranged as well. Therefore, aphasia is another example illustrating the dual aspect of sensorimotor processing. This is further illustrated by observations of deaf-mute patients using American Sign Language (ASL) for communication. The fact that a visual-gestural communication system can substitute for the auditory-vocal one shows the capacity of the human nervous system to deal with symbolic and iconic information in a context-specific way irrespective of the sensory modality or the motor subsystem involved. Patients with left hemisphere damage become sign-language aphasic because of a breakdown of the capacity to communicate by ASL, affecting comprehension and production.

The functional impairment selectively affects the linguistic components of sign language and does not reflect an underlying motor disorder of the capacity to express and comprehend symbols or of the production and imitation of representational and nonrepresentational movements. The patients are unable to produce the patterned arm and hand movements required to convey the linguistic information. Quantitative movement analysis of the arm trajectories combined with linguistic analysis illustrates how the brain controls movement at different levels: linguistic, symbolic, spatial, and motor. The errors for the spatially organized syntax for ASL stand in contrast to the flawless performance on a range of constructional tasks, including drawing, spatial construction, spatial attention, judgment of line orientation, and spatial discrimination. Conversely, deaf-mute ASL patients with damaged right hemispheres show gross impairment of constructional tasks contrasted by an immaculate performance of ASL.

Clinically, lesions of the right posterior parietal lobe frequently produce constructional apraxia, which is characterized by difficulty in putting one-dimensional units together to form two-dimensional figures or patterns. It appears in formative activities (e.g., arranging, building, or drawing), with the spatial part of the task being faulty, although the movement elements are normal. It is more frequently observed after lesions of the non-dominant side.

Apraxia and the Left Hemisphere

Unlike language organization, in which the minor hemisphere is virtually unable to maintain residual language functions after age 12 years, the right hemisphere is fully competent to conduct the whole movement repertoire for the opposite side of the body. Damage to the corpus callosum can produce an apraxia of the left hand, but only because language information is not available to that hemisphere. It is not clear why a left hemisphere lesion interferes with the otherwise normal control of left-sided motor behavior by the right hemisphere. It has been proposed that it reflects a disturbance of the priority of action control normally exerted by the left hemisphere.

Other Higher-Order Motor Disturbances

Motor impersistence refers to a patient's inability to sustain simple acts such as protruding the tongue, keeping the mouth open, or holding the eyelids shut (i.e., apraxia of lid closure). The syndrome is mostly transient, associated with other disturbances (e.g., neglect, sensory deficits, mental impairment), and more frequently observed in patients with right hemisphere lesions.

Neglect refers to situations in which a patient fails to report, respond to, or orient to novel or meaningful stimuli that are presented to the contralesional side. This failure cannot be attributed to sensory or motor deficits. It may affect different or all modalities and motor functions. Pure motor neglect is a clinical entity characterized by the following criteria:

1. Absence of paresis
2. Absence of muscle tone changes
3. Absence of pyramidal signs
4. Absence of spontaneous limb movements on the affected side
5. Limb movements of the affected side in response to tough encouragement
6. Absence of withdrawal of affected limbs from uncomfortable positions

Motor neglect can be associated with sensory neglect, but it can also be associated with hemiparesis, making the distinction between the components of such complex deficits difficult. Less severe varieties, which are characterized by a poverty rather than a lack of movements, have been called hemiakinesia or directional akinesia. Frequently, the head and eye deviate to the ipsilesional side. Directional akinesia may be detected by using a modification of the crossed response task. The examiner holds one hand in the patient's right visual hemifield and the other in the left visual hemifield. A patient who fails to look at the contralateral finger movement may be hemianopic or may have visual inattention or directional akinesia. These can be dissociated by instructing the patient to look to the side opposite the one that is stimulated. This is possible in the former two cases but not in patients with directional akinesia. The lesions can be located in different brain areas (i.e., premotor, parietal, subcortical). Positron emission tomography scans in such patients show widespread metabolic suppression in the thalamus and in the premotor, parietal, and cingulate cortex.

The alien hand syndrome, first described by Goldstein, is a condition in which the affected hand behaves in a fashion that is out of the patient's control. The movements are experienced as involuntary and contrary to the patient's stated intention. The other hand is frequently engaged in restraining the affected hand. The condition is different from rhythmic or spasmodic movements, which are often associated with the assumption of unusual postures. The neuropathologic substrate is damage to midline structures, the callosum, or both. In unilateral cases, left hemisphere lesions predominate. In frontal cases, the alien hand syndrome of the dominant hand is typically associated with reflexive grasping, impulsive groping, and compulsive manipulation of tools. In callosal cases, the syndrome affects the nondominant hand and bimanual interaction. This condition is also called diagnostic dyspraxia. The alien hand syndrome is of particular interest because its features are the reverse of hemiakinesia or akinetic mutism—another clinical syndrome caused by damage to the medial wall motor areas.

The most common brain lesions affect several functional zones. So far, the clinical sequelae of lesions restricted to certain functional zones have been described in order to outline their characteristic clinical features, but the most common types of brain lesions affect several areas with combined cortical and subcortical damage. Consequently, the ensuing deficits comprise different features determining the patients' residual motor capacity. In the majority of cases, hemiparesis is the initial sign. As previously described, damage to areas outside the precentral motor strip or its descending pyramidal fibers causes some weakness associated with the other features described. Two candidate mechanisms account for the paretic component. As shown in Figure 21-3, the medial wall motor areas and parietal cortex contribute substantially to the pyramidal projection.

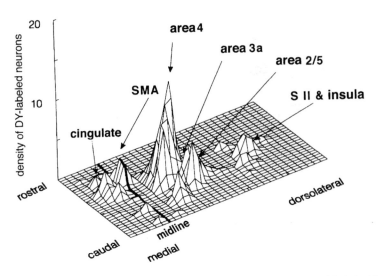

Figure 21-3. Three-dimensional maps of the corticospinal neuron soma distribution that were labeled with DY, a retrogradely transported tracer injected into the cervical spinal cord (C5–C7). The viewing angle is from above, behind, and medial to the central sulcus. Lamina V of the sensorimotor cortex has been unfolded to constitute the projection plane. Several clusters in the frontal motor areas (primary motor cortex [MI], ventral premotor cortex [PMv], supplementary motor area [SMA], cingulate motor area [CMA]) constitute approximately 70% of the contralateral corticospinal projection. The parietal projection also terminates in the intermediate zone and in the dorsal zone. Because no such data are available for humans, these data on the origin of the pyramidal tract are important for clinical neurology. (Reprinted with permission from MP Galea, I Darian-Smith. Multiple corticospinal neuron populations in the macaque monkey are specified by their unique cortical origins, spinal terminations, and connections. Cereb Cortex 1994;4:166.)

In addition, the premotor areas funnel parietal input and their own projection to the precentral cortex (Figure 21-4). A possible tuning effect of that input is suggested by experimental deactivation studies, in which the paresis occurring after precentral cooling recovers rapidly, but additional cooling of the postcentral gyrus abolishes the recovered function.

Detailed clinical analysis further shows lesion site–specific additional deficits such as hypokinesia, ataxia, apraxia, motor neglect, or other higher-order motor disturbances. Their relative proportion depends on lesion site and size and the actual impairment on their combined effect.

Recovery of Motor Function

Most recovery occurs during the first 4 weeks after acute brain damage. The severity of the initial deficit is the best predictor of outcome. Lesion size is poorly related to outcome, except for very large lesions. Fractionated finger movements can recover only when a minimum of approximately 20% of the pyramidal fibers are spared. Complex dysfunctions such as apraxias recover better, leaving only 20% of these patients with a permanent deficit, compared with 45% of persistent hemiparesis in stroke victims.

Several mechanisms underlying the restitution of function can be distinguished: *within-system recovery* depends on the preservation of part of a system and provides the best condition for restoration of function. This is shown by the excellent restitution of motor functions in patients with slight or moderate initial paresis or with preservation of magnet-evoked motor potentials. Compensation by ipsilateral components of the same system plays a major role in bilaterally organized systems (e.g., PM, SMA, CMA), so that the initial disturbances are mild and recover rapidly. The small ipsilateral component of the pyramidal sys-

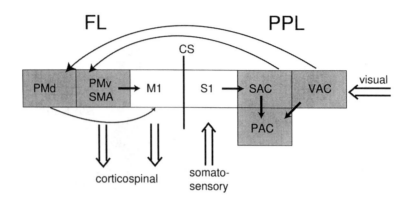

Figure 21-4. Simplified presentation of the major processing streams in the sensorimotor cortex. The incoming visual and somatosensory information is funneled to the posterior parietal unimodal (SAC = somatosensory association cortex, VAC = visual association cortex) and polymodal association cortex (PAC) before it reaches the primary motor cortex via the premotor areas. There is virtually no "reflex arc" from S1 to M1. (PMd = dorsal premotor cortex; PMv = ventral premotor cortex; SMA = supplementary motor area; FL = frontal lobe; PPL = posterior parietal lobe; CS = central sulcus.)

tem obviously contributes little in the adult nervous system. This is different in developmental lesions, which show remarkable plasticity so that even hemispherectomies are compensated to a degree that the patients can walk and use the arm and hand for synergistic movements. In the spinal cord, functional restoration is astonishingly rapid and good after unilateral transection of the pyramidal tract in adult patients with chordotomies. This is completely abolished by a second chordotomy on the other side, demonstrating that recovery was mediated by the ipsilateral pyramidal tract, possibly assisted by the propriospinal system. These important observations show that the contra-ipsilateral interactions are different in the cerebral and spinal cord levels of the pyramidal tract.

Dorsolateral premotor and medial wall areas (e.g., SMA, CMA), with their direct access to the spinal cord via the pyramidal tract but also via cortico-reticulo-spinal projections, are candidates for functional *substitution by related systems*. Imaging studies in patients with hemiparetic stroke show that sensorimotor areas outside the destroyed motor cortex become activated during the residual movements. Experimental infarcts in the motor cortical hand area cause an expansion of the dysfunctional zone with subsequent loss of further hand representation. This process can be modified by train-

ing, but only when performed within a particular time window. The investigation of use-dependent modification of cortical maps and the role of relearning, assumption of new strategies, and other specific therapeutic procedures are essential for new approaches in rehabilitative medicine.

It is not only the destroyed brain area itself that causes the resulting deficit, but also the effects of lesions on other parts of the network. In experimental infarcts, a surprisingly large perilesional area shows altered neuronal properties, widespread metabolic depressions and changes in receptor patterns. In addition, remote effects are frequently apparent, in particular in the thalamus and cerebellum. The development of dysfunctional and sometimes epileptogenic zones in the perilesional area and their influence on remote network components is a major issue for a better understanding of the pathophysiology of dysfunction. It is not only the initial period of tissue destruction, but also the subsequent period of plastic changes caused by these perilesional and remote processes that determine outcome.

There is a striking discrepancy between the effects of acute versus chronic lesions on function. For acute damage, within-system recovery is most effective. In slowly developing tumors, substitution of function plays a major role. Patients with tumors infiltrating the entire precentral gyrus often show no or minor deficits. Neuroimaging

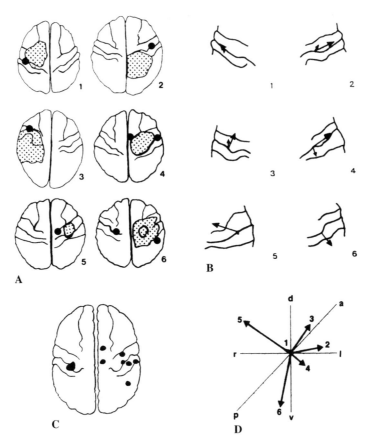

Figure 21-5. The pattern of reorganization of cortical motor activation sites in the vicinity of tumors infiltrating the motor cortex. (A) The increases in regional cerebral blood flow (rCBF) (*black dots*) did not occur in the tumor-affected (*shaded*) area. Right in the images corresponds to left in the patients. (B) The vectoral displacement of the central sulcus (*small arrows*) by the tumors, if present, was smaller and often in a different direction to the shift of the activation areas (*large arrows*). The spatial shift of the increases in rCBF varied among the patients but often followed the orientation of the central sulcus. (C) Superimposition of the mean increases in rCBF associated with finger movements of the normal (left) and affected hand (right) into stereotactic space. Finger movements of the affected hand showed a large spatial variability with no overlap of the peak rCBF increases, whereas for the normal hand a small area of overlap was observed in the middle portion of the central sulcus. The increase in rCBF in the supplementary motor area (patient 4) was included. (D) Three-dimensional vector displacement of the increases in rCBF in the affected cerebral hemisphere. The origin corresponds to the location of the motor hand area ($x = 35$ mm, $y = 20$ mm, $z = 50$ mm) as determined for the normal hand in stereotactic space. (a = anterior, p = posterior, d = dorsal, v = ventral, r = right, l = left, unit = 10 mm.) (Reprinted with permission from R Seitz, Y Huang, U Knorr, L Tellmann, et al. Large-scale plasticity of the human motor cortex. Neuroreport 1995;6:742.)

and intraoperative stimulation data show activations outside the infiltrated area (Figure 21-5). Consequently, tumor removal does not produce hemiparesis. This shows that related systems such as the medial wall motor areas, PM, or parietal cortex can substitute for the loss of the MI. This large-scale plasticity reveals the ability of the adult nervous system to adapt when it has time to reorganize slowly.

Suggested Reading

Balint R. Seelenlähmung des Schauens, optische Ataxie, räumliche Störung der Aufmerksamkeit. Monatsschr Psychiatr Neurol 1909;25:51.

Bellugi U, Poizner H, Klima ES. Language, modality and the brain. Trends Neurosci 1989;12:380.

Dum RP, Strick PL. Spinal cord terminations of the medial wall motor areas in macaque monkeys. J Neurosci 1996;16:6513.

Ebeling U, Schmid UD, Reulen HJ. Tumour surgery within the central motor strip: surgical results with aid of electrical cortical motor cortex stimulation. Acta Neurochir (Wien) 1990;101:110.

Foerster O. Motorische Felder und Bahnen. In H Bumke, O Foerster (eds), Handbuch der Neurologie (Vol 6). Berlin: Springer, 1936;1–357.

Freund HJ. Abnormalities of Motor Behavior After Cortical Lesions in Humans. In F Plum (ed), Handbook of Physiology, Section 1: The Nervous System (Vol V): Higher Functions of the Brain (Part 2). Baltimore: Williams & Wilkins, 1987;763–810.

Freund HJ. The Apraxias. In C Kennard (ed), Recent Advances in Clinical Neurology. New York: Churchill Livingstone, 1995;29–49.

Fulton JF. Definition of the motor and premotor areas. Brain 1935;58:311.

Galea MP, Darian-Smith I. Multiple corticospinal neuron populations in the macaque monkey are specified by their unique cortical origins, spinal terminations, and connections. Cereb Cortex 1994;4:166.

Glickstein M, May JG. Visual Control of Movement: The Circuits Which Link Visual to Motor Areas of the Brain with Special Reference to the Visual Input to the Pons and Cerebellum. In WD Neff (ed), Contributions to Sensory Physiology (Vol 7). New York: Academic, 1982;103–145.

Goldstein K. Zur Lehre der motorischen Apraxie. J Psychol Neurol 1908;11:169.

Heilman K. The Neuropsychological Basis of Skilled Movement in Man. In R Vandenburgh (ed), Handbook of Behavioral Neurobiology: Social Behavior and Communication (Vol 3). New York: Plenum, 1979;447–461.

Lawrence DG, Kuypers HGJM. The functional organization of the motor system in the monkey. I. The effects of bilateral pyramidal lesions. Brain 1968;91:1.

Lawrence DG, Kuypers HGJM. The functional organization of the motor system in the monkey. II. The effects of lesions of the descending brain-stem pathways. Brain 1968;91:15.

Liepmann H. Apraxie. Brugsch's Ergebnisse der gesamten Medizin. Berlin: Urban & Schwarzenberg, 1920;518–543.

Nathan PW, Smith MC. The rubrospinal and central tegmental tracts in man. Brain 1982;105:223.

Penfield W, Welch K. The supplementary motor area in the cerebral cortex of man. Trans Am Neurol Assoc 1949;74:179.

Seitz R, Huang Y, Knorr U, Tellmann L, et al. Large-scale plasticity of the human motor cortex. Neuroreport 1995;6:742.

Wise SP. What Are the Specific Functions of the Different Motor Areas? In DR Humphrey, HJ Freund (eds), Proceedings of the Dahlem Workshop on Motor Control: Concepts and Issues. Berlin, December 3–8, 1989. New York: Wiley, 1991;436–485.

Zilles K, Schlaug G, Matelli M, Luppino G, et al. Mapping of human and macaque sensorimotor areas by integrating architectonic, transmitter receptor, MRI and PET data. J Anat 1995;187:515.

Chapter 22
Aphasia

Atsushi Yamadori

Chapter Plan

Aphasia is operationally defined as a disorder of manipulation of spoken and written language secondary to brain damage. A developmental disorder of language is not included in the category of aphasia in the strict sense. A pure language disorder confined only to a single mode of operation, such as pure alexia involving only visual decoding of written material, may not be regarded as aphasia because internal language processing is not affected. Here, it is included in aphasia.

It is extremely difficult to assess the absolute incidence of aphasia. It depends on the total number of brain-damaged patients in a particular region, and the number varies depending on the preference of causes, as in the case of cerebrovascular diseases. However, relative incidence may be of some help. One recent study in the United States reported that aphasia was seen in 19.4% of men and 22.5% of women in the Stroke Data Bank. Another survey conducted in 1993 in Japan by the Japanese Association of Aphasiology estimated the percentage of aphasia seen in all brain-damaged patients receiving care at the time of the survey in 511 hospitals to be 4.2%. Although the latter study included all types of brain damage, the difference is still great, indicating a subtle difference of diagnostic criteria among countries concerned.

Methods of Clinical Evaluation

Evaluation of Spoken Language

Four abilities should always be evaluated in determining the status of spoken language: (1) spontaneous speech, (2) language comprehension, (3) word-finding, and (4) repetition.

The quality of spontaneous speech is evaluated in natural situations while engaging in free conversation and under structured conditions such as having patients explain the theme or content of a picture or narrate a well-known story. Among the many attributes of speech output, fluency-nonfluency is useful. Fluent aphasics produce larger numbers of uninterrupted chains of words in one utterance, whereas nonfluent aphasics produce a smaller number of words. According to pioneering studies, nonfluent aphasics rarely exceed three to four words per utterance. The presence or absence of production errors at the phonemic level (phonemic paraphasia) and word level (verbal paraphasia) should be noted. When a word is totally replaced by phonemic paraphasias, it is called *neologism*. When an utterance is replaced by paraphasias and neologisms and becomes unintelligible, it is called *jargon*. The status of articulation is also important. When articulatory deviation is regular and the content of utterances can be predicted, it is usually caused by disorders of articulatory organs and is called *dysarthria*. When no regularity is detected in articulatory distortion, it is interchangeably called *apraxia of speech*, *pure anarthria*, or *aphemia*. The ease or difficulty of initiating and maintaining speech, the prosodic quality, and the variety of words produced should also be noted.

The patient's ability to comprehend spoken language is evaluated in natural as well as structured conditions. Aphasics tend to comprehend sentences spoken in natural situations more easily than ones that are formally commanded or questioned by the examiner. Levels of difficulty in comprehension vary depending on the type of aphasia. Whenever possible, it must be determined whether the aphasia is at the level of phonemes, morphemes, lexicons, or sentences. A handy way to evaluate the level of comprehension at the bedside is by pointing. Five to seven common objects, such as a wrist watch and a pencil, are placed in front of the patient, and the examiner has the patient point to an appropriate item by saying the name of the object. Pointing becomes very difficult for aphasics as the number of words presented at a time increases.

Word finding is evaluated with or without a stimulus. The former is called *confrontation naming*, and the latter is called *word finding* in the narrower sense. When an object is present, it is usually easier to retrieve its name. In aphasia, the concept of the object itself is not impaired; this can easily be confirmed by having patients describe the object or gesture how it is used. Usually, retrieving a target name from a description is much more difficult for aphasics. Confrontation naming should be tested not only through vision but also through specific modalities such as audition or touch when necessary.

Exact repetition of an utterance is a very important capacity for language acquisition and operation. It is tested at word levels as well as sentence levels. This ability is unique in that it is independent of other capacities and its status is never known until it is tested. A seemingly normal patient might suddenly start to fumble when asked to repeat a sentence exactly, whereas a severely aphasic patient may repeat a long sentence without a flaw. Repetitive tendency may be automatic and compulsive (echolalia) or transformed to a certain degree as to be expressed as a patient's own speech (mitigated echolalia).

Language is organized in the brain based on anatomic rules. When we hear, linguistic signals carried through the air in the form of sound waves are decoded into neural impulses in the auditory receptive systems in the ears and transmitted to the auditory analyzer systems in the brain, where they are decoded into phonologic chains, and then to the associative areas, where they are experienced as meaningful events. When we speak, ideas are produced in the associative areas of the brain and are encoded into phonologic chains in the motor programming systems, and transmitted to the motor executive system in the brain to be encoded into patterns of neural impulses, which are again encoded into motor patterns of the articulatory muscles and emitted into the air as sound waves. This essential pattern of information flow is summarized in Figure 22-1. Although the terminology is different, the structure is essentially identical with Lichtheim's famous schema presented at the dawn of aphasiology.

Evaluation of Written Language

Written language is the secondary product of spoken language and evolved much later than spoken language. There still exist many isolated human races that have not developed writing systems. However, once established, written language becomes no less important than spoken language. In our modern society equipped with widely interconnected information systems, written language has become more and more important. In aphasia, writing disturbances usually parallel those of spoken language, but sometimes writing ability is separately affected or separately preserved, betraying its relative autonomy. Reading is evaluated with letters, words, and sentences. Because oral reading and comprehension show dissociation in many aphasics, both capacities should be evaluated separately. In countries in which nonalphabetic writing systems are used, the tests should be developed according to the characteristics of the system. In

Figure 22-1. The general framework of language processing in the brain. Speech sound is received by the auditory receptors (ears) and decoded into linguistic signs in the auditory-related analyzer systems in the brain, which are further decoded into meaning, probably activating several critical areas outside the auditory system (linguistic semantic system). In speaking, an idea evoked in the semantic system is encoded into linguistic signs, which are further encoded into articulatory patterns, which are emitted as sound waves.

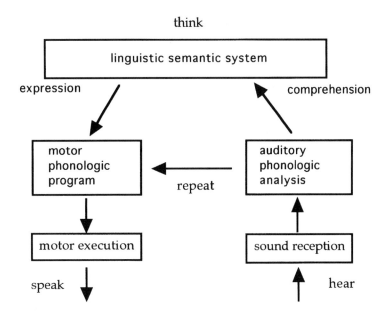

Japan, for instance, ideographic letters (kanji) and phonographic letters (kana) are used in combination and should be tested separately.

Writing ability is tested for spontaneity, dictation, and copying. Having the patient write his or her name and address is not enough. These automatic writing functions may be preserved in otherwise severely impaired agraphics. In testing a patient's capacity to copy letters, it should be noted whether the patient copies them piece by piece as figures or writes them down with his or her own penmanship as letters. The former indicates a visuoconstructive disturbance, whereas the latter is a usual pattern in aphasia. Writing is tested with the left hand when the right side is paralyzed. For right-handed writers, this may create clumsy writing, but the essential capacity to produce legible letters is not disturbed unless some pathologic condition is involved. In exceptional cases, only left-hand writing may be impaired, which suggests a callosal lesion.

Major Aphasic Syndromes

As suggested in the previous section, aphasia is a syndrome consisting of qualitatively different symptoms. Thus, to understand aphasia it is important to grasp the general pattern of impaired and preserved capacities of the different linguistic aspects in a particular patient. Because brain damage does not abide by the law of anatomy, symptoms of aphasia are more or less different in all patients. Also, language organization is subtly different in the non–right-handed population, and even in the right-handed majority there are cases in which the organization of language is exceptional. This leads to further complexity of aphasic symptomatology.

The following description of aphasic syndromes should be understood as a representative or model syndrome around which many deviant or actual syndromes are distributed.

Syndromes that Mainly Affect Spoken Language

Nonfluent Aphasia

The major impairment of nonfluent aphasia is in the domain of language production. The number of words produced in one utterance is invariably reduced. The capacity of comprehension and repetition differs depending on the subtypes.

Broca's Aphasia.   The amount of spontaneous speech is conspicuously reduced in Broca's aphasia. Occasional utterances are punctuated with pauses.

Effort is required to start speaking. Intended phrases do not come out and often are replaced by paraphasic, neologistic, or anarthric errors. In extreme cases, only a couple of syllables are produced, such as "tan tan" of the original Broca's patient, Leborgne. When a longer sentence is produced, it is often characterized by a lack of functional words or appropriate inflexion (agrammatism). Prosody is often disturbed (dysprosody). Word-finding ability is impaired on confrontation naming as well as during free recall. Repetition does not improve the output difficulty. Comprehension of spoken language, on the other hand, is relatively well preserved but is not normal in most of the cases. In unstructured conversation, patients seem to understand quite well. However, when exact comprehension is required, such as following an order expressed in a complex grammatical sentence or pointing to a series of objects in a required order, difficulty becomes apparent.

Writing ability is impaired to the same degree as spontaneous speech. Only a limited number of letters or words are produced. Oral reading ability is impaired, but reading comprehension may be fair.

Typical lesions are concentrated in the posterior portion of the inferior frontal gyrus and the lower portion of the central gyrus of the left hemisphere. Usually the lesions extend to the surrounding cortex and underlying deep white matter. The left posterior area of the inferior frontal gyrus, including the opercular and triangular region, has been called Broca's area. However, a small lesion restricted to Broca's area does not produce a typical Broca's aphasia. For Broca's aphasia to be produced, a more extended lesion is necessary.

Transcortical Motor Aphasia.   The clinical bedside impression of transcortical motor aphasia is that it resembles Broca's aphasia. The amount of speech is reduced. Patients tend to be taciturn even when spoken to. Essential differentiating points with Broca's aphasia are lack of anarthria and good repetition ability. Repetition ability may be extremely good. The patient may be able to repeat a fairly long sentence flawlessly; however, it is difficult to decide the absolute length of a phrase to be used as a criterion for repetition ability. Rather, it is a contrast between poor spontaneous speech and surprisingly good repetitive output that marks this syndrome. Comprehension of spoken language is fair if not completely normal. Confrontation naming is often easier than retrieval of a specific name without a stimulus. The ability to write is usually severely disturbed. Comprehension of written material is fair compared with the output disability. Oral reading ability varies. Often it is contaminated by misreadings (paralexia) or perseverative errors.

Typical lesions have been said to involve the left premotor area surrounding but sparing Broca's area. More recent studies indicate that if only the lower portion of the left precentral gyrus is spared, articulation and repetition ability would be spared.

Aphemia.   The core of the aphemia syndrome is speech output difficulty related to articulation. The quantity of utterances varies. Some patients may produce only a couple of connected words, whereas others may produce longer, dysprosodic utterances. Articulation is distorted, slurred, or aborted. It is essentially anarthric—that is, there is no apparent regularity in articulatory impairment. The patient may be able to clearly pronounce a correct sound at one time but not at other times. Patients may show visible efforts to produce correct target sounds and repeat self-correction without success. Repetition and naming ability remains at the same deficient level with spontaneous speech.

The most important aspect that differentiates aphemia from Broca's aphasia is preserved writing ability. In a very rare case of pure aphemia, no writing impairment was observed. In most other cases, however, some difficulty with writing is observed, such as omission, misplacement, or addition of letters.

Reflecting the relative purity of a syndrome confined to the articulatory domain, many names have been interchangeably used—that is, *aphemia, pure anarthria, subcortical motor aphasia*, and *apraxia of speech*. Lesions are regularly found in the middle to lower portion of the left precentral gyrus.

Fluent Aphasia

The major impairment of fluent aphasia is either in the domain of speech comprehension or in correct retrieval of phonemes and words for expression at the conceptual (premotor) level. The speech production mechanism in terms of articulatory realization and basic syntax construction seems not to be disturbed. However, because speech production requires constant monitoring from the auditory system as well as the conceptual system, the content of speech output may be strikingly abnormal. In other words, the output system as a vehicle of language expression remains intact, but linguistic materials in the vehicle may be wrongly loaded, hence, fluent speech output.

Wernicke's Aphasia.   Comprehension of spoken speech is invariably compromised in Wernicke's aphasia. In severe cases, even very simple conversation cannot be carried out. Simple auditory tasks, such as selecting a heard name from two or three candidate objects, may become impossible. In milder cases, conversational responses may be surprisingly successful. However, if a question is structured so that the answer must be precise, the deficit of comprehension becomes apparent. Matching of objects to spoken names rapidly deteriorates as the number of names to be presented auditorily or the number of stimulus objects to be selected is increased.

Spontaneous speech is produced without articulatory distortion or prosodic impairment. The number of words produced can be fairly large. However, the content would be vacant, with many clichés and circumlocutory expressions. It may be punctuated with neologisms and various types of paraphasias. In the most severe cases, all the output becomes unintelligible (jargon aphasia). In milder cases, fluent features may be less clear because output may be interrupted with frequent pauses with apparent effort in searching for a correct expression.

Word-finding ability is severely impaired in confrontation naming as well as in free recall. Repetition ability varies. In milder cases, some words or phrases may be repeated. In severe cases, even a syllable cannot be repeated. Disturbance of written language is usually proportional to that of spoken language, but in exceptional cases performance in written language is clearly superior.

The core lesion is always found in the posterior third of the left superior temporal gyrus—that is, Wernicke's area. When the lesion extends to surrounding areas of the inferior parietal lobule and middle temporal gyrus, the syndrome becomes more severe in degree.

Conduction Aphasia.   Spoken speech is contaminated with phonemic and to a lesser degree with verbal paraphasias. There is no articulatory or prosodic impairment. Words are well connected and produced in a long string. The content of speech is fairly intelligible, although there are many circumlocutory expressions. Comprehension is fair even with a complex sentence. Naming on confrontation is also contaminated with paraphasias, mainly of the phonemic type. Patients know the name to be produced but have difficulty producing it in a clear and correct sound sequence.

The most important characteristic of this type of aphasia is difficulty in repeating a heard word or sentence correctly. Although patients understand the meaning of a given stimulus, it is profoundly difficult for them to reproduce it correctly. They also immediately notice when they repeat it incorrectly and try to correct errors many times without success. Difficulty increases with the number of syllables contained in a stimulus. In some instances, paraphasias in spontaneous speech are not conspicuous, in which case failure in repetition ability may never be found even by a trained neurologist unless the task is given.

The ability to read orally is impaired in addition to the ability to write. In the latter, paragraphic errors are produced similar to those in spontaneous speech. However, comprehension of written language is well preserved, paralleling that of auditory comprehension.

Lesions most often involve the supramarginal gyrus and its subjacent white matter of the left hemisphere. A partial lesion of Wernicke's area may also produce this type of disorder. Classic theory maintains that the syndrome is a result of disconnection of the motor speech region in the frontal lobe from Wernicke's area by a cutting of the arcuate fasciculus, which is supposed to connect the posterior speech region with the anterior one. Because conduction aphasia affects all the output modalities of spontaneous speech, naming, and repetition, the mechanism disrupted probably involves not simply the subcortical fiber systems, but also cortical neural systems that subserve correct selection and sequencing of phonemes and syllables.

Transcortical Sensory Aphasia.   The essential feature of transcortical sensory aphasia is similar to that of Wernicke's aphasia. The main differential point is a preserved ability for repetition. Unlike Wernicke's aphasia, a fairly long phrase may be repeated easily. The contrast between poor auditory comprehension and excellent repetition of the same sentence is a hallmark of this syndrome. Word-finding ability is severely impaired. Oral reading ability may be preserved, again without comprehension. Writing ability is severely disturbed.

Anomic Aphasia. *Amnestic* and *nominal aphasia* are other terms designating anomic aphasia. Anomia, which is a difficulty in retrieving a correct name for a stimulus object, is a universal symptom across all types of aphasia. In anomic aphasia, difficulty with word-finding stands out against other symptoms. Naming a shown object becomes extremely difficult. Retrieval of appropriate words while engaging in free conversation is also difficult. Patients are acutely aware of this difficulty and try to circumvent it by periphrasis and frequent use of demonstrative or personal pronouns. Paraphasia is often produced in confrontation naming tasks but is conspicuously lacking in unstructured free speech. In rare cases of two-way anomic aphasia, not only retrieval of a specific name but also difficulty comprehending the same name are demonstrated.

In milder cases of anomic aphasia, it is usually difficult to pinpoint the responsible lesion. In severe cases, lesions are often identified in the middle to posterior portion of the left middle temporal gyrus or angular gyrus. Some studies suggest that names are organized in categories, and difficulty in retrieving the names in a specific category may be related to a specific lesion.

Pure Word Deafness. In pure word deafness, comprehension of spoken language is severely impaired but comprehension through reading remains intact. The basic capacity of hearing is normal. Comprehension of nonverbal sounds such as music or environmental sounds is relatively spared. A typical patient would complain that he or she can hear people talking but does not understand what they are saying. The ability to repeat spoken language and the ability to write dictation are also severely impaired. Because manipulative ability of written language is preserved, communication through writing is possible. Spontaneous speech is either unaffected or contaminated with mild paraphasia. Word-finding ability is preserved.

Lesions are usually found in the deep white matter in the posterior portion of the left superior temporal area disconnecting Wernicke's area from the left and right primary auditory areas. In cases of bilateral lesions, the superior temporal gyri are involved in various patterns, but at least Wernicke's area is spared in the left hemisphere.

Atypical Aphasia

The essential symptomatology of the groups of aphasic syndromes noted above had been well established by the end of the last century. Additional syndromes have been described relatively recently after the introduction of computed tomographic and magnetic resonance imaging scanning into clinical practice. Care should be taken that these are described in terms of location of lesions and not as a constellation of symptoms in classical types of aphasia.

Aphasia Caused by Supplementary Motor Area Lesions. Damage to the supplementary motor area in the left medial frontal lobe produces language disturbances of a peculiar nature. Spontaneous speech is extremely reduced. The voice is low. Encouragement and prompting are required to initiate and maintain speech. However, repetition and naming ability on confrontation are well preserved. Comprehension of spoken language is also surprisingly well preserved. Oral reading ability and comprehension of written language are also better preserved. However, writing ability is often severely impaired with many repetitive and perseverative errors. Essentially it belongs to the broad category of transcortical motor aphasia.

Aphasia Caused by Thalamic Lesions. Spontaneous speech is essentially fluent, but the overall quantity of speech is reduced, and the voice becomes low. Speech is contaminated with verbal paraphasias and perseveratory phrases. Comprehension is moderately or mildly disturbed. Word-finding ability is poor. Repetition ability is usually preserved. Written language is impaired in reading as well as writing.

Generally speaking, these aphasic syndromes are mild in degree and often show fluctuation during the day or between the test sessions, suggesting involvement of nonlinguistic factor, such as impairment of attention. They are often a transient symptom. The major differentiating point may be a complication of verbal memory disturbance. The presence of this symptom has been mentioned in all reported cases of thalamic aphasia.

Lesions are difficult to specify because the thalamus is a compact aggregate of a large number of nuclei. The anterior ventral (VA), lateral ventral (VL), medial (M), or intralaminar nuclear groups of the left thalamus have been suggested as being responsible for the aphasia. One autopsy case showed a major lesion in the pulvinar and the dorsal aspect of the lateral nucleus.

Aphasia Caused by Subcortical White Matter Lesions. Deeply seated lesions involving the putamen, white matter subjacent to the opercular cortices in the frontoparietal area, or the centrum semiovale of the left hemisphere often produce aphasia. The pattern of language disturbance varies depending on the size and location of lesions and is usually atypical. Many patients may show a unique articulatory impairment that gives an impression similar to mumbling, in which the bulk of utterances are produced in a hasty and dysarthric manner. Speech may sound unintelligible, but meaning is often discernible. The other feature often observed is fluctuation of aphasic status. Detailed analysis made it clear that the putamen is not responsible for the aphasia, but the white matter in the periventricular area, a portion of the internal capsule in the anterior limb, and the genu are critical.

Mixed Aphasia

When lesions are extensive or multiple, classification of a language deficit of a particular patient into one of the above mentioned syndromes becomes impossible. All the linguistic modalities are equally affected, resulting in mixed aphasia. In rare cases of mixed transcortical aphasia, spontaneous speech, comprehension, word-finding ability, and the ability to manipulate written language are all severely damaged with the exception of repetition ability. Rare autopsy reports show widely spread lesions are strategically placed, just sparing Wernicke-Broca's area and the intermediate regions.

In global aphasia, all aspects of language function are disturbed, leaving only a small number of utterances, which are either neologistic or perfectly intelligible. Comprehension is also severely compromised, but paralinguistic information seems to be comprehended surprisingly well. If no utter-

ances or signs of situational comprehension are observed in awake patients, other behavioral pathologic conditions such as akinetic mutism or psychiatric stupor should be considered. Widely distributed lesions involving the Broca-Wernicke core regions in the left hemisphere are the cause of this syndrome.

Syndromes that Mainly Affect Written Language

Alexia Without Agraphia

Alexia without agraphia shows selective difficulty in reading (oral reading ability as well as reading comprehension) against the background of preserved writing capacity as well as normal manipulation of spoken language. When a patient with this syndrome is assisted with the hand to write in the air the word that he or she cannot read visually, the patient is able to read it, indicating preserved graphemic imagery (kinesthetic reading). The syndrome is also characterized by isolated difficulty in reading with a preserved ability to recognize and name nonlinguistic visual materials.

Typical lesions are situated in the left occipital striate cortex and the splenium of the corpus callosum. Other often-reported lesions involve the white matter subjacent to the left angular gyrus. Both types of lesions effectively disconnect the visual letter from information generated in the intact occipital area from reaching the left angular gyrus area, which is responsible for letter processing.

Alexia with Agraphia

As the name suggests, patients with alexia and agraphia show prominent difficulty both in reading and writing. Oral reading ability and reading comprehension are disturbed to the same degree. Spoken language capacity is well preserved if not completely normal. Unlike alexia without agraphia, kinesthetic reading does not facilitate reading. The capacity for spontaneous writing and writing to dictation is equally impaired, but copying ability is usually preserved. Responsible lesions always involve the left angular gyrus area.

A unique type of alexia with agraphia has been reported in Japan—that is, selective difficulty of reading and writing ideograph letters (kanji) with a preserved ability to read and write phonographic letters (kana). Almost all the lesions reported conform to the area of the left posterior inferior temporo-occipital region. This is the area adjacent but inferior to the angular gyrus.

Pure Agraphia

A writing disturbance can occur as an isolated impairment without compromising the ability for reading or spoken language. It may occur either at the level of letter production or word production. In letter production agraphia, it should be made clear whether or not it is accompanied by difficulty in copying. If copying is impaired, chances are that it is related to motor apraxia or constructional impairment. If the ability to connect letters (word production) is disproportionally impaired, it is more likely caused by a difficulty of transcoding auditory word images into motor graphemic sequences.

Although it is still difficult to describe with confidence the lesions responsible for pure agraphia, representative cases so far reported point to lesions either in the posterior portion of the left middle frontal lobe or the left superior parietal lobule.

In Japan, a special type of pure agraphia limited to ideographs (kanji) has been described with lesions of the left inferior posterior temporal area. This area also causes alexia with agraphia limited to ideographs.

Anatomy of Aphasia

Lateralization of the Linguistic Function

Since Broca's time, it has been well established that language function is asymmetrically organized over the hemispheres. The other well-known asymmetric neural organization is handedness. The majority of the population is right handed, which implies that the organization of the motor implementation system is dominated by the left hemisphere. However, there are important exceptions. Most studies agree that roughly 10–12% of the population is non–right handed.

In most of the right handers, language is lateralized to the left hemisphere. In rare cases, lesions in the right hemisphere of the dextrals cause aphasia, which is called *crossed aphasia*. The incidence of this type of aphasia is estimated to be about 0.38% to 2.0% in the Euro-American literature. In non–Euro-American data, a Japanese study reported an incidence of 0.9%.

Left handers and ambidextrous persons demonstrate a slightly different lateralization pattern. Many show a left hemispheric dominance for language rather than a right hemispheric one. Thus, roughly 60% of aphasias are produced by damage to the left hemisphere and the rest by damage to the right hemisphere. Aphasia is generally less severe, and recovery tends to be better than right handed–left hemispheric aphasia. These facts led many scholars to speculate that language organization is less lateralized in non–right handers.

Language Organization Within the Hemisphere

In typical right-handed, left hemisphere–dominant persons, the core structure in auditory language comprehension is situated in the posterior third of the left superior temporal gyrus (Wernicke's area). For realization of speech, the posterior third of the inferior frontal gyrus (Broca's area), the lower portion of the precentral gyrus, and the anterior portion of the insular cortex are critical. The fiber systems connecting these anteroposterior regions—that is, the arcuate fasciculus, along with the supramarginal cortex situated in between, are also essential. Together, they constitute the most important axial language area dealing with phonology and syntax. The supplementary motor area and the thalamus are closely linked with this axial system. The relationship between these areas is shown in Figure 22-2 as a simplified schema.

The areas shown in the schema are not sufficient for language operation. Meaning, the most essential part of linguistic activity, is not generated within this axial system itself. The middle temporal gyrus, the angular gyrus, and regions of the frontal lobe overlying the anterior speech area are indispensable for mediating lexical and sentential meaning. Thus, a fairly large area of the left hemisphere functions as the organ of language.

From information deduced mainly from cases of crossed aphasia, it has been speculated that the language area in the right hemisphere is organized in an exact mirror pattern of the left hemisphere in some cases and in an anomalous pattern unpredictable from the standard syndrome in others.

Organization of written language in the left hemisphere is still difficult to delineate. The critical

Figure 22-2. An outline of the axial language area. The supplementary motor area and the thalamus work in coordination with Broca-Wernicke's area (*solid arrows*). Final articulatory commands are issued from the central gyrus (*broken arrow*). (L = left hemisphere; R = right hemisphere; Sm = supplementary motor area; Th = thalamus; B = Broca's area; C = lower portion of the pre- and post-central gyrus; SM = supramarginal gyrus; W = Wernicke's area.)

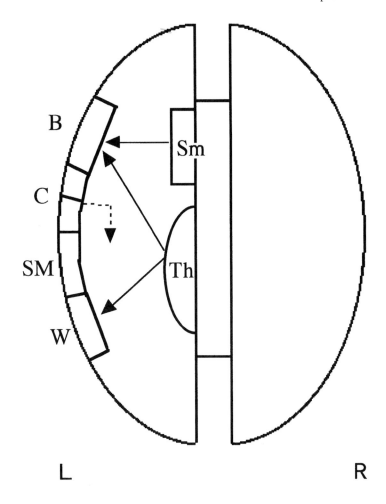

regions at least include the angular gyrus, the superior parietal lobule, and the posterior portion of the middle frontal gyrus of the left hemisphere in addition to the axial language areas. In cultures in which ideographic letters are used, a more inferiorly situated area than the angular gyrus (posterior inferior temporal area, for instance) may also play a role.

Suggested Reading

Alexander MP, Fischette MR, Fischer RS. Crossed aphasias can be mirror image or anomalous. Case reports, review and hypothesis. Brain 1989;112:953.

Alexander MP, Naeser MA, Palumbo CL. Correlations of subcortical CT lesion sites and aphasia profiles. Brain 1987;110:961.

Benson DF. Aphasia, Alexia and Agraphia. New York: Churchill Livingstone, 1979.

Crosson B, Parker JC, Kim AK, et al. A case of thalamic aphasia with postmortem verification. Brain Lang 1986;29:301.

Damasio AR. Aphasia. N Engl J Med 1992;326:531.

Dronkers NF. A new brain region for coordinating speech articulation. Nature 1996;384:159.

Geschwind N. Aphasia. N Engl J Med 1971;284:654.

Geschwind N. Disconnection syndromes in animals and man. Part I and II. Brain 1965;88:237,585.

Geshwind N, Quadfasel FA, Segarra J. Isolation of the speech area. Neuropsychologia 1968;6:327.

Goodglass H. Understanding Aphasia. San Diego: Academic, 1993.

Lichtheim L. On aphasia. Brain 1885;7:433.

Masdeu JC, Schoene WC, Funkenstein H. Aphasia following infarction of the left supplementary motor area. A clinicopathological study. Neurology 1978; 28:1220.

Mohr JP, Pessin MS, Finkelstein S, et al. Broca aphasia: pathologic and clinical. Neurology 1978;28:311.

Schiff HB, Alexander MP, Naeser MA, Galaburda AM. Aphemia. Clinical-anatomic correlations. Arch Neurol 1983;40:720.

Chapter 23

Sensory System Dysfunction

Jong Sung Kim

Chapter Plan

The sensory system receives information from the environment and transmits this information to the central nervous system. In this way, stimuli from the external world are perceived. Our sensory system also perceives information from the environment within the body: from blood vessels, the viscera, and the actions of the skeletal muscles. This sensory input is not consciously perceived and is used to regulate the autonomic functions such as maintenance of temperature, blood pressure, heart rate, and respiratory rate and to regulate our posture and voluntary movements. Thus, an intact sensory system is essential for maintaining life. In this chapter, the focus is on dysfunctions of sensory perception from the external world. Derangement of this system not only pro-duces impaired sensory input but also causes disturbing symptoms such as pain.

Anatomy of the Sensory Pathways

The most peripheral sensory organs are sensory receptors, which convert various forms of sensory stimuli into changes in membrane electric potentials. This electric information is then carried through the peripheral and the central nervous system. The individual sensory receptors are sensitive to a particular form of natural stimulation, although this specificity is not absolute. The receptors can broadly be classified as mechanoreceptors, which respond to mechanical stimulation; thermoreceptors, which respond to temperature changes; and nociceptors, which respond to noxious stimuli. Most mechanoreceptors are innervated by large myelinated axons, whereas thinly myelinated (A-delta) and nonmyelinated (C) fibers innervate thermoreceptors, nociceptors, and a few mechanoreceptors.

Sensory information from the periphery is conveyed to the spinal cord through afferent peripheral nerves. The afferent fibers of the first-order neurons enter the dorsal portion of the spinal cord as dorsal nerve roots, the cell bodies of which are located in the dorsal root ganglia (Figure 23-1). Thus, the peripheral axon of the neuron conveys afferent sensory information from the sensory receptors, whereas the central axon enters the spinal cord in the dorsal nerve roots. In the dorsal root entry zone

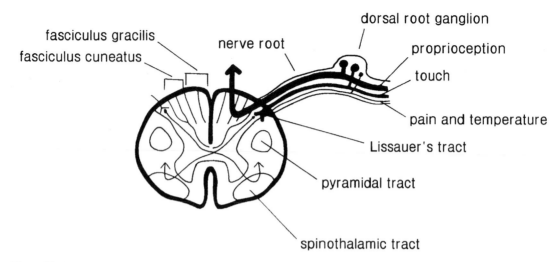

Figure 23-1. Anatomy of the dorsal root and spinal cord. Actually, fibers carrying pain and temperature sensation ascend up to two segments in Lissauer's tract before decussation.

of the spinal cord, the large, heavily myelinated proprioceptive fibers (medial division), the medium-sized fibers carrying tactile sensation (intermediate division), and the finely myelinated or unmyelinated fibers mediating pain and temperature sensation (lateral division) are located in a medial-to-lateral direction (see Figure 23-1). Some of the large-diameter fibers that do not ascend terminate directly in motor nuclei (lamina IX) and mediate stretch reflexes, whereas others ascend through the spinal cord.

There are two functionally and anatomically distinct ascending sensory systems (Figure 23-2). Fibers subserving proprioception, vibration, tactile discrimination, and some touch sensation turn upward in the posterior column (fasciculus gracilis and fasciculus cuneatus) up to the caudal medulla, where they synapse on the dorsal column nuclei neurons (nuclei of Goll's column and Burdach's column). From there, the tract decussates as the internal arcuate fibers and ascends through the opposite medial lemniscus, which is located medially in the medulla oblongata. This sensory system is called the *dorsal column–medial lemniscus system*. On the other hand, fibers carrying pain and temperature sensation, after entering the dorsal root entry zone, ascend a few segments at Lissauer's tract and then synapse at the dorsal horn. From there, some fibers ascend ipsilaterally, but the majority of the neurons cross the midline in the white commissure and ascend

toward the medulla as the spinothalamic tract in the opposite anterolateral column. In the medulla, the spinothalamic tract is located laterally and superficially. The spinothalamic tract mediates fast pain relayed by A-delta fibers. In addition, the spinoreticular and spinotectal tracts also carry pain and temperature sensation. The former is responsible for slow pain mediated by C fibers and ends on neurons in the reticular formation of the brain stem, which then relay information to the thalamus or mesencephalic periaqueductal gray matter. The spinotectal tract terminates in the tectum of the midbrain. These tracts carrying pain and temperature sensation are generally called the *anterolateral system*. A significant portion of the anterolateral system fibers ascend uncrossed, whereas tracts of the dorsal column–medial lemniscus system are strictly a crossed system. The differences between the dorsal column–medial lemniscal system and the anterolateral system are summarized in Table 23-1.

Facial (trigeminal) sensation is conveyed to the brain stem by the trigeminal nerve. The three divisions (ophthalmic, maxillary, and mandibular) are united as a single nerve and enter the lateral pons. The fibers carrying touch and tactile discrimination synapse at the principal trigeminal nucleus located in the lateral part of the pons. The secondary fibers (quintothalamic fibers) cross the midline and ascend to the thalamus. The fibers subserving pain and

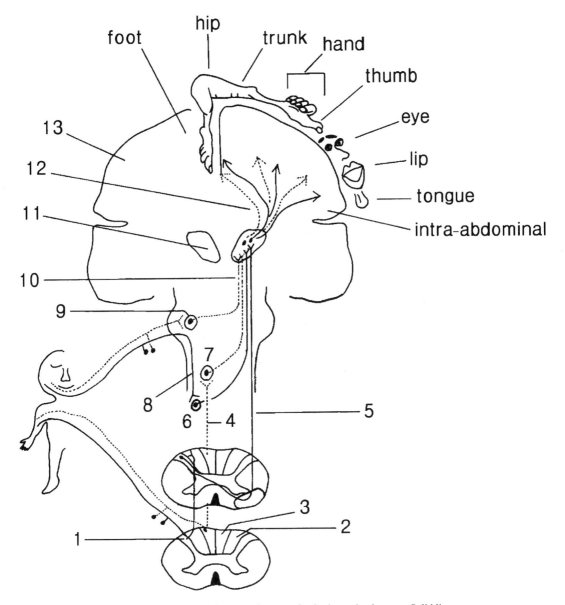

Figure 23-2. Diagram of the sensory tracts and sensory homunculus in the parietal cortex. Solid lines represent sensory fibers carrying pain and temperature and dotted lines represent fibers subserving tactile and proprioception. (1 = Lissauer's tract; 2 = fasciculus cuneatus; 3 = fasciculus gracilis; 4 = posterior column; 5 = spinothalamic tract; 6 = spinal nucleus of the trigeminal nerve; 7 = nucleus gracilis; 8 = spinal tract of the trigeminal nerve; 9 = principal trigeminal nucleus; 10 = medial lemniscus; 11 = thalamus; 12 = thalamoparietal projection; 13 = sensory cortex.)

thermal sensation do not synapse at the principal sensory nucleus. Instead, just after entering the pons, they run down as descending trigeminal roots and synapse at the trigeminal nuclei that form a long vertical structure extending far down to the second cervical cord, which is continuous with the posterior horn of the spinal gray matter. After synapsing, the fibers decussate and then ascend as the ascending trigeminal tract (trigeminal lemniscus) toward the thalamus (see Figure 23-2).

Sensory tracts of both systems as well as fibers carrying trigeminal sensation converge into the thal-

Table 23-1. Comparison Between the Anterolateral System and the Dorsal Column–Medial Lemniscus System

	Anterolateral System	Dorsal Column–Medial Lemniscus System
Modalities	Pain, temperature	Vibration, tactile, position
Nerves	Thinly myelinated, unmyelinated	Thickly myelinated
Spinal cord	Anterolateral column	Dorsal column
Decussation	Spinal cord, some ipsilateral projection	Caudal medulla, strict decussation
Termination	Brain stem reticular formation, midbrain tectal region, ventral posterior and other thalamic nuclei	Ventral posterior nucleus of thalamus

amus, which is a principal sensory relay station of the brain. The sensory relay nucleus, the ventralis posterolateralis, receives somatic sensation from the limbs and the trunk, and the ventralis posteromedialis receives sensory inputs from the face and oral area. In these nuclei, the sensory homunculus for the acral body parts (lip, fingers, and toes) are disproportionately large (Figure 23-3). Whereas the medial lemniscal tracts terminate mainly in the ventral posterior nucleus, fibers of the anterolateral system synapse in more diffuse areas, including the posterior nuclei, the intralaminar nuclei, and the ventral posterior nuclei.

From the thalamus, the impulses involved in sensation reach localized areas of the cortex through the thalamocortical projection (in the posterior limb of the internal capsule/corona radiata). The primary function of the sensory cortex is to discriminate sensation: appreciation and recognition of spatial relations, appreciation of similarity and differences of external objects, precise localization of the point touched, and identification of objects (stereognosis). The cortical area subserving general somatic sensation (superficial and deep) is located in the postcentral gyrus, Brodmann's areas 3, 1, and 2. Whereas six distinct histologic layers are preserved in Brodmann's areas 1 and 2, the layers II, III, and IV tend to fuse with each other in area 3. The various regions of the body are represented in specific portions of the postcentral gyrus (sensory homunculus), a pattern corresponding to that of the motor area. The area representing the face lies in the most lower part, after which areas for the hand, arm, trunk, leg, and foot are located in that order. The area for intra-abdominal structures is represented near the opercular surface of the

postcentral gyrus. Again, the cortical areas representing the mouth, face, hands (especially the thumb and index finger), and toes are disproportionately large (see Figure 23-2). There are observations that the somesthetic cortical area is not limited to the postcentral gyrus. Electrical stimulation of the precentral gyrus or the occurrence of small pathologic lesions in this region often produces sensory symptoms. Although the sensory cortex is primarily related to sensation of the contralateral body, stimulation of the cortex occasionally evokes bilateral sensory symptoms in the face, especially the perioral area.

Patterns of Sensory Dysfunction

Various disorders affecting the sensory pathway produce an impairment of sensory perception in a part of the body. In addition, patients often feel positive symptoms (subjective discomfort) over the affected area. Paresthesias mean spontaneous abnormal sensations that a patient experiences in the absence of specific stimulation; paresthesias are variably described as numbness, tingling, burning, cold, warm, crawling, and tightness. Dysesthesias are a patient's perverted interpretation of sensation, such as a burning feeling in response to tactile stimuli. For a complete understanding of sensory dysfunction, examination for various modalities of sensation should be performed; these include pinprick, temperature, touch, vibration, position, and other discriminative sensations. A careful examination of sensory dysfunction helps localize the lesions occurring in the nervous system. Because sensory dysfunction usually occurs in discrete patterns,

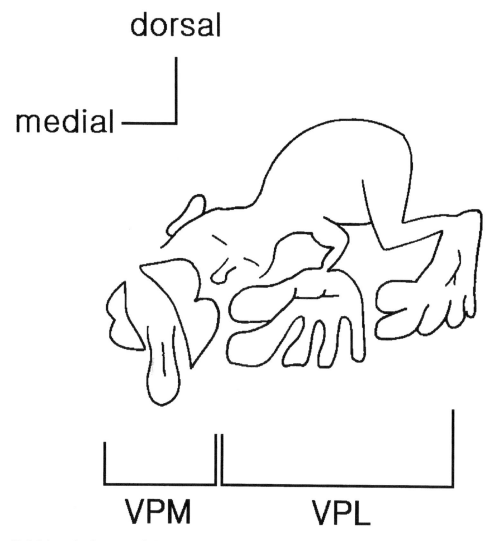

Figure 23-3. Schematic of somatotopic body representation in the ventral posterior nucleus of the thalamus in primates.

understanding these patterns is important in the assessment of a patient with neurologic diseases.

Peripheral Nerve Level

Figure 23-4 illustrates the cutaneous distribution of the major peripheral nerves. When a single nerve is damaged (mononeuropathy), a sensory deficit occurs in the focal area innervated by that particular nerve. For example, damage to the median nerve produces sensory symptoms over the thumb, index finger, middle finger, and the radial half of the ring finger, whereas ulnar nerve lesions induce symptoms over the little finger and the ulnar half of the ring finger (Figure 23-5). The common causes of mononeuropathy are various vasculopathies and local trauma. Carpal tunnel syndrome is a notable example of the latter and is commonly encountered in middle-aged women. It is caused by compression of the median nerve at the wrist by the thickened flexor retinaculum. When several peripheral nerves are involved simultaneously, it is called *multiple mononeuropathy* or *mononeuritis multiplex.*

A polyneuropathy occurs when numerous peripheral nerves are simultaneously involved. In this con-

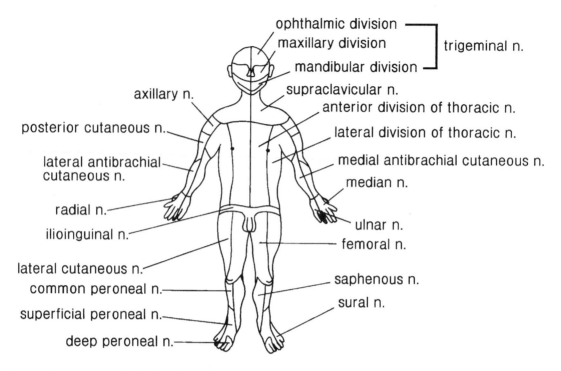

Figure 23-4. Cutaneous distribution of the peripheral nerves.

dition, nerves are usually involved symmetrically and the longest fibers tend to be most severely affected. Therefore, the feet and hands are commonly involved in a symmetric pattern producing a "glove and stocking" type of distribution (Figure 23-6). The abdomen, thorax, and face are spared except in the most severe cases. Although sensory and motor dysfunction is usually seen concomitantly in a patient with polyneuropathy, certain neuropathies preferentially involve either sensory or motor fibers. For example, although motor weakness is dominant in patients with Guillain-Barré

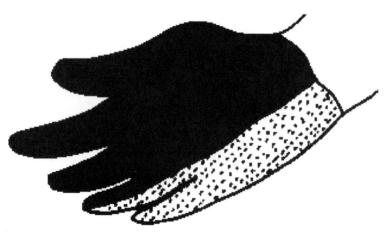

Figure 23-5. Topography of sensory loss secondary to damage to the median nerve (*black area*) and ulnar nerve (*dotted area*).

syndrome, sensory symptoms are major clinical features in diabetic neuropathy, alcoholic neuropathy, and amyloid neuropathy.

Root Level

The skin area supplied by a single root is called a *dermatome*. Although there is strict dermatomal or segmental distribution (Figure 23-7), there is a considerable overlap, and damage to a single root therefore may not produce an objective sensory deficit. Nevertheless, the occurrence of pain (radicular pain) or paresthesia in a particular dermatome helps localize the level of the lesion. The most common cause of radicular pain is a herniated intervertebral disc, usually in the lower lumbar area. The root involved by the herniated disc is generally one level below the spine level. For example, when a disc is herniated at the L5–S1 level, the root involved is usually S1. The radicular pain is characteristically exaggerated on maneuvers that stretch the root (e.g., straight leg raising) or increase the intraspinal pressure (e.g., coughing, sneezing).

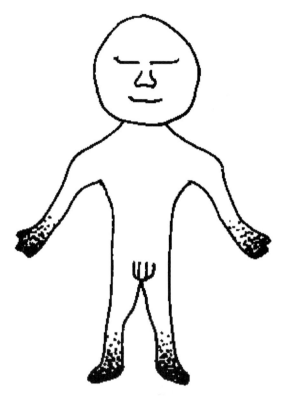

Figure 23-6. "Glove and stocking" type of sensory abnormality caused by polyneuropathy.

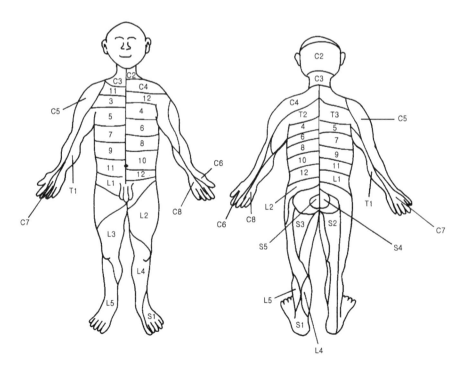

Figure 23-7. Cutaneous distribution of the spinal nerve roots.

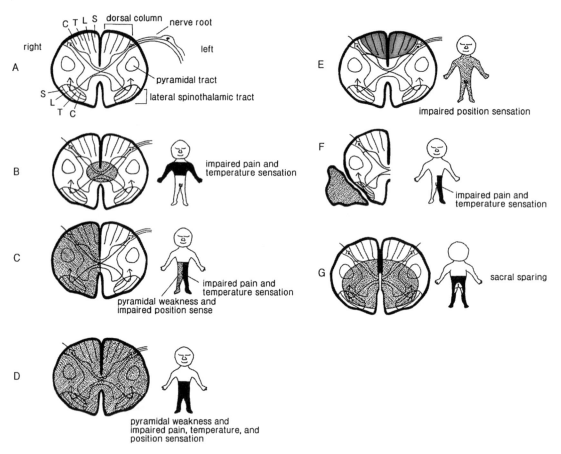

Figure 23-8. Various sensory syndromes caused by spinal cord lesions (shaded area). (T = thoracic; L = lumbar; C = cervical; S = sacral.)

Spinal Cord Level

Lesions affecting the spinal cord produce a variety of sensory syndromes according to their location as a result of distinctly arranged sensory tracts in this structure (Figure 23-8A). When the lesion involves the central region of the cord, loss of pain and thermal sensation over particular segments occurs because of bilateral interruption of the decussating second-order axons (Figure 23-8B). This so-called commissural sensory syndrome is caused by intra-axial spinal cord diseases such as syrinx, tumor, demyelinating diseases, or hemorrhages. As the lesion enlarges, other symptoms are added as adjacent structures are involved. A unilateral lesion affecting one-half of the cord would produce ipsilateral dorsal column sensory deficit and contralateral loss of pain and temperature

because of involvement of the already crossed spinothalamic tract and yet uncrossed dorsal column fibers (Figure 23-8C). Ipsilateral motor weakness also develops owing to involvement of the already crossed (at the caudal medulla) descending pyramidal tract. In clinical practice, however, this so-called Brown-Sequard syndrome is usually incomplete.

When the entire spinal cord is dissected, sensory loss of all modalities occurs below certain dermatomal levels and is associated with concomitant motor weakness below the level (Figure 23-8D). The sensory level is usually two segments below the actual lesion because pain and temperature fibers travel rostrally in Lissauer's tract for a few segments above their entry zone before decussating to the opposite spinothalamic tract (see Figure 23-2). A lesion preferentially affecting the dorsal column of the cord would produce a selective loss of lemniscal sensory modality (Figure 23-8E). Tabes dorsalis and subacute combined degeneration are notable examples. In the spinothalamic tract, the neurons are arranged in a way that fibers carrying sensation from the sacral, lumbar, thoracic, and cervical areas are located from outside to inward (see Figure 23-8A). Therefore, when a lesion is located extra-axially and compresses the cord from outside, the sacral area becomes most vulnerable and a sensory level may develop far below the actually involved site (Figure 23-8F). Examples are expanding bony lesions (e.g., tuberculoma) and various extra-axial tumors (e.g., meningioma, neurofibroma, and metastatic tumors). On the other hand, the sacral area becomes least vulnerable and tends to be spared in patients with a lesion expanding from inside the cord (e.g., syrinx, demyelinating diseases, and glioma) (Figure 23-8G).

Medulla Level

In the brain, the medulla oblongata is the only region where the tracts of two different sensory systems are widely separated: The medial lemniscus is situated medially and the spinothalamic tract is situated laterally. Therefore, a small medullary lesion usually results in a selective sensory deficit of one modality. In the lateral-dorsal area, descending trigeminal roots and nuclei are located. An infarction involving a dorsolateral part of the medulla (lateral medullary syndrome) is a relatively common type of stroke. The lesion often produces a characteristic ipsilateral trigeminal and contralateral body/limb sensory deficit as a result of concomitant involvement of the ascending spinothalamic tract and the ipsilateral descending trigeminal tract/nuclei (Figure 23-9A,B). This dissociated sensory pattern along with selective spinothalamic sensory impairment is nearly pathognomonic for lateral medullary lesions. However, lesions situated medially and ventrally would produce contralateral trigeminal sensory symptoms because of involvement of the secondary ascending trigeminal fibers (see Figures 23-9B,C). Large lesions involving both the ipsilateral descending and contralateral ascending trigeminal fibers may cause bilateral trigeminal symptoms (see Figure

23-9A–C). Lesions involving the most medial portion of the medulla (medial medullary syndrome) characteristically produce a dysfunction of lemniscal sensory modality (decreased position and vibration) because of selective involvement of the medial lemniscus (Figure 23-9D). Hemiparesis also develops because of involvement of the pyramidal tract. Sensory symptoms occur in the side contralateral to the lesion when the lesion is situated above the decussation (internal arcuate fibers). However, a lesion located below the crossing fibers may produce ipsilateral sensory symptoms.

Pons-Thalamus Level

In the pons and midbrain, the ascending trigeminal tract, the medial lemniscus, and the spinothalamic tract are located adjacently in the medial-lateral direction in the tegmentum (see Figure 23-9). Thus, lesions affecting the sensory pathway above the medulla usually result in sensory deficits of all modalities in the contralateral half of the body, including the face. A small stroke selectively involving the sensory pathway occasionally produces a pure hemisensory deficit without other neurologic dysfunction (pure sensory stroke). It is most commonly caused by a small infarction (lacuna) involving the VP nucleus of the thalamus (Figure 23-10). However, small lesions in the area of the pontine tegmentum or capsular-corona radiata can also produce pure sensory stroke. Although one-half of the body is usually affected, the sensory deficit may occur in only a part of the body when the lesion is very small. This restricted sensory syndrome most often, although not exclusively, occurs at the perioral area, the palm-fingers, and the toes, which may be explained by the proximity of areas representing the lips and fingers and the relatively large representation area of these acral body parts in the human sensory pathway (see Figures 23-2 and 23-3). The sensory symptoms limited to the perioral area and palm-fingers have been called *cheiro-oral syndrome.*

Cortical Level

Lesions involving the cortex characteristically produce an impairment of discriminative sensations that require cortical participation. Therefore,

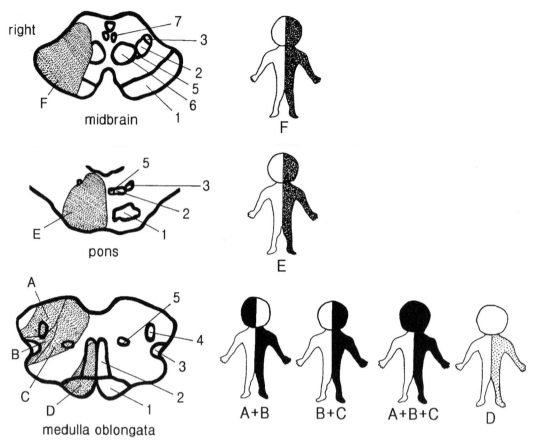

Figure 23-9. Patterns of sensory dysfunction caused by brain stem lesions (shaded area). (Black area = decreased spinothalamic sensation; lightly dotted area = decreased lemniscal sensation; heavily dotted area = decreased spinothalamic and lemniscal sensation; 1 = pyramidal tract; 2 = medial lemniscus; 3 = spinothalamic tract; 4 = descending trigeminal root/nuclei; 5 = ascending secondary trigeminal tract; 6 = red nucleus; 7 = oculomotor nucleus.)

patients with parietal lobe lesions typically show loss of position sense, elevation of the two-point discrimination threshold, and difficulties in localizing touch and pain stimuli (topagnosia). In addition, they fail to recognize the letters or numbers drawn on the skin (graphesthesia) and cannot appreciate the texture, size, and shape of objects by palpation (astereognosis) despite preserved perception of primitive sensation (pain, temperature, vibration). In some patients, however, primitive sensation is heavily affected and symptoms mimicking thalamic disease can be seen (pseudothalamic syndrome). Nevertheless, concomitant cortical symptoms such as aphasia, anosognosia, or acalculia are usually present in patients with cortical lesions. Because somatotopic representation of body parts is widely spread in the sensory cortex, small cortical lesions occasionally produce sensory symptoms in restricted areas of the arm, leg, or even a few fingertips that may lead inexperienced physicians to make a wrong diagnosis of a root or peripheral nerve disease. Finally, lesions of the sensory cortex may produce irritative symptoms such as sensory seizures.

Hysteria

Patients with hysteria often present with confusing sensory symptoms. Examples include sensory loss in distal parts of the limbs mimicking polyneuropathy and exact hemisensory changes simulating a thalamic lesion. Because routine sensory examination must rely on the subjective response of a patient, it is often difficult to differentiate hysteria from organic disorders. However, there are several clues to the diagnosis of hysteria. Generally, the sensory topography of the patient's complaints does not fit with anatomic knowledge. The area of sensory changes in the distal limbs usually has an abrupt line of demarcation between the normal and affected area, in contrast to peripheral neuropathy, where the sensory changes are gradual. More important, careful history taking almost always reveals that they have accompanying psychoneurotic symptoms that are associated with an intensely stressful environment.

Sequelae of Sensory Loss

When there is severe loss of pain and temperature sensation, the patient is prone to trauma or burning. Repeated injury to the anesthetic area may cause trophic ulcers and deformity of the hands or feet (Charcot's joint). A patient with loss of position sensation often has considerable difficulties in executing manual work despite normal motor strength because of deficient sensory feedback in the sensory-motor circuitry of the central nervous system. When stretching the arms devoid of position sense, the patient's fingers may wander or drift, especially when the eyes are closed. Sometimes, almost continuous purposeless movements are seen in the fingers (pseudoathetosis). Without proper position sense of the feet in relation to the ground, the subject tends to lift the feet unusually high and bang them down heavily (steppage gait). The subject also shows severe imbalance when the eyes are closed (Romberg's sign). When tested with meticulous tools, subtle discriminative sensory disturbances are commonly present in patients with cerebral lesions even when conventional sensory examination has shown normal findings. Discriminant sensory dysfunction of some modalities occasionally occurs bilaterally. This sensory deficit may be responsible, at least in part, for the clumsiness of these patients. Recent studies have provided evidence that sensory training can be of help in improving a patient's motor execution.

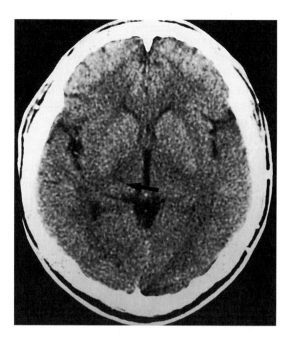

Figure 23-10. A computed tomographic scan showing a small infarct probably involving the ventral posterior nucleus of the right thalamus (*arrow*). The patient had a hemisensory deficit on the left side without other neurologic symptoms (pure sensory stroke).

One of the most troublesome sequelae of a sensory deficit resulting from a cerebral lesion is the gradual development of uncomfortable, distressful, sometimes painful paresthesias over the affected body parts. The exact pathogenesis for this symptom remains unclear. Although it has most often been described in patients with thalamic lesions (thalamic pain syndrome), nonthalamic lesions affecting the sensory pathway can also produce similar symptoms. Thus the term *central poststroke pain* is more appropriate. This distressing symptom may be modified by medications such as carbamazepine or amitriptyline but is occasionally intractable to any treatment.

Pain

Physiology

Pain is a common and disturbing example of sensory system dysfunction and deserves special mention. Although it is considered a warning signal against a danger, severe or long-lasting pain remains a great problem in medicine. What we call pain includes various sensations such as pricking, burning, aching, and soreness. The subjective intensity of pain is different among individuals, and even in the same individual it may vary widely according to circumstances. For example, the intensity of pain can be suppressed by joy and augmented by depression. Wounded soldiers often do not feel pain in the midst of the battle, but report pain afterward. Thus, what we perceive as pain is a combined effect of multiple and complex pain-provoking and pain-modulating pathways in the human nervous system rather than a dysfunction of a single sensory tract.

The peripheral receptors of pain are free nerve endings lying in the skin or other organs. The types of stimuli required to activate free nerve endings differ among individual organs: pricking, cutting, or freezing for skin, distension for abdominal viscera, and ischemia for skeletal muscles. Whatever the stimuli are, damaged tissues produce various chemical substances, including bradykinin, prostaglandin, and histamine, that stimulate free nerve endings. As described above, the thinly myelinated or unmyelinated fibers carrying pain sensation enter the lateral aspect of the dorsal horn (Lissauer's tract) and excite the secondary neurons. At this level, afferent impulses in the thick myelinated fibers exert an inhibitory effect on the same neurons via activation of inhibitory interneurons in the substantia gelatinosa. The interaction between the excitatory and inhibitory effects determines the activity of the second-order neurons of the spinothalamic pathways. This mechanism forms the theoretical base of the so-called gate control theory; a reduction and enhancement of the activities of the large myelinated fibers open and close the gate, respectively, and regulate the degree of pain sensation.

However, there also are many levels of modulation of pain in the central nervous system. Animal experiments have shown that electrical stimulation of particular regions of the brain (e.g., gray matter surrounding the third ventricle, cerebral aqueduct, and fourth ventricle) results in profound analgesia. Furthermore, neurons in the periventricular and periaqueductal gray matter in the midbrain make excitatory connections with the rostroventral medulla, a region encompassing the serotonergic nucleus raphe magnus and the nucleus reticularis paragigantocellularis. Because these anatomic regions correspond to the effective sites of morphine and neurons in these regions have been found to make inhibitory connections in laminae I, II, and IV of the dorsal horn, it is now considered that opioid analgesics produce analgesia by activating the descending pain modulatory pathways. Recently, a variety of endogenous opioid peptides (endorphins) have been identified, which include enkephalins, dynorphins, and substances of the pro-opiomelanocortin family. The presence of these opioids and their receptors in the central nervous system appears to be related to the emotional and behavioral aspects of pain.

Clinical Considerations

Intracranially, pain-carrying fibers are prominent in the dura, the large vessels in the subarachnoid space, the venous plexus, and the sinuses. Lesions primarily affecting these pain-sensitive structures produce headache and include meningitis, subarachnoid hemorrhages, and sinusitis. However, brain parenchyma does not contain pain fibers, and a focal intra-parenchymal lesion does not produce headache unless it produces expansion of the parenchyma to affect extraparenchymal pain-sensitive structures. Chronic headache is one of the most common illnesses of human beings. Patients with chronic headache most often do not harbor visible structural intracranial lesions. The two most common varieties of chronic headache are migraine and tension headache. The former is characterized by intermittent episodes of pulsating headache associated with nausea and vomiting often preceded by a visual aura, and is thought to be related to cyclic vasoconstriction-vasodilation cascades. On the other hand, tension headache is characterized by a relatively constant, dull headache probably associated with sustained muscle contraction. Neuralgia indicates an intermittent, brief, lancinating pain, and is characteristically seen in patients with herpes zoster infection (postherpetic neuralgia) or in patients with trigeminal neuralgia (tic douloureux). Chronic back (cervical or lumbar area) pain resulting from degenerative changes in the bony spine, ligaments, and disc is another problem very commonly encountered in neurology clinics.

Any injury to the nerve, root, or spinal cord may produce pain. *Causalgia* is a term for the particularly unpleasant, often burning pain that follows injuries in these structures. The involved skin area becomes shiny and shows various signs of autonomic dysfunction, suggesting that autonomic dysfunction may play a role in the pathogenesis of this yet poorly understood phenomenon. Sometimes patients may suffer from limb pain even after an amputation. They feel that the pain actually arises from a part of the missing limb (phantom limb pain), which suggests that a topographic image of the missing limb still exists in the brain. Finally, diseases of the viscera, especially distension of the organ, often produce pain in the skin area that has an identical dermatomal distribution. This so-called referred pain can be explained by the following: The visceral afferents converge on the same cells in the posterior horns as the somatic afferents, and the neurons subserving pain in the dorsal horn are more easily activated by skin afferents than visceral fibers. In clinical practice, an understanding of the source of referred pain is important in the diagnosis of visceral disorders. For example, intermittent pain felt at the inner side of the left arm (T1–T2) can be a signal of cardiac pain that arises from the T1–T4 dermatome.

Suggested Reading

Adams RD, Victor M, Ropper AH. Principles of Neurology (6th ed). New York: McGraw-Hill, 1997;127–166.

Bassetti C, Bogousslavsky J. Sensory Disturbances. In J Bogousslavsky, L Caplan (eds), Stroke Syndromes. New York: Cambridge University Press, 1995;15–29.

Calne DB. Vibratory sense: a critical review. Brain 1966;89:723.

Carey LM. Somatosensory loss after stroke. Crit Rev Phys Rehab Med 1995;7:51.

Devor M. Pain mechanisms. Neuroscientist 1996;2:233.

Haerer AF. DeJong's Neurological Examination (5th ed). Philadelphia: Lippincott, 1992;41–84.

Fisher CM. Pure sensory stroke and allied condition. Stroke 1982;13:434.

Martin JH, Jessell TM, et al. Sensory Systems of the Brain: Sensation and Perception. In ER Kandel, J Schwartz, TM Jessell (eds), Principles of Neural Science (3rd ed). London: Prentice-Hall, 1991;326–529.

Kim JS. Pure sensory stroke: clinical-radiological correlates of 21 cases. Stroke 1992;23:983.

Kim JS, Choi-Kwon S. Discriminative sensory dysfunction after unilateral stroke. Stroke 1996;27:677.

Kim JS. Restricted acral sensory syndrome following minor stroke: further observation with special reference to differential severity of symptoms among individual digits. Stroke 1994;25:2497.

Leijon G, Boivie J, Johansson I. Central post-stroke pain-neurological symptoms and pain characteristics. Pain 1989;26:13.

Parent A. Carpenter's Human Neuroanatomy (9th ed). Baltimore: Williams & Wilkins, 1996;325–420.

Schott GD. From thalamic syndrome to central poststroke pain. J Neurol Neurosurg Psychiatry 1995;61:560.

Woolsey CN. Organization of Somatic Sensory and Motor Areas of the Cerebral Cortex. In HF Harlow, CN Woolsey (eds), Biological and Biochemial Bases of Behaviors. Madison, WI: University of Wisconsin Press, 1958;63–81.

Chapter 24
Agnosia, Apraxia, and Amnesia

Patrik Vuilleumier

Chapter Plan

Agnosias

Agnosias are disorders at the higher level of perception. The term refers to an impaired recognition of what is perceived in the presence of relatively intact elementary sensory processes, memory, language, and other general cognitive functions. Teuber defined agnosia "in its purest form as a normal percept that has somehow been stripped of its meaning." Agnosia may affect any sensory modality independently. Visual, auditory, and tactile agnosias are best known, each being related to damage in distinct regions of the brain. However, deficits of odor recognition with preserved olfactory sensation occur with dysfunction of the medial temporal lobe or the caudal orbitofrontal cortex, such as in Alzheimer's disease, head trauma, temporolimbic epilepsy, or surgical resection, as well as with damage to the dorsal medial nucleus of the thalamus, such as in Korsakoff's syndrome or stroke. Gustation is impaired after damage to the parietal operculi or medial thalamic nuclei.

Visual Agnosias

Neurophysiology has shown that different parts of the brain deal separately with different basic properties of the visual world, such as shape and contours, color, or movement. Visual secondary cortical areas are schematically separated in two distinct anatomofunctional systems: Occipitotemporal areas are specialized in the discrimination and identification of visual patterns and objects (ventral "what" system), whereas occipitoparietal areas process the spatial location and orientation of objects (dorsal "where" system). In addition, in humans, each hemisphere has distinct specializations. It follows that brain damage can impair selective aspects of vision and leave others intact.

Disorders of Form and Object Recognition

Behavioral Aspects. Patients with visual agnosia are unable to identify visually presented objects or images of objects. Visual field defects are usually present, but careful ophthalmologic examination should exclude gross impairment of elementary visual perception in the spared fields, such as acuity or brightness and contrast discrimination. The deficit can be shown by the patient's inability to name or point to presented objects on request, to describe or demonstrate their use, to sort them according to categories or other characteristics, or to provide any other explicit response indicating that he or she knows what the object is. Recognition is often worse for line drawings than for photographs and worse for photographs than for real objects because more cues such as size, surface texture, or shadows are available in the latter. Conversely, the patient may indicate he or she has an intact knowledge about unrecognized objects by providing accurate verbal definitions or descriptions to their names and by immediately recognizing them through other sensory channels. For instance, the patient would fail to identify a visually presented bunch of keys, but immediately recognize it by touch or by hearing its characteristic sound.

Two forms of visual agnosia have been commonly distinguished, which are part of a continuum rather than single and independent disorders. In *apperceptive agnosia*, recognition fails because elementary features of objects are not derived properly nor combined in a structured whole. It is basically a disorder of *form* recognition. In most severe cases, even simple geometric shapes are not recognized, and the patient may fail at tasks of length, size, surface, or orientation discrimination (Figure 24-1). Such patients cannot copy simple drawings or match them to samples. Discrimination of a figure against the background and identification of incomplete figures are markedly abnormal. Recognition is sometimes facilitated by motion of the stimulus, probably because motion perception has distinct neural substrates that allow a global structure to be derived from the coherent displacements of local features. In severe cases, patients may complain that their vision is "blurred" or "foggy" or behave as if they were blind; others may be anosognosic and deny their difficulties.

By contrast, in *associative agnosia* structural encoding of elementary visual features is relatively preserved, although well-perceived shapes remain meaningless for the patient. It is a disorder of *object* recognition proper, or "pure" agnosia in Teuber's sense. Typically, the patient can copy complex visual stimuli, such as object drawings, even though he or she does not recognize them.

A

Figure 24-1. Examples of common tests of visual recognition. (A) The Efron (1968) test requires discrimination between pairs of simple shapes matched for total surface area and contrast. (B) The Street (1944) completion test examines the perceptual closure of fragmented pictures. (C) The Poppelreuter (1917) overlapping figures and (D) the Luria (1965) crossed-out masked figures assess both the ability to extract meaningful shapes from the interfering background and the ability to perceive more than one object at a time. (E) Similar tests use words as stimuli.

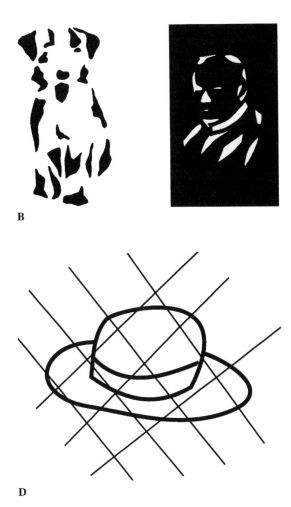

B

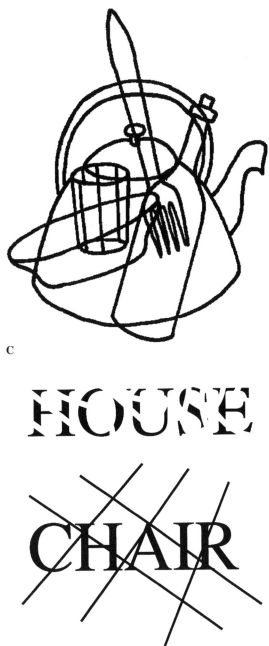

C

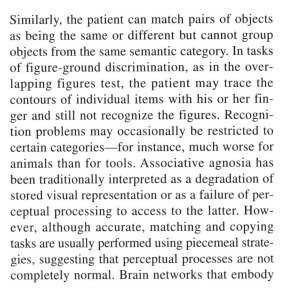

D

E

Similarly, the patient can match pairs of objects as being the same or different but cannot group objects from the same semantic category. In tasks of figure-ground discrimination, as in the overlapping figures test, the patient may trace the contours of individual items with his or her finger and still not recognize the figures. Recognition problems may occasionally be restricted to certain categories—for instance, much worse for animals than for tools. Associative agnosia has been traditionally interpreted as a degradation of stored visual representation or as a failure of perceptual processing to access to the latter. However, although accurate, matching and copying tasks are usually performed using piecemeal strategies, suggesting that perceptual processes are not completely normal. Brain networks that embody stored visual knowledge therefore might not be dissociated from those that subserve higher-level perceptual processing. *Visual mental imagery*, or the ability to conjure up visual images in the "mind's eye," also shares mechanisms and neural substrates with visual perception, and some patients show selective deficits in imagery (e.g., shapes, objects) that usually parallel their recognition disorder.

Associative visual agnosia must be distinguished from *optic aphasia*. In the latter, the patient is unable to name visually presented objects but can manifest that he or she recognizes them by correctly describing or mimicking their use. The ability to name objects through other sensory channels (e.g., touch or hearing) is preserved. The deficit can be interpreted as a disconnection between the left hemisphere lexicosemantic systems and the visual recognition systems, although the functional locus of the disconnection is still a matter of debate. In particular, the extent to which those patients may show an intact semantic knowledge of objects when they are presented visually is an unsettled question.

Anatomic and Etiologic Aspects.   Apperceptive agnosia is caused by widespread damage to the lateral and inferomedial aspects of the visual extrastriate cortices, most often after carbon monoxide poisoning, mercury intoxication, bilateral strokes in the territory of the posterior cerebral arteries, or anoxia after cardiac arrest. Many cases occur during recovery from cortical blindness. Rare cases are also associated with a slowly progressive posterior cortical atrophy caused by a focal variety of Alzheimer's disease or by another degenerative dementing disease without specific histologic features; most of those patients also eventually develop Balint's syndrome.

Associative agnosia may be caused by bilateral lesions as well as by unilateral left- or right-sided lesions involving the occipitotemporal regions, most often after a stroke in the territory of the posterior cerebral arteries or after herpes encephalitis. In unilateral cases, the fusiform, lingual, and parahippocampal gyri in the left medial occipitotemporal junction are commonly involved. This is consistent with positron emission tomography (PET) studies in normal subjects showing activation of the fusiform and middle temporal gyri on the left side as well as of the lateral occipitotemporal cortex on both sides during an object recognition task. Furthermore, it appears that the left hemisphere is specialized for processing local parts and the right hemisphere is specialized for processing global configurations of shapes. Whereas object recognition depends on a mixture of both types of representation, the former is most important for reading words and the latter for identifying faces, as revealed by unilateral damage that respectively leads to pure alexia or prosopagnosia.

Optic aphasia is seen with occipitotemporal or occipitoparietal lesions; a right homonymous hemianopia is always present, so that all visual information has to transit by the right hemisphere before accessing the left hemisphere language areas.

Disorders of Facial Recognition

Behavioral Aspects.   Perhaps because of their social relevance or their structural complexity and variety, faces have a special status in the visual environment and are processed by dedicated brain structures. In humans, whereas the left hemisphere plays a dominant role in language functions, the right hemisphere appears to be preferentially implicated in face processing.

Prosopagnosia represents an inability to recognize people by their face. The deficit may be unique to faces, or at least disproportionate with respect to other visual capabilities. It concerns faces previously known to the patient (e.g., close relatives, famous people, or his or her own face) as well as newly encountered faces (e.g., hospital staff). Knowledge about people and their biography, however, remains intact. The patient usually relies on nonfacial cues (e.g., the voice, gait, dress, wearing of eyeglasses) to recognize people he or she meets. Somehow schematically, as with object agnosia, two forms of prosopagnosia must be distinguished. In the apperceptive type, there is a deficit in the perceptual encoding of facial traits, and the patient cannot match pairs of faces (e.g., a same face pictured from different viewpoints or under different lighting). In the associative, or amnestic, type, there is either a disruption of the stored visual representation of known faces or a failure to activate them; the patient can match pairs of faces but cannot tell which are familiar from those that are not.

Perceptual encoding of facial traits is further fractionated in several independent components that appear to proceed in parallel pathways. Thus, although they fail in identifying or matching people's faces, most prosopagnosics can correctly discriminate their sex, race, and approximate age. Neither are they impaired in extracting facial information from lip-reading, perceiving the direction of gaze, and recognizing emotional expressions. Conversely, each of the latter capabilities may be selectively disturbed after focal lesions without concomitant prosopagnosia. The inability to recognize facial emotional expressions (in naming, pointing, or matching tasks) has been termed *prosopoaffective agnosia*, and it may occasionally predominate for some kinds of emotions rather than for others (e.g., happiness versus sadness or fear). In some cases, these deficits correlate with disturbances in subjective affective states or experiences.

A yet unexplained finding is that the behavior of some (but not all) prosopagnosics reveals an implicit recognition of familiar faces. For instance, even though patients deny they know anything about presented faces, they show differential electrodermal responses or evoked potentials to known and unknown faces and learn to associate a famous name with a face more successfully if the pairs are true than if they are untrue. However, forced-choice familiarity judgments are never above chance. Implicit recognition implies that stored visual representations of known faces are preserved but that the result of their activation does not reach awareness. Most often this has been observed in the apperceptive type of prosopagnosia, although exceptions exist.

Another issue is whether the deficit is really confined to faces or whether it extends to other visual categories made of a large number of individual exemplars that are perceptually similar. Some prosopagnosics are unable to recognize the various species of birds, dogs, flowers, trees, or makes of cars. Stock farmer patients have been reported who could no longer recognize their own cows. Because face recognition depends on the evocation of specific contextual memories related to one particular individual within a generic category, it has been argued that prosopagnosics were also unable to discriminate buildings with a unique individuality (e.g., the Kremlin or the Paris Pantheon) or their own belongings among other similar exemplars (e.g., one's glasses, razor, car). However, several studies supported the specificity of faces.

Anatomic and Etiologic Aspects.   PET studies in normal subjects showed that face identification activates the right parahippocampal gyrus as well as the fusiform and lingual gyri and the anterior temporal cortex on both sides. Accordingly, prosopagnosia is caused by bilateral or unilateral right-sided damage to the medial and inferior temporo-occipital cortex. Right-sided lesions are critical but explanatory only in some individuals. An interruption of association fibers in the inferior longitudinal fasciculus combined with damage to the inferotemporal cortex (areas 20/21/37) might be crucial in the associative type, whereas the lesions extend to more lateral parts of the right extrastriate visual cortices (areas 18/19) in the apperceptive type. Damage can be caused by posterior cerebral artery infarction, hematoma, trauma, tumor, encephalitis, or a rare progressive temporal atrophy of unknown origin. Some cases of congenital prosopagnosia have been reported.

The neural substrates of implicit recognition have not elucidated, but it has been argued that intact connections between the occipital cortex and the cingulate or ventromedial frontal areas might be required, perhaps via the dorsal occipitoparietal pathways. Damage to those connections in the presence of intact ventral occipitotemporal pathways might be present in delusional misidentification disorders, such as Capgras' syndrome or Frégoli's syndrome, in which facial discrimination is impaired and recognition preserved for identity but not familiarity.

Prosopoaffective agnosia is more frequent and severe after right hemisphere lesions, especially those involving the posterior temporal cortex in the vicinity of the superior temporal sulcus, but it is also found with damage to the amygdala or to the ventral frontal lobe, with Parkinson's disease and Huntington's disease, affective disorders, and schizophrenia. Neurons sensitive to gaze directions are found in the superior temporal sulcus and the amygdala in monkeys, and lesions to the latter structures may cause corresponding deficits in humans.

Disorders of Color Recognition

Behavioral Aspects.   Brain damage can result in a variety of disorders in color processing; see Table 24-1 for a summary of differential features.

Table 24-1. Characteristics of Color Processing Disorders

Tests	Achromatopsia	Color Imagery Disorder	Color Agnosia	Color Anomia
Color discrimination	↓	✓	✓	✓
Color categorization	↓	✓	(↓)	✓
Mental color comparisons	✓	↓	(↓)	✓
Colored objects fluency	✓	↓	↓	✓
Color names fluency	✓	✓	✓	(↓)
Color naming	↓	✓	✓	↓
Color pointing	↓	✓	✓	(↓)
Verbal-verbal color-object associations	✓	↓	↓	(↓)
Visual-visual color-object associations	↓	✓	↓	✓

↓ = performance typically impaired; ✓ = performance normal; (↓) performance variably impaired.

Central achromatopsia is a loss of color perception and must be distinguished from congenital (inherited) color blindness. Full-field achromatopsia is rare; most often color imperception affects only part of the visual field (a quadrant or hemifield). Patients usually report that objects appear in various shades of gray. Minor dyschromatopsia is a more frequent disorder in which fine color discrimination is impaired, and it can be shown in color-sorting tasks such as matching similar hues or arranging a smooth gradation of colors.

Many patients with achromatopsia (but not all) have an impairment in the *mental imagery of colors*—that is, an inability to imagine colors in their "mind's eye." They cannot answer questions about the color of well-known objects such as "What is the color of a watermelon?" Likewise, they cannot perform mental color comparisons such as "Do mint and parsley have the same or different color?" Mental imagery of other attributes of objects, such as their form, is intact, however, as is the recognition of correctly colored objects from improperly colored ones. Similar defects in color mental imagery may exist with unimpaired color perception.

In *color agnosia*, color perception is preserved but knowledge about color associations is impaired, such as knowing the usual color of objects. It has been also referred to as "color amnesia." This is best shown in visual-visual associative tests: The patient fails to match the appropriate colors to uncolored line drawings of objects or to point to the correct drawing out of a multiple choice of differently colored ones (e.g., choose between gray versus pink elephants). Verbal-verbal associative tests are also impaired (e.g., "What is the color of a watermelon?" or "What are some things that are green?"), but defects in color mental imagery or color naming can result in similar impairment. In some cases, color agnosia has also been used to describe an impairment in the *categorization of colors*—that is, an inability to sort different hues into a few groups of related colors in the absence of a disturbance in hue discrimination. The relationships between color agnosia, color imagery, and color categorization defects are still ill-defined.

Color anomia is a failure to label visually presented colors with their specific name; naming of mentally imagined colors and lexical fluency for color names (e.g., "say as many color words as you can") may be also impaired. However, color discrimination and knowledge about the color of objects are intact, at least as long as attempts to verbalize answers are avoided; the ability to name objects is preserved. It is therefore a selective visual-verbal disconnection. *Color aphasia* refers to similar patients who additionally fail to point to the correct colors when given their names. By contrast, the ability to name colors and comprehension of color names tend to be relatively preserved in most patients with aphasia.

Anatomic and Etiologic Aspects. The middle third of the lingual gyrus contralateral to the affected visual field is the most common site of damage in achromatopsia, which corresponds to the region activated by colored stimuli in PET studies of normal subjects and could represent the human homolog of area V4 in monkeys. Damage to the white matter immediately behind the posterior tip of the lateral ventricle is also common. Achromatopsia is often associated with prosopagnosia, topographic agnosia, or pure alexia. Minor forms of dyschromatopsia follow damage to other posterior cortical areas and tend to be more frequent with right-sided than with left-sided lesions.

Color anomia is caused by lesions in the left mesial occipitotemporal region centered on the anterior lingual and posterior parahippocampal gyri, just underneath the splenium of the corpus callosum, in such a way that they produce a right hemianopia by concomitant damage to the optic radiations and prevent the transfer of all visual color information to the left hemisphere's language areas. In cases of color anomia with pure alexia, there is additional damage in the deep paraventricular white matter of the left occipital lobe involving fibers from the inferior forceps major of the corpus callosum, whereas in the rare cases of pure alexia without color anomia, the left mesial occipitotemporal region appears to be spared.

Color agnosia and loss of color imagery are both caused by left inferior temporo-occipital damage, but precise anatomic correlations are lacking. PET studies in normal subjects have shown that evoking the colors of objects produces a left-predominant activation of fusiform gyri. Color anomia and color agnosia are commonly associated with pure alexia as well as one with the other. Besides cases with focal posterior lesions, such as in strokes or tumors, color agnosia may be part of a more global semantic disorder, as in Alzheimer's disease.

Related Disorders

Visuospatial disorders refers to a variety of disturbances in the perception of spatial locations and spatial relationships. These can be assessed by several tasks, such as having the patient judge the relative positions of objects or single points in space (e.g., single or multiple dots on cards) or discriminate the relative orientation of straight lines. Some spatial disorders are supramodal in nature and can be demonstrated in tactile and audi-tory modalities. They are strongly correlated with right parietal damage.

Akinetopsia is a selective impairment in the ability to recognize the motion of objects, which can be complete after bilateral damage to the parieto-temporo-occipital region at the junction between areas 19 and 37 (area MT or V5) or partial and ipsidirectional after unilateral damage. Visual acuity and other shape discrimination abilities are intact.

Topographical (or environmental) agnosia is an inability to recognize familiar places and find one's way in surroundings without a more global impairment of memory. This can arise from several mechanisms: a perceptual type, in which previously known buildings and landmarks cannot be discriminated; a specific mnesic type, in which familiar places cannot be recognized from unfamiliar places; and a spatial type, in which familiar places are recognized but their locations and relationships in space cannot be recalled or retained. Such disorders have been observed with a variety of lesions, specifically those involving the medial temporo-occipital lobe and the parahippocampal gyrus in the right hemisphere, the posterior parietal lobe, or the right cingulate cortex.

Auditory Agnosia

Behavioral Aspects

Patients with auditory agnosia are unable to recognize sounds even though they have adequate hearing and no significant audiometric loss. While tape-recorded material is required for precise assessment of basic auditory perception (i.e., click fusion, tone, pitch, and interval discrimination), bedside testing can use common objects or a portable tape player. Depending on the type of auditory material predominantly involved, four distinct syndromes can occur, either independently or in various combinations.

In *sound agnosia*, the patient is impaired in identifying common nonverbal environmental sounds, such as crumpling up a sheet of paper, shaking a bunch of keys, a telephone ringing, animal screams, and so on. Recognition can be tested by naming or matching pictures to heard sounds. As in visual agnosias, two forms are distinguished. In the acoustic-discriminative type, errors are made between acoustically related sounds (e.g., the sound of a cat meowing mistaken for the sound of a crying baby), whereas in the semantic-associative type, errors concern semantically related sound sources (e.g., the sound of a plane take-off mistaken for the sound of a train). The latter form is usually associated with language disturbances and part of a general semantic disorder, as it can be shown in other associative word-picture or picture-picture matching tasks.

Although music perception is impaired to some extent in most cases of auditory sound agnosia, a disproportionate difficulty in discriminating or recognizing melodies is referred to as *sensory (or receptive) amusia*. Music perception, however, is a multicomponent process. Two broad classes of abilities, at least, contribute to music recognition and each may be independently disrupted: These are "instant" perceptual processes, governing judgments of pitch, timbre, harmony, and intensity; and "sequential" time-dependent processes, governing judgments of rhythm and duration, as well as recognition of melody. Some investigators therefore have made the distinction between amelodia and arrhythmia. In normal subjects, the melodic contour is most determinant for tune recognition. Processing of musical information is clearly influenced by the individuals' pre-illness competencies, and musicians can use analytic strategies and local cues that are unavailable to nonmusicians. Expressive amusia, or an inability to sing, is not necessarily associated with a receptive disorder.

Pure word deafness is an auditory agnosia restricted to verbal material in the presence of otherwise intact language. The patient is unable to understand any spoken word but can read, speak, and write in a practically normal manner. The severely impaired comprehension in some cases of Wernicke's aphasia may represent a "nonpure" word deafness. Problems with temporal resolution and phonemic discrimination appear to be the prominent disturbance in these patients. They can, however, improve their comprehension with lip-reading, and some are unimpaired in understanding the paralinguistic aspects of speech, such as intonation (i.e., prosody) and vocal identity.

In contrast, disorders of auditory recognition can selectively affect paralinguistic aspects of speech. *Affective auditory agnosia* impairs the ability to understand the emotional prosody of speech (e.g., happiness) with no concomitant defect in understanding propositional content or grammatical intonations (e.g., interrogative tone). Similarly, *phonagnosia* impairs the discrimination or the identification of familiar known voices. However, it remains to be seen whether these disorders are truly agnosic in nature.

Anatomic and Etiologic Aspects

Sound objects are processed in distinct parallel systems. The right hemisphere deals with nonverbal sound patterns and seems to be specialized for fine perceptual discrimination abilities, whereas the left hemisphere is involved in decoding linguistic sounds and other sequentially organized material, and attributes meaning to perceived sounds. Environmental sound agnosia of the acoustic type occurs after unilateral right hemisphere damage, specifically centered on the posterior part of the superior temporal gyrus (areas 22/41/42)—that is, the primary and association auditory cortices. Sound agnosia of the semantic type can occur with unilateral damage of the homologous areas in the left hemisphere. Combined discriminative and semantic deficiencies have been found with unilateral right or bilateral lesions.

Both hemispheres contribute to the processing of music, with the right hemisphere dominant for "instant" sound patterns, such as pitch and timbre, and the left hemisphere dominant for rhythm patterns and intervals. In normal subjects, dichotic listening tasks show a left ear advantage in the identification of melodies for nonmusicians but more variable asymmetries for musicians. Whereas patients with amusia most often have bilateral temporal lesions, left hemisphere damage is more disruptive for recognition of the local and time-dependent aspects of melodies, while right hemisphere damage can impair recognition of both local aspects and global melodic contours.

Pure word deafness may result from two possible loci of damage. Most often, it is caused by bilateral cortical and subcortical lesions involving the anterior or the middle part of the superior temporal gyri of both hemispheres with some sparing of Heschl's gyri. Occasionally, it follows a single lesion in the dominant temporal lobe involving the primary auditory cortex or the ipsilateral auditory radiations from the medial geniculate nucleus, together with the callosal fibers from the contralateral auditory areas. Both instances result in a disconnection of Wernicke's language area from auditory input. Auditory affective agnosia and phonagnosia have both been described after damage to the right hemisphere in the temporoparietal junction region, somehow homologous to Wernicke's area. However, one PET study in normal subjects showed activation of the right prefrontal cortex during a task of emotional prosody discrimination.

Tactile Agnosia

As in other modalities, recognition of forms and objects by touch may fail in the absence of disturbances of elementary somatosensory perception (*astereognosis*) or even more complex somatosensory functions such as weight, size, texture, and simple shapes discrimination (*tactile agnosia*). These disorders result from damage to the primary and secondary somatosensory association cortices in the parietal lobe, respectively. Damage to the dorsomedial parietal lobe also impairs tactile recognition by disrupting skillful manipulative and exploratory movements (*palpatory apraxia*). The disorders above must be distinguished from tactile anomia—that is, an inability to name palpated objects that are nonetheless correctly recognized and handled, usually affecting the left hand and caused by callosal disconnection.

Apraxias

Apraxia refers to disorders of higher level motor behavior. It is defined as an inability to perform learned, skilled, and purposeful movements that is not caused by an elementary motor, sensory, extrapyramidal, or cerebellar dysfunction and not accounted for by severe attention or comprehension difficulties. However, in certain instances, apraxia may coexist with more elementary defects. There are several distinct apraxic disorders.

Limb Apraxia

Behavioral Aspects

Melokinetic (or kinetic) apraxia refers to a disproportionate difficulty in making precise or finely graded intentional movements of any kind (e.g., picking up a coin from the tabletop, producing a rhythm, moving a single finger up and down). The initiation of movement appears delayed and effortful, and its execution decomposed and awkward. There is no automatic-voluntary dissociation. Also termed "executional" or "motor" apraxia, kinetic apraxia probably represents impaired sequencing of elementary motor control. Therefore, it is sometimes disregarded as a "true" apraxia.

Ideomotor apraxia is by far the most important type of limb apraxia. It refers to a disruption of movements involved in specific purposeful gestures, dexterity being normal. It is tested by having the patient perform both meaningful and meaningless gestures (Table 24-2). Meaningful gestures can be transitive (i.e., using an object) or intransitive (i.e., symbolic or communicative signs). Meaningless gestures can be unimanual or bimanual. If possible, both the right hand and left hand should be tested independently. Testing should include the following conditions: pantomime made to a verbal request (e.g., "pretend to comb your hair"); imitation of pantomime performed by the examiner; pantomime in response to visually presented objects without actually using them (e.g., "pretend to use this"); and actual handling and use of objects (i.e., tactile presentation). Finally, recognition of pantomime performed by the examiner and discrimination between correct and incorrect gestures may be assessed. Ideomotor apraxia is frequently associated with aphasia. However, except in Wernicke's aphasia, the apraxic disorder is often disproportionate to the comprehension difficulties.

The hallmark of ideomotor apraxia is a failure to pantomime meaningful gestures to verbal requests with moderate or no improvement to imitation. Performance variably improves with use of actual objects, although the same gestures are typically performed flawlessly in the natural setting of daily life activities (automatic-voluntary dissociation). Imitation of meaningless gestures is usually similarly impaired; however, dissociation may occur, some patients being impaired on meaningless but not meaningful gestures and vice versa. Rarely, a patient may pantomime worse to imitation than to command (termed *conduction apraxia* in reference to conduction aphasia, in which repetition problems predominate) or worse to visually presented objects (*optic apraxia*). Various apraxic errors can be

Table 24-2. Examples of Gestures Used to Test Limb Apraxia*

Transitive Meaningful Gestures	Intransitive Meaningful Gestures	Meaningless Gestures
Comb one's hair	Wave good-bye	Unimanual
Brush teeth	Beckon "come here"	Hand under chin
Eat with a spoon	Cross oneself	Back of hand on ear
Drink with a glass	Gesture for silence, hush	Fist on head
Use a hammer	Military salute	Hand on shoulder
Use a screwdriver	Scold, threaten	Thumb to little finger
Use scissors	Thumb one's nose	Bimanual
Cut bread, saw a branch	Show someone is crazy	Double ring with fingers
Open a door with a key	Hitchhike	Backs of left and right hands next to each other
Open a bottle	Gesture that it is OK, all going well	Left- and right-hand fingers next to each other
		Left-hand forefinger to right-hand middle finger
		Butterfly-shaped crossed hands

*Apraxia of the lower limbs occasionally may also be tested with appropriate gestures (e.g., pedaling, shooting a ball, stubbing out a cigarette).

observed: substitutions or parapraxia (e.g., hammering instead of combing), perseverations, incorrect posturing or orientation of the hand, disrupted temporal sequencing, or body part used as an object (e.g., hammering with a clenched fist). Often, the intended goal and the axial-proximal part of the movement are recognizable, suggesting that the concept of the gesture is spared but cannot activate the appropriate motor program. Some normal subjects may make a few "body part as object" errors, which should be corrigible.

Ideational apraxia refers to two different disorders. In one, acceptation, it is a failure to carry out the correct sequence of acts in order to perform a given action. This can be assessed by having the patient pantomime familiar actions or execute them with actual objects (e.g., put a letter in an envelope, light a candle, prepare a cup of tea). Such patients also fail to arrange drawings that depict the steps of an action in a correct sequence. In the second acceptation, ideational apraxia is a disturbance in the knowledge of the use of real objects (conceptual apraxia, or agnosia of usage). The patient is unable to demonstrate correct gestures, to describe functions of tools, or to recall correct tool-object associations (e.g., nail with hammer rather than nail with screwdriver). It appears as a selective action–related semantic disorder. Ideomotor apraxia is commonly present, with predominant content or substitution

errors, and no improvement occurs with actual objects in comparison with pantomime.

Comprehension of mimicked gestures and matching drawings of objects with the associated typical gestures may be impaired with or without concomitant ideational or ideomotor apraxia (pantomime agnosia).

Anatomic and Etiologic Aspects

It is believed that representations of skilled and learned purposeful movements are stored in the brain as three-dimensional supramodal programs, or "formulas," which encode the specific spatiotemporal patterns of complex movements (also termed "visuokinesthetic engrams"), and that the left inferior parietal lobe in the vicinity of the supramarginal gyrus is the depository of those representations in most right-handed human subjects. To perform goal-directed gestures, formulas in the left parietal lobe have to be activated and transmitted to the supplementary motor areas and premotor cortices on both sides, which in turn mediate the programming and sequencing of corresponding innervatory inputs to the primary motor areas.

Anatomofunctional correlates of kinetic apraxia are unclear. It is usually unilateral and might be related to contralateral disturbances in the pathways connecting the supplementary motor and sensory areas, premotor cortex, and basal ganglia. It is common in corticobasal degeneration, in which it usually constitutes the presenting symptom. Some elements of kinetic apraxia are also found in other basal ganglia disorders (e.g., Parkinson's disease and Huntington's disease), and complex sensory loss after posterior parietal damage produces a similar disorder (corresponding to Luria's afferent kinesthetic apraxia).

Ideomotor apraxia is bilateral and, in right-handers, almost always caused by left hemisphere lesions. In patients with a right hemiparesis, it can be seen best on the left hand (ipsilateral sympathetic apraxia). Aphasia (any type) most often co-occurs, but the two disorders can be dissociated. The responsible lesions (e.g., stroke) can involve cortical and subcortical structures in the left suprasylvian/perirolandic region, the paraventricular white matter adjacent and superior to the body of the lateral ventricle, or the left medial frontal region including the supplementary motor area. Damage to associative fibers in the superior longitudinal (arcuate) fasciculus or the superior occipitofrontal fasciculus, respectively connecting posterior language and visual areas with anterior premotor areas, probably plays a critical role. Lesions confined to the basal ganglia without additional involvement of the white matter do not cause ideomotor apraxia, whereas thalamic lesions (in the lateral and posterior nuclei) might do so. It has been proposed that patients with parietal damage have both apraxia and impaired recognition of gestures because of a degradation in the "formula" representations, whereas patients with more anterior, subcortical, or frontal lesions have apraxia with preserved recognition of gestures. Parietal damage also results in mental imagery defects that are selective for hand movements (i.e., an inability to mentally simulate and predict the timing of gestures without other visual imagery impairment).

Ideomotor apraxia is common but usually occurs late in the course of Alzheimer's disease, whereas it is an early sign in corticobasal degeneration and other dementias with posterior focal cortical atrophy of unknown origin, specifically if there is a left-predominant parietal involvement. In the latter, occasional cases may present as an isolated slowly progressive apraxia.

Some patients with right hemisphere lesions are impaired in imitating meaningless but not meaningful gestures, which can be related to a right hemisphere contribution in the control of gestures or difficulties in spatial orientation. In left-handers, ideomotor apraxia is often caused by right hemisphere lesions.

Ideational apraxia of the conceptual type has been reported with focal lesions in the left posterior temporoparietal and angular gyrus region as well as in advanced Alzheimer's disease. Consistently, PET studies have shown an activation of the left posterior middle and superior temporal gyri when normal subjects evoke the action associated with a given object. Ideational apraxia of the sequential type is associated with widespread frontal damage (e.g., head trauma), confusional states, and also Alzheimer's disease.

Damage to the corpus callosum (genu or trunk) disconnects the right motor cortex from language and praxic networks of the left hemisphere and results in unilateral ideomotor apraxia of the left hand. It is most severe with verbal commands, may improve in imitation with genu lesions (disassociation apraxia) but not with trunk lesions, and may or may not be associated with a unilateral ideational-conceptual apraxia.

Orofacial Apraxia

Behavioral Aspects

As in ideomotor apraxia of the limbs, intentional and purposeful bucco-linguo-facial movements may be disproportionately impaired in the absence of elementary motor loss. Lip, tongue, face, or eyelid movements as well as respiratory movements are usually affected. As in limb apraxia, meaningless and meaningful, transitive and nontransitive movements must be tested to verbal command and to imitation (Table 24-3). Typically, patients produce only rough approximations of the requested action, substitutions, or perseverations. Automatic-voluntary dissociation is common—for instance, a patient who fails in pretending to blow out a match or blow a kiss may succeed when a match or the hand, respectively, is brought close to his or her mouth. Comprehension of orofacial gestures is rarely assessed but may be impaired. Ideomotor limb and orofacial apraxia are associated in one-third of the patients or they occur independently in another one-third each. Orofacial apraxia is fre-

Table 24-3. Examples of Gestures Used to Test Orofacial Apraxia

Transitive Meaningful Gestures	Intransitive Meaningful Gestures	Meaningless Gestures
Bucco-linguo-facial movements		
Blow out a match	Whistle	Open mouth
Suck on a straw	Yawn	Stick out tongue
Smoke a cigarette	Frown	Puff out cheeks
Kiss	Wink	Click tongue
Lick one's lip	Wrinkle forehead as if surprised	"Tut-tut"
Respiratory movements		
Sniff	Pant as if exhausted	Breathe in deeply
Cough	Clear throat	Breathe out fully

quently associated with nonfluent aphasia, occurring in 90% of Broca's aphasics, but, again, reciprocal dissociations are found. It is distinct from speech apraxia, a linguistic disorder of the articulation and sequencing of phonemes similar to anarthria.

Anatomic and Etiologic Aspects

Critical lesions (e.g., stroke, tumor, trauma) involve the frontal and central opercular cortex, the anterior insula, or the anterior paraventricular white matter. Focal cortical degenerative diseases (e.g., corticobasal degeneration, primary progressive aphasia) may present with a slowly progressive orofacial apraxia, usually accompanied by speech difficulties (anarthria). In children, orofacial apraxia and speech disturbances are seen in developmental dysplasia of the opercular cortex as well as in autosomal dominant or sporadic cases of rolandic epilepsy.

Orofacial apraxia must be distinguished from Foix-Chavany-Marie syndrome caused by bilateral anterior opercular damage, in which all voluntary orofacial movements are impaired although automatic movements are preserved.

Constructional Apraxia

Behavioral Aspects

Constructional (or visuoconstructive) disorders appear as a failure to organize component parts in a definite spatial relationship to each other in order to form a single structure. This can be tested by a vari-

ety of tasks: figurative drawings from memory or from a model (e.g., cube, house, clock); copying of nonfigurative drawings (e.g., Rey-Osterrieth complex figure); or arrangement of sticks, shapes, or blocks according to presented models.

Constructional performances require the integration of at least three distinct sets of abilities: visuospatial analysis of the reciprocal relations of elements, planning, and skilled movement behavior. Conceptual knowledge of the objects may be additionally required in figurative drawings. Therefore, although an impairment in visuospatial perception is usually the most important underlying causative factor, constructional apraxia is encountered in a variety of distinct conditions. However, some qualitative differences in performance can help to distinguish between them.

Anatomic and Etiologic Aspects

Constructional apraxia is most common and most severe after damage to the right posterior parietal lobe, which also results in the most important disorders of visuospatial perception; it appears in a rather "pure" form or together with left spatial neglect. Typically, drawings display a lack of global structure, piecemeal approach, rotated orientation, and too many strokes; they do not improve when the patient is provided with a model or guiding landmarks. Constructional apraxia is also found after left parietal damage and correlates with visuoperceptive difficulties, which are, however, less frequent than after right hemisphere damage; it does not correlate with ideomotor apraxia. Typically, drawings are oversimplified, display a preserved global structure, and improve with a model or guiding landmarks. In patients with frontal dysfunction of whatever origin (e.g., stroke, trauma, tumor, Parkinson's disease or Huntington's disease), constructional performance can be impaired as a result of defective planning but improves to normal when a structured program with sequential steps is provided as a model. Constructional apraxia is an early sign in Alzheimer's disease.

Related Disorders

Dressing apraxia refers to an inability to dress not caused by weakness, sensory loss, or disturbed recognition of garments. It is usually related to spatial disorders, such as unilateral sensory or motor neglect.

Diagonistic apraxia refers to an "alien hand" syndrome with intermanual conflict. It is seen after anterior callosal disconnection, with or without a concomitant dysfunction of medial premotor areas, and always involves the (left) nondominant hand.

Gait apraxia is characterized by a disproportionate difficulty to initiate and maintain the automatic sequences of walking. It is seen with extensive lesions in the white matter of the frontal lobes and presumably to basal ganglia connections, such as in vascular dementia or hydrocephalus.

Amnesias

Memory is not a unitary process. It encompasses the capacity to register, store, and retrieve various kinds of information over various spans of time. Depending on what, when, and how experiences are retained by the brain, several distinct types of memory can be involved, each linked to distinct but interrelated anatomofunctional systems.

Short-Term Memory

Behavioral Aspects

Short-term (or immediate) memory refers to the temporary retention of information (e.g., a telephone number), which can be used to perform other cognitive tasks (also termed "working memory"). This form of memory is both time- and capacity-limited and very sensitive to interference. It can be assessed in the auditory-verbal domain by having the patient repeat digit strings of gradually increasing length in the same or reverse order (forward and backward digit span); and in the visuospatial domain by similarly asking the patient to reproduce a sequence of spatial locations pointed to by the examiner (e.g., Corsi blocks). Introducing a brief delay or any activity interfering with rehearsal (e.g., counting backward by threes) between presentation and restitution will lead to a decrease in performance. Other working memory tasks require a subject to temporarily retain given stimuli for matching or detecting them in a series of subsequently presented probes.

Just as patients with a global amnestic syndrome have normal short-term memory (see below), patients may have severe deficits of short-term memory without being amnesic. That is, despite a memory span of two digits or two words, they can nevertheless show a normal long-term retention of lists of words. Deficits in short-term or working memory can be modality- (auditory, visual) or material- (verbal, visual, or spatial) specific. A marked impairment of auditory-verbal short-term memory is common in conduction aphasia.

Anatomic and Etiologic Aspects

Three major components of working memory are distinguished: (1) a verbal "phonologic loop," which consists of a passive buffer and an articulatory rehearsal process; (2) a visuospatial "sketchpad" system, which allows a person to set up and maintain imagistic information; and (3) a supramodal "central executive" system, which is responsible for coordinating the two modality-specific systems above (e.g., in simultaneous dual tasks) and for controlling attentional resources as well as other cognitive processes involved in strategy selection and reasoning.

Modality-specific components operate in conjunction with brain areas involved in perception and recognition through those modalities. Selective deficits of verbal short-term memory are observed after left hemisphere damage, specifically in the inferior parietal lobe, close to the supramarginal gyrus. PET studies in normal subjects suggest that the inferior part of the left supramarginal gyrus (area 40) and the adjacent superior temporal gyrus (areas 22/42) subserve the phonologic buffer storage, whereas Broca's area and the adjacent premotor cortex in the inferior frontal gyrus (areas 44/6) subserve the articulatory rehearsal process. Selective deficits of visuospatial short-term memory are observed after right hemisphere damage, specifically in the parietal-occipital junction. PET studies suggest that the right posterior parietal cortex (area 40) and superior occipital gyri (area 19) hold the more spatial aspects (i.e., locations), while bilateral occipital regions (areas 37/17/18) hold the more visual aspects (i.e., shape, color) of information, always in connection with activity of the prefrontal cortex (areas 6 and 46/47).

Finally, deficits of the "central executive" system are related to disturbances of frontal lobe functions and can be observed with focal brain lesions, head trauma, Alzheimer's disease, subcortical degenerative conditions such as Parkinson's disease and Huntington's disease, schizophrenia, confusional states, and to a slighter degree also in normal aging. A crucial role of the dorsolateral prefrontal cortex, specifically the middle frontal gyri (areas 9/46) on both the left and the right sides, has been suggested by several PET studies.

Long-Term Memory

Long-term memory is actually organized into a number of distinct systems (Table 24-4). These comprise a declarative-explicit type of memory and non–declarative-implicit type of memory, which are in turn divided into episodic and semantic and priming and procedural, respectively.

Declarative-Explicit Memory

Behavioral Aspects. *Long-term memory* refers to the ability to retain new information in more permanent stores, with a virtually unlimited capacity and a span of time ranging from minutes to years. Memory processes operate in three steps: (1) initial encoding of information, which is modulated by several factors, such as attention, motivation, and level of processing; (2) consolidation of traces, a still ill-defined mechanism by which new information is fixed and integrated with pre-existing knowledge; and (3) subsequent

retrieval, which can be elicited through varying conditions, such as intentional recall, recall cued by related stimuli (either external or internal), and recognition by confrontation. Intentional recall is more demanding than recognition because it requires the subject to internally generate his or her own cues and to plan appropriate search strategies in order to access the stored information.

Declarative memory comprises two systems concerned with facts known through previous experience and is explicit—that is, accessible to consciousness and deliberate use. *Episodic memory* is the record of personal experiences and events associated with a specific spatial and temporal context and thus represents memory in the common sense (e.g., "Last year, I visited Shanghai in China."). *Semantic memory* consists of general (conceptual) knowledge deprived of spatiotemporal context and personal relevance (e.g., "I know that Shanghai is in China."), although such knowledge may derive from specific episodes.

The *amnestic syndrome* is characterized by a global anterograde amnesia and variable retrograde amnesia in the episodic domain in the presence of intact short-term memory, normal attention, and preserved general semantic knowledge. Global *anterograde amnesia* means a failure to form new episodic memories through any modality (verbal, visual, tactile) and to learn new names, words, faces, or facts. The patient displays complete forgetfulness for delays exceeding a few minutes or even a few seconds—that is, exceeding his or her short-term memory span. The patient is disoriented in time and unable to describe his or her recent history. The memory deficit is exhibited on both recall and recognition as long as direct tests of memory are used and explicit recollection required. Learning of new semantic knowledge is hampered but nonetheless possible, particularly so through repetition, as revealed by the acquisition of new words or concepts (e.g., "AIDS"). In clinical practice, the full amnestic syndrome is a relatively rare condition, and milder forms of the disorder are more common.

Anterograde amnesia can be measured by presenting a list of stimuli (words, pictures) to the patient and then, after some delay, asking the patient to recollect as many items as possible (free recall) or to determine whether a given item was or was not in the previous list (recognition). On tasks of paired-associate learning, the patient is first presented with pairs of stimuli (e.g., the words "TABLE-DOLLAR") and then asked to recollect one item of the pair when given the other

Table 24-4. Divisions of Long-Term Memory and Patterns of Impairment in Neurologic Disorders

	Declarative, Explicit Memory (intentional-controlled access, with awareness)							Nondeclarative, Implicit Memory (unintentional-automatic access, without awareness)			
	Episodic memory (memory of events) — Autobiographical knowledge, Contextual, time and place						Semantic memory (memory of facts) — General knowledge, Noncontextual	Priming (facilitation of processing) — Perceptual/presemantic or semantic representations, Novel associations			Procedural learning (acquisition of skills) — Motor skills, Perceptual skills, Cognitive skills, Classical conditioning
	Encoding/consolidation	Retrieval/recall	Recognition	Retrograde memory	Source memory	Temporal order/recency		Meaning-based conceptual priming	Lexical-based word completion	Form-based perceptual priming	
Selective hippocampal damage	↓	↓	↓	✔	(✔)	(✔)	✔	✔	✔	✔	✔
Medial temporal lobe damage	↓	↓	↓	↓	(✔)	(✔)	✔	✔	✔	✔	✔
Thalamic damage	↓	↓	↓	(↓)	↓	↓	✔	✔	✔	✔	✔
Korsakoff's syndrome	↓	↓	↓	(↓)	↓	↓	✔	✔	✔	✔	✔
Frontal lobe dysfunction	✔	↓	✔	(↓)	↓	↓	✔	✔	✔	✔	✔
Parkinson's disease and Huntington's disease	✔	↓	✔	(↓)	↓	↓	✔	✔	✔	✔	↓
Alzheimer's disease	↓	↓	↓	↓	(↓)	(↓)	↓	↓	↓	✔	✔
Occipital damage (visual agnosia, alexia)	✔	✔	✔	✔	✔	✔	(↓)	✔	(↓)	↓	✔

↓ = performance typically impaired; ✔ = performance typically spared; (✔) = performance usually spared; (↓) = performance variably impaired.

associate as a cue (e.g., "TABLE-?"). Both verbal and nonverbal material must be assessed. Bedside testing may use the recall of three words paired with three simple drawings or the recall of three objects hidden in three different locations.

Retrograde amnesia means a failure to evoke memories acquired before brain damage. Although it is most often combined with anterograde amnesia, each disorder is, at least partially, independent, and severity of each disorder severity is not correlated. Rarely, retrograde amnesia occurs in isolation. Its extent is very variable, depending on the nature of the underlying cause, ranging from a few hours to many years, but a temporally graded loss is often found, with recent memories more affected than older ones. Remote memories from childhood and early adulthood are usually spared, presumably because they are integrated with some semantic knowledge about oneself. Retrograde amnesia can be assessed by questions about personal (autobiographical) and public (dated) information, such as knowledge of famous events or famous people across past decades (e.g., "Is X dead or alive? When did he die, and from what?").

Many patients are unaware of their memory impairment (anosognosia). Moreover, some of them produce *confabulations*—that is, false memories. Provoked confabulations are produced in response to questions or situations; these are plausible fabrications that may embody some real but distorted or transposed features (e.g., claiming to have visited a friend the day before) and correspond to episodic memory disturbances, specifically to a loss of contextual information. Spontaneous confabulations are either similar or can be fantastic fabrications that bear no relation to reality (e.g., claiming to have made a trip to the moon) and are often associated with superimposed semantic memory disturbances. Both types of confabulations frequently combine, but do not necessarily correlate, with a disturbance of frontal executive functions.

Anatomic and Etiologic Aspects.   The formation of new episodic memories and, at least to some extent, their subsequent retrieval depend on specific circuits that interconnect the medial temporal lobes with the diencephalon, the basal forebrain, and the prefrontal cortex (Figure 24-2). Amidst the former, the hippocampal formation and adjacent cortical areas play a pivotal role. Most of the input to the hippocampus consists of highly processed informa-

tion that is funneled through the entorhinal cortex (area 28), which receives, both directly and via the adjacent perirhinal and parahippocampal cortices (areas 35/36), extensive inputs from all modality-specific and associative areas of the brain. All these connections are reciprocal, the hippocampal formation projecting back to the entorhinal cortex, and from there to other neocortical areas. On the other hand, the hippocampus is part of the so-called Papez circuit, which projects (via the fornix) to the mamillary bodies, the anterior nucleus of the thalamus, and then (via cingulate and retrosplenial areas) back to the hippocampus. Another circuit connects the hippocampal formation to the basal forebrain, the cholinergic septal nuclei, the dorsomedial nucleus of the thalamus (via ventral amygdalofugal pathways), and the prefrontal cortex.

By the virtue of their strong reciprocal neocortical connections, the hippocampal system and adjacent areas of the medial temporal lobe probably subserve the binding and the consolidation of distinct sensory attributes of memories, which are ultimately represented and stored in a distributed fashion in dedicated areas of the neocortex (e.g., visual features in the occipitotemporal cortex, spatial features in the parietal cortex, auditory features in the superior temporal cortex, and so on). Over time, through prolonged consolidation processes, these neocortical representations may become directly associated with each other and their retrieval no longer depends on interaction with the hippocampal system.

The global amnestic syndrome is typically caused by bilateral damage to one or more structures within the above circuits, most often in the medial temporal lobe, diencephalon, or basal forebrain. Whereas defective consolidation accounts for anterograde amnesia, the gradual progression of consolidation over time also accounts for a moderate, temporally graded, retrograde loss that extends back to no more than 1–2 years in many cases. Patients with more extensive retrograde amnesia or no temporal gradient have additional deficits in retrieval processes, partly related to coexisting frontal executive dysfunction or degradation of memory traces themselves. Unilateral damage to this system leads to memory loss for verbal material in left-hemispheric cases and for nonverbal/visuospatial material in right-hemispheric cases, in keeping with other hemispheric specializations.

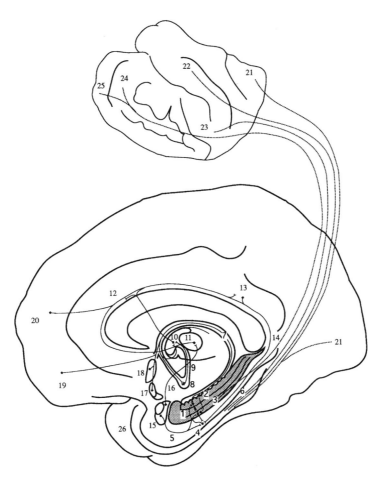

Figure 24-2. Neuroanatomy of the episodic memory system. The hippocampal formation comprises (1) Ammon's horn, (2) the dentate gyrus, and (3) the subiculum. Reciprocal connections with the neocortex are gated by (4) the entorhinal cortex (area 28), which receives from (5) the perirhinal cortex (area 34) and (6) the parahippocampal cortex (areas 35/36). The Papez circuit consists of projections from the subiculum to (7) the fornix, (8) the mamillary body, (9) the mamillothalamic tract, (10) the anterior nucleus of the thalamus, (12) the anterior cingulate (area 24), and (13) the posterior cingulate (area 23) gyri, and then via the cingulate bundle to (14) the retrosplenial cortex (areas 29/30) and back to the hippocampal region. Other subcortical pathways involve (15) the amygdala, (16) the ventral amygdalofugal fibers to (11) the dorsomedial nucleus of the thalamus, (17) the nucleus of the diagonal band of Broca and (18) the medial septal nuclei in the basal forebrain, (19) the orbitofrontal rectus gyri, and (20) the prelimbic areas (area 20) of the prefrontal cortex. Reciprocal neocortical connections involve (21) the occipital visual cortices, (22) the temporal auditory cortices, (23) the parietal associative cortices, (24) the dorsolateral (area 46) and (25) the polar (areas 9/10) regions of the prefrontal associative cortices as well as (26) the temporal polar cortex (area 38). (Adapted from R Nieuwenhuys, J Voogd, CHR van Huijzen. The Human Central Nervous System: A Synopsis and Atlas [3rd ed]. Berlin: Springer-Verlag, 1988.)

Damage restricted to the hippocampus is uncommon, occurring after anoxia caused by cardiac arrest, severe hypotension, or carbon monoxide poisoning, and leads to a rather mild, purely anterograde amnesia. Damage to the entorhinal and adjacent cortices is crucial for producing severe anterograde amnesia, together with a time-limited retrograde loss. This most often occurs with herpes simplex encephalitis, infarction caused by occlusion of inferotemporal branches from the posterior cerebral artery, trauma, or paraneoplastic limbic encephalitis, or in the early stage of Alzheimer's disease. It can also occur after temporal lobectomy for refractory epilepsy when surgery is performed on both sides or when the unoperated side is dysfunctional because of a bilateral hippocampal sclerosis.

Damage to diencephalic structures is implicated in Korsakoff's syndrome, which features both dense anterograde and retrograde amnesia. This syndrome is caused by vitamin B_1 (thiamine) deficiency. Although most often associated with chronic alcoholism, it is also seen in other disorders leading to nutritional insufficiency (such as in chronic gastrointestinal diseases, prolonged vomiting, bypass surgery, dialysis, or acquired immunodeficiency syndrome). The onset of amnesia usually follows an acute Wernicke encephalopathy, becoming apparent as the initial confusion clears. However, the acute stage may be of variable severity and at times go unnoticed. The critical lesions responsible for the amnesia are still debated, but involve the dorsomedial nuclei of the thalamus or the mamillary bodies. Similar memory disorders occur after focal thalamic lesions, such as stroke or (in unilateral cases) tumors that involve the anterior or medial nuclei. In these cases, combined damage to the mamillothalamic tract and the closely adjacent ventral amygdalofugal pathways in the inferior thalamic peduncle could be the critical lesion causing the amnesia. In cases with posterior cerebral artery occlusion, thalamic infarction may coexist and add to the clinical picture. Compared with amnesics with medial temporal lesions, patients with Korsakoff's syndrome or focal thalamic lesions have additional deficits in encoding, increased sensitivity to interference, and prominent difficulties in temporal order discrimination, which all appear to reflect superimposed deficits in frontal-related functions. These patients also frequently demonstrate anosognosia and (mostly provoked) confabulations.

Damage to the basal forebrain is chiefly encountered after rupture or surgical repair of aneurysms of the anterior communicating artery. Besides lesions to a number of nuclei and pathways in the basal and septal areas, unilateral or bilateral infarctions of the orbital-medial-frontal lobes in the territory of the anterior cerebral artery are frequently present as well as a disruption of rostral callosal fibers. The amnestic syndrome is characterized by a disproportionate deficit in retrieval processes with good recognition in relation to recall abilities, usually accompanied by marked (spontaneous/fantastic) confabulations, personality changes, and other frontal disorders. Degeneration of the basal forebrain cholinergic

nuclei also contributes to memory dysfunction in normal aging and Alzheimer's disease.

Damage to the pathways that interconnect the above three major structures within the hippocampal-related episodic memory system has ill-defined consequences on memory functions. Anterograde amnesia has been imputed to mamillary bodies lesions in a few cases with basal meningitis (e.g., tuberculosis or neoplasia), craniopharyngioma, or a penetrating selective injury. However, whether such restricted lesions are sufficient to cause a true amnestic syndrome is still a matter of debate. Several cases of anterograde amnesia have been documented after fornix lesions, such as tumor, trauma, or transcallosal surgery, but again, the role of fornicial connections remains disputed. Damage to the cingulate bundle and the retrosplenial cortex has also been implicated, leading to a circumscribed retrograde loss in addition to the anterograde amnesia.

Damage to the frontal lobes (e.g., stroke, trauma, tumor) or to their connections, such as seen in basal ganglia (Parkinson's disease, Huntington's disease) and subcortical white matter diseases, does not lead to an amnestic syndrome but impairs selective aspects of memory that are related to planning, problem solving, and other strategic organizational abilities. There is a prominent retrieval deficit with impaired recall but near normal recognition and a strong benefit from retrieval cues. Memory for contextual information such as source, temporal order, and recency discrimination, is disproportionately affected. Several PET studies found a differential involvement of the right prefrontal cortex in episodic memory retrieval and of the left prefrontal cortex in both episodic encoding and semantic retrieval, irrespective of the verbal/nonverbal nature of the material.

Pure retrograde amnesia without anterograde failure is very unusual but has been described after closed head injuries involving the anterior temporal lobes or the medial occipital lobes bilaterally, after herpes encephalitis, after diffuse anoxic damage, after thalamic infarction, after injury to the mesencephalic ventral tegmentum, or in some rare cases of transient global amnesia (TGA). An impairment in the reinstatement of old episodic memory traces, perhaps related to a disturbance in mental imagery and revisualization processes, has been hypothesized. This is consistent with PET studies that showed an activation of the precuneus associated with the retrieval of imageable episodic memories. Pure retrograde amnesia, however, is most typical of a psychogenic origin, in which a loss of personal identity and amnesia for autobiographical but not public events of the same period are common.

In closed head injury, recovery from loss of consciousness and initial confusion are commonly followed by a severe anterograde and retrograde amnestic syndrome. Although some patients have a permanent disorder, memory eventually recovers after a variable interval (a few hours to several months) in most cases. Typically, as registration of new ongoing events progressively improves, the initially extensive amnesia for events preceding the injury (e.g., months or years) shrinks to a far briefer but definitive retrograde loss (e.g., hours or minutes). *Post-traumatic amnesia* is defined as the interval between the last remembered event before injury and the first events that are recalled anew thereafter and has been repeatedly demonstrated as the strongest predictor of cognitive and socioprofessional outcome. In the chronic stage, residual memory disturbances represent the most common cognitive sequelae of head injuries. Amnesia probably results from a combination of damage to the frontal lobes and the hippocampal pathways together with diffuse axonal injury and lesions to other midline structures (e.g., fornices, diencephalon, and upper midbrain).

TGA refers to a common, benign disorder of unknown origin mostly affecting adults older than 50 years of age. Its typical presentation is the acute onset of a pure syndrome of anterograde and temporally graded (from a few months to a few years) retrograde episodic amnesia. It is sometimes triggered by emotion, exertion, coitus, pain, or a minor head trauma without loss of consciousness. Patients appear perplexed and repetitively ask questions. Spontaneous recovery occurs usually in less than 24 hours (mean, 6 hours), leaving a definitive gap in memory, and recurrence is uncommon. Single-photon emission computed tomography (SPECT) studies have shown hypoperfusion in the medial temporal or prefrontal lobes during the attack. A migraine history is frequent, and vascular risk factors are usually absent, although transient ischemic attacks or stroke may rarely present as TGA. This disorder must also be differentiated from temporal epilepsy with transient ictal or postictal amnesia, wherein subtle seizure signs may go unnoticed (e.g., automatisms) and attacks tend to be shorter (less than 1 hour) and recur. Other transient amnesias occur with benzodiazepine consumption, alcohol blackouts, hypoglycemia, vertebral arteriography, and electroconvulsive therapy.

Nondeclarative-Implicit Memory

Behavioral Aspects. The nonepisodic memory systems are intact in patients with typical amnestic syndrome. *Nondeclarative memory* refers to abilities acquired through previous experience and it is implicit, in that it can influence behavior without conscious explicit recollection of past learning. Simple examples are paradigms of *classical conditioning* (e.g., avoidance, or eye blink responses), which can be retained despite an inability to remember the previous exposure. *Procedural learning* means the acquisition of more complex skills and habits (e.g., playing the piano, typewriting), which can also be retained without explicit memory of the training episodes. Learning of perceptual motor skills can be assessed on a variety of tasks, such as drawing while viewing through a mirror, reading mirror-printed words, manual tracking and pursuit rotor tasks, or solving jigsaw puzzles. Learning of more elaborate cognitive skills, such as solving complex problems or applying abstract rules, can also be assessed. On each of the above tasks, amnesic patients have been shown to improve from one testing session to the other, as normal subjects do, even though they recall nothing about the task or the previous sessions. Such skills are retained over prolonged periods of time (i.e., at least several weeks or months). By contrast, procedural learning can be impaired without coexisting episodic amnesia.

Priming effects are another form of unconscious learning, corresponding to an item-specific facilitation of performance by prior exposure to the same material. Several levels of priming must be distinguished: perceptual (presemantic), conceptual (semantic), and associative. One example of perceptual priming involves showing the patient gradually more informative fragments of degraded pictures (or words) until identification is achieved;

when the same sequences are re-presented after a retention delay, saving is evidenced by the more rapid identification of previously seen pictures (or words) relative to new ones. Another example involves presenting the patient with a list of words (e.g., "MOTEL," "ABSENCE") and later asking him or her to complete word fragments (e.g., "MOT--," or "A-S---E") with the first solution that comes to mind; the completion rate is then found to be superior with studied than nonstudied words (although each fragment could be potentially completed with other, more common words). At the conceptual level, priming can be shown in tasks of word association or generation, where the subject is first presented with a list of stimuli (e.g., "EAGLE") and later asked, respectively, to produce free associations to related words (e.g., "FLYING-?") or to generate one exemplar from a given category (e.g., names of birds). Priming also occurs with nonverbal material, such as faces, pictures, or geometric shapes. Performance on such priming tasks is independent from explicit memory and patients with dense episodic amnesia show normal priming effects as long as the memory test is indirect and the instructions only require the subjects to give the first response that comes to mind. In addition, priming for novel material (e.g., nonwords) or novel associations (e.g., pairs of unrelated words) can be observed in normal subjects, but findings in amnesic patients are variable and still a matter of debate.

Most priming effects are transient—that is, lasting a few hours or days. They probably reflect the activation, or strengthening, of some representations stored in the dedicated brain modules normally involved in processing a specific type of information. For example, modality-specific priming for visual material (e.g., words) relies on the mechanisms implicated in normal visual recognition (e.g., reading) and thus is not dependent on the mechanisms necessary for episodic memory. Conversely, priming can be altered in disorders of perception or recognition (e.g., pure alexia, or agnosia).

Anatomic and Etiologic Aspects.   Procedural skill learning is subserved by the basal ganglia system. It is impaired in Parkinson's disease and Huntington's disease, progressive supranuclear

palsy, and with focal lesions to the caudate and putamen, independently from (frontal-related) deficits in explicit memory. Simple conditioning, such as the eye blink response, involves the cerebellum and can be unilaterally impaired, but more complex forms of conditional discrimination may also implicate the hippocampal system and the amygdala.

Priming effects are mediated by posterior associative cortices involved in perception, recognition, and semantic knowledge. Perceptual priming, but not conceptual priming, is impaired by lesions to temporo-occipital areas that also cause perceptual deficits, such as visual agnosia. Conversely, in Alzheimer's disease, perceptual repetition effects are intact but word-completion (lexical) priming and conceptual (semantic) priming are impaired, being correlated with other performances of verbal and lexical-semantic knowledge.

Suggested Reading

Agnosias

Caselli RJ. Ventrolateral and dorsomedial somatosensory association cortex damage produces distinct somesthetic syndromes in humans. Neurology 1993;43:762.

Damasio AR, Damasio H. The anatomic basis of pure alexia. Neurology 1983;33:1573.

Farah MJ. Visual Agnosias: Disorders of Object Recognition and What They Tell Us About Normal Vision. Cambridge, MA: MIT Press, 1990.

Grüsser OJ, Landis T. Visual Agnosia and Other Disturbances of Visual Perception and Cognition. London: Macmillan, 1991.

Martin A, Haxby JV, Lalonde FM, Wiggs CL, et al. Discrete cortical regions associated with knowledge of color and knowledge of action. Science 1995;270:102.

Sergent J, Ohta S, McDonald B. Functional neuroanatomy of face and object processing. A positron emission tomography study. Brain 1992;115:15–36.

Apraxias

Alexander MP, Baker E, Naeser MA, Kaplan E, et al. Neuropsychological and neuroanatomical dimensions of ideomotor apraxia. Brain 1992;115:87–107.

Benton A. Constructional Apraxia. In F Boller, J Grafman

(eds), Handbook of Neuropsychology. Amsterdam: Elsevier, 1989;387–394.

Heilman KM, Gonzalez-Rothi LJ. Apraxia. In KM Heilman, E Valenstein (eds), Clinical Neuropsychology (3rd ed). New York: Oxford University Press, 1993;141–163.

Pramstaller PP, Marsden CD. The basal ganglia and apraxia. Brain 1996;119:319.

Roy EA. Neuropsychological Studies of Apraxia and Related Disorders. Amsterdam: North Holland, 1985.

Sirigu A, Duhamel JR, Cohen L, Pillon B, et al. The mental representation of hand movements after parietal cortex damage. Science 1996;273:1564.

Memory

Fletcher PC, Shallice T, Frith CD, Frackowiak RSJ, et al. Brain activity during memory retrieval: the influence of imagery and semantic cueing. Brain 1996; 119:1587.

Parkin AJ, Leng NRC. Neuropsychology of the Amnesic Syndrome. Hove, United Kingdom: Lawrence Erlbaum Associates, 1993.

Salmon E, Van der Linden M, Collette F, Delfiore G, et al. Regional brain activity during working memory tasks. Brain 1996;119:1617.

Chapter 25
Neuropsychiatric Syndromes

Akira Sano, Naoko Tachibana, Manabu Ikeda,
and Hirotaka Tanabe

Chapter Plan

Delusions
Hallucinations
Anxiety
Obsessive-compulsive disorder
Depression
Mania
Personality alterations

Delusions

Delusions are false beliefs based on an incorrect inference about external reality that is held despite evidence to the contrary. They differ from overvalued ideas, which are not absolutely fixed. Delusions are the hallmarks of a paranoid illness, but they do occur in a variety of neurologic disorders. There is no specific delusional content that can be used to differentiate the background neurologic disorders and idiopathic disorders from psychiatric illnesses. The diagnostic criteria for a psychotic disorder according to the *Diagnostic and Statistic Manual of Mental Disorders (4th ed)* when it occurs in a general medical or neurologic condition is shown in Table 25-1. Various neurologic diseases that are often associated with delusions are dementia (e.g., Alzheimer's disease and vascular dementia), Huntington's disease, and Parkinson's disease after treatment with dopaminergic compounds. The pres-entation of the dementia of diffuse Lewy body disease often includes delusions or hallucinations.

Hallucinations

Hallucinations are sensory perceptions occurring in the absence of an adequate peripheral stimulus; they should be distinguished from illusions, which are misinterpretation of sensory perceptions. Hallucinations that occur with clear consciousness and no insight and that are incongruous with emotion are highly suggestive of schizophrenia. They are usually auditory, and generally auditory hallucinations are more typical of so-called functional patients with psychiatric disorders. The one notable exception is vivid auditory hallucinations in a fully oriented alcoholic patient. Hallucinations in other sensory modalities are less common than visual hallucinations in neurologic illnesses. Table 25-2 lists some of the common causes of various hallucinations. Hypnagogic and hypnopompic hallucinations occur in normal people when they are falling asleep and waking, respectively, and are also one of the features of narcolepsy. The treatment of delusions and hallucinations in a neurologic illness involves addressing the underlying illness as well. Both conditions may respond to antipsychotic agents or neuroleptics, but it should be kept in mind that all neuroleptics lower the seizure threshold.

Table 25-1. Diagnostic Criteria for Psychotic Disorders Caused by a General Medical Condition

1. Prominent hallucinations or delusions.
2. Evidence from the history, physical examination, or laboratory findings that the disturbance is the direct physiologic consequence of a general medical condition.
3. The disturbance cannot be accounted for by another mental disorder.
4. The disturbance does not occur exclusively during the course of a delirium.

Table 25-2. Common Causes of Various Hallucinations

Auditory hallucinations	Psychotic psychiatric disorders—schizophrenia, mania, psychotic depression
	Epilepsy (complex partial seizures)
	Ear disease
Visual hallucinations	Ocular disease
	Optic nerve disease—optic neuritis
	Brain stem disease—peduncular hallucinosis
	Cerebral hemispheric lesions—geniculocalcarine lesions, epilepsy (simple partial seizures)
	Medical illnesses—delirium
	Toxic disorders—withdrawal delirium, after ingestion of hallucinogens
	Psychotic psychiatric disorders
	Normal conditions—hypnagogic/hypnopompic hallucinations, sensory deprivation, sleep deprivation
Tactile hallucinations	Post–limb amputation
	Epilepsy (complex partial seizures)
	Drug withdrawal delirium
	After ingestion of hallucinogens
	Psychiatric disorders
Olfactory hallucinations	Epilepsy (complex partial seizures)
Gustatory hallucinations	Psychiatric disorders
Kinesthetic hallucinations	Psychiatric disorders

Anxiety

Anxiety suggests feelings of fear and apprehension, especially when these emotions seem to be unrelated to objective causes. Autonomic and somatic manifestations (e.g., tremor, palpitations, dry mouth, stomach churning) are common as a part of anxiety symptoms. When such symptoms occur in patients, the physician's ability to identify anxiety and perform a proper differential diagnosis is important. A paradigm change concerning anxiety disorders has taken place in psychiatry. Some anxiety disorders are no longer regarded as consequences of psychological conflicts and ineffective defenses but rather as disorders of their own and biological brain dysfunction. Although there are primary anxiety disorders, such as generalized anxiety disorder, panic disorder, posttraumatic stress disorder, and so on, anxiety symptoms also occur in a variety of neurologically or medically ill patients and can be caused by drugs. The comorbid presence of anxiety and depression is sometimes observed. Neurologic diseases such as cerebrovascular disease, brain trauma, brain tumor (especially in the temporal lobe), multiple sclerosis, Parkinson's disease, Huntington's disease, and Wilson's disease can be causes of anxiety symptoms. Medical conditions causing anxiety include hypoglycemia, hyperthyroidism, Cushing's disease, and pheochromocytoma. Drugs such as cocaine and amphetamine or withdrawal from alcohol and antianxiolytics are frequently associated with anxiety.

Obsessive-Compulsive Disorder

Obsessive-compulsive disorder (OCD) is an anxiety disorder that is characterized by a recurrent preoccupation with fixed images or thoughts or stereotyped repetitive behaviors that are often accompanied by symptoms of anxiety. OCD and neurology are closely linked. Neurologic diseases involving the basal ganglia are sometimes associated with OCD symptoms. These include Parkinson's disease, postencephalitic parkinsonism, carbon monoxide poisoning, Huntington's disease, Sydenham's chorea, and so on. More than one-half of patients with Gilles de la Tourette syndrome, in which abnormal function of the basal ganglia is assumed, have symptoms of OCD. Recent neuroimaging studies in patients with acquired OCD disclosed a variety of lesions involving exclusively the cerebral cortex (frontal, temporal, or cingulate regions), the basal ganglia, or both. A circuit linking the orbital cortex, the striatum, and the thalamus is thought to be involved in OCD symptoms. The treatment of OCD symptoms in such disorders depends on the underlying disease.

Depression

Depression is one of the common psychiatric disorders. Depressive symptoms are also recognized in patients with physical illness, including neurologic disorders. In some cases, the mood changes represent grief for lost function, a change in role or social status in life, or increased dependence. In many patients, however, secondary depression is more severe than anticipated for the functional disability. In those patients, the depression is a behavioral manifestation of the brain dysfunction. Neurologic diseases in which depression has been identified as a prominent symptom include cerebrovascular disorders, Parkinson's disease, Huntington's disease, Wilson's disease, idiopathic basal ganglia calcification, multiple sclerosis, encephalitis, neurosyphilis, epilepsy, brain tumor, and Alzheimer's disease. In patients with cerebrovascular disorders, the lesions have a marked left-sided anterior predominance. Endocrine disorders (e.g., hypothyroidism, Cushing's syndrome, Addison's disease, diabetes mellitus), infections (e.g., influenza, hepatitis, glandular fever), systemic illnesses (e.g., systemic lupus erythematosus, renal failure, carcinoma of the pancreas and lung), vitamin deficiencies (e.g., B_{12}, folate, niacin), a wide variety of medications (e.g., levodopa, barbiturates, reserpine, beta-blockers, methyldopa, oral contraceptives, corticosteroids), and drug withdrawal (e.g., benzodiazepines, amphetamines, alcohol) are also capable of inducing a depressive disorder. Depression in neurologic diseases usually responds to treatment.

Mania

Mania (secondary mania) is much less common than depression in the course of neurologic disorders. Manic symptoms have been observed in neurologic disorders such as Huntington's disease, Wilson's disease, idiopathic basal ganglia calcification, cerebrovascular disorders, trauma, multiple sclerosis,

neurosyphilis, viral encephalitis, and postencephalitis syndromes, frontal degenerative disorders, and after thalamotomy. A variety of medications also produce manic behavior, including steroids, triazolobenzodiazepines, dopaminergic agents, thyroid preparations, sympathomimetics, and stimulants. Antidepressants for a depressive disorder may precipitate manic episodes.

Structural lesions producing mania usually involve the basotemporal region, the parathalamic structures, and the inferior medial frontal lobe. When lateralized, the lesions have a marked right-sided predominance. The right-sided predominance of cerebral lesions associated with mania is supported by the finding that intracarotid sodium amobarbital injection preferentially elicits laughter and an elated mood after right-sided injections. The natural history of secondary mania is variable; patients may experience a single manic episode, recurrent mania, or alternating periods of depression and mania. The optimal treatment of secondary mania has not been determined. Tranquilization may be necessary in the acute phases of the manic episode; lithium, carbamazepine, clonazepam, and valproate may be used in the treatment of secondary mania; those agents may also be used prophylactically in patients who experience repeated episodes of manic behavior.

Personality Alterations

Personality changes in neurologic illness are the least explored area of neuropsychiatry. Few generalizations are currently possible. Frontal lobe lesions have profound effects on personality. Patients with the frontal convexity (dorsolateral frontal) syndrome show difficulty in problem solving, planning, cognitive flexibility, and judgment, whereas cases of the orbitofrontal syndrome are disinhibited, socially inappropriate, euphoric, and jocular. Patients with the dorsomedial frontal syndrome are apathetic, indifferent, or unmotivated. Large bilateral dorsomedial lesions may produce akinetic mutism. More often these three location-related syndromes appear in combination or in an incomplete form. Three distinct frontal lobe neurobehavioral syndromes also correspond to one of the currently recognized three prefrontal-subcortical circuits. The personality changes after frontal lobe lesions are recapitulated with lesions of subcortical member structures of the circuits, such as the striatum, globus pallidus, and thalamus. Not only does frontal lobe dementia such as Pick's disease exhibit marked personality alterations (e.g., disinhibition, impulsiveness, euphoria, and apathy), but also many subcortical dementia syndromes such as progressive supranuclear palsy cause apathy and indifference. Huntington's disease, which is associated with both atrophy of the frontal lobes and the caudate nucleus, combines marked irritability with impulsiveness, sometimes leading to aggression, violence, and suicide. Unilateral frontal lesions also cause neurobehavioral changes. As mentioned above, depression is common after left frontal lesions. After right prefrontal lesions, patients may exhibit blunted or labile affect, impersistence, and disinhibition. Limbic system lesions may also be associated with personality alterations.

Suggested Reading

Albert ML, Feldman RG, Willis AL. The sub-cortical dementia of progressive supranuclear palsy. J Neurol Neurosurg Psychiatry 1974;37:121.

American Psychiatric Association. Diagnostic and Statistical Manual of Mental Disorders (4th ed). Washington, DC: American Psychiatric Association, 1994;306.

Berthier ML, Kulisevsky J, Gironell A, Heras JA. Obsessive-compulsive disorder associated with brain lesions: clinical phenomenology, cognitive function, and anatomic correlates. Neurology 1996;47:353.

Breiter HC, Rauch SL, Kwong KK, et al. Functional magnetic resonance imaging of symptom provocation in obsessive-compulsive disorder. Arch Gen Psychiatry 1996;53:595.

Caine ED, Shoulson I. Psychiatric symptoms in Huntington's disease. Am J Psychiatry 1983;140:728.

Cummings JL, Mendez MF. Secondary mania with focal cerebrovascular lesions. Am J Psychiatry 1984;141:1084.

Cummings JL, Miller B, Hill MA, Neshkes R. Neuropsychiatric aspects of multi-infarct dementia and dementia of Alzheimer's type. Arch Neurol 1987;44:389.

Cummings JL. Frontal-subcortical circuits and human behavior. Arch Neurol 1993;50:873.

Hayden MR. Huntington's Chorea. New York: Springer-Verlag, 1981.

Kalra S, Bergeron C, Lang AE. Lewy body disease and dementia. A review. Arch Intern Med 1996;156:487.

Kertesz A. Frontal Lesions and Function. In A Kertesz (ed), Localization and Neuroimaging in Neuropsychology. San Diego: Academic Press, 1994;567.

Lee GP, Loring DW, Meador KJ, Flanigan HF. Emotional reactions and behavioral complications following intracarotid sodium amytal injection. J Clin Exp Neuropsychol 1988;10:83.

Pflanz S, Besson JA, Ebmeier KP, Simpson S. The clinical manifestation of mental disorders in Huntington's disease: a retrospective case record study of disease progression. Acta Psychiatr Scand 1991;83:53.

Rathbun JK. Neuropsychological aspects of Wilson's disease. Int J Neurosci 1996;85:221.

Ribstein M. Hypnagogic Hallucinations. In C Guilleminault, WC Dement, P Passouant (eds), Narcolepsy. New York: Spectrum, 1976;145.

Robinson RG, Starr LB, Kubos KL, Priced TR. A two-year longitudinal study of post-stroke mood disorders: findings during the initial evaluation. Stroke 1983;14:736.

Starkstein SE, Mayberg HS, Berthier ML, et al. Mania after brain injury: neuroradiological and metabolic findings. Ann Neurol 1990;27:652.

Starkstein SE, Robinson RG, Price TR. Comparison of cortical and subcortical lesions in the production of post-stroke mood disorders. Brain 1987;110:1045.

Stein MB, Heuser IJ, Juncos JL, Uhde TW. Anxiety disorders in patients with Parkinson's disease. Am J Psychiatry 1990;147:217.

Victor M, Hope JM. The phenomenon of auditory hallucinations in chronic alcoholism: a critical evaluation of the status of alcoholic hallucinosis. J Nerv Ment Dis 1958;126:451.

Section III
Neurologic Disorders

Chapter 26
Cerebrovascular Disorders

A. Ischemic Stroke

E. Bernd Ringelstein

Chapter Plan

Definition
Etiology
Pathophysiology (mechanisms of stroke)
Clinical findings
    Temporal aspects of stroke
    Topographic considerations
Diagnostic procedures
Treatment of ischemic stroke
    Basic management
    Specific therapy
    Decompressive surgery
    Preventive stroke treatment

Definition

An ischemic stroke is a clinical syndrome consisting of an acutely occurring, focal neurologic deficit that is caused by a circumscribed perfusion deficit in the brain. Ischemic stroke in the above sense should be delineated from ischemic encephalopathy, the latter being caused by diffuse hypoxic-ischemic brain damage after cardiac arrest, strangulation, suffocation, or carbon monoxide poisoning. Ischemic stroke syndromes are characteristic but not unequivocal. This forces the clinician to consider a broad spectrum of nonischemic diseases as potentially

underlying causes (Table 26A-1). Stroke that can be attributed to an ischemic brain lesion that is visible on computed tomographic (CT) or magnetic resonance imaging (MRI) scans or during postmortem examination is called an *ischemic infarct(ion)*. In contrast to completed strokes, the majority of transient ischemic attacks (TIAs)—that is, rapidly resolving ischemic strokes—are only rarely associated with a macroscopic brain infarction. Demonstration of an ischemic infarction depends on the duration of the TIA, as well as on the sensitivity of the imaging technique and its timing.

Etiology

The etiology of an ischemic stroke comprises a number of direct or indirect causal factors with varying clinical importance. The etiology remains undetermined in up to 25% of the cases. The majority of strokes are either caused by arteriosclerosis of the arteries supplying the brain or by embolic heart disease, including pericardiac sources of emboli, such as floating plaques in the ascending aorta or paradoxical embolism via a patent foramen ovale.

The degenerative changes of brain arteries called *arteriosclerosis* include a dilatative subtype of arterial degeneration leading to benign *kinking or coil-*

Table 26A-1. Differential Diagnosis of Ischemic Stroke

Intracerebral bleeding (CT)*

Hypoglycemia (immediate evaluation of blood glucose level)

Complicated migraine (individual and family history; abnormal EEG with normal CT findings)

SAH (lumbar puncture, CT, vasospasm with TCD)

Embolus from giant aneurysm (contrast enhanced CT, MRT, spiral-CT)

Vasospasm following unnoticed SAH (lumbar puncture; TCD)

Brain tumor (bleeding into glioma or metastasis) (CT)

Arteriovenous malformation (CT, angiography, MRT for cavernoma)

Congestive encephalopathy due to AV fistula (TCD, MRT, angiography)

Todd's paresis due to focal epilepsy (CT, MRT, EEG)

Encephalitis of various etiology (lumbar puncture, EEG, MRT)

Sinus venous thrombosis (MRT, angiography, MRA)

Multiple sclerosis (MRT, lumbar puncture)

Traumatic brain injury (history, CT)

Intoxication (ergotism, toxic vasculitis, serotonin antagonists)

Atrial myxoma mimicking vasculitis (TEE)

Neuro-acquired immunodeficiency syndrome (HIV serology)

Rare metabolic disorders, e.g., Fabry's disease, homocystinuria (specific metabolic tests)

Fat embolism (history; CT: air bubbles; MRI: white matter lesions)

Iatrogenic strokes (angiography, cardiac surgery, liposculpturing) (history, CT, MRT, vascular ultrasound, MRA)

Embolism from pulmonary vein thrombosis (thoracic CT, pulmonary arteriography)

Metastatic embolus from solid tumor (diagnosis of the underlying disease)

Psychogenic plegia, aphasia, blindness, etc. (psychiatric examination, clinical follow-up)

MRT = magnetic resonance tomography; CT = computed tomography; TCD = transcranial Doppler ultrasound; MRA = magnetic resonance angiography; TEE = transesophageal echocardiography; SAH = subarachnoid hemorrhage; EEG = electroencephalogram; AV = arteriovenous.

*The means by which diagnostic clarification can be achieved is given in parentheses.

Note: In case of stupor or coma as the primary presenting symptom, see Chapter 13 for differential diagnosis; in case of vertigo as the leading symptom, see Chapter 18 for differential diagnosis.

ing of the supra-aortic arteries. A much more hazardous variant localized to the basilar artery is called *megadolichobasilar artery,* which may lead to life-threatening strokes in the vertebrobasilar system. The *occlusive subtype* of arterial lesions refers to atheromatosis and atherothrombosis of the extracranial and intracranial large cerebral arteries (large vessel disease) or to not yet well-defined diseases of the thin and long penetrating brain arteries (i.e., cerebral small vessel disease). It mostly affects the lenticulostriate arteries from the middle cerebral artery (MCA) and the rami ad pontem from the basilar artery. The microscopically visible occlusive lesion has been termed *lipohyalinosis.* Both dilatation with kinking and coiling of the large arteries in the neck or the pial arteries and the occluding type of small vessel disease may be caused by long-standing arterial hypertension. Smoking and hyperlipidemia are additional important risk factors for the genesis of atheroma and plaque ulceration, particularly if combined with hypertension.

Other degenerative diseases of the large brain arteries have a strong genetic component. They should be differentiated from atherosclerosis. Such diseases are fibromuscular dysplasia (see below), Marfan's syndrome, and Ehlers-Danlos syndrome (fibrodysplasia elastica generalisata),which are caused by inborn abnormalities in the composition and network of the collagen involving the tunica elastica of the arterial walls. Additionally, a group of genetically defined, nonhypertensive cerebral microangiopathies may also cause strokes or stroke-like episodes (Table 26A-2). Most frequently, however, cerebral small vessel disease is the consequence of long-standing hypertension or hyperinsulinism. The diagnosis of cerebral small vessel diseases has a considerable clinical impact with respect to secondary prevention by risk factor modification, as well as to prognostic and genetic counseling. On CT or MRI scans, ischemic lesions mostly present as multiple, often confluent white matter lesions or as lacunar infarcts of the basal ganglia, internal capsule, or pons.

Approximately 50% of all cardiogenic cerebral emboli are caused by nonvalvular atrial fibrillation (NVAF) (including sick sinus syndrome), and 25% are caused by cardiac diseases resulting from coronary heart disease (e.g., ventricular thrombi after myocardial infarction; aneurysms of the myocardium). Approximately 10% of cerebral emboli are caused by congenital or acquired valve disease or by cardiomyopathies. Among the cryptogenic strokes, particularly in persons younger than 45 years of age, two major sources of pericardiac embolism have been identified: (1) floating or ulcerated atherothrombotic plaques of the ascending aorta, and (2) paradoxical embolism via a patent foramen ovale.

Table 26A-2. Cerebral Small Vessel Diseases

Term	Etiology	Pathogenesis	Clinical Findings	Diagnostic Procedures
Hypertensive cerebral microangiopathy (a) Lacunar state (b) Subcortical arteriosclerotic encephalopathy	Long-term hypertension, hyperinsulinemia Long-term hypertension	(a) Fibrinoid necrosis of lamina media of small penetrators (b) Like (a); additional hypothetical hemodynamic factors (?)	Age >60 yrs (a) Lacunar syndromes (see Table 26A-6) (b) Subcortical arteriosclerotic leukoencephalopathy with cognitive and motor deficits	(a) Physical examination, CT, MRT preferred (b) Same as (a)
CADASIL[a] (see text)	Autosomal dominant genetic abnormality; locus on chromosome 19p13	Specific thickening of endothelium; eosinophilic deposits in lamina media of small penetrators *and* small cortical arteries	Age <50 yrs, recurrent stroke, cognitive deficits, psychosis, progressive course, pseudobulbar palsy, migraine without aura	Multifocal leukoencephalopathy as typical, but nonspecific finding; autosomal dominant inheritance; linkage analysis[a]; specific electron-microscopic findings in skin or sural nerve
MELAS (see text)	Genetic deficit; point mutation of mtDNA (nucleotide 3243)	Endothelial swelling due to accumulation of enlarged mitochondria of small penetrators *and* small cortical recurring arteries	Age <40 yrs, hearing loss, deafness, epilepsy, myopathy, lactic acidosis, migraine, occipital lobe infarctions, cognitive deficits, cardiomyopathy, small stature	Parieto-occipital typical MRI findings; individual genetic diagnosis possible
Cerebral amyloid angiopathy	(a) Sporadic disease in the elderly (b) Rarely autosomal dominant inheritance; early onset: <20 yrs; late onset: >40 yrs (various mutations of amyloid precursor protein gene)	Mostly >70 (50) yrs, amyloidosis of lamina media and adventitia of small and middle-sized *cortical* arteries *and* veins; fibrinoid necrosis of vessel walls	Recurrent lobar bleeding; leukoencephalopathy, progressive dementia, psychosis	CT, MRT, brain biopsy
Susac's syndrome[b]	Unknown	Exclusively small cortical and retinal arteries involved; inflammation presumed, otherwise unknown	Only women up to 40 yrs, retinal infarctions, visual field defects, hearing loss, tinnitus, psychosis, small cortical or subcortical infarcts, epilepsy, pseudobulbar paralysis, headache	Fundoscopy, retinal angiography, MRT, ENT tests
Fabry's disease (α-galactosidase deficiency)	X-chromosomal mutation	Ceramide accumulation		
Vasculitides (SLE; IGA of CNS; collagenoses)	Unknown mostly	Inflammation and secondary thrombosis of small and middle-sized arteries		For further details see Moore 1994

mt = mitochondrial; SLE = systemic lupus erythematosus; IGA of CNS = isolated granulomatous angitis of the central nervous system.

[a] At the time of printing an individualized genetic diagnosis was not yet possible.

[b] Caution: Application of corticosteroids may cause exacerbation. ASA and nimodipine are recommended.

A still underestimated cause of ischemic infarction is dissection of the internal carotid and vertebral arteries, either spontaneous or after minor neck trauma. Every stroke patient younger than 50 years of age without vascular risk factors may be suspected of having suffered a dissection of a neck artery, particularly if associated with neck pain. In most cases, the underlying disease is fibromuscular dysplasia. Dissections may lead to an abrupt and complete occlusion of the internal carotid artery (ICA) with low-flow infarction if hemodynamic compensation via the circle of Willis is insufficient. Much more frequently, however, they lead to intracranial embolism of thrombotic material derived from the false lumen tunneled between the intimal flap and the tunica media of the dissected artery. Dissections of the vertebral arteries may occur after vigorous chiropractic manipulations of the neck with subsequent life-threatening embolism into the basilar distribution.

Vasculitides (i.e., angiitis, arteritis) of the brain are relatively rare causes of ischemic stroke (i.e., 1–2% in our stroke patients). Arteritis with secondary thrombotic occlusions of brain arteries is a frequent complication of bacterial meningitis, a complication of septic embolism resulting from endocarditis, a reflection of central nervous system (CNS) manifestations of collagenoses (e.g., arteritis temporalis, systemic lupus erythematosus, periarteritis nodosa, polyarthritis, Wegener's granulomatosis), or the result of allergic reactions to systemic infectious diseases. A few cerebral vasculitides constitute distinct etiologic entities, such as isolated granulomatous angiitis of the CNS, Churg-Strauss syndrome, Takayasu's disease, moyamoya disease, or Sneddon disease.

Several cerebral microangiopathies (see Table 26A-2) present with migraine as a leading or associated symptom. Common migraine with aura is a risk factor for stroke in women younger than the age of 35 years, particularly if combined with smoking, estrogen intake, or the presence of antiphospholipid antibodies.

Pathophysiology (Mechanisms of Stroke)

The relationship between various arterial diseases and ischemic infarctions of the brain has been explored in detail on the macroanatomic level.

Brain imaging techniques such as CT and MRI scanning (see Chapter 3) in conjunction with various techniques of cerebrovascular ultrasound (see Chapter 5) have provided important diagnostic findings. With the growing number of therapeutic options (see below), it has become more important to clarify the actual pathogenesis of the stroke in individual patients. The various manifestations of occlusive and embolizing diseases leading to ischemic stroke in the carotid distribution are depicted in Figure 26A-1. The strokes in the anterior circulation in approximately 80% of patients can unequivocally be attributed to one of the mechanisms indicated in this template, mostly to extracranial occlusive diseases or to cardiac embolism. These arterioarterial (i.e., artery-to-artery) or cardiogenic emboli lead to a territorial distribution of the infarction on CT or MRI images.

In the posterior (i.e., vertebrobasilar) circulation, intracranial arterial diseases predominate in stroke pathogenesis, particularly atherothrombosis of the distal segments of the vertebral artery, atherothrombosis of the basilar artery itself, and hypertension-induced occlusions of the pontine and mesencephalic penetrators (Figure 26A-2). Another important although neglected cause of stroke is dissection of a vertebral artery at the atlas loop or at the site of its dural penetration. Extracranial sources of embolism play a minor role, such as cardiac emboli migrating to the top of the basilar artery or extracranial stenoses and occlusions of the vertebral arteries causing artery-to-artery emboli.

Severe hemodynamic compromise of the cerebral circulation in areas particularly vulnerable to a critical drop in perfusion pressure (so-called border zones) is a rare event. In an individual patient, however, this aspect must be clarified with respect to the specific therapeutic options (e.g., induced hypertension). Very abrupt occlusions of the ICA, mostly acute dissections, may cause critical low flow in the brain and lead to infarctions in the terminal supply areas of the long penetrators in the centrum semiovale or in the cortical watershed areas (Figure 26A-3), provided that the circle of Willis is insufficient to compensate for the drop in perfusion pressure by cross-filling via its communicating arteries. Only in a few percent of normal beings are one or more of these communicating arteries lacking. In the posterior circulation, severe hemodynamic compromise resulting from a long-distance effect of proximal

Type of vascular disease

Cerebral small-vessel disease (microangiopathy)
- Lacunae
- Subcortical arteriosclerotic encephalopathy
- Branch occlusion of the basilar artery

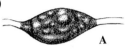

Noninvasive diagnostics

- Computed tomography
- Magnetic resonance imaging

Occlusive large-vessel
  disease of pial arteries

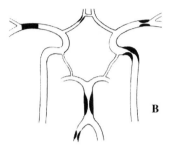

- Transcranial Doppler sonography
- Transcranial color-coded duplex
  sonography (with and without
  echocontrast)
- Spiral computed
  tomography–angiography
- Magnetic resonance angiography

Occlusive large-vessel disease of brain-
  supplying arteries in the neck

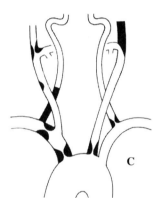

- Continuous-wave Doppler
  sonography
- B-mode sonography
- Duplex scanning
- Color-coded duplex
- Magnetic resonance angiography

Embolizing heart disease, including
  aortic plaques and right-to-left shunts

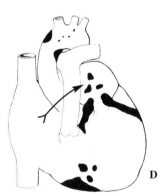

- Transthoracic echocardiography
  (TTE)
- Transesophageal echocardiography
  (TEE)
- Contrast echocardiography
  (by TTE or TEE)

Figure 26A-1. "The four floors" of manifestation of cerebrovascular diseases. (A) On the fourth floor, we find a disseminated occlusive disease of the small penetrating arteries leading to lacunar infarctions and subcortical arteriosclerotic encephalopathy. (B) On the third floor, we see large pial artery occlusive disease. (C) The second floor is characterized by the extracranial occlusive disease of the brain-supplying arteries in the neck. (D) On the first floor, a variety of embolizing heart diseases are operative, including paradoxical, transcardiac embolism and embolizing aortic plaques.

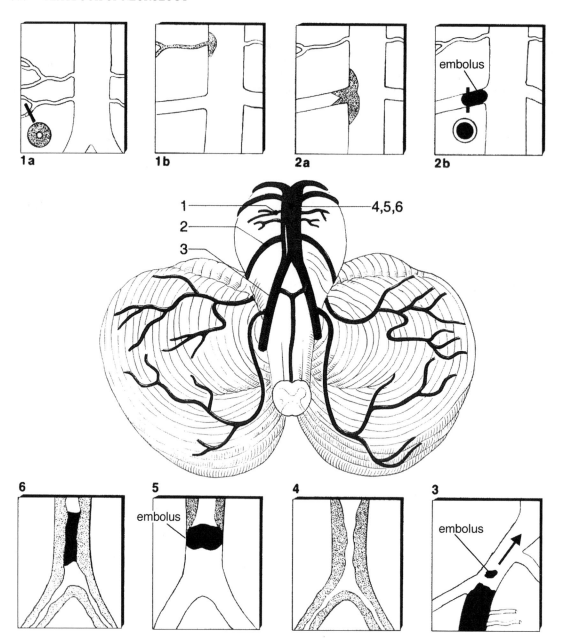

Figure 26A-2. Schematic diagram of various occlusive diseases in the vertebrobasilar system. (1a,b) Distal and proximal occlusion of one ramus ad pontem by small vessel disease (lipohyalinosis). (2a,b) Atherothrombotic or embolic occlusion of a cerebellar artery leading to cortical cerebellar infarctions. (3) Intracranial atherothrombosis (in situ thrombosis) of the distal vertebral artery (as depicted by *arrow*) (an important source of emboli to the top-of-the-basilar) and small vessel occlusions caused by blockage of vertebral artery branches supplying the medulla oblongata (leading to Wallenberg's syndrome). (4) Atheromatosis of the vertebrobasilar artery leading to multiple branch occlusions (see templates 1b and 2a). (5) Embolus sticking in the midbasilar artery at atheromatous plaques. (6) Autochthone (in situ) thrombosis of the basilar artery caused by ulcerated atheromatous plaques. (Modified from LR Caplan. Posterior Circulation Disease. Cambridge, MA: Blackwell Science, 1996.)

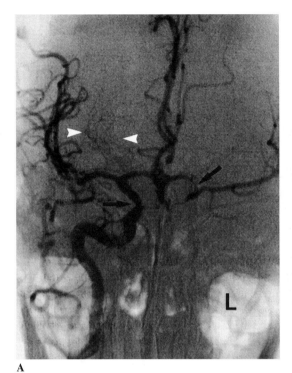 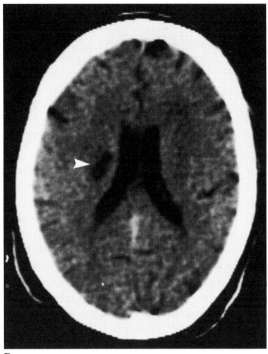

A   **B**

Figure 26A-3. Low-flow infarction in the corona radiata. (A) The patient had suffered a complete internal carotid artery occlusion on the left. Cross-flow via the circle of Willis (anterior communicating artery and anterior cerebral arteries) is severely hampered by contralateral siphon stenosis (*horizontal black arrow*) and ipsilateral severe stenosis of the anterior cerebral artery (ACA) (*oblique black arrow*). The severely reduced perfusion pressure in the left middle cerebral artery distribution prevents opacification of the lenticulostriate arteries on the left, as opposed to the right (*arrowheads*). (B) A low-flow infarction in the terminal supply area of the left lenticulostriate arteries is visible on a computed tomographic scan (*arrowhead*).

vascular lesions may be induced by the subclavian steal mechanism in high-grade stenosis or occlusion of the proximal subclavian artery (mostly on the left). This leads to a pendulum-like or retrograde flux in the basilar artery. The major complaint of these patients is brachial claudication when using the affected arm. By contrast, transient ischemic vertebrobasilar symptoms attributable to the steal mechanism are rare, and completed stroke caused by subclavian steal has never been proved.

A leading cause of ischemic stroke is the embolization of thrombotic material from athero-thrombotic stenoses or occlusions of the ICA in the neck (Figure 26A-4). The mechanism of embolism from high-grade stenosis is easily understood (see Figure 26A-4A), but embolism from complete, although acute ICA occlusion seems very improbable at first sight. It is a relatively common stroke

mechanism (see Figure 26A-4B,C). A very brittle "red" thrombus with its tail reaching up to the origin of the ophthalmic artery or retrograde cross-flow within the anterior cerebral artery from the contralateral ICA may produce emboli that finally lodge within the ipsilateral MCA. Although the ICA occlusion itself is hemodynamically compensated for by the circle of Willis, it is the embolic "occlusio supra occlusionem" that makes a patient suffer a stroke. This is why the acute obliteration of a symptomatic ICA occlusion is rarely ever beneficial to a patient.

Artery-to-artery embolism is also the main cause of severe strokes in the vertebrobasilar distribution, mostly from atherothrombosis or dissections within the distal vertebral artery (see Figure 26A-2, template 3). Emboli go into the middle basilar artery (see Figure 26A-2, template 5) and individual cerebellar arteries (see Figure 26A-2, template 2b) but mostly to the top of the basilar artery and into the posterior cerebral arteries.

At the molecular level, the pathologic mechanisms of cerebral infarction are very complex and not yet completely understood. In the core of the infarction, a cascade of destructive events occurs, starting with the excessive liberation of excitatory amino acids (as a direct consequence of the decrease in tissue PaO_2), with mainly two deleterious consequences: (1) The receptor-operated calcium channels of the surrounding neurons and glial cells—that is, the glutamate receptors and their subunits—are maximally opened, allowing massive calcium influx into the cells; (2) simultaneously, the large amount of excitatory neurotransmitters released leads to a strong depolarization of the neuropil, thus opening the voltage-operated calcium channels as well as exhausting the marginal energy reserves of the cells for repolarization. Several depolarizations and insufficient attempts to repolarize (so-called spreading depression) lead to a complete energy depletion of the neurons and cause a slowly centrifugal migration of severe ischemic damage from the core of the infarct to the still potentially viable periphery of the ischemic area, thus increasing the final infarction size. The initially viable tissue surrounding the irreversibly infarcted core is called the *penumbra*. This part of the ischemic lesion is the focus of interest for therapeutic intervention within the first hours after the ictus (see section on neuroprotective agents, below).

Overload of the cells with calcium ions leads to maximum activation of intracellular enzymes. This again consumes residual energy and finally leads to an autolytic destruction of the intracellular compartments—for example, the endoplasmic reticulum or the membranes of the mitochondria. Because of a lack of oxygen, mitochondria produce pathologic amounts of free radicals (OH–, H_2O_2, NO). They have an additional profound toxic effect on neuronal tissue and severely enhance the autolytic process and the destruction of the cell membranes. Drugs scavenging these free radicals have been developed.

Clinical Findings

Temporal Aspects of Stroke

Despite the introduction of an armamentarium of informative imaging techniques providing the

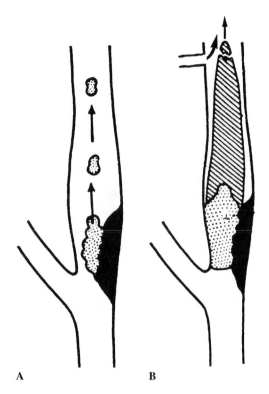

A   **B**

Figure 26A-4. Embolizing internal carotid artery plaque and occlusion. (A) As soon as an atheromatous plaque (*black*) ulcerates, a white thrombus (platelet thrombus; *dotted mass*) forms, which may embolize. (B) Complete occlusion may occur with a subsequent red thrombus (erythrocytes and fibrin; *hatched zone*) downstream and its tail reaching the next collateralizing artery (ophthalmic artery, *bowed arrow*). The brittle tail of the apposition thrombus may be removed as cerebral embolus (*arrow*). This event has been termed "occlusio supra occlusionem." (C) Postmortem specimen demonstrating the corresponding anatomic reality. (Part C reprinted with permission from JP Macadé, L Capron, P Amarenco. Images d'Athéro-Thrombose. Paris: Santé-Publishers, 1994.)

above synopsis of the stroke's angiologic background together with the resulting morphologic damage of the brain in the acute state, the clinical differentiation of transient strokes (TIAs), progressive strokes, or completed strokes is still a valuable guideline for (1) the urgency of the initial diagnostic workup, and (2) the initial differentiation of cerebral hemorrhages or tumors versus ischemia or other transient disorders. A careful evaluation of the patient's history with special attention to his or her transient symptoms

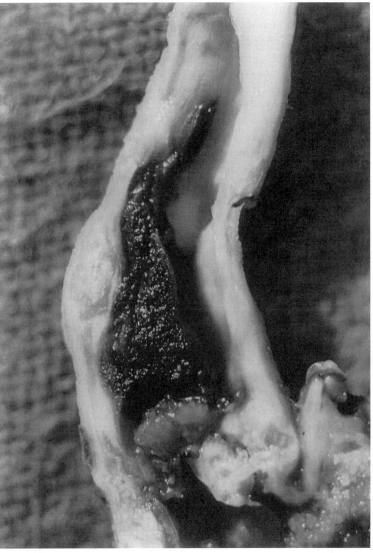

C

that are no longer present at the initial examination by the physician often gives clues to where to look for the underlying disease. Also, in certain circumstances, transient or minor strokes are accepted indications for surgical interventions, whereas completed strokes are not (e.g., carotid endarterectomy). On the other hand, the temporal features of a stroke (transient versus permanent) are basically nonspecific in terms of etiology or severity of the underlying cardiac or vascular diseases. This is why in every case, the TIA patient should be treated as a cerebrovascular emergency.

The threatening and dangerous character of even the slightest TIA is adequately described by the term *cerebrovascular accident*.

By arbitrary definition, a TIA is a stroke completely resolving by 24 hours at the latest. In clinical practice, most TIAs last only a few minutes, and the answer to the question of whether or not symptoms have completely resolved depends on the neurologic skill and care of the examiner. Every patient who has had a TIA within the preceding 6 months is at high risk to suffer subsequent recurring stroke. This risk is particularly high within the first few hours or days after an ischemic event. The lesion causing the stroke should be identified as rapidly as possible with the aim of subsequent specific treatment. The same holds true for minor strokes, which are strokes with a nearly complete resolution within 72 hours (also called *prolonged reversible ischemic neurologic deficit*).

If repetitive TIAs occur with an increasing tendency in duration, severity, or extension of the neurologic deficit or if a stepwise deterioration occurs within hours without intermittent complete resolution of the stroke symptoms, it is called a *progressive stroke.* These patients are emergency cases of the highest priority. If the underlying cause of the stroke is not identified and treated, progressive strokes nearly always produce a severe neurologic deficit. At least in some of the patients with progressive stroke symptoms, this disastrous course can be prevented by immediate and maximum diagnostic and therapeutic effort. In completed strokes, the neurologic deficit is or has become (nearly) stable at the end of the first 24 hours, leaving a neurologic deficit of dubious prognosis. Even then, clarification of the stroke's cause is helpful in preventing stroke recurrence, which would lead to death or even more severe neurologic handicap. Particularly within the first 2 weeks after an occlusion of the MCA caused by cardiac embolism, the recurrence rate is high (in the range of several percent). Particularly, there is the danger of the shedding of a second embolus into the anterior or posterior cerebral artery (PCA). Rarely can the resulting biterritorial infarction and excessive brain swelling be survived.

In the vertebrobasilar distribution, repetitive TIAs within several days or a week are highly suggestive of an evolving basilar artery thrombosis. Emergency treatment of these patients is a must because the prognosis of basilar thrombosis, once having occurred, is very poor. Strategically placed lacunar infarctions in the internal capsule or the pons may also present as a TIA, a crescendo TIA, or progressive stroke; however, as opposed to basilar artery thrombosis, each attack is characterized by a monomorphic and nearly identical symptomatology, and its prognosis is much better.

Ischemic infarctions involving the thalamus are a true challenge for clinicians specializing in stroke: (1) The allocation of the infarcts to the ante-

rior or posterior cerebral circulation is unequivocal (Figure 26A-5); (2) the above concept of small versus large vessel disease of the brain is no longer applicable; and (3) because of the large variety of stroke syndromes, they are difficult to diagnose by clinical characteristics alone (see below). The thalamus constitutes a group of gray matter nuclei operating as a key relay to and from the cerebral cortex. This is why its lesions give rise to a variety of stroke syndromes mostly mimicking cortical involvement.

The clinical findings in thalamic infarctions are characterized by sensory or sensorimotor hemideficits (or parts of one) with dissociated sensory loss, hemispasticity, or even severe impairment of position sense; segmental and focal dystonia with or without jerks; and abnormal dystonic posture of the affected hand (so-called thalamic hand). Infarctions of the anterior thalamic pole (polar artery) (see Figure 26A-5B) are characterized by neuropsychological deficits, with apathy, minor aphasic syndromes, and mnestic impairment. Bilateral lesions lead to severe mutism, abulia, and amnesia and have a poor prognosis. Infarctions of the posteromedial thalamus (thalamoperforate arteries) (see Figure 26A-5A) lead to vertical gaze palsies, impairment of vigilance (i.e., somnolence or even coma), or, if the patient is alert, psychosis with confabulations and amnesia. Again, bilateral paramedian infarctions may lead to severe, chronic neuropsychological deficits. Infarctions of the lateral thalamus (thalamogeniculate arteries) (see Figure 26A-5C) cause pure sensory stroke, which after weeks or even years may lead to central pain disease ("thalamic pain"). Sensorimotor stroke, focal dystonia, "thalamic hand," and hemiataxia are also common. Infarctions of the posterior pole and the pulvinar and lateral geniculate bodies of the thalamus (posterior choroidal arteries) (see Figure 26A-5D) cause defects in the visual field, mostly horizontal sectoranopias, but also aphasia and visual hallucinations.

Infarctions in the territory of the anterior choroidal artery have a distinct appearance on CT scans. Typically, the posterior limb of the internal capsule is infarcted, often also involving the anterolateral thalamus (Figure 26A-6). These infarcts cause a characteristic syndrome, with spastic hemiparesis, hemisensory loss, and hemiataxia. Sometimes this is accompanied by severe disturbances in

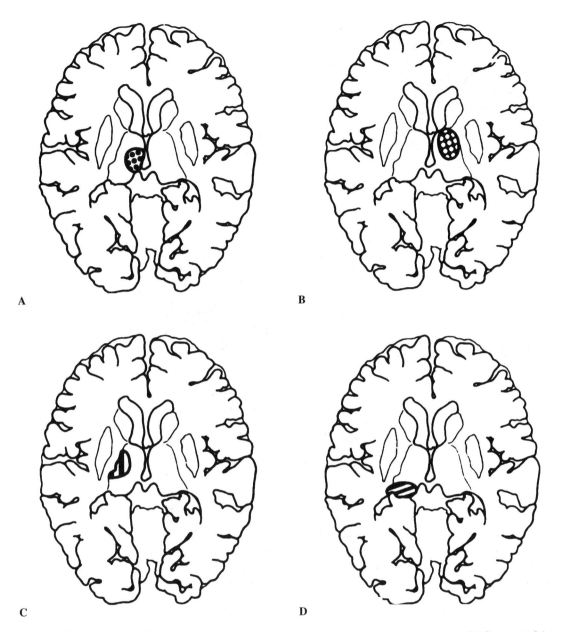

Figure 26A-5. Territories of the main thalamic arteries. (A) Core area of the thalamoperforate artery. (B) Core area of the polar artery. (C) Territory of the thalamogeniculate artery. (D) Distribution of the posterior choroidal artery. The thalamoperforate arteries on both sides may originate in one common pedicle. Thus, bilateral paramedian thalamic infarctions may be caused by one single vascular lesion (e.g., a top-of-basilar embolus). For correspondence of the territories to clinical syndromes see "Clinical Findings." (Modified from A Barth, J Bogousslavsky, L Caplan. Thalamic Infarcts and Hemorrhages. In J Bogousslavsky, L Caplan [eds], Stroke Syndromes. Cambridge, UK: Cambridge University Press, 1995.)

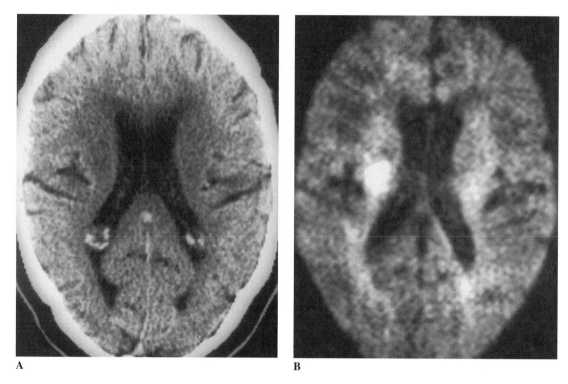

A   B

Figure 26A-6. Very early detection of brain infarction by diffusion-weighted imaging (DWI). The infarct corresponds to the territory of the anterior choroidal artery. (A) A computed tomographic (CT) scan of a patient with left-sided flaccid hemiplegia 2.5 hours poststroke was completely normal. (B) By contrast, DWI (EPI sequence; b-value = 1,000) 3 hours poststroke revealed a hyperintense lesion in the right corona radiata. (C) At the same site, the corresponding definite ischemic infarction could be seen 2 days later on a CT scan as well as on a T2-weighted magnetic resonance imaging (MRI) scan. (D) Conventional MRI is superior to CT in delineating the lesion. (Courtesy of Gerhard Schuierer, M.D., Neuroradiology, Münster, Germany.)

position sense of the affected hand and a specific type of visual field defect (i.e., homonymous hemianopia with sparing of the horizontal sector, also called quadruple sectoranopia). Despite the small size of the infarct, the resulting deficits are often strikingly severe and long-lasting. Bilateral infarctions in the territory of the anterior choroidal artery result in mutism, quadriparesis, and pseudobulbar palsy.

Topographic Considerations

In the vast majority of stroke patients, skilled neurologists are able to allocate the underlying vascular (or embolic) lesion to the *posterior* (i.e., vertebrobasilar) or *anterior* (carotid) circulation by means of a careful history and a thorough neurologic examination. Unfortunately, symptoms attributable to the PCA are equivocal because this artery is fed by the carotid artery in 15% of humans. This is why other associated symptoms may deliver key information about whether the stroke is attributable to the vertebrobasilar or the carotid distribution. The anterior/posterior differentiation of the stroke syndrome is of clinical value because it immediately gives an idea of the underlying disease and allows those emergency diagnostic procedures with the highest probability of positive findings to be prioritized. This approach helps to reduce the time between the onset of stroke symptoms and the beginning of treatment. Typical stroke symptoms of the carotid and the vertebrobasilar territory are listed in Tables 26A-3 and 26A-4. Each of the symptoms mentioned there may be transient (leading to the diag-

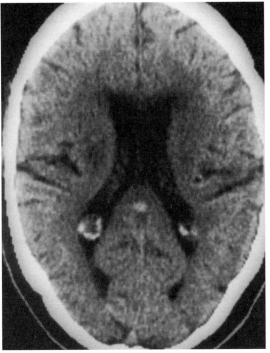

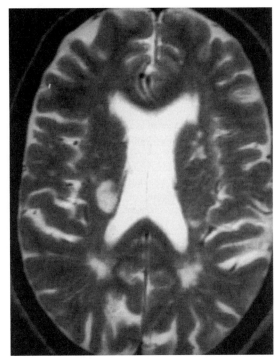

C   D

Table 26A-3. Typical Stroke Symptoms in the Carotid Distribution[a]

Ophthalmic artery
  Amaurosis fugax (note that the transient blindness is always monocular on the affected side)
  Spotlike permanent visual field defect on one side, abrupt onset (mostly retinal artery branch occlusion)
  Permanent monocular blindness with abrupt onset (mostly central artery occlusion)
  Chronic ischemic ophthalmopathy with gradual onset (an extremely reduced perfusion pressure in the ophthalmic artery
    caused by an internal carotid artery occlusion with an insufficient circle of Willis is a prerequisite)
Middle cerebral artery and its branches[b]
  Monoparesis of face, hand, or arm
  Distinct neuropsychological deficits (e.g., subtypes of aphasia with or without paresis)
  Motor aphasia, dysarthrophonia (anterior branch occlusion)
  Sensory motor palsy of upper quadrant, dysarthrophonia (middle branch occlusion)
  Global aphasia or Wernicke's aphasia, apraxia, neglect, hemianopia, quadrant anopia (posterior branch occlusion)
  Hemiplegia, global aphasia, severe apraxia, forced deviation (main trunk occlusion)
Anterior cerebral artery
  Crural monoparesis or evenly distributed motor hemiparesis
  Proximal limb paresis with limb kinetic apraxia
  Sensory deficits (in retrosylvian lesions)
  Transcortical motor aphasia (if left-sided)
  Hemineglect, mostly visual (in retrosylvian lesions)
  Activation of primitive reflexes like grasping, snout reflex, etc.
  Psychosis
Bilateral anterior cerebral artery[c]
  Mutism, grasping, incontinence, frontal ataxia, pseudoparaplegia
Posterior cerebral artery
  See vertebrobasilar symptoms in Table 26A-4.

[a]Occluding or embolizing lesions of the internal carotid artery can produce any of the symptoms listed.
[b]Symptoms cannot unequivocally be attributed to certain branches.
[c]With certain configurations of the circle of Willis, a single embolus can produce bilateral anterior cerebral artery infarctions.

Table 26A-4. Typical Stroke Symptoms in the Vertebrobasilar Distribution

1. So-called crossed palsies: deficits of cranial nerves ipsilateral to the lesion combined with contralateral deficits of sensory or pyramidal pathways[a]
2. Bilateral sensorimotor hemiparesis/paraparesis; tetraparesis; bilateral extensor plantar response
3. Hemianopia,[b] quadrant anopia, cortical blindness
4. Nystagmus if combined with long tract signs
5. Dysarthria (relatively unspecific)
6. Locomotor ataxia, ataxic gate and posture
7. Vertigo if combined with other signs
8. Somnolence, stupor, coma
9. Unspecific symptoms: dizziness, vertigo, headache, tinnitus, hearing loss

[a]The maximum deficit leads to a bilateral complete sensorimotor plegia (tetraplegia) with bilateral plegia of cranial nerves VI–XII. Consequently, the patient is tetraplegic and anarthric. He or she can see, hear, and move the eyes in vertical direction. This condition is called locked-in syndrome.
[b]Approximately 15% of patients have their posterior cerebral artery fed by the carotid artery. This is why these symptoms are not specific for the vertebrobasilar distribution.

Table 26A-5. Symptoms Not Typical for a Stroke

Stupor and coma without hemiplegia, or with normal vestibulo-ocular reflexes
Syncope
Amnesia
Dementia
Depression, irritability, mood disorder
Hallucinations, delirium
Disorientation

Note the following exceptions that frequently lead to a misdiagnosis:
    Cortical blindness with anosognosia
    Wernicke's aphasia with fluent jargon
Both conditions are often misinterpreted as disorientation or psychosis (see Chapter 25)

nosis of a TIA) or permanent (leading to the diagnosis of a completed stroke). In summary, the quality of the symptom and its temporal features must be taken into consideration. Table 26A-5 contains a list of complaints and symptoms that are *not* characteristic of stroke. These symptoms may occur as an adjunct to more specific stroke signs but most probably are caused by diseases other than stroke.

Another important clinical decision that should be made by the physician at the initial contact with the patient is the differentiation between strokes with and strokes without cortical symptoms. Cortical symptoms are mostly caused by emboli into the large pial arteries or their main branches. This is true for both the anterior and posterior circulation. Typical cortical symptoms are aphasia, apraxia, alexia, neglect, hemianopia, quadrantanopia, forced eye deviation, and other deficits of the visual cortex (see Chapter 9). Cortical strokes may be mimicked by thalamic infarctions (see above). Strokes with exclusively noncortical symptoms are often caused by cerebral small vessel disease. Symptoms such as sensory or motor hemiparesis, dysarthria, and hemiataxia are typical components of lacunar stroke syndromes (Table 26A-6). An experienced

clinician can pinpoint lacunar syndromes with a reliability of approximately 80%. They may be mimicked by small subcortical bleeding and other small focal brain lesions or by large striatocapsular infarctions, a subtype of territorial infarctions in the territory of the MCA caused by a rapidly lysed, or perfectly collateralized, embolic MCA occlusion.

Sensory or motor paresis of one limb or a part of one limb is termed *cortical monoparesis*, suggesting a small cortical infarction. These strokes are nearly always caused by an embolus into a distal pial artery branch. The same holds true for rare strokes with "pure" aphasia without paresis. A cortical monoparesis may, however, be mimicked by strategically placed lacunae in the pons, internal capsule, or corona radiata.

Crural motor monoparesis or hemiparesis with a clear crural preponderance is highly suggestive of an ischemic infarction in the distribution of the anterior cerebral artery, which, however, is only rarely the nidus of emboli. For angioarchitectural reasons, emboli from the ICA or the heart are preferably channeled into the MCA.

In the vertebrobasilar system, ischemic lesions are characterized either by massive, bilateral symptoms caused by basilar artery thrombosis or midbasilar embolic occlusion (the maximum symptomatology is seen in the locked-in syndrome; see Table 26A-4) or by a combination of deficits of the visual cortex (hemianopia, cortical blindness) with gaze palsies or

Table 26A-6. Lacunar Syndromes

Terminology	Clinical Findings	Site of Lesion
Pure motor stroke	Equally distributed, pure motor hemiparesis (sparing the face; minimal epicritical sensory loss may be present)	Lacuna at any level between medulla oblongata and corona radiata (posterior segment of internal capsule preferred)
Dysarthria-clumsy hand syndrome	Dysarthria, brachial monoparesis, facial palsy, hyperreflexia, extensor plantar response (dysphagia)	Anterior segment of inner capsule, basis pontis
Ataxic paresis (i.e., homolateral ataxia with crural paresis)	Crural hemiparesis, homolateral ataxia	Posterior segment of internal capsule, basis pontis, corona radiata
Pure sensory stroke	Sensory hemiparesis, dysesthesia (individual limbs may be spared)	Posterior ventral nuclei of thalamus, posterior segment of internal capsule, corona radiata
Hemichorea, hemiballism, segmental dystonia	Choreatic and ballistic movements of one limb or one side	Striatum, thalamus, subthalamic nucleus
Syndrome of the anterior choroidal artery[a]	Motor hemiparesis or hemiplegia, dysarthria (hemianopsia, mutism in bilateral lesions)	Posterior segment of internal capsule and periventricular corona radiata (uncus of temporal lobe, lateral geniculate body, optical tract, crus cerebri)
Syndrome of Heubner's recurrent artery[b]	Motor hemiparesis, mostly involving tongue and face (aphasia)	Anterior segment of internal capsule including frontal white matter, rostral caudate nucleus (putamen, pallidum)

[a,b]Syndromes mostly caused by small vessel disease, but also caused by (a) occlusions of carotid siphon or (b) occlusions of internal carotid bifurcation or proximal anterior cerebral artery.
Note: Symptoms or lesions in parentheses can occur but are not necessarily part of the syndrome.

long tract signs in patients with top-of-the-basilar embolus. The latter syndrome is extremely characteristic. Also very specific although relatively rare are crossed palsies (see Table 26A-4), which indicate a combined deficit of contralateral long-tract signs (sensorimotor hemiparesis, hyperreflexia) with ipsilateral cranial nerve involvement (oculomotor palsy: Weber's syndrome; facial palsy: Millard-Gubler syndrome; lateral gaze palsy or sixth nerve palsy: Foville's syndrome) (see Table 26A-4). In situ atherothrombosis of the intradural distal vertebral artery or posterior inferior cerebellar artery leads to Wallenberg's syndrome with ipsilateral Horner's syndrome, facial sensory loss, ipsilateral palatal palsy, and contralateral sensory loss for temperature and pain, sometimes with slight motor hemiparesis or merely hyperreflexia. These syndromes are highly specific for a brain stem lesion but not sensitive. Most brain stem strokes present with nonspecific minor stroke symptoms.

The largest proportion of the thalamus is supplied by the posterior circulation, but the anterolateral group of nuclei (adjacent to the posterior limb of the internal capsule), as well as parts of the pulvinar and lateral geniculate body, are supplied by the anterior choroidal artery, fed from the distal ICA. The bulk of the thalamic nuclei receive blood via the PCA and its perforating branches, as well as from the perforators of the posterior communicating artery. The thalamoperforating arteries, arising from the P1 segment, sometimes form a common pedicle, thus allowing bilateral thalamic infarction to be caused by a single vascular lesion (e.g., an embolus lodging in one proximal PCA stem). A unilateral infarct is shown in Figure 26A-5A. The polar artery arises from the posterior communicating artery, which is irrigated either way from the anterior circulation, the posterior circulation, or both (see Figure 26A-5B). The thalamogeniculate artery arises from the P2 segment of the PCA (see infarct in Figure 26A-5A), as does the posterior choroidal artery (see infarct in Figure 26A-5D). This particular vascular anatomy explains why thalamic infarctions visible on CT or MRI scans cannot unequivocally be attributed to small vessel disease (e.g., occlusion of one of these perforators) or to large vessel disease (e.g., an embolus lodging in the P1 or P2 segment of the PCA). Note that a thalamic lacune may indicate relatively benign small vessel disease but also be

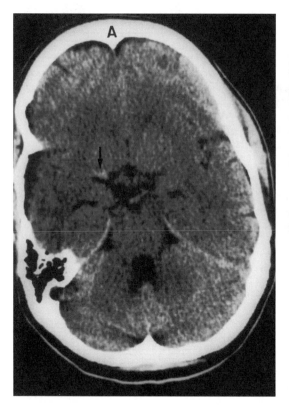
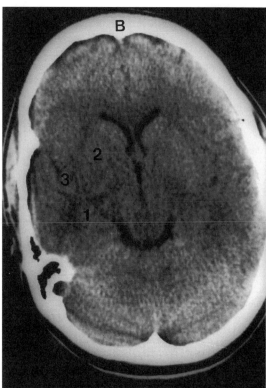

Figure 26A-7. Early infarct signs on computed tomography. (A) A 38-year-old woman with left-sided hemiplegia. The early computed tomographic (CT) scan 4 hours after stroke onset demonstrates "hyperdense media sign" (*arrow*) suggestive of an embolic occlusion of the middle cerebral artery (MCA). (B) Additional phenomena more rostrally: (1) Slight temporal hypodensity may be presumed; (2) the normal difference between the putamen and the external and internal capsule in the white-gray shadowing is strikingly diminished; (3) the sulci of the insular ribbon are reduced. All that suggests a large MCA infarction of the left. (C) 20 hours later, the large MCA infarction is clearly delineated (*white dots*). (D) Severe space occupation and midline shift are seen on the fourth day post-stroke. (Courtesy of Gerhard Schuierer, M.D., Neuroradiology, Münster, Germany.)

the consequence of life-threatening top-of-the-basilar embolism or thrombosis.

Diagnostic Procedures

After a history is obtained and a physical examination including a basic internal medical evaluation is performed, the first diagnostic procedure is either CT scanning or MRI (if immediately available). In patients in whom stroke symptoms are still present, this imaging is performed to check for intracranial bleeding. If the cerebral ischemia was transient, the neurovascular investigation of the patient by ultrasound has priority because it is expected that the

findings on the CT scan will be normal and thus inconclusive.

Within the first 6–12 hours after stroke onset, the underlying ischemic infarct is usually not clearly seen on CT images; nevertheless, this procedure is of importance with respect to the differential diagnosis (see Table 26A-1), as well as thrombolytic treatment (see below). Fibrinolysis with recombinant tissue plasminogen activator (rtPA) has been approved only if "early infarct signs on CT" are completely absent (Figure 26A-7). T2-weighted MRI scans permit a slightly earlier detection of the ischemic lesion. The main advantage of MRI, however, is the visualization of infratentorial infarctions (e.g., pontine lacunes) and small corti-

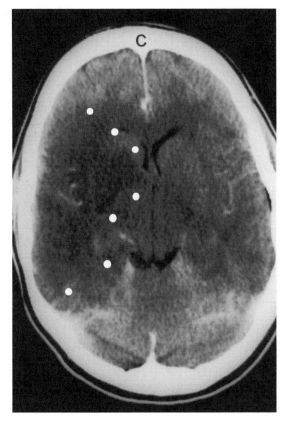

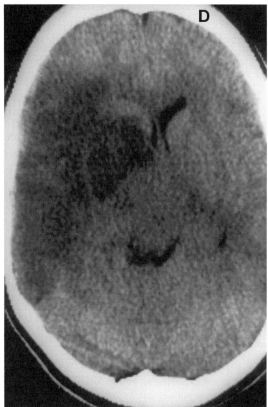

cal infarcts that are otherwise difficult to delineate from sulci (Figure 26A-8).

Equally important is a thorough extracranial and intracranial evaluation of the cerebral vasculature by ultrasound. This includes a continuous-wave Doppler sonographic study of the arteries in the neck that supply blood to the brain (usually with the frequency analysis of the flow signal presented as an audiosignal and displayed on the screen); a duplex scan of the extracranial carotid and vertebral arteries, usually performed with color-coded duplex sonography; and transcranial Doppler sonographic examination via various ultrasound windows in the skull. With transcranial Doppler ultrasound, every large pial artery is evaluated. These arteries include the distal vertebral artery, the basilar artery, the retromandibular ICA, the carotid siphon, the mainstem of the MCA (M1), the main branches of the MCA (M2 segments), the P1 and P2 segments of the posterior cerebral artery, the A1 segment of the anterior cerebral artery, and the ophthalmic artery. Intracranial anatomic orientation can be considerably facilitated and accelerated by using a color-coded transcranial duplex device. In case of insufficient ultrasound windows in the temporal skull, the cerebral arteries can be visualized by echocontrast agents injected into an antecubital vein. These tests not only detect stenoses or occlusions of the pial arteries, but also vasospasm, collateral pathways, or hyperperfusion occurring after spontaneous or therapeutically induced lysis of embolic occlusions or in intracranial arteriovenous malformations and fistulas. Also, transcranial Doppler ultrasound is the only method for detecting microemboli shed from various upstream embolic sources located in either the major cerebral arteries or the heart. This promising technique helps to differentiate embolically active but clinically silent vascular lesions (e.g., ulcerated plaques with superimposed thrombosis) from inactive ones (e.g., healed plaques). Detection of microemboli allows the actual source of emboli to be localized and differentiated from the innocent

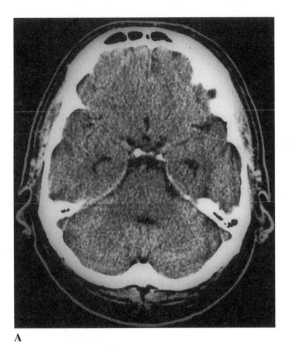

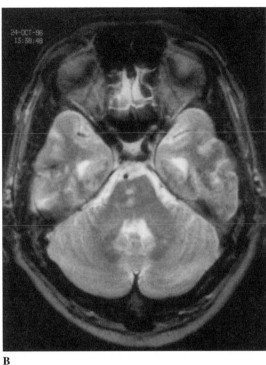

A   B

Figure 26A-8. Patient with a paramedian pontine infarction. (A) Whereas the computed tomographic (CT) scan shows normal findings, the simultaneously performed magnetic resonance imaging (MRI) scan (T2-weighted images) (B) clearly demonstrates two adjacent ovoid, paramedian lesions in the basis pontis, demonstrating the superiority of MRI scanning in the posterior fossa.

bystander if multiple, potentially embolizing lesions are present.

Other noninvasive imaging techniques of the cerebral vasculature such as magnetic resonance angiography or spiral CT scanning have not yet been validated convincingly but appear to be very promising. Their advantage is that they can be performed as a rapid adjunct to CT or MRI examination of the brain once the patient is in the machine.

If the above diagnostic tests do not demonstrate the causative vascular lesion of the stroke or if an intracranial (presumably embolic) arterial occlusion has been found but not the upstream embolic source, the next most important diagnostic step is echocardiography. For reasons of preciseness and sensitivity, transesophageal echocardiography (TEE) is the key procedure. The left atrium and its appendix and the ascending aorta are the most frequent sources of cardiac embolism, both of which cannot readily be visualized transthoracically. The rate of positive findings with TEE is two to three times greater than with the

transthoracic approach. Contrast echocardiography should always be added to check for right-to-left shunts at the atrial level (e.g., patent foramen ovale).

Single-photon emission computed tomography and positron emission tomography are nuclear medical imaging techniques for measuring (semi-)quantitatively cerebral blood flow or cerebral glucose consumption, respectively. These techniques play an important role in clinical science because they provide better insight into the pathophysiology of stroke, but they are of little practical value in routine patient care. Presumably, complete perfusion deficits in the entire MCA territory in a young stroke patient, as well as biterritorial profound perfusion deficits, evaluated a few hours after stroke onset may serve as a key finding to subject these patients to decompressive surgery of the ipsilateral skull (Figure 26A-9).

A much greater diagnostic gain will be achieved in the near future by ultrafast MRI-based sequences imaging of the brownian movement of water mole-

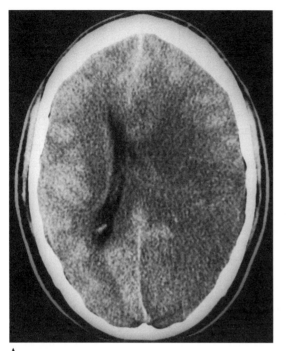

A

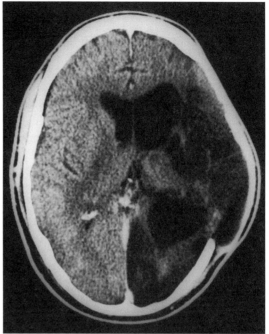

B

Figure 26A-9. Decompressive surgery in a 26-year-old man with malignant middle cerebral artery–territory infarction. (A) On early computed tomography, the delineation of the left-sided infarct and the space-occupying swelling is visible. Note additional involvement of the distribution of the left posterior cerebral artery. (B) A large hemicraniectomy prevented the infarct from life-threatening tentorial herniation. (C) Six months later, the skull had been reimplanted and the final pseudocystic lesion became delineated. The patient can walk again and speak, although still dysphasic.

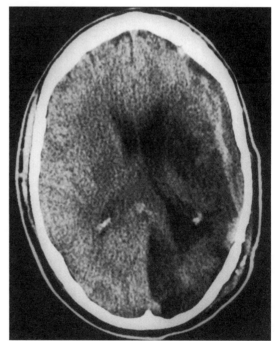

C

cules (diffusion-weighted imaging [DWI]), or the altered magnetic field in the brain tissue if a bolus of contrast medium passes it (perfusion imaging). DWI (see Figure 26A-6) can visualize cerebral ischemia a few minutes after stroke onset and is quite comparable with but more detailed than the electrocardiogram in myocardial infarction. Perfusion imaging could become a decisive guide for early therapeutic interventions, such as thrombolysis or induced hypertension, because it shows the extent of the momentary misery perfusion or its modifications by treatment, respectively.

Selective cerebral digital subtraction angiography (DSA) by a transfemoral catheter is a potentially harmful procedure that has an approximate risk of iatrogenic stroke of 1% in patients with cerebrovascular disease and a 0.1% risk in nonvascular patients. DSA should be reserved for patients with suspected vasculitis or other special indications. Before subjecting patients to carotid endarterectomy, a DSA may be required by the surgeon because it presently is the most precise imaging technique. In patients suffering from arteriovenous malformations or aneurysms and in patients with cerebral artery dissections, DSA may be necessary if ultrasound or MRI findings are equivocal. In general, arteriography should be restricted to patients in whom selective cerebral angiograms could deliver additional diagnostic information leading to potentially therapeutic consequences.

Treatment of Ischemic Stroke

The number of therapeutic options for ischemic stroke victims (including TIAs) has increased considerably during the last decades, and individually tailored therapeutic regimens have already become reality. The direct treatment, that is, stoppage or reduction of the ischemic infarct itself, however, still remains a dream in managing patients, although it has already become a fact in experimental animals.

Basic Management

Awareness of stroke symptoms and the emergency character of an ischemic event among the general population or among the ambulance services is a prerequisite for the patient's rapid contact with a local medical center experienced in modern stroke treatment. The slogan "time is brain" refers to the fact that the extension of an ischemic infarction can be reduced only if specific treatment is initiated within the first 3 hours (or 6?) after stroke onset. The individual time window for efficacious therapy varies considerably depending on the pathogenesis of the stroke, the spontaneous lysis of embolic clots, the compensatory recruitment of collateral blood flow, and the patient's general metabolic situation. The emergency physician should avoid aspiration in the patient, supply the patient with oxygen insufflation via a nasal tube (2 liters per minute), establish an intravenous (IV) line for treatment of complications, and place the patient in a decubitus position with a slight upward tilt (approximately 30 degrees) for prevention of brain swelling. During patient transport, the blood glucose level, temperature, and arterial blood pressure should be measured and should be corrected as necessary. Severe hypoglycemia can mimic any stroke syndrome, whereas hyperglycemia increases the volume of the final infarction. An increased body temperature must be lowered as soon as possible. Congestive heart failure should be treated with diuretics and angiotensin-converting enzyme inhibitors. A rapid drop in arterial pressure, however, may be deleterious. In patients with respiratory distress, endotracheal intubation should be performed without delay, and the patient should be hyperventilated slightly to a Pco_2 of approximately 35 mm Hg. A systolic blood pressure of more than 200 mm Hg and a diastolic one of more than 120 mm Hg should actively be lowered, preferably with intravenously administered alpha-blockers. The use of cortisone is now obsolete.

Specific Therapy

The neuroangiologic approach to acute stroke patients aims at improving perfusion pressure and microcirculation in the penumbra. A general hemodilution by plasma expanders or starch solutions is no longer used because fluid overload led to increased mortality. In individual patients with spontaneously low arterial pressure (lower than 140/80 mm Hg), and particularly in those in whom carbon dioxide–dependent cerebrovascular reactivity is exhausted (see section on severe hemodynamic compromise), induced hypertension is recommended, either by hypervolemia, the application of catecholamines, or both. Although prospective trials are lacking, this approach seems reasonable in selected cases. Only rarely does a subtotal ICA stenosis or pseudo-occlusion cause a drop in perfusion pressure so severe that transient ischemic cerebral symptoms or ischemic ophthalmopathy occur for hemodynamic reasons. This latter constellation is a good indicator for carotid endarterectomy (eventually in conjunction with the treatment of secondary glaucoma), although controlled trials are again lacking.

In complete ICA occlusions, extracranial-intracranial bypass surgery has not turned out to be beneficial to the patient. There are strong opinions, however, that a small, highly selected subgroup of patients would benefit from this procedure as long as valid selection criteria are applied. So far, proof in a randomized trial is still lacking, presumably because of the rareness of these patients.

The antithrombotic approach aims at stopping thrombus formation and subsequent in situ occlusion or distal embolism. Acetylsalicylic acid (ASA) is one of the most frequently used compounds in this respect; its efficacy, however, is low—that is, the rate of long-term prevention of recurring strokes is approximately 15–20%. There is still worldwide controversy about the optimal dose. In Europe, doses of 40–325 mg per day are preferred; in the United States, 325–1,300 mg per day is advocated. We use 300 mg per day. Ticlopidine is another thoroughly investigated platelet-antiaggregant agent that shows an approximately 10% greater efficacy in stroke prevention than ASA. This holds particularly true for secondary prevention of ischemic events after completed stroke, where ASA has not yet been proved to be beneficial. Clopidogrel is another antiplatelet agent presently being approved for secondary prevention in cerebrovascular and cardiovascular disease. It is similar to ticlopidine but has the advantage of having fewer undesired side effects. New compounds or combinations of antiaggregant medications are being developed but their efficacy is not yet established.

There is another worldwide controversy about the superiority of anticoagulation over platelet antiaggregant agents in the very acute state of stroke, particularly with respect to heparin. Some stroke centers in Europe and United States advocate initial intravenous (IV) heparin treatment with a partial thromboplastin time (PTT) 1.5–2.0 times normal control values (1) in patients with cardiogenic brain

Table 26A-7. Rules for the Selection of Patients for Carotid Endarterectomy

1. Only symptomatic carotid artery stenoses should be operated on. Symptomatic means transient or minor stroke within the last 6 months.
2. The degree of stenosis documented on a two-plane intra-arterial digital subtraction arteriogram must be at least 70% according to NASCET criteria and at least 82% according to ECST criteria. Patients with lower-grade stenoses would not benefit from surgery.
3. Check the artery under study for complete occlusion immediately before surgery.
4. Check the patient for concomitant coronary heart disease and other severe disorders arguing against carotid endarterectomy.
5. Check the complication rate of the operation team. The upper limit of 30-day perioperative stroke or death in symptomatic stenoses must be less than 5%.
6. Optimal outcome can only be achieved with simultaneous consequent treatment of vascular risk factors and simultaneous treatment with antiplatelet agents.

ECST = European Carotid Surgery Trial; NASCET = North American Symptomatic Carotid Endarterectomy Trial.
Note: If these rules are considered, approximately one stroke can be avoided in the postoperative year if 10 patients are operated on.

embolism (this indication is widely accepted); (2) in acutely symptomatic, high-grade ICA stenoses until carotid endarterectomy is performed (not generally accepted); (3) in intracranial, surgically nonaccessible distal vertebral artery, carotid siphon, and pial artery stenoses (accepted by the majority); and (4) in acute ICA or vertebral artery dissections (not generally accepted, but advocated by this author). The known contraindications against anticoagulation should be considered. The risk of intracerebral bleeding with therapeutic heparin treatment within the first 2–3 weeks after an acute ischemic stroke is in the range of 1–2%. This risk is particularly high in patients with peaks of critically high blood pressure and in those with cerebral small vessel disease, particularly with diffuse white matter lesions.

A very effective antithrombotic treatment is the surgical removal of symptomatic plaques in the carotid bifurcation. Patients must be carefully selected for this procedure, according to generally accepted standard criteria (Table 26A-7). In asymptomatic ICA stenoses with lumen reductions of more than 60%, the absolute risk reduction by endarterectomy is only 1% per year, compared with

Table 26A-8. Risk Factors and Concomitant Cardiovascular Diseases Underlying Ischemic Stroke: Costs of Stroke Prevention

RF or Concomitant Cardiovascular Disease	Risk of Stroke	Preventive Measure	Costs of Treatment to Avoid One Stroke (DM = Deutsche Mark)
Hypertension	2.5- to 6.3-fold	Antihypertensive treatment	2,000 DM
Smoking	2(1.9–3.4)-fold	Stop smoking	Nil
Diabetes	2- to 4-fold	?	?
Increased low-density lipoprotein cholesterol	4-fold	Lowering cholesterol by diet	Nil
		Lowering cholesterol by drugs	2,200 DM
Obesity	1.5-fold	Weight reduction by fasting	Nil
Lack of physical activity	1.5-fold	Sports activities	Nil
Nonvalvular atrial fibrillation	6(2–17)-fold	Low-dose anticoagulation	2,200 DM
CHD/MI	?	?	?
Asymptomatic ICA stenosis >60% (asymptomatic)	Approximately 1% per year	Antiplatelet therapy presumably not effective	300 DM
	1–2% per year	Carotid endarterectomy (85 operations necessary to avoid one stroke per year)	1,770,000 DM
Symptomatic ICA stenosis	2- to 15-fold (?), 2–30% per year depending on degree of stenosis	Antiplatelet therapy	300 DM
		Carotid endarterectomy (23 operations necessary)	480,000 DM
Oral contraceptives (premenopausal)	2- to 3-fold	Stop intake	Not only nil but even cost reduction

RF = risk factor; ICA = internal carotid artery; CHD/MI = coronary heart disease/myocardial infarction.
Source: Adapted from the findings of NASCET Collaborators. Beneficial effect of carotid endarterectomy in symptomatic patients with high-grade carotid stenosis. N Engl J Med 1991;325:445; R Shinton, G Beevers. Metaanalysis of relation between cigarette smoking and stroke. BMJ 1989;298:789; R Bonita, R Beaglehole. Does treatment of hypertension explain the decline in mortality from stroke? BMJ 1986;292:191; MG Marmot, NR Poulter. Primary prevention of stroke. Lancet 1992;339:344; European Atrial Fibrillation Trial (EAFT) Study Group. Secondary prevention in non-rheumatic atrial fibrillation after transient ischemic attack or minor stroke. Lancet 1993;342:1255; PA Wolf, B D'Agostino, AJ Belanger, WB Cannel. Probability of stroke: a risk profile from the Framingham Study Group. Stroke 1991;22:312; Hankey (Perth), oral communication, 1995; PROCAM (personal communication by G. Assmann, M.D., Münster, Germany).

an absolute stroke risk of 2% per year with medical treatment. To avoid one disabling stroke in carriers of high-grade asymptomatic ICA stenoses, at least 67 patients have to be operated on. This is an extremely expensive type of primary stroke prevention (see also economical aspects in Table 26A-8). Furthermore, the surgical procedure has to be done by very skilled surgeons to guarantee a positive risk-benefit ratio. Only in rare cases does carotid endarterectomy for asymptomatic carotid stenosis seem beneficial, provided that the patient is free of coronary heart disease. We advocate surgery if the stenosis is hemodynamically severely compromising (90% or more in conjunction with an insufficient circle of Willis) or if the lesion shows rapid progression during sequential ultrasound investigations. The role of microembolus detection by transcranial ultrasound in this context has not yet been evaluated but seems promising. In clinical practice, it is more important to teach patients with asymptomatic ICA stenoses about the characteristics and the emergency character of TIAs and to make them seek immediate medical and surgical care as soon as an ischemic event has been noted (i.e., as soon as his or her asymptomatic ICA stenosis has become a symptomatic one). Even more important is the consequent treatment of the patient's vascular risk factors.

Fibrinolysis is a new treatment for dissolving occluding emboli lodged in the large pial arteries.

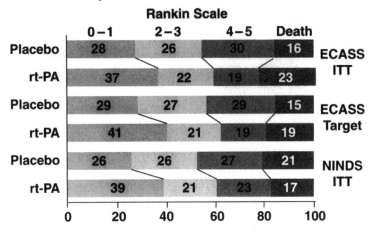

Figure 26A-10. Harm and benefit of recombinant tissue plasminogen activator (rtPA) in acute ischemic stroke. Results of the modified ranking scale in the European Cooperative Acute Stroke Study (ECASS) and the National Institute of Neurological Disorders and Stroke (NINDS) rtPA Stroke Study. The ECASS results are given for both the intention-to-treat (ITT) and the target populations (Target). Note that the positive effects (increase in number of patients with ranking score 0–1) are similar in both trials, whereas mortality ("Death") in the ECASS is higher among patients treated with intravenous rtPA. (Courtesy of Werner Hacke, M.D., Heidelberg, Germany.)

Two recently published trials demonstrate the feasibility and even the efficacy of systemic treatment with recombinant tissue plasminogen activator (rtPA) within the first 3 hours after stroke onset (Figure 26A-10). It is believed that its efficacy is based on the rapid removal of the occluding thrombus and on early reperfusion of the penumbra. However, additional effects may also be operative, such as prevention of thrombus propagation or keeping the transcortical leptomeningeal anastomoses patent. It is mandatory to exclude cerebral hemorrhage before starting treatment with 0.9 mg/kg rtPA via an antecubital vein. Its use is related to to the complete absence of early infarct signs on CT scans, such as circumscribed swelling of the cortex and a minimal territorial hypodensity or radiolucent homogeneity of the gyri, the underlying white matter, the adjacent internal capsule, and the basal ganglia (see Figure 26A-7). If the above prerequisites are not strictly considered, thrombolytic treatment will worsen the patient's prognosis through an excess of intracranial hemorrhages. Further trials are under way for a better selection of patients and a wider opening of the therapeutic time window.

The idea underlying the neuroprotective approach is to stop the biochemical digestion of the brain tissue within the core ischemic area and to prevent propagation of the ischemic necrosis into the penumbra. Neuroprotective agents are compounds that prevent or limit ischemia-induced brain damage and reduce infarct size. Consequently, a reduced mortality and an improved functional outcome are expected. Neuroprotectants are highly unlikely to affect cerebral bleeding adversely, which gives them the tremendous advantage in that they are applicable immediately after the ictus and to all patients with suspected stroke. Many of the neuroprotective agents have been highly effective in animal models of focal cerebral ischemia, but so far none of them has been effective in clinical trials. At present, the most relevant therapeutic principles of the available compounds are (1) free radical scavenging, (2) blockage of calcium channels, (3) blockage of excitatory amino acids, (4) inhibition of NO synthase, (5) inhibition of endothelial adhesion molecules, (6) enzymatic defibriogenation, and (7) the combination of the above compounds with or without fibrinolysis (so-called cocktails). A battery of further ideas has been issued, and new agents are still under development.

Decompressive Surgery

Large, acute, lobar infarctions of the cerebellum resulting from embolic or thrombotic occlusions of single pial cerebellar arteries (mostly the posterior inferior cerebellar artery) may produce ataxia and vertigo in an alert patient that is often misinterpreted as peripheral vestibular disorder. This situation is life-threatening because within a few hours the swelling of the cerebellar infarction may compress the patient's brain stem and the aqueduct, with subsequent occlusive hydrocephalus, stupor, coma, or even respiratory failure. Transcerebral drainage of the lateral ventricle or even surgical removal of the infarcted tissue via a suboccipital bur-hole will save the patient's life. As a rule, this surgical procedure does not lead to permanent neurologic deficits.

In large, space-occupying infarctions of the MCA distribution, particularly in a young patient with less subarachnoid space—so-called malignant MCA infarction—timely removal of the hemi-skull and slitting of the dura with a large patch of autologous fascia may be life-saving (see Figure 26A-9). A prospective randomized trial is under way. Preliminary findings are very promising, not only with a dramatic improvement of mortality, but also with an impressive reduction in the final neurologic deficit and the patient's handicap. One might speculate whether this type of treatment qualifies as "reperfusion therapy," in that decompression allows the ischemic tissue to be optimally perfused via collateral pathways, or whether decompression constitutes a mechanical and thermic type of neuroprotection, in that compression of the brain is released and the temperature of the exposed hemisphere is lower than contralaterally. Of course, a severe midline shift and tentorial herniation of the temporal lobe are immediately prevented by this heroic procedure. Our personal experience with decompressive surgery is very encouraging.

Preventive Stroke Treatment

Two principles of primary prevention are generally accepted and highly effective: (1) the avoidance and treatment of vascular risk factors (see Table 26A-8), and (2) low-dose anticoagulation in nonvalvular (non-rheumatic) atrial fibrillation. Among the risk factors for stroke (as well as other cardiovascular diseases), cessation of smoking is the most cost-effective primary preventive measure. With respect to stroke, the treatment of arterial hypertension is most important and has also turned out to be highly effective in the elderly with either isolated systolic or combined systolic and diastolic hypertension. Optimal treatment of diabetes and hyperinsulinemia (particularly in syndrome X); body weight normalization; regular physical conditioning; and lowering of high levels of low-density lipoprotein (LDL) cholesterol by a healthy lifestyle, medication, or both are also important. Atherosclerosis of the carotid bifurcation and the intracranial large arteries is strongly dependent on the patient's fat metabolism. In the latter context, the physician should keep in mind that coronary heart disease itself and its consequences on the myocardium are a frequent cause of cardioembolic stroke as well.

Considerable therapeutic progress in terms of primary stroke prevention has been made in patients with NVAF. In the general population of Western countries, the prevalence of NVAF is less than 1%, but it is as high as 12% in persons older than 75 years of age. The annual risk of severe ischemic stroke strongly depends on concomitant risk factors: arterial hypertension, congestive heart failure, previous cardiogenic embolism, age older than 60 years, or a thrombotic mass detected by ultrasound within the left atrium or its appendix. If several of these risk factors are present, the cumulative annual stroke risk reaches nearly 20%. This risk can be reduced by approximately 70% if the patient is subjected to anticoagulation with warfarin (Coumadin) or coumarin derivatives, with the ideal international normalized ratio (INR) value being 2.5–3.5. This low-dose anticoagulation provides a minimum of both ischemic strokes and cerebral or extracerebral bleeding.

A randomized trial could not demonstrate a beneficial, primary preventive effect of antiplatelet therapy in asymptomatic ICA stenoses, although many physicians prescribe such agents as soon as they become aware of the patient's cerebrovascular occlusive disease.

Prevention of thrombotic complications (e.g., deep venous thrombosis) and secondary stroke in the acute stage of ischemic stroke with heparin or subcutaneous application of low-molecular-weight heparins and early treatment with ASA is a therapeutic approach. The latter seems to have only a very limited effect in the acute phase, in the 0.1% range, but is strongly promulgated by British trialists because of its low costs and its low risk of bleeding.

In the subacute or chronic state of secondary prevention—that is, approximately 2–3 weeks poststroke—oral anticoagulation is restricted to specific embolizing cardiac diseases (e.g., dilatative cardiomyopathy, mechanical heart prosthesis, parietal thrombus of the ventricle, atrial fibrillation). There is a strong controversy about whether secondary prevention of cervical artery dissection or intracranial pial artery stenosis should preferably be treated with oral anticoagulation, with antiplatelet agents, or with both. Several trials are under way addressing this particular issue. In our department, we prefer low-dose oral anticoagulation in these latter conditions for a limited period of 6–24 months, depending on ultrasound follow-up findings at the dissected or otherwise stenosed intracranial arteries.

Compared with a placebo, both ASA and ticlopidine have been proven to significantly prevent major stroke and vascular death after a TIA or minor strokes from other than the above reasons or of cryptogenic origin. The absolute risk reduction by means of 40–325 mg per day ASA is approximately 15% but amounts to approximately 25% for ticlopidine at 2×250 mg per day. Clopidogrel, a derivative of ticlopidine with fewer side effects and a better efficacy than ASA, is presently being approved in Europe and the United States. Another trial demonstrated that the combination of 2×50 mg ASA per day plus 2×200 mg dipyridamole per day provided a nearly twofold efficacy than either of the compounds alone at the same dosage. However, there are no data about combinations with higher ASA doses. At present, this combined medication is also in the approval process.

Suggested Reading

Antiplatelet Trialists' Collaboration. Collaborative overview therapy. I: Prevention of death, myocardioinfarction, and stroke by prolonged antiplatelet therapy in various categories of patients. BMJ 1994;308:81.

Barnett HJM, Eliasziw M, Meldrum HE, Tailor DW. Do the facts and figures warrant a 10-fold increase in the performance of carotid endarterectomy on asymptomatic patients? Neurology 1996;46:603.

Barth A, Bogousslavsky J, Caplan L. Thalamic Infarcts and Hemorrhages. In J Bogousslavsky, L Caplan (eds), Stroke Syndromes. Cambridge, UK: Cambridge University Press 1995;276–283.

Bogousslavsky J, Regly F, Uske A. Thalamic infarcts: clinical syndromes, etiology and prognosis. Neurology 1988;38:837.

Caplan LR. Binswanger's disease—revisited. Neurology 1995;45:626.

CAPRIE Steering Committee. A randomised, blinded trial of clopidogrel versus aspirin in patients at risk of ischaemic events (CAPRIE). Lancet 1996;348:1329.

Carolei A, Marini C, DeMatteis G, and the Italian National Research Council Study Group on Stroke in the Young. History of migraine and risk of cerebral ischemia in young adults. Lancet 1996;347:1503.

Castaigne P, Lhermitte F, Gautier JC, et al. Arterial occlusions in the vertebrovasilar system. A study of 44 patients with post mortem data. Brain 1973;96:133.

Diener HC, Cunha L, Forbes C, et al. European stroke prevention study 2. Dipyridamole and acetylsalicylic acid in the secondary prevention of stroke. J Neurol Sci 1996;143:1.

European Atrial Fibrillation Trial (EAFT) Study Group. Secondary prevention in non-rheumatic atrial fibrillation after transient ischemic attack or minor stroke. Lancet 1993;342:1255.

European Carotid Surgery Trialists' Collaborative Group. Endarterectomy for moderate symptomatic carotid stenosis: interim results from the MRC European Carotid Surgery Trial. Lancet 1996;347:1591.

Fisher CM. Lacunar strokes and infarcts: a review. Neurology 1982;32:871.

The French Study of Aortic Plaques in Stroke Groups. Atherosclerotic disease of the aortic arch as a risk factor for recurrent ischemic stroke. N Engl J Med 1996;334:1216.

Hacke W, Kaste M, Fieschii D, et al. for the ECASS Study Group. Intravenous thrombolysis with recombinant tissue plasminogen activator for acute hemispheric stroke. The European Cooperative Acute Stroke Study Group (ECASS). JAMA 1995;174:1017.

Kay R, Wong KS, Yuh YL, et al. Low-molecular-weight heparin for the treatment of acute ischemic stroke. N Engl J Med 1988;318:1148.

NASCET Collaborators. Beneficial effect of carotid endarterectomy in symptomatic patients with high-grade carotid stenosis. N Engl J Med 1991;325:445.

Ringelstein EB. Ultrasound Evaluation of the Posterior Cerebral Circulation. In B Hofferberth, GG Brune, G Sitzer, HD Weger (eds), Vascular Brainstem Disease. Basel: Karger, 1990;174–198.

Ringelstein EB, Koschorke S, Holling A, et al. Computed tomographic patterns of proven embolic brain infarctions. Ann Neurol 1989;26:759.

Ringelstein EB, Biniek R, Weiller C, et al. Type and extent of hemispheric brain infarctions and clinical outcome in early and delayed middle cerebral artery recanalization. Neurology 1992;42:289.

B. Intracranial Hemorrhage

Steven M. Greenberg

Chapter Plan

Pathophysiology
    Intracranial aneurysm
    Hypertensive vasculopathy
    Cerebral amyloid angiopathy
    Vascular malformations
    Hemorrhagic transformation of ischemic stroke
        and hemorrhage after anticoagulant/throm-
        bolytic therapy
    Other causes of hemorrhage
Clinical presentation
Diagnosis
Treatment
Prognosis and preventative treatments

Intracranial hemorrhage constitutes approximately 20% of all strokes, divided about equally between intracerebral hemorrhages (ICH) in the brain parenchyma itself and subarachnoid hemorrhages (SAH). Acute mortality after hemorrhage is high (greater than 30%), emphasizing the need for improvements in both prevention and treatment. The incidence of intracranial hemorrhage will likely be swelled by the growing use of anticoagulant and thrombolytic agents, further underscoring the need for improved understanding of this entity.

Intracranial hemorrhage, like ischemic stroke, represents the end result of several distinct pathophysiologic pathways. Many principles of management apply to all types of hemorrhage. It is nevertheless important to maintain the distinctions among the different pathogenic processes in assessing treatment and prevention strategies.

This chapter discusses nontraumatic causes of intracranial hemorrhage. The term *hemorrhagic stroke* causes some confusion, because it is variously applied either to primary cerebral hemorrhage or to hemorrhagic conversion of an ischemic infarction. For the purposes of this chapter, this term is avoided in favor of the terms *ICH* and *SAH* to describe primary intracranial hemorrhages.

Pathophysiology

Intracranial Aneurysm

Rupture of an intracranial saccular aneurysm is the most common cause of primary nontraumatic SAH. Saccular aneurysms are outpouchings of vessel walls in which the media layer is thin or nonexistent, leaving only the intima and adventitia to protect the integrity of the vessel. Saccular aneurysms typically occur outside the brain parenchyma and are thus generally associated with SAH rather than with primary ICH. Their most common sites are at branching points of large intracranial vessels such as the junctions of the internal carotid and posterior communicating arteries (Figure 26B-1), the anterior cerebral and anterior communicating arteries, or the vertebral and posterior inferior cerebellar arteries, and at the bifurcations of the middle cerebral or basilar arteries (Figure 26B-2).

Although the precise steps that lead to formation of intracranial aneurysms have not been identified, both genetic and environmental risk factors appear to have a role. The genetic component is highlighted by the common presence (up to 20%) of asymptomatic or symptomatic aneurysms in first-degree relatives of patients with SAH. Among defined familial syndromes related to saccular aneurysms are the collagen-vascular diseases, polycystic kidney disease, and neurofibromatosis type I. Environmental risks for aneurysms include tobacco use and possibly hypertension and heavy alcohol

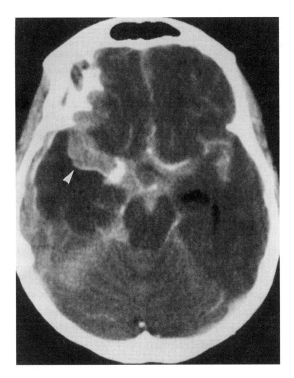

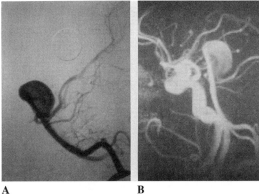

A   B

Figure 26B-2. Saccular aneurysm. An aneurysm of the tip of the basilar artery is demonstrated by digital subtraction contrast angiography (A) and magnetic resonance angiography (B). Also seen on the magnetic resonance imaging scan are the carotid arteries in lateral view. (Courtesy of Pamela W. Schaefer, M.D., Department of Radiology, Massachusetts General Hospital, Boston.)

Figure 26B-1. Subarachnoid hemorrhage. This contrast-enhanced computed tomographic scan demonstrates extensive subarachnoid hemorrhage and a large aneurysm of the right internal carotid artery (*arrowhead*) at the level of the sylvian fissure. (Courtesy of Pamela W. Schaefer, M.D., Department of Radiology, Massachusetts General Hospital, Boston.)

use. Estrogen has been suggested as a possible protective environmental factor.

Most aneurysms do not rupture, as demonstrated by the high frequency of asymptomatic, unruptured aneurysms at postmortem examination. Aneurysms appear at highest risk for rupture when large (more than 1.0 cm), growing, multiple, part of a familial syndrome, or present in a patient with a previous SAH. Rebleeding from a previously ruptured aneurysm is very common and represents one of the most important considerations in therapy.

Hypertensive Vasculopathy

Hypertension, despite generally improving control, remains the major environmental risk factor for nontraumatic ICH. Hypertension may play a limited role in the formation of saccular aneurysms, but its major pathologic effects are on middle and distal segments of deep penetrating arterioles within the brain parenchyma. The pathologic changes that appear to lead directly to vessel rupture and hemorrhage are necrosis and replacement of the vessel media with lipohyalinotic or fibrinoid material.

Hypertensive vasculopathy and hemorrhage favor areas where arterioles branch off of large-caliber vessels and are thus exposed to high pressures relative to their thin lumens. The most common locations for hypertensive hemorrhages are in the putamen, thalamus (Figure 26B-3), pons, and cerebellum, and they often rupture into the ventricles. Unlike vessels with ruptured saccular aneurysms, vessels that have ruptured from hypertensive changes appear to be at low risk for recurrent hemorrhage. Multiple small hemorrhages have been detected elsewhere in brains with a large hypertensive hemorrhage, however, suggesting that hypertensive vasculopathy can occur concurrently in separate locations within a brain.

Whereas *chronic* hypertension appears to be the strongest risk factor for ICH, *acute* hypertension may also cause vasculopathy and hemorrhage in some instances. In hypertensive encephalopathy, for example, there is radiologic and pathologic evidence for petechial cerebral hemorrhages as well as ischemic damage. ICH has also been reported in nonhypertensive patients with sudden rises in blood

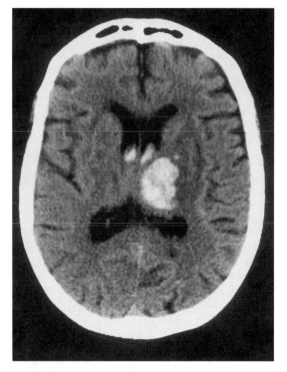

Figure 26B-3. Hypertensive hemorrhage. The computed tomographic scan shows a hemorrhage in the left thalamus, one of the deep regions typically affected by hypertensive vasculopathy.

pressure such as during extreme stress or with use of a sympathomimetic drug.

Cerebral Amyloid Angiopathy

Cerebral amyloid angiopathy (CAA) is defined as the deposition of a particular type of insoluble material in medium- and small-sized vessels in the leptomeninges and cortex. The deposited material has the characteristic staining properties of amyloid, including the ability to generate green birefringence when stained with Congo red and exposed to polarized light. Although the amyloid in cerebral vessels is closely related to the amyloid that comprises neuritic plaques in Alzheimer's disease (AD), it is entirely unrelated to the protein deposits in the systemic amyloidoses. Amyloid deposition in CAA is strikingly restricted to vessels of the leptomeninges and gray matter, often appearing to stop abruptly when a penetrating ves-

sel reaches the junction of the cortex and subcortical white matter.

Deposition of amyloid in cerebral vessels is common in the elderly and is generally asymptomatic. Certain pathologic changes appear to characterize the subset of CAA that is sufficiently severe to cause hemorrhage. These vasculopathic changes include cracking and fibrinoid necrosis in vessel walls. Hemorrhages in CAA typically occur in the cortex or at the gray-white junction (lobar hemorrhages) and may extend to subcortical white matter and subarachnoid space (Figure 26B-4).

Like AD, CAA and CAA-related hemorrhage are highly dependent on age. Other identified risk factors for CAA, such as the accompanying presence of AD and the presence of the e4 allele of the apolipoprotein E gene, further highlight the close relationship between CAA and AD. It is important to note that, although AD occurs at increased frequency in patients with CAA, the majority of individuals with CAA-related hemorrhage appear *not* to have a history of dementia at the time of presentation.

Vascular Malformations

The most common types of vascular malformations in the central nervous system are arteriovenous malformations (AVMs), cavernous malformations (CMs), venous malformations, and telangiectasias. These vascular malformations are congenital and have no known environmental risk factors.

AVMs, as the only of the malformations with an arterial component, present the largest risk of clinically severe ICH. AVMs consist of tufts of arterial and venous vessels with intervention of dilated shunting channels but no true capillary bed. They can occur in the brain parenchyma or, less commonly, in the dura, where they can produce symptoms by hemorrhage or by mass effect. Although AVMs can occur multiply or as part of a familial syndrome, they appear to have less of a genetic component than intracranial aneurysms.

CMs (tufts of large, thin-walled vessels without intervening brain parenchyma), venous malformations (abnormal aggregates of veins with interspersed brain tissue), and telangiectasias (aggregates of dilated capillaries with intervening brain tissue) are more often silent than symptomatic. The widespread use of magnetic resonance imaging (MRI),

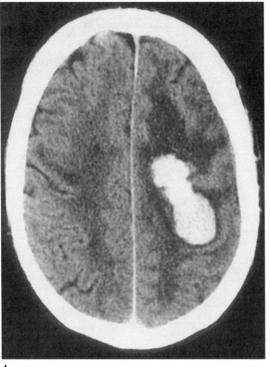
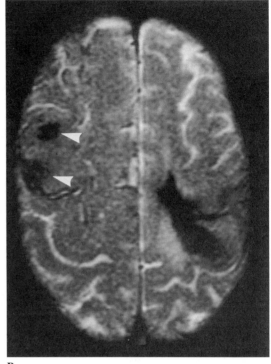

A   B

Figure 26B-4. Probable cerebral amyloid angiopathy–related hemorrhage. Computed tomographic scan (A) shows an acute left frontoparietal hemorrhage. Gradient-echo magnetic resonance imaging scan (B) performed 1 week later demonstrates this lesion as well as several other areas of hypointense signal (*arrowheads*) at the border of the cortical gray and white matter. The presence of multiple hemorrhages confined to this region is suggestive of cerebral amyloid angiopathy (see text).

however, has led to increased recognition of CMs in particular as a source of clinical symptoms via leakage of small volumes of blood. Improved detection of CMs has also provided increasing evidence for familial occurrence of multiple malformations, suggesting a significant genetic component. CMs can coexist with venous malformations and telangiectasias and appear to increase their likelihood of hemorrhage in these instances.

Hemorrhagic Transformation of Ischemic Stroke and Hemorrhage After Anticoagulant/Thrombolytic Therapy

Hemorrhagic transformation commonly occurs during the first few days after ischemic infarction. The region of hemorrhagic transformation typically consists of scattered petechial hemorrhages

within necrotic tissue and has little or no clinical consequence. Even the less common appearance of a frank hematoma within infarcted tissue (Figure 26B-5) is often well tolerated by the brain, but in severe cases produces mass effect and clinical deterioration.

Hemorrhagic transformation appears to arise from reperfusion of damaged vessels within a necrotic region of brain. The major risk factor for hemorrhagic transformation is a large volume of infarcted tissue, whereas blood pressure seems not to correlate with risk. Strokes that occur by the relatively uncommon mechanism of cerebral vein or sinus thrombosis also commonly undergo petechial hemorrhage, presumably a result of the infarction occurring at arterial pressures.

Hemorrhagic transformation is the most important complication of acute thrombolysis for cerebral infarction. Hemorrhage has been observed in

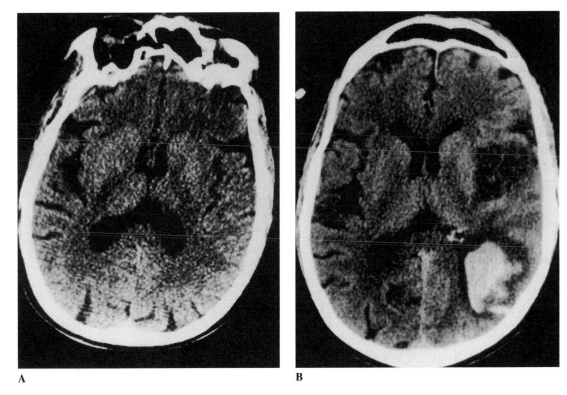

A   B

Figure 26B-5. Hemorrhagic transformation of an ischemic infarction. Shown are two unenhanced computed tomographic scans of a 79-year-old man who presented with the acute onset of global aphasia and right face and hand weakness, within hours after the onset of symptoms (A), and 2 days later (B), at a time when the patient was clinically stable or improving. The patient did not receive anticoagulant treatment during his hospitalization.

approximately 10–20% of patients treated with tissue plasminogen activator for acute stroke, many of these hemorrhages associated with clinical deterioration or death. Hemorrhagic transformation after thrombolysis, like spontaneous hemorrhagic transformation, appears related to reperfusion within necrotic tissue. Risks for hemorrhage include large size of stroke with major neurologic deficits at the time of treatment, the appearance of mass effect or edema related to the stroke on initial CT scans, and possibly a longer (i.e., more than 3-hour) interval between symptom onset and thrombolysis. It is unclear whether controlling blood pressure may lower the risk of this complication. Use of anticoagulant agents after acute stroke appears to have relatively little effect on the overall risk of hemorrhagic transformation. Their use, however, probably does increase the likelihood of severe transformation with formation of hematoma and clinical worsening.

The majority of intracranial hemorrhages related to anticoagulant or thrombolytic therapy do not arise in the setting of ischemic stroke, but instead happen spontaneously during use of the medication. Because of the very poor prognosis associated with these events, their occurrence can tip the risk-to-benefit analysis toward or away from treatment. The likelihood of intracranial hemorrhage from warfarin is increased by advancing age and degree of anticoagulation, with significantly elevated risk at international normalized ratios greater than 4.0–5.0. Thrombolysis-associated hemorrhage also appears related to dose of medication and has been decreasing in incidence with the trend toward lower doses of thrombolytic agent. Both types of hemorrhage typically occur in the brain parenchyma or subdural space, with a suggestion of increased representation of lobar ICHs in this group.

Postmortem studies have demonstrated that at least some apparently "spontaneous" hemorrhages

Table 26B-1. Nontraumatic Causes of Intracranial Hemorrhage According to Most Common Locations

Subarachnoid	Lobar	Deep
Saccular aneurysm	AVM, CM	Hypertensive vasculopathy
Extension from lobar hemorrhage	CAA	CM
	Hemorrhagic tumor	
	Hemorrhagic transformation of ischemic infarction	
	Coagulopathy, thrombolysis	
	Infective endocarditis	
	Extension from deep hemorrhage	

AVM = arteriovenous malformation; CM = cavernous malformation; CAA = cerebral amyloid angiopathy.

from warfarin or thrombolysis in fact arise from an underlying vasculopathy such as CAA. Diagnosis of underlying risks for hemorrhage thus represents a promising approach toward improving outcomes of thrombolysis and anticoagulation.

Other Causes of Hemorrhage

There are a variety of other potential causes of nontraumatic cerebral hemorrhage (Table 26B-1), some of which are discussed elsewhere in this volume. Hemorrhagic tumors can be primary or metastatic. They consist of both those tumors with a particular tendency for hemorrhage (e.g., metastatic melanoma, choriocarcinoma, renal cell cancers, oligodendrogliomas) and tumors that bleed at a lower rate but are present in the brain with an overall greater frequency (e.g., metastatic breast and lung tumors, glioblastoma multiforme).

Both systemic (most notably polyarteritis nodosa and systemic lupus erythematosus) and primary central nervous system vasculitides can cause ICH. These syndromes typically cause ischemic infarction as well as ICH. A similar mix of ischemic and hemorrhagic lesions can result from the multifocal vasospasm related to sympathomimetic drugs such as amphetamines or cocaine. Still another mechanism for hemorrhage related to sympathomimetic drugs is the unmasking of a previously silent lesion such as an AVM.

Intracranial hemorrhage (ICH or SAH) occurs in approximately 5% of patients with infective endocarditis. Hemorrhage in these patients can result from a variety of mechanisms, including formation of mycotic aneurysms in cerebral vessels, hemor-

rhagic transformation of ischemic infarction, and infective vasculitis. The high risk of clinically significant hemorrhage generally precludes use of anticoagulants in patients with endocarditis.

Several epidemiologic risk factors are associated with intracranial hemorrhage. There is a consistent tendency for patients with low serum cholesterol levels to demonstrate higher rates of ICH. The mechanism underlying this relationship has not been established, and there is no rationale at this time to avoid cholesterol-lowering treatments in patients for whom they are otherwise indicated. Excessive alcohol use also appears to raise the risk for hemorrhage, in part because of its association with hypertension and coagulopathy.

Clinical Presentation

The ready availability of CT scanning has served to de-emphasize the clinical differentiation between ischemic stroke and ICH. This is indeed a fortunate development, as distinction between the two on clinical grounds alone can at times prove difficult or impossible. Clinical diagnosis of intracranial hemorrhage nonetheless remains an important challenge, particularly for those syndromes in which either CT scanning is not perfectly sensitive (e.g., SAH) or when an imaging study may not initially be suggested by the presenting complaint (e.g., cerebellar hemorrhage).

Certain clinical features, although not sufficiently sensitive to detect all cases of hemorrhage, strongly suggest this diagnosis. Hemorrhage that involves the subarachnoid space or ventricles produces severe headache ("worst of my life") with or

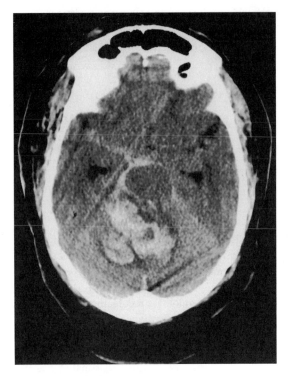

Figure 26B-6. Cerebellar hemorrhage. (Courtesy of Pamela W. Schaefer, M.D., Department of Radiology, Massachusetts General Hospital, Boston.)

without vomiting and meningismus. Hemorrhages that are wholly contained in the brain parenchyma, however, can present entirely without headache. Similarly, a history of neurologic symptoms that smoothly progress over minutes or hours favors the diagnosis of hemorrhage, but often cannot be elicited. Another clinical feature that suggests SAH or cortical ICH is the occurrence of seizures at the time of symptom onset.

ICH typically causes focal signs or symptoms in a pattern that reflects the location of the hemorrhage. *Lobar hemorrhages* can produce weakness of a single limb or disturbances of language, spatial perception, or visual field. Their relationship to the cortex and subarachnoid space make these hemorrhages more likely to cause seizure or headache. *Putaminal hemorrhages* typically cause contralateral weakness of the face, arm, and leg together with variable degrees of sensory loss, ataxia, visual field loss, and (depending on the side involved) aphasia or visuospatial neglect. Clinical signs in *thalamic hemorrhages* can include con-

tralateral sensory loss and weakness caused by involvement of sensory nuclei and the adjacent internal capsule. Thalamic hemorrhages that extend to or compress the superior midbrain can also cause a decreased level of consciousness and midbrain eye signs such as loss of upward gaze. *Pontine hemorrhages* often result in severe impairments in consciousness, bilateral motor function, and pontine cranial nerve function.

Prompt recognition of *cerebellar hemorrhage* (Figure 26B-6) can be life-saving. Whereas the clinical features of headache and vomiting might be mistaken for benign conditions such as gastroenteritis, the presence of focal neurologic findings such as ataxia of gait, trunk, or limb and palsies of horizontal gaze or facial movements are strong indications for acute neuroimaging.

The clinical diagnosis of *SAH* also remains of vital importance, particularly as it can be missed on CT scans (see later). SAH is characterized by the sudden onset of extremely severe headache with or without acute loss of consciousness. The release of blood under arterial pressure into the subarachnoid space presumably accounts for both the acute loss of brain perfusion (often causing sudden loss of consciousness) and the presence in some patients of subhyaloid hemorrhages on funduscopic examination. Focal symptoms are often absent.

Some of the pathophysiologic processes that underlie intracranial hemorrhage can present clinically before major hemorrhage has occurred. The increasing availability of preventative treatments and avoidable risk factors for hemorrhage lend greater importance to identification of these early presentations. Neuroimaging studies performed for unrelated reasons may detect unruptured saccular aneurysms or vascular malformations. In addition, dilated aneurysms can compress cranial nerves as they exit the brain stem or traverse the cavernous sinus. Large AVMs can cause mass effect, and small hemorrhages that occur around vascular malformations often give rise to seizures.

Petechial hemorrhages related to CAA have been identified as a cause of recurrent stereotyped neurologic spells that can be confused with transient ischemic attacks (TIAs). These CAA-related spells typically consist of weakness, numbness, or paresthesias that spread across adjacent body parts over a period of minutes. The smoothly spreading progression, together with their sensitivity to anti-

Table 26B-2. Radiographic Appearance of Intracranial Hemorrhage

Duration After Hemorrhage	Minutes–Hour	Hours–Days	Days–Week	Weeks	Years
Source of Radiographic Signal	Extravascular Blood	Deoxyhemo-globin	Intracellular Methemoglobin	Extracellular Methemoglobin	Ferritin/ Hemosiderin
Imaging Technique					
CT scan	↑↑	↑↑	↑↑	↑, ↔	↓, ↔
MRI: T1-weighted	↓, ↔	↓, ↔	↑↑	↑↑	↓, ↔
MRI: T2-weighted	↑	↓↓	↓↓	↑↑ + dark rim	↓
MRI: gradient-echo					↓↓

CT = computed tomographic; MRI = magnetic resonance imaging; ↑ or ↑↑ = hyperintense signal; ↓ or ↓↓ = hypointense signal; ↔ = isointense signal.

convulsant treatment and the absence of critical vascular stenosis on diagnostic evaluation, differentiates these spells from true TIAs—and thus allows antiplatelet or anticoagulant therapy to be avoided.

Diagnosis

CT scanning has transformed the diagnosis of acute intracranial hemorrhage into a relatively straightforward task. Extravascular blood appears hyperdense on non–contrast-enhanced CT scans acutely (see Figures 26B-1, 26B-3, 26B-4, 26B-5, and 26B-6) and remains so for several weeks after hemorrhage, allowing detection of ICH with nearly complete sensitivity. It is essential to note that CT scanning is only approximately 90–95% sensitive for SAH, probably less so for those patients with small SAHs and relatively mild symptoms. These considerations highlight the need for emergent lumbar puncture in virtually any patient suspected of SAH not demonstrable on CT scans.

The MRI image of ICH evolves in a complex fashion according to a variety of physical and chemical factors (Table 26B-2). These include the initial deoxygenation and subsequent chemical breakdown of hemoglobin into methemoglobin, the dissolution of the erythrocyte cell membrane, and finally the formation of iron-containing hemosiderin deposits. The sensitivity of high–field-strength MRI to detect these changes makes this technique complex to interpret but ultimately of great use for evaluation of subacute and chronic hemorrhage. Of most practical importance are the

high signal intensity on T1-weighted images produced by methemoglobin in the subacute phase of hemorrhage followed by the hypointensity on T2-weighted images caused by ferritin and hemosiderin deposits during the chronic stage. The latter effect can be accentuated by gradient-echo MRI (see Figure 26B-4). This technique, which requires no additional MRI hardware or software, offers the greatest radiologic sensitivity for even small chronic ICHs.

The most helpful information for determining the cause of hemorrhage is typically the demographic characteristics of the patient and the radiographic location and appearance of the hemorrhage. Among important demographic characteristics are age, family history, and the presence of risk factors such as hypertension, systemic cancer, coagulopathy, or AD. Age, for example, can be useful in discriminating lobar hemorrhages caused by CAA (which rarely present in patients younger than age 50 years) from those caused by an AVM (which typically cause symptoms before this age). Laboratory testing is useful in pursuing less common causes of hemorrhage such as vasculitis or infectious endocarditis.

Table 26B-1 shows causes of hemorrhage according to their favored locations in the brain: subarachnoid, lobar (primarily affecting the cortex and subcortical white matter), or deep (primarily involving basal ganglia, thalamus, brain stem, or cerebellum). It should be noted that the various pathologic entities do not invariably respect anatomic boundaries and can occur outside their typical regions. Also, the location of origin for a hemorrhage may be difficult to trace from the radi-

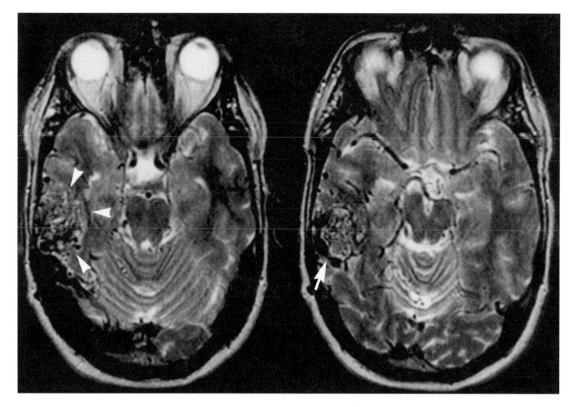

Figure 26B-7. Arteriovenous malformation. This T2-weighted MRI scan demonstrates multiple areas of flow-void (*arrowheads in left image*) in the right temporal lobe representing the nidus of the malformation. There is also a dilated linear region of flow-void (*arrow in right image*) that is likely a draining vein. There is no evidence for hemorrhage arising from this lesion. (Courtesy of Pamela W. Schaefer, M.D., Department of Radiology, Massachusetts General Hospital, Boston.)

ographic image. Thus, it is not unusual for a putaminal hemorrhage to extend to subcortical and cortical regions and thus simulate lobar hemorrhage, or for an anterior communicating artery aneurysm to bleed into the frontal lobes simulating primary ICH.

Other radiographic features characterize particular types of ICH. AVMs are demonstrated by conventional angiography or MRI studies as clusters of vascular channels with rapid flow (Figure 26B-7). MRI and angiography studies have to some degree supplanted conventional angiography for AVMs because of their ability to demonstrate the relationship of the lesion to surrounding brain structures and to detect previous hemorrhage. CMs, which are typically undetectable by conventional angiography, appear on MRI scans as small areas of hemorrhage without associated dilated vessels. The characteristic "target" appearance (Figure 26B-8) is created by a central region of mixed signal surrounded by a ring of decreased signal produced by hemosiderin and ferritin deposits. Hemorrhagic tumors (Figure 26B-9) can also contain complex mixtures of increased and decreased signal related to the presence of viable tumor, necrotic tissue, calcification, and variously aged hemorrhages. Tumor is suggested when the lesions are multiple, are strongly (sometimes heterogeneously) enhancing, have clear nonhemorrhagic components, or are surrounded by excessively large areas of edema. The tendency of CAA-related hemorrhages to be multiple and recurrent leads to a distinctive pattern of multiple hemorrhages of various sizes entirely restricted to the lobar regions. This pattern, best demonstrated by gradient-echo MRI (see Figure 26B-4), is highly suggestive of CAA in elderly patients without other known causes for ICH. Hem-

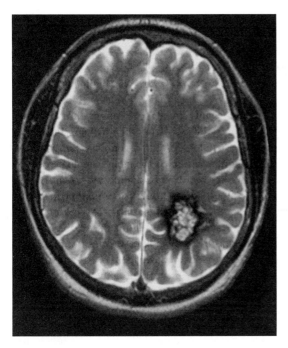

Figure 26B-8. Cavernous malformation. This lesion was identified in a 44-year-old woman with a seizure disorder since childhood. The T2-weighted magnetic resonance imaging scan demonstrates the "target" appearance characteristic of cavernous malformations. Typical features include the complete ring of hemosiderin (producing decreased signal) and the absence of associated edema. (Courtesy of Pamela W. Schaefer, M.D., Department of Radiology, Massachusetts General Hospital, Boston.)

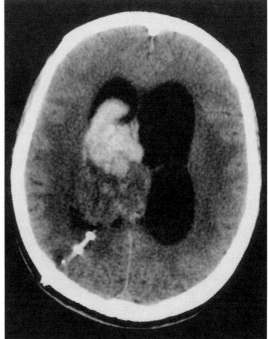

Figure 26B-9. Hemorrhagic tumor. This unenhanced computed tomographic scan demonstrates a heterogeneous mass in the region of the right lateral ventricle with a large hemorrhagic component. The pathologic diagnosis of this mass has not been determined.

orrhagic transformation of an ischemic infarction is often demonstrated by the emergence of hemorrhage after clinical symptoms are already present from the underlying infarction (see Figure 26B-5). Cerebral vasculitis can be suggested by the concurrent appearance of ischemic and hemorrhagic lesions.

Examination of cerebrospinal fluid is essentially 100% sensitive for detection of SAH. Problems of interpretation arise in distinguishing SAH from traumatic lumbar puncture. The finding of xanthochromia in the spinal fluid is most helpful in this regard, appearing several hours after SAH and persisting in spectrophotometrically detectable amounts for several weeks. Conventional angiography remains the primary technique for detection of saccular aneurysms in patients with SAH (see Figure 26B-2A). MRI and MR angiography are also sensitive for all but the smallest aneurysms (see Fig-

ure 26B-2B) and can be helpful in monitoring aneurysms after surgical clipping. (Aneurysm clips in current use are nonmagnetic.) MRI is not sensitive for the detection of acute SAH and has no role in its diagnosis.

The presence of recent hemorrhage and thrombus can obscure underlying structural lesions such as a saccular aneurysm, AVM, or tumor. Thus, it is often helpful to repeat brain or blood vessel imaging weeks to months after acute hemorrhage. Repeat MR or conventional angiography is of particular importance in patients with SAH and negative findings on the initial angiogram, as approximately 5% will subsequently disclose a saccular aneurysm.

Hemorrhagic tumors tend to evolve differently on follow-up MRI scanning from the pattern described for primary hematomas (see Table 26B-2), a result of differences in blood-brain barrier and tissue oxygenation related to the tumor.

Table 26B-3. Factors Regulating Intracranial Pressure and Cerebral Perfusion After Intracranial Hemorrhage

Intracranial pressure
 Hematoma volume
 Edema
 Volume of surrounding brain
 Cerebral blood volume
 Hydrocephalus
Cerebral perfusion
 Cerebral perfusion pressure (i.e., mean arterial
  pressure – intracranial pressure)
 Local mass effect (intracerebral hemorrhage)
 Vasospasm (subarachnoid hemorrhage)

Treatment

Tissue damage after intracranial hemorrhage results from both the local effects of the hematoma and its generalized effects on intracranial pressure (ICP) and cerebral perfusion. No treatments have yet emerged to retard the destructive effects of the hematoma on surrounding tissue. Also, while there is good evidence that ICHs can continue to grow during the hours after their onset, it is unclear whether treatment can affect either the rate of growth or (with the exception of SAH; see later) the risk of acute recurrence.

Acute treatment for hemorrhages with significant mass effect is thus largely focused on limiting the effects of increased ICP on healthy brain tissue. Some of the principles that guide medical management of ICP and cerebral perfusion are listed in Table 26B-3. Increases in ICP threaten healthy brain tissue by several mechanisms. Massively increased ICP can cause the well-known syndromes of brain herniation and mechanical damage to essential brain structures or vessels. Elevated ICP also lowers the cerebral perfusion pressure (CPP), which is the difference between the arterial and ICPs (see Table 26B-3), and thus increases the risk of ischemia to other parts of the brain.

Treatments of increased ICP include removal of exacerbating factors (e.g., fever, hypoventilation, and seizures) and institution of therapies (e.g., hyperventilation and osmotic agents). Hyperventilation (targeting the P_{CO_2} to approximately 30–35 mm Hg) causes cerebral vasoconstriction in normal areas of the brain, thus decreasing cerebral blood volume and ICP. Hyperventilation can serve as a bridge to longer-lasting treatments of ICP, as its effects begin within minutes but typically last only several hours. Osmotic agents such as mannitol (typically given at doses of 0.25–1.0 g/kg, aiming for a serum osmolarity of 310–320 mOsm/liter) lower ICP by reducing the volume of normal brain tissue. The effect of osmotic agents on ICP can be detected in less than an hour and persists for several days. Greater degrees of hyperventilation or osmotic agent can further reduce ICP, although with the risk of producing metabolic derangements or rebounds in ICP when the values are allowed to return towards normal. Corticosteroids have no clear role in the treatment of elevated ICP after ICH.

ICP can be measured continuously through a subarachnoid pressure transducer or intraventricular catheter. External monitoring of ICP is most helpful when the clinical signs of neurologic deterioration cannot be adequately followed, such as in a sedated or anesthetized patient.

Another medical issue that arises is whether and how to treat elevations in blood pressure. Hypertension can raise the ICP (via increased cerebral blood volume) or potentially increase the risk of persistent or recurrent hemorrhage (although a relationship of hematoma expansion to blood pressure has yet to be demonstrated). Balancing potential concerns about hypertension after ICH is the risk that hypotension might lower CPP (see Table 26B-3), particularly in those areas adjacent to the hematoma where local ICP might be highest. A second concern with antihypertensive treatment is that many agents are cerebral vasodilators and thus will *increase* cerebral blood volume and ICP. In the absence of clear evidence from interventional clinical trials, a reasonable practice might be to treat only systolic blood pressures of more than 180 mm Hg or mean arterial pressures more than 125 mm Hg. On theoretical grounds, preferred antihypertensive agents would be those drugs with the least tendency to cause cerebral vasodilation. These agents include alpha- and beta-blocking antiadrenergic agents such as labetalol, diuretics, and angiotensin converting enzyme inhibitors. Because of their ability to decrease cerebral blood volume as well as ICP, barbiturates offer the possibility of controlling blood pressure without reducing CPP, although at a cost of depressing global neurologic function.

Coagulopathies should be rapidly reversed after ICH. Among patients with ICH on warfarin, the very high short-term mortality (approximately 60%) generally argues for reversal of the coagulopathy in precedence to the original indications for anticoagulation. The risk of seizure in medically or neurologically unstable patients supports acute use of anticonvulsant agents in patients with cortical involvement. Seizures generally do not occur when the cortical gray matter is spared.

The precise indications for acute surgical removal of an intracerebral hematoma remain to be defined. Surgery appears to offer little benefit either to patients with minor deficits only (who will typically do well with conservative treatment) or patients with devastating neurologic deficits (who are unlikely to achieve good functional outcomes regardless of therapy). The factors that favor hematoma resection are (1) acute neurologic deterioration while in the hospital, suggesting that some deficits may be reversible; (2) surgical accessibility of the lesion, such as in cerebellar or cortical locations; (3) location in the posterior fossa, which is more sensitive to mass effect than the supratentorial compartment; and (4) younger patient age, suggesting potentially better functional prognosis (see later). Ongoing advances in surgical methods, such as enzymatic lysis of intracerebral hematomas and use of stereotactic techniques for evacuation, promise to expand the indications for surgical treatment. It should be noted that despite reported instances of recurrent bleeding after resection of CAA-related hematomas, the body of clinical experience with CAA suggests that surgery can be performed with no greater incidence of complications than in other types of hemorrhage.

Clinical deterioration after ICH can occur by several mechanisms. These include increased edema and mass effect surrounding the hemorrhage, hydrocephalus, seizure, and (least commonly) recurrent hemorrhage. Hydrocephalus can occur within the first few days after hemorrhage (because of obstruction of the ventricular system by clot) or during the subsequent days or weeks (often the result of decreased cerebrospinal fluid resorption by the hemosiderin-laden arachnoid villi). Deterioration related to hydrocephalus typically responds well to prompt ventricular drainage.

Several specific considerations apply to the management of SAH. Acute recurrent hemorrhage is unusual in ICH but common and potentially devastating after rupture of a saccular aneurysm. Acute treatment is therefore focused on early radiographic identification and surgical clipping of the underlying aneurysm. In the absence of factors predisposing to cerebral ischemia (e.g., hydrocephalus, cerebral vasospasm, or significant mass effect), blood pressures are typically kept in a somewhat lower range in hopes of preventing early rebleeding. In addition to the mechanisms for neurologic deterioration noted earlier, patients with SAH can undergo cerebral vasospasm and ischemic stroke. The risk of vasospasm is greatest in patients with large volumes of hemorrhage in close apposition to cerebral vessels. The risk is decreased by treatment with the calcium channel blocker nimodipine (60 mg every 4 hours, avoiding hypotension).

Prognosis and Preventative Treatments

Mortality during the first days and weeks after either SAH or ICH is approximately 30–40%, a range considerably higher than that of ischemic stroke. Among survivors of ICH, however, functional outcome appears comparable to that for ischemic stroke. High mortality and poor functional outcome after ICH are predicted by the occurrence of a large hemorrhage (particularly those greater than 60–70 cm^3) and low level of consciousness at presentation (Glasgow Coma Scale score of less than 8). Other baseline factors such as elevated blood pressure and intraventricular extension of the hematoma have also been suggested as poor prognostic indicators. Advanced age appears to have relatively little effect on short-term survival but is associated with worse functional outcome.

Despite prospects for better treatments, the devastating nature of intracranial hemorrhage highlights the need for improved prevention. A variety of surgical treatments are available for presymptomatic treatment of aneurysms and vascular malformations. In addition to surgical resection or clipping, these include endovascular placement of material into the abnormal vessels or, for vascular malformations, obliteration by external radiation. Given the availability of preventive treatments for SAH, it is reasonable to use cranial MRI to screen for unruptured aneurysms in individuals with a positive family history (two or more relatives with saccular aneurysms) and possibly those with a predisposing medical illness (such as a collagen vascular disease or polycystic kidneys).

Preventive strategies for other types of hemorrhage are focused on control of risk factors. Marked reductions in the incidence of hypertensive hemorrhage have been achieved through improved control of blood pressure in the general population. Unfortunately, no similar strategy has emerged for prevention of CAA-related hemorrhage, an entity likely to increase in prevalence as the population ages.

Suggested Reading

Brott T, Broderick J, Kothari R, et al. Early hemorrhage growth in patients with intracerebral hemorrhage. Stroke 1997;28:1.

Caplan LR. Intracerebral hemorrhage revisited. Neurology 1988;38:624.

Daverat P, Castel JP, Dartigues JF, Orgogozo JM. Death and functional outcome after spontaneous intracerebral hemorrhage. A prospective study of 166 cases using multivariate analysis. Stroke 1991;22:1.

Diringer MN. Intracerebral hemorrhage: pathophysiology and management. Crit Care Med 1993;21:1591.

Fisher CM. Pathological observations in hypertensive cerebral hemorrhage. J Neuropathol Exp Neurol 1971;30:536.

Greenberg SM, Vonsattel JP, Stakes JW, et al. The clinical spectrum of cerebral amyloid angiopathy: presentations without lobar hemorrhage. Neurology 1993;43: 2073.

Hylek EM, Singer DE. Risk factors for intracranial hemorrhage in outpatients taking warfarin. Ann Intern Med 1994;120:897.

Kase CS, Caplan LR. Intracerebral Hemorrhage. Boston: Butterworth–Heinemann, 1994.

Ropper AH. Treatment of Intracranial Hypertension. In AH Ropper (ed), Neurological and Neurosurgical Intensive Care. New York: Raven, 1993;29–52.

Schievink WI. Intracranial aneurysms. N Engl J Med 1997; 336:28.

Sloan MA, Price TR, Petito CK, et al. Clinical features and pathogenesis of intracerebral hemorrhage after rt-PA and heparin therapy for acute myocardial infarction: the Thrombolysis in Myocardial Infarction (TIMI) II Pilot and Randomized Clinical Trial combined experience. Neurology 1995;45:649.

Thulborn KR, Atlas SW. Intracranial Hemorrhage. In SW Atlas (ed), Magnetic Resonance Imaging of the Brain and Spine. Philadelphia: Lippincott–Raven, 1996; 265–314.

Tuhrim S, Dambrosia JM, Price TR, et al. Intracerebral hemorrhage: external validation and extension of a model for prediction of 30-day survival. Ann Neurol 1991;29:658.

Vinters HV. Cerebral amyloid angiopathy. A critical review. Stroke 1987;18:311.

Chapter 27
Cognitive Disorders

A. *Degenerative Dementias*

David A. Drachman and Joan M. Swearer

Chapter Plan

Dementia is defined as "the decline of memory and other cognitive functions in comparison with the patient's previous level of function as determined by a history of decline in performance and by abnormalities noted from clinical examination and neuropsychological tests." The deficits "must be sufficiently severe to cause impairment in occupational and social functioning. . . ." Circumscribed impairment of cognitive function, such as aphasia, does not satisfy the definition of dementia, nor can dementia be diagnosed in a patient whose cognitive performance is compromised by delirium, drowsiness, stupor, or coma. Limited intellectual endowment or mental retardation may be confused with dementia, especially in patients examined for the first time, but the *absence of decline* from a previous higher level of function distinguishes mental retardation from dementia.

The course of dementia may be either *static* or *progressive*. Static dementia, which is produced by a single, circumscribed event such as head trauma, encephalitis, anoxia, or a stroke, is the result of major damage incurred by the brain resulting in loss of memory and intellect; the deficits remain fixed over time. Because the cause is usually obvious and the loss of cognitive function a direct consequence, it is rarely considered in the same context or clinical setting as progressive dementia. By contrast, progressive dementias frequently present as diagnostic unknowns, the underlying cause to be discovered only after careful evaluation of the entire array of possible causes. The pace of progression varies from a subacute course over several weeks or months (as may be seen with Creutzfeldt-Jakob disease or an expanding subdural hematoma) to a chronic course over years, as is more typical of Alzheimer's disease. In this chapter we consider a subset of the progressive dementias: the *degenerative* dementias.

Degenerative dementias are of uncertain mechanism (as contrasted with symptomatic dementias, e.g., those caused by infection, trauma, or stroke), are increasingly common with advancing age, likely to result from acceleration or exaggeration of "normal" senescent processes that often occur benignly with aging, may occur with or without a genetic predilection or etiology, and usually evolve over years. As the molecular mechanisms of these dementias are elucidated, however, we can expect some "degenerative" dementias to be removed from this category and placed among the "symptomatic" dementias.

Although the definition of dementia requires only global impairment of memory and other cognitive functions, additional behavioral and neurologic symptoms and signs are often associated with the degenerative dementias as they progress. "Obstreperous behaviors" seen in Alzheimer's disease, for example, can include aggressive and assaultive behaviors (from yelling to hitting), mechanical and motor behaviors (from manipulating papers to wandering), ideational disorders (paranoid ideas, hallucinations), and abnormal vegetative behaviors (weight loss, incontinence). Movement disorders, including chorea (Huntington's chorea), myoclonus (Alzheimer's disease), and tremors (Lewy body dementia, parkinsonism) may occur, and rigidity is common in late stages. Many other neurologic signs may occur as the degenerative dementias progress, and an end-stage pattern of an immobile, mute patient bedridden and curled into a fetal posture with pyramidal, extrapyramidal, and frontal release signs is common.

The degenerative dementias are among the most common neurologic disorders. Most degenerative dementia occurs among the elderly, the frequency increasing exponentially with age; the extended life expectancy in modern developed countries has contributed greatly to the number of individuals affected by dementia. Epidemiologic studies in the United States show that approximately 10% of those over the age of 65 years are demented, increasing to 50% of those over the age of 85 years, with 20% totally incapacitated by their dementia. In the oldest old—those older than 90 years—the *incidence* continues to rise, but the *prevalence* of dementia levels off below 60% because of the limited number of years of life expectancy (with or without dementia) at that advanced age. In a healthy middle-aged adult with no known genetic risk factors, the lifetime risk of Alzheimer's disease is approximately 15%; the risk of any progressive dementia is between 15% and 20%. Progressive

dementia is an important cause of death in addition to disability: In the United States, Alzheimer's disease is the fourth most common cause of death after heart disease, cancer, and stroke.

Diagnosis of progressive dementia depends on demonstrating not only a decline from previously higher cognitive performance, but also that the decline is continuing over time—either by history or on repeated examinations. Most progressive dementias advance gradually, with no sudden worsening or improvement; however, situational changes, such as the death of a supportive spouse or a change from a familiar to an unfamiliar environment, may produce an apparent rapid decline in function.

Early in the course of progressive dementias, differentiating the dementia from normal aging or depression may be extremely difficult. In many older individuals, early dementia is not suspected or recognized; screening tests may be helpful in identifying those with mild changes. In some individuals, a reliable history of functions lost, and a bedside mental status examination may be most valuable; in others, detailed psychometric examination is more useful. Psychometric testing over an interval of at least 6 months to 1 year provides an objective means of demonstrating whether increasing loss of cognitive ability is evolving over time.

Evaluating patients and distinguishing among the large array of possible causes of dementia might seem to be an overwhelming task, but by using a clinically based strategy, it is possible to sort them into a manageable order (Figure 27A-1):

1. Progressive dementias (those that continue to deteriorate over time) are separated from static dementias (those that do not progress over time and are caused by a single event such as head trauma or a major stroke).
2. Among the progressive dementias, symptomatic dementias (those resulting from a recognized cause, identifiable usually by laboratory tests, e.g., brain tumors, hydrocephalus, hypothyroidism, syphilis) are separated from degenerative dementias.
3. We then divide the degenerative dementias into four clinical groups: (a) Alzheimer's disease (AD), including pure AD and "Alzheimer's plus" (e.g., AD combined with vascular disease); (b) extrapyramidal dementias: Lewy body

Figure 27A-1. This flow diagram indicates the sequence of steps necessary to distinguish the degenerative dementias from other symptomatic progressive dementias, and to establish specific diagnoses.

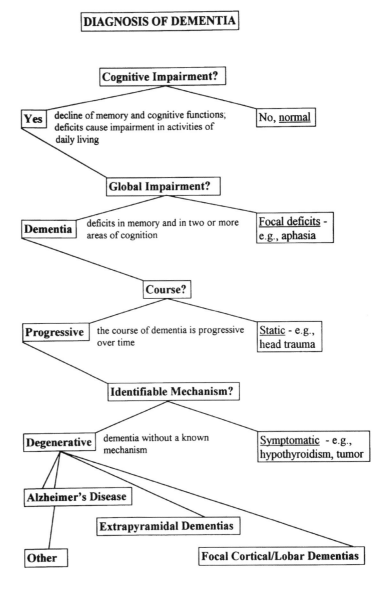

DIAGNOSIS OF DEMENTIA

Cognitive Impairment?

Yes | decline of memory and cognitive functions; deficits cause impairment in activities of daily living | **No, <u>normal</u>**

Global Impairment?

Dementia | deficits in memory and in two or more areas of cognition | **<u>Focal deficits</u> - e.g., aphasia**

Course?

Progressive | the course of dementia is progressive over time | **<u>Static</u> - e.g., head trauma**

Identifiable Mechanism?

Degenerative | dementia without a known mechanism | **<u>Symptomatic</u> - e.g., hypothyroidism, tumor**

Alzheimer's Disease

Extrapyramidal Dementias

Other

Focal Cortical/Lobar Dementias

dementia, Huntington's disease (HD), and so forth; (c) dementias of focal cortical or lobar origin: Pick's disease, frontal dementia, temporal dementia, and so forth; (d) Other: (i) dementia occurring as a minor problem as part of another degenerative disorder, such as myotonic dystrophy; (ii) dementia lacking distinctive histologic features; and (iii) *pseudodegenerative* dementias—conditions of known cause, such as vascular dementia, that mimic degenerative dementias in their course and manifestations.

Specific diagnostic tests for causes of symptomatic progressive dementias or for conditions contributing to the severity of degenerative dementias are indicated in Table 27A-3, and elaborated for the degenerative dementias in the discussion of each disease entity. We believe that everyone with a progressive dementing disorder should undergo a neurologic evaluation and comprehensive diagnostic testing to determine whether a treatable condition is either causing or contributing to the dementia.

Table 27A-1. Progressive Degenerative Dementias

Alzheimer's disease
   Pure Alzheimer's disease
   Alzheimer's plus
      Vascular dementia ("mixed dementia")
      Lewy body dementia
Extrapyramidal dementias
   Lewy body dementia
   Parkinson's disease with dementia
   Huntington's disease
   Progressive supranuclear palsy
   Cortical-basal ganglionic degeneration
Dementias of focal cortical/lobar origin
   Pick's disease
   Frontotemporal dementias
   Primary progressive aphasia
Other degenerative dementias
   Degenerative disorders with minor dementia
   Dementia lacking distinctive histology
   "Pseudodegenerative" dementias

In summary, Alzheimer's disease is the most common cause of progressive degenerative dementia, its pure form causing at least 50–65% of all cases. Combined with vascular damage in the form of small or lacunar strokes, it accounts for another 15–20%. The role of vascular disease in causing dementia remains controversial. In some patients, multiple inapparent strokes may produce a dementing disorder—multi-infarct dementia. In most patients who have cognitive loss resulting from vascular disease, however, mental impairment has been caused by one or two fixed major strokes; the patient presents to the clinician with aphasia or some other focal cognitive deficit rather than global dementia, and the cognitive impairment is not progressive. Small, inapparent strokes may combine with underlying age-related or AD-related cognitive losses to produce significant impairment. As the primary cause of progressive dementia, however, vascular dementia makes up only approximately 10% of cases. The effects of uncontrolled hypertension or generalized cerebrovascular disease may account for some cases of progressive dementia without actual strokes, but the precise role of this entity and the criteria for the diagnosis remain uncertain.

Among the extrapyramidal dementias, Lewy body dementia, a disorder in which the cytoplasmic eosinophilic inclusions typical of Parkinson's disease are found in cortical and subcortical neurons, is an increasingly recognized cause of dementia. More common is the *Lewy body variant of AD,* a combination of typical Alzheimer's disease with extrapyramidal features. In parkinsonism itself, however, dementia may eventually develop in one-third of those affected, often in association with the pathologic features of AD. HD and progressive supranuclear palsy (PSP) also produce dementia in association with movement disorders.

In some degenerative dementias, only limited parts of the cortex and underlying white matter are affected, at least early in their course, producing asymmetric focal lobar atrophy with the concomitant cognitive and behavioral disorders. Pick's disease has long been recognized as a cause of severe temporal and frontal atrophy, seen at autopsy, with microscopic Pick bodies found in neurons. More recently, progressive dementias with a focal onset but lacking Pick bodies at autopsy have been named *frontotemporal dementia, frontal lobe dementia,* or *temporal lobe dementia,* but likely are variants of Pick's disease. Many other conditions, ranging from multiple system atrophy to olivopontocerebellar atrophy, can also produce progressive dementia, as listed in Table 27A-1.

Alzheimer's Disease

Alzheimer's disease (AD) is the most common of the degenerative dementias, accounting for at least one-half of the cases in autopsy studies of demented patients. The onset of symptoms is insidious and incremental, beginning between 40 and 90 years of age, but is most common after 65 years. The prevalence of AD is approximately 1–2% at age 65 years, but doubles every 5 years at least to age 90 years. Estimates vary, but by the age of 85 years some 35–50% of those surviving to that age have AD, and 20% are severely incapacitated by their dementia. The disease is gradually progressive, with an average life expectancy of 8–12 years.

The cause of AD is unknown in the vast majority of cases. Approximately 5% of patients with AD have an early-onset, dominantly inherited form of familial AD (EODI FAD), which usually begins before age 50 years; the remainder are considered to have sporadic AD (SAD), although genetic risk factors may modify their chances of developing the dementia.

In EODI FAD patients, genetic abnormalities have been found, most often as the presenilin 1 gene on chromosome 14; in an extended group of individuals with Volga German ancestry as the similar presenilin 2 gene on chromosome 1; and rarely involving the amyloid precursor protein (APP) gene on chromosome 21. The abnormalities of the APP gene are believed to contribute to the inappropriate processing of APP and the resulting accumulation of amyloid, which is a neuropathologic hallmark of AD, both in senile (neuritic) plaques and in the walls of cerebral blood vessels (amyloid angiopathy). At the time of this writing, the normal and deranged functions of the presenilin 1 and 2 genes are not known.

SAD is 20 times as common as EODI FAD, and its etiology is not clearly understood. We do know that age, apolipoprotein E4, and being female are important risk factors for the development of SAD. Increasing age is by far the most powerful risk factor for SAD: At age 85 years, the annual incidence of SAD is 20–30 times greater than at age 65 years. This suggests that an exaggeration or acceleration of processes that occur normally with aging may be among the most important causes of AD. It is also known that inheritance of one of the three isoforms of the apolipoprotein E allele—ε4 (*APOE ε4*)—is associated with an earlier age of disease onset, and a 2- to 4-fold increase in the lifetime risk of developing AD. Women have a higher age-adjusted incidence of AD than men; combined with their longer life expectancy, this results in a much higher number of elderly women than men with AD. Other factors that may increase the risk of AD include significant head trauma, hypertension, or cardiovascular disease.

Clinical Features and Neurologic Findings

The onset of AD is usually gradual and insidious. Memory impairment is the cardinal clinical feature of AD and is usually one of the earliest deficits observed. Over months, or at most a year or two from onset, the memory and cognitive deficits become increasingly obvious and interfere with the patient's ability to perform his or her usual activities: work, household duties, social relations, card games, driving, and so forth. As cognitive functions decline further, the patient develops difficulty finding words, recalling even familiar events, reading, writing, and following movies or television shows. With further global impairment, the patient becomes dependent on others for self-care—help with dressing, bathing, toileting, feeding. Such dependence usually develops within 3–6 years after the initial diagnosis. In the terminal stages the patient becomes mute, incontinent, and bed-bound. Bronchopneumonia is a common cause of death.

Behavioral disturbances are a frequent feature of AD as well as other degenerative dementias, affecting most patients at some time during the course of the illness. The types of abnormal behaviors that are exhibited by demented patients are variable but can be classified into four categories: (1) aggressive and assaultive behaviors (e.g., physical and verbal attacks); (2) disordered ideation (e.g., hallucinations, delusions, paranoia); (3) mechanical or motor abnormalities (e.g., pacing, wandering, repeatedly handling small objects); and (4) vegetative disorders (e.g., incontinence, hyposexuality, and sleep disturbances). A convenient mnemonic for the behavioral disorders that are often most troublesome to caregivers is "SWID": *S*leep disorders, *W*andering, *I*ncontinence, and *D*angerousness (to self or others). We have found that when patients develop three or more of the "SWID features," they are often placed in nursing homes; similarly, when patients develop incontinence combined with aggressive behaviors, more than 60% are placed in nursing homes within a year.

Early in the course of AD, the physical and neurologic examination results are usually entirely normal, except for memory and cognitive functions, and the patient's usual personal manners may be preserved, often remaining superficially gracious. At this stage, it may be impossible to distinguish between usual age-associated memory impairment (AAMI) in the elderly and AD. We recommend the routine use of simple cognitive screening tests in those older than 75 years of age to evaluate cognitive function and to establish a baseline of performance. As AD evolves, the history and cognitive evaluation provide incontrovertible evidence of rapid decline in cognition, and the evolution of decline frequently is the only reliable way to resolve the question of AAMI versus AD. With further advance of the process, primitive reflexes such as grasping, sucking, and the glabellar reflex are not uncommon, and extrapyramidal rigidity (but rarely tremor) may develop. When rigidity and a parkinsonian gait occur relatively early—that is, when the dementia is still mild—this may suggest the Lewy body variant of AD. Even in later stages of AD, while the patient continues to live in the community, neurologic abnormalities remain confined to cognitive changes, extrapyramidal rigidity, and primitive reflexes. In very advanced AD—often when the patient is in a nursing home—random myoclonic jerks and seizures may develop. In the end stages of AD, patients become mute, develop rigid flexion of limbs, impaired swallowing and cachexia, and become confined to bed. The use of phenothiazines or haloperidol may accelerate the development of immobility dramatically, especially in those patients with the Lewy body variant of AD. Death usually results from intercurrent pneumonia.

Diagnosis

A diagnosis of probable AD is made during life by exclusion in patients with a gradually progressive dementing disorder, in whom all other symptomatic or other identifiable causes of progressive dementia have been ruled out. Definitive confirmation of the diagnosis is possible only by neuropathologic examination of the brain, where the typical neurofibrillary tangles, neuritic plaques, and amyloid angiopathy are seen. It is important to understand, however, that the diagnosis of AD cannot be made at autopsy in the absence of clinical dementia during life. Although the neuropathologic changes (and the absence of other pathologic lesions) confirm the clinical diagnosis, 30%–40% of cognitively normal elderly individuals over age 65 years may show similar findings at postmortem. Presently, laboratory tests specifically for diagnosing AD are unreliable. In those uncommon patients with a known hereditary form of FAD, molecular genetic studies can establish whether a family member has inherited the genetic defect that would inevitably lead to AD by the 50s, but whether the patient has developed dementia requires clinical demonstration. In SAD, although the cerebrospinal fluid tau protein may be elevated and the β-amyloid-42 levels reduced, the specificity of these findings is not sufficient to establish the diagnosis of AD. The fact that the pathologic changes of AD evolve over decades, and the observation that many normal elderly individuals show pathologic changes indistinguishable from AD, suggest that it is unlikely that any single, simple diagnostic test will be both sensitive and specific.

Laboratory studies are exceedingly valuable, however, in ruling out all other possible causes of dementia, and diagnostic criteria for AD have been developed. These criteria have been shown to have high sensitivity and specificity in clinicopathologic studies and are listed in Table 27A-2.

Laboratory Studies

Whenever the diagnosis of Alzheimer's disease is considered, a comprehensive laboratory evaluation should be carried out to examine alternative causes of dementia that may be treatable or additional conditions that may contribute to the degree of dementia (Table 27A-3).

The findings on routine laboratory studies of blood (complete blood cell count and differential count, electrolytes, survey 12, thyroid function studies, vitamin B_{12} level, serologic test for syphilis) and urine are normal in AD and are performed to rule out a variety of metabolic disorders that may produce cognitive impairment (e.g., hypothyroidism, hepatic encephalopathy, pernicious anemia, uremia, hyponatremia) and the now rarely seen cases of tertiary syphilis. The electroencephalogram (EEG) shows few abnormalities early in AD, but with progression there is usually a slowing of the background alpha rhythm. As the disease progresses, frontally predominant delta activity occurs and fast activity is lost. The EEG pattern in AD contrasts with the typical intermittent periodic bursts seen in Creutzfeldt-Jakob disease but does not distinguish AD from other degenerative dementias. Neuroimaging in AD by computed tomography (CT), or preferably, by magnetic resonance imaging (MRI), is used primarily to rule out structural lesions, such as subdural hematomas, brain tumors, strokes, or other vascular changes that may impair cognitive function. Scans may appear normal for age at the onset of AD; later, cerebral atrophy occurs, with resulting enlargement of the ventricles and widening of cortical sulci. Volumetric measurements often (but not always) show a reduction in size of the medial temporal lobes in AD (Figure 27A-2); some shrinkage is also seen in normal aging. Localized severe frontal lobe

Table 27A-2. The NINCDS-ADRDA Criteria for Clinical Diagnosis of Alzheimer's Disease

I. The criteria for the clinical diagnosis of *probable* Alzheimer's disease include
- dementia established by clinical examination and documented by the Mini-Mental Test, Blessed Dementia Scale, or some similar examination, and confirmed by neuropsychological tests;
- deficits in two or more areas of cognition;
- progressive worsening of memory and other cognitive functions;
- no disturbance of consciousness;
- onset between ages 40 and 90, most often after age 65; and
- absence of systemic disorders or other brain diseases that in and of themselves could account for the progressive deficits in memory and cognition.

II. The diagnosis of *probable* Alzheimer's disease is supported by
- progressive deterioration of specific cognitive functions such as language (aphasia), motor skills (apraxia), and perception (agnosia);
- impaired activities of daily living and altered patterns of behavior;
- family history of similar disorders, particularly if confirmed neuropathologically; and
- laboratory results of:
  normal lumbar puncture as evaluated by standard techniques,
  normal pattern or nonspecific changes in the electroencephalogram (EEG), such as increased slow-wave activity, and
  evidence of cerebral atrophy on computed tomographic (CT) scans with progression documented by serial observation.

III. Other clinical features consistent with the diagnosis of *probable* Alzheimer's disease, after exclusion of causes of dementia other than Alzheimer's disease, include
- plateaus in the course of progression of the illness;
- associated symptoms of depression, insomnia, incontinence, delusions, illusions, hallucinations, catastrophic verbal, emotional, or physical outbursts, sexual disorders, and weight loss;

- other neurologic abnormalities in some patients, especially with more advanced disease and including motor signs such as increased muscle tone, myoclonus, or gait disorder;
- seizures in advanced disease; and
- CT scans normal for age.

IV. Features that make the diagnosis of *probable* Alzheimer's disease uncertain or unlikely include
- sudden, apoplectic onset;
- focal neurologic findings such as hemiparesis, sensory loss, visual field deficits, and incoordination early in the course of the illness; and
- seizures or gait disturbances at the onset or very early in the course of the illness.

V. Clinical diagnosis of *possible* Alzheimer's disease:
- may be made on the basis of the dementia syndrome, in the absence of other neurologic, psychiatric, or systemic disorders sufficient to cause dementia, and in the presence of variations in the onset, in the presentation, or in the clinical course;
- may be made in the presence of a second systemic or brain disorder sufficient to produce dementia, which is not considered to be the cause of the dementia; and
- should be used in research studies when a single, gradually progressive severe cognitive deficit is identified in the absence of other identifiable cause.

VI. Criteria for diagnosis of *definite* Alzheimer's diseases are
- the clinical criteria for probable Alzheimer's disease, and
- histopathologic evidence obtained from a biopsy or autopsy.

VII. Classification of Alzheimer's disease for research purposes should specify features that may differentiate subtypes of the disorder, such as
- familial occurrence;
- onset before age of 65 years;
- presence of trisomy-21; and
- coexistence of other relevant conditions such as Parkinson's disease.

NINCDS-ADRA = National Institute of Neurological and Communicative Disorders and Stroke-Alzheimer's Disease and Related Disorders Association.
Source: Reprinted with permission from G McKhann, DA Drachman, M Folstein, et al. Clinical diagnosis of Alzheimer's disease: report of the NINCDS-ADRDA Work Group under the auspices of Department of Health and Human Services Task Force on Alzheimer's Disease. Neurology 1984;34:939–944.

atrophy is more suggestive of Pick's disease or frontal lobe dementia than of AD. Functional neuroimaging using positron emission tomography (PET) or single-photon emission CT (SPECT) often shows bilaterally reduced metabolism and decreased cerebral perfusion in the temporoparietal regions, but is generally too nonspecific to be diagnostic of

AD. In atypical cases of dementia, these studies are occasionally of use in identifying unusual asymmetries that may suggest Pick's disease or areas of hypoperfusion that may indicate a vascular dementia.

Where normal pressure hydrocephalus is a serious consideration in the differential diagnosis, lumbar puncture may be done to instill an indium or

Table 27A-3. Diagnostic Evaluation
of Progressive Dementia

Laboratory studies
    Blood studies
        Complete blood count
        Erythrocyte sedimentation rate
        Serum electrolytes
        Chemistry screen
        Serologic test for syphilis
        Free thyroxine index
        Serum vitamin B_{12}, folate
    Urinalysis
    Electrocardiogram
    Chest roentgenogram
    Magnetic resonance imaging of brain
    Psychometric testing
    Electroencephalogram
    Duplex scan of carotid/vertebral arteries
Optional studies
    Single-photon emission computed tomography/positron
        emission tomography
    Cerebrospinal fluid examination
    Indium cisternogram
    Genetic analysis for familial Alzheimer's disease,
        Huntington's disease, etc.

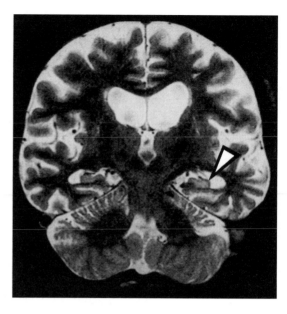

Figure 27A-2. A T2-weighted magnetic resonance imaging scan of a patient with Alzheimer's disease at a moderately advanced stage. Note the enlarged lateral ventricles, atrophy of the cortex, and small hippocampal complexes (*arrowhead*).

technetium isotope for cisternography. The usual cerebrospinal fluid tests (i.e., cell count and differential, protein, glucose, serology, culture) produce normal results in AD and may be performed to rule out another disorder, such as an indolent meningitis.

Although the presence of *APOE ε4* has been clearly associated with the increased risk of occurrence of AD and an earlier age at onset, testing for its presence or absence in a demented patient is of minimal value, and is not useful for predicting the future occurrence of AD. Even those individuals with an *APOE ε4* allele have a lifetime risk of developing AD of less than 30%, suggesting that the *APOE ε4* allele is neither necessary nor sufficient for the development of AD.

AD is easily diagnosed when the symptoms, clinical course, and absence of other conditions that may contribute to dementia follow the pattern described. The clinical diagnosis may be difficult when AD presents in an atypical pattern, such as with focal deficits or impairment of cognitive functions other than memory; when it occurs before age 60 years in patients without a family history of EODI FAD; when it progresses either extremely

rapidly or unusually slowly; or if it occurs in association with another known serious disease.

Treatment

There are more than 75 compounds that have been tried or are currently under study for the treatment of AD, but only two have been approved at the time of this writing by the U.S. Food and Drug Administration. Tetrahydroaminoacridine or tacrine (Cognex) and donepezil hydrochloride (Aricept) are cholinesterase inhibitors that reportedly improve memory and cognitive function in AD; tacrine is little used because of its hepatic toxicity. The rationale for studying cholinomimetic agents stems from the central cholinergic deficit in AD and the role the cholinergic system plays in learning and memory. The neurons of origin of the cholinergic system (in the nucleus basalis of Meynert) are not the only neurons that degenerate in AD, however, and the cholinergic system is not the only neurotransmitter system affected by AD. This likely accounts for the variable and modest

Figure 27A-3. A coronal section of brain from a patient with advanced Alzheimer's disease. The brain is atrophic, with widened sulci and shrunken gyri. Note the marked atrophy of the hippocampi (*arrowhead*).

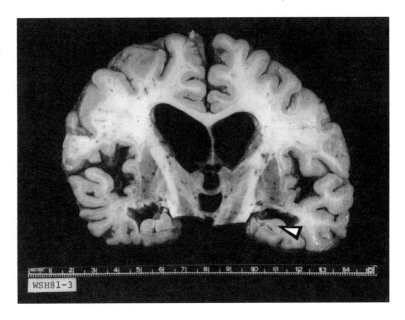

benefits described for this class of drugs. At present, there is no available treatment that alters the course of the disease.

Behavioral disturbances pose significant management problems in AD and, in many cases, may be treated with drugs and nonpharmacologic techniques. Neuroleptics such as phenothiazines and haloperidol are frequently used, often in large doses, despite the lack of empiric evidence regarding efficacy and the high incidence of disabling extrapyramidal side effects in this population. Newer antipsychotic drugs such as olanzapine (Zyprexa) and risperidone (Risperdal) have fewer extrapyramidal side effects; their role in controlling behavioral symptoms in AD remains to be established. We have found doxepin, 25 mg three times a day, to be useful in reducing the incidence of behavioral symptoms without inducing troublesome side effects, and small doses of lorazepam (Ativan), 0.5–1.0 mg every 6 hours as needed, may be added if necessary. Ambien, 5 mg at bedtime, or chloral hydrate, 500 or 1,000 mg, may be helpful in inducing sleep.

Neuropathology

The gross brain in AD is usually atrophic at autopsy, weighing between 950 and 1,200 g. Atro-

phy of the frontal, temporal, and parietal cortical gyri with sulcal enlargement is common (Figure 27A-3). The ventricles are enlarged and the hippocampal complex is often shrunken. On microscopic examination there is neuronal cell loss, especially of the entorhinal cortex of the temporal lobe, and involving the nucleus basalis of Meynert—the site of origin of the cholinergic fibers. The locus ceruleus is typically largely depigmented. Neuritic (senile) plaques with amyloid cores are seen throughout the cortex (Figure 27A-4), and silver-stained neurofibrillary tangles are present in many cortical neurons (Figure 27A-5); these are the hallmark features of AD. Blood vessels in affected cortical areas show amyloid angiopathy when stained appropriately (Figure 27A-6), and granulovacuolar degeneration may be seen in hippocampal neurons.

Extrapyramidal Dementias

A number of progressive degenerative dementias are characterized by the occurrence of movement disorders during the course of the dementing process, the abnormal movements developing in varied time relations to the dementia: in anticipation, concurrently, or after the onset of the demen-

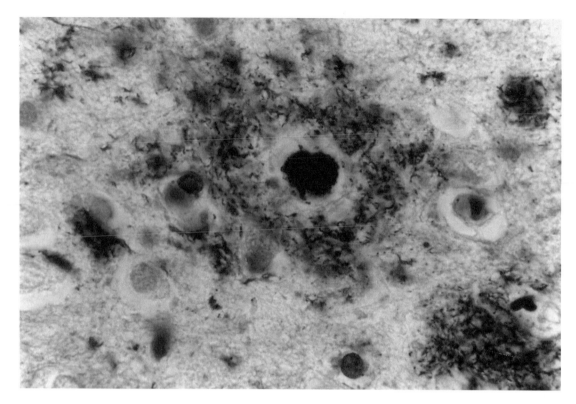

Figure 27A-4. Silver stain of neuritic (senile) plaque in a patient with Alzheimer's disease. Note the central amyloid core and the surrounding degenerating fragments of axons and dendrites. (250× magnification.)

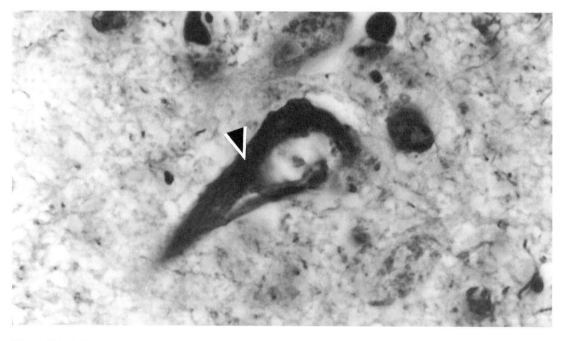

Figure 27A-5. Silver stain of the neurofibrillary tangle within a neuron in a patient with Alzheimer's disease. The thickened tangle is composed of paired helical filaments containing abnormally phosphorylated tau protein. (250× magnification.)

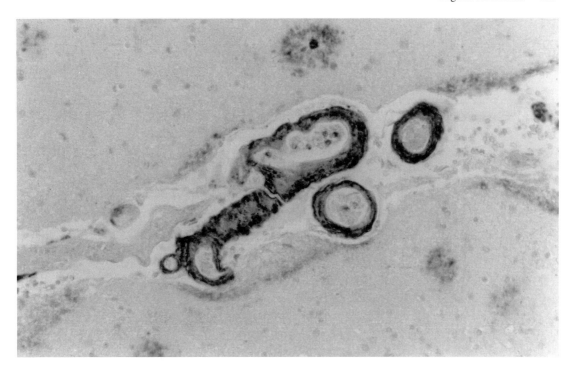

Figure 27A-6. Cerebral blood vessels from the brain of a patient with Alzheimer's disease, stained with immunohisto-chemical stain for β-amyloid, showing typical amyloid angiopathy. (20× magnification.)

tia. Of these, the most common are the Lewy body dementias (LBDs); the plural is used because LBD may occur as a pure entity or as a variant in combination with AD or Parkinson's disease. Other extrapyramidal dementias include HD, PSP, multiple system atrophy (Shy-Drager syndrome) and cortical-basal ganglionic degeneration (CBGD).

Lewy Body Dementias

Lewy bodies were first described in parkinsonism in 1913 by the German neuropathologist, F.W. Lewy, almost 100 years after Parkinson's description of the "shaking palsy." Lewy and subsequent neuropathologists found these hyaline, eosinophilic concentric intracytoplasmic inclusions in the neurons of the brain stem substantia nigra and locus ceruleus nuclei in patients dying with parkinsonism (Figure 27A-7). For years, Lewy bodies were considered to be diagnostic of parkinsonism. Seventy years later, neuropathologists and neurologists became aware that cortical Lewy bodies could also be found in some

cases of dementia. With greater awareness of this entity, and the use of immunohistochemical staining of ubiquitin (which is present in Lewy bodies) to visualize these pathologic findings, LBD has become an increasingly recognized, recognizable, and therefore a more common dementing disorder.

Confusion arises from the observation that cortical Lewy bodies can be found in patients with clinical and neuropathologic findings of AD, Parkinson's disease, a combination of both, or, more rarely, neither. In fact, at postmortem examination some cortical and subcortical Lewy bodies are found in the brains of 13% of elderly demented patients. There has been much discussion about the exact nomenclature of progressive degenerative dementias with extrapyramidal signs and the neuropathologic finding of cortical Lewy bodies. Hansen and Samuel observed, "There is no nosologic consensus concerning dementia with Lewy bodies."

We believe that the finding of Lewy bodies in association with dementia is evidence of alteration of neuronal proteins that have been targeted for repair or degradation, rather than a unique signature

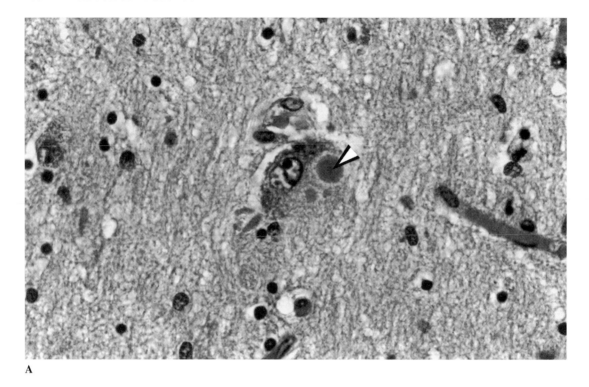

A

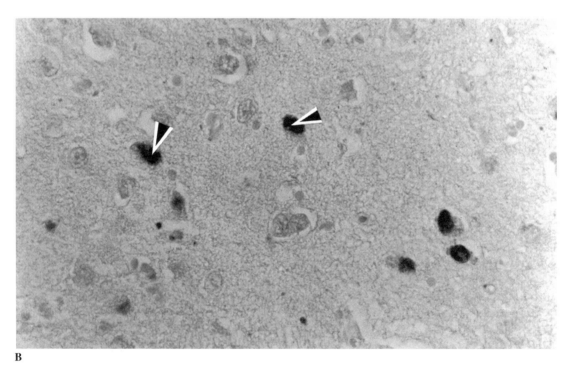

B

Figure 27A-7. Lewy bodies. (A) The typical intracytoplasmic inclusion body in the nucleus basalis of a patient with Parkinson's disease combined with Alzheimer's disease. (Hematoxylin and eosin stain; 100× magnification.) (B) A cortical Lewy body in a patient with Lewy body dementia. (Anti-ubiquitin immunohistochemical stain; 100× magnification.)

of a specific disease; ubiquitin is a "chaperone" protein, capable of these functions. Nevertheless, certain relatively distinctive clinical characteristics have been identified in some patients with degenerative dementia who are found to have neocortical Lewy bodies at postmortem examination. Therefore, for clinical purposes, we divide LBDs into three entities: diffuse LBD (DLBD), Lewy body variant of Alzheimer's disease (AD/LBD), and Parkinson's disease with dementia (PDD).

Diffuse Lewy Body Dementia

In the relatively uncommon form of dementia known as *diffuse Lewy body dementia* (DLBD), Lewy bodies are found in neurons in neocortical (frontal, temporal parietal lobe), allocortical (hippocampal complex, entorhinal cortex), and subcortical structures (substantia nigra, locus ceruleus), in the absence of the quantity of senile plaques, neurofibrillary tangles, or amyloid angiopathy typical of AD. DLBD affects middle-aged or elderly men more than women and tends to be more rapidly progressive than AD, with severe disability often within 5 years. The clinical characteristics include progressive dementia with relatively little memory impairment at first but poor attention and executive functions; fluctuating cognitive performance with surprisingly good performance on occasions; frequent and striking visual hallucinations early in the course, usually of people or animals; extrapyramidal features, including rigidity, retropulsion, impaired balance, and hypophonia, but less commonly tremor; and marked sensitivity to neuroleptic medications. Hallucinations and delusions may antedate parkinsonian features. The unusual sensitivity to neuroleptics such as phenothiazines, haloperidol, Risperdal, and olanzapine are such that management of the patients' bizarre ideation and hallucinations may present a problem. These patients are also thought to show more improvement with centrally active anticholinesterase medications (e.g., donepezil, tacrine) than patients with AD, and some of the extrapyramidal features may respond to levodopa-carbidopa, although not as consistently as with parkinsonism.

Lewy Body Variant of Alzheimer's Disease

In AD/LBD, which is a far more common progressive dementia, the initial pattern of clinical findings is typical of AD, as described earlier. After several years, however, extrapyramidal rigidity, hypophonia, and visual hallucinations may develop; the extrapyramidal features typically suggest the diagnosis. At postmortem examination, the pathologic features are typical of AD, with the addition of some cortical or brain stem Lewy bodies. The number of neocortical neurofibrillary tangles may be less than in AD without Lewy bodies, and cortical measurements of the phosphorylated form of the microtubule-associated protein, *tau*, may be less as well. The possibility that this is a further manifestation of advanced but typical AD is supported by the observation that, in some patients with FAD resulting from the presenilin 1 gene, Lewy bodies may be seen at postmortem examination. It is likely that, in many patients with typical AD, progression of the disease eventually involves brain stem nuclei, with resulting extrapyramidal clinical features and some Lewy bodies at autopsy.

Parkinson's Disease with Dementia

Between 20% and 30% of patients with PD eventually develop dementia, although estimates vary widely. Patients who develop PD after the age of 70 years have a higher risk of developing dementia than patients with an earlier age of onset. The majority of PD patients who eventually develop dementia show the typical pathologic changes of AD at autopsy in addition to those of PD. As with AD, age is a significant risk factor for developing dementia in PD. Although the possibility has been raised that the development of dementia in PD is a coincidental concurrence of two common conditions, the incidence and prevalence rates of dementia are higher in patients with PD than in others of similar age in the population who do not have PD. Virtually all patients with parkinsonism have Lewy bodies in the basal ganglia, and some also have cortical Lewy bodies. Thus, PDD—with or without the additional pathology of AD—is included in the group of LBDs.

Bradykinesia and bradyphrenia are characteristic features of all three forms of LBD. The extrapyramidal features of typical PD include resting tremor; cogwheel rigidity of the limbs; increased axial tone; bradykinesia; masked facies; and disturbances of posture, gait, and equilibrium. Tremor is common only in those patients whose LBD begins with a

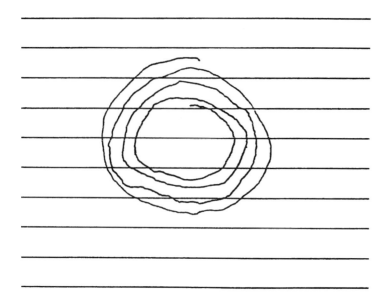

Figure 27A-8. Archimedes' screw drawn by a patient with early parkinsonism. The patient attempts to draw a closely lined spiral from outside in. Note the tremulous areas most prominently in the 2-o'clock and 7-o'clock diagonal regions.

parkinsonian clinical picture. Speech volume is usually reduced (hypophonia) and prosody is flat. Micrographia is common, and the handwriting (or especially drawing the spiral of Archimedes' screw) is tremulous (Figure 27A-8). Neuro-ophthalmologic abnormalities (e.g., decreased volitional up-gaze, impaired convergence) are also frequent. In pure parkinsonism, deficits in effortful cognitive processing may occur, and depression is a common clinical feature. In all three forms of LBD, psychometric studies are very useful in documenting the presence and extent of dementia, but less useful for distinguishing among DLBD, AD/LBD, or PDD.

Differential Diagnosis

The differential diagnosis among DLBD, AD/LBD, and PDD is controversial, but is primarily clinical during life and based on the presenting features early in the course. LBD can be strongly suspected by the clinical criteria given above, but definitive diagnosis at the present time requires pathologic examination. DLBD typically presents with prominent hallucinations and postural instability together with dementia, and at times may be easily confused with delirium. Clinical criteria for antemortem diagnosis have been proposed and require at least two of the following features for a diagnosis of probable LBD (one feature for a diagnosis of possible disease): (1) fluctuating cognition, attention, and alertness; (2) visual

hallucinations; and (3) extrapyramidal signs. Supportive features (not required for diagnosis) include repeated falls, syncope, transient loss of consciousness, neuroleptic sensitivity, systematized delusions, and hallucinations in other modalities. AD/LBD begins with dementia, similar to typical AD, with the extrapyramidal features developing late. In PDD, the motor findings of extrapyramidal disease are prominent early on, the dementia occurring only after 1 or more years.

Pathogenesis of Dementia in Lewy Body Dementia

Whatever the etiologies of these conditions may be, it is clear that the combination of two degenerative dementing pathologic features often causes considerably more clinical impairment than either alone. Patients with only moderate changes of AD at autopsy but combined with a moderate number of cortical Lewy bodies may be severely demented. This is similar to the observation that, when modest neuropathologic changes of AD (senile plaques, neurofibrillary tangles, amyloid angiopathy) are combined with a few small infarcts or lacunes in the basal ganglia or thalamus, dementia may result.

Laboratory Studies

Laboratory studies, including MRI and CT, show the expected findings for AD in those patients with

AD/LBD, whereas neuroimaging findings in PD may be normal or show mild atrophy with sulcal dilatation and ventricular enlargement. In PD, SPECT may show a picture that differs from the typical appearance in AD: In addition to the diffuse cerebral hypometabolism with marked declines in association areas, there may also be hypoperfusion in occipital association cortex and primary visual cortex, with relative sparing of subcortical structures. Diffuse cerebral hypometabolism can be demonstrated on PET scans. The findings in DLBD do not distinguish among the conditions in this group. Other laboratory studies are of value to rule out other contributing medical conditions, as in the evaluation of AD.

Treatment

Treatment is directed at the specific symptoms that predominate in each patient with LBD. Where the dementia is prominent, donepezil or tacrine may be of some benefit; carbidopa/levodopa, dopamine agonists, and monoamine oxidase B inhibitors can provide symptomatic improvement for motor abnormalities; and the hallucinations and other behavioral symptoms may be treated cautiously with very small doses of neuroleptic drugs that have minimal extrapyramidal side effects (e.g., olanzapine, 1.25–5.00 mg/day), or minor tranquilizers (e.g., oxazepam, 10 mg every 6 hours, or lorazepam, 0.5–1.0 mg every 6 hours). Balance problems are resistant to treatment; physical therapy and the use of easily steered rolling walkers with four large wheels and hand brakes (such as the Noble Walker, Pittsburgh, PA) can be helpful.

Neuropathology

On microscopic examination, the substantia nigra shows severe pathologic changes involving extensive neuronal loss in the pars compacta. Other brain stem and diencephalic nuclei are also involved. Lewy bodies—eosinophilic cytoplasmic inclusions found in neurons—are present (see Figure 27A-7), and as noted above, in some cases there are extensive pathologic features of AD in the cortex, with senile plaques and neurofibrillary tangles. In patients with the pathologic changes of AD, vacuolar change may be seen in the temporal lobes, at times resembling the spongiform change seen in Creutzfeldt-Jakob disease but more limited in anatomic distribution (Figure 27A-9).

Other Movement Disorders with Cognitive Impairment

Huntington's Disease

HD is an autosomal dominant disorder whose clinical manifestations include dystonic and choreiform movements, dysarthria, dementia, and personality and behavioral changes. The genetic defect occurs in the coding region of the huntingtin gene, which is on the short arm of chromosome 4, and consists of variable expansion of triplet repeats of the CAG sequence in this region. Men and women are equally affected with an average age of onset in the late 30s and early 40s, although both childhood and late onset forms are observed. The age of onset is largely dependent on the number of trinucleotide repeats in the huntingtin gene, occurring at advanced ages in those individuals with 35–39 repeats and early ages in those with 45–50 repeats. The average duration from onset to death is 15–20 years.

Clinical Features and Neurologic Findings. Personality changes of increased irritability and apathy frequently occur before the onset of chorea, and some patients may present with increasing depression or schizophrenia-like symptoms, such as flattened affect, excessive religiosity, or tangential thinking. Early in the disease, choreiform movements appear and include transient grimacing, head nodding, and delicate superimposed movements of the hands and hips when walking, leading to the descriptive term, *chorea* (literally, "the dance"). Cognitive deficits become apparent soon after the chorea begins, and the dementia at this stage is characterized by slowness of thought without aphasia or agnosia. As the disease progresses, movements of the face, neck, limbs, and torso increase, and the hands may alternate between extension-supination and flexion-pronation postures. In advanced stages, there are continuous athetotic or dystonic movements, whereas in the terminal stage there is fixed double hemiplegic posture with little involuntary movement. Neurologic examination reveals a number of helpful signs, such as the *pronator sign*, in which the hands, which are held with palms facing and the arms extended over the head, move involuntarily to a more pronated posture; the *milking sign*, in which the patient's grip on the examiner's hand simulates milking by gripping and releasing; impersistence, demonstrated by the limited

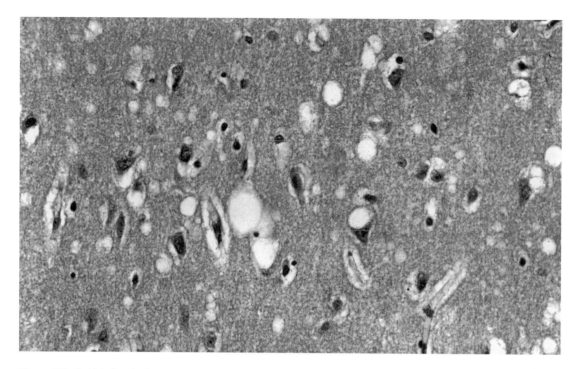

Figure 27A-9. Alzheimer's disease combined with Lewy body dementia. Spongiform changes are typically found in the temporal regions in this variant of Alzheimer's. (Hematoxylin and eosin stain; 50× magnification.)

ability of the patient to maintain the tongue protruded for a prolonged time; and superimposition of choreic gasps on a prolonged "aaah" vowel sound.

Laboratory Studies.   Routine laboratory studies are unremarkable in HD. Molecular genetic testing for the CAG repeat expansion of the huntington gene is definitive, and reveals abnormally high numbers of repeats in essentially all patients with HD. CT or MRI scans demonstrate atrophy of the caudate nuclei and dilatation of frontal horns. On T2-weighted MRI scans, decreased signal in the globus pallidus and putamen may be seen. EEGs appear normal in presymptomatic cases, whereas low voltage and poorly developed or absent alpha activity may be seen in symptomatic patients. Decreased caudate glucose metabolism and diminished caudate perfusion are found on PET and SPECT studies.

Diagnosis.   Chorea, dementia, and a history of dominant familial occurrence of a similar disorder are suggestive of HD. Abnormal CAG repeat expansion confirms the clinical diagnosis of the disease.

Treatment.   The choreiform movements can be reduced with major tranquilizers, especially haloperidol. Depression can be treated with antidepressants of the selective serotonin-reuptake inhibitor class, such as sertraline (Zoloft); there is no effective treatment for the dementia.

Neuropathology.   The brain is atrophic, with marked atrophy of the striatum and virtual loss of the heads of the caudate nuclei. Small neurons in the basal ganglia are affected first. The exact nature of the neurotransmitter abnormalities remains unclear, although levels of γ-aminobutyric acid have been consistently shown to decline.

Progressive Supranuclear Palsy (Steele-Richardson-Olszewski Syndrome)

PSP is an uncommon disorder in which dementia is variable and usually not present at onset. Onset is in late middle or late life, typically in the 60s, and survival ranges from 5 to 10 years. PSP occurs more frequently in men than in women.

Postural instability and falls are the most frequent initial manifestations, together with difficulty initiating voluntary vertical gaze. An inability to look down is characteristic of PSP and is not seen in other conditions where up-gaze may be limited (such as Parkinson's disease or advanced age). An akinetic-rigid parkinsonian-like condition characterized by bradykinesia and axial rigidity is frequently present and is not relieved by levodopa. Pseudobulbar palsy and frontal release signs may be seen. The dementia, occurring a year or so after the onset of postural instability, is characterized by symptoms typical of frontal lobe disorders, including decreased verbal fluency and concrete thought. Apathy and depression are common.

Routine laboratory studies of blood and urine show normal results in PSP. MRI scans may show enlargement of the cerebral aqueduct and enlargement of the perimesencephalic cisterns, caused by midbrain atrophy, and strongly support the diagnosis; diffuse cortical and subcortical atrophy may also be seen. Hypoperfusion, especially in frontal regions, may be found on SPECT or PET studies, and differ from the findings in AD. The diagnosis of PSP is clinical, supported by imaging studies. Consensus research criteria for the diagnosis of PSP were published in 1996.

In PSP, there is gross atrophy of the midbrain, with enlargement of the cerebral aqueduct and third ventricle. Gliosis and neuronal loss are seen in the substantia nigra, globus pallidus, striatum, and subthalamic nucleus, with neurofibrillary degeneration of neurons in these areas.

Cortical-Basal Ganglionic Degeneration

CBGD was first described by Rebeiz and colleagues in 1968 as "corticodentatonigral degeneration with neuronal achromasia," a disorder involving the motor (perirolandic) cortex, basal ganglia, and cerebellar nuclei with predominantly motor manifestations, involving limb apraxia and impaired balance. In the three cases originally described, cognitive impairment occurred only after a number of years and was considered to have been mild. In subsequent cases, fewer than half have been found to have dementia. The clinical symptoms of CBGD suggest a movement disorder, but one that is asymmetric, and with prominent "alien limb" symptoms, or limb-kinetic apraxia, in which the patient treats his or her arm as if it belongs to someone else. As the disorder evolves, oculomotor apraxia may occur, producing diagnostic confusion with PSP. Because of the prominent movement disorder and the fact that dementia is a late and usually mild development, it is unlikely to be confused with AD or AD/LBD. The pathologic appearance is striking, with focal atrophy of the perirolandic gyri, which are generally uninvolved in other dementias. The appearance of achromasia in ballooned neurons shares a similar appearance with cases of Pick's disease and other focal, cortical, or lobar dementias described later. The presence of abnormal phosphorylated *tau*-containing neurofilaments provides another link between this degenerative disorder and other degenerative dementias, although the neurofilaments are straight rather than helical and paired, as in AD.

Clinical features of CBGD early in the disease include limb dystonia, asymmetric extrapyramidal rigidity, ideomotor and limb-kinetic apraxia (the alien limb syndrome), and the absence of dementia until late. Balance and gait disturbances become prominent later in the course of the disease, and patients become bedridden. Imaging studies (CT, MRI) may show asymmetry of sulci in the anterior parietal region and pontine atrophy; PET and SPECT may show asymmetry of cortical and subcortical metabolism and perfusion of parietal cortex and basal ganglia. Diagnosis is based on neuropathologic findings, but can often be made clinically by recognition of the characteristic limb apraxia or alien limb syndrome in a patient with parkinsonism plus. This condition is not likely to be confused with other dementing disorders, unless patients are seen late in the course, with little information on the earlier manifestations. Treatment is ineffective. The motor abnormalities do not respond to levodopa or other medications, and the disorder progresses relentlessly.

The neuropathologic features are characteristic and consist of atrophy of perirolandic cortical areas with neuronal loss and achromasia in affected cortical areas, the cerebellar nuclei (dentate, roof nuclei), and the substantia nigra.

Dementias of Focal, Cortical, or Lobar Onset: Pick's Disease and Others

Among the progressive degenerative dementing disorders where extrapyramidal features are absent and no other underlying cause can be identified (e.g., vascular disease, brain tumors), a number turn out *not* to have the pathologic changes of AD at autopsy. Instead, there are focal or limited areas of marked gross brain atrophy at autopsy, often asymmetric; frequently ballooned chromatolytic neurons (which stain with neurofilament-derived antibodies) in the atrophic areas; and in some cases, Pick bodies, which are silver-staining inclusions containing neurofilaments (different from those in AD) that are found in hippocampal and neocortical neurons. Some of these patients have clinical patterns that can be distinguished from AD; some are indistinguishable from AD. The presence or absence of Pick bodies does not seem to differentiate clinically among these disorders; the clinical manifestations vary primarily as a result of the specific area or areas of brain involved in the degeneration.

These conditions should be considered when (1) the onset of dementia is before age 60 years in an individual without a family history of FAD; (2) onset is with behavioral changes, and memory impairment is not prominent early; (3) the patient develops progressive aphasia (primary progressive aphasia) in the absence of other evidence of dementia; and (4) there is a pure progressive impairment of memory (verbal learning) remaining as an isolated disturbance for more than a year.

Pick's Disease

Pick's disease is a rare degenerative dementia that occurs in fewer than 5% of demented patients according to autopsy studies. As noted, it is diagnosed by the autopsy finding of focal degeneration of the frontal or temporal lobes (or both) and the characteristic Pick bodies seen microscopically in affected neurons. Pick bodies cannot always be demonstrated, however, and despite their absence, in some patients the diagnosis is made when typical lobar "knife-edge" degeneration of the frontal or temporal lobes is seen.

Clinical Features and Neurologic Findings

The clinical diagnosis of Pick's disease, like that of AD, requires exclusion of alternative treatable disorders. The age of onset of symptoms is often somewhat earlier, averaging about 60 years, with a survival of 6–12 years after onset. The cause of Pick's disease is unknown in the majority of cases, although an autosomal-dominant pattern of inheritance has been described in a few families; the locus or loci of the genetic deficit or deficits is not known. Personality changes and behavioral disturbances are often among the first clinical features of Pick's disease and may include apathy or impulsivity, sexual disinhibition, environmental exploration or roaming, and hyperorality. Patients with Pick's disease may demonstrate signs of frontal lobe impairment, losing the "executive ability" to follow directions or make decisions, with impaired expression of usual social behaviors and emotional niceties. The dementia syndrome is characterized by early dysfunction of expressive speech, including decreased verbal output and echolalia, as well as impairment of judgment and executive functions. Global memory and cognitive deficits occur in late stages, with terminal mutism. Frontal release signs such as grasp reflexes may be present; aside from the mental changes, the findings on neurologic examination are not distinctive.

Diagnosis

There are few clinicopathologic studies of Pick's disease, and the clinical features that have been reported are based on retrospective case studies. No specific clinical criteria have been established. Onset before age 60 in the absence of a family history of AD, early occurrence of personality and behavioral changes, language disturbances, frontal release signs, and focal frontal or temporal atrophy on CT or MRI are suggestive of Pick's disease.

Laboratory Studies

Routine blood and urine studies produce normal findings in Pick's disease. The EEG is normal until late in the disease, when diffuse slowing or focal frontal or temporal slow-wave activity may occur. CT or MRI studies may be characteristic, however, if they demonstrate marked frontal or temporal atrophy. The caudate nuclei may be shrunken with enlargement of the frontal horns of the ventricles, and lateral ventricular dilation may be seen. Frontotemporal hypometabolism and hypoperfusion are found in PET and SPECT studies.

Treatment

There is no treatment for Pick's disease. Supportive care is warranted as in other degenerative dementias. As with AD, both pharmacologic and nonpharmacologic interventions may be helpful in the treatment of behavioral disturbances.

Neuropathology

On external examination of the brain, there is severe frontal or temporal cortical atrophy rather than the diffuse cerebral atrophy usually observed in AD (Figure 27A-10). Microscopic examination demonstrates cortical neuronal cytoplasmic inclusions (Pick bodies, Figure 27A-11), ballooned neurons with achromasia, the absence of neurofibrillary tangles or neuritic plaques (other than those expected for age), and astrocytic hyperplasia and microglial cell proliferation in affected cortical regions.

Frontotemporal Dementia

Progressive dementias have been identified in which frontal, temporal, or frontotemporal atrophy may be seen without Pick bodies (frontal, temporal, or frontotemporal dementia). The clinical presentation of these conditions overlaps considerably with Pick's disease, and it is unclear whether this is actually "Pick's disease *sine* Pick bodies," or another condition. Like Pick's disease, onset is often before age 60, although cases with earlier and later onset have been reported. Reported survival rates vary from 2 to 10 years. Prevalence rates are unknown; with increasing reports, the true prevalence may be higher than once believed.

Clinical Features and Neurologic Findings

Several clinical patterns have been described in frontotemporal dementia depending on the focal area or areas of atrophy and degeneration. Early in the course of disease there may be a personality change, poor insight and judgment, and disinhibition, and hyperorality may occur. Some patients, however, may present with the syndrome of primary progressive aphasia (see later), in which impaired language function far exceeds any other manifestation of dementia for some years. Some patients become

hyperkinetic and ritualistic in behavior; others become apathetic and inert. Executive functions of abstraction and planning are often impaired. Primitive reflexes may be present early. As the disease progresses, memory becomes impaired, and eventually extrapyramidal symptoms, rigidity, and dysarthria may emerge. At later stages, the patient may become apathetic, aphasic, and amimiac. In a few patients, where mesial temporal (hippocampal complex) degeneration occurs in the absence of frontal atrophy, memory impairment may occur in excess of other manifestations of dementia.

The syndrome of primary progressive aphasia, described in 1982 by Mesulam, should be readily identifiable, and deserves a more complete description. Typically, these patients present with nonfluent aphasia, and do not develop a global dementia until late in the disease. Speech production is nonfluent and effortful, hesitant, and with paraphasic errors. Repetition, oral reading, and writing abilities are impaired. Comprehension is intact until late in the disease. Nonlanguage cognitive functions are preserved but become untestable when communication is severely impaired. Social graces and insight usually remain intact, although some patients may develop behaviors characteristic of frontal lobe dementia in the later stages of disease. The neurologic examination is usually unremarkable.

Laboratory Studies

Routine laboratory studies are unremarkable and EEGs appear normal. CT and MRI scans appear normal in most cases early in the course, but eventually may show focal frontal lobe atrophy similar to more typical Pick's disease. SPECT scans may demonstrate decreased blood flow in the frontotemporal regions or in the dominant hemisphere in primary progressive aphasia.

The diagnosis and management of frontotemporal dementia is similar to that of more typical Pick's disease and the distinction may be merely a neuropathologic one.

Neuropathology

Just as the clinical presentation of frontal lobe dementia is heterogeneous, so too are the reported neuropathologic features. Focal atrophy of the

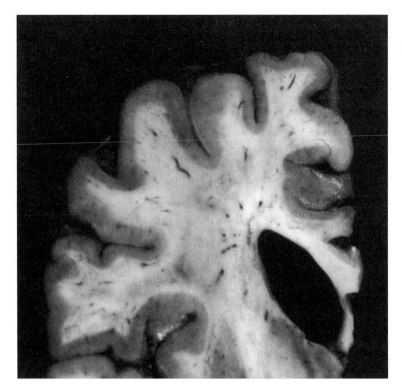

Figure 27A-10. Coronal brain section of a patient with Pick's disease shows the marked degree of lobar atrophy involving the medial frontal, inferior temporal, and hippocampal regions. The lateral frontal and superior temporal gyri are relatively spared.

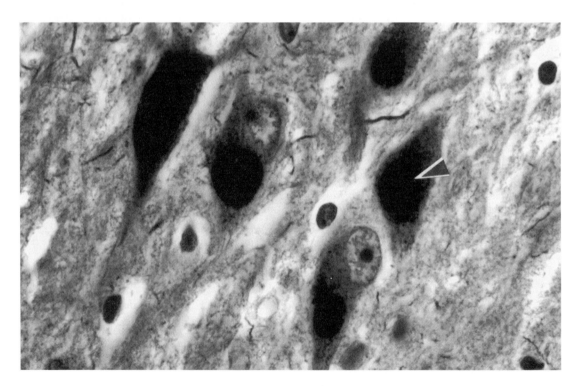

Figure 27A-11. Pick bodies in a case of Pick's disease. These intracytoplasmic silver-staining bodies may balloon surviving neurons; there is loss of neurons in the affected lobar areas of the brain. (250× magnification.)

frontal or temporal lobes may be seen; microscopically there is neuronal cell loss in affected areas, often with ballooned achromasic neurons, but without Pick bodies or the findings of typical AD. Astrocytosis and microvacuolation occur in the frontal and temporal cortices, with variable limbic and subcortical involvement. In patients with the syndrome of primary progressive aphasia, these findings may be confined to or predominantly in the dominant hemisphere in the frontal and temporal lobes.

Other Dementias

Three other groups of dementing disorders may be considered for completeness (Table 27A-4): degenerative disorders with minor dementia, dementias lacking distinctive histology (DLDH), and pseudodegenerative dementias.

Degenerative disorders with minor dementia are degenerative neurologic disorders that produce some cognitive impairment but as a secondary manifestation compared with the more striking features of the disease process. Included in this group are olivopontocerebellar atrophy, myotonic dystrophy, and striatonigral degeneration.

DLDH are true degenerative dementias, but at postmortem examination show no distinctive neuropathologic findings. Some of these disorders involve cortical areas and may present with primary progressive aphasia or other cortical manifestations; some may present with thalamic degeneration and some with motor neuropathy.

"Pseudodegenerative" dementias are disorders of known etiology, not degenerative in origin, but with manifestations that may be confused with the degenerative dementias already described. The most important members of this group are vascular dementias, Creutzfeldt-Jakob disease, and normal pressure hydrocephalus.

Conclusion

There are many degenerative dementing disorders, most of which produce their manifestations more commonly with advancing age. The characteristics that result in inclusion in this group are the progressive course of the disorders and the lack of an

Table 27A-4. Other Progressive Dementias

Progressive dementias with a known etiology
  Vascular dementias
    Multiple infarctions
    Binswanger's disease
    Other vascular dementia (long-standing hypertension, postcoronary bypass surgery, etc.)
  Viral, prion, and infectious diseases
    Creutzfeldt-Jakob disease
    Syphilis
    Human immunodeficiency virus encephalopathy
    Cryptococcosis, fungal, etc.
  Normal-pressure hydrocephalus
  Wilson's disease
  Leukodystrophies: metachromatic leukodystrophy
  Metabolic and endocrine disturbances
    Recurrent hypoglycemia
    Hypothyroidism
    Hyponatremia
    Hypercalcemia
    Uremia
    Hepatic encephalopathy
    Cushing's disease
  Toxic dementias
    Drugs: anticholinergic, psychotropic, antihypertensive, anticonvulsants, antineoplastic, polydrug use
    Alcohol
    Metals: lead, mercury, aluminum, gold, tin
    Industrial compounds: toluene, methyl chloride, organophosphate insecticides, jet fuels
Degenerative disorders with minor dementia
  Myotonic dystrophy
  Shy-Drager syndrome
  Striatonigral degeneration
  Olivopontocerebellar atrophy
  Other spinocerebellar degeneration
Dementia lacking a distinctive histology

identified metabolic, vascular, or infectious mechanism. Clinically, it is important to consider for every patient the large array of medical and neurologic conditions that may mimic or contribute to degenerative dementias. We strongly support the concept that no patient with a suspected degenerative dementia should be diagnosed as such without benefit of a comprehensive evaluation for these identifiable and treatable conditions. Failure to diagnose a subdural hematoma, hypothyroidism, combined systems disease with vitamin B_{12} deficiency, or any of the many other possible causes or contributors to cognitive decline in the elderly can be avoided by obtaining a complete battery of laboratory tests.

As the mechanisms by which the degenerative dementias produce their neuronal loss and cognitive decline become better understood, some of the members of this group may be removed from the category of the "degenerative dementias." The mechanisms by which Alzheimer's disease or Pick's disease result in neuronal death, for example, are likely to be deciphered during the next decade. These late-onset disorders may be caused in part by exaggeration or acceleration of the mechanisms of senescence that produce declines in brain functions during normal aging. An understanding of these processes—from oxidative stress to conformational change in structural proteins, from apoptosis to a decline in mitochondrial function—is likely to illuminate the causes and potential treatments for what we now know as the degenerative dementias.

Acknowledgments

We are grateful to Dr. Thomas Smith for kindly providing Figures 27A-3 through 27A-7 and 27A-9 through 27A-11, as well as to Dr. John Knorr for kindly providing Figure 27A-2. This chapter was supported in part by NIA Grant #P50AG05134; the Sterling Morton Neurological Research Fund; and the Stanley and Harriett Friedman Research Fund.

Suggested Reading

Adams RD, Fisher CM, Hakim S, et al. Symptomatic occult hydrocephalus with "normal" cerebrospinal fluid: a treatable syndrome. N Engl J Med 1965;273:117.

Drachman DA. Aging and the brain: a new frontier. Ann Neurol 1997;42:819.

Drachman DA. New criteria for the diagnosis of vascular dementia. Do we know enough yet? Neurology 1993; 43:243.

Drachman DA, Leavitt J. Human memory and the cholinergic system. Arch Neurol 1974;30:113.

Feany MB, Mattiace LA, Dickson DW. Neuropathic overlap of progressive supranuclear palsy, Pick's disease and corticobasal degeneration. J Neuropathol Exp Neurol 1996;55:53.

Hagnell O, Ojesjö L, Rorsman B. Incidence of dementia in the Lundby study. Neuroepidemiology 1992;11 (Suppl 1):61.

Huntington's Disease Collaborative Research Group. A novel gene containing a trinucleotide repeat that is expanded and unstable on Huntington's disease chromosomes. Cell 1993;72:971.

Jorm A, Korten A, Henderson A. The prevalence of dementia: a quantitative integration of the literature. Acta Psychiatr Scand 1987;76:465.

Katzman R. The prevalence and malignancy of Alzheimer's disease: a major killer. Arch Neurol 1976;33:217.

Kirschbaum WR. Jakob-Creutzfeldt Disease. New York: American Elsevier, 1968.

Knopman D. The Non-Alzheimer Degenerative Dementias. In JC Morris (ed), Handbook of Dementing Illnesses. New York: Marcel Dekker, 1994;265.

Mayeux R, Denaro J, Hemenegildo N, et al. A population-based investigation of Parkinson's disease with and without dementia. Relationship to age and gender. Arch Neurol 1992;49:492.

McKeith IG, Galasko D, Kosaka A, et al. Consensus guidelines for the clinical and pathological diagnosis of dementia with Lewy bodies: report of the CDLB international workshop. Neurology 1996;47:1113.

McKhann G, Drachman DA, Folstein M, et al. Clinical diagnosis of Alzheimer's disease: report of the NINCDS-ADRDA Work Group under the auspices of Department of Health and Human Services Task Force on Alzheimer's Disease. Neurology 1984;34:939.

Mirra SS, Markesbery WR. The Neuropathology of Alzheimer's Disease: Diagnostic Features and Standardization. In ZS Khachaturian, TS Radebaugh (eds), Alzheimer's Disease: Cause(s), Diagnosis, Treatment, and Care. Boca Raton, FL: CRC Press, 1996;111.

National Institute on Aging/Alzheimer's Association Working Group. Apolipoprotein E genotyping in Alzheimer's disease position statement. Lancet 1996; 347:1091.

O'Donnell BF, Drachman DA, Barnes HJ, et al. Incontinence and troublesome behaviors predict institutionalization in dementia. J Geriatr Psychiatry Neurol 1992;5:45.

Roman GC, Tatemichi TK, Erkinjuntti T, et al. Vascular dementia: diagnostic criteria for research studies. Report of the NINDS-AIREN International Workshop. Neurology 1993;43:250.

St. George-Hyslop P, Haines J, Rogaev E, et al. Genetic evidence for a novel familial Alzheimer's disease locus on chromosome 14. Nat Genets 1992;2:330.

B. Vascular Dementia

Richard K.T. Chan and Vladimir Hachinski

Chapter Plan

Etiology and pathogenesis
Symptoms and signs
Diagnosis
Differential diagnosis
Treatment and prevention

Vascular dementia is the second most common cause of cognitive decline in Western societies. It affects 1–20% of people aged 65 years or older. The prevalence is likely to increase as life expectancy increases for a greater proportion of the population. Vascular dementia is fast becoming a problem affecting the aging society. At the individual level, it is associated with a decline in the quality of life. At the societal level, it increases health care costs. Intensive research efforts are under way to better prevent and treat this condition.

Etiology and Pathogenesis

As the name implies, the cognitive decline of vascular dementia is secondary to some form of vascular injury to the brain. The vascular insult can take the form of an infarct or parenchymal hemorrhage. Cerebral infarcts are caused by occlusion of intracranial or extracranial arteries supplying the brain matter. Atherosclerosis of the carotid artery or its branches is the most common cause of cerebral infarct in the Western world. Atheromatous plaques in the vessel wall may become denuded, leading to local thrombosis and distal embolization. Emboli may also arise from more proximal sources, such as the heart or the aorta.

Cerebral infarct may also be caused by small vessel disease. The vessel walls of the small arter-

ies or terminal arterioles supplying the cerebral structure become thickened from various causes. The lumen then becomes occluded by the thickened vessel wall, local thrombosis, or distant emboli. The small cylinder of neural tissue supplied by the affected vessels becomes infarcted. Hypertension can lead to such small vessel changes; under the microscope, the vessel wall shows changes of lipohyalinosis. Diabetes mellitus may also be associated with small vessel disease. Small, deep gray matter or white matter infarcts are commonly seen in elderly patients, although it is uncertain if old age alone causes small vessel changes. Whether the infarct is caused by thrombosis, embolization, or small vessel disease, the result is the same. The lack of oxygen and essential nutrients leads to death of the neurons in the cortex or the neural fibers in the white matter. With time, the infarcted tissue is replaced by glial cells.

Primary intracerebral hemorrhages are secondary to rupture of a small artery or arteriole within the brain substances. In most cases, this is the result of some abnormality in the vessel wall (e.g., amyloid deposit within the vessel wall in congophilic angiopathy, Charcot-Bouchard aneurysm in hypertensive microangiopathy, or arteriovenous malformation). Normal appearing vessel wall may also rupture if there is excessive systemic blood pressure. The extravasated blood forms a clot immediately adjacent to the artery, pushing away the neural element in its path. With time, the clot organizes itself and is gradually resorbed by the body, leaving a cavity in its place. Loss of neurologic function is the result of the pressure effect of the blood clots as well as interruption of nutrient supplies secondary to the elevated pressure locally and within the intracranial cavity.

The neurons are highly specialized cells that cannot replicate themselves. Recovery of neurologic function can only be achieve by reorganization at the cellular and subcellular levels—a property of the brain called *plasticity*. Plasticity enables those functions normally served by the affected tissues to be taken over by collateral pathways. The reorganization is seldom complete. In cases where the infarct volume is large or if the affected tissue serves a highly specialized function, functional recovery may not be possible.

How does vascular injury lead to dementia? A simplistic approach is to conceptualize cognition as a sum total of neurologic function. The more neurologic function is affected, the worse is the cognitive status. Within this model, there are areas where the deficit is especially critical. Examples of these include the memory function served by the mesial temporal lobes and limbic system, personality traits that reside in the frontal lobes, and language ability in the dominant hemispheres. When the sum of the impaired neurologic function leads to impaired social functioning of an individual, the result is dementia.

Symptoms and Signs

The symptoms reported by the affected patients or their families are not unlike those of degenerative dementia. Forgetfulness, disorientation, nocturnal confusion, and personality changes are common. Some individuals may have more subtle affections. Individuals who previously functioned at a high level may complain that they need more time to complete a familiar task or have difficulty in dealing with abstract ideas. Family members and coworkers may notice a slowdown in performance. In classic cases, these complaints appear within 3 months after a cerebrovascular event. Sometimes the cerebrovascular events are clinically silent. Episodes of sudden worsening of cognitive function with or without subsequent improvement may be the only clue to the underlying cerebrovascular disease.

Vascular dementia is a heterogeneous condition, and clinical manifestations vary according to the size and location of the cerebrovascular lesions. Patients with overt hemiplegia or aphasia present little challenge in determining the cause of their cognitive decline. In some patients the abnor-

mality may be more subtle, such as asymmetric tendon reflexes, unilateral or bilateral Babinski's sign, a homonymous segmental visual field cut, agnosia, or apraxia. Primitive reflexes or release phenomena such as the grasp response, suck reflex, rooting reflex, and palmomental reflexes may be present, but they are not specific for vascular dementia.

Diagnosis

As the name implies, patients with vascular dementia must have a clinically significant cognitive defect (dementia), a history of cerebral infarct or intracerebral hemorrhage, *and* a potential causal link between the vascular event or events and the cognitive decline. Several diagnostic criteria are in use. None of the diagnostic criteria had been shown to be superior to the other.

All the current diagnostic criteria of vascular dementia require that the affected individuals have a deficit in at least two cognitive domains. Recognized cognitive domains are memory (i.e., immediate recall, recent memory, remote memory), orientation, language, praxis, attention, visualspatial skills, problem solving, judgment skill, and social function. To avoid overdiagnosis, the criteria also require that the cognitive deficit not be the result of the effect of the stroke alone. For example, a patient who has suffered a dominant cerebral hemispheric stroke with dysphasia cannot be considered to have a deficit in the language domain. On the other hand, if the same patient had worsening of his or her language ability but without another cerebrovascular event, the patient would be considered to have a defective language function. Folstein's bedside Mini-Mental Status Examination is particularly useful in screening for deficits in various cognitive domains.

A cerebrovascular event can be frequently inferred by careful history taking from the patient or family members as well as a detailed neurologic examination. When there is no obvious history of cerebrovascular disease and neurologic examination only revealed subtle findings, a computed tomographic (CT) or magnetic resonance imaging (MRI) study of the brain is needed before the diagnosis of vascular dementia is given. Between the two neuroimaging techniques, MRI is more sensitive in picking up abnormalities with reasonable specificity. It may not be universally available and is contraindicated in patients with implanted metallic or electronic devices. A CT scanner is more widely available, although it will miss small subtle changes of old infarction or hemorrhage.

It is easy to establish a history of cerebrovascular events and easy to establish that a patient is demented. Demonstration of a cause-and-effect relationship is not quite as straightforward. The patient may have an underlying cognitive problem that has nothing to do with the cerebrovascular event. A cause-and-effect relationship can be inferred when a clear temporal relationship between the onset or worsening of cognitive decline and cerebrovascular event can be established. When the temporal relationship is not as clear-cut, involvement of critical brain structures or involvement of a large volume of cerebral structures can also infer a cause-effect relationship. There is no consensus about how much brain tissue must be lost before one can attribute the cognitive decline to the cerebrovascular event. As a general tool, small (<1.0 cm) discrete lesions seldom lead to cognitive decline.

Once vascular dementia is suspected, the clinician should proceed to rule out other conditions that can mimic vascular dementia or worsen the cognitive deficit.

Differential Diagnosis

The most important conditions in the differential diagnosis of vascular dementia are Alzheimer's disease or other degenerative dementias. There is no definitive treatment available for degenerative dementia and it carries a worse prognosis. Most patients suspected of having vascular dementia are elderly individuals in whom degenerative dementia is also prevalent. A CT or MRI scan of the brain that is free from or shows only minimum vascular events makes the diagnosis of vascular dementia very unlikely.

Patients who have suffered a stroke are at high risk of developing depression. This is particularly true if the left cerebral hemisphere is affected. Cognitive decline may be attributed to depression alone (pseudodementia). A therapeutic trial of antidepressants should always be considered in patients with

Table 27B-1. Screening Tests for the Common Treatable Dementias

Etiology	Screening Test
Vitamin B_{12} deficiency	Serum vitamin B_{12} level
Neurosyphilis	Serum and cerebrospinal fluid treponema antigen/antibody tests
Hypothyroidism	Serum thyrotropin and free thyroxine levels
Normal-pressure hydrocephalus	Computed tomographic or magnetic resonance imaging scans of the brain
Chronic subdural hematoma, intracranial tumor	Computed tomography or magnetic resonance imaging of the brain

suspected vascular dementia and symptoms of depression.

Treatable concomitant conditions that cause or worsen cognitive decline should also be excluded. These conditions are listed in Table 27B-1.

Treatment and Prevention

The currently available diagnostic criteria make vascular dementia sound like an all-or-none phenomenon. As most readers would appreciate, patients do not develop dementia overnight. Patients who have recent stroke and started showing symptoms and signs of cognitive decline may not fulfill the criteria of dementia. It would be wrong to do nothing about these patients, waiting for them to become demented before intervention is planned. We have termed this phase between normal cognitive state and vascular dementia "vascular cognitive impairment." Patients with vascular cognitive impairment should be managed as aggressively, if not more so, as those with vascular dementia.

There is no proven therapy that can reverse the neurologic damage suffered by the patients. Likewise, there is no treatment available that can reverse the cognitive deficit. It may be possible to prevent worsening of cognitive function and possibly to retard the rate of cognitive decline by preventing more strokes from occurring.

Patients with a history of cerebral infarcts are prone to recurrent infarctions. The risk of recurrent strokes can be substantially reduced by aggressive treatment of hypertension, treatment of hypercholesterolemia, better control of diabetes mellitus, and the cessation of cigarette smoking. The use of antithrombotics such as acetylsalicylic acid (ASA), ticlopidine, and warfarin sodium is associated with a reduction of risk of recurrent cerebral infarction. The optimal dose of ASA in stroke prevention is still a controversial subject. We prefer to prescribe ASA at a dose of 1,300 mg daily, or 325–650 mg daily in patients who are unable to tolerate the higher dose. Patients who have recurrent cerebral ischemic episodes while taking a sufficient dose of ASA may be treated with either ticlopidine or warfarin sodium. Ticlopidine is usually given as 250 mg twice daily. Warfarin sodium is the preferred antithrombotic when a cardioembolic source is suspected. The dose of warfarin should be adjusted constantly to maintain an international normalized ratio of 2.0–3.0.

In patients with recent cerebral ischemia and ipsilateral severe internal carotid artery stenosis, carotid endarterectomy substantially reduces the risk of recurrent stroke. The role of carotid endarterectomy in patients with silent cerebral infarct is not clear. Most studies report no difference in the risk of stroke in patients with asymptomatic carotid artery stenosis with or without carotid endarterectomy. In one study, the stroke risk was statistically different in favor of those who had carotid endarterectomy, but it is not certain if the difference was clinically relevant.

In patients whose cerebrovascular events were intracerebral hemorrhages, the key to preventing future events is good blood pressure control. Whatever the underlying vessel wall abnormality, sustained high blood pressure increases the risk of recurrent hemorrhage. If the initial hemorrhage was related to an arteriovenous malformation, selected embolization or resection of the abnormal tissue can reduce the risk of recurrent hemorrhage. No treatment is available to reverse the vessel wall defect of amyloid angiopathy.

Patients diagnosed as having vascular dementia may have underlying depression that can worsen the cognitive deficit. As mentioned in the previous section, a trial of antidepressants is often helpful. If there is no clear cut improvement in the cognitive status after a good trial of an antidepressant, the drug can be safely discontinued. In most cases, it is necessary for the patient and the family to develop coping strategies to minimize the effect of cognitive decline. This might include a shift in family responsibility, a change in daily routine, and use of memory aids. When a patient becomes so demented that safety cannot be guaranteed at home, placement in a monitored environment is often necessary.

Vascular dementia is not truly "reversible." It is potentially treatable. What is more important, it is also preventable. Vascular dementia will not occur if we can prevent the first stroke from happening. Epidemiologic and interventional studies have suggested that better treatment or control of hypertension, hyperglycemia, and hypercholesterolemia, cessation of smoking, use of antithrombotics, and timely surgical intervention can reduce the risk of stroke. These same interventions also lead to a lower incidence of cardiac disease and other vascular disease. This is a worthwhile effort in which every developed country should invest. In the long run, this will reduce the health-care costs of the society.

Suggested Reading

Ballard C, Bannister C, Solis M, et al. The prevalence, associations and symptoms of depression amongst dementia sufferers. J Affect Disord 1996;36:135.

Bowler JV, Hachinski V. Vascular cognitive impairment: a new approach to vascular dementia. Baillieres Clin Neurol 1995;4:357.

Censori B, Partziguian T, Manara O, et al. Dementia after first stroke. Stroke 1996;27:1205.

Hachinski V. Vascular dementia: a radical redefinition. Dementia 1994;5:130.

Hebert R, Brayne C. Epidemiology of vascular dementia. Neuroepidemiology 1995;14:240.

Vascular dementia: an updated approach to patient management. A roundtable discussion: part 3. Geriatrics 1994;49:39.

Verhey FR, Rozendaal N, Lodder J, Jolles J. Comparison of seven sets of criteria used for the diagnosis of vascular dementia. Neuroepidemiology 1996;15:166.

Chapter 28
Parkinson's Disease and Related Movement Disorders

Pierre Pollak

Chapter Plan

Definition and Etiology of Parkinsonism

Parkinsonism is a clinical syndrome dominated by disorders of movement consisting of akinesia, rigidity, tremor, and postural abnormalities. The use of the term *akinesia* often encompasses akinesia itself (loss of movement), bradykinesia (slowness of movement), and hypokinesia (reduced movement). Parkinsonism can be classified into two major categories: idiopathic Parkinson's disease (PD) and atypical parkinsonian disorders. PD consists of a typical parkinsonian syndrome related to specific pathologic features (see "Pathology and Biochemistry"). Atypical parkinsonian disorder can be caused by neurodegenerative disorders or various secondary causes (Table 28-1).

All these disorders have in common either a lesion of the basal ganglion or functional disturbance in that structure. The prevalence of most of these parkinsonian disorders has not yet been estimated, but they are rare in clinical practice. PD is the most commonly encountered disorder, followed by drug-induced parkinsonism. Among the neurodegenerative causes of parkinsonism other than PD, we will focus on multiple system atrophy (MSA), progressive supranuclear palsy (PSP), and corticobasal degeneration (CBD) because they are the most common and the most frequently misdiagnosed.

Parkinson's Disease

Epidemiology

The incidence rates for PD range from 4.5 to 21.0 per 100,000 population per year. Reports of prevalence are also variable, with a mean estimated at about 120 per 100,000 persons. PD represents the second most common cause of motor handicap in adults after stroke. The peak age of onset is 55–60 years; over 65 years, 1 in 100 of the population is affected. The disease is rare before age 50 years, although onset before 40 years is possible, but not before 20 years. Despite the advent of levodopa, which is a

Table 28-1. Causes of Atypical Parkinsonism

Neurodegenerative Disorders	Secondary Causes
Multiple system atrophy	Drug-induced (antidopaminergic drugs)
Progressive supranuclear palsy	Arteriosclerotic pseudoparkinsonism
Corticobasal degeneration	Hydrocephalus
Dementia with Lewy bodies	Postencephalitis
Alzheimer's disease	Post-trauma
Pallidal degeneration	Space-occupying lesions
Huntington's disease, rigid variant	Toxin-induced: MPTP, carbon monoxide, manganese
Pick's disease	Post-anoxic encephalopathy
Parkinson dementia complex of Guam	Wilson's disease

MPTP = 1-methyl-4-phenyl-1,2,3,6-tetrahydropyridine.

highly effective therapeutic agent, the life expectancy of PD patients is still mildly reduced.

Etiology

The cause of PD is unknown. The disease could result from the combination of an inherited genetic predisposition and an environmental toxin. The genetic change could involve the detoxification systems. Because the injection of 1-methyl-4-phenyl-1,2,3,6-tetrahydropyridine (MPTP), a heroin-like substance, induced a parkinsonian syndrome that resembled PD, environmental toxins, especially pesticides and herbicides, were actively researched but with conflicting results. PD exists worldwide but is less frequent in China and Africa, whereas the prevalence is the same between American blacks of African origin and American whites, which favors the potential role of an environmental factor. Among individual risk factors, the sex ratio slightly favors men. PD patients more frequently have a history of head trauma, smoke less than the control population, and exhibit a more rigid personality. Rare family cases of PD have been reported with an autosomal dominant transmission. In such a family, genetic markers were found on chromosome 4 q21–q23 linked to the PD phenotype, which does not mean that the usual sporadic PD is linked to the same markers.

Pathology and Biochemistry

Neuropathologic examination shows a selective neuronal cell loss of pigmented brain stem nuclei, especially the substantia nigra pars compacta, with the presence of spherical eosinophilic intraneuronal inclusions called *Lewy bodies* in the remaining neurons. The lesions of the dopaminergic system include the neurons of the substantia nigra pars compacta, which project to the striatum (caudate nucleus and putamen), and the neurons of the mesencephalic ventral tegmental area, which project to the frontal cortex and the limbic system. The dopaminergic cell loss is heterogeneous, with the main lesion located in the ventrolateral part of the substantia nigra. In the striatal projection areas, dopamine levels are more diminished in the putamen than in the caudate. The lesional map is different from one patient to another, which explains the variability in symptoms. The activity of remaining neurons of the substantia nigra is increased, and this compensation is at the origin of a latent phase of the illness, as the symptoms occur after a 50–70% loss of nigral neurons. Striatal dopaminergic receptors of the D_1 or D_2 types (linked or not linked to adenylate cyclase, respectively) are unchanged in keeping with the normality of the striatal neurons where they are located. In the substantia nigra, the cell death is accompanied by the formation of free radicals and the occurrence of oxidative stress, which may play a role in the lesional process. Changes are noted in iron metabolism and mitochondrial function, especially a decrease in complex I activity and the loss of antioxidative defenses such as a decrease in glutathione levels.

Apart from the major dopaminergic disturbances, other variable neurotransmitter defects are found. In parallel with the cell loss, norepinephrine activity is decreased in the locus ceruleus as

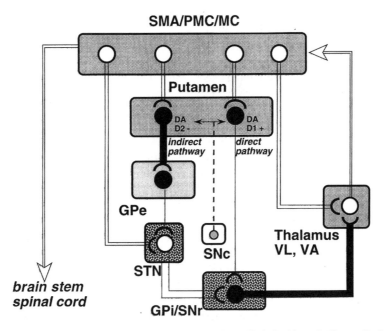

SMA/PMC/MC

Figure 28-1. Schematic representation of the functioning of the basal ganglia in Parkinson's disease. In the basal ganglia, filled lines correspond to inhibitory gamma-aminobutyric acid (GABA)ergic pathways, open lines correspond to excitatory glutamatergic pathways, and the dotted line corresponds to the lesioned dopaminergic pathway. Thin lines correspond to hypoactivity and thick lines to overactivity. Mottled nuclei are overactive. (DA = dopamine; D1 = D_1 dopaminergic receptors activated by dopamine; D2 = D_2 dopaminergic receptors inhibited by dopamine; GPe = globus pallidus external; GPi = globus pallidus internal; MC = motor cortex; PMC = premotor cortex; SMA = supplementary motor area of the cortex; SNc = substantia nigra pars compacta; SNr = substantia nigra pars reticulata; STN = subthalamic nucleus; VL, VA = ventrolateral and ventral anterior nuclei of the thalamus.)

well as serotonin activity in the raphe nuclei and their areas of projection both upward to the telencephalon and downward to the spinal cord. The cholinergic pathway is normal in the mesostriatal system but can be altered in the innominate-cortical system. The numerous striatal neurons that project to the pallidum and the substantia nigra pars reticularis are normal as are their gamma-aminobutyric acid (GABA)ergic and peptidergic activities.

Pathophysiology

Motor symptoms of PD are related to the dopaminergic lesions as demonstrated by the occurrence of a typical parkinsonian syndrome after intoxication by MPTP, which selectively injures the dopaminergic nigrostriatal system. In particular, the degree of akinesia parallels the loss of nigral dopaminergic neurons and the decrease in the striatal dopamine concentrations.

The major afferent to the basal ganglia arrives in the striatum from the predominantly cerebral cortex, with motor components projecting to the putamen and sensory and associative components to the caudate nucleus. The striatum integrates all these messages, which are layered somatotopically to the output structures of the basal ganglia. This function is properly carried out through the modulation of the nigrostriatal dopaminergic pathway. The outputs of the striatum converge to the internal pallidum (GPi) and the substantia nigra pars reticulata (SNr) using, schematically, either a direct pathway with a single neuron or an indirect pathway composed of three neurons passing through the external pallidum (GPe) and the subthalamic nucleus (STN) (Figure 28-1).

Thus, the STN plays a key role in the function of the basal ganglia because it is connected reciprocally with the entire output of the basal ganglia and receives other direct inputs, especially from the motor cortex. This STN-GP/SNr pathway is glutamatergic and excitatory, whereas the other connections from the striatum to the GP and the thalamus are GABAergic and inhibitory. Finally, the outputs from the basal ganglia project to the thalamus (ventrolateral and ventroanterior nuclei) and return to the cerebral cortex in the motor, premotor, and supplementary motor areas, completing the corticobasal ganglia-cortical loop. Another output pathway from the basal ganglia goes down to brain stem nuclei and beyond to the spinal cord.

In PD, the loss of striatal dopaminergic modulation leads to an overactivity of the GPi through both the direct and the indirect pathways. The disinhibition of the subthalamopallidal structures excessively brakes the thalamus, which delivers an underactive message to the frontal cortex. The latter cannot provide adequate motor information to the spinal cord, which may account for the akinesia.

The mechanisms underlying rigidity are less well known. The exteroceptive polysynaptic reflexes are abnormal and the tonic muscular response to slow and sustained stretch exaggerated. This long latency stretch reflex reflects the influence of abnormal supraspinal information on the spinal cord neuronal machinery. The overactive pathway descending directly from the GPi could be the cause of this change.

Parkinsonian rest tremor is also related to the dopaminergic defect, perhaps because of a subpopulation of dopaminergic mesencephalic neurons located in the perirubral region. As a result, phasic neuronal activities synchronous to tremor occur in the GPi, STN, and the thalamus (ventral lateral and ventral intermediate nuclei) as well as the motor cortex. The latter sends to the spinal cord the rhythmic activities as revealed by the arrest of tremor after a cortical or internal capsular stroke.

A lesion of the nondopaminergic system is thought to play a role in the occurrence of nonmotor symptoms. For example, the noradrenergic and cholinergic lesions would be involved in dementia and the serotonergic lesion in depression. The various dysautonomic symptoms would be related to the lesions of the dorsal motor nucleus of the vagus nerve, the intermediolateral cell column of the spinal cord, and even the myenteric plexus.

Clinical Manifestations

The role of the physician is substantial in three clinical domains of the disease. First, he or she must recognize subtle signs or symptoms at the onset of the disease that are often overlooked or misdiagnosed, leading to incorrect treatment. Second, the physician must know the full clinical spectrum of PD, which extends beyond the typical motor manifestations. Third, levodopa, the drug taken by most PD patients during the course of their disease, has had such an impact that it has created a new disease; PD treated with levodopa develops new symptoms mixed with those belonging to the disease itself. This must be clearly recognized in order to provide adequate treatment.

Disease Onset

The onset of PD is insidious and almost always unilateral, so patients are aware early of a slight clumsiness when it occurs in their dominant hand. The more frequent manifestations are tremor and slowness, stiffness, or clumsiness of one upper limb. Numb, painful muscles are reported, as well as fatigue, lack of vital energy, depression, and unexplained weight loss. One of these features may be the sole complaint for many months. At this stage, one should endeavor to acknowledge the parkinsonian nature of these symptoms and eliminate other diagnoses. The most common misdiagnoses are to interpret tremor as physiologic or essential tremor, stiffness or aches as rheumatism, and loss of energy as depression. The general and neurologic examination must be normal.

Resting tremor of the hand, which is characteristic of PD, may be absent or intermittent. It is typically elicited or worsened by stress, mental calculation, repetitive movement of another part of the body, or walking. The resting parkinsonian tremor may disappear at the beginning of the contraction of muscles involved in tremor.

Activation maneuvers, called *Froment's sign,* cause the appearance or aggravation of *rigidity.* To demonstrate this, the patient is asked to perform rotating movements of the upper limb around the shoulder contralateral to the wrist examined by passive movements, or to stand up and bend the trunk forward as if to catch an object with the contralateral hand.

Akinesia appears in activities of daily life during tasks that require repetitive or fine movements such as brushing the teeth, scrubbing, beating eggs, buttoning clothing, lacing shoes, and writing. Examination determines how well the patient performs 10–20 repetitive movements of opposing the thumb to the forefinger, alternating pronation and supination of the wrist while tapping with the foot. In case of PD, these movements show a progressive slowness and require an unusually high degree of concentration; if normal, some difficulties may be brought out when the patient is asked to do repetitive movements of the affected hand while squeezing the fist with the other hand or simultaneously performing other repetitive movements. Walking enables the physician to note a decrease in the arm swing.

Cardinal Manifestations

Tremor.   The classic tremor involves rhythmic oscillating movements at 4–6 Hz of a body part at rest. The hand, which is the most frequent location of tremor, mimics the classic "pill-rolling" movement, with an alternating opposition of the thumb and fingers. Tremor occurs mainly in the distal part of the limbs. The lower limb and the perioral region (lips, chin, and tongue) may be involved. Moderate tremor abates when the involved muscles are activated in the performance of a task for hand tremor, speaking for face tremor, or walking for leg tremor. This explains why tremor is usually not very disabling as opposed to akinesia. When tremor is severe, the proximal part of the limbs may be concerned and tremor may recur during postural or kinetic action after a short dampening period at the onset of movement. Tremor disappears in sleep and worsens with stress and anxiety. In addition to rest tremor, most patients exhibit a postural and kinetic tremor of low amplitude and high frequency, which can be felt internally. This fine action tremor, albeit frequent in parkinsonism, is not representative of what is meant by parkinsonian tremor, which only makes reference to rest tremor.

Rigidity.   Rigidity is noted as increased resistance to passive movement of a limb segment or the neck. This resistance is almost the same throughout the entire range of movement and is not clearly influenced by the speed or force of the movement, which distinguishes it from spasticity. When rigidity is constant, it resembles a lead pipe or wax, but some brief and irregular arrests of movement are often superimposed and are called the *cogwheel phenomenon*. Tremor may be partly responsible for the cogwheeling. The predominance of rigidity of the flexors participates in the global appearance of PD patients with all joints slightly flexed, elbows against the sides of the body, a flexed neck, and a stooped posture, often with pronounced kyphosis and varying degrees of scoliosis.

Akinesia.   Akinesia is usually the most disabling symptom because it limits most of the activities of daily living such as hygiene, dressing, walking, arising from a chair, turning over in bed, or eating. There is a global poverty and slowness of movement, a lack of strength, and nonexpressiveness in the face; blinking is rare, which contrasts with the exaggeration of the inability to inhibit blinking in response to a tap over the glabella. The unilaterality of the symptoms, noted from the onset of the disease, persists over time in the form of asymmetry, which then becomes less and less marked. Neurophysiologic studies show a moderate increase in reaction time in motor initiation. Movement time is greatly increased and accounts for bradykinesia and a decrease in movement amplitude. During a ballistic—that is, a brisk movement—this prolongation in movement time is caused by a reduction in the initial electromyographic burst of the agonist muscle by lack of muscular energy. These defects are increased when simultaneous and successive sequential movements are performed. Akinesia is proportional to the complexity of the motor task, which frequently involves the coordination of several motor programs. As the disease worsens over the years, the initiation of any movement may become impossible (start hesitation) or the completion of the movement may be arrested for many seconds, a phenomenon called *freezing*. An unusual external stimulus such as a phone ringing or a stressful event may trigger a freezing episode, whereas sensory guidance, in particular one that is rhythmic in nature, helps to continue the task. Any movement can also be arrested if the patient does not concentrate specifically on its completion or try to initiate another task simultaneously. However, at moments of great motivation or in circumstances of extreme happiness or sudden fright, the patient is capable, albeit briefly, of effecting movements such as running or dancing.

Postural Instability and Gait Impairment.   Gait impairment is mainly caused by akinesia. When the disease is asymmetric, the patient often drags a leg. Afterward, the step shortens and walking becomes reduced to a shuffle. There are no accompanying synergic movements of the rest of the body, which remains inert in the flexed posture mentioned earlier. The stooped posture associated with short steps may induce a transient acceleration of gait called *festination*. Finally, walking is impossible and the patient seems statuesque and claims that the soles of the feet are stuck to the floor or the legs are too heavy to lift. Start hesitation and freezing of gait are characteristic of parkinsonism and can cause falls. They are triggered by obstacles, door frames, or changes in direction and relieved by watching a nondangerous obstacle put just in front of the patient's foot or colored stripes regularly spaced on the floor. Freezing of gait disappears, usually when the patient moves using another motor program such as climbing up stairs or walking backward or sideways like a crab.

Loss of orthostatic stability generally occurs only in advanced PD and in the elderly. Although the gait is unsteady, the base is minimally or not at all widened, and truncal ataxia is absent. The patient can lose balance in any direction but a tendency toward retropulsion seems more frequent. It is assessed by the pull test on the patient's shoulders with the patient's eyes open. The patient is unable to perform the postural adjustments to avoid falling or cannot even move one leg at all and would fall en bloc if not retained by the examiner. This imbalance is accompanied by falls, which cause broken limbs and eventually a bedridden invalid.

Secondary Manifestations

Mental Dysfunction.   The mental status is roughly normal during the first years of evolution of PD, with the exception of depression, which may be the initial symptom and affects approximately 50% of patients whatever the stage of the disease. However, higher-order cognitive disturbances suggestive of frontal lobe dysfunction are extremely common in nondemented patients. Specific neuropsychological tests show mild to moderate disturbances such as slowed thinking (bradyphrenia), visuospatial impairment, attentional set-shifting difficulties, memory deficits only for recall, and poor executive functions. The tests usually carried out to demonstrate these deficits are the Wisconsin Card Sorting Test, the Stroop test, the Grober and Buschke memory test, verbal fluency tests, and imitation behavior tests. However, this impairment does not prevent patients from managing most activities of daily life. But approximately one-third of patients develop true dementia of the subcortical type at the late stage of the disease when they are older than 70 years. Because of deficient diagnostic precision for both PD and dementia, it is difficult to assess the specific role of PD in the genesis of this cognitive decline. The association of Alzheimer's disease, multi-infarct dementia, dementia with Lewy bodies, or other dementing diseases may play a contributory role. Although dementia is of major concern in old PD patients, we must keep in mind that true dementia almost never occurs in young-onset PD until the patient becomes considerably older.

Autonomic Dysfunction.   The most frequent complaints are bowel and bladder symptoms. The reduced colonic mobility may lead to severe constipation and intestinal pseudo-obstruction. Urinary urgency and increased frequency are usually related to the hypertonia of the detrusor muscle of the bladder. Sexual dysfunction is frequent and related to multiple factors. Episodic sweating and abnormal sensations of heat or cold occur in some patients. Seborrhea of the face can lead to dermatitis. Severe orthostatic hypotension and syncope are uncommon and generally the result of medication.

Other Manifestations

Some manifestations actually represent special cases of rigidity and akinesia. Speech is monotonic, hypophonic, and inarticulate. Dysarthria may become so severe that the patient is incomprehensible or only whispers.

Pharyngeal akinesia leads to dysphagia only later in the disease. Consuming a meal takes an inordinately long time. Finally, dysphagia may induce choking and aspiration pneumonia and prove life-threatening. Excessive saliva and drooling are reported by the majority of patients, which is presumed to be the result of a decrease in the swallowing of saliva.

Oculomotor function is usually almost normal, but limitation of upgaze is common, as in the normal elderly. Weakened convergence may result in blurred vision and difficulty in reading. Dopaminergic loss in the retina is responsible for defects in the vision of contrasts, which can only be assessed with a special examination. A decrease in the olfactory function is common but rarely a complaint.

Pain and sensory symptoms are common and take the form of paresthesia, numbness, burning, or muscle cramps. Akinesia and rigidity favor arthralgia, entrapment neuropathies, and musculoskeletal deformities. In advanced disease, the hand displays ulnar deviation with flexion of the metacarpophalangeal joints, the toes are curled but the big toe is often extended, and curvature of the spine leads to kyphosis and generally concave scoliosis contralateral to the most affected side.

Sleep disturbances affect almost all patients but not during the first years of the disease. Patients report that sleep is disrupted by frequent awakenings from many factors, especially the need to urinate, together with motor and sensory symptoms. Rapid eye movement (REM) sleep behavior disorder, consisting of purposeful behaviors such as kicking or hitting during REM sleep, occur in many patients with advanced disease.

Levodopa-Induced Motor Complications

Phenomenology. Levodopa profoundly changed the appearance of PD, intermingling new signs and symptoms with those of the disease. These manifestations can be separated into levodopa-induced motor complications and other complications. The latter will be dealt with separately regarding each drug.

After a honeymoon period of motor benefit for 1–10 years (mean, 3–6 years), chronic levodopa therapy induces two types of motor complications, motor fluctuations and dyskinesias, in approximately 60% of patients after 5 years of treatment and in 90% after 10 years. Motor fluctuations are related to the appearance of the levodopa-induced short-duration response in conjunction with the

Table 28-2. Levodopa-Induced Motor Fluctuations

Wearing-off
    End-of-dose deterioration or akinesia
    Nocturnal akinesia
    Early morning akinesia
On-off phenomenon
    Sudden unpredictable fluctuations (if levodopa doses
        are small and frequent)
    Sudden predictable fluctuations (if levodopa doses are
        high and spaced by more than 3 hours)
    Yo–yoing
Increased latency to dose response
No response
Meal-associated, delayed response, or no response
Rebound superparkinsonism

progressive worsening of the disease, which results in a greater disability during the periods of recurrence of parkinsonian syndrome. These periods of parkinsonism are named "off-motor periods" in comparison with the periods of levodopa-induced motor improvement named "on-motor periods." Off-motor periods occur at approximately 4- to 6-hour intervals, close to the time of the next levodopa dose. With the progression of the disease, this interval tends to be reduced to less than 2 hours, even to a few minutes. The various types of motor fluctuations are listed in Table 28-2 and dyskinesias are listed in Table 28-3. All types of dyskinesias may occur, but some are more characteristic: dystonic inversion of the foot with extension of the great toe, internal rotation of the upper limb backward while walking, rotation of the neck, and grimacing. Abnormal movements can be so severe that they interfere with tasks, speech, and balance. Most patients prefer the dyskinesias, even when severe, to the parkinsonian off-periods.

The temporal pattern of dyskinesias after a single levodopa dose can help in their classification and, to some degree, in understanding their mechanisms. A complete examination of a fluctuating patient requires the assessment of the various phases of the disease, at least the worst "off," the worst dyskinetic, and the best "on" periods. This is difficult to obtain even by multiple consultations and can necessitate a levodopa test in the morning after an overnight fasting with multiple successive evaluations during the 2–4 hours of

Table 28-3. Levodopa-Induced Dyskinesias

Off-period dystonia (usually fixed and painful dystonia in
feet, more rarely paraspinal region)
    Early-morning dystonia
    After abatement of benefit
Off-period akathisia
On-period dyskinesias (generally increased by voluntary
action)
    Peak-dose dyskinesias (occurring at presumed time of
maximal dopaminergic stimulation corresponding to
maximal blood levels of levodopa)
        Chorea, dystonia, rarely ballism, usually mildly
or moderately disabling, patient not even
aware if mild; all parts of the body may be
involved
    Diphasic dyskinesias or beginning and/or end-of-dose
dyskinesias (occurring at intermediate dopaminergic
stimulation at onset and end of dose-related benefit)
        Dystonia, ballism, rarely chorea, usually dis-
abling even if mild in amplitude; onset generally in feet, more frequent in lower limbs and
trunk and neck but all parts of the body may
be involved
    Square-wave dyskinesias (occurring throughout dura-
tion of benefit)
Other dyskinesias (rare): myoclonus, asterixis, tics

response. During in-between periods, some parts of the body can be dyskinetic while other parts are parkinsonian. In fact, the clinical aspect of the patient changes frequently according to the level of the dopaminergic stimulation and the psychic state and motor activity. This explains why a levodopa test using a suprathreshold dose of levodopa may be necessary in some fluctuating patients to assess both the type of dyskinesias and the full dopaminergic response, especially of imbalance and freezing of gait.

Mechanisms. The relationship between the dopaminergic activation by intravenous levodopa infusion and the motor response has been studied in four groups of PD patients representative of the evolution of the levodopa effect over time: de novo untreated patients, patients with a stable motor response, patients with wearing-off effect, and patients with on-off effect. The occurrence and the loss of the optimal antiparkinsonian response follow a continuum. In the initial phases of treatment, the effect is slow and progressive over several days. At the later stages of the on-off

effect, the benefit occurs and disappears suddenly on either side of a given threshold of dopaminergic activity. The response is of the all-or-none type—that is, absent below this threshold and straightaway maximal above it. Because this threshold rises with the duration of the treatment, the duration of the response becomes shorter and shorter (Figure 28-2).

The dyskinetic effect is absent at the start of the treatment and develops progressively after several months to years of continuous levodopa intake, more typically if the drug is given intermittently. The development of this response is partly reversible as demonstrated experimentally by drug holidays or continuous infusions of levodopa for a few days or weeks.

At the beginning of treatment, the dopaminergic lesions are moderate, with persistence of striatal dopaminergic presynaptic endings of a sufficient amount to buffer the fluctuations of the dopamine levels resulting from intermittent oral levodopa. At the stage of the wearing-off phenomenon, this buffering effect is lost, and the motor response becomes sinusoidal, with striatal extracellular dopamine levels parallel with the fluctuations of blood levodopa levels. The pharmacokinetics of levodopa with an elimination half-life of approximately 90 minutes explains to a great extent these fluctuating effects. To explain the suddenness of the motor changes at the stage of on-off effect, pharmacodynamic factors are added to pharmacokinetic factors, which are not altered during long-term levodopa therapy. Dyskinesias result from the conjunction of both the dopaminergic lesions and the chronic levodopa administration. The more severe the parkinsonian syndrome, the more intense and early the onset of the levodopa-induced motor complications. Off-period dystonia is a relative exception to this rule, as the dystonic foot is not always located on the side of predominance for akinesia.

The mechanism of peak dose dyskinesia is relatively easy to understand. Maximal concentrations of striatal dopamine induce an excessive dopaminergic receptor response. These dyskinesias are simultaneous with the maximal improvement in parkinsonian syndrome. However, the mechanisms at the origin of diphasic dyskinesias are unknown. They may result from a partial stimulation of the dopaminergic receptors inducing a dysequilibrium

Figure 28-2. Modifications of the dopaminergic response over time. The curve indicates the intensity of dopaminergic activation induced by levodopa intake. The antiparkinsonian effect threshold tends to rise and the dyskinesia effect threshold tends to lower. When these thresholds coincide, the motor response is of the all-or-none type and corresponds to the on-off phenomenon.

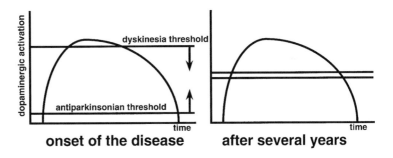

of the striatal output pathways. Some pharmacodynamically reversible changes of the dopaminergic response, in particular a progressive hyposensitivity, may develop over several hours during the day, which explains why the worst parkinsonism and the worst dyskinetic periods occur late in the afternoon. The best levodopa response is usually obtained after the first intake in the morning. On awakening, most patients, generally not the most severe, exhibit a sleep benefit of undetermined mechanism for 1–2 hours.

Clinical Types

Patients with PD can be categorized according to symptom dominance and age of onset. Rest tremor, albeit highly characteristic of PD, is not a constant feature, since only approximately 80% of patients are affected with tremor from the onset of the disease. When rest tremor represents the main symptom and disability, we call this form the *tremor-dominant type* of PD. It usually follows a more slowly progressive, benign course than the opposite form of PD, called the *akinetic-rigid–dominant type*.

Young-onset (before age 40 years) PD patients tend to show an excellent response to levodopa but early development of levodopa-induced motor complications. These patients retain a pure parkinsonian syndrome for many years. Patients with an onset of PD after 70 years of age tend to show an initial moderate to good response to levodopa, develop late and moderate levodopa-induced motor complications, and are prone to be disabled by cognitive dysfunction, postural instability, and dysautonomia. Patients with the onset of PD in between these age extremes have an intermediate evolution of the disease.

Diagnosis and Investigations

Because there is no specific test, the diagnosis of PD is clinical. A definitive diagnosis is pathologic, and some other causes of parkinsonism occur in at least 15% of cases clinically diagnosed as PD by experienced neurologists. The difficulty is to distinguish PD from the many parkinsonian syndromes, in particular those caused by other degenerative diseases or by neuroleptics.

All neuroleptics or other drugs with antidopaminergic properties can induce parkinsonism. Flunarizine, cinnarizine, and calcium-channel blocking agents can also be involved. If the intake of neuroleptics is easy to assess in psychotic patients, more effort is needed to disclose the administration of neuroleptics or neuroleptic-like drugs prescribed for insomnia, nausea or emesis, vertigo, or any psychosomatic manifestations. Patients with neuroleptic-induced parkinsonism usually exhibit bilateral symptoms and a fine action tremor more frequently than the classic pill-rolling rest tremor. Levodopa therapy is ineffective. When symptoms have lasted for many months or years, there is no progressive worsening of symptoms, and orofacial dyskinesias may be associated. Parkinsonism appears generally during the first 3 months of the neuroleptic treatment, and parkinsonism slowly abates after the discontinuation of the drugs. After 3 months of drug arrest, 90% of patients are no longer parkinsonian, but the syndrome may last up to 1 year. Neuroleptic-induced parkinsonism is moderately improved by anticholinergics or amantadine. Maintaining the neuroleptic therapy at the lowest effective dose must be attempted, in addition to discontinuation periods according to the evolution of psychotic symptoms. In case of disabling parkinsonism, clozapine, an

Table 28-4. Criteria for the Diagnosis of Parkinson's Disease

Bradykinesia	Tremor	Asymmetry	Levodopa Effect	Pure Sporadic Parkinsonian Syndrome
Obligatory criterion	Classic rest tremor	Unilateral onset Progressive persistent asymmetry	Excellent (>70%) response to levodopa Continued response to levodopa Levodopa-induced dyskinesias Exclusion criterion if no response to levodopa	No more than one affected relative No early dementia No early postural imbalance and falls No early dysautonomia No significant abnormality of eye movements No cerebellar signs No pyramidal signs

atypical neuroleptic drug, can be used to replace the offending agent but must be used in conjunction with regular monitoring of the leukocyte count because of the possibility of agranulocytosis. If parkinsonism lasts more than 3–12 months after stopping neuroletpic drugs, underlying idiopathic PD is possible, and a levodopa challenge for at least 3 months is worthwhile.

Normal-pressure hydrocephalus can create a parkinsonian gait and postural instability but without tremor and with cognitive and urinary impairments. Brain imaging supports the diagnosis.

Arteriosclerotic parkinsonism is caused by a series of lacunar infarcts in the region of the basal ganglia or by Binswanger's disease. The medical history of the patient, brain magnetic resonance imaging (MRI) findings, corticospinal tract signs, and levodopa resistance help the diagnosis.

Essential tremor and other causes of postural tremors may mimic the tremor-dominant type of PD, especially in the elderly. However, tremor amplitude is greater in action than in the position of repose, head and voice tremors are often involved, and rigidity or akinesia is slight or absent.

Clinical features specific to various degenerative causes of parkinsonism may be lacking during the first years of evolution, thus raising the percentage of misdiagnosis of PD at this initial stage. Table 28-4 shows the criteria proposed to improve the success rate in the diagnosis of PD. They were obtained on the basis of autopsy findings.

In typical cases, neither brain imaging nor laboratory tests are useful. If the patient is younger than 35 years of age, a serum ceruloplasmin deter-mination and a slit-lamp examination for the Kayser-Fleischer ring allow Wilson's disease to be ruled out. In atypical parkinsonism, these tests should be carried out if the age of onset is below 50 years. In other atypical parkinsonisms, standard laboratory tests (complete blood cell count, chemistry analysis, tests of liver and thyroid function) are useful in detecting other diseases that can induce fatigue, general slowness, or postural tremor. Brain imaging is useful in all cases of atypical parkinsonism, in particular when the parkinsonian syndrome is not pure or is unresponsive to levodopa. MRI scanning, is preferable to computed tomographic (CT) scanning because it is more sensitive for the visualization of both atrophy (sagittal plane for brain stem and cerebellar vermis) and abnormalities of basal ganglia intensities using a T2-weighted sequence. Positron emission tomography is currently of no diagnostic use. It was developed essentially for research, it is costly, and it is not widely available. Decreased uptake in striatal ^{18}F-fluorodopa (a functional marker of the nigrostriatal pathway) or a ligand of the presynaptic endings associated with a normal striatal postsynaptic dopaminergic receptor uptake is highly suggestive of PD but not specific.

Pharmacologic Treatments

Dopaminergic Agents

Since 1968, levodopa has been regarded as the gold standard of pharmacotherapy. Levodopa is the pre-

Table 28-5. Antiparkinsonian Drugs

Substance Group	Generic Name	Most Frequent Trade Name and Dosage (Not Exhaustive)
Levodopa	Levodopa + benserazide ratio, 100 mg/25 mg	Madopar, Modopar, Prolopa, 62.5 mg, 125.0 mg, 250.0 mg, dispersible 125.0 mg CR or depot or HBS or LP or Retard, 125 mg
	Levodopa + carbidopa ratio, 100 mg/10 mg or 100 mg/25 mg	Sinemet, Nacom, 50 mg, 100 mg, 250 mg Sinemet CR or depot or LP or Nacom ret 100/25 mg, 200/50 mg
Dopamine-receptor agonists	Apomorphine	Apomorphin, Apokinon, 10 mg/ml Apokinon penject, 30 mg/3ml
	Bromocriptine	Parlodel, 2.5 mg, 5.0 mg, 10.0 mg
	Lisuride	Dopergin, 0.2 mg, 0.5 mg
	Pergolide	Celance, Parkotil, Permax, 0.05 mg, 0.25 mg, 1.0 mg
	Piribedil	Trivastal, 20 mg, 50 mg
	Ropinirole	Requip, 0.25 mg, 0.5 mg, 1.0 mg, 2.0 mg, 5.0 mg
Adamantanamine	Amantadine	Symmetrel, Mantadix, Amantadin, PK-Merz, 100 mg
MAO B inhibitors	Selegiline	Deprenyl, Eldepryl, Jumex, Movergan, 5 mg
Anticholinergics	Benztropine	Cogentin, 1 mg, 2 mg
	Biperiden	Akineton, 2 mg, 4 mg
	Bornaprin	Sormodren, 4 mg
	Mexiten	Tremaril, Trest, 1 mg, 5 mg
	Orphenadrine	Disipal, Norflex, 50 mg, 100 mg
	Procyclidine	Kemadrin, 5 mg
	Trihexyphenidyl	Artane, 2 mg, 5 mg
	Tropatépine	Lepticur, 10 mg
Antihistaminergics	Diphenhydramine	Benadryl, 25 mg, 50 mg

CR = controlled release; HBS = hydrobalanced system; LP = libération prolongée; MAO = monoamine oxidase.
Note: The diversity of preparations and trade names available in different countries are reported in WH Oertel, RC Dodel. International guide to drugs for Parkinson's disease. Mov Disord 1995;10:121.

cursor of the neurotransmitter dopamine, which does not cross the blood-brain barrier. Levodopa supplies the dopamine defect after transformation by the aromatic amino acid decarboxylase (AAAD) enzyme. To avoid the formation of excessive dopamine outside the brain, levodopa is almost always given with a peripheral AAAD inhibitor, which does not enter the brain (either benserazide or carbidopa). These drugs are named *combined levodopa* and are referred to as *levodopa* for the remainder of the chapter. Because at least 25 mg of carbidopa three times a day is necessary to inhibit the peripheral synthesis of dopamine, a higher proportion of carbidopa (1:4 instead of 1:10) is useful in the case of a low daily dose of Sinemet or peripheral adverse effects. The various forms of levodopa are shown in Table 28-5. Before entering the brain, levodopa passes through several steps: solubilization in the stomach, passing the pylori, crossing the jejunal bar-

rier by amino acid transporters in competition with the other amino acids from feeding, and crossing the brain-blood barrier by the same transporters. Therefore, the various forms of levodopa have different absorption properties. The absorption is the fastest with the liquid form (dispersible Madopar or crushed Sinemet in water) on an empty stomach. Standard Madopar or Sinemet is also well or less well absorbed according to the accompanying feeding. Large meals and proteins slow down the gastric emptying and decrease barrier crossings, whereas mild liquid and sweetened feeding improve absorption. Controlled (slow)-release forms of levodopa delay absorption from 1 to 3 hours. Moreover, absorption is random and bioavailability is decreased, evaluated at 70% of the standard form but with high interindividual variability.

Levodopa must be titrated slowly, with an initial individual dose of 50 mg or even lower using divis-

Table 28-6. Management Options of Motor Complications in Treated Parkinson's Disease Patients

Complications	Management
Dyskinesias	
Peak dose	Reduce unitary levodopa dose; L-dopa retard; stop selegiline; add/increase dopaminergic agonist; use continuous drug delivery; neurosurgery
Diphasic	Increase unitary levodopa dose, avoid slow-release preparations or give very low levodopa doses with high doses of dopaminergic agonists; apomorphine injections; neurosurgery
Early morning and off-period dystonia	Add/increase dopaminergic agonist; bedtime slow-release levodopa or nocturnal levodopa; botulinum toxin injection into dystonic muscles; ?baclofen, lithium
Nocturnal myoclonus	Bedtime clonazepam
	Eliminate last evening levodopa dose
Gait freezing (levodopa responsive or unresponsive)	Readaptation using rhythmic internal routines and external visual cues
Motor fluctuations	
Predictable or unpredictable	Decrease interval between levodopa doses; increase levodopa dose; add/increase dopaminergic agonist; add selegiline (if no disabling dyskinesias); move to slow-release levodopa or combine slow-release and standard levodopa; levodopa 30 minutes before meals; small meals and low-protein diet; apomorphine injections or infusion; neurosurgery
No-response levodopa dose	Increase unitary levodopa dose taken before low protein meals; dispersible Madopar or liquid Sinemet

ible tablets of standard levodopa. A total daily dose of 300–600 mg is reached over a few weeks or months in three to four intakes. In the long term, rare patients can receive doses of more than 1,000 mg per day up to 2,000 mg per day.

Adverse effects are related to the activation of dopaminergic systems. Nausea and vomiting occur mainly at the start of treatment and are induced by the stimulation of D_2 dopaminergic receptors of the area postrema, which contains the chemical trigger zone for vomiting located on the posterior surface of the medulla oblongata. Because this region is barrier-free, the association of domperidone, a peripheral dopaminergic receptor antagonist, prevents levodopa-induced vomiting without interfering with the central beneficial antiparkinsonian effect. Orthostatic hypotension is caused by the stimulation of dopaminergic receptors located both on the splanchnic and renal arteries responsible for vasodilatation and on the presynaptic sympathetic noradrenergic terminals responsible for a vegetative sympathetic inhibition. Sleep can be disturbed by vivid dreams. Diurnal sedation and mental confusion can occur, especially in old patients. Illusions, hallucinations of any type, and paranoid delirium can be induced by high doses. These psychotic disorders could be related to the excessive stimulation of corticolimbic dopaminergic receptors.

After several years of continuous levodopa therapy, adverse motor effects definitely occur. A permanent motor improvement is no longer possible whatever the therapeutic strategy and all types of dyskinesias occur both spontaneously and especially during voluntary movements such as eating or speaking.

A sudden cessation of levodopa for a few days may induce a syndrome of dopaminergic deprivation similar to the neuroleptic malignant syndrome. It includes fever, diffuse rigidity, and mental confusion, and is life-threatening in the absence of an immediate resumption of levodopa, sometimes by nasogastric tube or by subcutaneous infusion of apomorphine. The management of drug-induced adverse effects is summarized in Table 28-6.

Dopaminergic agonist drugs work similarly to dopamine by stimulating dopaminergic receptors directly. Dopaminergic receptors are classified into two main types: type D_1 (D_1 and D_5), linked to adenylate cyclase, and type D_2 (high- and low-affinity D_2, D_3, and D_4), not linked to this enzyme. Most dopamine agonists activate predominantly or solely the D_2 dopaminergic receptors, and apomorphine activates both D_1 and D_2 receptors such as dopamine. Bromocriptine is the drug of reference, and depending on the country, other dopamine agonist drugs are available or under development. Long-acting drugs such as pergolide or cabergoline have theoretical advantages in the control of motor fluctuations and drugs such as ropinirole or pramipexole, which are nonergot derivatives, do not expose the patient to the risks of serous effusion or fibrosis. Apomorphine is the sole drug of this class commercially available in many countries and is given by subcutaneous injections, either continuously with portable minipumps or intermittently with pen-type autoinjectors as soon as a severe off-motor period occurs. The latency for motor benefit is 10 minutes on average, the dose range per injection is 2–8 mg, and the duration of the effect lasts less than 1 hour. This last form of administration therefore represents a rescue treatment added to the usual therapy in a minority of patients severely disabled by off-motor symptoms. Apomorphine administration requires association with domperidone, 60 mg per day given at least 2 days before the first injection, continued for a few weeks and on demand thereafter in case of nausea. All dopamine agonist drugs should be titrated progressively over weeks to limit the occurrence of adverse effects. These are similar to those induced by levodopa but occur more frequently, especially nausea, orthostatic hypotension, and psychosis. The transient association with domperidone started 2 days before the dopaminergic agonist can prevent the possible orthostatic syncope induced by the first pill. Given as monotherapy, the dopaminergic agonists do not induce dyskinesia, but the antiparkinsonian effect is less powerful than that of levodopa and tends to decrease after a few years. Thus dopaminergic drugs are generally associated with levodopa and both are given at moderate dose, approximately 20 mg per day of bromocriptine or equivalent and 400 mg per day of levodopa. This allows a limitation of levodopa-induced motor complications and dopaminergic agonist–induced adverse effects.

Nondopaminergic Agents

Selegiline is a selective inhibitor of the monoamine oxidase type B. Selegiline mildly improves the response to levodopa by partly blocking the central metabolism of dopamine. Given as the sole drug, selegiline induces a slight symptomatic benefit with few adverse effects. Therefore, selegiline

delays for some months or longer the requirement of levodopa, as would other antiparkinsonian drugs. It has not been proved that selegiline slows down the evolution of PD, although the induced blocking of the dopamine oxidative metabolism would theoretically exert a neuroprotective effect. When associated with levodopa, selegiline increases all the dopaminergic adverse effects. The dyskinesias can be worsened. The use of selegiline in the long-term management of PD has not been clearly demonstrated. The usual dose of selegiline is 5 mg twice a day.

Amantadine was developed as an antiviral agent and has demonstrated some antiparkinsonian effect. Dopamine release is favored by amantadine, but its precise action is not well known. Amantadine has a weak antiglutamate property. Some but not all patients are sensitive to amantadine administration at a dose of 100–300 mg per day. Adverse effects include dopaminergic side effects, edema, and livedo reticularis of the lower limbs, which can require drug arrest in case of functional disability. Amantadine can decrease levodopa-induced dyskinesias in some patients.

Anticholinergics used as antiparkinsonian drugs are muscarinic receptor blockers that penetrate into the brain. They are effective for rest tremor, mildly effective for rigidity, but not for akinesia. The adverse effects are the result of the peripheral and central atropinic effects and include dry mouth, constipation, blurred vision, urine retention, confusion, memory loss, hallucinations, and psychosis. These latter relatively contraindicate the use of anticholinergics in patients older than 65 years of age, with few exceptions, and require a very low titration—for example, 2 mg per day of trihexyphenidyl the first week, increased by 1 mg per day every week up to a moderate dose of 4–10 mg per day. Some antihistaminergic drugs are used as antiparkinsonian drugs because of their central anticholinergic properties.

Catechol-*o*-methyl-transferase (COMT) inhibitors are now being marketed. Because COMT is the principal enzyme of levodopa and dopamine metabolism, COMT inhibitors potentiate all levodopa-induced effects. The peripheral metabolism of levodopa can explain the greatest part of their action. The elimination half-life and area under the curve of levodopa are increased, whereas its blood concentration at peak is unchanged. This pharmacologic class is rep-

Table 28-7. Management of Nonmotor Complications in Treated Patients with Parkinson's Disease

Complications	Management
Nausea, vomiting	Slower increase in dopaminergic drugs; drug intake at the end of meals; domperidone at least 30 minutes before each meal
Symptomatic orthostatic hypotension	Compressive stockings; increase salt in meals; sleep in semi-sitting position; high-dose domperidone (90 mg/day), ?indomethacin; alpha$_1$-agonist drug such as midodrine; mineralocorticoids (fludrocortisone, 50–100 µg/day)
Psychosis or mental confusion	Withdraw anticholinergics, amantadine, selegiline, dopaminergic agonists, psychotropic agents; minimum effective dose of levodopa; slow-release levodopa; atypical neuroleptics such as clozapine (if psychosis only)
Sedation	Minimum effective dose of levodopa or slow-release preparations; coffee no later than 4 PM

resented by tolcapone and entacapone, which are always combined with levodopa.

Treatment of Secondary Manifestations

Symptomatic treatments can be applied to the various secondary manifestations of PD (Table 28-7). Depression, if not improved by levodopa, can be treated by tricyclic antidepressants, which exert a more or less anticholinergic action—for example, beneficial for drooling or urinary emergency and deleterious for constipation. Specific serotonin reuptake blockers are also effective for depression and may occasionally aggravate parkinsonism or improve dyskinesias. Their combination with selegiline must be done cautiously because of the risk of a serotonergic crisis.

Sialorrhea can be decreased by peripheral anticholinergics. Constipation is usually improved by dietary means and cisapride (Propulsid), a prokinetic gastrointestinal drug. Urinary emergencies if related to detrusor hypertonia can be relieved by a peripheral anticholinergic drug such as oxybutynin.

Nonpharmacologic Treatments

Nonpharmacologic treatments of PD include motor and speech physiotherapy and surgery. Because PD and other causes of parkinsonism mainly disrupt motor function, any motor rehabilitation process, such as daily walking, keep-fit exercises, balneotherapy, speech therapy, balance training, and expert physical therapy, should be encouraged.

Neurosurgical treatment was common in the 1960's but is presently applied to selected patients. Up to 1992, surgical treatment of PD was aimed at lesioning or stimulating at high frequency the ventral intermediate nucleus of the thalamus involved in tremor. Stimulation induced the same effect as a lesion, with the advantage of being adjustable over time, reversible, and thus applicable bilaterally if necessary with low morbidity rates. Tremor that disappears during action, however, is rarely disabling. Only the tremor-dominant type of PD, characterized by severe disability and relative pharmacoresistance, has been subjected to thalamic surgery. The demonstration that akinesia was related to an overactivity of the subthalamopallidal pathway aroused interest in the surgical treatment of PD by lesioning the ventrolateral part of the GPi (pallidotomy) or stimulating the same target or stimulating the STN. Lesioning the STN is hazardous because of the risk of contralateral hemiballism, which is difficult to manage in PD. GPi and STN surgery improves all of the motor symptoms of parkinsonism in the same way as levodopa but without motor fluctuations or dyskinesias. Levodopa-induced dyskinesias are improved either directly in the surgical disruption of the GPi neuronal activity or indirectly owing to the improvement in parkinsonian symptoms responsible for a major decrease in levodopa dose. This is the case in particular after STN stimulation, which seems to decrease akinesia more markedly and constantly than GPi surgery. The latter induces a dramatic effect on levodopa-induced dyskinesias.

The criteria for the surgical treatment of parkinsonism are the following: levodopa-responsive parkinsonism with severe motor complications, either disabling off-motor periods, dyskinesia, or both; persistence of a good but transient levodopa response; good general health; no dementia or severe depression; and findings on brain imaging in the normal range.

Striatal transplantations of fetal tissue are aimed at ameliorating the dopamine deficiency. The grafts were shown to release dopamine in the long-term with some motor improvement. Given the lack of available fetuses, the moderate benefit, the complexity of the method, and ethical reasons, striatal transplantation remains experimental.

Practical Treatment Decisions

The management of PD is based on the principles shown in Table 28-8. The main principle is the individualization of treatment according to the degree of discomfort and disability (mainly for social and professional activities), the clinical type of PD, the age of onset of the disease, its rate of decline, and the personality of the patient, including his or her potential compliance to drugs. Treatment decisions can be simplified by studying two opposite clinical cases. The first case concerns a 47-year-old patient who develops over a few years a severe form of PD that hampers his professional life. Because the main risk factors for fluctuations appear to be the duration and dosage of levodopa treatment, the severity of the PD, and the young age of onset of the disease, the date of starting levodopa is delayed and the first treatment is selegiline, amantadine, or an anticholinergic drug in the case of tremor or a dopamine agonist drug for rigidity and akinesia. Because of a relative lack of efficacy, however, levodopa therapy is soon given at low dose three to five times a day or in a slow-release preparation. If this low dose is insufficiently effective, a dopamine agonist is used if not already done. Ten to 15 years later, the severity of off-motor periods necessitates multiple daily levodopa intakes, then subcutaneous multiple apomorphine injections or, exceptionally, continuous infusion. Surgical treatment is discussed.

The second case concerns a 73-year-old patient who is disabled by some imbalance and cognitive slowness from the onset of PD. It is common that this type of patient has already suffered from other medical or surgical disorders. Levodopa is recommend as the sole drug with physiotherapy from the start of the disease. Other treatments would have a negative benefit-to-risk ratio.

Table 28-8. Principles of Pharmacotherapy in Parkinson's Disease

- So far, only a symptomatic effect induced by drugs has been demonstrated.
- The aim of the treatment is not to make the parkinsonian symptoms disappear but to allow the patient to cope with the activities of daily living.
- Levodopa toxicity has never been proved in vivo.
- Levodopa is the most effective drug.
- Levodopa and other dopaminergic drugs are always titrated slowly and given at the lowest possible dose.
- The narrower the therapeutic window between the antiparkinsonian effect and the dyskinesias, the more difficult the use of slow-release levodopa preparations.
- Dopaminergic agonist drugs induce more adverse effects (nausea, orthostatic hypotension, psychosis) than levodopa but no motor complications when given as a monotherapy.

Atypical Parkinsonian Disorders

General Considerations

The clinical examination of a patient with parkinsonism during the first years of evolution of the disease should endeavor to search for nonparkinsonian signs, which are highly suggestive of degenerative diseases other than PD when they are present from the onset or during the first years of the disease. The difficulty arises from the fact that most of these signs may occur in PD with the difference that they are generally mild to moderate and appear late in the course of the disease and mainly in PD patients older than 70 years of age. These signs, called *red flags*, caused by lesions outside the dopaminergic pathways, include the following: severe frontal lobe syndrome or dementia or apraxia, hallucinations or delirium unrelated to dopamine agonist drugs or anticholinergics, postural imbalance and falls, cerebellar ataxia, inability to produce vertical saccades, pyramidal signs, severe speech or swallowing difficulties, urinary incontinence, and orthostatic hypotension unrelated to dopaminergic drugs. Although great progress has been made in suggesting correct diagnoses before death, definitive diagnosis remains neuropathologic.

Dementia associated early with parkinsonism suggests the various causes of frontal lobe dementia including Alzheimer's disease and dementia with Lewy bodies. The association of parkinsonism that is sometimes levodopa-responsive and dementia with fluctuating cognition and recurrent hallucinations is highly suggestive of the latter.

Currently, the only medications we have to treat the various parkinsonian syndromes are those specifically designed for PD. Therefore, making a precise diagnosis may not be critical from a therapeutic point of view, but is important when giving a clearer prognosis. The following three degenerative disorders have in common a rapidly evolving parkinsonian-type syndrome, other suggestive associated features, and a poor or transient response to levodopa. Their treatment is mainly symptomatic and their prognoses are poor.

Multiple System Atrophy

MSA is a sporadic entity that is a grouping together of three degenerative diseases. The variability of both the clinical symptoms and the neuropathologic findings is a result of a topographic predominance, but the nature of the disease seems to be unique. The neuropathologic lesions include oligodendroglial argyrophilic cytoplasmic inclusions; neuronal loss; gliosis and pigment deposition in the striatum, substantia nigra, and many other structures (e.g., the inferior olives, the pons, the cerebellum, and the intermediolateral cell columns and Onuf's nucleus of the spinal cord). The severity of these lesions is variable and underlies the three main clinical presentations, which can overlap between patients and in the same patient during the evolution of the disease. When parkinsonism predominates, the disease has been called *striatonigral degeneration* by Adams, Van Bogaert, and Van der Eecken. When cerebellar signs predominate, the condition has been called *olivopontocerebellar atrophy*, described originally by Dejerine and Thomas. *Shy-Drager syndrome,* described by these two authors, corresponds to the third condition when dysautonomic features predominate.

The onset of MSA is between the ages of 33 and 76 years (mean, 53 years). Almost all patients develop parkinsonism, which can be asymmetric but with an action tremor or a mixed resting-action tremor. Only one-third of patients may respond to levodopa, but usually only during the first years of the disease. These patients may exhibit dyskinesias that are atypical, mostly dystonic in the face and neck, and rarely accompanied by the functional motor improvement seen in PD. Cerebellar signs are dominated by postural instability with a wide base and the impossibility of tandem walking. Typical cerebellar gait ataxia, limb ataxia, and nystagmus occur more rarely. The most common dysautonomic feature is male impotence, which is often the earlier symptom. Urinary incontinence occurs more frequently than retention. It is frequent that patients have undergone ineffective prostatectomies. Orthostatic hypotension is symptomatic in approximately one-half of MSA patients, with recurrent syncopes in some that are not due to other causes, especially drugs. Pyramidal signs also develop in approximately one-half of patients. Other symptoms, less frequent but suggestive of MSA, are cold, red hands with poor circulatory return, inspiratory stridor, irregular myoclonic jerks of the fingers mimicking tremor, limb contracture, and severe speech and swallowing difficulties. Cognitive functioning is variable, ranging from almost normal to frontal lobe or cortical dementia, and cannot be used to differentiate MSA from PD. Death occurs after a mean duration of 6–9 years but with a wide range.

Cardiovascular dysautonomia can be documented by specific functional tests (cardiac beat-to-beat variability during breathing or during a Valsalva's maneuver) and bladder disturbance by external sphincter electromyography. Cerebellar and brain stem atrophy can be visualized by CT or MRI scanning (Figure 28-3), but rarely from the onset of MSA. High-field T2-weighted MRI scans may show putaminal hypointensity and slitlike hyperintensities in the lateral border of the putamen. Isotope scanning using dopamine receptor ligands may show decreased uptake, whereas it is normal in PD.

Progressive Supranuclear Palsy

Steele, Richardson, and Olzewski described PSP, which is characterized neuropathologically by neuronal loss, gliosis, and neurofibrillary tangles and neuropil threads. All of these abnormalities are located in some areas of the basal ganglia and

Figure 28-3. A T1-weighted magnetic resonance imaging scan of a sagittal view of the brain showing severe brain stem and cerebellar atrophy.

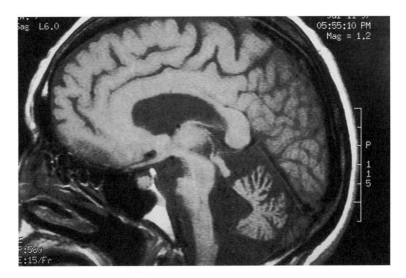

brain stem, mainly the pallidum, subthalamic nucleus, substantia nigra, pons, striatum, and oculomotor complex. PSP has a mean age of onset of 63 years and never starts before age 40. The typical patient with PSP presents with postural instability and falls, supranuclear vertical gaze palsy, parkinsonism, pseudobulbar palsy, and fronto-subcortical dementia. Marked slowing of vertical gaze commonly precedes the limitation of vertical gaze that enables the diagnosis to be made. A staring expression is characteristic. Blepharospasm and apraxia of eyelid opening can occur. Axial rigidity is severe with a tendency to retrocollis, a more erect posture than in PD, and backward falls. The frontal lobe symptomatology is severe and characteristic. MRI is of little help but may show atrophy of the midbrain, a large third ventricle, a thinning of the quadrigeminal plate, and abnormalities of signal in the periaqueductal region.

Corticobasal Degeneration

As its name tells us, CBD, or corticobasal ganglionic degeneration, neuropathologically shows frontoparietal or lobar atrophy of the cerebral cortex and basal ganglia. Neuronal loss and gliosis are severe in the cortex, and spongiosis, ballooned cells, and achromatic neurons can be found. Basophilic, argyrophilic, and tau-positive inclu-

sions are present in the basal ganglia, subthalamic nucleus, and sometimes along the dentatorubrothalamic tracts. Neuropathologically, Pick's disease is closely related, but the lesions are less extensive and characterized by neuronal inclusions called *Pick bodies*. The typical patient with CBD presents a parkinsonian syndrome associated with unilateral apraxia of an upper limb. Postural instability, difficulty walking, dystonia or contracture, reflex myoclonus, and cortical sensory deficits of the affected limb are frequent, as is dysarthria. The alien limb syndrome, aphasia, supranuclear oculomotor difficulties, and action tremor can occur. Although focused on one limb, the symptoms spread eventually to the other limbs, and the cognitive failure may be more global. CBD never starts before age 45 years and has a mean age at onset of 61 years. Death usually occurs 4–8 years after symptom onset. CT or MRI scans show asymmetric frontoparietal atrophy contralateral to the predominant symptoms and isotope scans also appear asymmetric.

Suggested Reading

Agid Y, Ruberg M, Raisman R, et al. The Biochemistry of Parkinson's Disease. In GM Stern (ed), Parkinson's Disease. London: Chapman and Hall, 1990;99.

Alexander GE, Crutcher MD. Functional architecture of basal ganglia circuits: neural substrates of parallel processing. Trends Neurosci 1990;13:266.

Ben Shlomo Y. How far are we in understanding the cause of Parkinson's disease? J Neurol Neurosurg Psychiatry 1996;61:4.

Brown RG, Marsden CD. Cognitive function in Parkinson's disease: from description to theory. Trends Neurosci 1990;13:21.

Hughes AJ, Daniel SE, Kilford L, Lees AJ. Accuracy of clinical diagnosis of idiopathic Parkinson's disease: a clinico-pathological study of 100 cases. J Neurol Neurosurg Psychiatry 1992;55:181.

Jenner P, Schapira AHV, Marsden CD. New insights into the cause of Parkinson's disease. Neurology 1992;42:2241.

Limousin P, Pollak P, Benazzouz A, et al. Effect on parkinsonian signs and symptoms of bilateral subthalamic nucleus stimulation. Lancet 1995; 345:91.

Litvan I, Agid Y, Calne D, et al. Clinical research criteria for the diagnosis of progressive supranuclear palsy (Steele-Richardson-Olszewski syndrome): report of the NINDS-SPSP international workshop. Neurology 1996;47:1.

Lozano A, Lang A, Galvez-Jimenez N, et al. Effect of GPi pallidotomy on motor function in Parkinson's disease. Lancet 1995;346:1383.

Marsden CD. Parkinson's disease. J Neurol Neurosurg Psychiatry 1994;57:672.

Marsden CD. Neurophysiology. In GM Stern (ed), Parkinson's Disease. London: Chapman and Hall, 1990;57.

Montastruc JL, Rascol O, Senard JM. Current status of dopamine agonists in Parkinson's disease management. Drugs 1993;46:384.

Mouradian MM, Chase TN. Improved Dopaminergic Therapy of Parkinson's Disease. In CD Marsden, S Fahn (eds), Movement Disorders 3. Oxford, UK: Butterworth–Heinemann, 1994;181.

Nutt JG, Holford NHG. The response to levodopa in Parkinson's disease: imposing pharmacological law and order. Ann Neurol 1996;39:561.

Quinn N. Multiple System Atrophy. In CD Marsden, S Fahn (eds), Movement Disorders 3. Oxford: Butterworth–Heinemann, 1994;262.

Chapter 29
Cerebellar and Spinocerebellar Disorders

Alessandro Filla and Giuseppe De Michele

Chapter Plan

Congenital cerebellar ataxias
Metabolic ataxias
    Intermittent metabolic ataxias
    Progressive metabolic ataxias
    Ataxias associated with defective DNA repair
Degenerative ataxias
    Early-onset inherited ataxias
    Late-onset inherited ataxias
    Idiopathic late-onset cerebellar ataxias

Congenital Cerebellar Ataxias

Maturation of the cerebellum and its pathways may not be complete until the third year of life. This makes it difficult to assess cerebellar function in a young child. Delayed motor milestones are usually the earliest signs of developmental disorders of the cerebellum. Ataxia is usually not progressive, and improvement has been observed in some cases during the course of the disease. Mental retardation is frequent. Congenital ataxic syndromes are rare. Inheritance is autosomal recessive in most cases, but dominant and X-linked inheritance has also been reported. Sporadic patients are misdiagnosed as having cerebral palsy in most instances.

Cerebellar hemisphere hypoplasia, granule cell layer hypoplasia, pontocerebellar hypoplasia, granular cell hypertrophy, and dysequilibrium syndrome have rather nonspecific clinical presentations with motor and mental retardation sometimes associated with spasticity and microcephaly. Nystagmus and intention tremor can be observed before ataxia becomes evident. Inheritance is autosomal recessive in some cases.

Peculiar clinical and pathologic features are present in Joubert's syndrome (episodes of hyperpnea and apnea, abnormal eye movements, and agenesis of the vermis) and Gillespie's syndrome (partial aniridia). These syndromes have an autosomal recessive inheritance. The inheritance is X-linked in Paine's syndrome, which is characterized by microcephaly, myoclonic jerks, generalized seizures, optic atrophy, and spasticity. Necropsy shows hypoplasia of the cerebellum, pons, and olives.

Metabolic Ataxias

Cerebellar ataxias with specific biochemical abnormalities may be divided into intermittent and progressive forms according to Harding. They are rare and usually have an autosomal recessive inheritance and early onset. The main causes of intermittent ataxia are hereditary urea cycle disorders and disorders of amino acid or pyruvate metabolism. The main causes of progressive ataxia are disorders associated with vitamin E deficiency, mitochondrial encephalomyopathies, and storage diseases. Ataxia may be also present in other metabolic and storage disorders, such as metachromatic and globoid-cell leukodystrophy, adrenoleukomyeloneuropathy, sphingomyelin lipidoses, ceroid lipofuscinosis, sialidosis, and Wilson's disease, which are not treated in this chapter. Details on metabolic ataxias can be found in Scriver, et al.

Intermittent Metabolic Ataxias

Deficiency of Urea Cycle Enzymes and Hyperornithinemia

The most frequent metabolic abnormality associated with intermittent ataxia is hyperammonemia. It is usually caused by a deficiency of urea cycle enzymes and hyperornithinemia. The most common urea cycle enzyme defect is a deficiency of ornithine transcarbamylase, which is a mitochondrial enzyme that catalyzes the synthesis of citrulline from carbamyl phosphate and ornithine. A deficiency of this enzyme leads to hyperammonemia and hyperglutaminemia. The disease is X-linked and presents in males as a dramatic hyperammonemic encephalopathy that is often fatal in the neonatal period. The clinical picture in females is highly variable and ranges from apparent normality to profound neurologic impairment. Symptoms include irritability, episodic vomiting, ataxia, lethargy, coma, developmental delay and delayed physical growth, mental retardation, and seizures. Variable expression may be explained either by the proportion of hepatocytes in which the active X chromosome bears the mutant allele or by different mutations. The episodes are precipitated by high-protein meals or intercurrent infections. Treatment consists of low-protein diet, citrulline, and fluid administration during attacks. Drugs that increase waste-nitrogen excretion (sodium benzoate, sodium phenylbutyrate) decrease the occurrence of hyperammonemic episodes and reduce the risk of further cognitive decline. Enzyme activity can be measured in the liver, jejunal mucosa, and leukocytes. It is usually absent in affected males and varies from very low to normal in carrier females. Missense and nonsense mutations and exon deletions have been associated with different levels of disease severity.

The other urea cycle enzyme deficiencies have a similar clinical picture and are transmitted as autosomal recessive traits. Point mutations and exon deletions have been described in citrullinemia (argininosuccinate synthetase deficiency, chromosome 9); in argininosuccinicaciduria (argininosuccinase deficiency, chromosome 7); and in argininemia (arginase deficiency, chromosome 6). They are rare and clinically heterogeneous diseases. Hyperammonemia in hyperornithinemia-hyperammonemia-homocitrullinuria syndrome is not caused by a urea cycle enzyme deficiency, but by a defective transport of ornithine into mitochondria.

Disorders of Amino Acid Metabolism

Intermittent branched-chain ketoaciduria is a variant of maple syrup urine disease. It is caused by branched-chain alpha-ketoacid dehydrogenase deficiency, a multienzyme complex associated with the inner mitochondrial membrane. The disease presents in children as attacks of ataxia, vomiting, lethargy, metabolic acidosis, coma, and large urinary excretion of ketoacids, which are responsible for the characteristic odor.

In Hartnup disease, the defect involves the intestinal and renal transport of monoamino-monocarboxylic acids. Approximately one-third of patients with the amino acid abnormality are asymptomatic. The main features are a pellagra-like light-sensitive rash, cerebellar ataxia, psychiatric disturbances, and aminoaciduria. Skin lesions usually precede ataxia. Episodes of ataxia are precipitated by infections, stress, poor diet, and drugs. Some patients also show mental retardation. Therapy is oral nicotinamide and a high-protein diet. Both intermittent branched-chain ketoaciduria and Hartnup disease have autosomal recessive inheritance.

Disorders of Pyruvate and Lactate Metabolism

For energy production, the brain depends on glucose metabolism through oxidative decarboxylation of pyruvate via the pyruvate dehydrogenase enzyme complex (PDH). This is a complex of three enzymes: pyruvate decarboxylase, dihydrolipoyl transacetylase, and dihydrolipoyl dehydrogenase. This enzyme complex has a critical level in the anterior vermis in animals, which possibly explains the cerebellar features in partial deficiency of the enzyme. PDH deficiency is a rare disorder that is transmitted as an X-linked dominant or autosomal recessive trait. When the deficiency is below 15% of normal, infantile lactic acidosis, severe mental retardation, seizures, and early death occur. Patients with higher enzyme activity present with intermittent ataxia and choreoathetosis, and increased levels of blood pyruvate, lactate, and alanine. A ketogenic diet may be useful.

Progressive Metabolic Ataxias

Disorders Associated with Vitamin E Deficiency

Bassen and Kornzweig reported abetalipoproteinemia in 1950. The disorder is recessively inherited and more prevalent in Ashkenazi Jews. The initial symptoms are those of malabsorption with steatorrhea and failure to thrive. Celiac disease may be suspected. A progressive ataxia begins in the first or second decade and is associated with areflexia and proprioceptive loss resembling Friedreich's ataxia. Other features include extensor plantar response; ptosis; external ophthalmoplegia; loss of touch, pain, temperature sensation; scoliosis; pes cavus; and cardiomyopathy. Night blindness and poor vision resulting from pigmentary retinal degeneration may develop before ataxia. Heart failure is a frequent cause of death. Laboratory findings show thorny red blood cells (acanthocytosis); a marked reduction in levels of plasma cholesterol, other circulating lipids, and vitamins A, D, E, and K; and absent apoprotein B. The disease is caused by mutations in the gene coding for one subunit of the microsomal triglyceride transfer protein. Defects in this subunit result in impaired formation and secretion of very low–density lipoproteins (VLDLs) by the liver. VLDLs are the transport molecules for vitamin E. Therefore, vitamin E delivery to peripheral tissue is impaired. Large oral doses of vitamin E may improve the neurologic symptoms. Additional vitamin A and K are required.

Hypobetalipoproteinemia is an autosomal dominant disorder that is characterized by decreased levels of low-density lipoproteins, cholesterol, and triglycerides. The association between this biochemical entity and neurologic disease is uncertain in heterozygotes. Homozygotes have lipid profiles identical to those found in abetalipoproteinemia and a similar clinical picture. Heterozygotes have hypocholesterolemia in hypobetalipoproteinemia and are normal in abetalipoproteinemia.

Ataxia with isolated vitamin E deficiency (AVED) is a rare autosomal recessive disorder that is more frequent in north Africa. Serum vitamin E levels are very low or undetectable, whereas those of the other fat-soluble vitamins are normal. Patients have a normal gastrointestinal absorption of dietary α-tocopherol, the most biologically active form of vitamin E, and normal incorporation in chylomicrons, but they have an impaired ability to incorporate α-tocopherol into VLDLs secreted by the liver. Incorporation of vitamin E in VLDLs is thought to be mediated by the α-tocopherol transfer protein (α-TTP). Frame-shift mutations in the α-TTP gene on chromosome 8 with truncation of the protein are the most frequent mutations. Point mutations are usually rarer and less severe. The onset is in the first or second decade with progressive ataxia, absence of tendon reflexes, decreased vibration sense and proprioception, weakness, and Babinski's sign. Scoliosis, pes cavus, head titubation, fasciculations of the tongue, and cardiomyopathy may also be present. The patients eventually become wheelchair bound in the third or fourth decade. Pathologic studies have shown that vitamin E deficiency causes a dying-back neuropathy in sensory neurons that is more severe in the centrally directed fibers than in peripheral axons. Neurophysiologic studies show decreased amplitude of the sensory response with normal velocity in the peripheral nerve and delayed central conduction of somatosensory evoked responses. Supplementation with vitamin E (600 IU twice daily) raises plasma concentrations to normal. Treatment may stop disease progression or even improve the neurologic syndrome. Serum vitamin E and molecular tests can be used to differentiate AVED from Friedreich's ataxia.

Mitochondrial Encephalomyopathies

Mitochondrial diseases are genetically heterogeneous and are caused by defective nuclear or mitochondrial genes. Manifestations are highly variable because mitochondrial dysfunction can affect virtually all organ systems. Ataxia is a common feature. Kearns-Sayre syndrome is a form of sporadic chronic progressive external ophthalmoplegia that begins before the age of 20 years and is characterized by pigmentary retinopathy, elevated levels of cerebrospinal fluid protein, ataxia, and heart block. Most of the patients die in the third or fourth decade. Almost all patients have large, single deletions in mitochondrial DNA.

Myoclonic epilepsy with ragged-red fibers (MERRF) is characterized by action myoclonus, myoclonic epilepsy, cerebellar ataxia, weakness, and short stature. Dementia and hearing loss may be present. Age at onset varies from the first to the fifth decade. Maternal inheritance may be evident and maternal relatives may have partial clinical syndromes. Plasma pyruvate, lactate, alanine, and creatine phosphokinase levels are increased and muscle biopsy shows accumulation of abnormal subsarcolemmal and intermyofibrillar mitochondria (ragged-red fibers). Pathogenetic point mutations have been shown in the lysine transfer RNA of the mitochondrial DNA. Neuropathy, ataxia, and retinitis pigmentosa is a maternally inherited multisystem disorder characterized by developmental delay, retinitis pigmentosa, dementia, seizures, ataxia, and sensory neuropathy. It is associated with a point mutation in the ATPase 6 gene of mitochondrial DNA. The same mutation when abundant may cause maternally inherited Leigh syndrome (LS), also called *subacute necrotizing encephalomyelopathy*. LS is clinically and genetically heterogeneous. Cytochrome *c* oxidase deficiency is the most commonly reported biochemical abnormality, followed by deficiencies of NADH dehydrogenase, pyruvate dehydrogenase, or pyruvate carboxylase. They have mendelian inheritance. Symptoms usually begin in early infancy, but juvenile and adult-onset cases have been described. Pathologic findings are distinctive and consist of focal, symmetric necrotic lesions extending from the thalamus to the pons, the inferior olives, and the posterior columns in the spinal cord. Microscopically there is vascular proliferation, astrocytosis, and neuronal changes. The clinical features vary according to age at onset and include developmental delay, vomiting, respiratory abnormalities, psychomotor regression, ataxia, seizures, optic atrophy, ophthalmoplegia, peripheral neuropathy, weakness, dystonia, choreoathetosis, and dementia.

Storage Diseases

Hexosaminidase deficiency causes GM_2 gangliosidosis. There are three hexosaminidase enzymes: A, B, and S. Hexosaminidase A is a multimer composed of alpha and beta subunits. The gene encoding for the alpha chain is located on chromosome 15 and the beta encoding gene is on chromosome 5. Hexosaminidase A deficiency causes classic infantile Tay-Sachs disease. Later-onset forms with prominent

cerebellar ataxia have been reported in Jewish patients. Onset usually is in the first or second decade and may be as late as age 30 years. Features include early cerebellar signs, followed by development of upper and lower motor neuron signs. Dementia, psychosis, and ophthalmoplegia are also present. There is considerable variability between and within families. Neuroradiologic investigations show cerebellar and brain stem atrophy. Lamellar cytoplasmic inclusions are found in rectal biopsy specimens.

Niemann-Pick type C is an autosomal recessive lysosomal storage disease distinct from the primary sphingomyelinase disorders. Impaired esterification of exogenous cholesterol is present in cultured fibroblasts. Neurologic dysfunction may appear from 6 months to 18 years and comprises constant ataxia, mental impairment, supranuclear vertical gaze paralysis, dystonia, seizures, pyramidal signs, severe late dysphagia, organomegaly, and pulmonary involvement. Lipid-laden macrophages (foam cells) are present in the bone marrow aspiration and liver biopsy specimens. It is genetically heterogeneous, and one form has been mapped to chromosome 18.

Cerebrotendinous xanthomatosis (cholestanolosis) is a rare lipid-storage disease transmitted in an autosomal recessive fashion. Onset is in childhood. Xanthomata, especially of the Achilles tendon, and cataracts appear early, and neurologic impairment develops later. The most prominent neurologic feature is spastic ataxia associated with pseudobulbar palsy, dementia, palatal myoclonus, and peripheral neuropathy. Deposits of cholesterol and cholestanol are found particularly in tendons, brain, and lungs. Serum cholesterol levels are normal, but cholestanol (a metabolite of cholesterol) is increased. The defect resides in sterol 27-hydroxylase, an enzyme involved in the bile acid synthesis pathway. Mutations resulting in single amino acid substitution have been found in the gene, which maps to chromosome 2. Treatment with chenodeoxycholic acid decreases cholestanol levels and improves the neurologic features.

Ataxias Associated with Defective DNA Repair

Ataxia Telangiectasia

The autosomal recessive disorder ataxia telangiectasia bears the eponym of Louis Bar, who described it in 1941. However, the association between the neurologic disease and the ocular dilated blood vessels (telangiectases) had been reported previously. The disease is probably underdiagnosed. The estimated prevalence is 0.5–1.0 per 100,000.

Ataxia telangiectasia is characterized by a triad of clinical manifestations: a complex, progressive neurologic syndrome, telangiectases, and immunologic deficiency. Cerebellar ataxia begins when the child starts walking. Dysarthria, intention tremor, head titubation, choreoathetosis, impassive facies, and drooling are present. On attempting to look at objects, the patient turns his or her head excessively and the eyes follow slowly (oculomotor apraxia). Rotatory nystagmus in primary position may be present in older patients. In the course of the disease, weakness and sensory loss develop, whereas tendon reflexes disappear. Most patients are unable to walk independently at puberty, and death occurs during the second or third decades from intercurrent bronchopulmonary infections or neoplasms.

Telangiectases usually develop by the age of 3–6 years and are most evident in the conjunctivae, the "butterfly area" of the face, the pinnae, and the ears and they are also evident on the neck, arms, and legs. Progeria and endocrine disturbances (hypogonadism and abnormal glucose test) are present. Height and mental performances are usually below average.

Patients have deficiencies in both humoral and cellular immunity. Immunoglobulin levels (particularly IgA) are decreased; the thymus, lymph nodes, and tonsils are atrophic. Respiratory infections are recurrent, leading to bronchiectasis. Patients have an increased occurrence of lymphoreticular malignancies, carcinoma, and glioma. Heterozygous carriers of the gene may have an increased risk for cancer, particularly of the breast. Lymphocytes and fibroblasts show hypersensitivity to ionizing radiation and radiomimetic drugs and increased chromosome breaks.

High levels of α-fetoprotein are a useful laboratory test. Neuroradiologic investigations show cerebellar atrophy in the early stages of the disease and cerebrocerebellar atrophy in the advanced cases. Nerve conduction studies reveal a mainly sensory axonal neuropathy. Necropsy studies show loss of cells in the cerebellar cortex and nuclei and loss of myelinated fibers in the spinocerebellar tracts, posterior columns, and peripheral nerves.

Mutations causing truncation or deletion of amino acids of the protein product have been found in the ATM gene, which maps to chromosome 11. The protein has one domain resembling phosphoinositol-3 kinase, a signal transduction mediator, and another similar to yeast proteins involved in DNA repair. Radiotherapy seems to be contraindicated in malignancies because of the risk of radiodermatitis and ulcerative lesions.

Xeroderma Pigmentosum

Xeroderma pigmentosum is transmitted in an autosomal recessive fashion and it is genetically heterogeneous. It primarily presents as a skin disorder. Patients show abnormal sensitivity to sunlight, freckles, keratoses, telangiectases, and skin cancer (melanomas, squamous and basal cell carcinomas). The association with severe neurologic signs defines the De Sanctis-Cacchione syndrome. The features of this syndrome are variable and include mental retardation and dementia, peripheral neuropathy, ataxia, choreoathetosis, seizures, spastic tetraplegia, deafness, microcephaly, short stature, and hypogonadism. Skin lesions appear in infancy and neurologic symptoms usually develop before the age of 30 years. Death may occur because of metastatic cancer in the second decade. Survival is normal in milder cases. Necropsy shows cell loss in the cerebrum, cerebellum, and brain stem. Repair of DNA damaged by ultraviolet light is deficient.

Cockayne's Syndrome

The autosomal recessive disorder known as Cockayne's syndrome is characterized by growth retardation and mental retardation, microcephaly, ataxia, extrapyramidal features, deafness, pigmentary retinopathy, photosensitive dermatitis, and peripheral neuropathy. Onset is in late infancy. Patients have characteristic facies with sunken eyes, a prominent nose, large ears, and prognathism. Death usually occurs before the age of 20 years. Neuroradiologic investigations show basal ganglia calcification. A small brain and leukodystrophy are reported at necropsy.

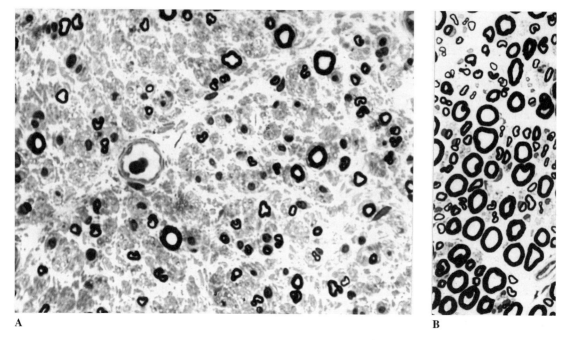

A   B

Figure 29-1. (A) Semithin transverse section of the sural nerve of a 24-year-old patient with Friedreich's ataxia showing marked loss of large myelinated fibers. (B) Control. (Toluidine blue stain; × 680.) (Courtesy of Professor F. Barbieri and the Department of Neurological Sciences, Federico II University, Naples, Italy.)

Degenerative Ataxias

Most degenerative ataxias are hereditary. Harding distinguished two main groups according to onset before or after 20 years. Early-onset disorders are transmitted mainly in an autosomal recessive fashion and late-onset disorders mainly in an autosomal dominant fashion. The nonhereditary degenerative ataxias usually have a late onset.

Early-Onset Inherited Ataxias

Friedreich's Ataxia

Friedreich's ataxia (FA) is an autosomal recessive, spinocerebellar degeneration. Friedreich described the disease in 1863, differentiating it from tabes dorsalis. This entity was not immediately accepted. Charcot considered the patients described by Friedreich as affected by multiple sclerosis. FA is the most common form of hereditary ataxia, comprising approximately 50% of cases in the largest series. The prevalence ratio ranges from 1.0 to 2.1

per 100,000 in Europe and carrier frequency from 1/110 to 1/70.

Spinal involvement is more marked than that of the brain stem and cerebellum. The most relevant pathologic finding is atrophy of the long ascending and descending spinal tracts (dorsal columns, spinocerebellar and pyramidal tracts), with shrinkage in the cross-section of the cord. Atrophy of the gracile and cuneate nuclei as well as of other lower brain stem nuclei has been frequently reported. Loss of Purkinje cells and atrophy of the nucleus dentatus and of the superior and middle cerebellar peduncles are present. Loss of Betz cells and degenerative changes in the optic nerves have been reported. Neurons are reduced in number in the dorsal root ganglia and Clarke columns. The peripheral nerve shows a marked loss of the large myelinated fibers (Figure 29-1). Cardiomegaly with ventricular hypertrophy is found. The histologic changes are interstitial fibrosis and degeneration of the cardiac muscle cells.

Several biochemical abnormalities of mitochondrial enzymes, fatty acid metabolism, and taurine urinary excretion have been reported in FA. None is constant, specific, and of sufficient amplitude to be considered the primary defect of the disease.

The FA locus (*FRDA*) maps to chromosome 9. The defective gene (*X25*) encodes a 210-amino acid protein of unknown function called *frataxin*. Frataxin is located in mitochondrial membranes and is involved in homeostasis and respiratory funcion. Frataxin m-RNA levels are decreased in FA patients. An expanded unstable trinucleotide guanine-adenine-adenine (GAA) repeat is present in the X25 first intron on 95% of FA chromosomes. Normal chromosomes contain 6–36 units, whereas FA chromosomes carry 120–1,400 repeats. The length of the GAA expansion correlates with the age of onset and disease severity and determines the presence of cardiomyopathy and diabetes. Rare point mutations have been found in the remaining affected alleles.

Mean age of onset is 14 years (range, 2–36) in a personal series. Eighty percent of patients develop the disease within the age of 20 years and 95% within the age of 30 years. The most frequent presenting symptom is gait ataxia, followed by lower limb weakness and clumsiness. Occasionally, the disease becomes evident after a febrile illness. Gait and stance ataxia is a constant finding. Ataxia has both a cerebellar and a spinal component. Closure of the eyes may cause the patient to fall (Romberg's sign). Ataxia also affects the trunk and the limbs. Dysarthria may be absent at the beginning, but it always appears in the course of the disease. Speech becomes slow, slurred, explosive, and finally difficult to understand. Eye movement abnormalities, consisting of fixation instability, flutter, jerky smooth pursuit, and saccade dysmetria, are almost always present. Nystagmus on lateral gaze occurs in about one-third of patients. Lower limb reflexes are usually absent but may be retained or even exaggerated in 4% of cases. Corticospinal involvement, demonstrated by proximal weakness more marked in the lower limbs and extensor plantar response, is evident in 50% of patients at the beginning and eventually in all. Coexistence of lower limb areflexia and Babinski's sign strongly suggests the diagnosis of FA. Muscle tone is usually reduced, but spasticity may be found rarely. Decreased joint position and vibration sense, more evident in the lower limbs, are present in most patients at the onset and eventually become constant. Distal wasting is a late feature. Skeletal deformities are present in 90% of patients and may precede the onset of ataxia. Scoliosis may

be severe, impairing cardiopulmonary function (Figure 29-2). The most frequent foot deformities are pes cavus and equinovarus deformity (Figure 29-3). Dysphagia, usually for liquids, and cold extremities with peripheral cyanosis are common. Urinary urgency occurs in 20%. Deafness and visual loss are rarely reported features. Cognitive function is normal, even in advanced disease.

Progressive impairment of cerebellar function and the corticospinal pathways mainly account for the worsening of the disease, whereas the sensory neuropathy is severe at an early stage and shows only slight further progression. Weakness, which is initially mild, eventually leads to virtual total paralysis. The mean age of becoming wheelchair bound is 26 years (range, 12–49 years). Median survival is 36 years from onset. Prognosis has probably improved over the years because of better therapy of disease complications. The presence of diabetes increases the risk of death by approximately threefold and that of hypertrophic cardiomyopathy by twofold. On the other hand, patients with onset after 20 years of age keep independent walking for a longer time, are usually employed, and are married with children.

Electrocardiographic changes are present in 80% of patients. They are not specific and vary in the course of the disease. Repolarization abnormalities, consisting of nonspecific ST segment changes and T-wave inversion, are the most common findings (Figure 29-4). Left or right ventricular hypertrophy, supraventricular arrhythmias, and conduction abnormalities are also found. Echocardiographic abnormalities are less frequent (40%) and more specific. The most frequent finding is concentric left ventricular hypertrophy (Figure 29-5).

Diabetes mellitus, which is present in 17% of patients, is caused by both decreased insulin secretion and increased insulin resistance. The mean age of appearance of diabetes is 29 years (range, 9–42 years) in patients who are usually wheelchair bound.

Magnetic resonance imaging (MRI) demonstrates cervical cord atrophy, frequent and slight involvement of the brain stem and cerebellum, and rare cortical atrophy. A marked pontocerebellar atrophy argues against the diagnosis of FA. Peripheral nerve conduction studies show a mainly sensory axonal neuropathy. Conduction velocities are normal or slightly reduced and sensory evoked responses are absent or markedly reduced in ampli-

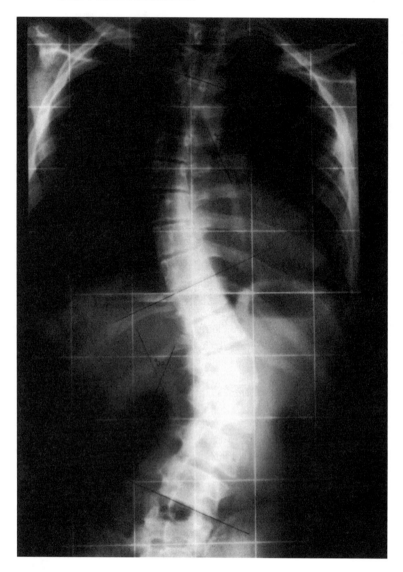

Figure 29-2. Scoliosis in a 28-year-old patient with Friedreich's ataxia.

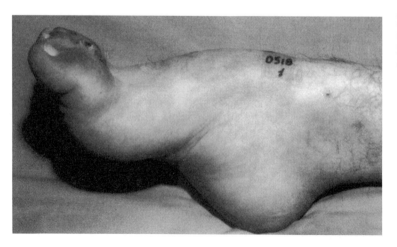

Figure 29-3. Pes cavus and equinovarus deformity in a 28-year-old patient with Friedreich's ataxia.

Figure 29-4. Electrocardiographic recordings of an 18-year-old patient with Friedreich's ataxia showing T-wave inversion in the inferior (II, III, aVF) and precordial leads (V3–6).

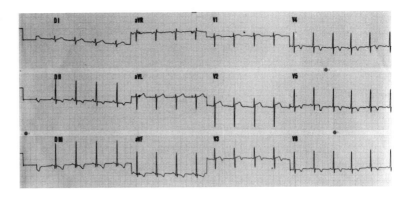

Figure 29-5. Two-dimensional echocardiographic frame of an 18-year-old patient with Friedreich's ataxia showing a marked increase of diastolic thickness of both the interventricular septum (IVS) and left posterior wall (PW) (concentric left ventricular hypertrophy). (AO = aorta; LA = left atrium; LV = left ventricle.)

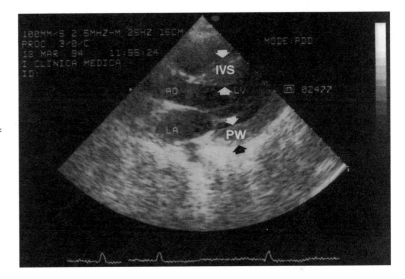

tude. Somatosensory evoked potentials show a constant impairment of central conduction. Brain stem and central motor evoked potentials may be normal in early stages of the disease and become eventually abnormal in all patients. Abnormal visual evoked potentials are found in 60% of patients.

A possible differential diagnosis is with hereditary motor and sensory neuropathy (HMSN) type I, which sometimes may be sporadic or recessive. Ataxia may occur in HMSN type I, but dysarthria and Babinski's sign are extremely rare, and hypertrophic cardiomyopathy has not been reported. Conduction velocities are severely reduced in HMSN type I. Normal serum vitamin E and α-fetoprotein exclude ataxia with isolated vitamin E deficiency or ataxia-telangiectasia. Molecular tests confirm the clinical diagnosis in typical cases and settle it in atypical ones. Prenatal diagnosis is possible, and a carrier test may be performed on relatives of patients.

As in other degenerative ataxias, no satisfactory treatment is available. Trials of choline chloride, lecithin, physostigmine, gamma-vinyl GABA, 5-hydroxytryptophan alone or associated with benserazide, thyrotropin-releasing hormone, and amantadine hydrochloride have been reported with conflicting results. Diabetes may be treated initially with oral hypoglycemic drugs, but all patients eventually require insulin. Heart failure and arrhythmia require specific treatment. Surgery for foot deformity and scoliosis may benefit selected patients provided that bed rest is restricted to a minimum.

Early-Onset Cerebellar Ataxia with Retained Tendon Reflexes

Harding in 1981 described early-onset cerebellar ataxia with retained tendon reflexes (EOCA) as the second most common form, after Friedreich's ataxia, among the early-onset inherited ataxias. EOCA differs from Friedreich's ataxia mainly in preservation of knee jerks. Other distinguishing features are a better prognosis and absence of severe skeletal deformities, cardiomyopathy, and diabetes mellitus. Onset is with progressive ataxia starting in the first two decades. Gait ataxia is constant. Dysarthria, dysmetria, and nystagmus are present in most patients. Increased knee jerks, spasticity, and Babinski's sign are frequent. Vibration sense is decreased in most patients. Progression of the disease is slow and patients may remain ambulant until their 40s or longer.

MRI shows cerebellar atrophy in almost all cases, associated with brain stem or spinal cord atrophy in some. An axonal sensory neuropathy is present in 40% of patients. Brain stem evoked potentials are impaired in most patients, whereas somatosensory and central motor evoked potentials are abnormal in 50%.

EOCA is genetically and clinically heterogeneous. Inheritance is autosomal recessive in most cases. One form with infantile onset, described in Finland, maps to chromosome 10. Some EOCA patients may have atypical Friedreich's ataxia and carry frataxin mutation.

Cerebellar Ataxia with Hypogonadism

In 1907, Gordon Holmes described a family in which three brothers and one sister developed progressive ataxia in the fourth decade. The three brothers also had hypogonadism. The postmortem examination of a patient showed a very small cerebellum with atrophy greatest in the superior part of the vermis and hemispheres. Atrophy of the inferior olives was also present. Inheritance appeared to be autosomal recessive. Despite this, there has been a tendency to apply the label of "Holmes type" of cerebello-olivary degeneration to dominantly inherited ataxias in absence of genital abnormalities purely on the basis of similar pathologic findings.

The age at onset and the clinical picture are extremely variable. Onset may occur until the fourth decade. Corticospinal signs, dementia, peripheral axonal neuropathy, and deafness are variably associated with the cerebellar features. Hypogonadism is of hypogonadotrophic origin in most

patients, and a hypothalamic defect has been suggested. In a few cases a deficiency of cytochrome *c* oxidase has been shown.

Progressive Myoclonic Ataxia

In 1921, Ramsay Hunt described a heterogeneous group of six patients under the title "dyssynergia cerebellaris myoclonica—primary atrophy of dentate system." Four cases were not familial, had myoclonus and epilepsy before the age of 20 years, and later developed progressive cerebellar ataxia. The other two were twins with a neurologic syndrome resembling Friedreich's ataxia, with onset in early childhood followed by myoclonus and epilepsy in the third decade of life. The term *Ramsay Hunt syndrome* has caused confusion in literature, largely because of the inappropriate use. Patients may be divided into two broad categories: progressive myoclonic epilepsy (PME) and progressive myoclonic ataxias (PMA), depending on the prevalence of epileptic seizures or ataxia. However, the limits between the categories are ill defined. Members of the same family may present with PME or PMA, and PMA may evolve into a typical PME syndrome.

The syndrome of PMA comprises myoclonus, progressive cerebellar ataxia with infrequent or absent epileptic seizures, and little or no cognitive dysfunction. Possible causes are spinocerebellar degeneration, Unverricht-Lundborg disease, MERRF, Lafora's disease, celiac disease, neuronal ceroid lipofuscinosis, and sialidoses. However, a specific diagnosis often cannot be reached.

Unverricht-Lundborg disease is an autosomal recessive disorder with myoclonus, tonic-clonic seizures, cerebellar signs, and mild dementia. The onset is at the ages of 6–15 years and course is progressive. Mutations in the gene encoding cystatin B on chromosome 21 are responsible for the disease.

Other Early-Onset Ataxias

Behr's syndrome is characterized by optic atrophy, spasticity, ataxia, and mental retardation. It is probably a heterogeneous entity. Marinesco-Sjögren syndrome comprises mental retardation, cerebellar ataxia, cataracts, short stature, and delayed sexual development. Other rare early-onset ataxias include those associated with pigmentary retinal degeneration, optic

Table 29-1. Classification of the Autosomal Dominant Cerebellar Ataxias

				Number of Repeats	
Ataxia	Gene	Chromosome	Gene Defect	Normal Alleles	Expanded Alleles
ADCA type I (with ophthalmoplegia,	SCA1	6p	(CAG)n	6–39	41–81
dementia, pyramidal or extrapyramidal	SCA2	12q	(CAG)n	17–29	37–50
features, optic atrophy, amyotrophy)	SCA3/MJD	14q	(CAG)n	12–37	62–84
	SCA4	16q	Unknown		
ADCA type II (with pigmentary retinal dystrophy)	SCA7	3p	(CAG)n	7–17	38–130
ADCA type III (pure cerebellar of	SCA5	11cen	Unknown		
later onset)	SCA6	19p	(CAG)n	4–18	21–30
Dentatorubropallidoluysian atrophy	DPRLA	12p	(CAG)n	8–35	54–79
Periodic ataxias: EA-1	KCNA1	12p	Missense mutations		
EA-2	CACNL1A4	19p	Truncating mutations		

ADCA = autosomal dominant cerebellar ataxia; EA = episodic ataxia; p = short arm of the chromosome; q = long arm; cen = centromere.

atrophy, deafness, and extrapyramidal features. All the above syndromes are autosomal recessive.

A few families have X-linked inheritance. They have a consistent phenotype with onset in childhood or adolescence and with spastic paraparesis preceding ataxia and dysarthria. A differential diagnosis has to be considered with adrenoleukomyeloneuropathy.

Late-Onset Inherited Ataxias

Adult-onset cerebellar ataxias are transmitted in autosomal dominant fashion or have a sporadic occurrence. Autosomal recessive inheritance is extremely rare.

The first observation of an autosomal dominant cerebellar ataxia (ADCA) was made by Menzel in 1891. The patient had progressive ataxia with onset at 28 years, increased tendon jerks in the legs, and choreiform movements. Postmortem study showed olivopontocerebellar atrophy and marked degeneration of the long tracts of the spinal cord.

Several classifications have been proposed for ADCA mainly on pathologic grounds. Harding's classification based on clinical criteria is now widely accepted (Table 29-1). ADCA type I is by far the most frequent and is characterized by progressive cerebellar ataxia, variably associated with ophthalmoplegia, dementia, optic atrophy, amyotrophy, and pyramidal or extrapyramidal features. ADCA type II is characterized by a pigmentary

macular dystrophy, and ADCA type III is a "pure" cerebellar ataxia of later onset.

Autosomal Dominant Cerebellar Ataxia Type I

The prevalence ratio for ADCA type I ranges from 0.3 to 1.2 per 100,000 in Europe. Much higher figures have been reported in the Azores, Holguin (Cuba), and Calabria (southern Italy), probably because of a founder effect.

Pathologic heterogeneity is well recognized in ADCA because olivopontocerebellar atrophy, cerebello-olivary degeneration, and parenchymatous cerebellar cortical atrophy may be found. Olivopontocerebellar atrophy, the most frequent pattern, is characterized by atrophy of the middle cerebellar peduncle; shrinkage of the ventral part of the pons (which appears wedge-shaped); and atrophy of the inferior olives, the cerebellar cortex, and the nuclei pontis. Degeneration of spinal tracts, especially the dorsal columns and spinocerebellar tracts, is almost constant. Myelin staining shows pallor of transverse fibers in the ventral half of the pons and of cerebellar white matter. Loss of both granular and Purkinje cells varies from case to case, and loss of neurons in the substantia nigra and in the corpus striatum has been reported in a considerable number of cases.

Mean age at onset is 34 years (range, 4–63 years) in our experience. Fifty percent of the patients have onset in the third or fourth decade.

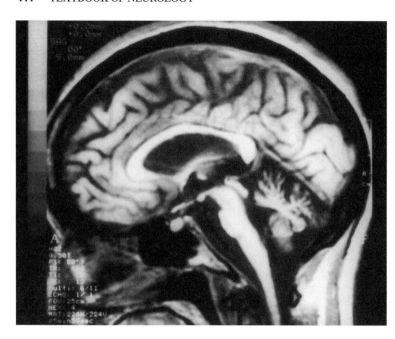

Figure 29-6. T1-weighted sagittal magnetic resonance imaging scan of a 45-year-old patient with ADCA type I (SCA2) showing marked atrophy of the cerebellum and pons.

Approximately 10% have onset before 20 years, and 95% of the patients become symptomatic by the age of 56 years. Anticipation—that is, an earlier onset in more recent generations usually associated with a more severe phenotype—is common and more pronounced in paternal transmission.

Onset age and clinical picture are highly variable between and within families. The most frequent presenting symptom is gait ataxia. The clinical picture is characterized by constant gait ataxia, almost constant dysarthria, and very frequent dysmetria. Abnormal eye movements are found in more than 70% of the patients. Supranuclear ophthalmoplegia initially affects upward gaze and may eventually lead to complete absence of eye movements. Slow saccades are frequent. Nystagmus is found in about one-third of patients. Corticospinal signs (increased knee jerks, spasticity, and Babinski's sign), mild cognitive impairment, dysphagia (mainly for liquids), sphincter disturbances (usually urinary urgency), and decreased vibration and position sense are frequent. Perioral fasciculations, cramps, and amyotrophy are sometimes observed. Extrapyramidal features, which include facial impassivity, cogwheel rigidity, choreiform and athetoid movements, and dystonia, are rare in large series of patients. Optic atrophy is a rare and late feature. The majority of patients are unable to walk independently 15–20 years from onset. Life expectancy is shortened, and the mean age of death is 56 years (range, 20–93 years).

MRI shows constant cerebellar atrophy usually associated with brain stem atrophy, mainly of the ventral pons, reflecting the pathologic process of olivopontocerebellar atrophy (Figure 29-6). In T2-weighted images, the transverse pontine fibers show increased signal in most patients. Atrophy of the supratentorial structures and cervical cord is frequently found. Brain stem and lower limb somatosensory and central motor evoked potentials are impaired in approximately 80% of patients. Visual evoked potentials are abnormal in 50% of cases. Electrophysiologic signs of a mainly sensory axonal neuropathy are present in approximately 60% of patients.

The label of Machado-Joseph disease (MJD) applies to an autosomal dominant disorder first reported in North American families of Portuguese-Azorean descent and subsequently in families of diverse ethnic origins on different continents. The clinical picture comprises progressive cerebellar ataxia, ophthalmoplegia, pyramidal signs, dystonia, distal amyotrophy, eyelid retraction, and faciolingual fasciculation. Pathologically the disease is characterized by involvement of dentate and substantia nigra and sparing of the inferior olives and Purkinje cells. According to Harding, this syndrome may be included in ADCA type I.

Genetic heterogeneity has been recognized within ADCA type I, in which at least four different loci have been recognized (see Table 29-1). The *SCA1* locus is linked to chromosome 6; *SCA2* to chromosome 12; *SCA3/MJD* to chromosome 14; and *SCA4* to chromosome 16. The disease-causing genes have been found for spinocerebellar atrophy type 1 (SCA1), SCA2, and SCA3/MJD. Orr et al. reported an expanded trinucleotide cytosine-adenine-guanine (CAG) repeat within the coding sequence of SCA1-affected alleles. The same mutational mechanism is responsible for SCA2 and SCA3/MJD. There is an inverse correlation between repeat number and age of onset of symptoms. Expanded trinucleotide repeats are unstable—that is, they have tendency to further expansion on meiosis. This is the molecular mechanism of anticipation. Male gametogenesis is more likely to result in repeat expansion, which explains why earlier onset and more severe phenotypes more often result from paternal transmission. The CAG repeat is translated into a polyglutamine tract. The elongation of the polyglutamine tract provides the protein with a new function that is ultimately toxic to specific neuronal cells (gain of function hypothesis).

Because ADCA type I is characterized by a great clinical and pathologic variability both between and within families, only molecular genetics allow a definite diagnosis of subtype. It has been suggested that some clinical features may be more frequently associated with a given genotype: signs of corticospinal impairment are early features in SCA1; supranuclear ophthalmoplegia and peripheral neuropathy are more frequent in SCA2; extrapyramidal features are prominent in SCA3/MJD; and axonal sensory neuropathy is prominent in SCA4. The occurrence of the mutations differs in different populations. SCA3/MJD is prevalent in Portuguese, French, and American populations, whereas it has not been described in Italy. Altogether, SCA3/MJD is found in one-fourth of the ADCA type 1 families and SCA2 has a similar value, whereas SCA1 has a lower occurrence in large series.

Autosomal Dominant Cerebellar Ataxia Type II

ADCA type II is characterized by the presence of pigmentary macular dystrophy. Pathologic findings are those of olivopontocerebellar atrophy. Some obligate carriers are asymptomatic. Incom-

plete penetrance is not described in other types of ADCA. Age at onset may vary from 6 months to 60 years, and it is usually earlier than in ADCA type I. Patients with childhood onset have a rapidly progressive phenotype and early death. Anticipation is marked in offspring of affected males. The most common presenting symptom is ataxia. Visual failure may precede ataxia in approximately one-third of patients. The clinical picture is otherwise not specific, and it is characterized by ataxia, pyramidal signs, supranuclear ophthalmoplegia, slow saccades, occasional choreiform movements, and, rarely, dementia. Visual symptoms consist of reduced central acuity, with relative preservation of peripheral vision, which eventually progresses to blindness. Funduscopic examination shows coarse granulation of pigment at the macula and fine pigment epithelial changes in the peripheral retina. Optic atrophy is present in late stages. The ADCA type II (also called *SCA7*) locus has been mapped to chromosome 3. The disease is associated with the expansion of a trinucleotide CAG repeat in the coding region of the responsible gene.

Autosomal Dominant Cerebellar Ataxia Type III

ADCA type III may be more common in Japan. Pathologic findings are those of cerebellar cortical atrophy. Age at onset is later than for the other ADCAs and it occurs most commonly in the fifth and sixth decade, but may be delayed to the eighth decade. Anticipation, if present, is slight. The picture is that of a pure cerebellar ataxia without ophthalmoplegia, amyotrophy, extrapyramidal features, or dementia. Sensation and tendon reflexes are usually normal. Pyramidal signs may be present. Mild course and normal life expectancy are usual, but clinical and genetic heterogeneity is probably present, because a rapidly progressive form has been described. SCA5 and SCA6 usually present as mild and slowly progressive cerebellar ataxia. SCA5 has been mapped to chromosome 11 and SCA6 to chromosome 19. A very small CAG expansion within the α_{1A} voltage-dependent calcium channel (CACNL1A4) gene is associated with SCA6. Different mutations in the same gene are also responsible for familial hemiplegic migraine and episodic ataxia type 2. Only one SCA5 family has been reported, whereas occurrence of SCA6 varies from 2% to 31% in ADCA series.

Other Autosomal Dominant Cerebellar Ataxias

Dentatorubropallidoluysian atrophy (Haw River syndrome) has been reported in sporadic cases without a family history, but it is predominantly found as an inherited condition that is particularly prevalent in Japan. Neuropathologic changes consist of combined degeneration of the dentatorubral and pallidoluysian system. Onset age ranges from the first to the seventh decade. Anticipation is present, especially when the disease is transmitted paternally. The disease is characterized by various combinations of progressive myoclonus, epilepsy, ataxia, choreoathetosis, and dementia. Patients with onset before 20 years have a phenotype of PME characterized by myoclonus, epileptic seizures, dementia, and ataxia, whereas the later onset form exhibits cerebellar ataxia, choreoathetosis, and dementia, sometimes indistinguishable from Huntington's disease. A CAG expansion on chromosome 12 is associated with the disease.

Hereditary periodic ataxia is a rare disorder that is transmitted in an autosomal dominant fashion and characterized by sudden attacks of limb and gait ataxia. In the majority of cases, the age at onset ranges from early childhood to adolescence. The attacks are often precipitated by physical and emotional stress, fatigue, exercise, alcohol, and menstrual periods. The patients usually respond to acetazolamide. A clinical and genetic heterogeneity has been recognized. Episodic ataxia type 1 is caused by point mutations in the voltage-gated K$^+$ channel gene (*KCNA1*) on chromosome 12 and is characterized by brief episodes of ataxia lasting from seconds to minutes. Neurologic examination during and between attacks shows myokymia in periorbital muscles or hands. Mutations disrupting the reading frame of CACNL1A4 gene on chromosome 19 cause episodic ataxia type 2 (EA-2). Attacks tends to last hours to days and are associated with vertigo, nausea, and headache. Interictal nystagmus and a progressive cerebellar syndrome are also present. Cerebellar and brain stem atrophy has been shown in some patients.

Gerstmann-Sträussler-Scheinker disease is a rare autosomal dominant prion disease, but its occurrence may be underestimated. At necropsy, diffuse atrophy of the cerebral hemispheres and cerebellum is observed. The neuropathologic diagnosis is based on the presence of amyloid deposits immunoreactive with antibodies to prion protein, which are present throughout the brain and are particularly abundant in the cerebellar cortex. Spongiform degeneration is an inconstant finding. In some families, neurofibrillary tangles indistinguishable from those found in Alzheimer's disease are present in the cerebral cortex and in several subcortical nuclei. The original case reported by Gerstmann in 1928 was that of a 25-year-old woman with progressive ataxia, severe intention tremor, dysarthria, nystagmus, decreased reflexes at lower limbs, Babinski's sign, and dementia, who died 6 years after the onset of symptoms. The clinical spectrum is wide. Onset may vary from the third to the sixth decade. Ataxia, spastic paraparesis, extrapyramidal features, and dementia may be the dominant clinical presentation. Mean disease duration is 5 years. Point mutations and insertions have been described in the prion protein gene on chromosome 20, which result in amino acid substitution or a truncated protein. Different mutations may be associated with different pathologic pictures. Inoculation of brain homogenates from patients with mutation at codon 102 resulted in spongiform encephalopathy in animals.

Idiopathic Late-Onset Cerebellar Ataxias

In 1900, Dejerine and Thomas first introduced the term *olivopontocerebellar atrophy* in reporting the pathologic findings in two patients with disease onset in middle age whose clinical features were impassive facies, dysarthria, cerebellar ataxia, and increased tone. In 1922, Marie, Foix, and Alajouanine reported cortical cerebellar atrophy, a normal pons, and atrophy of the inferior olives in four patients with markedly ataxic gait and mild disturbances of speech and upper limb coordination. The age of onset ranged from 40 to 78 years. Harding suggested the term *idiopathic late-onset cerebellar ataxia* (ILOCA) for all sporadic cases of late-onset cerebellar ataxia with unknown origin. These cases are not rare and they are probably underdiagnosed. The frequency of occurrence is not far from that of the dominant ataxias in our experience. Diagnosis of ILOCA is dependent on the exclusion of known causes of acquired cerebellar degeneration, such as alcoholism, chronic anticonvulsant therapy, malignancy, and hypothyroidism.

Onset is in the fifth or sixth decade in most patients, but it varies from the fourth to the eighth. A preponderance in males has been reported. Gait ataxia, which is constant, is the most frequent presenting symptom. Limb incoordination is almost constant and dysarthria very frequent. Knee jerks may be normal, brisk, or depressed and ankle jerks are absent in one-third of patients. Extensor plantar response is present in approximately 50%. Vibration sense is frequently impaired. Some patients have intention or postural tremor, nystagmus, dysphagia, cognitive impairment, and sphincter disturbances. Parkinsonian features, choreiform movements, amyotrophy, and supranuclear ophthalmoplegia are rare. Optic atrophy and pigmentary retinal degeneration are absent.

The disease is progressive and the ability to walk is lost after 5–20 years from onset. Life expectancy is reduced. Patients with pure cerebellar syndrome might have a better prognosis than those with additional features.

MRI shows almost constant atrophy of the cerebellar hemispheres and vermis associated with brain stem or cerebral atrophy in about one-half of patients. White matter lesions are a frequent finding. Neurophysiologic investigation may show peripheral and central pathway impairment.

Absence of family history, later onset, and rarer ophthalmoplegia differentiate ILOCA from ADCA type I. CAG expansions within the *SCA1* and *SCA3* genes have not been found in ILOCA. It may be difficult to distinguish ILOCA from multisystem atrophy, which is characterized by a combination of cerebellar, pyramidal, extrapyramidal, and dysautonomic features. Signs of autonomic failure or a pathologic sphincter electromyographic examination are required for the clinical diagnosis of multisystem atrophy. Finding glial cytoplasmic inclusions at necropsy makes the diagnosis certain. Prognosis in multisystem atrophy is poorer than in ILOCA because of severe incapacity and more limited survival.

Acquired cerebellar degeneration should be considered in the differential diagnosis. The most common cause of cerebellar degeneration is alcoholism, in which there is a history of alcohol abuse, subacute onset, and prominent ataxia of gait associated with polyneuropathy and features of Wernicke-Korsakoff encephalopathy. Chronic phenytoin toxicity may cause irreversible cerebellar ataxia, nystagmus, and dysarthria. Cancer of the lung or ovary, non-Hodgkin's lymphoma, or Hodgkin's disease may be associated with a subacute cerebellar syndrome. The diagnosis of the primary cancer may occur years after the presentation of the cerebellar syndrome. Treatment with thyroid hormones, vitamin E, and antigliadin and antiendomysial antibodies exclude hypothyroidism, chronic fat malabsorption, and celiac disease, which are other possible causes of a progressive and treatable cerebellar syndrome. MRI can differentiate ILOCA from ataxia secondary to benign and low-grade malignant posterior fossa tumors, communicating or obstructive hydrocephalus, and chronic progressive multiple sclerosis. Cerebellar ataxia may be a prominent feature in prion disease, which is usually characterized by marked dementia, rapid course, pyramidal and extrapyramidal signs, and myoclonic jerks.

Suggested Reading

Barbeau A. Friedreich's ataxia 1979: an overview. Can J Neurol Sci 1979;6:311.

Campuzano V, Montermini L, Moltò MD, et al. Friedreich's ataxia: autosomal recessive disease caused by an intronic GAA triplet repeat expansion. Science 1996;271:1423.

Di Mauro S, Moraes CT. Mitochondrial encephalomyopathies. Arch Neurol 1993;50:1197.

Dürr A, Brice A. Genetics of movement disorders. Curr Opin Neurol 1996;9:290.

Filla A, De Michele G, Cavalcanti F, et al. The relationship between trinucleotide (GAA) repeat length and clinical features in Friedreich ataxia. Am J Hum Genet 1996;59:554.

Harding AE. The Hereditary Ataxias and Related Disorders. Edinburgh: Churchill Livingstone, 1984.

Lowe J, Lennox G, Leigh PN. Disorders of Movement and System Degenerations. In DI Graham, PL Lantos (eds), Greenfield's Neuropathology (6th ed). London: Arnold, 1997;281.

Orr HT, Chung M, Banfi S, et al. Expansion of an unstable trinucleotide CAG repeat in spinocerebellar ataxia type 1. Nature Genet 1993;4:221.

Rosenberg RN. Machado-Joseph disease: an autosomal dominant motor system degeneration. Mov Disord 1992;7:193.

Scriver CR, Beaudet AL, Sly WS, Valle D. The Metabolic and Molecular Bases of Inherited Disease (7th ed). New York: McGraw-Hill, 1995.

Chapter 30
Multiple Sclerosis

Aaron Miller

Chapter Plan

Epidemiology
Clinical features
Diagnosis
Magnetic resonance imaging
Course of multiple sclerosis
Etiology and pathogenesis
Treatment

Epidemiology

Multiple sclerosis (MS) is an acquired inflammatory demyelinating disease of central nervous system white matter, principally affecting young adults between the ages of 20 and 50 years. Approximately 10% of cases begin after age 50 years, whereas initial symptoms before age 10 years are rare. Women are affected somewhat more commonly than men, as is typical for other presumed autoimmune-based disorders. MS is more common in temperate than tropical climates. Interestingly, people who move from a relatively high prevalence region to one of low prevalence after puberty carry their enhanced risk with them; individuals moving in the opposite direction carry a lower risk. Several "point epidemics" of substantially increased incidence have occurred with a subsequent return to baseline incidence, suggesting the introduction of a causative agent into a susceptible population. These epidemiologic observations must be acknowledged when theories about the pathogenesis of MS are proposed.

Clinical Features

When it presents in classic fashion, the diagnosis of MS is straightforward. However, the disorder has protean manifestations that may challenge the diagnostician. Furthermore, a variety of other neurologic disorders may pose diagnostic dilemmas. The clinical hallmark of MS is the dissemination of symptoms and signs in time and space. Thus, the illness typically begins with discrete attacks, episodes of varying central nervous system dysfunction lasting days to weeks or months. Early in the illness, these attacks generally resolve with little or no sequelae.

The second critical feature requires evidence that two or more *noncontiguous* areas of central nervous system white matter be involved. For example, a patient may show signs of both optic nerve and spinal cord abnormality. Alternatively, brain stem symptoms such as diplopia or vertigo may occur on one occasion, and signs of myelopathy on another.

The most frequent initial manifestations of MS involve somatosensory symptoms, motor weakness, or visual disturbance. Sensory abnormalities may actually be the most common initial symptoms, but these problems are often not reported to a physician; they should, however, be carefully sought when a history is obtained. Sensory symptoms include numbness or paresthesias, sometimes with a painful quality (dysesthesias). Patients may feel as if a garment is covering an unclothed body part. A typical pattern is to experience ascending numbness beginning in the toes and eventually reaching the abdomen or thorax. Such a pattern indicates a spinal cord lesion and in many cases is not associated with weakness or sphincter disturbance. Sometimes the area just "feels funny" or "different," and the patient cannot offer a more precise description. Strange itching may at times herald the illness.

If the patient with sensory symptoms does present to a physician, the examination is often unhelpful. The patient's symptoms may not be accompanied by any altered or reduced sensation on examination of the affected body part. Frequently, the physician may be perplexed by the fact that the patient's area of sensory complaint does not seem to follow the pattern of spinal dermatomes or peripheral nerves.

Although somatosensory symptoms may involve any part of the body, certain patterns occur more commonly. Frequently, patients complain of numbness or paresthesias involving one or both legs or arms distally. Sometimes, a girdlelike tightness or peculiar sensation around the midriff is described, suggesting involvement of spinal sensory nerves as they exit through the white matter at a particular spinal level.

Motor weakness, which most often results from corticospinal tract lesions within the spinal cord, is another common initial manifestation of MS. This most typically affects one or both legs. Less often, a hemiparesis occurs. With corticospinal tract weakness in the leg, flexors are generally much more paretic than extensors. Thus, the iliopsoas (hip flexors), hamstrings (knee flexors), and anterior tibialis (foot dorsiflexors) are typically weaker (often dramatically so) than the glutei (hip extensors), quadriceps (knee extensors), and gastrocnemius (foot plantar flexors) muscles. The patient's gait will be affected, leading to circumduction at the hip or a foot-drop pattern distally. Whereas motor deficits are the most common cause of gait abnormalities in MS patients, sensory and cerebellar abnormalities may also contribute to the development of this most important source of disability. A Babinski's sign often accompanies even early corticospinal tract weakness, whereas hyperreflexia, although extremely common later, may not be apparent with new symptoms.

Visual disturbance in early MS usually results from optic neuritis and presents as complaints of monocular visual blurring, frequently accompanied by pain on eye movement and photophobia. The range of severity is great. Patients may experience involvement so mild that only color desaturation is evident. Conversely, complete unilateral visual loss may occur. Typical episodes are intermediate between these extremes, usually resulting in a central scotoma on visual field examination and a moderate decrease in visual acuity. Examination of the fundus at the acute stage of optic neuritis is most often normal (retrobulbar neuritis). However, a minority of cases may demonstrate swelling of the optic nerve (papillitis). A helpful sign of optic nerve involvement, even of a subclinical degree, is the afferent pupillary defect, as demonstrated by the swinging flashlight test. To elicit this sign, the physician shines a bright flashlight first in the *affected* eye. This produces pupillary constriction both ipsilaterally and contralaterally. The flashlight is then moved to the normal eye and continued pupillary constriction is observed. However, when the flashlight is rapidly swung back to the affected eye, that pupil paradoxically dilates (the afferent pupillary defect), because the stimulus for pupillary constriction is now perceived less intensely than was the stimulus in the contralateral eye, which thus produced a greater degree of consensual constriction.

Visual complaints do not always result from optic neuritis. Less commonly, symptoms may result from brain stem disease. Thus, patients may complain of diplopia, oscillopsia (movement of visual images), or simply blurry vision. Examination may reveal internuclear ophthalmoplegia (INO), either unilaterally or bilaterally, which is an almost pathognomonic sign of MS in young people. This sign results from a lesion of the median longitudinal fasciculus, a myelinated tract that connects the sixth nerve nucleus (for the lateral rectus) on one side of the pons with the third nerve nucleus (for the medial rectus) on the other side of the midbrain. In an INO, one eye fails to adduct properly, while the other eye fully abducts and typically demonstrates horizontal nystagmus. MS patients may also develop bilateral horizontal, vertical, or rotatory nystagmus or a variety of extraocular motility disturbances (e.g., sixth nerve palsy).

Cerebellar symptoms represent a less common presentation of the illness but are not rare. Patients may present with an unsteady gait, upper limb ataxia, or intention tremor. Cerebellar dysfunction may occur in isolation or with other evidence of central nervous system dysfunction. In occasional MS patients, the cerebellar abnormalities lead to severe and difficult-to-manage disability.

Other brain stem symptoms, such as trigeminal neuralgia (jabs of lancinating facial pain) or, rarely, hearing loss may be an initial or later symptom. Very characteristic of MS is Lhermitte's sign, which is, in fact, a symptom. Patients, usually on flexing the neck, experience electrical shock–like jabs down the back or into the extremities. This implies a lesion in the posterior columns of the cervical spinal cord but is not specific for MS.

Disturbances of micturition, although very common during the course of MS, may occasionally be the sentinel symptom. Most typically, the patient develops urinary retention, although at times the presenting complaint may be urinary urgency or incontinence. Both hyperactive and hypoactive disturbances of bladder function occur in MS and differentiation on clinical grounds can be difficult. For patients who are experiencing noticeable bladder dysfunction, urologic referral and dynamic studies of bladder function are indicated. Bowel dysfunction is much less common, but bowel urgency and incontinence are very troubling symptoms.

Diagnosis

The key to the diagnosis of MS is evidence that the disease is disseminated in time and space. The former criterion is usually satisfied when the patient has had two or more attacks (neurologic symptoms that have persisted for at least 24 hours). The requirement may also be met by progression of symptoms or signs for more than 6 months. *Dissemination in space* means that there must be evidence of two or more lesions that are not anatomically contiguous.

Most published diagnostic criteria are variations on those established by Schumacher et al. Their criteria are as follows:

1. Age of onset between 10 and 50 years
2. Evidence of white matter disease
3. Objective signs on neurologic examination
4. Two or more attacks or progression for more than 6 months
5. Two or more lesions that are not anatomically contiguous
6. No better clinical explanation

According to Schumacher et al., a patient could be considered to have clinically definite MS if at least five of these criteria, always including the last, are met.

In 1983, a committee published diagnostic criteria that made several important modifications. In addition to attacks consisting of symptoms lasting at least 24 hours, patients who experienced brief recurrent (paroxysmal) symptoms over a period of days or weeks were regarded as having an attack. Examples of such symptoms would include trigeminal neuralgia or Lhermitte's phenomenon. This group recognized the possibility that one of the required lesions in their diagnostic scheme could be evident by paraclinical means—that is, neuroimaging studies or evoked response testing. The latter provides an electrophysiologic means of demonstrating subclinical lesions in the optic nerve, spinal cord, or, less commonly, the brain stem.

The committee also recognized the importance of cerebrospinal fluid (CSF) examination, which typically demonstrates immunologic abnormalities in patients with MS. The CSF may show oligoclonal bands in the immunoglobulin region. Alternatively, evidence of increased IgG synthesis or elevated IgG levels (in the presence of normal total CSF protein levels) may be found. A category of laboratory-supported diagnosis of MS was included, which allowed a diagnosis of the disease when there are two attacks and one lesion, or one attack and two lesions, accompanied by typical abnormalities in the CSF. Table 30-1 demonstrates the so-called Poser classification scheme and illustrates a widely used current approach to the diagnosis of relapsing-remitting MS.

Magnetic Resonance Imaging

The advent of magnetic resonance imaging (MRI) in the early 1980s has contributed greatly not only to the diagnosis of MS, but also to an understanding of the biology of the disease. In well-established

Table 30-1. Diagnostic Criteria for Multiple Sclerosis

Category	Attacks	Clinical Evidence		Paraclinical Evidence	CSF OB/IgG
Clinically definite (CD)					
CDMS A1	2	2			
CDMS A2	2	1	and	1	
Laboratory-supported definite (LSD)					
LSDMS B1	2	1	or	1	+
LSDMS B2	1	2			+
LSDMS B3	1	1	and	1	+
Clinically probable (CP)					
CPMS C1	2	1			
CPMS C2	1	2			
CPMS C3	1	1	and	1	
Laboratory-supported probable (LSP)					
LSPMS D1	2				

MS = multiple sclerosis; CSF = cerebrospinal fluid; OB/IgG = oligoclonal bands or increased IgG; + = present.
Source: CM Poser, DW Paty, L Scheinberg, et al. New diagnostic criteria for multiple sclerosis: guidelines for research protocols.
Ann Neurol 1983;13:227, reproduced with permission.

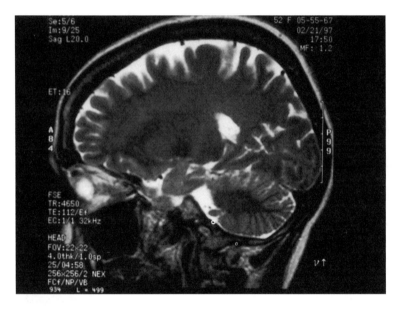

Figure 30-1. Magnetic resonance image demonstrating hyperintense lesions in the corpus callosum consistent with multiple sclerosis.

cases of MS, approximately 90% will have evidence of white matter lesions on brain MRI scans. Even at the time of monosymptomatic presentations, such as optic neuritis, partial transverse myelopathy, or isolated brain stem syndromes, 50–60% will have abnormal findings on brain imaging. The brain lesions have a number of characteristic features, including a typical periventricular location (Figure 30-1). Often these lesions have an ovoid appearance, with the long axis directed perpendicular to the body of the lateral ventricles.

Another feature on MRI studies in MS patients is involvement of the corpus callosum, which can be particularly well demonstrated with T2-weighted or proton density images in the sagittal plane. Finally, infratentorial lesions lend greater specificity to the MRI findings in MS. Spinal cord lesions are also quite common, although imaging this structure is considerably less sensitive than studying the brain.

Several investigators have performed serial MRI scans on patients at various stages of the disease, typically imaging monthly for 6–12 months. Such studies have indicated that MS is much more active, as evidenced on MRI scans, than clinically recognized. Active lesions occur five to ten times more frequently on brain MRI scans than are apparent symptomatically. The most sensitive marker of new lesions on MRI scans is gadolinium enhancement, which persists, on average, for approximately 4 weeks.

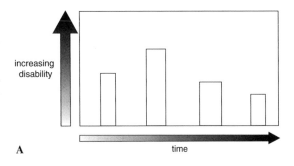

Course of Multiple Sclerosis

The temporal profile of MS is quite variable. Recently, investigators have attempted to establish a more uniform descriptive nomenclature to describe the course of the disease (Figure 30-2). Approximately 85% of patients begin with relapsing-remitting disease. In this stage, symptoms develop or worsen over a relatively short time (usually days to weeks). The attack then plateaus or improves, often to normal in the beginning of the illness. The key to this stage of MS is that the neurologic baseline remains stable between attacks. Approximately 15% of patients have primary progressive MS in which the disease steadily worsens (perhaps with an occasional plateau) from the onset. Among patients who begin with relapsing disease, the majority (50–65%) evolve into secondary progressive disease, in which the disease steadily worsens, with or without continued relapses. Finally, a rare course of the disease is labeled *progressive-relapsing*, in which an initially progressive course changes to one of relapses and remissions.

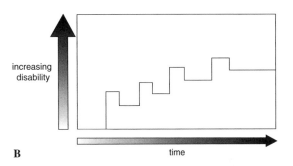

Figure 30-2. Courses of relapsing-remitting (A,B), primary-progressive (C,D), secondary-progressive (E,F), and relapsing-progressive (G,H) course of multiple sclerosis. (Reprinted with permission from FD Lublin, SC Reingold. Defining the clinical course of multiple sclerosis: results of an international survey. Neurology 1996;46:907.)

Etiology and Pathogenesis

Current evidence strongly suggests that MS is an autoimmune disorder, most likely occurring in individuals genetically predisposed to the illness. The importance of a genetic influence is emphasized by the fact that approximately 25% of monozygotic twins are concordant for the disease. Furthermore, siblings or children of affected parents are at a 20- to 50-fold increased risk for MS. The 75% discordancy rate in monozygotic twins indicates the likelihood of environmental factors, however.

Support for such an acquired exogenous precipitant comes from a series of epidemiologic studies that strongly suggest that the risk of MS is acquired during childhood, although clinical disease is not expressed until substantially later, typically in young adulthood. The disease is several times more common in temperate latitudes than in subtropical or tropical latitudes, with such data being particularly robust in the northern hemisphere. Furthermore, studies of immigrant populations demonstrate that those emigrating from areas of high prevalence to areas of low prevalence retain the higher rate of disease if they emigrate after the age of 15 years, but acquire the lower rate of their new country if they move at an earlier age.

These migration studies as well as extensive study of an epidemic in the Faroe Islands after World War II spurred the hypothesis that MS might be caused by a specific viral agent. Despite numerous claims over the years, to date no convincing

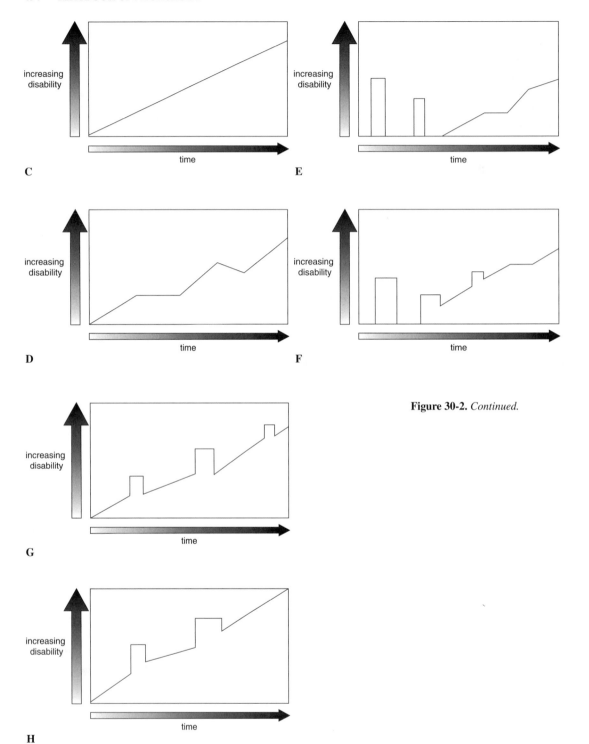

Figure 30-2. *Continued.*

evidence for a particular pathogen has been established. However, the possibility remains and is not inconsistent with the currently postulated autoimmune nature of the disease.

Pathologically, the disease is characterized by perivenular infiltration of mononuclear cells, particularly in periventricular locations. Evidence indicates that Th1 lymphocytes are recruited into the central nervous system, attracted to an as yet undetermined antigenic component of myelin. They then unleash an immunologic cascade, with the resulting inflammation and edema causing neurologic symptoms and signs. Persistent clinical deficits result from permanently damaged myelin and probably axonal damage as well.

Treatment

Therapy for MS may be divided into three rubrics: treatment for acute exacerbations; chronic therapy to influence the long-term natural history of the disease; and, finally, symptomatic treatments that may improve the quality of life but do not alter the course of the disease. The first treatment proved to be beneficial in ameliorating acute exacerbations was adrenocorticotrophic hormone, now called *corticotropin*. Intramuscular administration of corticotropin was shown in the late 1960s to shorten the duration of an acute exacerbation, although it did not appear to produce more complete recovery. During the 1970s and 1980s, corticosteroid use gradually replaced corticotropin. Today, most experts regard a short course (3–7 days) of high-dose intravenous methylprednisolone to be the most effective therapy for an acute attack.

The first of a series of parenterally administered immunomodulatory agents partially effective in the chronic therapy of patients with relapsing/remitting MS was approved in 1993. Interferon β_{1b} and interferon β_{1a} are recombinant interferons, differing somewhat in their protein chemistry and route and frequency of administration. Both decrease the attack frequency by approximately 30%, and both probably slow the progression of disability. A third agent, glatiramer acetate, is a synthetic polypeptide that may divert the immune system's attack on a natural myelin antigen or may induce suppression of that attack.

It too reduces relapse rate by approximately 30% and may slow progression. Each of these agents has advantages and disadvantages and none has yet proved to be more effective than the others.

Symptomatic treatments may be helpful for a variety of the clinical manifestations of MS and can contribute greatly to improvement in the patient's quality of life. Spasticity may be helped by the oral drugs baclofen, tizanidine, or dantrolene. Occasionally, surgical approaches are useful. Fatigue may be improved by amantadine or pemoline. The nature of urinary complaints must be investigated in order to determine the appropriate type of treatment. When indicated, anticholinergic medications (e.g., oxybutynin, propantheline, imipramine) may improve frequency, urgency, and incontinence. Patients who tend to retain residual urine may be taught to perform intermittent self-catheterization. Men with erectile dysfunction may be able to perform sexual intercourse through the use of intracorporeal injection or intraurethral administration of prostaglandin. Depression, a very common symptom in patients with MS, often responds to selective serotonin reuptake inhibitors or tricyclic antidepressants.

Finally, the importance of physical medicine interventions should not be underemphasized, particularly for patients with gait impairment. Selection of the proper gait aid and training in its use is critical. The correct choice of a brace may also be extremely helpful. For those patients who are no longer able to walk or can do so for only very limited distances, choosing the best mobility aid (e.g., scooter or wheelchair) may make an enormous difference in quality of life.

Suggested Reading

Lublin FD, Reingold SC. Defining the clinical course of multiple sclerosis: results of an international survey. Neurology 1996;46:907.

Miller A. Current and investigational therapies used to alter the course of disease in multiple sclerosis. South Med J 1997;90:367.

Miller AE. Clinical Features. In SD Cook (ed), Handbook of Multiple Sclerosis (2nd ed). New York: Marcel Dekker, 1996.

Poser CM, Paty DW, Scheinberg L, et al. New diagnostic criteria for multiple sclerosis: guidelines for research protocols. Ann Neurol 1983;13:227.

Pryse-Phillips W. The Epidemiology of Multiple Sclerosis. In SD Cook (ed), Handbook of Multiple Sclerosis (2nd ed). New York: Marcel Dekker, 1996.

Schapiro RT. Symptom Management in Multiple Sclerosis (2nd ed). New York: Demos Publications, 1994.

Schumacher GA, Beebe G, Kubler RF, et al. Problems of experimental trials of therapy in multiple sclerosis: report by the panel on the evaluation of experimental trials of therapy in multiple sclerosis. Ann NY Acad Sci 1965;122:522.

Weinshenker BG, Bass B, Rice GPA, et al. The natural history of multiple sclerosis: a geographically based study. I. Clinical course and disability. Brain 1989;112:133.

Chapter 31
Spinal Cord Disorders

Adolf Pou Serradell

Chapter Plan

Anatomic considerations for the spinal cord
Myelopathies and their causes
    Myelitis and nontumoral myelopathies
    Spondylogenic myelopathies
    Intraspinal tumors
    Syringomyelia
    Vascular myelopathies

Spinal cord (SC) disorders are frequent and often severe, and they raise special problems in diagnosis. A certain number of distinctive syndromes resulting from the different lesions of the SC are related to special physiologic and anatomic features of the cord, some of which are considered here.

Anatomic Considerations for the Spinal Cord

The SC extends from the medullary cervical junction at the foramen magnum to the level of the body of the first lumbar vertebra. The spinal roots exit in relation to their corresponding vertebral body. Because of the presence of eight cervical segments and only seven cervical vertebrae, the route of exit for spinal nerves from the vertebral canal varies according to the cord level. The first seven cervical nerves exit above the vertebral body, and the eighth exits below C7. The remainder of the spinal roots exit below their corresponding vertebral body. The spinal roots are increasingly longer the more caudal their origin and the elongated roots of the lumbar and sacral spine nerves are collectively referred to as the *cauda equina*. The cervical SC is somewhat elliptic in cross section, whereas the thoracic cord appears more round. The conus medullaris has a diamond-shaped enlargement before it terminates in the cauda equina. The normal conus in adults ends typically at the L1–L2 level. This so-called adult position is attained during the first few months of life and varies little thereafter. In contrast to the gray matter, the quantity of white matter increases progressively from the sacral through the cervical regions because of the larger number of tracts, both ascending and descending at higher levels. Cross-sections of the SC delineate the centrally placed gray matter and the surrounding white matter. The gray matter forms a butterfly-shaped column in the center of the cord containing the cell bodies of many of the motor, sensory, and autonomic neurons. These neurons are grouped into various zones (Rexed's laminae) depending on their function. Surrounding the gray matter are the white matter pathways, or long tracts, which carry ascending and descending information throughout the cord. The most important long tracts in the SC, their location, and their function are reflected in the diagram of the axial section of the SC shown in Figure 31-1. The major special physiologic and anatomic features of the SC are (1) prominent function in sensorimotor conduction and relatively primitive reflex activity;

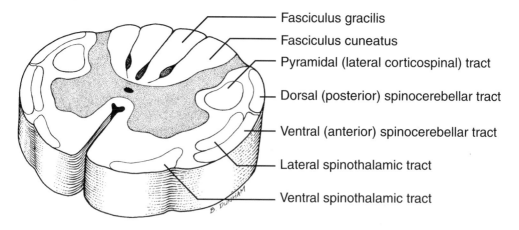

Long tracts in the spinal cord

Tract	Location	Function
Gracile	Medial dorsal column	Proprioception from the leg
Cuneate	Lateral dorsal column	Proprioception from the arm
Spinocerebellar	Superficial lateral column	Muscular position and tone
Pyramidal	Deep lateral column	Upper motor neuron
Lateral	Ventrolateral	Pain and thermal
Spinothalamic		

Figure 31-1. The major long tracts of the spinal cord.

(2) its long, cylindrical shape; (3) its tight envelopment by the meninges; (4) the peripheral location of medullary fibers, next to the pia; (5) the special arrangement of its blood vessels; and (6) its particular relationship to the vertebral column.

Myelopathies and Their Causes

A myelopathy is any pathologic process that affects primarily the SC and causes neurologic dysfunction. Woolsey and Young estimated that there are approximately 30 diseases known to affect the SC, of which half are seen with regularity. These diseases express themselves by a number of readily recognized syndromes, and according to the characteristics of the syndrome, a certain disease is preferentially invoked. Thus, the major syndromes to be considered are (1) a transverse sensorimotor myelopathy, which may be related to trauma, infection, vasculitis, or other processes; (2) a hemicord (Brown-Séquard) syndrome, which may reflect a cord compression, especially by disc herniation, benign intraspinal tumor, or some other entity; (3) a ventral cord syndrome, sparing posterior column function, that is related to an anterior spinal artery (ASA) occlusion or some other process; (4) a central cord or syringomyelic syndrome as a manifestation of primary (foraminal) syringomyelia, cervical ependymoma, or some other process; (5) a syndrome of the cauda equina related to a narrowness of the lumbar canal or another entity; and (6) a dorsal cord syndrome, sparing all functions except proprioception, as a possible manifestation of a para-neoplastic or inflammatory (multiple sclerosis [MS]) myelopathy.

The most common types of myelopathies and their causes are discussed in the following sections.

Myelitis and Nontumoral Myelopathies

Transverse Myelitis

Transverse myelitis is a condition that is generally encountered in the younger age groups. It consti-tutes a syndrome of multiple causes and it devel-ops characteristically as a rapidly progressing myelopathy, interrupting both motor and sensory tracts at one level, usually thoracic. It typically begins with localized back or radicular pain fol-lowed by bilateral paresthesias of the legs, an ascending sensory level, and a paraparesis that often progresses to paraplegia. Bladder and bowel involvement occurs early and is a prominent fea-ture. Generally, the myelitis usually regresses, par-tially or completely, in 1 or 2 months, although in some cases a severe neurologic deficit may per-sist. Patients with rapid progression and flaccid-ity below the level of the lesion have the worst prognosis. In many cases, transverse myelitis is related to a viral infection: enterovirus (groups A and B Coxsackie virus, poliomyelitis, others), herpes zoster, Epstein-Barr virus, cytomegalovirus (CMV), rabies, B virus, human T-cell lymphotropic virus (HTLV-1) (tropical spastic paraparesis [TSP]), or human immunodeficiency virus. Her-pesviruses occur in the cord in two forms: herpes simplex (HSV) types 1 and 2. The first more com-monly causes an acute limbic encephalitis, rarely a myelitis, and the second causes an acute lum-bosacral radiculopathy. The varicella-zoster virus causes a primary ganglionic infection with pain and a vesicular eruption in a corresponding distribution, and sometimes this can be followed by an acute myelitis when the eruption is thoracic. Immuno-compromised patients are at special risk. Less fre-quently a transverse myelitis may be related to systemic lupus erythematosus, Sjögren's syndrome, or another vasculitis, or to MS. Obviously, it is important to exclude cord compression by epidural abscess or tumor, bacterial or fungal infections, and vasculitic diseases. Reports of magnetic resonance imaging (MRI) in transverse myelitis emphasize diffuse cord enlargement but describe conflicting signal characteristics of the cord on T2-weighted sequences, which frequently make it difficult to differentiate it from SC lesions of MS.

Postinfectious and Postvaccinal (Autoimmune) Myelopathies (Measles, Varicella, Rubeola, Smallpox)

Myelitides (the name reserved for postinfectious and postvaccinal myelopathies) are basically leukomyelitides (lesions of the white matter), but the clinical picture (usually monophasic) is that of an acute transverse myelitis. There is often associ-ated encephalitis leading to the concept of acute demyelinating encephalomyelitis (ADEM). ADEM and MS are both demyelinating diseases, may coexist in members of the same family, and appear to be the same disease that evolution must con-firm. There are neither specific clinical nor MRI findings for ADEM. Its diagnosis must be mainly supported by the clinical course and findings on serial MRI scans.

On the basis of the clinical features of dissemi-nated postinfectious encephalomyelitis and an experimental autoimmune model, postinfectious myelitis is presumed to be autoimmune in nature, reflecting an attack that preferentially affects SC myelin. In general, the prognosis is better than the initial symptoms might suggest.

Acute Transverse Necrotizing Myelitis

Some cases of myelitis, usually without a detectable cause, run a particularly rapid and severe course. They are termed *acute transverse necrotizing myelitis* because pathologically necrosis with hem-orrhages is associated or predominate over demyeli-nation. Some of these cases are associated with unilateral or bilateral involvement of the optic nerves (Devic's neuromyelitis optica).

Subacute Necrotizing Myelitis

Subacute necrotizing myelitis occurs as a progres-sive myelopathy over several months or years, affecting mostly the lumbosacral cord, preferen-tially in men, and corresponds to the description given by Foix and Alajouanine. An early spastic paraplegia evolves after a few months or longer into a flaccid one associated with sensory loss, at first dissociated and then complete, and loss of sphincter control. Postmortem examination in some cases reveals abnormalities in the intramedullary small vessels (angiodysplasia). We are inclined (see section on vascular malformations), as others, to consider this myelopathy to be an arteriovenous malformation (AVM). Adams, Victor, and Ropper suggest that only when the abnormal vessels involve the surface and adjacent parenchyma of the cord does the disorder deserve to be designated Foix-Alajouanine myelopathy. The remaining cases are of the necrotizing type or are caused by vasculitis.

Subacute Paraneoplastic Necrotizing Myelopathy

Subacute paraneoplastic necrotizing myelopathy is an unusual disorder that can be associated with lung carcinoma and solid lymphomas. The clinical syndrome consists of a rapidly progressive loss of motor and sensory tract function, usually with sphincter disorder. The lesions are of a necrotic type and impair the gray and, preferentially, the white matter. In some cases, lesions are limited to the posterior and lateral funiculi and often are associated with a diffuse loss of Purkinje cells. This syndrome is selectively related to ovarian carcinoma and to Hodgkin's disease. There is also a paraneoplastic disorder in which anterior horn cells selectively disappear (paralymphomatous).

Myelopathies Related to Human Retrovirus Infection

A variety of acute myelopathies have been reported in HIV-infected patients, including those caused by identifiable viruses (e.g., herpes simplex, CMV), transverse myelitis of obscure origin, and seroconversion. Subacute or chronic myelopathies with pyramidal and posterior column signs are more frequent, particularly vacuolar myelopathy, probably related to direct injury of the neurons by the HIV. Nevertheless, the existence of a similar syndrome in patients with other diseases suggests that it is not specific to HIV infection. Clinically, we have observed that there is leg weakness, often symmetrical and developing over a period of weeks, to which the signs of deep sensory involvement and sphincteric disorder are added. A coexisting peripheral neuropathy is sometimes present, and it must be suspected if the ankle jerks are often unilaterally absent. This association may closely resemble subacute combined degeneration as seen in vitamin B_{12} deficiency. The signs may remain static or progress over a few months or years to a severe spastic paraplegia. The involvement of the SC seems to progress from the lumbar to the thoracic cord. The cerebrospinal fluid (CSF) is usually normal. There is no treatment. Some patients benefit from antispastic drugs.

Tropical Spastic Paraparesis

TSP (due to HTLV-1) was described first in the Caribbean island of Martinique and corresponds to the term *HTLV-1–associated myelopathy* used by Japanese investigators. TSP is a neurologic disorder endemic in many tropical and subtropical countries that is characterized by a slowly progressive spastic paraparesis. Disorder of sphincter control is usually an early change, and sensory function is variably affected. MRI studies reveal a normal brain but thinning of the SC. Beyond clinical differences, MRI is the most useful technique in distinguishing TSP from forms of MS affecting the cord. Neuropathologic studies reveal an inflammatory myelopathy with focal spongiform demyelinating and perivascular infiltrates. Treatment to date has been disappointing.

Myelitis Caused by Other Infectious Agents (Bacterial, Fungal, Parasitic, and Granulomatous Diseases)

Bacterial diseases may cause myelopathies as part of a systemic disease. Only rarely does the process involve the cord, such as SC abscess from *Mycoplasma pneumoniae* or *Listeria monocytogenes*. Osteomyelitis whether acute (*Staphylococcus aureus*, gram-negative organisms, or anaerobes) or subacute (tuberculosis of the spine [Pott's disease] or brucellosis) can similarly cause cord infarction but also may compress the cord from the mass of the abscess itself. Fungal infections are a cause of epidural lesions from hematogenous dissemination from neighboring vertebral lesions. The main causes are *Actinomyces, Coc-*

cidiodes, *Blastomyces*, and *Aspergillus* organisms. Parasitic myelitis may occur with types of *Schistosoma*. *Toxoplasma gondii*, which is the frequent cause of cerebral lesions in patients with acquired immunodeficiency syndrome (AIDS), rarely causes myelitis. A spectrum of peripheral and central nervous system disorders can occur after infection with *Borrelia burgdorferi* (Lyme disease); frequently, the clinical presentation is dominated by painful radiculopathy with mental confusion and in some patients a spastic paraparesis with exclusively thermalgesic sensory impairment develops as part of Lyme disease, presumably related to a vasculitic occlusion of the ASA, and patients may experience a spontaneous recovery. A number of granulomatous conditions may cause an intrinsic or, more often, a compressive myelopathy. Sarcoid may present, exceptionally, as an intramedullary SC tumor.

Nutritional, Metabolic,
and Endocrine Myelopathies

The term *subacute combined degeneration of the SC* is customarily reserved for vitamin B_{12} deficiency and serves to distinguish it from several other types of SC disease that rarely involve the posterior and lateral columns (e.g., niacin deficiency, or pellagra; alcoholism; diabetes; MS; adhesive spinal arachnoiditis; malnourishment). This disease is now infrequent in Western countries because of the treatment of pernicious anemia (the hematologic effects of vitamin B_{12} deficiency). The hematologic and neurologic manifestations of vitamin B_{12} deficiency occasionally complicate other malabsorptive disorders (e.g., celiac sprue, extensive gastric or ileal resections, conditions resulting in intestinal stasis, infestation with cobalamin-metabolizing fish tapeworm). Clinical manifestations include a demyelination in the posterior and lateral column leading to sensation of pins and needles in the legs with loss of vibration and proprioceptive sensation and weakness and spasticity with an unsteady gait. A polyneuropathy may exist in advanced stages of the disease, and then deep tendon reflexes may be absent. Mental signs are frequent. Visual impairment may result from a coexistent optic neuropathy. The blood may not show the typical changes of pernicious anemia, and bone marrow specimens

must be obtained. Low levels of serum cobalamin support the diagnosis (Schilling test). Serum levels of less than 100 pg/ml are usually associated with neurologic symptoms and signs. Immediate and lifelong treatment with vitamin B_{12} injections is necessary. Recovery is possible with the early lesions. Folate, given alone, can cure the anemia but not the myelopathy.

Progressive, chronic, spastic, or spastic-ataxia paraparesis may also develop in conjunction with chronic, decompensated liver disease. Portocaval myelopathy presents, characteristically, as a spastic paraparesis in patients with portal hypertension in whom a surgical portosystemic anastomosis has been undertaken. It is considered that the primary lesion involves Betz cells in the precentral gyrus; thus, the term *encephalomyelopathy* may be more appropriate.

Lathyrism is an acquired spastic paraplegia related to the prolonged consumption of *Lathyrus sativus* (chickling vetch, or grass pea). The toxic nature of this disease is a neuroexcitatory amino acid, beta-*N*-oxalyl-aminoalanine. This amino acid may induce corticospinal dysfunction in monkeys. The disease is still common in some parts of India, Africa, and Catalonia. In individuals exposed to periods of famine (e.g., during the civil war in Spain) who consume a diet of flour made of the grass pea, a gradual weakening of the legs with spasticity and cramps occurs, leading to a very chronic (four decades) spastic paraparesis often associated with a secondary spondylotic myelopathy or cauda equina syndrome related to degenerative changes in the spine. The symptoms are not always progressive, and most patients live out their natural life span.

Another myelopathy that closely resembles lathyrism or TSP is subacute myelo-optic neuropathy. It has been attributed to use of iodochlorhydroxyquin to treat traveler's diarrhea. This kind of myelopathy has been observed specifically in Japan. Several intrathecally injected chemotherapeutic agents, among them methotrexate and cytarabine, can cause an acute myelopathy. A transverse myelopathy has also been reported with chemonucleolysis by chymopapain, as have fatal allergic reactions.

Adrenomyeloneuropathy is a related X-linked leukodystrophy with relatively later onset and a slow course. The majority of these patients have adrenal insufficiency (Addison's disease) beginning in childhood and usually in the second or third decade develop neurologic symptoms with progressive spastic paraparesis and, in some cases, peripheral neuropathy. Most patients are male but there may also be symptomatic heterozygotes—that is, a female carrier. A definitive diagnosis can be made by demonstrating high levels of very long chain fatty acids in plasma, leukocytes, or cultured fibroblasts. Adrenal replacement therapy may prolong life and occasionally effects a partial neurologic remission.

Myelopathies Caused by Physical Agents

Electric Currents and Lightning.   Among acute physical injuries to the SC, those caused by electric currents and lightning should be mentioned because the cord is specifically vulnerable to electric shocks. Significant factors associated with the extent of injury are the amount of amperage (not voltage), duration of contact, resistance of skin (less resistance when covered with water), and path of the current (the cord is particularly at risk with an arm-to-arm path). After electrical or lightning injuries, an immediate disturbance of sensorimotor function of a limb or of all the limbs may occur. It usually disappears within 12–24 hours, but in some instances it may persist. Delayed (weeks or months) myelopathy may also occur resembling amyotrophic lateral sclerosis (ALS).

Radiation Myelopathy.   Radiation myelopathy is an uncommon complication of radiation therapy of the spine when the treatment plan does not allow for protection of the SC. Its incidence correlates positively with the total radiation dose, dose per fraction, and length of the SC irradiated. The latent period of radiation myelopathy has two distinct peaks: One is 12–14 months and the other 24–28 months. The histopathologic features of radiation myelopathy consist primarily of a white matter parenchymal lesion, a primary vascular lesion, or a combination of both. The gray matter is rarely involved. Clinically, the onset is insidious and painless, usually with sensory symptoms and weakness of one or both lower extremities. It progresses at first rapidly and then more slowly, but later the syndrome is that of a transverse myelopathy. It must be stressed that radiation myelopathy is an iatrogenic disease and is therefore preventable. Treatment for radiation myelopathy has been disappointing, but steroids have been helpful in some patients.

Caisson Disease (Decompression Sickness). Caisson disease derives its name from the French word *caisson* (for "wooden boxes"). This disease impairs individuals subjected to high underwater pressure. Lesions of an ischemic type are mainly observed in the white matter of the upper thoracic cord, preferentially in the posterior columns. The clinical features are extreme pain, paraplegia, and involuntary flexion of the trunk ("the bends"). Treatment requires immediately placing the patient in a hyperbaric chamber; later treatment of neurologic residuals is the same as for similar defects from other causes.

Spinal Epidural Abscess, Pott's Disease

Spinal epidural abscess is uncommon, but it is important to be aware of this disease process because early diagnosis improves outcome. MRI appears to greatly facilitate the diagnosis. *Staphylococcus aureus* is the most frequent etiologic agent and usually is a complication of direct extension from a vertebral osteomyelitis or discitis. Chronically, granulation tissue rather than frank pus is typically present. At first, the suppurative process, with or without fever, presents with back pain or with nuchal rigidity when the location is cervical or even with a selective rotational limitation of the head when the location is at the highest cervical level (C1) or at the odontoid process. After several more days with motor weakness, sensory loss in the extremities and sphincter disturbances may appear. Percussion of the spine elicits tenderness over the site of the infection. An acute form can progress over an interval of 24 hours to a few days, and rapid diagnosis is obviously very important because timely treatment and decompression can save neurologic function. The CSF contains a small number of white cells (usually fewer than 100 per µl), the protein content is high (200–300 mg per 100 ml or more), and the glucose level is normal. MRI is the most sensitive technique for detecting spinal epidural abscesses. The sagittal image is the most useful for demonstrating disc space or adjacent vertebral body involvement (Figure 31-2). Osteomyelitis may not be seen early on in standard x-ray films, and bone scans and MRI are more sensitive. Antibiotics in large doses must be given. Surgical treatment by drainage (by laminectomy or through an anterolateral approach) must be carried out. Definitive treatment depends on the nature of the underlying disease and the general condition of the patient.

The diagnosis of a subacute pyogenic infection and granulomatous infections (tuberculous or others) depends on the demonstration of a partial or complete block of the spinal canal on MRI scans. Tuberculosis is the most common cause of vertebral body infection particularly in Third World countries. Currently, AIDS is responsible for a reappearance of tuberculosis in developed countries. The SC may be affected in a number of ways during the course of a tuberculous infection. SC symptoms may accompany vertebral caries (Pott's paraplegia) and are then caused by compression by an epidural mass of granulation tissue or by a mechanical effect of angulation of the spine. The treatment of tuberculous meningomyelitis consists of the administration of a combination of drugs—isoniazid; rifampin; and a third drug, which may be ethambutol, ethionamide, or preferably pyrazinamide. Corticosteroids should be used only in life-threatening situations.

Tabes Dorsalis (Tabetic Neurosyphilis)

Tabes dorsalis, the tabetic type of neurosyphilis, usually develops 15–20 years after the onset of the infection. Syphilis is caused by a slender, spiral motile organism, *Treponema pallidum*. Tabes dorsalis can occur as an isolated form of tertiary syphilis affecting the SC. It is a myelopathy associated with atrophic, degenerated, and demyelinated dorsal nerve roots and posterior spinal column. A triad of symptoms (lightning-like pains, dysuria, and ataxia) and a triad of signs (Argyll-Robertson pupil, areflexia, and loss of proprioception) are characteristics of this disorder. Diagnostic confirmation of neurosyphilis is based on a positive serum fluorescent treponeural antibody absorption test, CSF pleocytosis, elevated CSF protein levels, and a positive CSF Venereal Disease Research Laboratory (VDRL) test. MRI may reveal hyperintensities on T2-weighted images involving the posterior third of the thoracic and lumbar SC (Figure 31-3). Symptoms of tabetic neurosyphilis are often not influenced by treatment with penicillin, the drug of choice for all varieties of neurosyphilis. Lightning-like pains may respond to phenytoin or to carbamazepine.

Multiple Sclerosis

MS clinically begins in many patients as a myelopathic syndrome. The most common symptoms and signs attributable to SC MS can be separated into two main categories, according to motor and sensory disturbances:

1. An asymmetric spastic paraparesis is the most common motor abnormality. The predominant findings are of upper motor neuron dysfunction (spasticity, extensor plantar responses, hyperreflexia). Loss of muscle stretch reflex may occur from demyelination at the dorsal root. These motor forms predominate in men.
2. Ataxic paraparesis and an asymmetric proprioceptive sensory deficit in the limbs are probably the most common manifestations of MS affecting the SC, and purely spinal involvement may occur with no clinical signs being found outside of the SC. Examination of the sensory system is sometimes difficult, but it is useful to establish a sensory level when possible. Posterior column function loss can also be established clinically or after somatosensory evoked potential testing. Quantifying and localizing pain and thermal sensation are more problematic (or not possible).

The clinical forms that involve selectively the posterior columns at the cervical level, preferentially at the cuneatus fasciculi unilaterally or bilaterally, seem to be much more frequent in young women, and according to our experience, they present a clear tendency to spontaneous clinical reversibility with a remaining good state for a long time.

MRI is the best imaging modality for directly visualizing intramedullary demyelinating plaques in MS. Correlation between the location of the plaque in sagittal and axial sections on MRI scans and clinical myelopathic findings are good (Figure 31-4).

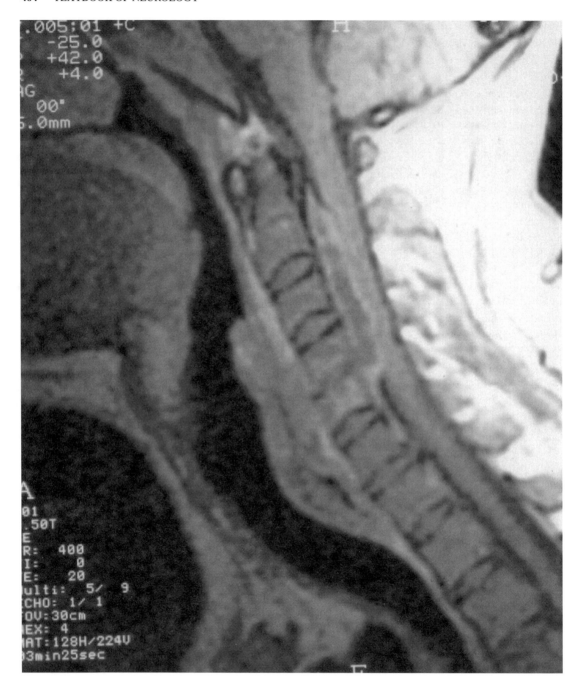

Figure 31-2. Epidural abscess. Pyogenic cervical vertebral osteomyelitis with associated epidural abscess. A 48-year-old man with diabetes mellitus and a 3-week history of cervical pain, and mild left hemiparesis. A magnetic resonance imaging scan of the midsagittal cervical spine (1.5T; SE 400/20) demonstrated loss of height at the C4–C5 interspace. An epidural soft tissue mass produces mild compression of the cervical cord. Anteriorly there is a large prevertebral mass. The patient underwent surgery with a good result. He is asymptomatic at present.

Figure 31-3. Tabes dorsalis. A T2-weighted magnetic resonance imaging scan of the SC showing a hypersignal symmetrically located in the posterior aspect of the thoracic spinal cord. Note the reduced volume of the parenchymal cord tissue compared with the high signal of the surrounding cerebrospinal fluid.

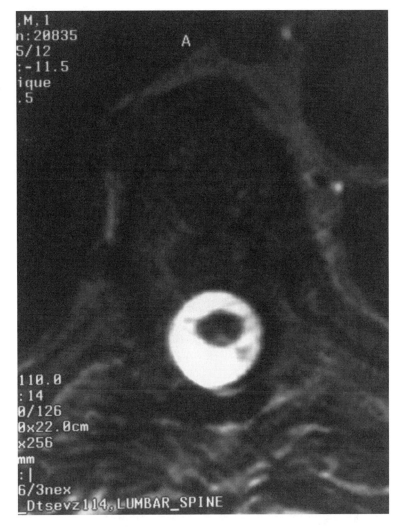

This correlation allows an approximate prognosis to be established, especially when plaques are dorsally located at the cervical level (good prognosis), when MRI shows cord atrophy (poor prognosis), or when segmental fusiform enlargement of the cord is present (unpredictable prognosis).

System Degeneration

System degeneration of the SC includes pure motor syndromes, especially hereditary spastic paraplegia (HSP), spinal muscular atrophies (SMAs), and ALS. System degenerations also include sensorimotor degenerative diseases, the syndrome complex of Friedreich's ataxia being the best known. The SC syndrome component features (initiated in childhood) include developing ataxia, dysarthria, areflexia, and loss of position sense. The sporadic form of ALS, a disease of middle and late life, is the most common pure motor syndrome seen in everyday practice. Classically, it begins with cramps and atrophy of the small muscles of the hand, appearing first asymmetrically, within months of evolution. Atrophy, fasciculations, and weakness appear later in the shoulders, arms, tongue, and other muscles. A rare but distinctive syndrome of primary lateral

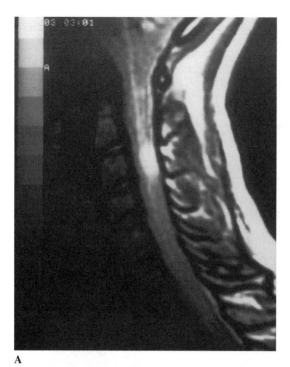

A

Figure 31-4. Multiple sclerosis in the acute phase. A 21-year-old woman with known cerebral multiple sclerosis lesions presented with a deafferentation of both upper limbs as the only clinical manifestation. The magnetic resonance imaging (MRI) study shown here was done in 1993. Sagittal (A) and axial (B) T2-weighted scans show the acute plaque located at the C3 level and occupying the dorsal part of the cord. In 1997, the patient was asymptomatic and the MRI findings of the cord were normal.

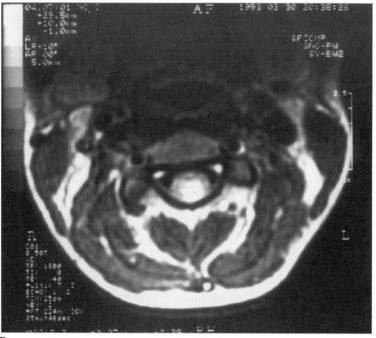

B

sclerosis (when evidence of lower motor neuron deficit is not present within 2 years of the onset of symptoms) features exclusively spastic weakness. SMAs are motor neuron diseases that affect only the lower motor neuron (alpha motor neuron), and they must be differentiated into generalized forms, focal forms, and secondary forms. HSP is a heterogeneous syndrome that affects the corticospinal tracts alone. All these systemic degenerations are treated extensively in other parts of this textbook (Chapter 43).

Spondylogenic Myelopathies

The SC is obviously vulnerable to any vertebral disease or maldevelopment that encroaches on the spinal canal or compresses its arteries, which supply nutrients. The most frequent of these circumstances are spondylosis and disc herniations.

Cervical Myelopathy

The term *cervical myelopathy* refers to the chronic medullary complications of cervical spinal stenosis as the main cause of cervical spondylosis (CS).

Historical Note.   The first cases of "CS with paraplegia" were described at the end of the last century by Strümpell (1888), Pierre Marie (1898), and Betcherew (1899). Later on, interest was devoted to the acute ruptured disc. Russell Brain (1948) was the first to establish the difference between cervical disc herniation and chronic SC compression consequent on disc degeneration, associated osteophytic bars, and thickening in the surrounding joint and ligaments. Payne and Spillane (1957) emphasized the importance of narrowing in the genesis of myelopathy in patients with CS and we pointed out the main clinical signs of the disease. A model reference of the natural history of CS myelopathy is given by Rowland (1992).

Cervical Spondylotic Myelopathy.   The term *cervical spondylotic myelopathy* (CSM) is given to the cervical myelopathy produced by the bony and soft tissue changes of CS. CSM is the most common cause of myelopathy in patients older than 55 years of age and is more common in men than in women. Long tract involvement resulting from cord compromise may be associated with radicular features.

Pathogenesis.   There is no consensus about the nature of cord injury in CSM. Initially, compression was thought to be the primary mechanism of CS injury (repeated compression). Vascular factors were also implicated (arterial insufficiency caused by stretching of intramedullary vessels during flexion). Narrowing of the cervical spinal canal, acquired or congenital, seems to be necessary for CSM (the range of narrowing that produces CSM is 7–12 mm, the normal values being 17–18 mm). The current literature supports a combined mechanism (repeated compression, narrow canal, vascular insufficiency).

Symptomatology.   The classic presentation of CSM consists of varying combinations of a stiff and painful neck and shoulder, numb hands, and, the most characteristic, spastic leg weakness (spastic paraparesis) with unsteadiness of gait. Each of these components may occur separately (especially spastic paraparesis), or they may occur in several combinations. Motor findings are myelopathic (spastic paraparesis, hypertonia in both lower limbs), but they may also be radicular (arm weakness, muscle atrophy, fasciculations). Urinary urgency or hesitancy is relatively rare. Sensory findings are variable. Decreased posterior column function in the lower extremities and a positive Romberg's sign may be significant in some cases. Lhermitte's sign is relatively uncommon. Reflexes tend to reflect the radiculopathy or the myelopathy (changes in the tendon reflexes in the arms, briskness of reflexes in the legs, Babinski's sign). An interesting study has shown that a positive Hoffmann's sign during neck flexion, a "dynamic Hoffmann's" could be a specific finding in CSM. Spread of reflexes appears regularly in the upper extremities of patients with CSM. Reflexes may also be inverted in the arms, as in the case of a lesion of the sixth or seventh cervical segments; here, the brachioradialis and the triceps reflexes are abolished and only the finger flexors and the biceps, whose reflex arcs are intact, respond to the radial or tricipital tap. Disease progression is not well defined; CSM sometimes progresses intermittently with long periods of relatively unchanging symptomatology.

Diagnosis. Imaging is essential in the diagnosis of CSM. MRI provides excellent visualization of the SC and extradural compression caused by spondylosis. On high-quality T2-weighted images, intrinsic cord changes may be demonstrated. MRI is helpful in differentiating CSM from tumors, vascular malformations, and epidural abscesses of the spine. Other intrinsic lesions of the cord are not so easily distinguished by conventional imaging. Included in this group are ALS, MS, neurosyphilis, and subacute combined system diseases (vitamin B_{12} deficiency). Appropriate screening tests are available for the majority of these diseases. ALS may raise major difficult questions. Nevertheless, ALS has seldom been a diagnostic problem: Very few patients with CSM present with an absolutely pure motor syndrome (impairment of vibratory sense in the legs; sensory symptoms in the arms must be sought through a careful history, physical examination, or electrophysiologic studies). A pure spastic paraparesis is more likely to be a manifestation of MS, HSP, multiple infarctions in the brain stem (signs of palmomental reflex would be present), liver failure, and adrenoleukodystrophy.

Treatment. Treatment constitutes the major area of controversy in this disease. The use of a soft collar to restrict anteroposterior motions of the neck and anti-inflammatory medication seems reasonable. Patients who do not improve after 5 months of conservative therapy do not show any improvement after longer periods. When the disease progresses, with a significantly narrowed canal and severe neurologic compromise, surgical treatment is usually indicated with two aims: The first is to decompress the SC and nerve roots, the second is to slow progression of the disease by reducing the hypermobility of the cervical spine. There are two surgical approaches: the posterior approach (cervical laminectomy, with difficulty in removing anterior osteophytes), and the anterior approach (decompressing the cervical spine with direct removal of the offending tissues and interbody fusion). With more widespread osteophytic overgrowth, the anterior approach has given better results and carries less risk.

Cervical Disc Herniation with Spinal Cord Compression. Disc herniation in the cervical spine can cause compression of the SC and nerve roots in two ways. A disc herniation can evolve acutely (soft disc herniation) or as an osteophyte (hard disc herniation). Disc herniation most commonly involves a single level but involves two levels in 6% of cases. Cervical herniations most commonly (90%) occur at the C5–C6 or C6–C7 levels. The clinical symptoms include various combinations:

1. Isolated radiculopathy (45%)
2. Isolated myelopathy (24%) with the following rare possibilities: quadriplegia, bilateral arm weakness, quadriparesis, Brown-Séquard syndrome, hemiparesis, hemiplegia, isolated paraparesis/paraplegia, ataxia, or amyotrophy
3. A combination of radiculopathy and myelopathy (25%)

The evolution can be acute, subacute, or chronic. Typically, the clinical picture of soft disc herniation is that of a young man with an acute radiculopathy after cervical trauma. Rarely, the clinical picture can be dominated by myelopathy. Nevertheless, signs of motor radicular deficit (amyotrophy, brachial, radial, or triceps decreased reflexes) associated with spastic paraparesis constitute the classic symptomatology. Sometimes the clinical findings of cervical disc herniation resemble those of degenerative disease, but a careful history and physical examination associated with good radiologic investigations usually help to establish the correct diagnosis. MRI is the examination of choice in patients with disc herniation, because it displays on sagittal images as well as axial images (Figure 31-5) the relationship between the disc herniation and the subarachnoid space and the SC. The best results after surgical treatment are obtained with an anterior surgical approach when dealing with soft disc herniations. If the herniation is laterally located, a posterior approach usually leads to a good result.

Thoracic Disc Herniation and Thoracic Spinal Stenosis

Herniated discs in the thoracic region are being increasingly recognized because of the ease of scanning the thoracic spine with MRI. A thoracic herniated disc may present exclusively as back pain but usually presents with some form of a Brown-

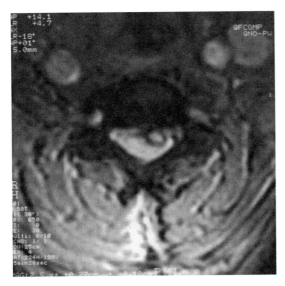

Figure 31-5. Left paramedial C5–C6 disc herniation. A 64-year-old man with a short neck and presumably narrow cervical spinal canal presented with a subacute left Brown-Séquard syndrome. The axial magnetic resonance imaging (MRI) section through C5 and C6 shows a high-intensity signal posterior and lateral to vertebral body. It was consistent with soft disc material found at surgery. The herniation was completely removed and the patient became asymptomatic.

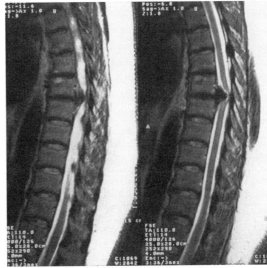

Figure 31-6. Calcified T8–T9 disc herniation. This 52-year-old woman presented with Brown-Séquard syndrome, left lower extremity weakness, spasticity, and thermalgesic disturbances in her contralateral lower extremity. Sagittal T2-weighted magnetic resonance imaging scans, left paramedial and medial, show how the calcified disc herniation compressing the cord at the level of T8–T9 has very low intensity. Surgical treatment was postponed for the moment.

Séquard syndrome. The patient is typically middle aged with a history of a stepwise, slowly progressive, midthoracic anterior hemicord syndrome manifesting as hemianalgesia below the affected segment followed by contralateral lower limb spasticity that develops into an asymmetric paraparesis with sparing of dorsal column sensation. Because of the normal dorsal kyphotic curvature, the thoracic cord is positioned close to the vertebral bodies, and therefore a small disc herniation can produce a significant myelopathy. Large herniations of a calcifying nucleus pulposus also occur in the thoracic region (Figure 31-6), making their removal a neurosurgical challenge. A congenital stenosis of the thoracic canal is rare and may be associated with achondroplasia or mucopolysaccharidosis. Acquired stenosis may be related to thickening and ossification of the ligamentum flavum. Clinical symptoms range from simple radicular or back pain to neurogenic claudication when walking. A mixture of pyramidal signs and peripheral neuropathy are found when the stenosis is localized to lower

levels, between T10 and T12. Other causes of non-tumoral stenosis that may lead to a thoracic cord compression are Paget's disease (Figure 31-7) and epidural lipomatosis. Epidural lipomatosis consists of increased epidural fat within the spinal canal, and this condition is related to patients with an underlying endocrinopathy or being treated chronically with steroids.

Lumbar Stenosis

Lumbar stenosis is another spondylotic abnormality related to the cauda equina syndrome that results from a congenitally narrowed canal, spondylosis, or both. It is frequent in older people, and the clinical features are often characteristic. After a long period of walking, especially downhill, painful paresthesias appear in both legs, often asymmetrically, sometimes ascending up to the buttocks. They can force the patient to stop and sit. The ankle reflex may disappear and reappear. This neurogenic claudication must be differentiated from vascular claudication. In contrast to

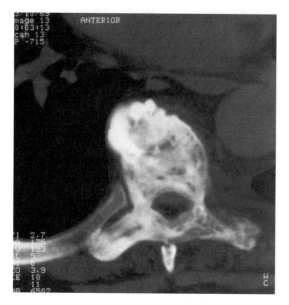

Figure 31-7. Paget's disease of the thoracic spine. A 40-year-old man presented with a slight but progressive spastic paraparesis. Hypertrophy of several vertebral bodies and of the corresponding neural arches resulting in central canal stenosis was apparent. Surgical treatment (decompressive laminectomy) was carried out and the patient improved dramatically.

vascular claudication, those with lumbar stenosis typically lack the acute pain, and stopping does not bring about a complete relief of symptoms; relief is better obtained by flexing the spine. Plain films and computed tomographic and MRI scans are mandatory for correctly studying a narrow lumbar canal. Electromyography may show radicular lumbosacral abnormalities and allows other polyneuropathies to be excluded. When the syndrome progresses (when the amount of walking before symptoms appear becomes shorter and shorter), surgical treatment must be considered, but each particular case requires an accurate evaluation in order to promote the best tactical and technical therapeutic approach.

When the acquired narrowing of the lumbar canal is caused by a spondylolisthesis (spondylolisthesis is the forward slippage of a vertebral body relative to the vertebral body beneath it, whatever its cause), the choice of treatment becomes more difficult.

Anomalies at the Craniocervical Junction

Among the skull base anomalies, the most frequent consist of a congenital fusion, partial or total, of the

atlas and axis with the occipital bone. The size of the foramen magnum then may be reduced (critical minimal diameter, 19 mm) with evidence of cord compression. The base of the skull may also be flattened (platybasia) and there may be an ascension of the bony structures (basilar impression or invagination).

The clinical syndrome may feature vestibular or cerebellar or brain stem disturbances (MS-like) or cord syndromes from local compression, sometimes mimicking ALS (a combination of lower cranial nerve involvement with signs attributed to a pyramidal tract lesion). The cord syndrome appears, especially in cases of atlantoaxial dislocation, related to a cruciate or alar ligament lesion that may be congenital (hypoplasia), acquired (inflammatory), or traumatic. If the upper cervical cord is compressed, the odontoid process must be removed and C1–C2 decompressed and stabilized.

Intraspinal Tumors

SC tumors are histologically similar to brain tumors, but they occur considerably less frequent than tumors that involve the brain. The relationship of the SC to its meninges (extensive meningeal surface covering a relatively small amount of parenchymal tissue) is the inverse of that between the brain and its meninges (voluminous mass of glial tissue being surrounded by a relatively reduced surface of meninges), and this explains the higher frequency of meningeal tumors in the spinal region as opposed to the frequency of tumors of glial origin in this same region. Thus, the majority of intraspinal tumors are benign and produce their effects mainly by compression of the SC rather than by invasion. Metastases are typically extradural, whereas brain metastases are generally intracerebral. In accordance with the origins of these neoplastic lesions, intraspinal tumors fall into three large categories (Figure 31-8): extradural neoplastic tumors, intradural extramedullary neoplastic tumors, and intramedullary tumors (ITs). This classification is based on the topographical relationship between the spine and spinal cord (see Figure 31-8A).

Extradural neoplastic tumors (see Figure 31-8D) are the most frequent intraspinal tumors. The tumors are predominantly metastatic, usually an extension of nearby neoplasms, and most often malignant (carcinoma, lymphoma, myeloma). They arise from hematogenous dissemination or extension of tumors from the vertebral bodies or paravertebral tissues via intervertebral foramina. The spine is a favorite site for metastasis from primary tumors of the lung, breast, thyroid, and prostate. The involvement of the vertebral body or pedicle often causes backache before evidence of disturbance in cord function, and a long time (months) may pass between the appearance of back pain and the signs of a compressive myelopathy. Limb weakness, paresthesias in the distribution of a nerve root, and bowel or bladder dysfunction suggest a neurologic emergency that requires prompt evaluation and treatment. MRI is the most sensitive technique for the detection of spinal osseous metastasis. Radiotherapy has become the preferred form of therapy for most patients with spine metastasis. High-dose corticosteroids and fractionated radiation are as effective as surgery. Sometimes, with a rapidly growing tumor, laminectomy and decompression are necessary. When a posterior decompressive laminectomy is used, postoperative radiotherapy is mandatory.

Much more uncommon neoplasms of the spine are the benign osteogenic and chondrogenic tumors. Some of them may result in SC compression. Also, a disc herniation may represent a benign cause of extradural SC compression (see Figure 31-6).

Intradural extramedullary neoplastic tumors (see Figure 31-8C) arise from supporting structures: meninges (meningiomas), nerve sheath (neurofibromas), or Schwann cells (schwannomas or neurinomas). They are usually benign. Meningiomas are more common in aged women and are often in the thoracic region (Figure 31-9). Schwannomas and neurofibromas appear predominantly in the cervical and lumbar regions. They are often associated (when they are multiple) with neurofibromatosis type I (neurofibromas) or more frequently with neurofibromatosis type II (schwannomas). The attachment site is especially in the dorsal nerve root and in some cases they may extend into the extradural space through the neural foramina (dumbbell-shaped tumors). When these tumors are large, they may displace the cord. Typically the syndrome of SC compression is associated with radicular pain, which radiates in a distal direction and is intensified by coughing, sneezing, or straining. Other segmental signs, particularly sensory ones, may precede the signs of SC compression by months.

Uncommon causes of extramedullary tumors include dermoid or epidermoid tumors (predilection for the lumbosacral region), lipomas (frequently

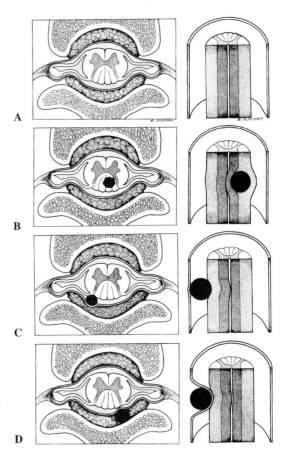

Figure 31-8. Diagrammatic representation of spinal tumors and their location with respect to the spinal canal and its contents. (A) Anatomy of the spine and the spinal cord in the axial plane. (B) Intramedullary tumor. (C) Intradural extramedullary tumor. (D) Extradural tumor. The black round image represents the location of the tumor.

attached to the posterior aspect of the SC), arachnoid cysts, and others. All these tumors should be removed as soon as possible after their discovery.

ITs (see Figure 31-8B) and tumors of the cauda equina (CE) comprise 2–4% of all central nervous system tumors and 20% of all adult intradural spinal tumors. Ependymomas that also can arise from the filum terminale represent approximately 60% of cases, astrocytomas approximately 20%, and the remainder (20%) consist of a diverse group of tumors: lipomas that are usually not amenable to a complete resection, epidermoids, hemangioblastomas, ependymomas (often from the filum terminale), and astrocytomas. The most common initial symptom is pain adjacent to the affected spinal

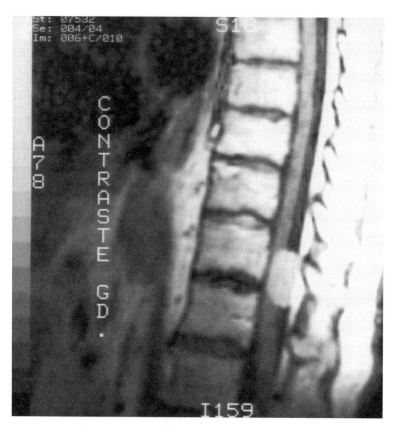

Figure 31-9. Thoracic intraspinal tumor (meningioma) at T9–T10. A 70-year-old woman had proprioceptive sensory disturbances referred to her lower extremities and a progressive ataxic gait for the preceding 2 years. A magnetic resonance imaging scan with gadolinium contrast shows in this sagittal section an oval tumor with distinct borders that is slightly enhanced by the contrast. The tumor, located posteriorly, intradurally, and extramedullary, displaces the spinal cord forward. After the tumor was removed, the patient became asymptomatic.

region with a tendency to be diffuse depending on the level of the tumor and worse at night. Some patients report paresthesias that tend to extend caudally with time. A smaller group of patients present with weakness. At the cervical level, SC tumors may cause wasting confined to the patient's hands. The classic sensory deficit is a dissociated suspended sensory level that descends with time. Incontinence is usually a late manifestation and appears coincident with paralysis of the legs. Patients rarely present with sudden neurologic deficits secondary to a hemorrhage into the tumor (hemangioblastomas). In children, back pain, scoliosis, and spasm of the paravertebral muscles are often the prominent symptoms in the early stages of intramedullary SC tumors. Because of this unusual clinical presentation, SC tumors in this age group may be overlooked.

Pain is also the most common presenting symptom of the tumors of the CE and may precede weakness or sphincter disturbances by several years. Pain is more severe at night or when the patient assumes a recumbent position, and pain is mitigated when the patient stands or sits up.

Patients occasionally present with papilledema, which is presumably the result of an increase of spinal fluid protein. Surgery has been reported to be successful in removing approximately 50% of mixopapillary ependymomas. Hemangioblastomas have a propensity to appear on the dorsum of the SC and can be identified by the tortuous vessels and varices emerging from their surface. One-third of patients with hemangioblastomas present with von Hippel-Lindau disease. There is a frequent association between intramedullary gliomatous or nongliomatous tumors and syringomyelia, the hemangioblastomas being by far the tumors in which this association is most frequent. The basis of this relationship probably depends on disturbances in the interstitial intramedullary fluids created by the tumor that block the subarachnoid spaces at the level of the tumor in those cases with an added disturbance in hydrodynamics of the CSF. Among the secondary ITs, intramedullary metastasis is not as rare as is generally believed. Diagnosis is sometimes difficult. Because of its high sensitivity, MRI can demonstrate the presence

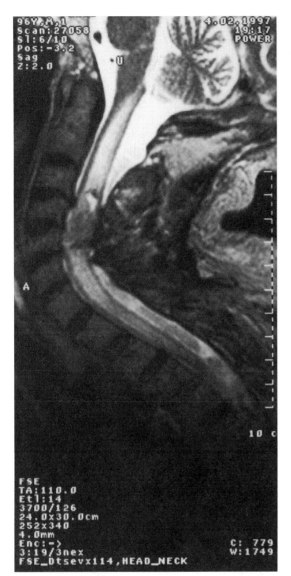

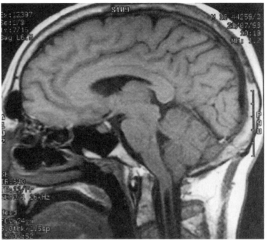

Figure 31-11. Syringomyelia associated with Chiari type-1 malformation. A sagittal magnetic resonance imaging scan. The cervical syrinx cavity extended cephalad to C1–C2. Note the Chiari type-1 malformation (cerebellar tonsils located below the foramen magnum) and the narrowness of the cisterna magna and platybasia. There is no communication between the syrinx and the ventricular system.

Syringomyelia

In 1824, Ollivier d'Angers first used the term *syringomyelia* (from de Greek *syrinx*, meaning "pipe" or "tube" and *muelos* meaning "cord") to describe a chronic progressive degenerative disorder of the SC presenting with intramedullary cavities unconnected with the central canal. Simon suggested in 1875 that the term *syringomyelia* be reserved for such cavities and that the term *hydromyelia* be restricted to simple dilatation of the central canal. Imaging modalities cannot always distinguish syringomyelia from hydromyelia and so the terms *hydrosyringomyelia* and *syringomyelia* are more frequently used. Frequently, there are associated abnormalities of the spine (thoracic scoliosis), the base of the skull (platybasia, reduced dimensions of the posterior fossa, stenosis of the foramen magnum), and the cerebellum and medulla oblongata, which extend caudally through the foramen magnum (Chiari type-1 malformation) (Figure 31-11). Approximately 90% of cases of syringomyelia have Chiari type-1 malformation: The term *primary (or foraminal) syringomyelia* is reserved for those cases of syringomyelia in which

Figure 31-10. Intramedullary metastasis from bronchogenic carcinoma. A 78-year-old man with bilateral brachialgia for several weeks and recent paraplegia. A sagittal T2-weighted magnetic resonance imaging scan shows a hypointense tumor nodule at C4–C5 surrounded by extensive hyperintense areas caused by edema.

of intramedullary metastasis (Figure 31-10). Radiation therapy should be used in those cases before paraplegia appears. The treatment of intramedullary gliomas should consist of laminectomy, decompression, and excision with aid of an operating microscope and radiotherapy.

no other abnormalities except a Chiari type-1 malformation are found. The Chiari type-1 malformation may be the consequence of the reduced dimensions of the posterior fossa. Exceptionally, the foramen magnum is obstructed by a lesion other than a Chiari type-1 malformation (dural cyst, occipitoatlantal fusion, basilar invagination). The term *secondary syringomyelia* is reserved for those cases in which syringomyelia is associated with other diseases of the SC or spine, such as SC tumors, usually intramedullary and especially hemangioblastoma traumatic myelopathy, or arachnoiditis or even spondylosis with a narrow spinal canal. The term *idiopathic syringomyelia* is reserved for an intramedullary cavity not associated with bony or neural malformation at the craniocervical junction, or with tumor, trauma, or infection. Idiopathic syrinx is rare, and an MRI scan with gadolinium is mandatory to rule out a tiny tumor nodule.

Pathogenetic Hypothesis

It is now accepted that primary syringomyelia can appear after a hydrodynamic disturbance of the CSF related with a congenital or acquired obstruction of the foramen magnum. Using dynamic MRI studies, it has been possible to demonstrate in patients with Chiari type-1 malformation the disappearance of the rapid to-and-fro movement of CSF in the subarachnoid space across the obstructed foramen magnum and the flow of CSF rostrally in the sylvian aqueduct during systole. At the same time, the tonsils are the object of an abrupt caudal movement.

The pistonlike effect of this movement imparts an accentuated systolic pressure wave to the spinal subarachnoid CSF (partially isolated from the cranial subarachnoid space). This acts on the posterior surface of the SC (1) to propel the fluid into the cord, particularly at the entrance of the posterior roots (Lissauer's zone)—this explains the preferential location of the lesion in the posterior horns in the majority of syringomyelias; and (2) the increase sometimes of the bulk movement of CSF in the cord. This may represent the mechanism for maintaining the syrinx and even explain its progression. Thus, progression of the syrinx cavity is the result of hydrodynamic mechanisms. The cavitation is nearly always located in a sym-

metric or asymmetric position in the cervical portion of the cord. It generally occupies the gray matter, where it produces damage preferentially in the sensory tract (in the posterior horns) or in the motor neurons (of the anterior horns). This may interrupt the crossing pain and temperature fibers at the anterior commissure, and when the cavity enlarges, it may extend into the lateral and posterior funiculi of the cord. Occasionally, the cavity may extend into the medulla oblongata, dissecting the descending tract of the fifth cranial nerve so that the facial sensory loss does not necessarily mean syringobulbia.

The current classification of syringomyelia, modified from Barnett and related to extensive experience with the disease and the pathogenetic mechanism of the disease is as follows:

I. Primary (or foraminal) syringomyelia with obstruction of the foramen magnum with abnormalities at the craniocervical junction (the great majority being related to Chiari type-1 malformation).

II. Secondary syringomyelia related to other diseases of the SC:
Intraspinal tumors (intramedullary or not)
Spinal chronic arachnoiditis
Traumatic myelopathy related to spine injury
Chronic vascular myelopathy related to cord compression (spondylosis, narrow canal, arachnoidal cysts, tumor).

III. Idiopathic syringomyelia without obstruction of the foramen magnum and without any other intraspinal recognizable lesion.

IV. Pure hydromyelia associated or not with hydrocephalus.

These different types have been listed according to their frequency of presentation in clinical practice: The great majority are primary or foraminal syringomyelias.

Clinical Symptoms

The syringomyelic cavity generally develops very slowly over years or decades and is more common in men (64%) than in women (36%). Exceptionally, the cavity may developed abruptly. The disease may be discovered at any age, but it is most frequent in the third decade of life. The initial clinical manifestations of syringomyelia are protean:

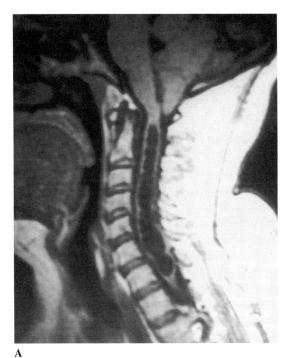
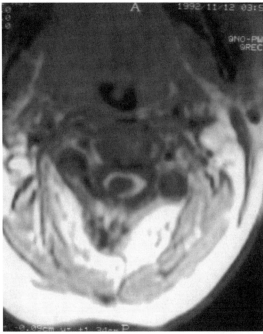

A   B

Figure 31-12. Primary (foraminal) syringomyelia. A 48-year-old woman with right chronic cervicobrachialgia. (A,B) Presurgical magnetic resonance imaging (MRI) scans. (A) Sagittal section. The voluminous cervical syrinx cavity extending cephalad to C1–C2. (B) Cervical axial section. The cavity communicates with the subarachnoid space at the posterolateral level through the posterior horns.

1. Pain is not a rare condition and may be the first symptom. The pain is usually unilateral and can mimic chronic brachialgia or arthritic shoulder pain. Sometimes the symptoms consist only of paresthesias and are preceded by posterior occipitocervical pain intensified by coughing, laughing, or sneezing and may appear syncope-like. Pain in syringomyelia appears clearly related in some cases to damage of the posterior horns (Figure 31-12A and B).
2. Sometimes, patients consult a doctor because they have lost the normal feeling of hot and cold, they have burned a finger without noticing it, or they have trophic disorders of the hand presenting as an arthropathy, especially in the shoulder or in the elbow.
3. Sometimes an atrophy of the hand is discovered accidentally. Other motor disorders, such as proximal paresis in the upper limb or even an atrophy of muscles innervated by the eleventh cranial nerve, may represent the first sign of the disease.

4. Thoracic kyphoscoliosis or other skeletal abnormalities leading to a suspected cervico-occipital or even cranial malformation (short neck, low hairline, turricephaly) are present long before the actual clinical manifestations of syringomyelia in some patients. Familial antecedents of syringomyelia or coexistence of the disease in two siblings is very rare but does exist.

The neurologic examination shows a characteristic "dissociated" syndrome not always associated with additional abnoramalities more distally. The characteristic dissociated or segmental syndrome consists of the loss of pain, cold, and heat sensations with sparing of touch and positional and vibratory sensations (syringomyelic dissociation). At the onset, the sensory disorder is generally asymmetric, unilateral, and may involve the face because the sensory root of the trigeminal nerve runs down low in the cervical cord. The sensory loss may have a cape or hemicape distribution. Loss of tendon reflexes usually involves all

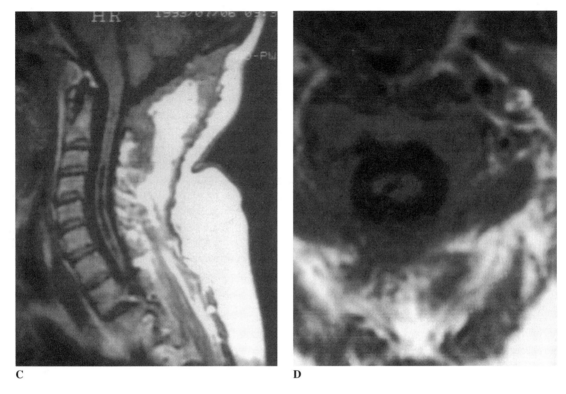

C   D

Figure 31-12. *Continued.* (C,D) Postsurgical MRI findings 8 months later. (C) After fossa posterior and posterior upper cervical decompression, the syrinx cavity appears dramatically reduced in its volume. (D) The size of the communication is also clearly diminished. The patient improved after interventions and 3 years after surgery was free of symptoms.

reflexes of the upper limb; sometimes the areflexia is one-sided, located on the same side where temperature sensation has been lost. Atrophy involves mainly the muscles of the hand, and the hand in long-standing cases often assumes a particular position ("preacher's hand," "simian hand"). Other muscles may be involved at the upper limbs and sometimes a Horner's syndrome may result because of the ipsilateral involvement of the intermediolateral cell column at C8–T1 level (Budge's center). Exceptionally there is no sensory loss in the presence of amyotrophy. There are usually few or no fasciculations.

Below the lesion there is often a very slight spastic paraparesis and, in rare cases, there is weakness and ataxia of the legs from involvement of the posterior columns in the cervical regions. There are few or no sphincter disorders.

The course of the disease is extremely variable and makes treatment decisions difficult. MRI is the best tool for demonstrating the lesion in most

instances and for allowing follow-up of the characteristics of the syrinx after the patient has undergone surgical treatment.

Treatment

The only therapy of value for primary or foraminal syringomyelia is decompression of the foramen magnum and upper cervical canal. Of course, the unpredictable course of the disease makes it difficult to establish the indications for surgical treatment. For patients whose clinical course is relentlessly progressive and whose main clinical problems are chronic pain or other subjective sensitive disturbances, surgical treatment must be done. The results are excellent in some cases (Figure 31-12C and D). Where there is hydrocephalus, ventricular shunting must precede any other type of treatment. Syringostomy, or shunting of the cavity, has been performed with good results (relief of pain) in patients with post-traumatic syringomyelia. In cases of syringomyelia with tumor, it is enough in the majority of cases to excise the tumor.

Vascular Myelopathies

It is very important to know the blood supply of the SC under normal conditions to be able to understand pathogenetic mechanisms, clinical manifestations, and even prognostic aspects in patients suffering from myelopathies related to vascular disorders.

Just as there is an extracranial and an intracranial portion of the arteries to the brain, so too is there an extraspinal and intraspinal arterial system for the cord. Pial arteries on the surface of the cord constitute three longitudinal systems, of which the main arterial system is the anterior-midline ASA. The two smaller systems are the paramedial posterior spinal arteries (PSAs), and between the PSAs and the ASA, there is a coronal system around the cord with poor anastomotic flow. The ASA originates from the confluence of two branches that emerge from each vertebral artery at the intracranial level. The ASA runs caudally to the conus medullaris, where it anastomoses with the PSAs. The ASA supplies blood to the anterior two-thirds of the cord after giving off the sulcal arteries, which enter the anterior median fissure (at the cervical and thoracic levels) of the cord and alternately turn to the right and to the left, which explains the frequent asymmetry of infarctions in those spinal regions. The PSAs supply most of the posterior columns. Rostrocaudally, the arteries to the cord are derived from the vertebral arteries and branches of the aorta that through the radicular vessels feed the ASA and PSAs after dividing into ascending and descending rami that join to form the ASA and PSAs. The radicular arteries that pass through the intervertebral foramina are very reduced in number in adults. Eventually, few remain significant. There are five to eight or even less that supply the ASA, usually one at the C6–C7 level attached to the C7 root, more often on the right side, one or two small ones in the thoracic region, and one to three in the lumbosacral region, the most significant of those being the great radicular artery (or arteria radicularis magna) of Adamkiewicz, which is found on one side only, more often on the left. It passes more often at the T11–T12 level, but its origin varies widely anywhere from T8 to L2. When its origin is higher, it

exists as a supplementary circulation for the conus medullaris related to the existence of an ascending recurrent unilateral radicular artery attached to S1. When its origin is low, the entire lumbosacral cord is fed by this great radicular artery of Adamkiewicz. This artery in any case is an artery of great clinical significance.

The blood supply of the cord has two critical zones (watershed, dernier-prés, campo-limitante): One is intramedullary and located at the junction of the territories of the ASA and PSAs (selectively located in the place occupied by the crossed pyramidal tract and anterior horns), the other is intermedullary between the blood supply of the cervical and thoracic zones (at the T3–T4 level) and between the thoracic and lumbar zones (at L1–L2). Thus, in cases of critically low blood flow, the most selective vulnerability is located in the upper and lower thoracic cord.

Spinal veins drain into the longitudinal venous channels that are in continuity, rostrally, with the cranial dural sinuses. The longitudinal channels are drained by radicular veins to the extradural venous plexus, and because these systems have no valves, the blood can change direction, reflecting pressure in the neck, chest, or abdomen. It is perhaps for these anatomophysiologic reasons that venous infarctions of the SC are so rare. Also, the anastomoses with pelvic plexi could be implicated in the vertebral metastases of prostatic carcinoma or in the cerebral thrombophlebitis in gynecologic infections.

Of all vascular disorders of the SC infarction, bleeding and AVMs are the only ones that occur with any regularity.

Vascular Malformations

SC vascular malformations are usually caused by SC AVMs. AVMs of the SC are relatively rare, but in our experience, the correct diagnosis is often not made. This point is of relevance because AVMs may be treated successfully by surgery and embolization. SC AVMs first must be distinguished (Figure 31-13) from spinal dural arteriovenous fistulas or dural arteriovenous fistulas (dAVFs) fed by dural branches of the radicular arteries and drained by perimedullary veins and second from intradural arteriovenous fistulas (iAVFs) fed by arteries supplying the SC and drained by perimedullary veins.

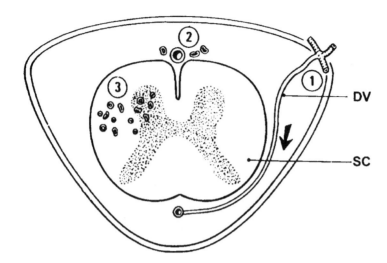

Figure 31-13. Diagrammatic representation of different vascular malformations of the spinal cord. (1) Spinal dural arteriovenous fistula. (2) Spinal perimedullary intradural arteriovenous fistula. (3) Spinal cord arteriovenous malformation with a nidus or with an arteriovenous fistula (direct fistula). (DV = dural vein; SC = spinal cord.)

Table 31-1. Clinical Symptoms of Spinal Cord Arteriovenous Malformations and Spinal Dural Arteriovenous Fistulas

Type	SC AVMs	dAVFs	iAVFs
Incidence	40%	50%	10%
Mean age (years at time of diagnosis)	35	60	45
Sex (M/F)	2/2	4/1	0/1
Location (cervical/thoracolumbar)	3/1	0/4	0/1
Back/radicular pain	25%	80%	0
Paresis			
Initially	75%	20%	Claudication to walk (Dejerine's sign)
At diagnosis	100%	80%	
Sensory changes	75%	80%	—
Sphincter disturbances			
Initially	25%	0	0
At diagnosis	75%	80%	0
Hemorrhages	50%	0	0
Evolution	Acute	Progressive	Progressive or relapsing
Flow	High +++	Low	High +

SC AVM = spinal cord arteriovenous malformation; dAVF = dural arteriovenous fistula; iAVF = intradural arteriovenous fistula.

Distinctive features of SC AVMs and AVFs (both dAVFs and iAVFs), including incidence, age, sex, location, and clinical symptoms, are presented in Table 31-1 (based on our personal experience of 10 cases: 5 dAVFs, 4 SC AVMs, and 1 iAVF). SC AVMs are frequent and usually are seen in young patients. Paresis is the initial symptom in nearly two-thirds of cases, sometimes preceded by a slight trauma. Once hemorrhage occurs, the recurrence rate within 1 year is nearly 40%. MRI shows an excavated cord when the nidus is intramedullary (Figure 31-14A). Spinal angiography demonstrates the size of the nidus and the caliber of the feeders and the draining veins (Figure 31-14B).

Spinal dAVFs (or radiculomeningeal AVMs) are the most common type of vascular malformations of the SC. By definition, the vascular nidus of these lesions lies embedded in the dura of a nerve root sleeve or adjacent spinal dura. Patients with dAVFs have a higher mean age than those with iAVFs (approximately 60 versus 45 years) and are more often male. No case of spinal hemorrhage has been reported in dAVFs. Dural AVFs are almost always located in the thoracolumbar region, whereas iAVFs are also found in the cervical segments. Pain, sensory abnormalities, sphincter disturbances, and signs of both upper and lower motor neurons are common in dAVF. Typically, dAVFs present with a slowly progressive myelopathy leading to paraparesis, sometimes mimicking the clinical picture of *myélite nécrotique subaiguë* described by Foix and Alajouanine and sometimes

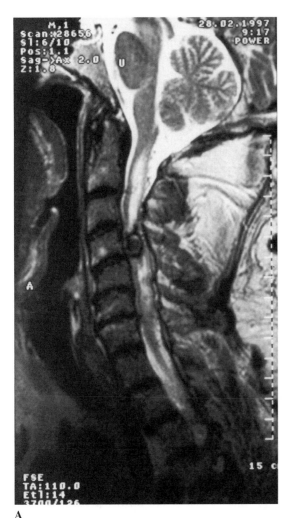

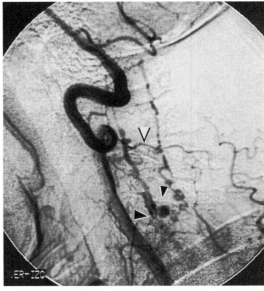

B

Figure 31-14. Cervical spinal cord arteriovenous malformation (AVM) with intramedullary hematoma. A 53-year-old man presented with cervical and unilateral brachial pain and a partial Brown-Séquard syndrome. (A) A sagittal T2-weighted magnetic resonance imaging scan shows a round area of void signal within the cord representing central cord hematoma. (B) Lateral vertebral angiography. The nidus of the AVM is supplied by anterior radiculomedullary branches from C4 and C5 (*arrows*). Hypertrophied veins with ectasias drain mainly cranially. Note the transmedullary vein (*open arrow*).

mimicking SC tumor or peripheral neuropathies such as chronic polyradiculoneuropathies. Although symptoms are commonly aggravated by activity or postural changes, dramatic *spinal transient ischemic attacks* are rarely described. Spinal iAVFs usually present as a progressive myelopathy with a very slow progression and initially may correspond to a myelopathic claudication (Dejerine). MRI can be used to identify in dAVFs serpentine linear or round low-intensity vessels around the dorsal surface of the SC. Positive MRI findings sometimes need spinal angiography to determine the type and extent of the vascular malformation. Myelography is occasionally mandatory in iAVFs to identify the presence of an abnormal vessel in the surface of the SC (Figure 31-15).

Infarction of the Spinal Cord and Spinal Cord Ischemia

SC ischemia occurs much less frequently than ischemia in the brain. The spinal arteries are not susceptible to atherosclerosis, and emboli rarely lodge there. However, clinical manifestations are similar: often abrupt in onset, dramatic in scope, and frequently disabling. Acute SC infarction (ASCI) may have many and diverse causes (Table 31-2) and occurs particularly in the territory of the ASA. The diagnosis of ASCI and particularly ASA syndrome can be confirmed nowadays by MRI scans, whereas in the past only necropsy confirmation was possible. The clinical manifestations of ASA occlusion will, of course, vary with the

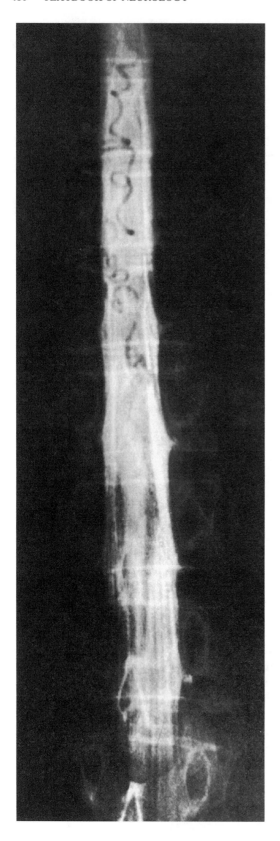

level but usually involve the territory of the ventral two-thirds of the SC to a variable vertical extent. The first description of this syndrome is attributed to Preobraschenski in 1904. It consisted of motor paralysis, usually bilateral (as a result of interruption of the pyramidal tracts). Onset is abrupt and includes initial flaccid paralysis and depression of tendon reflexes. As time progresses, the reflexes become hyperactive with Babinski's sign. Muscle atrophy of the upper extremities, particularly the extensors of the elbow and wrist preferentially on the right side, may occur when the infarction involves the cervical cord. The motor symptoms are associated with a loss of pain and temperature sensations (because of interruption of the spinothalamic tracts), but vibration and position sense, two-point discrimination, and judgment of degree of pressure are preserved (because the blood supply of the posterior columns depends on the PSAs). Bowel and bladder paralysis are common. Recovery after an ASA syndrome tends to be dependent on the severity of the initial deficit. At the cervical level, clinical and MRI findings argue in favor of extrinsic selective compression of the C7 right radiculomedullary artery as one of the main causes responsible for the ASA syndrome. At a thoracic level, the artery preferentially occluded for an ASA syndrome is related to an extrinsic selective compression. Besides the extrinsic selective compression of the radicular arteries as a cause of ASA syndrome, atherosclerosis and other occlusive diseases of the aorta and its branches must be considered. In the rare documented cases of ischemic myelopathy secondary to atherosclerosis, a progressive ischemic myelopathy is described. Atherosclerosis also has been related to the syndrome of SC claudication, a syndrome distinct from neurogenic claudication. Patients experience intermittent exercise-induced painless lower extremity weakness sometimes accompanied by

Figure 31-15. Spinal perimedullary intradural arteriovenous fistula. A 48-year-old woman presented with claudication on walking as the exclusive clinical symptomatology. The myelogram with water-soluble contrast shows dilated tortuous vessels at the level of the thoracolumbar enlargement. The spinal angiogram confirmed the diagnosis and embolization led to the disappearance of clinical symptomatology.

sphincter disturbances. Spontaneous aortic dissection may also be a cause of acute or chronic SC ischemia, the clinical presentation of SC deficits being variable. Dissecting aneurysms of the aorta usually are characterized by intense interscapular or chest pain, but some reports have stressed that they can occur without pain. The motor deficits in all pathologically proved cases of ischemic myelopathy are bilateral. The mechanism of cord ischemia appears to be occlusion of the mouths of segmental spinal arteries by the dissection. Thromboemboli as a cause of SC infarction have rarely been documented. Fibrocartilaginous embolization is described as a cause of ischemic cord infarcts, and 25 cases have been reported. SC ischemia has been recognized to occur with cardiovascular surgery, being most common in surgery involving the thoracic aorta or the abdominal aorta below the level of the renal arteries. Other iatrogenic causes of SC ischemia are intra-aortic balloon counterpulsation, continuous epidural or spinal anesthesia, and catheterization of the thoracic or abdominal vessels.

The frequency of these complications was greatly reduced by the introduction of less toxic contrast media. Infarction in the lumbosacral SC may very considerably. Lesions are determined by the different patterns in the lumbosacral arterial supply.

Treatment of all forms of spinal ischemia can be symptomatic or focus on preventing progression or recurrence. The removal of risk factors is most helpful in reducing the incidence as well as the mortality and morbidity of cord infarcts. Specific treatment measures include care of the bladder, bowel, and skin, anticoagulation in some cases, and naloxone and steroids may also be indicated.

Hematomyelia

The identifying features of hematomyelia are an apoplectic onset of medullary symptoms associated with blood in the CSF. It is usually attributed to a vascular malformation or bleeding, particularly after the administration of anticoagulants. Advances in selective spinal angiography and microsurgery have allowed the visualization and treatment of vascular lesions with a precision not imaginable a few decades ago.

Table 31-2. Causes of Ischemia and Infarction in the Territory of the Anterior Spinal Artery

Extrinsic selective compression of radiculomedullary arteries
Sprain of the cervical spine
Intervertebral disc herniation
Temporary cervical subluxation
Atherosclerosis
Hypertension
Diabetes
Fibrocartilaginous embolism
Giant cell arteritis
Arteritis related to systemic diseases (systemic lupus
    erythematosus, polyarteritis nodosa)
Isolated granulomatous angiitis
Other arteritis (related or not to spinal meningitis)
Radiation
Hypotension
    Cardiac arrest
    Traumatic rupture of aorta
    Dissection of ascending aorta
Aneurysm of the abdominal aorta
Spontaneous epidural hemorrhage
Sickle cell anemia
Syphilis
Angiography (vertebral, renal, aortic)
Surgery for aortoiliac occlusive disease
Mitral valve disease and multiple embolism
Caisson disease (decompression sickness)

Cavernous Malformation

Spinal cavernous malformation may produce an acute, recurrent, or progressive myelopathy that probably results from hemorrhage. The diagnosis of cavernous malformation is achieved with MRI (a central area of mixed signal intensity surrounded by a hypointense rim of hemosiderin). Improvement or stabilization of neurologic function can generally be anticipated. Surgical treatment must be reserved for patients with symptomatic malformations.

Suggested Reading

Adams RA, Victor M, Ropper AH. Principles of Neurology (6th ed). New York: McGraw-Hill, 1997;1227.

Armstrong RM. Myelopathies. In LA Rolak (ed), Neurology Secrets. Philadelphia: Hanley & Befus, 1993.

Casademont J, Pou Serradell A, Casademont M. Hernias discales dorsales. A propósito de cinco observaciones. Rev Esp Reumat 1988;61:1479.

Herbreteau D, Casasco A, Houdart E, et al. Malformations vasculaires vertébromédullaires: clinique, imagerie, traitment. Editions Techniques. Encycl Méd Chir (Paris), Neurologie 1995;17-067-C-10:12.

Jomin M, Lesoin F, Lozes G, Clarisse J. Les hernies discales cervicales. Deux cent trente observations. Semin Hop Paris 1985;61:1479.

Linden D, Berlit P. Spinal arteriovenous malformations: clinical and neurophysiological findings. J Neurol 1996; 243:9.

Oldfield EH, Muraszko K, Shawker TH, Patronas NJ. Pathophysiology of syringomyelia associated with Chiari I malformation of the cerebellar tonsils. J Neurosurg 1994;80:3.

Pou Serradell A (ed). Enfermedades de las neuronas motoras. Neurología 1996;11(Supp 5):1.

Pou Serradell A. Myélopathies aiguës d'origine ischémique. Infarctus médullaires. Étude clinico-évolutive et IRM de 8 cas. Rev Neurol (Paris) 1994;150:22.

Pou Serradell A, Aragones JM, Oliveras C, et al. Infarctus de la moelle lombosacrée. Données de l'imagerie par résonance magnétique. Rev Neurol (Paris) 1990;146: 293.

Pou Serradell A, Casademont M. Manifestaciones clínicas y aspectos radiológicos de las malformaciones congénitas occipito-cervicales. Med Clín 1969;3:191.

Pou Serradell A, Marés R. Corrélations clinico-morphologiques par IRM dans la syringomyélie (étude de 22 cas). Rev Neurol (Paris) 1988;144:181.

Pou Serradell A, Marés R, Lamarca J. Hémangioblastome médullaire associé à une syringomyélie dans un cas de maladie de Hippel-Lindau: étude pathologique. Rev Neurol (Paris) 1988;144:456.

Pujol J, Roig C, Capdevila A, et al. Motion of the cerebellar tonsils in Chiari type I malformation studied by cine-phase contrast MRI. Neurology 1995; 45:1746.

Shinhof E. Arteriosclerosis of the spinal cord. Acta Psychiatry Scand 1954;29:139.

Chapter 32
Motor Neuron Disorders

C.M. Ellis and P. Nigel Leigh

Chapter Plan

The purpose of this chapter is to consider disorders in which there is a relatively selective degeneration of the motor systems. The disease can involve the upper motor neurons, the lower motor neurons, or both. Although the World Federation of Neurology classification lists more than 120 disorders involving motor neuron degeneration, only the more common diseases are discussed.

Anatomic Considerations

Disorders of the motor neurons can occur as a result of disease in any part of the motor system, from the motor cortex down to the peripheral nerves. The majority of the fibers of the corticospinal and corticobulbar tracts, the pathways relaying the motor fibers from the cerebral cortex, originate in the precentral area. There is a predominance of pyramidal cells, including the giant pyramidal cells known as *Betz's cells*. The precentral area is divided into the posterior region, the primary motor area, and the anterior region, the premotor area. No Betz's cells are found in the premotor area. The area of the cortex controlling movement in a particular part of the body is proportional to the skill involved in performing the movement and therefore more area is devoted to the face and hands than to the trunk or legs. The arrangement over the precentral area forms a homunculus, with the face situated inferiorly and the lower limbs superiorly on the medial surface of the hemisphere.

Fibers originating predominantly from the precentral gyrus form the corticospinal tract. The descending fibers of these upper motor neurons converge in the corona radiata and then proceed through the posterior limb of the internal capsule. The tract continues via the midbrain and pons, and in the medulla forms the pyramid. At the junction of the medulla oblongata and the spinal cord, the majority of the fibers cross the midline and descend down the spinal cord as the lateral corticospinal tract, with fibers terminating in the anterior gray column of all the spinal cord segments. Most of the fibers synapse with interconnecting neurons, although some connect directly to the anterior horn cells of the lower motor neurons.

The anterior horn cells are the cell bodies of the lower motor neurons that supply the voluntary skeletal muscle. A motor unit consists of one motor neuron and the muscle fibers it supplies. For intricate movements, such as fine finger movements, the motor unit would have only a small number of muscle fibers, whereas for large muscles, a single motor nerve may innervate many hundreds of muscle fibers.

Upper Motor Neuron Disorders

Hereditary Spastic Paraparesis

Hereditary spastic paraparesis (HSP) is characterized by spasticity of the lower limbs with little loss of power, the upper limbs being slightly or not at all affected. Pure and complicated forms are recognized clinically. The pure form is often autosomal dominant in inheritance, with families tending to vary in age of onset but having a similar clinical course. The dominant pure HSP has been further subdivided into disease in which the age of onset is before 35 years (type 1) and in which the age of onset is after 35 years (type 2). In type 1 cases, spasticity of the lower limbs tended to be more marked than weakness, with a slowly progressive and variable clinical course. In the type 2 group, muscle weakness, urinary symptoms, and memory loss were more common. The complicated form of HSP is more frequently autosomal recessive and is associated with other neurologic disorders, such as optic atrophy, extrapyramidal features, epilepsy, and mental retardation.

Clinical Features

Seventy-five percent of patients present with difficulty in walking and gait abnormalities. They may be asymptomatic at diagnosis, being brought to medical attention by an affected family member. Less commonly, weakness, sensory disturbance, or urinary symptoms may predominate. Examination reveals spasticity of the lower limbs, with hyperreflexia and extensor plantar responses. Early in the disease, plantars may be flexor and abdominal reflexes increased. The finding of pes cavus may point to the chronic nature of the disease. Proprioception and vibration may be reduced distally. Slight ataxia of gait and clumsiness of the upper limbs are noted in some cases of otherwise pure HSP. It is difficult to differentiate the clumsiness of early pyramidal involvement from a true cerebellar component, and thus it is reasonable to include such patients in the pure group.

Clinical Course

The rate of progression of HSP is generally extremely slow. In autosomal dominant HSP, type 1 is generally less severe, although the age of losing independent mobility tends to be lower than in the type 2 group because of the younger onset of disease. The recessive forms may be more severe and shorten life expectancy.

Investigations

Investigations are performed to exclude other potentially treatable conditions, such as demyelination, cervical spondylosis, spinal tumors, and vitamin B_{12} deficiency. In the presence of a strong family history, detailed investigations are seldom indicated.

Pathology

Degeneration of the lateral corticospinal tracts and posterior columns is typical. There may be involvement of the spinocerebellar and anterior corticospinal tracts with some loss of Betz's cells in the motor cortex. The remainder of the nervous system is usually spared in uncomplicated disease.

Management

Although the genetic basis of HSP is firmly established, the cause remains unknown. Examination of other family members will help in providing accurate genetic counseling. Treatment is symptomatic, aimed mainly at reducing the spasticity. Oral baclofen can decrease the symptoms, and in severe cases, the use of intrathecal baclofen delivered via an indwelling pump has proved successful. Physiotherapy and the use of aids may also be helpful.

Progressive Lateral Sclerosis

Progressive lateral sclerosis (PLS) is considered to be a variant of motor neuron disease affecting only the upper motor neurons. It usually presents between the ages of 50 and 60 years and is characterized clinically by progressive spasticity leading to involvement of the upper and lower limbs. Pseudobulbar dysarthria and dysphagia also occur and may be the presenting feature. In contrast to amyotrophic lateral sclerosis (ALS) the rate of progression in PLS is very slow, with a course of 25 years or more being reported. Patients do not develop lower motor neuron features. Pathologically, degeneration of the corticospinal and corticobulbar tracts is found with loss of Betz's cells in the motor cortex.

Treatment is symptomatic. Baclofen, delivered orally or intrathecally, reduces the limb spasticity. Both physiotherapy and occupational therapy play a major role in the management of severe PLS. In patients with pseudobulbar features, aids for speech may be necessary, and if swallowing is impaired, alternative feeding methods can be used (see Motor Neuron Disease, Management).

Tropical Spastic Paraparesis

Tropical spastic paraparesis is caused by the human T-cell lymphotrophic virus (HTLV)-1 and encompasses a slowly progressive spastic paraparesis with variable sphincter disturbances, lumbar pain, and paresthesia. Both the viral infection and the host immune responses are implicated in the pathologic mechanisms. HTLV-1 is endemic in a number of tropical regions, such as parts of Africa, southern India, and South America. The seroprevalence in blood donors in Europe is less than 0.03%, and most cases seen there are first- or second-generation immigrants from endemic regions. However, rare cases have been reported in European-born subjects. Diagnosis is based on detecting antibodies to HTLV-1 in the serum and cerebrospinal fluid.

Neurolathyrism and konzo are endemic or epidemic toxic parapareses resulting from the consumption of *Lathyrus sativus* (chickling, or grass pea) or unprocessed cassava, respectively. Both conditions are seen more commonly in times of famine or drought. The toxin responsible for neurolathyrism is thought to be β-oxalyl-amino-L-alanine, which is a potent excitotoxin. Konzo is related to ingestion of cyanogenic glucosides from bitter cassava. Protein deficiency may be an important contributory factor.

Upper and Lower Motor Neuron Disorders

Motor Neuron Disease

Motor neuron disease is a progressive, degenerative condition affecting predominantly the motor neurons. Different presentations are recognized. ALS describes the classic combination of upper and lower motor neuron signs secondary to degeneration of the corticospinal tract neurons in the motor cortex and brain stem and the anterior horn cells of the spinal cord. Progressive bulbar palsy (PBP) describes the predominant bulbar onset with dysarthria and dysphagia; progressive muscular atrophy (PMA) encompasses a lower motor neuron presentation with weakness and wasting of the limbs in the absence of upper motor neuron signs and symptoms. This occurs in approximately 10% patients with motor neuron disease and tends to be associated with a better prognosis.

Epidemiology

The incidence of motor neuron disease is relatively constant worldwide at 2 per 100,000 population per year, with a prevalence of 4–6 per 100,000. The majority of cases are sporadic, with a mean age of onset of 60 years and a male-to-female ratio of 1.5 to 1. Five percent of patients have a family history, usually with autosomal-dominant inheritance. The male-to-female ratio in familial motor neuron disease is 1 to 1, with a mean age of onset of approximately 50 years. The phenotypes of ALS—PBP, and PMA—have been found within the same family, suggesting that the pathogenesis of the conditions are closely linked.

A syndrome of ALS, extrapyramidal features, and dementia is found with high incidence in the western Pacific, for example, the island of Guam. The cause is unknown, and both genetic and environmental theories have been proposed. Current evidence points toward an environmental cause. The incidence of this complex appears to be decreasing.

Pathology and Pathogenesis

Although macroscopic examination of the brain may produce normal findings, microscopy reveals degeneration of the anterior horn cells of the spinal cord and the brain stem motor nuclei, the corticospinal tracts, and pyramidal cells of the motor cortex. Accumulation of neurofilaments in the proximal axons of motor neurons is a common finding, and cytoplasmic eosinophilic inclusions (Bunina bodies) and ubiquinated inclusions can be detected in the brain stem motor nuclei and anterior horn cells.

The cause of motor neuron disease is unknown in the majority of cases. Twenty percent of familial cases are caused by a point mutation in the Cu/Zn superoxide dismutase gene, leading to the suggestion that free radicals and oxidative damage contribute to motor neuron death.

Excitotoxicity secondary to glutamate excess has been proposed as a causative factor because of the finding of excessive extracellular glutamate in motor neuron disease. The accumulation of neurofilaments suggests a possible defect in axonal transport. Mutations in one of the neurofilament genes have been detected in a few patients with sporadic motor neuron disease. Autoimmune theories have been posed, although drugs aimed at modifying the immune system have not affected the course of motor neuron disease. Environmental toxins, pesticides, and viral agents have been implicated, but their role is unproved. It seems likely that motor neuron disease is a heterogeneous disorder. Genetic risk factors are likely to be important, and the role of environmental triggers remains undefined.

Clinical Features

Seventy-five percent of patients present with symptoms in the limbs. This is most commonly an asymmetric weakness of one limb occurring either proximally, causing difficulty rising from a chair or raising an arm, or distally, causing stumbling secondary to a footdrop or difficulty with the fine hand functions such as unscrewing bottle tops or holding a knife and fork. The arms are affected first in 35% cases and the legs in approximately 40%. The remaining 25% present with slurring of the speech, often first noted by friends or relatives, or with swallowing disorders. Fasciculations may be noted by the patient and muscle cramps are common, often preceding the weakness and wasting. Although sensory symptoms such as distal numbness may be described by the patient, on examination, formal sensory testing usually produces negative results. Bladder and bowel involvement is uncommon and would suggest an alternative diagnosis.

Clinical examination reveals the typical combination of upper and lower motor neuron features. In the cranial nerves, eye movements are usually normal, reflecting the fact that the oculomotor nerves are rarely affected. There may be weakness of the lower facial muscles and a wasted, fasciculating tongue with slow, spastic movement. The gag and cough reflexes may be reduced, but the jaw jerk is often brisk. The dysarthria may be predominantly bulbar, with a nasal speech, or pseudobulbar, with spastic speech. Frequently there is a combination of the two. A reduced vital capacity may indicate ventilatory failure caused by involvement of the diaphragm, and a weak cough may signify weakness of the abdominal wall muscles. In the upper and lower limbs, fasciculations, wasting, and weakness are often found in combination with spasticity and brisk tendon reflexes. The plantar responses may be extensor or flexor, even in the presence of marked spasticity of the legs.

Differential Diagnosis

Many conditions should be considered in the differential diagnosis of motor neuron disease, particularly early in the course of the condition, as signs may be ill-defined and mistaken for localized lesions (Table 32-1 lists some of the conditions to be considered).

Investigations

There is no specific test for motor neuron disease, and therefore it remains a diagnosis of exclusion. In all patients, a hematologic and biochemical screening should be performed, with an erythrocyte sedimentation rate, autoantibody profile, thyroid function tests, protein electrophoresis, vitamin B_{12} and folate, and syphilis serologic determinations. These will exclude diseases both causing motor neuron disorders and co-existing with motor neuron disease.

Magnetic resonance imaging of the head and spinal cord will help exclude compressive lesions. High-signal intensity white matter lesions in the cortex, internal capsule, brain stem, and spinal cord indicate extensive corticospinal tract involvement, although often the magnetic resonance imaging scan appears entirely normal.

Electromyography and nerve conduction studies reveal widespread anterior horn cell damage with denervation and reinnervation outside the distribution of a single peripheral nerve or root. This is manifested as a reduction in the number of motor unit action potentials with an increase in amplitude and duration. Fibrillation and fasciculation are found in affected muscles. Motor conduction velocity is seldom low enough to suggest demyelination, and conduction block is not a feature of motor neuron disease but would suggest a demyelinating neuronopathy such as multifocal motor neuropathy (MMN). The conduction of sensory nerve fibers is normal.

Occasionally, more specific investigations may be warranted: levels of antiganglioside antibodies (which may be elevated in immune-mediated damage to motor neurons), hexosaminidase A and B activity, and lead levels in the blood and urine. Kennedy's disease can be excluded by looking for the androgen receptor gene mutation. In cases of motor neuron disease where a family history is present, a screening can be done for point mutations in the Cu/Zn superoxide dismutase gene on the long arm of chromosome 21. Any genetic screening should only be undertaken after proper counseling.

Course and Prognosis

Motor neuron disease is a progressive condition with a median survival of approximately 3.5 years. Older age of onset, bulbar onset, and female sex are associated with a worse prognosis. Ventilatory impairment is one of the most robust predictors of poor outcome. Death usually occurs as a result of respiratory failure or associated chest infections. It is increasingly recognized that certain variants of motor neuron disease are associated with a longer survival, for example, monomelic amyotrophy with an asymmetric upper limb onset and very slow progression, and lower motor neuron forms of motor neuron disease.

Management

The management of motor neuron disease involves a multidisciplinary approach. The diagnosis should ideally be given with a spouse or close friend present and should take place in privacy. The information retained by the patient may be only a fraction of that given, and therefore early follow-up and close liaison with the patient's general practitioner are advised. Written information may be useful, and contact with a local motor neuron disease association to provide practical support and advice is valuable.

Early referral to a dietitian, physiotherapist, occupational therapist, and speech therapist allows problems to be recognized and dealt with appropriately. The treatment strategies for motor neuron disease can be divided into those aimed at relief of

Table 32-1. Conditions to Be Considered in the Differential Diagnosis of Motor Neuron Disease

Structural lesions of brain and spinal cord
    Tumors
        Primary (e.g., glioma)
        Secondary (e.g., carcinoma)
        Hematologic (e.g., lymphoma)
    Arteriovenous malformation
    Cervical spondylotic myelopathy and other lumbosacral
        radiculopathies
    Syrinx
Heredofamilial disorders
    Kennedy's syndrome
    Late-onset spinal muscular atrophy
    Hexosaminidase A and (rarely) B deficiency
    Adrenoleukodystrophy
Metabolic disorders
    Thyrotoxicosis
    Hyperparathyroidism
    Diabetic amyotrophy
Autoimmune mechanisms
    Multifocal motor neuropathy
    Monoclonal gammopathy
    Lymphoma
    Paraneoplastic
Infections
    Human immunodeficiency virus–associated
    Human T-cell lymphotrophic virus 1
    Syphilis
Neuromuscular disorders
    Myasthenia gravis
    Lambert-Eaton syndrome
    Certain myopathies (e.g., inclusion body myositis)
Toxins
    Lead
    Manganese
    Mercury

symptoms and those intended to alter the progression of the disease.

Symptomatic Treatment.   Dysphagia and dysarthria are managed in conjunction with the speech-language therapist and dietitian. Dietary advice and the use of food thickeners are useful early measures; later in the disease process, percutaneous endoscopic gastrostomy can be performed to supplement nutrition. This should be performed before significant weight loss has occurred. Dysarthria may require the use of specific communication aids.

As the muscles of ventilation become weaker, a problem aggravated at night when lying flat, noninvasive nasal intermittent positive pressure ventilation has been demonstrated to improve symptoms and quality of life in motor neuron disease patients. Benzodiazepines and opiates provide symptomatic relief from breathlessness.

Excess salivation can be treated with suction devices and medications to dry up the saliva. Anticholinergics or antidepressants are appropriate. If uncontrolled by these methods, the use of local radiotherapy to the parotid glands has been successful.

Muscle cramps are relieved by quinine, and spasticity by baclofen or dantrolene. Other symptoms commonly occurring include dyspepsia (often a result of esophageal reflux), constipation, poor sleep, and depression. These respond to standard treatments. Early referral to a local hospice allows a further channel of support, initially perhaps as a day case and later for respite care and finally terminal care.

Specific Therapy.   It seems likely that different therapies may be appropriate at different stages of the disease process. In the familial form of motor neuron disease caused by the superoxide dismutase 1 mutation, this results in free radical formation and oxidative stress and therefore theoretically may be helped by antioxidants such as vitamins E and C and selenium. Trials of growth factors such as insulin-like growth factor are continuing, but to date, the only medication that has been shown to alter the progression of motor neuron disease is riluzole, a glutamate release inhibitor. The effect is modest, however, and patients may experience side effects such as fatigue and gastrointestinal upset.

Some patients develop transient abnormalities of liver function or a leukopenia, and therefore blood chemistry and liver function should be monitored.

Chronic Juvenile Amyotrophic Lateral Sclerosis (Tunisian Disease)

The familial disorder known as chronic juvenile ALS (Tunisian disease) has an increased incidence in Tunisia and appears to be inherited as an autosomal recessive disorder. It is characterized clinically by weakness with atrophy and fasciculation in the upper limbs and sometimes lower limbs, with bilateral upper motor neuron features. Bulbar involvement can also occur.

Brown-Vialetto–van Laere and Fazio-Londe Syndromes

The Brown-Vialetto–van Laere syndrome presents in the second decade with bilateral sensorineural hearing loss and progressive lower cranial nerve palsies. The limb muscles are affected later in the course of the disease, and death occurs, usually due to ventilatory failure, before the age of 40 years. The inheritance was thought to be autosomal recessive, although a dominant transmission may occur.

The Fazio-Londe syndrome presents in the first decade with a progressive bulbar palsy without deafness. Multiple cranial nerves become involved and death occurs secondary to respiratory failure. The median survival is 18 months.

Postpolio Syndrome

Postpolio syndrome (PPS) is characterized by a functional deterioration many years after developing acute poliomyelitis. Patients present with fatigue, weakness, and pain involving the muscles and joints. Breathing and swallowing difficulties can occur. It is important to show progression after a period of stability, often for many years. The muscular atrophy seen in typical PPS results from lower motor neuron degeneration. A few reports have described patients developing upper and lower motor neuron features, but it is controversial whether this represents a PPS or whether they would have developed motor neuron disease despite their previous polio.

Lower Motor Neuron Disorders

Spinal Muscular Atrophy

The spinal muscular atrophies (SMAs) are a group of genetically inherited disorders affecting only the lower motor neurons. The gene locus for types I–III has been mapped to chromosome 5q, and abnormalities have been found in the *SMN* and *NAIP* genes at that locus. Muscle weakness with atrophy occurs secondary to degeneration of the anterior horn cells, whereas upper motor neurons are unaffected. Bulbar symptoms are uncommon.

Type I SMA (Werdnig-Hoffman disease) presents at birth or in early infancy with hypotonia, reduced movements, proximal weakness and wasting, and hyporeflexia. The condition is autosomal recessive in the majority of cases and is progressive, leading to death by 3 years of age, with a median survival of 7 months.

Type II SMA is also usually autosomal recessive. The condition presents between 6 months and 5 years of age with hypotonia and delayed motor milestones. There may be involvement of the bulbar muscles. The course is more protracted, with death occurring between 5 and 10 years of age.

Type III SMA (adult-onset SMA) presents between the second and fifth decades with weakness and wasting of the proximal lower limb muscles, and may be confused with the progressive muscular atrophy variant of motor neuron disease. The progression is very slow with periods of apparent stabilization. Lifespan can be normal or only slightly reduced.

Distal forms of SMA are also described, with juvenile and adult onsets. As with type III SMA, the disease tends to progress very slowly and may stabilize.

X-Linked Recessive Bulbospinal Muscular Atrophy (Kennedy's Disease)

X-linked recessive bulbospinal muscular atrophy, or Kennedy's disease, is a rare disorder that presents in males between the ages of 20 and 50 years. It affects the lower motor neurons, leading to dysarthria and a wasted, fasciculating tongue in the region of the cranial nerves, and proximal weakness and wasting with fasciculations peripherally. Tremor is an early feature, and reflexes are reduced or absent. Endocrine abnormalities include gynecomastia, maturity-onset diabetes mellitus, and reduced fertility. The abnormality has been identified as a trinucleotide repeat expansion in exon 1 of the androgen receptor gene on the X chromosome. Genetic testing is therefore possible.

Multifocal Motor Neuropathy

MMN presents clinically with an asymmetric, lower motor neuron distal weakness and wasting, usually of the upper limb, in the absence of sensory symptoms. The progression is very slow. The detection of multifocal conduction block on electrophysiologic testing is considered essential in differentiating this syndrome from other lower motor neuron disorders, although it must be appreciated that conduction block occurring proximally can be difficult to detect. IgM antibodies against ganglioside GM_1 may be present at high titers. Intravenous human immunoglobulin (HIG) therapy is now established as an effective treatment of MMN, but the benefit is short lived. Steroids are not usually helpful and may exacerbate weakness. Cyclophosphamide and other immunosuppressants may help, but their role is unproved. Although the pathogenesis is unknown, the clinical improvement after HIG treatment suggests an immune-mediated neuronopathy.

Suggested Reading

Bensimon G, Lacomblez L, Meininger V, and the ALS/Riluzole Study Group. A controlled trial of riluzole in amyotrophic lateral sclerosis. N Engl J Med 1994;330:585.

Bouche P, Moulonguet A, Younes-Chennoufi AB, et al. Multifocal motor neuropathy with conduction block: a study of 24 patients. J Neurol Neurosurg Psychiatry 1995; 59:38.

Harding AE. The Hereditary Ataxias and Related Disorders. Edinburgh: Churchill Livingstone, 1984.

Harding AE. Hereditary "pure" spastic paraplegia: a clinical and genetic study of 22 families. J Neurol Neurosurg Psychiatry 1981;44:871.

Harding AE. Classification of the hereditary ataxias and paraplegias. Lancet 1983;1:1151.

Haverkamp LJ, Appel V, Appel SH. Natural history of amyotrophic lateral sclerosis in a database population: validation of a scoring system and a model for survival prediction. Brain 1995;118:707.

Lacomblez L, Bensimon G, Leigh PN, et al. Dose ranging study of riluzole in amyotrophic lateral sclerosis. Lancet 1996;347:1425.

Leigh PN, Ray Chaudhuri K. Motor neuron disease. J Neurol Neurosurg Psychiatry 1994;57:886.

Ray Chaudhuri K, Leigh PN. Genetics of motor neuron disease. Adv Clin Neurosci 1994;4:267.

Roos RR, Siddique T, Tainer JA. Summary of "superoxide dismutase (SOD) and free radicals in amyotrophic lateral sclerosis and degeneration" conference. Neurology 1995;45:1779.

Rothstein JD. Excitotoxic mechanisms in the pathogenesis of amyotrophic lateral sclerosis. Adv Neurol 1995;68:7.

Rothstein JD. Excitotoxicity hypothesis. Neurology 1996;47 (Suppl 2):S19.

Van den Berg LH, Franssen H, Wokke JHJ. Improvement of multifocal motor neuropathy during long term weekly treatment with human immunoglobulin. Neurology 1995;45:987.

Zeman S, Lloyd C, Meldrum B, Leigh PN. Excitatory amino acids, free radicals and the pathogenesis of motor neuron disease. Neuropathol Appl Neurobiol 1994;20:219.

Chapter 33
Nerve Root and Plexus Disorders

David A. Chad

Chapter Plan

Anatomic Considerations

Nerve Roots

Nerve roots are delicate structures bathed in cerebrospinal fluid and surrounded by a rigid bony canal. Figure 33-1 shows dorsal and ventral nerve rootlets uniting just beyond the spinal ganglion (dorsal root ganglion) to form a short mixed spinal nerve that almost immediately divides into a thin dorsal ramus and a much thicker ventral ramus. The dorsal ramus innervates the deep posterior muscles of the neck and trunk (the paraspinal muscles) and the overlying skin. The ventral or anterior branches contribute to the cervical, brachial, or lumbosacral plexus and thereby supply the limb muscles. Nerve root fibers together with their meningeal coverings occupy up to 50% of the cross-sectional area of an intervertebral foramen. The remaining space is occupied by loose connective tissue, fat, and blood vessels. On computed tomographic (CT) and magnetic resonance imaging (MRI) scans, the fat acts as an excellent natural contrast agent that defines the thecal sac and nerve roots, allowing nerve root compromise to be detected.

The dorsal roots contain sensory fibers that are the central processes of the unipolar neurons of the dorsal root ganglia. On reaching the spinal cord, these fibers either synapse with other neurons of the posterior horn or pass directly into the posterior columns. The ventral root is comprised of alpha and gamma motor fibers. Of interest, approximately 30% of the total population of ventral root axons are unmyelinated afferent fibers that originate in the dorsal root ganglion.

There are 31 pairs of spinal nerve roots running through the intervertebral foramina of the vertebral column: eight cervical, 12 thoracic, five lumbar, five

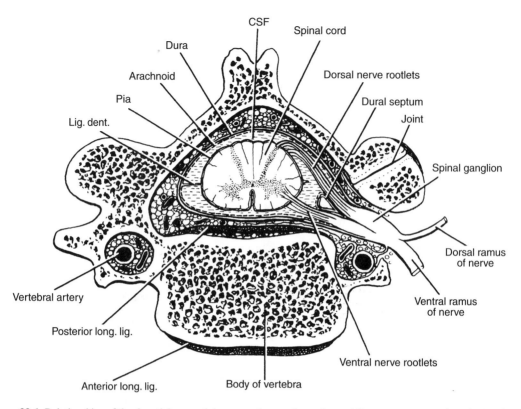

Figure 33-1. Relationships of the dura to bone and the roots of nerve shown in an oblique transverse section. On the right, the relationships between the emergent nerve and the synovial joint are seen, but the joint between the vertebral bodies is not in the plane of the section. The dorsal and ventral roots meet at the dorsal root ganglion in the intervertebral foramen to form the mixed spinal nerve. The small dorsal ramus is the most proximal branch of the mixed spinal nerve and serves the cervical paraspinal muscles (not shown). The dura becomes continuous with the epineurium of the mixed spinal nerve at the intervertebral foramen. The posterior longitudinal ligament helps to contain the intervertebral disk (not shown), preventing protrusion into the spinal canal. (CSF = cerebrospinal fluid; Lig. Dent. = dentate ligament; Long Lig. = longitudinal ligament.) (Reprinted with permission from M Wilkinson. Cervical Spondylosis: Its Early Diagnosis and Treatment. Philadelphia: Saunders, 1971.)

sacral, and one coccygeal (Figure 33-2). An anatomic feature of clinical relevance is that as the lumbar and sacral roots leave the spinal cord and make their way to their respective dorsal root ganglia to form spinal nerves, they descend caudally beside and below the spinal cord, forming the cauda equina, a multiplicity of nerve roots concentrated in a confined area, an anatomic arrangement that makes this structure vulnerable to various pathologic processes.

Brachial Plexus

The brachial plexus is formed by five ventral rami (C5–T1), each of which carries motor, sensory, and postganglionic sympathetic fibers to the upper limb. Figure 33-3 shows the five ventral rami uniting to form the upper, middle, and lower trunks of the plexus above the clavicle. Beneath the clavicle, each trunk divides into anterior and posterior divisions. Three cords (lateral, posterior, and medial) lie below the pectoralis minor muscle. Major upper limb nerves originate from the cords. After contributing a branch to the formation of the median nerve, the lateral cord continues as the musculocutaneous nerve. After it makes its contribution to the median nerve, the medial cord continues as the ulnar nerve. The posterior cord divides into a smaller axillary nerve and a much larger radial nerve. Some important nerve branches originate from the most proximal portion, or root level, of the brachial plexus. For example, the long thoracic nerve derives from roots C5, C6, and C7 to supply the serratus anterior, and the dorsal scapular nerve arises from C5 to supply the rhomboids.

Lumbosacral Plexus

The lumbar plexus is formed within the psoas major muscle by the anterior primary rami of lumbar spinal nerves L1, L2, L3, and L4. It is connected to the sacral plexus in the true pelvis by the anterior division of L4 (Figure 33-4). The branches of major clinical significance include the lateral femoral cutaneous nerve of the thigh originating from the posterior divisions of L2 and L3, the femoral nerve formed from the posterior divisions of L2, L3, and L4, and the obturator nerve formed by the anterior divisions of L2, L3, and L4.

The lumbar plexus communicates with the sacral plexus via the anterior division of L4 which joins with L5 to form the lumbosacral trunk. The sacral plexus, derived from the anterior rami of spinal nerves L4, L5, S1, S2, and S3, forms in front of the sacroiliac joint. The anterior division of the sacral plexus contributes to the tibial portion of the sciatic nerve, while the posterior division contributes to the peroneal portion of the sciatic nerve. The sciatic nerve per se leaves the pelvis through the greater sciatic notch. Branches of major clinical importance coming from the sacral plexus in the pelvis include the superior and inferior gluteal nerves that supply the gluteus medius and minimus muscles and the gluteus maximus, respectively. The pudendal nerve originates from the undivided anterior primary rami of S2, S3, and S4 and extends into the gluteal region via the greater sciatic foramen.

Nerve Root Disorders

Root Avulsion

Because spinal roots have about one-tenth the tensile strength of peripheral nerves, they are the weak link in the spinal root–spinal nerve–plexus complex. Nerve root avulsion from the spinal cord may result from severe traction injury, and ventral roots are more vulnerable to avulsion than dorsal, probably

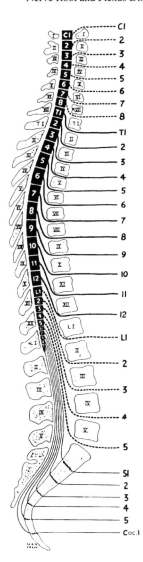

Figure 33-2. The relationship of spinal segments and nerve roots to the vertebral bodies and spinous processes in an adult. The cervical roots (except C8) exit through foramina above their respective vertebral bodies, and the other roots issue below these bodies. The spinal cord is much shorter than the spinal column, ending between vertebral bodies L1 and L2. The lumbar and sacral roots form the cauda equina and descend caudally, beside and below the spinal cord, to exit at the intervertebral foramina. (Reprinted with permission from W Haymaker, B Woodhall. Peripheral Nerve Injuries [2nd ed]. Philadelphia: Saunders, 1953.)

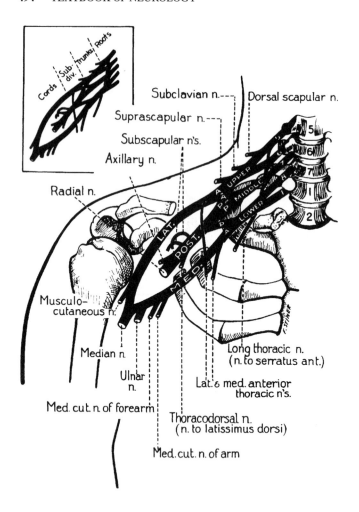

Figure 33-3. Brachial plexus. The components of the plexus have been separated and drawn out of scale. The five ventral rami (C5–T1) unite to form the upper, middle, and lower trunks of the plexus above the clavicle. Beneath the clavicle each trunk divides into anterior (A) and posterior (P) divisions. Three cords (lateral [lat.], posterior [post.], and medial [med.]) lie below the pectoralis minor muscle (not shown). Major upper limb nerves originate from the chords. (n. = nerve; ant. = anterior; cut. = cutaneous.) (Reprinted with permission of the authors and publisher from W Haymaker, B Woodhall. Peripheral Nerve Injuries [2nd ed]. Philadelphia: Saunders, 1953.)

because of the interposition of the dorsal root ganglia and a thicker dural sheath along dorsal roots. The vast majority of root avulsions occur in the cervical region.

Clinical Features

Two distinct clinical syndromes have been described. When there is avulsion of the C5 and C6 roots, Erb-Duchenne palsy results wherein the arm hangs by the patient's side internally rotated and extended at the elbow. When the C8 and T1 nerve roots are avulsed, the resulting Dejerine-Klumpke palsy is characterized by weakness and wasting of the hand with a characteristic claw deformity. One encounters the Erb-Duchenne palsy syndrome in the setting of injuries causing a sudden, severe increase in the angle between the neck and shoulder, whereas Dejerine-Klumpke palsy is seen when

the limb is elevated beyond 90 degrees and tension falls directly on the lower trunk of a plexus. Motorcycle accidents are perhaps the most common cause of these palsies.

At the onset of root avulsion, flaccid paralysis and complete anesthesia develop in the myotomes and dermatomes served by the ventral and dorsal roots, respectively. A clinical clue to the presence of a T1 root avulsion is an ipsilateral Horner's syndrome caused by damage to preganglionic sympathetic fibers as they traverse the ventral root to their destinations in the superior cervical ganglion.

Diagnosis

Electromyographic (EMG) studies are extremely helpful in localizing nerve root lesion. In the face of clinical evidence of sensory loss, preservation of sensory nerve action potentials indicates that

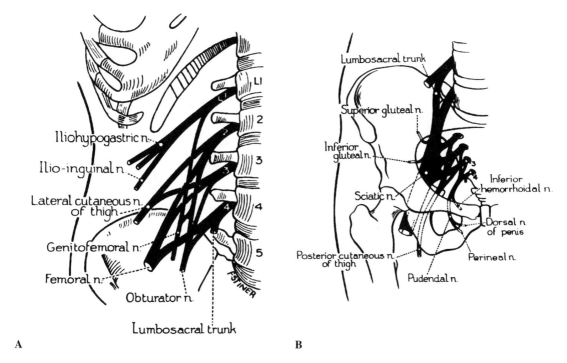

Figure 33-4. (A) The lumbar plexus is formed by anterior primary rami of lumbar spinal nerves L1, L2, L3, and L4. Note the branches that arise from the plexus. (B) The sacral plexus is connected to the lumbar plexus by the lumbosacral trunk. Note the branches that arise from the plexus in the pelvis. (n. = nerve.) (Reprinted with permission of the authors and publisher from W Haymaker, B Woodhall. Peripheral Nerve Injuries [2nd ed]. Philadelphia: Saunders, 1953.)

peripheral axons in the dorsal root ganglia sensory neurons are intact despite proximal sensory root damage. Needle EMG testing of cervical paraspinal muscles permits assessment of ventral root fibers because the posterior primary ramus, which arises just beyond the dorsal root ganglion and proximal to the plexus, is the first branch of the spinal nerve to innervate these muscles. Thus, cervical paraspinal fibrillation potential activity supports the diagnosis of root avulsion. MRI scanning usually demonstrates an outpouching of the dura filled with cerebrospinal fluid (CSF) at the level of an avulsed root.

Disc Degeneration and Spondylosis

Degeneration of the intervertebral discs occurs with age. The mucoid central portion of the disc, the nucleus pulposus, desiccates and shrinks and fibers of the annulus fibrosus that surround the nucleus lengthen and weaken, allowing the disc to bulge posteriorly. In this setting, relatively minor trauma leads to further tearing of annular fibers and ultimately to herniation of disc material. Most lumbar disc herniations are posterolateral, compressing nerve roots in the lateral recess of the spinal canal (Figure 33-5). On occasion, the degenerative process is particularly severe, leading to large rents in the annulus and permitting disc material to herniate into the spinal canal as a free fragment with the potentially damaging capacity to compress two or more nerve roots of the cauda equina. Most cervical disc herniations are also posterolateral. On occasion, disc herniations are far lateral, compressing the nerve root in the foramen per se and are known as foraminal protrusions.

The degeneration of a disc is part of a larger condition of spondylosis characterized by osteoarthritic degenerative changes in the joints of the spine. This condition leads to compromise of the spinal cord in the spinal canal and of the nerve roots in the intervertebral foramina. Restriction in the dimensions of these bony canals is exacerbated by thickening and

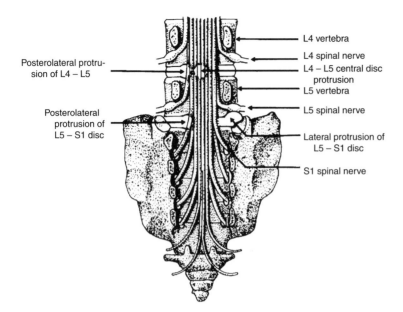

Posterolateral protru-
sion of L4 – L5

Posterolateral
protrusion of
L5 – S1 disc

L4 vertebra

L4 spinal nerve

L4 – L5 central disc
protrusion

L5 vertebra

L5 spinal nerve

Lateral protrusion of
L5 – S1 disc

S1 spinal nerve

Figure 33-5. Dorsal view of the lower lumbar spine and sacrum, showing the different types of herniations and how different roots and the cauda equina can be compressed. (Reprinted with permission from JD Stewart. Focal Peripheral Neuropathies [2nd ed]. New York: Raven, 1993.)

hypertrophy of spinal ligaments, which is especially detrimental in patients with congenital cervical or lumbar canal stenosis.

Clinical Features

Root compression from disc herniation gives rise to a rather characteristic group of symptoms and signs. Radicular pain, paresthesias, and sensory loss in the dermatome are accompanied by weakness in the myotome (defined as muscles innervated by the same spinal cord segment and nerve root; Table 33-1) and diminished deep tendon reflex activity at a segmental level subserved by the nerve root in question. Nerve root pain is described as knifelike or aching and is widely distributed, projecting to deep structures such as muscles and bones innervated by the affected nerve root. Typically, the radicular pain is aggravated by coughing, sneezing, and straining at stool, actions that produce a Valsalva's maneuver and raise intraspinal pressure. Accompanying the pain are paresthesias referred to the specific dermatome, especially to the distal regions of the dermatome; indeed, these sensations strongly suggest that the pain has its origin in compressed nerve roots rather than spondylotic facet joints. Sensory loss caused by the compromise of a single root may be difficult to

ascertain because of the overlapping territories of adjacent roots, although loss of pain is usually more easily demonstrated than loss of light touch.

Nerve root compromise by herniated disc and spondylotic change occurs in the lumbosacral and cervical regions. Thoracic disc herniations are exceedingly rare. In the lumbosacral region, 95% of disc herniations occur at the L4–L5 or L5–S1 levels. As Figure 33-5 illustrates, the lumbar roots emerge beneath the pedicle of their like-numbered vertebral bodies. For example, the L4 root exits beneath the pedicle of the L4 vertebra through the L4–L5 foramen. Because of this anatomic relationship of nerve root exiting above the level of the intervertebral disc, a posterolateral disc herniation will be too low to affect that exiting nerve root. For example, in Figure 33-5, note that the posterolateral protrusion of the L4–L5 disc leaves the exiting L4 spinal nerve root unscathed. Note, however, that the L4–L5 posterolateral disc herniation involves the L5 nerve root as it begins to exit the spinal canal below the pedicle of the L5 vertebra. Therefore, most L4–L5 and L5–S1 disc herniations produce L5 and S1 radiculopathies, respectively. Figure 33-5 also demonstrates that when the disc herniation is far lateral, the spinal nerve root may be compromised as it exits its intervertebral foramen. Far lateral disc herniations probably occur in no more than 10% of cases.

Table 33-1. The Distribution of Weakness and Clinical Presentation of Commonly Occurring Radiculopathies

Radiculopathy	Muscles Weakened	Classic Presentation
C6	Supraspinatus, infraspinatus, deltoid, serratus anterior, biceps	Shoulder girdle weakness, atrophy
C7	Triceps, flexors and extensors of wrist	Arm and forearm weakness
C8	Finger extensors, hand intrinsics	Clumsy, atrophic hand
L4	Hip flexors, quadriceps, thigh adductors	Knee buckling (instability)
L5	Tibialis anterior and posterior, glutei, hamstrings	Footdrop
S1	Gastrocnemius, foot intrinsics, glutei, hamstrings	Calf and foot atrophy

In an L5 radiculopathy, the pain radiates to the buttock and down the back of the leg, with paresthesias generally felt over the dorsum of the foot and the outer portion of the calf. The ankle reflex is typically normal, but there may be reduction of the medial hamstring reflex. Weakness may be found in muscles innervated by two or more nerves carrying L5 motor fibers. For example, one might find weakness in the extensor hallucis longus or tibialis anterior (muscles supplied by the peroneal nerve), the tibialis posterior (supplied by the tibial nerve), and the gluteus medius (supplied by the superior gluteal nerve).

In an S1 radiculopathy, the distribution of pain is similar to what one encounters in L5 radiculopathy. Paresthesias are generally felt on the plantar and outer surfaces of the foot. The ankle reflex is generally diminished or lost, and weakness may be detected in two or more nerves containing S1 motor fibers. For example, there is commonly weakness in the long toe flexors and gastrocnemius muscles (served by the tibial nerve), and the gluteus maximus (served by the inferior gluteal nerve). Positive findings on the straight leg raising test are a sensitive indicator of nerve root irritation. The test is deemed positive when the patient complains of pain radiating from the back into the buttock and thigh with elevation to less than 60 degrees. The test is positive in 95% of patients with a proven disc herniation at surgery. Less sensitive but highly specific is the cross straight leg raising test, when the patient complains of radiating pain on the affected side with elevation of the contralateral leg.

L4 radiculopathy is less common than L5 and S1 radiculopathies and characterized by pain and paresthesias along the medial aspect of the knee and lower leg. The knee jerk is diminished. Weakness is seen in muscles innervated by two or more nerves containing L4 motor fibers, such as the iliopsoas and quadriceps (supplied by the femoral nerve) and the adductor longus (supplied by the obturator nerve).

When large herniations occur in the midline at either the L4–L5 or L5–S1 levels, all the nerve roots below that level may be compressed, producing the cauda equina syndrome, consisting of bilateral radicular pain, paresthesias, weakness, attenuated reflexes below the disc level, and urinary retention.

In the cervical region, nerve roots emerge above the vertebra that shares the same numerical designation. Therefore, C7 exits between C6 and C7 and spondylotic changes with or without additional acute disc herniation would be expected to compress the C7 nerve root. Similarly, disc degeneration at C5–C6 and C7–T1 would compress the C6 and C8 roots, respectively. Because of the greater mobility at levels C5–C6 and C6–C7, earlier and more extensive cervical disc degeneration and subsequent spondylosis occur at these levels, and hence the most frequently encountered cervical radiculopathies are C6 and C7, whereas C5 and C8 are somewhat less common.

C6 radiculopathy is associated with pain at the tip of the shoulder, radiating into the upper part of the arm, the lateral side of the forearm, and the thumb. Paresthesias are felt in the thumb and index finger. The brachioradialis and biceps reflexes are attenuated or lost. Weakness may occur in muscles supplied by two or more nerves carrying C6 motor fibers such as the biceps (supplied by the musculocutaneous nerve), the deltoid (supplied by the axillary nerve), and the pronator teres (supplied by the median nerve). In C7 radiculopathy, pain radiates in a wide distribution to include the shoulder, chest, forearm, and hand. Paresthesias involve the dorsal surface of the middle finger. The triceps reflex is usually reduced or absent. A varying degree of weakness usually involves two or more nerves carrying C7 motor fibers such as the triceps (supplied by the radial nerve), the flexor pollicis longus (supplied by the median nerve), and the flexor carpi ulnaris (supplied by the ulnar nerve). The less commonly encountered C5 radiculopathy is fairly similar to the C6 radiculopathy except that the rhomboids and supra- and infraspinatus muscles may be weakened. C8 radiculopathy involves paresthesias in the fourth and fifth digits and weakness in a distribution similar to C7 radiculopathies except that there is often involvement of the intrinsic hand muscles supplied by both median and ulnar nerves.

Diagnosis

The mainstay of diagnosis of cervical and lumbosacral radiculopathy is neuroimaging. Although plain radiography is not helpful in the identification of a herniated disc per se, in both the cervical and lumbar areas it will reveal spondylotic changes when present and may be useful in the identification of less common disorders that produce radicular symptoms and signs, such as bony metastases, infection, fracture, and spondylolisthesis.

In the cervical region, the best method for assessing the relationship between neural structures and their fibro-osseous surroundings are CT-myelography and MRI scans. The latter is probably the only imaging study necessary to define the pathologic anatomy in patients with cervical disc disease. In the lumbosacral region, CT scanning is an effective noninvasive method of evaluating disc disease, with an accuracy rate up to 93%. When available, however, MRI is considered superior because of excellent resolution, multiplanar imaging, the ability to see the entire lumbar spine including the conus medullaris, and the absence of ionizing radiation.

Electromyography, including motor and sensory nerve conduction studies, late responses, and needle electrode examination, is a powerful physiologic technique that complements neuroimaging in localizing radiculopathy, assessing its severity, and contributing to prognostic assessments. As alluded to in the early discussion on nerve root avulsion, discogenic or spondylotic radiculopathy should spare sensory action potentials. Motor evoked responses may be diminished if there has been extensive loss of motor axons. Needle electromyography would be expected to disclose fibrillation potential activity in paraspinal muscles and in muscles innervated by the same root via different peripheral nerves. Fibrillation potentials are not usually seen until 2–3 weeks after nerve root injury. Beginning at about a month after nerve root compromise, collateral reinnervation occurs in partially denervated muscles, and this leads to a change in the morphology of remaining motor unit potentials, which become increased in amplitude and duration and tend to be polyphasic or complex in appearance.

Treatment

For cervical spondylotic radiculopathy, the mainstay of treatment is conservative management—a combination of several days of bed rest, a soft cervical collar, low-weight cervical traction, and anti-inflammatory agents. Most patients improve, even those with mild to moderate motor deficits. However, a surgical approach may be warranted in certain instances: (1) if there are clinical and radiologic signs of an accompanying myelopathy; (2) if there is unremitting pain despite an adequate trial of conservative management; or (3) if there is progressive weakness in the territory of a compromised nerve root.

In the lumbosacral region, disc herniation and spondylotic changes can be managed conservatively in more than 90% of patients. There are three situations, however, in which surgical referral is indicated: (1) in patients with the cauda equina syndrome (in which surgery may be required urgently); (2) if the neurologic deficit is severe or progressing; or (3) if severe radicular pain is compromising lifestyle and continues after 6–8 weeks of conservative management.

The centerpiece of conservative management is rest. For most patients, lying on a firm mattress eases pain almost immediately. After a few days of bed rest, patients should be encouraged to begin to stand and walk for short periods inside the house and then return to bed. A program of increasing low-level activity (walking) seems to be effective for many patients. When patients are out of bed, discomfort should be controlled with nonsteroidal anti-inflammatory drugs and, if necessary, low doses of narcotic agents such as codeine or oxycodone. Attention to bowel hygiene is essential because any activity that produces a Valsalva's maneuver will greatly increase the pain of lumbosacral disc disease. A high-fiber diet, stool softeners, and laxatives should be prescribed.

Many clinicians recommend a course of oral corticosteroids consisting of 7–10 days of a tapering regimen of prednisone. Others have had excellent results with two or three epidural corticosteroid injections. There are, however, no controlled studies documenting the efficacy of either of these treatments.

The best indication that acute radiculopathy is improving is the lessening of pain and the ability of the patient to tolerate increasing nerve root stretch as documented—for example, by the straight leg raising test for evaluation of lumbosacral nerve root compression.

Diabetic Polyradiculopathy

Diabetics are susceptible to different types of neuropathy, including a distal symmetric polyneuropathy and an asymmetric focal or multifocal neuropathy. Examples of the latter include cranial mononeuropathies and the conditions to be discussed in this section—the thoracoabdominal and lumbosacral polyradiculopathies.

When there is predominant involvement of the thoracic roots, the presenting symptoms are generally the rapid onset of pain and paresthesias in the abdominal and chest wall. Trunk pain may be severe, described variably as burning, sharp, aching, and throbbing, and may mimic the pain of acute cardiac or intra-abdominal medical emergencies. Such pain also simulates disc disease, but the rarity of thoracic disc protrusions and the usual development of a myelopathy in the setting of thoracic disc disease help to exclude this diagnosis. In diabetic thoraco-abdominal polyradiculopathy, there is heightened sensitivity to light touch over affected regions; patches of sensory loss on the anterior, lateral, or posterior aspects of the trunk; and unilateral abdominal swelling caused by localized weakness of the abdominal wall muscles.

Diabetic lumbosacral polyradiculopathy involves the legs, especially the anterior thighs, with pain, dysesthesias, and weakness reflecting the major involvement of upper lumbar roots. This condition has also been called *diabetic amyotrophy*, *proximal diabetic neuropathy*, *diabetic lumbosacral plexopathy*, *diabetic femoral neuropathy*, and *Bruns-Garland syndrome*. Because it is likely that the brunt of nerve disease falls on the nerve roots, it is generically designated diabetic polyradiculoneuropathy.

In most patients, the onset is fairly abrupt, with symptoms developing over days to a couple of weeks. Early in the course of the condition, clinical findings are usually unilateral and include weakness of muscles supplied by the L2–L4 roots (the iliopsoas, quadriceps, and hip adductors), a reduced or absent patellar reflex, and mild impairment of sensation over the anterior thigh. As time passes, there may be spread of weakness to involve more distal muscles of the affected extremity as well as the contralateral limb. Worsening may occur in a steady or stepwise fashion. Progression from onset of the disease to maximum involvement averages approximately 6 months, with a range between a couple of weeks and 18 months. At its peak, weakness varies in severity and extent from mild unilateral thigh weakness to a profound degree of bilateral and extensive leg weakness.

The condition typically affects diabetics in the sixth or seventh decades of life who have had diabetes of several years' duration. It has been described in insulin-treated diabetics, diabetics taking oral hypoglycemic agents, and those controlled with diet alone. In up to 50% of patients, the disorder is preceded by substantial weight loss of 30–40 pounds. Occasionally, it may be the first manifestation of diabetes, unlike diabetic polyneuropathy, which most often takes 10 or more years to develop and is usually a long-term complication of the disease.

The natural history of diabetic polyradiculopathy is that of gradual improvement, although recovery (often incomplete) may take as long as 18 months. Therapy is usually directed at ameliorating the severe pain of this condition: The tricyclics such as desipramine or amitriptyline, anticonvulsants such as carbamazepine or clonazepam, baclofen, clonidine, mexiletine, intravenous lidocaine, and topical capsaicin may all have a role separately or in combination.

Neoplastic Polyradiculopathy

Neoplastic polyradiculopathy usually occurs in patients known to have an underlying neoplasm, although meningeal symptoms may be the first manifestation of malignancy. The clinical features include radicular pain, dermatomal sensory loss, areflexia, and weakness of the lower motor neuron type. Often the distribution of the sensory and motor deficits is widespread and simulates a severe sensory motor polyneuropathy. There are often associated clinical manifestations that result from infiltration of the meninges, such as nuchal rigidity, confusion, and cranial polyneuropathies. A wide variety of neoplasms spread to the leptomeninges, including carcinoma of the breast, lung and melanoma, non-Hodgkin's lymphoma, and leukemias.

The most revealing diagnostic procedure is lumbar puncture (LP), which almost always discloses some abnormality such as elevated protein levels, reduced glucose levels, mononuclear pleocytosis, or the presence of malignant cells on cytologic examination. The latter abnormality may not be detected on the first, second, or even third LP, and four or more LPs may be required to establish a definitive diagnosis. A spinal MRI scan, especially with gadolinium enhancement, is probably the test of choice in a cancer patient in whom leptomeningeal involvement is suspected. Approximately 50% of patients with neoplastic meningitis and spinal symptoms have abnormalities on this study. Gadolinium-enhanced MRI scanning of the brain discloses contrast enhancement of the basilar cisterns or cortical convexities and hydrocephalus. Standard therapy for neoplastic meningitis includes radiotherapy to sites of symptomatic disease, intrathecal chemotherapy, and optimal treatment of the underlying malignancy.

Infectious Polyradiculopathy

Several infectious diseases affect the nerve roots. These include tabes dorsalis, human immunodeficiency virus (HIV) infection, Lyme disease, and herpes zoster.

Tabes dorsalis is the most common form of neurosyphilis. After 10–20 years of infection, damage to the dorsal roots is severe and extensive, producing lightning pains, ataxia, bladder disturbance, Argyll Robertson pupils, areflexia, and loss of proprioceptive sense. Lancinating or lightning pains are brief, sharp, and stabbing and are more apt to occur in the legs than elsewhere. Sudden visceral crises characterized by abrupt onset of epigastric pain that spreads around the body or up over the chest occur in up to 20% of patients. The brunt of the pathologic involvement is in the posterior roots, wherein there is destruction of proprioceptive fibers and partial loss of small myelinated and unmyelinated fibers.

The diagnosis is established by demonstrating abnormalities in the CSF. Fifty percent of patients have a mononuclear pleocytosis, more than 50% have a mild protein elevation, and 72% have positive serologic findings. In all cases of neurosyphilis, antibodies specific for *Treponema pallidum* are found, and the preferred treatment is aqueous penicillin G, 2–4 million units intravenously every 4 hours for 10–14 days with careful follow-up through CSF examination. CSF examination 6 months after treatment should demonstrate a normal cell count and a reduction in protein content. If not, a second course of therapy is indicated. CSF examination should be repeated every 6 months for 2 years until the fluid is normal.

In HIV-infected patients, cytomegalovirus polyradiculopathy is a rapidly progressive opportunistic infection that occurs late in the course of HIV infection when the CD4 count is very low (less than 200 per μl) and an acquired immunodeficiency syndrome–defining infection is present. Presentation is marked by the rapid onset of pain and paresthesias in the legs and perineal region associated with urinary retention and progressive ascending weakness of the lower extremities. There is a flaccid paraparesis; absent deep tendon reflexes in the legs; reduced or absent sphincter tone; and variable loss of light touch, vibration, and joint position sense. The CSF shows elevated protein levels, depressed glucose levels, and polymorphonuclear pleocytosis.

Left untreated, this polyradiculopathy is rapidly fatal within about 6 weeks of onset. Antiviral nucleoside treatment leads to improvement over weeks to months.

Lyme radiculoneuropathy is caused by the spirochete *Borrelia burgdorferi* transmitted by the tick *Ixodes dammini*. Nerve root and peripheral nerve abnormalities occur early and late in the course of Lyme disease. Days to weeks after the onset of the characteristic rash of erythema chronica migrans, a combination of aseptic meningitis, cranial neuropathy, and radiculoneuropathy may occur. The clinical features of nerve root involvement include severe radicular pain followed by weakness, sensory loss, and hyporeflexia in the territory of the involved roots. The CSF profile discloses protein elevation and mononuclear pleocytosis. This radiculopathy improves without treatment, although antibiotics hasten recovery. Clinical improvement occurs in three-fourths of patients treated with intravenous ceftriaxone.

Herpes zoster, also known as shingles, is a common painful vesicular eruption occurring in a segmental or radicular distribution. It most often occurs in thoracic dermatomes, less often in the cervical, and rarely in the lumbosacral segments. Zoster may also present in one of the divisions of the trigeminal nerve and cause herpes zoster ophthalmicus.

For several days before the rash, patients usually complain of radicular pain, sometimes accompanied by fever and malaise. The rash presents as grouped, clear vesicles on an erythematous base. Pain usually disappears as vesicles fade, but 20% develop severe postherpetic neuralgia. This is most likely to develop in the elderly and occurs in 50% of the patients older than age 60. An uncommon complication of cutaneous herpes zoster is segmental motor weakness, which occurs in approximately 5% of patients.

In an immunologically normal host, dissemination of the virus is rare, occurring in less than 2% of patients. In immunocompromised patients, dissemination occurs in up to 50% of patients. Most often, spread is to distant cutaneous sites, but involvement of the viscera may occur.

The major goal of treatment is to relieve local discomfort, prevent dissemination, and reduce the severity of postherpetic neuralgia. In immunocompromised patients, acyclovir should be administered intravenously. Oral acyclovir is indicated for an immunocompetent patient older than age 50 with herpes zoster because the antiviral agent speeds clearing of the lesions and leads to immediate reduction in pain.

Acquired Demyelinating Polyradiculopathy

Acquired demyelinating polyradiculopathy has two major forms. One develops acutely and is known as the *Guillain-Barré syndrome*; the other is chronic progressive or relapsing and remitting and is designated *chronic inflammatory demyelinating polyradiculoneuropathy*. In these conditions, pathologic changes may be pronounced in the spinal nerve roots, especially the ventral roots. The predilection for root involvement helps to explain certain features of these disorders, including the CSF formula wherein there is an albuminocytologic dissociation (high protein level and normal or mildly elevated cell count); some neurophysiologic findings, including abnormalities in the late responses; and disturbances in autonomic function that may be especially problematic in patients with Guillain-Barré syndrome. Another consequence of root involvement is the prominence of proximal muscle weakness in these disorders.

Disorders of the Brachial Plexus

Clinical Features and Diagnosis

Patients with a brachial plexopathy present with a variety of patterns of weakness, reflex changes, and sensory loss depending on whether the whole or a portion of the plexus is disturbed. In a panplexopathy, there is paralysis of muscles supplied by segment C5–T1. The arm hangs by the side except that an intact trapezius allows shrugging of the shoulder. The limb is flaccid and areflexic with complete sensory loss below the shoulder. Lesions of the upper trunk produce weakness and sensory loss in a C5 and C6 distribution. The patient is unable to abduct the arm at the shoulder or flex at the elbow. The arm will hang at the side internally rotated at the shoulder with the elbow extended and the forearm pronated in a "waiter's tip" posture. The biceps and brachioradialis reflexes are diminished or absent, and sensory loss is found over the lateral aspect of the arm, forearm, and thumb. Lesions of the lower trunk produce weakness, sensory loss, and reflex changes in a C8 and T1 distribution. Weakness is present in intrinsic hand muscles supplied by both the median and the ulnar nerves and in the medial finger and wrist flexors. There is sensory loss over the medial two fingers and the medial aspect of the hand and forearm.

EMG studies are extremely helpful in confirming the diagnosis of brachial plexopathy. Because the lesion in plexopathy is by definition distal to the origin of the dorsal primary rami, needle examination of cervical paraspinal muscles produces normal results, and in the face of sensory loss, sensory nerve action potentials are reduced or absent in contrast to the situation in radiculopathy. The needle examination in classic plexopathy shows sparing of paraspinal muscles with involvement of upper extremity muscles innervated by at least two cervical segments and two different peripheral nerves.

Neuroimaging is helpful in finding the presence of a cervical rib or long transverse process of C7, in demonstrating a pulmonary apical lesion, and in permitting a CT-guided biopsy, which can be used to obtain cytologic or histologic material for precise diagnosis.

Traumatic Plexopathy

The most common traumatic plexopathy is caused by stretch-contusion, usually secondary to motorcycle crashes, but sporting accidents and football, cycling, skiing, and equestrian events are also important. The brachial plexus may also be injured by a heavy rucksack or backpack pressed to the shoulders and exerting pressure in the region of the upper trunk of the plexus and leading to weakness in a C5 and C6 distribution.

Neurogenic Thoracic Outlet Syndrome

Neurogenic thoracic outlet syndrome is much diagnosed but is a rare entity in the experience of most neurologists, being seen only once or twice per year in a busy EMG laboratory. In the classic case, the patient is typically a younger woman who presents with pain along the inner aspect of the arm. Tingling sensations are also felt along the inner aspect of the forearm and in the hand. The majority of patients note slowly progressive wasting and weakness of the hand muscles. The examination discloses muscle weakness and atrophy most marked in the lateral part of the thenar eminence, and in a small number of patients there is mild atrophy and weakness in the forearm muscles. Sensory loss is present along the inner side of the forearm. Vascular symptoms per se are rather uncommon in true neurogenic thoracic outlet syndrome.

In most instances, cervical spine films disclose small, bilateral cervical ribs or enlarged downcurving C7 transverse processes. Electrodiagnostic studies are essential for diagnosis and show reduction in the amplitude of the median motor response, a reduced ulnar sensory response, a mildly reduced ulnar motor response, and a usually normal median sensory response.

The site of involvement is the lower trunk of the brachial plexus. In most patients, a fibrous band extends from the tip of a rudimentary cervical rib to the scalene tubercle of the first rib, causing angulation of either the C8 and T1 roots or the lower trunk of the brachial plexus. Surgical division of the fibrous band can be expected to relieve pain and paresthesias and arrest muscle wasting and weakness.

Metastatic and Radiation-Induced Brachial Plexopathy

Damage to the brachial plexus in patients with cancer is usually secondary to either metastatic plexopathy or radiation-induced injury. Lung and breast carcinoma are the tumors most frequently metastasizing to the brachial plexus; lymphoma, sarcoma, melanoma, and a variety of other types are less common. Tumor metastases spread via lymphatics and the area most commonly involved is adjacent to the lateral group of axillary lymph nodes.

The hallmark of metastatic plexopathy is severe pain located in the shoulder girdle with radiation to the elbow, the medial portion of the forearm, and the fourth and fifth digits of the hand. In many patients, weakness is referable to the lower plexus in its divisions and more than half the patients have Horner's syndrome. Some patients have signs indicating involvement of the entire plexus.

One cause of a neoplastic plexopathy described by Pancoast is a tumor spreading from the pleural surface of the apex of the lung and growing into the paravertebral space and posterior chest wall, invading extraspinal roots, sympathetic chain, and stellate ganglion.

Radiation-induced plexopathy is unlikely to occur if the dose is less than 60 Gy. If more than 60 Gy is given, the interval between the end of radiation treatment and the onset of symptoms ranges between 3 months and 26 years, with a mean interval of 6 years. Pain is a relatively minor aspect of the presenting symptom complex. Paresthesias and swelling are present in approximately half the patients and are more common than pain. Weakness is usually most prominent in muscles innervated by the branches of the upper trunk, but involvement of the entire limb from damage to the upper and lower portions of the plexus can also occur.

A diagnostic dilemma arises when symptoms and signs of brachial plexopathy develop in a patient known to have had cancer and radiation in the region of the brachial plexus. A painful lower trunk lesion with Horner's syndrome is strongly suggestive of metastatic plexopathy, whereas a relatively painless upper trunk lesion with lymphedema is highly suggestive of radiation-induced plexopathy. Needle EMG testing is often helpful because in radiation-induced plexopathy it discloses myokymic discharges. Sometimes the only way to establish a diagnosis is exploration of the involved region and biopsy by direct visualization.

Idiopathic Brachial Plexopathy

Arm pain and weakness are the cardinal features of idiopathic brachial plexopathy. Men are affected two to three times more often than women, and there appears to be a higher incidence among athletic individuals. In approximately one-half of the cases, there is an antecedent event such as an upper respiratory infection, a flulike illness, an immunization, or a surgical procedure. The disorder is probably immunologically mediated.

The illness begins with intense pain located in the shoulder scapular area and arm. Pain usually lasts from hours to weeks and gradually abates. Lessening of pain is associated with evolving weakness, which peaks in 2–3 weeks in most patients. Pain generally subsides but may continue for several weeks after weakness has reached its peak.

On examination, about one-half of patients have weakness in muscles of the shoulder girdle and one-third have weakness referable to the upper and lower parts of the plexus. In a small number of patients, weakness is referable to the lower plexus alone. In many patients, weakness seems to result from involvement of individual peripheral nerves such as the suprascapular, axillary, long thoracic, median, and anterior interosseous. One-third of cases are

bilateral and a small percentage have diaphragm weakness. In a small number of cases, there appears to be an underlying axonal polyneuropathy.

In the acute stage of the disorder, a narcotic analgesic may be necessary to control pain. Some clinicians use a short course of corticosteroids. The vast majority of patients improve and in one series 90% had recovered by 3 years after onset.

Lumbosacral Plexopathy

Clinical Features and Diagnosis

Lumbar plexopathy produces weakness, sensory loss, and reflex changes in segments L2–L4, whereas sacral plexopathy leads to similar abnormalities in segments L5–S3. Characteristic findings in lumbar plexopathy include weakness and sensory loss in the territories of both the obturator and femoral nerves. There is weakness of hip flexion, knee extension, and hip adduction with sensory loss over the anteromedial aspect of the thigh; the knee jerk is absent or depressed. This combination of hip flexor and adductor weakness marks the disorder as either a plexopathy or radiculopathy and more precise localization depends on laboratory studies including needle EMG testing and CT and MRI scanning.

Findings in sacral plexopathy include weakness and sensory loss in the territories of the gluteal (motor only), peroneal, and tibial nerves. There is extensive leg weakness involving the hip extensors and the abductors, knee flexors, and ankle plantar flexors and dorsiflexors. Sensory loss is found over the posterior aspect of the thigh, the anterolateral and posterior aspects of the leg below the knee, and the dorsolateral and plantar surfaces of the foot. Weakness of the gluteal muscles points to involvement of fibers proximal to the piriformis muscle, that is, the sacral plexus per se in the true pelvis or at a more proximal sacral root level. As in lumbar plexopathy, accurate diagnosis often depends on electrodiagnostic studies and neuroimaging.

As in brachial plexus lesions, EMG studies are very helpful in diagnosis. Reductions in the amplitude of the sensory and motor action potentials are expected, and needle EMG testing shows fibrillation potential activity and motor unit potential changes of remodeling (resulting from reinnervation) in muscles innervated by at least two lum-

Table 33-2. Clues to the Nature of a Plexopathy

Structural disorders
    Past history or presence of malignancy
    Hemophilia or treatment with an anticoagulant
    Pelvic trauma
    Known atherosclerotic vascular disease and hyperten-
      sion (aneurysm)
    Pregnancy, labor, delivery
    Abdominal (pelvic) surgery
Nonstructural disorders
    Diabetes mellitus*
    Vasculitis
    Previous pelvic radiation

*Diabetics may develop a polyradiculopathy that will simu-
  late a lumbosacral plexopathy.

bosacral segmental levels and involving at least two different peripheral nerves. Classically, in plexopathy the EMG examination of paraspinal muscles produces normal results.

Neuroimaging, including CT and MRI scanning through the abdomen and pelvis from a rostral point at the level of L1–L2 to a caudal point below the level of the symphysis pubis, allows the regional anatomy of the entire lumbosacral plexus to be scrutinized. A CT scan may provide guidance for percutaneous needle biopsy as well.

Differential Diagnosis

The differential diagnosis for lumbosacral plexopathy includes spinal root disorders such as lumbosacral radiculopathy, polyradiculopathy, and the cauda equina syndrome, anterior horn cell disorders, and myopathic conditions. Radiculopathies are usually painful, and the distribution of the pain follows a predictable radicular distribution, as we have seen. Weakness is usually found in several muscles supplied by the same root, and needle EMG studies demonstrate paraspinal muscle involvement. As noted earlier, it is sometimes difficult to separate plexopathy from radiculopathy on clinical grounds alone, especially if several roots are involved.

Anterior horn cell disorders give rise to painless, progressive weakness with atrophy and fasciculations in the absence of sensory loss. Myopathies are rarely confused with lumbosacral plexopathy: although a painful, focal myositis can occur, absence of sensory loss, elevation of muscle enzyme levels, and myopathic features on both needle EMG examination and muscle biopsy point away from plexopathy.

Structural Plexopathy

The structural plexopathies include hematoma, abscess, aneurysm, trauma, neoplasia, and the compression of elements of the plexus that occur during pregnancy (Table 33-2).

Hematoma

Patients with hemophilia and those receiving anticoagulants are at risk of developing hemorrhage in the iliopsoas muscle complex. This will give rise to involvement of the femoral nerve and sometimes to the obturator nerve as well. Severe pain is usually the first manifestation of a retroperitoneal hematoma. It is present in the groin and radiates to the thigh and leg and is associated with gradually increasing paresthesias and weakness. When the femoral nerve is involved, weakness and sensory loss occur in its territory; when other components of the plexus are involved, changes are more extensive and conform to the territories supplied by involved branches of the plexus.

Diagnosis is generally established with neuroimaging, especially CT scanning. Psoas abscess was common when tuberculosis was prevalent, but neurologic complications such as lumbar plexopathy and femoral neuropathy were rare. In the case of acute nontuberculosis psoas infection, nerve compression appears uncommonly, probably because the psoas fascia is relatively distensible.

Aneurysm

Back and abdominal pain is often an early manifestation of abdominal aortic aneurysms. An expanding abdominal aortic aneurysm may compress the iliohypogastric or ilioinguinal nerves (see Figure 33-4) and lead to pain in the lower abdomen and inguinal areas. Pressure on the genitofemoral nerve will produce pain in the inguinal area, testicle, and anterior thigh. Compression of nerve trunks L5–S2, which lie directly posterior to the hypogastric artery, may give rise to sciatica. Unexplained back pain, leg pain, or pain radiating in the distribution of cutaneous nerves coming from the lumbar plexus should raise the suspicion of an aneurysm of the aorta or its major branches. The presence of a pulsatile mass felt while palpating the abdomen and rarely on rectal examination strongly suggests the presence of an aneurysm. The diagnosis can be confirmed by abdominal sonographic or CT scanning.

Trauma

Because of its relatively protected position, the lumbosacral plexus is not commonly affected by traumatic lesions. A fracture of the pelvis, acetabulum, or femur or surgery on the proximal femur and hip joint may injure the lumbosacral plexus.

Pregnancy

The lumbosacral trunk may be compressed by the fetal head during the second stage of labor. This tends to occur in prolonged labor with mid-forceps rotation in a short-primigravida mother carrying a relatively large baby. A day or so after delivery, when the patient gets out of bed, she notes difficulty walking because of foot dorsiflexor weakness. There is weakness in both dorsiflexion and inversion with reduced sensation over the lateral aspect of the leg and the dorsal surface of the foot. The prognosis for recovery is good.

Neoplasms

The lumbosacral plexus may also be involved by tumors that invade the plexus, either by direct extension from intra-abdominal neoplasms or by metastases. Most tumors involve the plexus by direct extension while metastases account for only one-fourth of cases. Neoplastic plexopathy typically has an insidious onset over weeks to months. Pain is a prominent early manifestation. Weeks to months after pain begins, numbness, paresthesias, weakness, and leg edema develop. Neuroimaging with CT or MRI scanning usually establishes the diagnosis of neoplastic plexopathy. Because pelvic neoplasms may extend into the epidural space, most often below the conus medullaris, an MRI scan of the lumbosacral spine is indicated in most patients.

Nonstructural Plexopathy

Nonstructural plexopathic disorders include radiation plexopathy, vasculitis, and an idiopathic lumbosacral plexopathy.

Radiation Plexopathy

Slowly progressive, painless weakness is an early manifestation of radiation plexopathy. Pain develops in approximately one-half of patients but is not a major problem. Most patients eventually develop bilateral weakness, which is often asymmetric and affects predominantly the distal muscles in the L5–S1 distribution. The latent interval between radiation and the onset of neurologic manifestations is between 1 and 31 years with a median of 5 years. In most patients, radiation plexopathy is gradually progressive and results in significant or severe disability. Neuroimaging is typically normal. A clue to the diagnosis comes from needle EMG examination, which discloses myokymic discharges.

Vasculitis

Vasculitic neuropathy has generally been associated with a pattern of mononeuritis multiplex, but other neuropathic syndromes have also been described. It is likely that mononeuritis multiplex evolves into a pattern of overlapping multiple mononeuropathies (simulating polyneuropathy), but the pattern of plexopathy has also been described.

Idiopathic Lumbosacral Plexopathy

In some patients, lumbosacral plexopathy occurs in the absence of a recognizable underlying disorder. In this way, it can be considered a counterpart of idiopathic brachial plexus neuropathy. It usually begins with the abrupt onset of pain, followed days later by weakness, which usually progresses for a few days or weeks and then stabilizes. Both upper and lower portions of the lumbosacral plexus appear to be involved in 50% of cases, major involvement in the territory of the upper portion in 40% of cases, and changes confined to the lower portion in only 10% of patients. Most patients recover over a period of months to 2 years, although recovery is often incomplete. Some patients respond to high-dose intravenous gamma globulin.

Suggested Reading

Deyo RA, Loeser JD, Bigos SJ. Herniated lumbar intervertebral disc. Ann Intern Med 1990;112:598.

Donaldson JO. Neurology of Pregnancy (2nd ed). London: Saunders, 1989.

England JD, Sumner AJ. Neurologic amyotrophy: an increasingly diverse entity. Muscle Nerve 1987;10:60.

Harati Y. Frequently asked questions about diabetic peripheral neuropathies. Neurol Clin 1992;10:783.

Haymaker W, Woodhall B. Peripheral Nerve Injuries (2nd ed). Philadelphia: Saunders, 1953.

Jaeckle KA. Nerve plexus metastases. Neurol Clin 1991;9:857.

Logigian EL, Steere AC. Clinical and electrophysiologic findings in chronic neuropathy of Lyme disease. Neurology 1992;42:303.

Simon RP. Neurosyphilis. Arch Neurol 1985;42:606.

Simpson DM, Olney RK. Peripheral neuropathies associated with human immunodeficiency virus infection. Neurol Clin 1992;10:685.

Stewart JD. Focal Peripheral Neuropathies (2nd ed). New York: Raven, 1993.

Tsairis P, Dyck PJ, Mulder DW. Natural history of brachial plexus neuropathy. Arch Neurol 1972;27:109.

Wilbourn AJ. True neurogenic thoracic outlet syndrome. Muscle Nerve 1982;7:3.

Wilbourn AJ, Aminoff MJ. The electrophysiologic examination in patients with radiculopathies. Muscle Nerve 1988;11:1099.

Wilson DW, Pezzuti RT, Place JN. Magnetic resonance imaging in the pre-operative evaluation of cervical radiculopathy. Neurosurgery 1991;28:175.

Chapter 34
Peripheral Nerve Disorders

Gerard Said and Jean-Marc Guglielmi

Clinical Approach to Peripheral Nerve Disorders

The diagnosis of peripheral neuropathy requires careful clinical examination. Information about the course of the illness provides important data. The clinical course ranges from acute (days) to subacute (weeks) to chronic (months). If a relapsing-remitting course is associated with inflammatory demyelinating neuropathies, attention should be paid to exposure to toxins. For patients with chronic neuropathies, a specific family history must be obtained.

Most neuropathies produce motor, sensory, and sometimes autonomic dysfunction that result in symptoms that have positive or negative effects:

- Loss of muscle strength is the predominant negative symptom and can be caused by axonal degeneration or by conduction block.
- Cramps, myokymia, fasciculations, and neuropathic tremor are positive motor symptoms and

may be the earliest manifestations of disease of the motor fibers.

- Sensory fibers are represented by a full range of size diameters. Most neuropathies involve nerve fibers of all sizes, but sometimes selective damage to large or small fibers predominates. Ataxia and loss of reflexes reflect loss of large fibers. Loss of temperature and pain sensation reflects involvement of small fibers, as in diabetic polyneuropathy or amyloidosis.
- Autonomic dysfunction is a feature of neuropathies affecting the unmyelinated fibers.

Examination of the distribution of lesions permits a classification of a patient's neuropathy:

- Mononeuropathy indicates damage to individual peripheral nerves.
- Multiple neuropathies are characterized by involvement of several nerves. The distribution is asymmetric and progression in time is irregular.
- Polyneuropathies are characterized by symmetric and distal involvement.
- Cranial nerves are predominantly involved in Guillain-Barré syndrome and sarcoidosis.

Electrodiagnostic studies, including motor and sensory nerve conduction studies combined with needle examination, provide information about the localization of nerve lesions and give information on the underlying mechanisms—axonal or demyelinating. Cutaneous nerve biopsy should be performed in specific situations: vasculitis, leprosy or amyloidosis, and chronic inflammatory demyelinating neuropathy.

Focal Neuropathies

Focal neuropathies may be caused by compression resulting from external pressure or entrapment, which results in damage to the nerve because of mechanical constriction within an anatomic canal. It should be added that the effects of local pressure are increased in some generalized neuropathies:

- The hereditary neuropathy liable to pressure palsy known as *tomaculous neuropathy*
- Diabetic nerves show increased susceptibility to compression at entrapment sites
- Hereditary and acquired demyelinating hypertrophic neuropathy
- Leprosy

The electrophysiologic hallmarks of entrapment neuropathy or compression are conduction blocks or marked slowing across the entrapment site. In severe cases there also are features of wallerian degeneration. Changes that occur in acute and chronic compression have been studied experimentally and found in large myelinated fibers. There is evidence of intussusception of the terminal myelin of the node under the myelin of the internode. Ischemia is not a significant factor.

Median Nerve at the Wrist

For many years, the occurrence of a burning, pins-and-needles sensation at night in the fingers was known as the *acroparesthesia syndrome*. MacArdle in 1949 suggested that this syndrome could be caused by compression of the median nerve in the carpal tunnel. Clinical features of carpal tunnel syndrome (CTS) include sensory and motor deficits in the hand. Nocturnal exacerbation of the paresthesia is common. Pain may radiate up to the forearm or even the shoulder. Examination may reveal flattening of the lateral aspect of the thenar eminence and sensory signs.

The diagnosis is usually obvious clinically, but it is important to confirm this with electrophysiologic studies: Digital sensory median nerve potentials are of low amplitude or absent. Median nerve motor conduction is abnormal less often than is sensory conduction. Distal latencies are prolonged, and sometimes a reduced compound muscle action potential (CMAP) amplitude is present, indicating an axonal loss. Conservative therapy includes splinting or local injection of steroids. Surgery is indicated when conservative therapy fails.

Median Nerve at the Elbow

On rare occasions the median nerve may be compressed as it passes under the bicipital aponeurosis between the two parts of the pronator teres muscle. This condition produces pain in the forearm and weakness of median-innervated muscles including the pronator teres. The anterior interosseous nerve is a pure motor branch arising in the forearm supplying the flexor pollicis longus, the flexor digitorum profundus for the second and third digits, and the pronator quadratus. Damage to this nerve produces loss of grip between the thumb and the second finger.

Ulnar Nerve

The ulnar nerve is susceptible to acute compression or chronic entrapment as it passes behind the elbow in the ulnar groove and less commonly at the wrist in the cubital tunnel (Guyon's canal) by osteophytes. The ulnar nerve is also vulnerable in the axilla. Entrapment neuropathy of the ulnar nerve in the forearm is rare.

Examination reveals muscle wasting in the hypothenar eminence, but most often it is more pronounced in the first dorsal interosseous; weakness involves ulnar-innervated muscles proximal or distal depending on the level of injury. Sensory changes are found over the fifth finger. Diagnosis should be confirmed by nerve conduction testing. Measuring conduction velocity gives the best chance of localizing a segmental lesion between the axilla and the elbow or the elbow and the wrist.

Differential diagnosis of ulnar neuropathy includes thoracic outlet syndrome (TOS). Although TOS is not an entrapment neuropathy, the lower trunk of the brachial plexus may be stretched over an extra rib at the level of the seventh cervical vertebra or by an abnormal fibrous band running between the clavicle and a cervical rib. A patient may develop pain in the arm and hand. There is weakness of all intrinsic hand muscles, and sensory loss is marked in the inner side of the forearm and of the hand. Diagnosis is made by neurophysiologic and radiologic studies.

Radial Nerve

The radial nerve is more often susceptible to damage by external compression in the upper arm at the level of the spiral groove. Clinically, there is a wrist and fingerdrop with weakness of the brachioradialis muscle and reduction of the brachioradialis reflex. An entrapment neuropathy localized in the forearm may occur when the posterior interosseous branch of the radial nerve penetrates the arcade of Frohse. Clinically, the patient complains of an ache in the forearm and may develop weakness of the finger extensors sparing the extensor carpi radialis.

Sciatic Nerve

The sciatic nerve is formed by branches from the lumbosacral plexus and the upper sacral roots. The nerve can be damaged by stretching or direct trauma during hip surgery, a neoplasm of the pelvis, or intramuscular injection. Compression of the proximal sciatic nerve where it passes under the piriformis has been claimed, but this entrapment is poorly validated. Clinically, there is weakness of the hamstrings and all muscles below the knee. Sensory changes involve the dorsum and the sole of the foot and the lateral part of the lower leg.

Common Peroneal Nerve

Entrapment of the common peroneal nerve is the most frequent entrapment neuropathy in the leg and occurs at the fibular head. Entrapment caused by a fibrous band at the origin of the peroneus longus can occur but is rare. Rare compressive causes include a popliteal aneurysm, Baker's cyst, or a ganglion. A clinically painless footdrop may develop, with weakness in dorsiflexion and eversion of the foot on clinical examination. Usually there is numbness of the lateral part of the foreleg.

Posterior Tibial Nerve

The posterior tibial nerve may be affected by cyst or lesion of the lower leg. Clinically, there is weakness of plantar flexion of the foot.

Femoral Nerve

A femoral nerve injury produces weakness of the quadriceps and the iliopsoas if the lesion is more proximal. Sensory loss may be present in the anterior and lateral aspect of the leg. The nerve may be injured by bleeding or traumatic injury.

Inflammatory Demyelinating Polyradiculoneuropathies

Guillain-Barré Syndrome

Guillain-Barré syndrome (GBS) is an acute inflammatory, predominantly demyelinating neuropathy usually presenting as an areflexic paralysis. Early diagnosis is important because good supportive care and immunoglobulin therapy or plasmapheresis can decrease morbidity. It is not a benign illness because the overall mortality is approximately 5%. GBS affects people of all ages. In a large number of cases, an upper respiratory or intestinal infection occurs several weeks before the onset of the syndrome. Several viruses or bacteria have been implicated. Weakness affects the lower extremities and spreads up to the trunk, the upper limbs, and muscles innervated by the cranial nerves. Progression of the weakness is maximal by 3–4 weeks in the majority of patients. Pain is a frequent complaint. Sensory symptoms and signs are much less frequent. Areflexia is the rule. Autonomic neuropathy affecting the sympathetic and the parasympathetic nerves is common: sinusal tachycardia, cardiac arrhythmia, hypertension, and sweating dysfunction are the most noticeable. Recovery begins within 2–4 weeks after the plateau. GBS variants include the Miller-Fisher syndrome with ataxia, ophthalmoplegia, and areflexia, and a pandysautonomic neuropathy. The cerebrospinal fluid (CSF) protein level is characteristically increased, with no increased cellularity. When GBS is associated with human immunodeficiency virus (HIV) infection, CSF cellularity is usually increased. Electrophysiologic studies are helpful in confirming the diagnosis. Monitoring in an intensive care unit, plasma exchange, or intravenous immunoglobulin are the usual treatments in more severely affected patients.

Chronic Inflammatory Demyelinating Polyradiculoneuropathy

Chronic inflammatory demyelinating polyradiculoneuropathy (CIDP) represents an important acquired condition because it is often an undiagnosed neuropathy and patients may respond to immunosuppressive therapy. The diagnosis of CIDP is supported by the clinical features and findings on laboratory studies. Typically, patients with CIDP show progressive muscular weakness involving distal and proximal muscles of both the upper and lower extremities. Deep tendon reflexes are depressed or lost. Sometimes patients have ataxia, indicating proprioceptive loss. Sensory symptoms are variable. The CSF study shows a characteristic elevated level of CSF protein without a high cell count. Nerve conduction studies show features suggesting demyelination of the peripheral nerves: focal motor conduction block, segmental reduction in nerve conduction velocities, prolonged distal latencies, and prolonged or absent F waves. Nerve biopsy is an important part of the laboratory evaluation and shows demyelinated or thinly myelinated axons with various degree of myelinated fibers. Mononuclear cells are present in some instances.

Most patients with CIDP will improve initially, but the possibility of relapse is high, and some patients undergo a chronic progressive course. Plasma exchange, corticosteroids, and human immunoglobulin therapy are used with variable results in CIDP.

Neuropathies Caused by Systemic Disorders

Vasculitis

Vasculitic disorders are characterized by inflammation and damage or destruction of blood vessel walls, causing ischemic lesions in the distribution of the damaged vessels. Vasculitis may occur as primary vasculitic syndromes (polyarteritis nodosa, Wegener's syndrome) or as part of an underlying process such as cryoglobulinemia, rheumatoid arthritis, infections, or malignancies. It is generally assumed that immune complex deposition and cell-mediated immune reactions are the main determinants according to experimental models, but in fact, little is known about the pathogenesis of most vasculitic disorders encountered in humans. Neuropathies associated with necrotizing arteritis can be observed in apparent isolation (35%) or in the context of multisystemic disorders (65%) with involvement of the skin, kidneys, and central nervous system.

Onset of neuropathy is abrupt and the deficit is partial. Focal or multifocal neuropathies are the most common presentation of systemic vasculitis, but distal symmetric sensorimotor neuropathy resulting from an overlapping mononeuritis multiplex can occur in 25%. The nerves affected most often are the peroneal, tibial, ulnar, median, and radial. Clinically, peripheral nerve vasculitis involves sensory and motor function and can be accompanied by pain. Recovery takes months because of the axonal lesions.

Careful electrophysiologic examination will demonstrate axonal nerve damage in a multifocal distribution. Nerve and muscle biopsies are the best way to confirm the diagnosis by demonstrating the characteristic lesions of muscular and epineurial arteries; nerve ischemia induces acute axonal degeneration of large diameter fibers; asymmetry of lesions between and within nerve fascicles is also common. Steroids and cyclophosphamide are the main treatments of vasculitic neuropathies.

Diabetic Neuropathies

Diabetic neuropathies may complicate adult-onset diabetes mellitus and represent the most common cause of peripheral neuropathy in industrialized countries. The prevalence of the neuropathy increases with the duration of diabetes and the poor control of hyperglycemia. Pirart, in a large prospective outpatient clinic, showed that 8% of diabetics had neuropathy at the time of diagnosis and 50% had the condition after 25 years of diabetes. However, others factors are involved; on rare occasions very severe diabetic neuropathy develops in the 2–3 years after the onset of diabetes.

Diabetic peripheral neuropathy can take several forms, and it is important to remember that in diabetic patients not all neuropathies are caused by diabetes.

Symmetric Polyneuropathy

The most common type of neuropathy that occurs in diabetic patients is a symmetric distal polyneuropathy that involves mainly sensory function. Numbness and tingling start in the distal regions of the lower limbs. Later, the upper limbs are affected. Most often, small sensory fiber involvement is more pronounced than large fiber involvement, so there is a predominant loss of pain and temperature over joint position sense. Foot ulcera-

tion and neuropathic joint degeneration affecting the feet may develop.

Acute Painful Diabetic Neuropathy

The patient experiences intense burning pain day and night, mainly in the lower limbs. This syndrome may develop in poorly controlled diabetic patients demonstrating severe weight loss. There is a contrast between mild sensory loss on examination and a very marked hyperesthesia of the skin.

Autonomic Neuropathy

Autonomic neuropathy usually accompanies a distal symmetric sensory polyneuropathy. A wide variety of symptoms may develop: resting tachycardia resulting from vagal denervation; abnormal cardiovascular reflexes, which can induce severe postural hypotension; impotence in men, which is one of the earlier autonomic manifestations in diabetes; and gastroparesis with nocturnal diarrhea, which can be severe.

Focal Neuropathies

Focal and sometimes multifocal neuropathies occur in diabetes more often in the elderly. The main clinical locations of mononeuropathies are the cranial nerves, trunk, and proximal lower limbs.

Among the cranial nerves, an acute third nerve palsy is the most common. The onset is acute and painful, with complete oculomotor dysfunction and, typically, sparing of pupillary function. The sixth nerve is also often involved. Evidence for involvement of other cranial nerves is rare. Pathologic data indicate an ischemic origin; however, it has recently been shown that the lesions are not always in the nerve itself but also in the midbrain. Recovery is spontaneous, taking 2 or 3 months on average, and repeated palsies may occur but are rare.

Lesions of limb nerves also occur. These are located at common entrapment or external compression sites such as the median nerve at the wrist, the ulnar nerve at the elbow, or the peroneal nerve at the fibula head. A thoracoabdominal neuropathy is an acute unilateral pain syndrome with a radicular distribution that occurs in older diabetic patients.

Asymmetric or unilateral lower limb proximal motor neuropathy is characterized by unilateral or bilateral proximal weakness and muscle atrophy with a variable degree of sensory loss and pain, often at night. The onset of proximal diabetic neuropathy is acute or subacute. Patients complain of burning pain that is worse at night and numbness or hyperesthesia of the anterior thigh. Weakness is pronounced in the iliopsoas and quadriceps muscles. Amyotrophy is an early and common phenomenon. The patient's condition improves after months. Recent reports have demonstrated inflammatory changes, including evidence of vasculitis in biopsy specimens of cutaneous nerve of the thigh.

Uremic Neuropathy

Polyneuropathy as a complication of end-stage chronic renal failure has been recognized for 30 years. The main risk factor for the appearance of neuropathy is the duration and the severity of renal failure. In all the clinical studies, the incidence in males is higher than in females. Initially, sensory symptoms predominate: "Burning feet" and distal dysesthesia are common early symptoms. The polyneuropathy is distal and symmetric, mainly a sensory disturbance affecting the legs more than arms. On early neurologic examination, ankle jerks are lost, and vibratory sensation is impaired. Pain and temperature modalities are less involved. There is a considerable variation in the severity of the neuropathy from one patient to another.

Electrophysiologic study has shown that conduction is slowed in motor and sensory fibers. Clinicopathologic studies suggest two types of neuropathy: acute and axonal, and a slowly progressive, demyelinating neuropathy. With successful renal transplantation, progressive improvement is the rule.

Isolated mononeuropathy syndromes occur in patients with renal failure. The two most frequent are CTS and monomelic neuropathy secondary to a vascular shunt.

Sarcoidosis

Sarcoidosis is a multisystem granulomatosis disorder that should be considered in patients with mul-

tiple mononeuropathies involving cranial or limb nerves or polyneuropathy associated with eye or skin lesions and hilar lymphadenopathy. Facial nerve palsy is the most common neurologic manifestation, and the palsy is usually complete. Incomplete recovery and bilateral involvement is common. Peripheral nervous system manifestations include multiple mononeuropathies, polyradiculitis, and a symmetric polyneuropathy. The natural history of sarcoid neuropathy is uncertain. Nerve conduction studies show evidence of axonal degeneration. Muscle biopsy is more helpful than nerve biopsy in making the diagnosis. Granulomas are situated in the perineurium and can extend into the endoneurium of cranial and spinal nerves. Steroids are justified in some patients.

Peripheral Neuropathy Associated with Monoclonal Gammopathy

Searching for the presence of monoclonal gammopathy is an important part of the evaluation of patients with peripheral neuropathy. One group found that 10% of patients with idiopathic peripheral neuropathy have a monoclonal gammopathy. Immunofixation is the most efficient and cost-effective method of screening for monoclonal gammopathy. A very small proportion of those patients have amyloidosis or underlying malignancy (multiple myeloma or lymphoma). The other patients are described as having a monoclonal gammopathy of undetermined significance (MGUS), which occasionally progresses to malignancy.

Neuropathy Associated with Monoclonal Gammopathy of Undetermined Significance

Mean age at onset of symptoms of MGUS is approximately 56 years. Men are more frequently affected than women. Typical initial symptoms are sensory: paresthesias, loss of feeling, and unsteadiness. Later, most patients develop motor signs. The distal segments of the lower limbs are more affected than the upper limbs. Most patients have a sensory motor polyradiculoneuropathy. Sensory loss, upper limb tremor, and gait ataxia predominate in the immunoglobulin (Ig)M group compared with those with elevations of IgG or IgA. The course of this neuropathy is slowly progressive over years. Electrophysiologic studies show features of axonal degeneration and demyelination. Motor nerve conduction velocities are in the demyelinating range with a marked increase of the distal motor latency related to forearm or leg motor conduction delay in IgM-MGUS. An important part of the laboratory evaluation is to look for reactive monoclonal IgM antibodies against myelin-associated glycoprotein (50% of patients with IgM-MGUS). Nerve biopsy specimens show loss of large myelinated fibers with segmental demyelination and remyelination on testing. Clinical responses to prednisone, cyclophosphamide, azathioprine, chlorambucil, and cyclosporine have been described in uncontrolled trials involving small numbers of patients.

Neuropathy Associated with Multiple Myeloma

Usual neurologic manifestations of multiple myeloma (MM) are root and cord compression from a lytic vertebral lesion. In MM, peripheral neuropathy may be caused by several entities: direct root compression, a toxic effect of the treatment, and amyloidosis. Amyloid deposition is responsible for a symmetric polyneuropathy with marked initial sensory symptoms, "burning," and autonomic features. Diagnosis depends on nerve biopsy results. In osteosclerotic myeloma, most patients initially described were from Japan and developed lymphadenopathy or hepatosplenomegaly, diabetes, hypothyroidism, gynecomastia in men, amenorrhea in women, and skin changes (hypertrichosis and hyperpigmentation). The type of neuropathy associated with osteosclerotic myeloma is a diffuse polyradiculoneuropathy.

Neuropathy Associated with Lymphoma

In patients with neuropathy associated with lymphoma, nerve root and meningeal infiltration can result in a generalized polyradiculoneuropathy and cranial neuropathies. The course is progressive, and the diagnosis is established by finding malignant cells in the spinal fluid or a nerve biopsy specimen.

Malignancy-Associated Neuropathy

Compression and infiltration of peripheral nerve roots and cranial nerves are the most common

effects of malignancy. However, the frequency of peripheral neuropathy depends on the type of investigation used and varies from 5% of a clinically symptomatic neuropathy to 50% when electrophysiologic criteria are used.

The sensory neuropathy associated with oat cell carcinoma of the lung was described in 1948 and is the most distinctive. Its recognition is important because it may develop before the recognition of the cancer. Patients experience paresthesia and ataxia. Pathologic data indicate neuronal degeneration of the dorsal root ganglia.

In addition, a mixed sensorimotor distal neuropathy is much more common than the sensory neuropathy. Primary carcinomas of the lung, breast, colon, uterus, and pancreas are associated with this type of neuropathy. The course is variable; acute-onset and relapsing neuropathy have been described. Electrophysiologic studies show evidence of axonal neuropathy. Pathologically, axonal degeneration is the most frequent abnormality.

Inherited Peripheral Neuropathies

Hereditary Motor and Sensory Neuropathy

Charcot-Marie-Tooth neuropathy is a heterogenous group of disorders and the classification became easier after the systematic use of nerve conduction studies, nerve biopsies, and, recently, molecular genetic studies.

Hereditary Motor and Sensory Neuropathy Type 1

Hereditary motor and sensory neuropathy type 1 (HMSN-1) is a chronic neuropathy with onset in the first decade and mainly motor impairment, which is usually symmetric. Weakness and atrophy are found in intrinsic foot and anterior compartment muscles of the legs. Foot deformities include pes cavus and clawing of the toes. Weakness and wasting of the hands begin some years after the lower extremity involvement. Sensory loss is not a prominent feature of this condition. Deep tendon reflexes are almost always absent. Peripheral nerves are thickened. Progression of the disease is gradual. Autosomal dominant inheritance is most common, although some recessive inheritance is observed.

Electrodiagnostic studies show marked uniform slowing along the nerve. Nerve biopsy specimens in most cases reveal onion bulb formations, various degrees of fiber loss, and demyelination and remyelination. There are three genetic variants characterized by genetic linkage and gene analysis. Charcot-Marie-Tooth disease type 1a (CMT-1a) is the most common variant mapped to chromosome 17p. Patients have been found to have duplication at 17p11.2–12 or a point mutation in the peripheral myelin protein 22. Charcot-Marie-Tooth disease type lb (CMT-lb) maps on chromosome 1; point mutations in the human myelin protein gene *Po* have been found. Charcot-Marie-Tooth disease type 1c (CMT-1c) represent patients unlinked with chromosome 1 and 17, and they have no current known genetic abnormalities.

Hereditary Motor and Sensory Neuropathy Type 2

HMSN-2 is much less common than HMSN-1. Onset of symptoms is most often in the second decade or even later. Clinical features, course, and prognosis are similar to those of HMSN-1 except nerve thickening does not occur. Inheritance is usually autosomal dominant and rarely recessive. Motor and sensory nerve conduction are in the normal range or mildly reduced. On the basis of genetic linkage, two types have been found: one group maps to the short arm of chromosome 1 and the other to the long arm of chromosome 3. No candidate gene has been identified.

Hereditary Motor and Sensory Neuropathy Type 3

HMSN-3 is a rare condition that begins in infancy and is characterized by its severity. Weakness appears in a distal lower extremity and the upper extremities are involved soon afterward. Enlarged peripheral nerves can be palpated. Abnormal pupillary responses to light are seen. Severe skeletal abnormalities are also present. Conduction velocity is very slow, less than 10 meters per second. The pattern of inheritance of CMT-3 is more often autosomal recessive. Point mutations have been found in the *PMP22* gene and *Po* (as above).

*X-Linked Hereditary Motor
and Sensory Neuropathy*

An X-linked pattern of inheritance has been described in some families with Charcot-Marie-Tooth disease. Females are affected less often than males. Nerve conduction studies show moderate slowing. Linkage studies localized the *CMTX* gene on the proximal part of the long arm of the X chromosome. Different types of mutations have been described in connexin 32 gene.

*Hereditary Neuropathy with Liability
to Pressure Palsy*

Also designated "tomaculous neuropathy," hereditary neuropathy with liability to pressure palsy is characterized by the observation that patients develop sudden and painless symptoms as a result of external pressure. Nerves affected are those associated with compressive lesions: the peroneal nerve at the head of the fibula, the median nerve at the wrist, the ulnar nerve at the elbow, and the radial nerve in the spiral groove. The majority of the patients have their initial episode in the first decade; complete recovery usually follows, but on occasion generalized neuropathy may also be present. Electrophysiologic studies show demyelinating features, especially at entrapment sites. Nerve biopsy specimens show focal thickening of myelin described as a "sausage." The genetic abnormality maps to the short arm of chromosome 17, with a large deletion of the *PMP22* gene. Inheritance is autosomal dominant.

Familial Amyloid Polyneuropathy

Amyloid polyneuropathies may be inherited or acquired. It is important to remember that many different proteins can be deposited in tissue as amyloid. In plasma cell dyscrasias, immunoglobulin light chains represent the protein-forming amyloid deposits. In familial amyloid polyneuropathy inherited as an autosomal dominant trait, the majority of cases are associated with transthyretin protein deposition but in a smaller number of cases apolipoprotein or gelsolin are involved. Typically, clinical manifestations start with sensory impairment, including dysesthesia and distal sensory loss affecting more selectively pain and temperature sensation. Autonomic participation includes impotence, orthostatic hypotension, and sphincter disturbances. Patients suspected of having familial amyloid polyneuropathy can undergo DNA testing that looks for a specific mutation.

Refsum's Disease

Demyelinating polyneuropathy is a cardinal feature of Refsum's disease associated with hearing loss, retinitis pigmentosa, anosmia, and cardiomyopathy. This disease has been reported in people of northern Europe and is inherited in an autosomal recessive manner. Diagnosis is confirmed by demonstrating high serum phytanic acid levels.

Fabry's Disease

Fabry's disease is an X-linked disorder that first appears in childhood or early adult life. Most patients have angiokeratoma with a very specific distribution. Strokes and cardiovascular and renal failure are common. Pain is the hallmark of the disease, and the neuropathologic data show selective loss of small myelinated and unmyelinated fibers. Diagnosis is made by measuring the concentration of leukocyte lysosomal alpha galactosidase.

Porphyric Neuropathy

Porphyrias are a group of rare hereditary disorders. Some are associated with peripheral nerve and mental symptoms. Porphyric neuropathy occurs as an acute episode of proximal and distal weakness associated with abdominal pain and psychosis, often induced by drugs or nutritional factors.

Neuropathies Associated with Infection

Leprosy

Leprosy represents a chronic granulomatous and treatable infection by *Mycobacterium leprae* and is one of the main causes of neuropathy in the world. Leprosy occurs in tropical and subtropical developing countries, mainly in Africa and Asia. The manifestations of leprosy depend on the patient's immunologic status. The lepromatous form is associated with low cell-mediated immunity and the tuberculoid form is associated with high cell-mediated immunity.

Sensory loss is the cardinal and most constant feature of leprous neuropathy. Sensory loss is variable in distribution and is caused by cutaneous nerve damage involving at first pain and temperature modalities leading to trophic changes and painless trauma. Joint position and tendon reflexes are preserved. Sensory loss may demonstrate a nerve root pattern when an intense inflammatory response affects a nerve trunk (tuberculoid leprosy). Nerve hypertrophy occurs in approximately one-third of patients with leprosy. The auricular nerve in the neck and the ulnar nerve above the elbow are common sites. The peroneal nerve and radial cutaneous nerve at the wrist are often enlarged. Motor disturbance is a late event in the course of the disease, involving the ulnar and median nerves in the upper limb and the peroneal nerve in the lower limb. Facial palsy with lagophthalmos is a classic feature.

Spontaneously or during treatment an acute generalized systemic reaction may occur in response to an alteration of the immunity. A reversal reaction (type I) appears during the first year of therapy, which is characterized by general malaise, fever, pain, and swelling of nerve trunks with sensory and motor deficit. Pathologic features include endoneural granuloma, giant cells, vasculitis, and perineuritis. Erythema nodosum leprosum type II occurs in a proportion of patients with the lepromatous form, which responds to antibacterial treatment. This causes an acute painful neuritis accompanied by fever and arthritis. Pathologic features include inflammatory infiltrates in the nerve.

Nerve conduction studies are not specific. They show reduced amplitude of sensory nerve action potentials (SNAPs) and CMAPs with focal conduction slowing. For diagnosis and management, a nerve biopsy is useful.

Prolonged treatment is given with rifamycin and Dapsone for tuberculoid forms and with clofazimine for lepromatous forms. Corticosteroid treatment is useful for reactions.

Peripheral Neuropathies in Human Immunodeficiency Virus Infection

Peripheral nerve disorders are common complications of HIV infection. Symptomatic neuropathy affects 5–10% of HIV-infected patients. Early recognition and treatment of polyneuropathies are very important because they can improve the overall well-being of the patient. Different types of neuropathies have been observed in the course of HIV infection: inflammatory polyneuropathy of the GBS type, multifocal neuropathy, acute bilateral facial palsy, and meningoradiculoneuritis.

Guillain-Barré Syndrome

The GBS variant can be observed at the time of seroconversion to HIV or later. The prognosis is usually good, with a spontaneous recovery. Relapsing forms are occasionally observed. A more pronounced inflammatory reaction is seen in the CSF: lymphocytic pleocytosis and an elevated protein level. Electrophysiologic testing results are identical to those of acute inflammatory demyelinating polyradiculpathy. Nerve biopsy specimens show evidence of a variety of lesions: macrophage-mediated demyelination, mixed axonal and demyelinating lesions, or axonal lesions. Inflammatory infiltrates are usually mild.

Subacute Multifocal Neuropathy

Subacute multifocal neuropathy is the most common cause of neuropathy observed in HIV patients before cellular immunosuppression. The clinical picture may be multiple sensory motor deficits with paresthesias and pain involving either the lower or upper limbs. Involvement of the cranial nerves may occur. The facial nerve is the most commonly affected nerve, followed by the trigeminal nerve. The outcome of the neuropathy is usually good; patients do improve spontaneously or with immunomodulating therapy.

The CSF shows an increase in protein and a mild pleocytosis. Electrophysiologic data show multifocal involvement, and nerve biopsy specimens show mixed axonal and demyelinating lesions of the nerve fibers with inflammatory infiltrates. In a few (10%) patients, necrotizing arteritis has been found in the nerve and muscle.

Distal Symmetric Polyneuropathy

Distal symmetric polyneuropathy is the most common type of neuropathy seen at the later stages of HIV infection. The main complaint is "burning feet" affecting both lower limbs and associated with painful contact dysesthesias. Motor involvement is moderate. Nerve biopsy specimens show marked axonal lesions. The specific etiology is unknown.

Autonomic Neuropathy

Abnormalities of autonomic function may occur in HIV patients, and cases of pandysautonomia have been reported.

Lymphoma

Lymphoma associated with HIV infection may induce focal or multifocal nerve lesions by invading spinal roots or nerve trunks.

Cytomegalovirus Infection

Cytomegalovirus (CMV) infection is one of the most common viral opportunistic infections in acquired immunodeficiency syndrome, affecting 15–35% of the patients, and is amenable to specific treatment. There are different patterns of CMV neuropathies: a polyradiculopathic pattern developing within a few days or weeks of infection, and a multifocal pattern that includes lesions of spinal roots, nerve trunks, and cranial nerves. Abnormalities of the CSF are specific, including high protein content, low glucose levels, and cellular reaction with predominant polymorphonuclear leukocytes. Nerve lesions are specific, showing scattered cytomegalic cells and endothelial cells of endoneurial capillaries.

Lyme Borreliosis

Lyme disease is a multisystem illness caused by a tick-transmitted spirochete, *Borrelia burgdorferi,* that affects skin, joints, heart, and the nervous system. This disease can be divided into three clinical stages. Stage 1 follows the tick bite and is characterized by erythema chronicum migrans and general symptoms such as myalgia, fatigue, fever, and arthralgia caused by the general dissemination. Stage 2 occurs within weeks to months or later. Neurologic signs develop in 15–20% of patients. Meningitis is the most common abnormality. CSF examination reveals a lymphocytic pleocytosis; the glucose level is usually normal. Spirochetes can be isolated using special staining methods. Cranial neuritis, most often facial palsy, is present in 50% of patients and usually resolves spontaneously within weeks or months. Peripheral neuropathy occurs in 30–50% of patients. Signs and symptoms suggest a multifocal sensorimotor involvement of the peripheral nervous system. Nerve conduction studies show focal or multifocal, predominantly axonal degeneration; less commonly, demyelinating changes are noted. Pathologically, axonal degeneration is the predominant feature and lymphocytic and plasma cell inflammatory infiltrates are located around the perineural and endoneural vessels. Stage 3 is characterized by the occurrence of asymmetric arthritis. Various syndromes affecting the central nervous system have been described, but there is no convincing evidence for central nervous system complications of Lyme disease.

The diagnosis of Lyme disease is confirmed by testing for the presence of antibodies against *Borrelia burgdorferi* in the serum and the CSF. False-positive and false-negative results may occur. Neurologic manifestations respond to ceftriaxone or high doses of intravenous penicillin G.

Toxic and Drug-Induced Peripheral Neuropathies

Alcoholic Neuropathy

Alcoholic neuropathy one of the most common causes of peripheral neuropathy. Some patients have asymptomatic loss of ankle jerks and distal sensory loss over the feet. In more severely affected patients, complaints of pain in the calf, lower limb paresthesia, distal weakness, and a stocking-glove symmetric pattern of sensory loss involving all modalities occur. In addition, alcoholic patients can develop focal compressive peripheral nerve lesions affecting generally the radial, ulnar, or common peroneal nerves.

Electrodiagnostic studies typically show evidence of an axonal sensory motor neuropathy. Sural nerve biopsy shows loss of nerve fibers affecting large myelinated fibers. Axonal lesions are more marked than demyelinating lesions. The pathogenesis of alcoholic neuropathy includes nutritional deficiency and the direct toxic effect of ethanol. Improvement does occur with long-term abstinence. It is important to know that disulfiram therapy for alcoholism can induce an axonal sensorimotor neuropathy.

Drugs

Vinca Alkaloids

Vinca alkaloids are used in the treatment of lymphoma and leukemia. The peripheral neuropathy is initially sensory, and the distribution of weakness is peculiar, involving the ankles and extensor muscles of the fingers and wrists.

Cisplatin

A predominantly sensory neuropathy developed in patients after cumulative dose of 225–500 mg per m^2 cisplatin. There is involvement of large sensory myelinated fibers. Symptoms and signs may start after the last dose of cisplatin. SNAPs are decreased; motor conduction is normal.

Taxol

Used in human breast cancer, taxol produces sensory neuropathy in doses exceeding 200 mg per m^2.

Perhexiline

Used in the treatment of angina and cardiac arrhythmias, perhexiline induces a subacute sensorimotor neuropathy. Nerve biopsy specimens show segmental demyelination.

Metronidazole

A large-fiber–type sensory neuropathy may occur in patients with inflammatory bowel disease with the prolonged administration of metronidazole with a total dose of at least 30 g.

Nucleoside Neuropathies

Nucleosides are used to treat acquired immunodeficiency syndrome. These are responsible for a subacute distal axonopathy characterized by intense burning sensation.

Heavy Metals

Lead, thallium, and arsenic are classic causes of neuropathy. Thallium neuropathy is characterized by the loss of hair.

Suggested Reading

Bolton CF, Young GB. Neurological Complications of Renal Disease. Boston: Butterworths, 1990;59–74.

Gilliatt RW, Harrison MJG. Nerve Compression and Entrapment. In AN Asbury, RW Gilliat (eds), Peripheral Nerve Disorders. Boston: Butterworth, 1984; 243–286.

Harding AE, Reilly MM. Molecular Genetics of Inherited Neuropathies. In AN Asbury, PK Thomas (eds), Peripheral Nerve Disorders II. Boston: Butterworth–Heinemann, 1995.

Hughes RAC. Guillain-Barré Syndrome. Heidelberg: Springer-Verlag, 1990.

Said G. Inflammatory Neuropathies Associated with Known Infection (HIV, Leprosy, Chagas disease, Lyme disease). In JG McLeod (ed), Inflammatory Neuropathies. London: Tindall-Baillières, 1994;149–171.

Said G. Diabetic neuropathy: an update. J Neurology 1996;243:431.

Said G, Lacroix-Ciaudo C, Fujimura H, et al. The peripheral neuropathy of necrotizing arteritis: a clinicopathologic study. Ann Neurol 1988;23:461.

Stewart JD. Focal Peripheral Neuropathies. New York: Raven Press, 1993.

Thomas PK , Ochoa J. Clinical Features and Differential Diagnosis. In PJ Dyck, PK Thomas, J Griffin, J Posdulo (eds), Peripheral Neuropathy (3rd ed). Philadelphia: Saunders, 1993;749–774.

Thomas PK. The Peripheral Nerves as a Target for Toxic Subtances. In PS Spencer, H Schaumburg (eds), Experimental and Clinical Neurotoxicology. Baltimore: Williams & Wilkins, 1980;35–47.

Victor M, Adams RM, Collins GH. The Wernicke-Korsakoff Syndrome and Related Neurologic Disorders Due to Alcoholism and Malnutrition. Contemporary Neurology Series. Philadelphia: Davis, 1989.

Chapter 35
Autonomic Disorders

Christopher J. Mathias

Chapter Plan

The autonomic nervous system supplies and influences virtually every organ in the body. Additionally, it is involved in major integrative processes such as control of blood pressure and body temperature. It has many intricate pathwaysand uses a wide range of neurotransmitters; thus, there is considerable flexibility and capability in its actions. Autonomic disorders have many causes, affecting one or more sites and involving single or multiple organs. These disorders are seen in neurologic and general medical practice, and additionally in specialties ranging from cardiology and endocrinology to ophthalmology and urology.

This chapter outlines the basic principles behind the functioning of the autonomic nervous system, followed by a classification of autonomic disorders, a description of the key components on clinical assessment and investigation, and finally, a brief description of the major disorders seen in clinical practice.

Basic Principles

The autonomic nervous system has two major divisions: the parasympathetic, with a cranial and sacral spinal outflow, and the sympathetic, with a thoracolumbar spinal outflow (Figure 35-1). These efferent pathways are influenced by a variety of afferents involving virtually every sensory pathway. There are many centers within the brain controlling autonomic function, with key centers in the hypothalamus, the midbrain, and the brain stem. Neurons within the spinal cord include the intermediolateral cell mass for sympathetic control and the nucleus of Onufrowicz (Onuf's nucleus) in the sacral segments for urinary sphincter function. Preganglionic efferent pathways from the brain and spinal cord synapse in ganglia, with postganglionic pathways to target organs; in the parasympathetic system, these are usually close to the target organ, unlike the sympathetic system where the ganglia are paravertebral and thus usually some distance away.

The major neurotransmitters in ganglionic and postganglionic autonomic function are outlined in Figure 35-2; additionally there are numerous amines, peptides, and purines involved in neurotransmission and neuromodulation.

The postganglionic autonomic nerve terminals and their interphase with effector cells are where

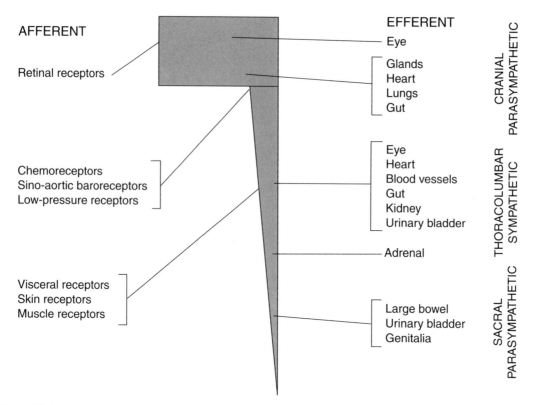

Figure 35-1. Schema indicating the major afferent pathways that influence the major autonomic efferent outflows from the brain and spinal cord (the cranial and sacral parasympathetic and the thoracolumbar sympathetic) that supply various organs.

complex activity occurs. In sympathetic nerve terminals a series of processes result in the formation of the major neurotransmitter, noradrenaline. After its release, it has both presynaptic and synaptic effects, and the overflow into the circulation can be measured. Circulating levels of noradrenaline often are used as an index of sympathetic activation, although there are limitations in certain circumstances. Muscle and skin sympathetic neural activity may be measured from peripheral nerves using percutaneous microneurographic techniques.

Classification

Autonomic disorders may be classified in a number of ways. Some affect localized areas (Holmes-Adie pupil), whereas others have widespread effects involving many systems (multiple system atrophy [MSA]). Classification under the site of the lesion (e.g., spinal cord transection) or the specific biochemical deficit (e.g., dopamine β-hydroxylase deficiency) provides a further approach. Many autonomic disorders complicate well-described diseases (e.g., diabetes mellitus and liver failure). A number do not easily fit into one category and could belong to multiple groups. Moreover, with increasing knowledge, there are regular additions to the list, with the description of autonomic dysfunction in otherwise well-documented diseases (e.g., human immunodeficiency virus infection) or in new disorders (e.g., the prion disease, fatal familial insomnia). The main approach to the classification used here is under primary disorders where the cause is not known, and secondary disorders resulting from lesions at known sites, definitive causes, or disease associations (Table 35-1). There are two additional important categories: neurally mediated syncope in which the disorder usually is intermittent, and autonomic dysfunction resulting from drugs (Table 35-2). Finally, although the majority of autonomic disorders result from underactivity and failure, there are disorders in which autonomic overactivity

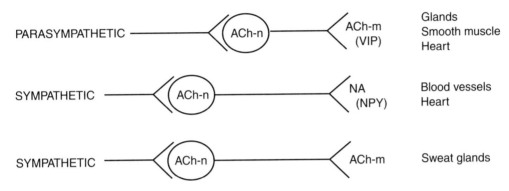

| GANGLIA | | TARGET ORGAN |

Figure 35-2. Outline of the major transmitters at autonomic ganglia and postganglionic sites on target organs supplied by the parasympathetic and sympathetic efferent pathways. The acetylcholine (ACh) receptor at all ganglia is of the nicotinic subtype (ACh-n). Ganglionic blockers such as hexamethonium thus prevent both parasympathetic and sympathetic activation. Atropine, however, acts only on the muscarinic (ACh-m) receptor at postganglionic parasympathetic and sympathetic cholinergic sites. The cotransmitters, along with the primary transmitters, are also indicated (NA = noradrenaline; VIP = vasoactive intestinal polypeptide; NPY = neuropeptide Y).

Table 35-1. Classification of Disorders Resulting in Autonomic Dysfunction

Primary (etiology unknown)
Acute/subacute dysautonomias
  Pure cholinergic dysautonomia
  Pure pandysautonomia
  Pandysautonomia with neurologic features
Chronic autonomic failure syndromes
  Pure autonomic failure
  Multiple system atrophy (Shy-Drager syndrome)
  Autonomic failure with Parkinson's disease
Secondary
Congenital
  Nerve growth factor deficiency
Hereditary
  Autosomal dominant trait
    Familial amyloid neuropathy
    Porphyria
  Autosomal recessive trait
    Familial dysautonomia—Riley-Day syndrome
    Dopamine β-hydroxylase deficiency
    Aromatic L-amino acid decarboxylase deficiency
  X-linked recessive
    Fabry's disease
Metabolic diseases
  Diabetes mellitus
  Chronic renal failure
  Chronic liver disease
  Vitamin B_{12} deficiency
  Alcohol-induced
Inflammatory
  Guillain-Barré syndrome
  Transverse myelitis

Infections
  Bacterial: tetanus, leprosy
  Viral: human immunodeficiency virus infection
  Parasitic: Chagas' disease
  Prion: fatal familial insomnia
Neoplasia
  Brain tumors—especially of the third ventricle or
    posterior fossa
  Paraneoplastic, to include adenocarcinomas—lung,
    pancreas, and Lambert-Eaton syndrome
Connective tissue disorders
  Rheumatoid arthritis
  Systemic lupus erythematosus
  Mixed connective tissue disease
Surgery
  Regional sympathectomy—upper limb, splanchnic
  Vagotomy and drainage procedures—"dumping
    syndrome"
  Organ transplantation—heart, kidney
Trauma
  Spinal cord transection
Neurally mediated syncope
Vasovagal syncope
Carotid sinus hypersensitivity
Micturition syncope
Swallow syncope
Associated with glossopharyngeal neuralgia
Drugs
See Table 35-2

Table 35-2. Drugs/Chemicals/Poisons/Toxins

Decreasing sympathetic activity
  Centrally acting
    Clonidine
    Methyldopa
    Reserpine
    Barbiturates
    Anesthetics
  Peripherally acting
    Sympathetic nerve ending (guanethidine, bethanidine)
    Alpha-adrenoceptor blockade (phenoxybenzamine)
    Beta-adrenoceptor blockade (propranolol)
Increasing sympathetic activity
  Amphetamines
  Releasing noradrenaline (tyramine)
  Uptake blockers (imipramine)
  Monoamine oxidase inhibitors (tranylcypromine)
  Beta-adrenoceptor stimulants (isoprenaline)
Decreasing parasympathetic activity
  Antidepressants (imipramine)
  Tranquilizers (phenothiazines)
  Antidysrhythmics (disopyramide)
  Anticholinergics (atropine, propantheline, benztropine)
  Toxins (botulinum)
Increasing parasympathetic activity
  Cholinomimetics (carbachol, bethanechol, pilocarpine, mushroom poisoning)
  Anticholinesterases
    Reversible carbonate inhibitors (pyridostigmine, neostigmine)
    Organophosphorous inhibitors (parathion)
Miscellaneous
  Alcohol, thiamine (vitamin B_1 deficiency)
  Vincristine, perhexiline maleate
  Thallium, arsenic, mercury
  Cyclosporin
  Mercury poisoning ("Pink" disease)
  Cignatera toxicity
  Jellyfish and marine animal venoms

Table 35-3. Some Clinical Manifestations of Autonomic Dysfunction

Cardiovascular	
Postural hypotension	Supine hypertension
Lability of blood pressure	Paroxysmal hypertension
Tachycardia	Bradycardia
Sudomotor	
Hypohidrosis or anhidrosis	Hyperhidrosis
Gustatory sweating	
Hyperpyrexia	Heat intolerance
Alimentary	
Xerostomia	Dysphagia
Gastric stasis	Dumping syndromes
Constipation	Diarrhea
Urinary	
Nocturia	Frequency
Urgency, retention	Incontinence
Sexual	
Erectile failure	Ejaculatory failure
Retrograde ejaculation	
Eye	
Pupillary abnormalities	Ptosis
Alacrima	Abnormal lacrimation with food ingestion

is a major problem (e.g., cardiac vagal overactivity in neurally mediated syncope, and autonomic dysreflexia in spinal cord injury).

Clinical Features

In autonomic disorders, the spectrum of clinical manifestations is wide (Table 35-3). Briefly, sympathetic adrenergic failure can result in orthostatic hypotension and ejaculatory failure; sympathetic cholinergic failure can cause anhidrosis; and parasympathetic failure can result in a fixed heart rate, a sluggish urinary bladder, and large-bowel and erectile failure. Autonomic hyperactivity may cause the reverse, and in some there may be a combination of the two. In the generalized disorders, the presenting features depend on which organ or system is initially involved and the ensuing functional deficit. This may be even more complicated in those with progressive disorders, such as MSA. Because the clinical features often overlap with those that occur in a number of other diseases, there often are difficulties with the diagnosis of autonomic disorders.

In localized disorders, the description itself may provide the diagnosis, as in primary palmar hyperhidrosis or gustatory sweating. The latter, however, may be a harbinger of more widespread autonomic impairment because it may complicate diseases such as diabetes mellitus. In the generalized disorders, a cardinal feature may be symptoms resulting from orthostatic (postural) hypotension (Figure 35-3) that classically results from impaired perfusion, especially to vital organs (Table 35-4). With long-standing orthostatic hypotension, however, improvements in cerebral

Figure 35-3. Blood pressure and heart rate measured by a noninvasive technique (with the Finapres), in two patients with autonomic failure. In the upper panel, blood pressure falls to extremely low levels; the patient, however, could maintain head-up tilt with a low blood pressure for more than 20 minutes with few symptoms. This patient had autonomic failure for many years and could tolerate such levels, unlike the patient in the panel below, who had to be put back to the horizontal position fairly quickly. She developed severe postural hypotension soon after surgery. (Reprinted with permission from CJ Mathias. Disorders Affecting Autonomic Function in Parkinsonian Patients. In L Battistin, G Scarlato, T Caraceni, S Ruggieri [eds], Advances in Neurology [Vol. 69]. Philadelphia: Lippincott–Raven, 1996;383–391.)

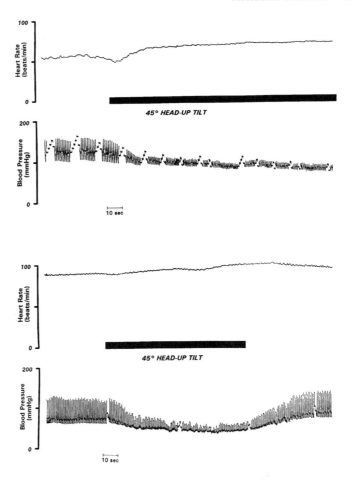

autoregulation increase orthostatic tolerance, and there may be few or nonspecific symptoms. These nonspecific symptoms include generalized weakness, lethargy, and fatigue and thus may be unhelpful or even misleading. Various factors in daily life may influence orthostatic hypotension (Table 35-5). Also, presyncopal symptoms or syncope may be unrelated to postural change. In neurally mediated syncope, there may be a history of a relationship of syncope with neck movements (in carotid sinus hypersensitivity) or with psychological trauma and fear (in vasovagal syncope). A history of impaired sweating (and temperature intolerance), urinary disturbances, sexual dysfunction (in men), or gastrointestinal abnormalities (e.g., constipation), especially in combination, should alert one to the possibility of a generalized autonomic disorder.

Other aspects in the history may be of relevance. Infants with Riley-Day syndrome (familial dysautonomia) usually have a history of consanguinity and usually are of an Ashkenazi Jewish origin. A family history may be elicited in vasovagal syncope. Obtaining a detailed drug history to include exposure to chemical agents, toxins, and poisons is essential because many substances directly or indirectly cause autonomic dysfunction.

The general examination may provide clues to an autonomic disorder. Pupillary and associated abnormalities occur in Horner's syndrome (Figure 35-4). Blood pressure should be measured while the patient is lying flat and after standing to assess the presence of orthostatic hypotension, which is defined as a decrease in systolic blood pressure of more than 20 mm Hg. A small decrease or even no change in blood pressure on postural change in the presence of appropriate symptoms does not exclude autonomic dysfunction because orthostatic hypotension may be unmasked or enhanced by other situations, such as food ingestion and exer-

Table 35-4. Some of the Symptoms Resulting from Orthostatic (Postural) Hypotension and Impaired Perfusion of Various Organs

Cerebral ischemia
    Dizziness
    Visual disturbances
        Blurred vision
        Tunnel vision
        Scotoma
        Graying out
        Blacking out
        Color defects
    Loss of consciousness
Muscle ischemia
    Paracervical and suboccipital ("coat-hanger") ache
    Lower back/buttock ache
    Calf claudication
Cardiac ischemia
    Angina pectoris
Spinal cord ischemia
Renal ischemia
    Oliguria
Nonspecific
    Weakness, lethargy, fatigue

Table 35-5. Factors that Influence the Degree of Orthostatic Hypotension

Speed of positional change
Time of day (worse in the morning)
Prolonged recumbency
Warm environment (hot weather, central heating, hot bath)
Raising intrathoracic pressure—micturition, defecation, or coughing
Food and alcohol ingestion
Physical exertion
Physical maneuvers and positions (bending forward, abdominal compression, leg crossing, squatting, activating calf muscle pump)*
Drugs with vasoactive properties (including dopaminergic agents)

*These maneuvers usually reduce the postural fall in blood pressure, unlike the others.

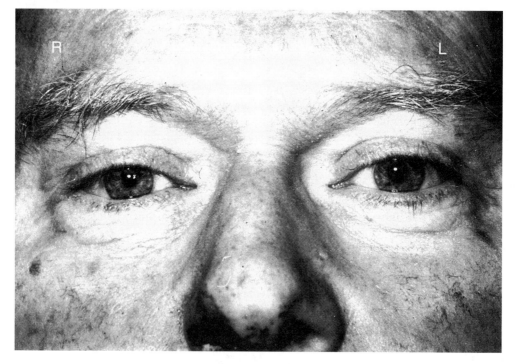

Figure 35-4. Partial ptosis and miosis, on the right, in a patient who presented with epistaxis. He had poorly controlled hypertension and neurologic features consistent with thrombosis of the posterior inferior cerebellar artery (the lateral medullary, Wallenberg's syndrome).

Figure 35-5. Intravenous digital subtraction angiogram of the carotid vessels in a patient with hypertension and widespread atherosclerosis. She had symptoms of cerebral ischemia associated with postural change. These occurred despite a small blood pressure fall of approximately 10 mm Hg. In the presence of left carotid artery stenosis, as demonstrated, this was sufficient to induce symptoms. She benefited from a reduction in her antihypertensive therapy, which abolished the small orthostatic fall in blood pressure.

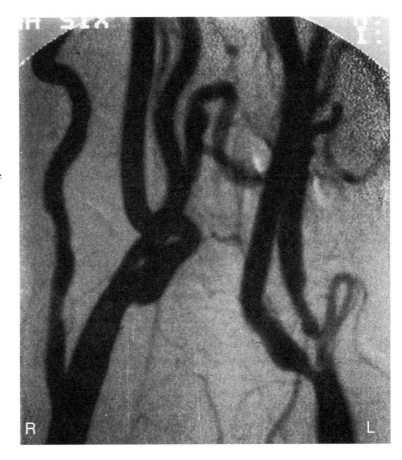

cise. Furthermore, in the presence of cardiovascular disease (e.g., carotid artery stenosis), even a small decrease in blood pressure may cause hemodynamically induced cerebral ischemia (Figure 35-5). The examination may provide information about associated diseases, such as liver cirrhosis and diabetes mellitus. The neurologic examination may indicate a specific deficit, such as a peripheral neuropathy in familial amyloidosis and parkinsonian/cerebellar lesions in MSA. Basic bedside testing for glycosuria in diabetes mellitus or proteinuria in systemic amyloidosis may provide important diagnostic information.

Investigation

When an autonomic disorder is suspected, the first step should be to determine if autonomic function is normal or abnormal. Autonomic screening tests are a useful initial means but have their limita-

tions. These have been best directed toward cardiovascular assessment, mainly utilizing noninvasive approaches, although a number of tests are now available, or being developed, for many of the other systems (Table 35-6). Normal screening test results do not necessarily exclude an autonomic disorder; this is where the clinical history and examination is of particular importance. An example is in neurally mediated syncope, where carotid sinus massage will be needed to diagnose carotid sinus hypersensitivity.

If the autonomic screening test results are abnormal, then further evaluation is needed to determine the site and extent of the lesion, the functional deficit, and whether it is a primary or secondary disorder. This is essential for an accurate diagnosis, for prognosis, and for management. The tests that are used to determine the site and extent of the lesion depend on the systems involved and the condition suspected (see Table 35-6). Some investigations may provide the diagnosis (see Figures 35-5, 35-6);

526 TEXTBOOK OF NEUROLOGY

Table 35-6. Outline of Investigations in Autonomic Failure

Cardiovascular
  Physiologic
    Head-up tilt, standing; Valsalva's maneuver
    Pressor stimuli: isometric exercise, cutaneous cold pressor, mental arithmetic
    Heart rate responses: deep breathing, hyperventilation, standing, head-up tilt, liquid meal challenge
    Exercise testing
    Carotid sinus massage
  Biochemical
    Basal plasma noradrenaline, adrenaline, and dopamine levels
    Plasma noradrenaline: supine and standing
    Basal urinary catecholamines
    Plasma renin activity
    Plasma aldosterone
  Pharmacologic
    Noradrenaline: alpha-adrenoceptors, vascular
    Isoprenaline: beta-adrenoceptors, vascular and cardiac
    Tyramine: pressor and noradrenaline response
    Edrophonium: noradrenaline response
    Clonidine: growth hormone response
    Atropine: heart rate response
Sweating
  Thermoregulatory: increase core temperature by 1°C
  Sweat gland response to intradermal acetylcholine
  Sympathetic skin response
Gastrointestinal
  Barium studies, videocinefluoroscopy, endoscopy, gastric-emptying studies, anal sphincter electromyography
Renal function and urinary tract
  Day and night urine volumes and sodium/potassium excretion
  Urodynamic studies, intravenous urography, ultrasound examination, urethral sphincter electromyography
Sexual function
  Penile plethysmography
  Intracavernosal papaverine
Respiratory
  Laryngoscopy
  Sleep studies to assess apnea/oxygen desaturation
Eye
  Schirmer's test
  Pupillary function: pharmacologic and physiologic

Source: Adapted from CJ Mathias, R Bannister. Investigation of Autonomic Disorders. In R Bannister, CJ Mathias (eds), Autonomic Failure: A Textbook of Clinical Disorders of the Autonomic Nervous System (3rd ed). Oxford, UK: Oxford University Press, 1992;255–290.

others may be valuable in certain disorders (Figure 35-7). Assessing the functional deficient may be of particular importance for therapy; an example is the 24-hour, noninvasive, ambulatory measurement of blood pressure and heart rate (Figure 35-8A,B) and the effects of various stimuli in daily life (e.g., food ingestion, exercise). A variety of tests may be needed for diagnosing or excluding underlying diseases. These may include neuroimaging studies (e.g., computed tomographic [CT] and magnetic resonance imaging [MRI] brain scans), sural nerve biopsy (and specific staining with monoclonal antibodies), and genetic testing. These need to be combined with other non-neurologic investigations depending on the clinical disorder suspected.

Management

Management varies considerably depending on the autonomic disorder, the functional autonomic deficit, and whether it is primary or secondary. In secondary disorders in particular, the management must involve the underlying condition, as its treatment may worsen certain autonomic features. In certain situations, simple procedures may help, such as withdrawal of an offending drug or the unblocking of a urinary catheter (to prevent autonomic dysreflexia in spinal cord injuries). Complex procedures may be needed, such as hepatic transplantation to reduce levels of variant transthyretin in familial amyloid polyneuropathy. Quality of life is often substantially improved by reducing orthostatic hypotension, overcoming urinary incontinence, alleviating gastrointestinal disturbances, and treating sexual dysfunction.

Description of Autonomic Disorders

Localized Disorders

Localized disorders are described separately from the generalized disorders (Table 35-7). Some may be discovered incidentally, such as the Holmes-Adie pupil. This usually is a benign condition in which the pupil is large and responds sluggishly to light; documentation is of value to avoid further

Figure 35-6. Plasma noradrenaline, adrenaline, and dopamine levels (measured by high-pressure liquid chromatography) in normal subjects (controls) and patients with multiple system atrophy (MSA) (Shy-Drager syndrome), pure autonomic failure (PAF), and two siblings with dopamine β-hydroxylase deficiency (DBH). Measurements were taken while subjects were supine and after head-up tilt to 45 degrees for 10 minutes. The asterisk indicates levels below the detection limit, which are less than 5 pg/ml for noradrenaline and adrenaline and less than 20 pg/ml for dopamine. Bars indicate ±SEM. (Reprinted with permission from CJ Mathias, R Bannister. Investigation of Autonomic Disorders. In R Bannister, CJ Mathias [eds], Autonomic Failure. A Textbook of Clinical Disorders of the Autonomic Nervous System [3rd ed]. Oxford, England: Oxford University Press, 1992;255–290.)

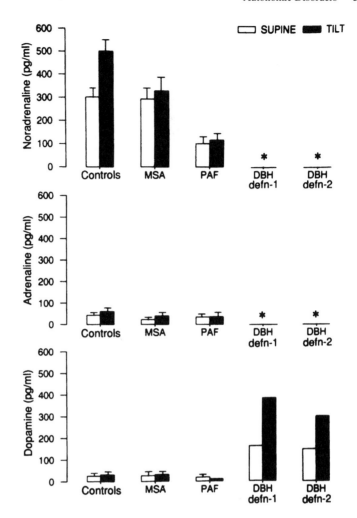

investigation and concern. Occasionally, it may be associated with anhidrosis and hyperhidrosis (Ross's syndrome) and less frequently with dry cough, diarrhea, or orthostatic hypotension. When associated with absent tendon reflexes, the term *Holmes-Adie syndrome* is used. The prognosis in this condition usually is favorable. This may not be so in other localized disorders affecting pupillary function, such as in Horner's syndrome where there is impairment of the facial sympathetic causing partial ptosis, miosis, facial cutaneous vasodilatation, and anhidrosis. Few complain of, or present with, this abnormality, which can be a harbinger of serious underlying disease (Figure 35-9).

Certain localized disorders may present with specific features, and the diagnosis can be ascertained readily on examination. Examples are the syndrome of crocodile tears and gustatory sweating; these result from aberrant reinnervation of the lachrymal glands in the former, and facial glands in the latter, as a result of trauma or surgery. A peripheral neuropathy, with denervation followed by reinnervation, may occur in systemic diseases such as diabetes mellitus, which also may cause gustatory sweating. Distressing localized disorders include hyperhidrosis of the palms, soles, and axillae of unknown etiology that may be associated with, or caused by, psychological disorders. Ascertaining the psychological component and its management may be important, as percutaneous endoscopic transthoracic sympathectomy, which is usually successful in abolishing sweating of the arms and palms, may

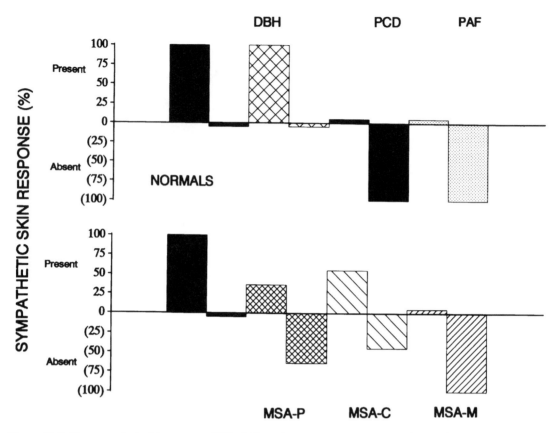

Figure 35-7. The sympathetic skin response (SSR), indicated as a percentage present or absent. The upper panel indicates responses in normal subjects and in different groups with peripheral autonomic failure. In peripheral disorders the SSR is of value; it is present in dopamine β-hydroxylase deficiency (DBH; where there is sympathetic adrenergic failure but sparing of the sympathetic cholinergic system) and is absent in pure cholinergic dysautonomia (PCD) and in pure autonomic failure (PAF). The lower panel indicates responses in the central disorder of multiple system atrophy (MSA). The SSR is present in a variable number of the parkinsonian (MSA-P) and cerebellar (MSA-C) forms, despite all having definite sympathetic adrenergic failure. In the multiple/mixed form (MSA-M) the SSR is absent in all subjects; this is consistent with MSA being a progressive disorder that in this form is probably more advanced than in MSA-P and MSA-C. It also indicates that in MSA, sympathetic adrenergic failure may occur before, or independently of, sympathetic cholinergic failure.

result in compensatory hyperhidrosis affecting the trunk and lower limbs (Figure 35-10). In some patients this may be worse than the original complaint.

In reflex sympathetic dystrophy, the debate continues about the role of the sympathetic nervous system in the cause or continuation of the disorder. It may be that postsynaptic adrenoceptors or the associated release of noncatecholamine neurotransmitters are responsible. It may follow trauma or surgery and cause severe pain that in some patients responds to regional guanethidine blocks, while in others is refractory to whatever therapy is used.

Disorders of the gut may affect a small segment, as in Hirschsprung's disease, which involves the intrinsic autonomic innervation, or may be localized to specific components, as in Chagas' disease,

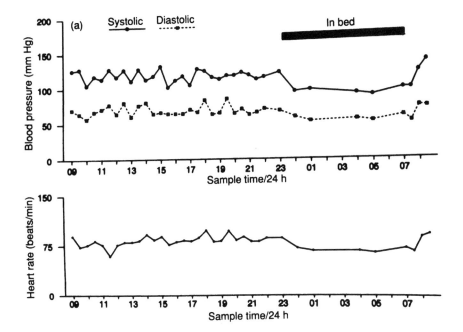

A

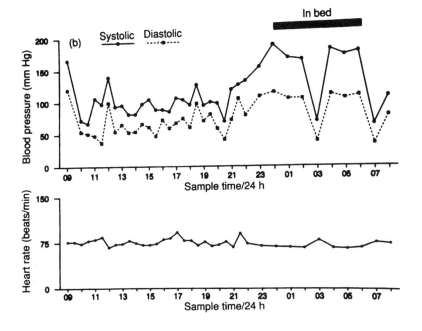

B

Figure 35-8. Twenty-four-hour noninvasive ambulatory blood pressure and heart rate profiles showing systolic and diastolic blood pressure and heart rate at intervals throughout the day and night. The horizontal axis depicts a 24-hour time scale. (A) Changes in a normal subject; showing an expected circadian fall in blood pressure while asleep. (B) Marked fluctuations in blood pressure in a subject with pure autonomic failure. The falls were usually the result of postural changes, either sitting or standing. Supine blood pressure, particularly at night, was elevated, with a reversal of the normal circadian fall in blood pressure. Rising to micturate caused a severe fall in blood pressure (at 0300 hours). There were relatively small changes in heart rate considering the marked fluctuations in blood pressure. (Reprinted with permission from CJ Mathias, R Bannister. Investigation of Autonomic Disorders. In R Bannister, CJ Mathias [eds], Autonomic Failure. A Textbook of Clinical Disorders of the Autonomic Nervous System [3rd ed]. Oxford, England: Oxford University Press, 1992;255–290.)

Table 35-7. Examples of Localized Autonomic Disorders

Holmes-Adie pupil
Horner's syndrome
Crocodile tears (Bogorad's syndrome)
Gustatory sweating (Frey's syndrome)
Reflex sympathetic dystrophy
Idiopathic palmar/axillary hyperhidrosis
Hirschsprung's disease (congenital megacolon)
Chagas' disease (trypanosomiasis)
Surgical procedures*
    Sympathectomy: regional
    Vagotomy and gastric drainage procedures in "dumping
        syndrome"
    Organ transplantation: heart, lungs

---

*Surgery may cause some of the disorders listed above (e.g., Frey's syndrome after parotid surgery).

where infection by the parasite *Trypanosoma cruzi* affects millions of South Americans and kills thousands each year. In the latter, there is targeting, probably on an immunologic basis, of the intrinsic plexuses in the heart and gut, resulting in cardiac conduction abnormalities, megaesophagus, megaduodenum, and megacolon. Although a generalized disease initially, it has been included here because of highly localized autonomic damage.

Various surgical procedures can cause autonomic dysfunction. This may be intentional, as in sympathectomy for hyperhidrosis. Vagotomy with gastric drainage procedures may cause the dumping syndrome, either early or late, with a number of systemic effects. The most recent addition to the list of localized autonomic disorders is organ transplantation.

Primary Autonomic Failure Syndromes

Primary autonomic failure syndromes may be subdivided into the acute/subacute dysautonomias and the chronic autonomic failure syndromes.

Acute/Subacute Dysautonomias

The acute/subacute dysautonomias include pure cholinergic dysautonomia, pure pandysautonomia, and pandysautonomia with neurologic features. They are characterized by an onset ranging from a few

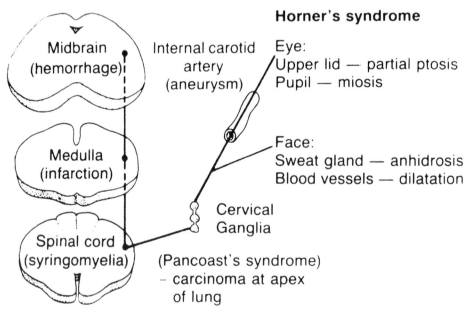

Figure 35-9. Some causes of Horner's syndrome, occurring at different sites of the central and peripheral sympathetic pathways to the face. (Reprinted with permission from CJ Mathias. Autonomic dysfunction. Br J Hosp Med 1987;38:238–243.)

Figure 35-10. Schematic representation showing the posterior and anterior surface of a subject who had undergone percutaneous endoscopic upper thoracic sympathetic ganglia ablation for palmar hyperhidrosis. The blank areas indicate lack of sweating during thermoregulatory testing when the body temperature was raised by 1°C. The hatched areas indicate excessive sweating (compensatory hyperhidrosis) over the trunk and inner thighs.

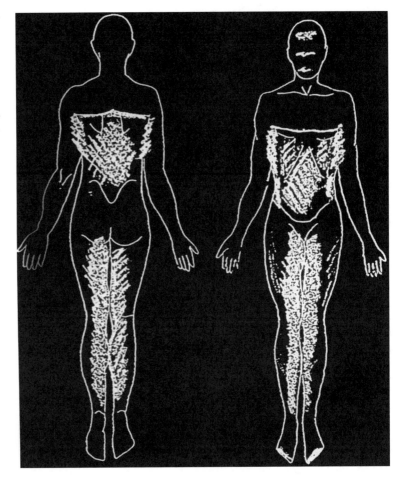

hours to a few days. In pure cholinergic dysautonomia, described mainly in children and young adults, there are features of widespread parasympathetic failure that include blurred vision, dry eyes, xerostomia, dysphagia (involving mainly the lower esophagus), constipation, and urinary retention. The term *cholinergic* is more appropriate than parasympathetic, as the sympathetic cholinergic pathways to sweat glands are also affected, resulting in anhidrosis and a tendency to hyperthermia. The clinical findings include dilated pupils, an elevated heart rate, dry and warm skin, a distended abdomen, and a palpable urinary bladder. Sympathetic vasoconstrictor function is preserved, and orthostatic hypotension does not occur. Recovery is not usual, and supportive therapy, especially in the initial stages, is needed to ensure an adequate fluid intake (especially in the presence of paralytic ileus) and to prevent hyperthermia.

Barium meal examinations should be avoided (Figure 35-11). The differential diagnosis includes exposure to anticholinergic drugs, poisons, and toxins that have similar effects. In jimsonweed (*Datura stramonium*) seed poisoning, there are similar autonomic features, but usually with hallucinations, hyperreflexia, and clonic jerking movements. Recovery often occurs in a few days. A variant of botulism (botulism B) affects cholinergic pathways with sparing of the motor pathways; substantial recovery often occurs within 3 months.

The pandysautonomias affect both sympathetic and parasympathetic pathways, and in addition to the cholinergic features, postural hypotension is a problem. There may be additional neurologic features, which are usually indicative of a peripheral neuropathy. The prognosis is variable, and in some there may be a substantial recovery. In addition to

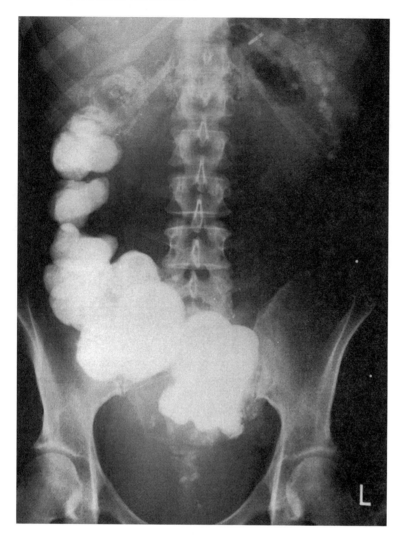

Figure 35-11. Radiograph showing inspissation of barium in the colon, 3 months after administration for the investigation of dysphagia at the onset of symptoms, when the diagnosis of pure cholinergic dysautonomia was not known. Because of large-bowel atony, it was not possible to dislodge the barium, and ultimately a colostomy was needed.

supportive therapy, immunoglobulin administration has been used with success in a few, favoring the possibility of an immunologic basis for some of these disorders.

Chronic Autonomic Failure Syndromes

The two well-recognized groups of chronic autonomic failure syndromes consist of pure autonomic failure (PAF) and MSA (Shy-Drager syndrome). In the former there are no additional neurologic features, unlike the latter. There is an additional rarer group with drug responsive idiopathic Parkinson's disease (IPD) and autonomic failure (Figure 35-12).

The majority of PAF patients are older than age 50 years at presentation, although with increasing awareness, younger patients are being diagnosed. The presenting features are variable and the majority are diagnosed when orthostatic hypotension is detected (Table 35-8). The diagnosis may not be made for a prolonged period, as the onset may be insidious and compensatory means may be used, often unwittingly, to reduce the symptoms. Even in those with the characteristic features of orthostatic hypotension and syncope, the diagnosis can be missed for years, as alternative diagnoses ranging from epilepsy to a psychiatric disorder may be considered erroneously. In males, impotence is common. Nocturia (rather than the other urinary

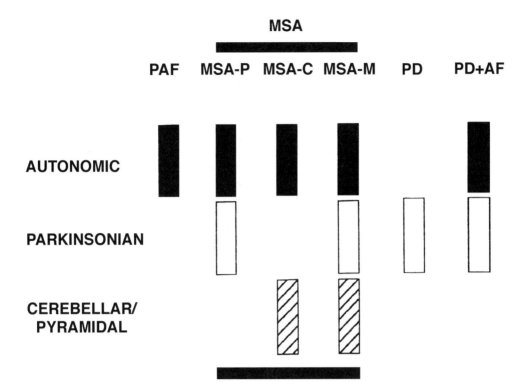

Figure 35-12. Schematic representation indicating the major clinical features in primary chronic autonomic failure syndromes and Parkinson's disease (PD). These include pure autonomic failure (PAF), the three major neurologic forms of multiple system atrophy (MSA), the parkinsonian form (MSA-P; synonymous with striatonigral degeneration), the cerebellar form (MSA-C; the olivopontocerebellar degeneration form), and the mixed form (MSA-M; with both features), and the rarer subgroup with Parkinson's disease and autonomic failure (PD + AF). (Adapted from CJ Mathias. Autonomic disorders and their recognition. N Engl J Med 1997;336:721.)

Table 35-8. Some Clinical Manifestations in Patients with Primary Autonomic Failure

Body System	Clinical Manifestation
Cardiovascular system	Orthostatic (postural) hypotension
Sudomotor system	Anhidrosis, heat intolerance
Alimentary tract	Xerostomia, oropharyngeal dysphagia, constipation, occasionally diarrhea
Urinary system	Nocturia, frequency, urgency, incontinence, retention
Reproductive system	Erectile and ejaculatory failure (in men)
Respiratory system	Stridor, involuntary inspiratory gasps, apneic periods
Ocular	Alacrima, anisocoria, Horner's syndrome
Nervous system	Parkinsonian, cerebellar, and pyramidal signs

symptoms listed in Table 35-8) is frequent. Constipation is often present. Impairment of sweating may not be recognized in temperate climates, although heat intolerance and collapse may occur in tropical areas. The clinical and laboratory features include the effects of widespread sympathetic failure, usually with parasympathetic deficits. The physiologic and biochemical tests indicate a peripheral autonomic lesion, consistent with limited but definitive neuropathologic data. The man-

Table 35-9. Some of the Approaches Used in the Management of Postural Hypotension, Especially in Patients with Chronic Autonomic Failure

Avoid
>   Sudden head-up postural change, especially in the morning
>   Straining during micturition and defecation
>   Heat
>   Large meals, especially with carbohydrate and fat
>   Alcohol
>   Drugs with vasodepressor properties

Physical methods
>   Elastic stockings
>   Abdominal binders
>   Antigravity suits
>   Head-up tilt

Drugs
>   Reducing salt loss/plasma volume expansion
>   Mineralocorticoids (fludrocortisone)
>   Reducing nocturnal polyuria
> V_2-receptor agonists (desmopressin)
>   Sympathetic vasoconstrictors
>   Directly on resistance vessels (midodrine, phenyle-
>   phrine, noradrenaline, clonidine) and capacitance
>   vessels (dihydroergotamine)
>   Indirectly (ephedrine, tyramine with monoamine
>   oxidase inhibitors, yohimbine)
>   Prodrug (L-dihydroxyphenylserine)
>   Nonsympathomimetic vasoconstrictors
> V_1 receptor agents: terlipressin
>   Preventing vasodilatation
>   Prostaglandin synthetase inhibitors (indomethacin,
>   flurbiprofen)
>   Dopamine receptor blockade (metoclopramide,
>   domperidone)
>   Beta$_2$-adrenoceptor blockade (propranolol)
>   Preventing postprandial hypotension
>   Adenosine receptor blockade (caffeine)
>   Peptide release inhibitors (somatostatin analog:
>   octreotide)
>   Increasing red cell mass (erythropoietin)
>   Increasing cardiac output (pindolol, xamoterol)

agement of orthostatic hypotension is usually of utmost importance, as the symptoms contribute to morbidity and may result in injuries (Table 35-9). Control of bowel and bladder function, and, in males, sexual function, may need to be addressed. The overall prognosis in PAF is good, with a life expectancy not dissimilar to those individuals of an equivalent age.

The most common neurodegenerative condition affecting the autonomic nervous system is MSA. Its prevalence and incidence are not known. It is a nonfamilial and sporadic disorder with autonomic, parkinsonian, cerebellar, and pyramidal features that occur in any combination over a varying time scale (see Figure 35-12 and Table 35-8). It is a progressive disorder, which adds to its complexity and difficulties in diagnosis. The majority of patients with MSA have parkinsonian features; thus, it may be difficult to distinguish MSA from IPD, especially in the early stages. In various series up to 25% of patients diagnosed as having IPD in vivo were found to have the characteristic features of MSA at postmortem examination. Depending on the ensuing disabilities (see Table 35-8), patients initially may consult a range of specialists from neurologists and cardiologists to urologists and psychiatrists. The eponym *Shy-Drager syndrome* was often used to describe MSA in combination with autonomic abnormalities. Autonomic dysfunction, affecting in particular the genitourinary and cardiovascular systems, is an integral part of MSA, and *Shy-Drager syndrome* is now accepted as being interchangeable with *MSA*.

The neurologic features in MSA have led to recognition of three major subgroups: those with parkinsonian features (MSA-P), those with cerebellar or pyramidal features (MSA-C), and those with a combination of these neurologic features (the mixed form; MSA-M) (see Figure 35-12). It is likely that the neuropathologic findings in MSA-M include striatonigral degeneration, in MSA-C olivopontocerebellar degeneration, and in MSA-M a combination of the two. The presence of intracytoplasmic argyrophilic inclusions in oligodendrocytes within the brain and spinal cord is thought to be a specific feature of this condition. Cell loss is observed in various brain stem nuclei (including those of the vagus), the intermediolateral cell mass in the thoracic and lumbar spinal cord, and Onuf's nucleus in the sacral spinal cord; cell loss in these regions may account for the various autonomic abnormalities. In MSA, the paravertebral ganglia and the visceral (enteric) plexuses appear to be spared.

In MSA, the neurologic features alone may not distinguish the condition from overlapping neurologic syndromes, especially in the early stages. In the parkinsonian forms, the onset of bradykinesia and rigidity is often bilateral and with minimal or no tremor, unlike PD. The lack of a motor response to L-dopa alone is not helpful, as two-thirds of patients may respond initially, although side effects and diminution in responsiveness with time lowers this

Figure 35-13. A normal anal sphincter electromyograph (A) compared with an abnormal one (B) from a subject with MSA. In the MSA subject there are polyphasic and prolonged motor units indicative of denervation and reinnervation. (Courtesy of CJ Fowler. Reprinted with permission from CJ Mathias. Gastrointestinal dysfunction in multiple system atrophy. Semin Neurol 1997;16:251.)

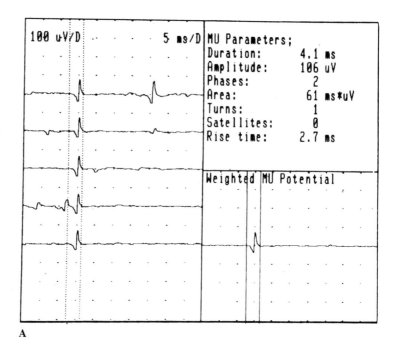

A

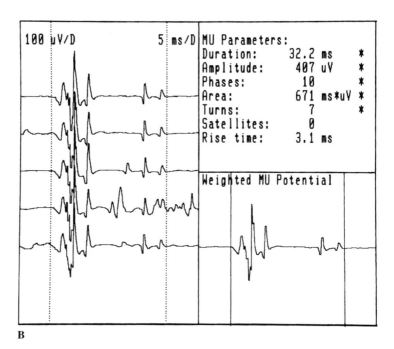

B

to one-third or less. The presence of autonomic failure (especially cardiovascular and genitourinary), however, should alert one to the possibility of MSA. Respiratory abnormalities together with oropharyngeal dysphagia favor MSA, although these may occur later, as the disease progresses. Autonomic abnormalities on cardiovascular testing and abnormal urethral/anal sphincter electromyographic findings (Figure 35-13) in conjunction with the characteristic clinical features are virtually confirmatory of MSA.

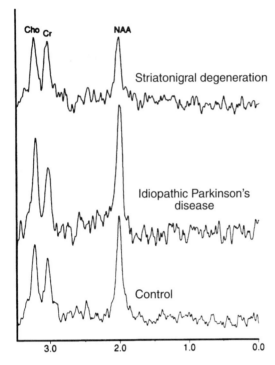

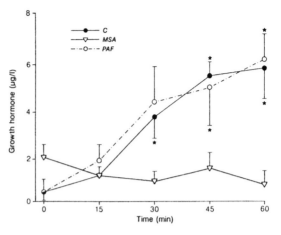

Figure 35-15. Plasma growth hormone concentration before (0) and 15, 30, 45, and 60 minutes after administration of clonidine (1.5 μg/kg) in normal subjects (controls, C) and in subjects with multiple system atrophy (MSA) and pure autonomic failure (PAF). The arrow bars indicate ±SEM. (Reprinted with permission from T Thomaides, KR Chaudhuri, S Maule, et al. The growth hormone response to clonidine in central and peripheral primary autonomic failure. Lancet 1992;340:263.)

Figure 35-14. Proton magnetic resonance spectroscopy in three subjects: from bottom to top, a normal subject (control), idiopathic Parkinson's disease, and striatonigral degeneration (the parkinsonian form of multiple system atrophy). The choline (Cho) and creatinine (Cr) ratio in comparison with *N*-acetyl aspartate (NAA) is abnormal in the subject with MSA. NAA is a chemical that is selective to neurones. (Reprinted with permission from CA Davie, GK Wenning, GJ Barker, et al. Differentiation of multiple system atrophy from idiopathic Parkinson's disease using proton magnetic resonance spectroscopy. Ann Neurol 1995;37:204.)

Diagnosis is difficult, especially in the early stages of the disease. Noninvasive tests ranging from CT and MRI to positron emission tomography brain scanning and proton magnetic resonance spectroscopy of the basal ganglia (Figure 35-14) have been used to help distinguish MSA from other extrapyramidal disorders, such as IPD and progressive supranuclear palsy. A recent noninvasive approach that is sensitive, specific, and patient acceptable for repeat studies is clonidine–growth hormone (GH) testing. The centrally acting alpha-2 adrenoceptor agonist clonidine normally raises levels of GH (Figure 35-15), probably through stimulating hypothalamic GH releasing hormone

(GHRH), which then acts on the anterior pituitary to release GH. After administration of clonidine there is a rise in levels of GH in IPD and PAF (with peripheral autonomic failure) that is similar to the size observed in normal subjects. However, GH levels after clonidine remain unchanged in the different forms of MSA (with central autonomic failure). When another GH secretagogue, L-dopa, is given to MSA patients, levels of both GHRH and GH rise, indicating that the clonidine-GH abnormality is not the result of widespread neuronal fallout and probably indicates a specific hypothalamic alpha-2 adrenoceptor deficit. The GH-clonidine test therefore may form the basis of an early means to distinguish MSA from other parkinsonian and peripheral autonomic syndromes, and additionally may provide a means of determining in vivo the various central neurotransmitter abnormalities in MSA.

The prognosis in MSA is poor compared with IPD and PAF, because motor and autonomic deficits usually worsen. The majority of MSA patients have parkinsonian features that in due course become

Figure 35-16. A still from a videocinefluoroscopic examination indicating oropharyngeal dysphagia and showing penetration of the larynx with the potential to lead to tracheal aspiration. (Reprinted with permission from CJ Mathias. Gastrointestinal dysfunction in multiple system atrophy. Semin Neurol 1997;16:251.)

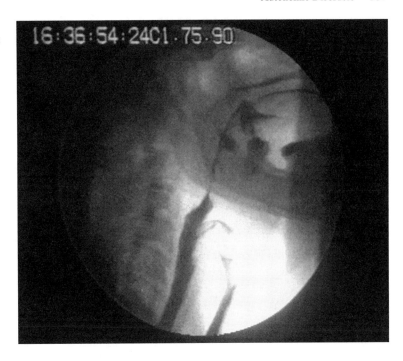

refractory to antiparkinsonian drugs; they may also develop side effects, including orthostatic hypotension, which reduce the therapeutic efficacy of these agents. Increasing rigidity impairs their mobility and ability to communicate. In the cerebellar forms, worsening truncal ataxia may result in falls and an inability to stand upright. Incoordination in the upper limbs, speech defects and nystagmus add to their disability.

In MSA, oropharyngeal dysphagia may enhance the risk of aspiration (Figure 35-16), especially because such patients are prone to vocal cord abnormalities. A percutaneous feeding gastrostomy may be needed. Respiratory abnormalities, which include an obstructive apnea (due to laryngeal abductor cord paresis) and central apnea, may necessitate a tracheostomy. In the majority of MSA patients, there is no active means of reversing the neurologic decline; thus, supportive therapy is an important component in management and should incorporate the family and community. The outlook for the autonomic deficits is more promising. Orthostatic hypotension may be a severe problem in some, and the difficulties may be compounded by the motor deficits. However, orthostatic hypotension it is more likely to respond to therapy in MSA than in PAF. The management of bowel and bladder dysfunction,

and, if appropriate, sexual dysfunction, is important in improving the quality of life.

A less-well-described group are those with classic IPD (often successfully treated with L-dopa for many years) who later develop features of autonomic failure, often with severe postural hypotension. Therefore, they differ from the majority of patients with IPD, in whom autonomic deficits, if present, are relatively mild and may be compounded by drug therapy. Pharmacologic approaches, and, more recently, positron emission tomography cardiac scanning studies, favor the autonomic lesions being peripheral and thus similar in nature to those of PAF. The etiology is unknown. It remains unclear whether classic IPD is a coincidental association of a common condition (IPD) with an uncommon disease (PAF); an indication of vulnerability to autonomic degeneration in a subgroup of IPD; linked to increasing age, chronic drug therapy, or an inherent metabolic susceptibility; or a result from a combination of these factors. Data on the natural history and prognosis of these patients are limited, probably because their age precludes long-term follow-up. However, they appear not to suffer from many of the characteristic complications of MSA, and therefore clinically they differ from them in many ways.

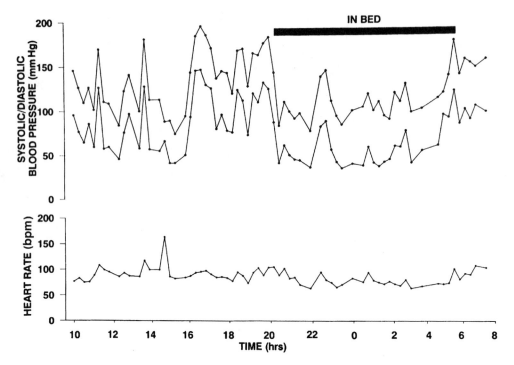

Figure 35-17. The 24-hour ambulatory blood pressure and heart rate profile in a subject with the Riley-Day syndrome (familial dysautonomia). There are fluctuations in blood pressure with a fall in blood pressure at night, as in normal subjects and in contrast to autonomic failure as shown in Figure 35-8. (Reprinted with permission from CJ Mathias. Autonomic Disorders in Childhood. In B Berg [ed], Principles of Child Neurology. New York: McGraw-Hill, 1996;413–436.)

Secondary Disorders

Hereditary

Riley-Day Syndrome (Familial Dysautonomia).
Familial dysautonomia should be considered in a child of Ashkenazi Jewish extraction with absent fungiform papillae, lack of corneal reflexes, decreased deep tendon reflexes, and a diminished response to pain. An abnormal intradermal histamine skin test (with an absent flare response) and pupillary hypersensitivity to cholinomimetics confirm the diagnosis. The genetic abnormality in this condition is linked to chromosome 9 (*q31*), with sufficient DNA markers to enable prenatal diagnosis

A variety of symptoms resulting from both autonomic underactivity and overactivity may occur, including a labile blood pressure with hypertension and postural hypotension (Figure 35-17), and parasympathetic abnormalities with periodic vomiting,

dysphagia, constipation, diarrhea, and urinary bladder disturbances. Neurologic abnormalities, associated skeletal problems (scoliosis), and renal failure previously contributed to a poor prognosis. The ability to anticipate complications and provide adequate support and therapy has changed this, with a number of children now reaching adulthood.

Familial Amyloid Polyneuropathy. In familial amyloid polyneuropathy, symptoms usually occur in adulthood. There are sensory, motor, and autonomic abnormalities caused by the deposition in peripheral nerves of variant transthyretin, which is produced in the liver. Symptoms of motor and sensory neuropathy often occur initially in the lower limbs. The cardiovascular system, gut, and urinary bladder can be affected at any stage. The disease progresses relentlessly at a variable speed. There may be a dissociation of autonomic symptoms from functional deficits; this is of importance, as evaluation of cardiovascular autonomic abnormalities may be essential in prevent-

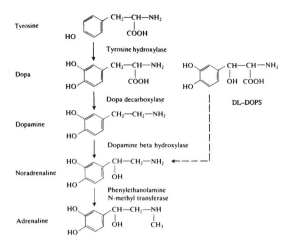

Tyrosine

Dopa

Dopamine

Noradrenaline

Adrenaline

Tyrosine hydroxylase

Dopa decarboxylase

DL–DOPS

Dopamine beta hydroxylase

Phenylethanolamine
N-methyl transferase

Figure 35-18. Biosynthetic pathways in the formation of noradrenaline and adrenaline. The structure of DL-threo-dihydroxyphenylserine (DL-DOPS) is indicated on the right. The enzyme dopa-decarboxylase, which is present both intraneuronally and extraneuronally, converts it to noradrenaline, thus bypassing the hydroxylation step, which depends on the enzyme dopamine β-hydroxylase. (Reprinted with permission from CJ Mathias, R Bannister, P Cortelli, et al. Clinical autonomic and therapeutic observations in two siblings with postural hypotension and sympathetic failure due to an inability to synthesize noradrenaline from dopamine because of a deficiency of dopamine beta hydroxylase. QJ Med [New Series 75] 1990;278:617.)

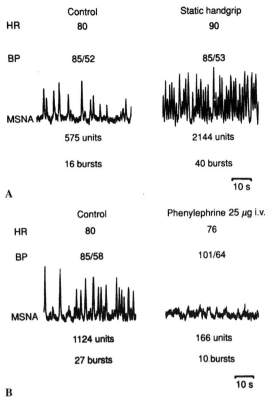

Figure 35-19. Heart rate (HR), blood pressure (BP), and muscle sympathetic nerve activity (MSNA) recorded from the peroneal nerve in a patient with dopamine β-hydroxylase (DBH) deficiency before (control) and during isometric exercise (static handgrip) (A), and during injection of phenylephrine (B). Isometric exercise increases MSNA and phenylephrine decreases MSNA, indicating that baroreflex pathways are intact. (Reprinted with permission from R Rea, I Biaggoni, RM Robertson, et al. Reflex control of sympathetic nerve activity in dopamine beta-hydroxylase deficiency. Hypertension 1990;1:107.)

ing morbidity and mortality, especially when surgical intervention, such as hepatic transplantation, is performed. Currently this is the only way to reduce levels of variant transthyretin, and it appears either to reverse the neuropathy or prevent its progression. It may be of greater value if performed before substantial nerve damage occurs.

Dopamine β-Hydroxylase Deficiency. Dopamine β-hydroxylase deficiency is a rare disorder, first recognized in the mid-1980s, currently with seven patients (two of whom are siblings) described in detail. The presentation often is in childhood, although in all these cases an autonomic disorder was not considered until they became teenagers, when postural hypotension was first recognized. Whether the symptoms at this stage become more prominent or are easier to detect is unclear. The clinical features indicate sympathetic adrenergic failure with sparing of sympathetic cholinergic and parasympathetic function. Sweating is preserved and urinary bladder

and bowel function are normal; in one of the males erection was possible but ejaculation was difficult to achieve. The diagnosis may be made from basal levels of plasma catecholamines; noradrenaline and adrenaline levels are undetectable, whereas dopamine levels are elevated (see Figure 35-6 and Figure 35-18). The enzymatic defect is highly specific, with the sympathetic nerve pathways and terminals otherwise intact, as has been demonstrated by electron microscopy, immunohistochemical studies, and the measurement of muscle sympathetic nerve activity using microneurography (Figure 35-19). These subjects therefore form a unique model of

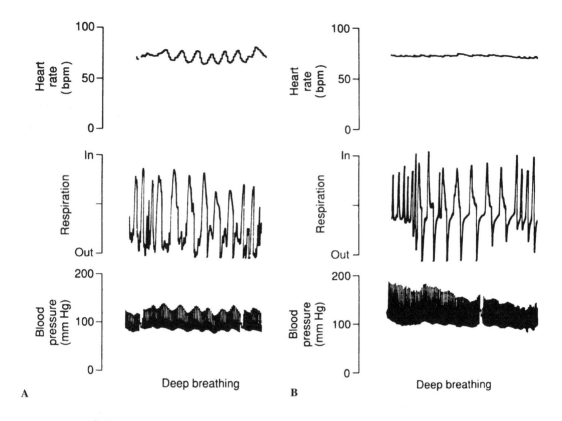

Figure 35-20. Heart rate, respiration, and blood pressure in a normal subject (A) and in a subject with cardiac vagal denervation (B) before and during deep breathing. The sinus arrhythmia seen in the normal subject does not occur in the denervated subject. (Reprinted with permission from CJ Mathias, R Bannister. Investigation of Autonomic Disorders. In R Bannister, CJ Mathias [eds], Autonomic Failure. A Textbook of Clinical Disorders of the Autonomic Nervous System [3rd ed]. Oxford, England: Oxford University Press, 1992;255–290.)

superselective sympathetic adrenergic failure. The deficit can be satisfactorily treated with the pro-drug DL- or the active isomer, L-dihydroxyphenylserine (see Figure 35-18), which has a structure similar to noradrenaline except for a carboxyl group that is acted on by the enzyme dopadecarboxylase, which is abundantly present in extraneuronal tissues such as the liver and kidneys, thus transforming it into noradrenaline. This drug is effective in reducing orthostatic hypotension and has resulted in remarkable improvements in their ability to lead active lives.

Diabetes Mellitus.   There is a high incidence of both peripheral and autonomic neuropathy, especially in older, long-standing diabetics on insulin therapy. Their morbidity and mortality are considerably higher than in those without a neuropathy.

Diabetic autonomic neuropathy initially often involves the vagus, with characteristic features of cardiac vagal denervation (Figure 35-20). There may be involvement of the gastrointestinal tract (gastroparesis diabeticorum) and the urinary bladder (diabetic cystopathy). Damage to other organs may occur through non-neuropathic factors peculiar to diabetes itself, and may compound the problems caused by the neuropathy. An example is the heart, where the lack of control exerted by vagal denervation may occur in conjunction with partial preservation of cardiac sympathetic nerves; this may predispose diabetics, many of whom have ischemic heart disease, to sudden death from cardiac dysrhythmias. In some diabetics, sympathetic failure may cause severe orthostatic hypotension, which may be enhanced by insulin. Other than maintaining normoglycemia, there is no known

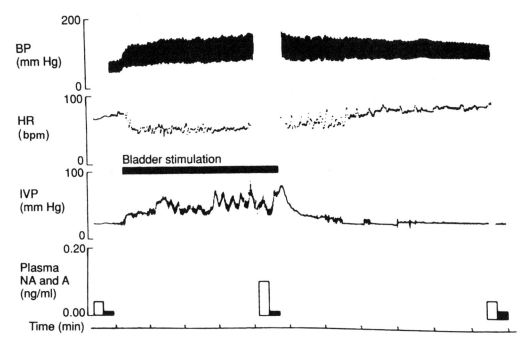

Figure 35-21. Blood pressure (BP), heart rate (HR), intravesical pressure (IVP), and plasma noradrenaline levels (NA, open histograms) and adrenaline (A, filled histograms) in a tetraplegic patient before, during, and after bladder stimulation induced by suprapubic percussion of the anterior abdominal wall. The rise in BP is accompanied by a fall in heart rate as a result of increased vagal activity in response to the rise in blood pressure. Levels of plasma NA but not A rise, suggesting an increase in sympathetic neural activity independent of adrenomedullary activation. (Reprinted with permission from CJ Mathias, H Frankel. The neurological and hormonal control of blood vessels and heart in spinal man. J Auton Nerv Syst 1986;[Suppl]:457.)

means to prevent and reverse the neuropathy except, possibly, by pancreatic transplantation.

Autonomic Disorders with Both Underactivity and Overactivity

Guillain-Barré syndrome is an autonomic disorder in which there is both underactivity and overactivity; tachycardia and hypotension may alternate with bradycardia and hypertension. The precise mechanisms are unclear; the possibilities should be anticipated, as appropriate drugs may be needed to prevent one or the other complication. Cardiovascular disturbances of a similar nature may occur in tetanus, especially in those who need skeletal muscle relaxants and are on assisted respiration. In cervical and high thoracic spinal cord lesions, orthostatic hypotension results from the inability of the brain to activate efferent sympathetic pathways despite preservation of baroreceptor afferent and central connections. In these subjects the reverse, paroxysmal hypertension along with large bowel and urinary bladder contraction as part of the mass reflex, may occur in the syndrome of autonomic dysreflexia (Figure 35-21). This is the result of isolated spinal cord reflex activity (without the restraint of cerebral control) and can be induced by a variety of stimuli, from cutaneous, skeletal muscle, or visceral sources below the level of the lesion. In the acute phase after injury, such patients may have a different set of clinical problems because of "spinal shock" and the absence of even isolated spinal sympathetic activity; some of these result from parasympathetic overactivity because the cardiac vagi are not opposed by the sympathetic nervous system and other factors (Figure 35-22).

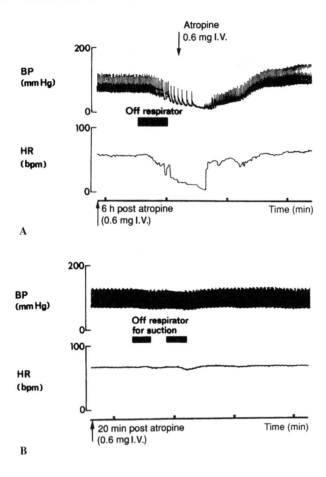

Figure 35-22. (A) The effects of disconnecting the respirator (as required for aspirating the airways) on the blood pressure (BP) and heart rate (HR) of a recently injured tetraplegic patient (C4–5 lesion) in spinal shock, 6 hours after the last dose of intravenous atropine. Sinus bradycardia and cardiac arrest (also observed on the electrocardiograph) were reversed by reconnection, intravenous atropine, and external cardiac massage. (Reprinted with permission from HL Frankel, CJ Mathias, JMK Spalding. Mechanisms of reflex cardiac arrest in tetraplegic patients. Lancet 1975;2:1183.) (B) The effect of tracheal suction 20 minutes after atropine. Disconnection from the respirator and tracheal suction did not lower either heart rate or blood pressure. (Reprinted with permission from CJ Mathias. Bradycardia and cardiac arrest during tracheal suction—mechanisms in tetraplegic patients. Eur J Intens Care Med 1976;2:147.)

Neurally Mediated Syncope

Neurally mediated syncope is characterized by intermittent cardiovascular autonomic abnormalities resulting in loss of consciousness. An increase in cardiac parasympathetic activity causes severe bradycardia or cardiac arrest, and sympathetic neural withdrawal results in hypotension. The two may occur separately, as the cardio-inhibitory or vasodepressor forms, or together, as the mixed form. Between episodes there may be no abnormalities detected on routine autonomic testing. In the young, the more common condition is vasovagal syncope (Figure 35-23), in which there may be a familial tendency. Vasovagal syncope may be induced by a range of stimuli, from fear and the sight of blood to venipuncture and, at times, even discussion of venipuncture. Modified testing, which includes prolonged tilt-table testing, and, in some, the application of a provocative stimulus

(including venipuncture or pseudovenipuncture), may be needed to induce an attack. The management includes reducing or preventing exposure to precipitating causes; in some patients, especially in those with phobias, behavioral psychological approaches are needed. The cause may be unclear and attacks recurrent, with injury in a proportion of patients, who are sometimes described as having *malignant vasovagal syncope.* Cardiac conduction disorders and other causes of syncope need to be excluded. A diet high in salt content and various drugs, such as fludrocortisone, vasopressor agents, and antidepressants (including the serotonin-uptake release inhibitors), have been used with success in individual cases. The long-term prognosis is favorable.

In the elderly, carotid sinus hypersensitivity may be more common than previously thought. There may be a classic history of syncope induced by head movements or collar tightening; in many, the precip-

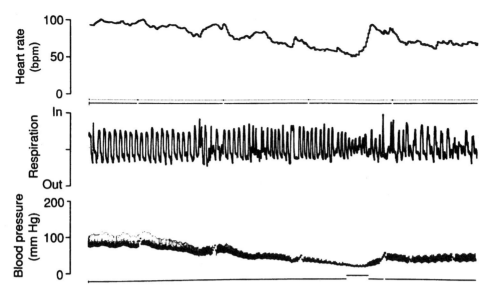

Figure 35-23. Blood pressure changes toward the end of a period of head-up tilt in a patient with recurrent episodes of vasovagal syncope. Blood pressure, which was previously maintained, begins to fall. There is also a fall in heart rate. There initially are relatively minor changes in respiratory rate, which can be derived from the time signal above it, each minor dot indicating a second and the bolder mark indicating a minute. The patient was about to faint and was put back to the horizontal (indicated by elevated time signal below) and then to 5-degree head-down tilt. Blood pressure and heart rate recover but still remain lower than previously. This patient had no other autonomic abnormalities on detailed testing. Blood pressure was measured noninvasively by the Finapres. (Reprinted with permission from CJ Mathias, R Bannister. Investigation of Autonomic Disorders. In R Bannister, CJ Mathias [eds], Autonomic Failure. A Textbook of Clinical Disorders of the Autonomic Nervous System [3rd ed]. Oxford, England: Oxford University Press, 1992;255–290.)

itating factors are unclear. The investigation should include carotid sinus massage. This should be performed in the laboratory with requisite precautions, ideally using a beat-by-beat continuous blood pressure and heart rate recording device (Figure 35-24). Carotid massage also should be performed with the subject tilted head-up, as hypotension is more likely to occur in situations when sympathetic nerve activity is needed. The diagnosis may be difficult to make but is of importance, because it may be a major cause of unexplained falls. The management in the cardioinhibitory form includes a cardiac demand pacemaker. The vasodepressor forms are more difficult to treat and various pressor agents have been used. In some, denervation of the carotid sinus may be needed. Rarer causes of neurally mediated syncope include those associated with glossopharyngeal neuralgia (and often induced by swallowing), micturition, defecation, coughing, and even laughing.

Drugs, Chemicals, Toxins

Drugs may cause autonomic dysfunction through their pharmacologic effects; these may be well-recognized actions of drugs, such as the sympatholytic agents. Autonomic dysfunction may result from a drug side effect that becomes clinically prominent when the drug is used in high dosage or over a prolonged period (such as the anticholinergic effects of antidepressants), or when deficits are unmasked or induced in susceptible individuals (Figure 35-25). Examples of the latter category include L-dopa worsening orthostatic hypotension in MSA, the ability of pressor agents to cause severe hypertension in certain autonomic disorders because of denervation supersensitivity (Figure 35-26), and the antiarrhythmic disopyramide inducing urinary retention in subjects with benign prostatic hypertrophy. Certain drugs or substances,

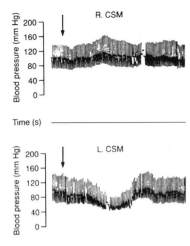

Figure 35-24. Continuous noninvasive recording of finger arterial blood pressure (Finapres) before, during, and after carotid sinus massage on the right (R. CSM) and left (L. CSM). The fine dots indicate the time marker in seconds. The arrow indicates when stimulation began. Stimulation on the right for 10 seconds did not lower blood pressure and heart rate. On the left, carotid sinus massage caused a substantial fall in both systolic and diastolic blood pressure, during which the patient felt light-headed and had graying-out of vision. There was only a modest fall in heart rate. The syncopal attacks were abolished by left carotid sinus denervation. (Reprinted with permission from CJ Mathias, A Armstrong, N Browse, et al. Value of non-invasive continuous blood pressure monitoring in the detection of carotid sinus hyperintensity Clin Auton Res 1991;1:157.)

The Initiating or Facilitating Role of the Autonomic Nervous System in Various Diseases

There is increasing evidence from a variety of both experimental and clinical research sources that the autonomic nervous system may play either an initiating or a facilitating role in various medical diseases. An example is primary (essential hypertension), where the sympathetic nervous system is thought to be an important etiologic factor in both the development and maintenance of hypertension. In secondary forms of hypertension, such as renal hypertension and, more recently, gestational hypertension, pharmacologic and physiologic studies also favor this possibility. In other states, such as cardiac failure, the sympathetic nervous system and its altered responsiveness are thought to play a contributory role. There are thus major disease states not classified directly under autonomic disorders, where knowledge of the role of the autonomic nervous system is important both for understanding the pathophysiologic basis of the condition and for their management.

such as perhexiline maleate, vincristine, and alcohol, may cause an autonomic neuropathy.

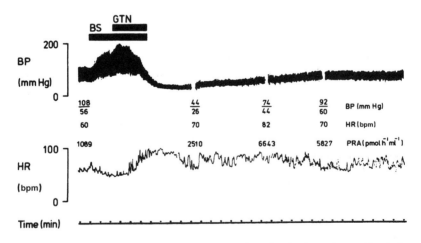

Figure 35-25. Blood pressure (BP) and heart rate (HR) in a tetraplegic patient in the supine position before, during, and after bladder stimulation (BS) induced by suprapubic percussion of the anterior abdominal wall; this causes bladder contraction, micturition, and a marked rise in blood pressure. Sublingual glyceryl trinitrate (GTN), used in a standard dose of 0.5 mg, rapidly reverses the hypertension, elevates the heart rate, and causes substantial hypotension, despite only 3.5 minutes of use. The breaks in the record indicate when plasma renin activity (PRA) was measured; this rises markedly as the pressure falls and may contribute, albeit slowly, to the recovery in blood pressure. (Reprinted with permission from CJ Mathias, HL Frankel. Cardiovascular control in spinal man. Ann Rev Physiol 1988;50:577.)

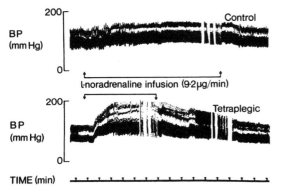

Figure 35-26. The effect of a similar dose infusion rate of L-noradrenaline on the blood pressure (BP) of a paraplegic control (lesion below T12–L1 and therefore a nearly intact sympathetic nervous system) and a tetraplegic patient with a complete cervical lesion. There is a marked pressor response in the tetraplegic. These pressor responses are observed over a wide dose infusion range and apply not only to noradrenaline, but also to a number of other vasopressor agents. (Reprinted with permission from CJ Mathias, HL Frankel, NJ Christenson, JMK Spalding. Enhanced pressor response to noradrenaline in patients with cervical spinal cord transection. Brain 1976;99:757.)

Suggested Reading

Bannister R, Mathias CJ (eds). Autonomic Failure: A Textbook of Clinical Disorders of the Autonomic Nervous System (3rd ed). Oxford, UK: Oxford University Press, 1992.

Kenny RA (ed). Syncope in the Older Patient. London: Chapman and Hall, 1996.

Korcyzn AD (ed). Handbook of Autonomic Nervous System Dysfunction. New York: Marcel Dekker, 1995.

Low P. Clinical Autonomic Disorders. Boston: Little, Brown, 1993.

Mathias CJ. Disorders of the Autonomic Nervous System in Childhood. In B Berg (ed), Principles of Child Neurology. New York: McGraw-Hill, 1996;413–436.

Mathias CJ. Disorders of the Autonomic Nervous System. In WG Bradley, RB Daroff, GM Fenichel CD Marsden (eds), Neurology in Clinical Practice (2nd ed). Boston: Butterworth–Heinemann, 1996;1953–1981.

Robertson D, Low PA, Polinsky RJ (eds). A Primer on the Autonomic Nervous System. San Diego: Academic Press, 1996;230–236.

Also note the series of books on basic and clinical aspects of the autonomic nervous system, edited by G Burnstock, Harwood Academic Publishers, Chur, Switzerland, from 1992.

Chapter 36
Neuromuscular Junction Disorders

Kerry H. Levin

Anatomy of the Neuromuscular Junction

The neuromuscular junction (NMJ) is the synapse between the distal nerve terminal of a motor nerve and the muscle fiber that it innervates. The signal for muscle fiber contraction passes across the NMJ in the form of the neurotransmitter acetylcholine (ACh). ACh is synthesized in the endoplasmic reticulum of the nerve terminal and is packaged into vesicles, each containing approximately 10,000 molecules. Vesicles of ACh attach to active release sites at the nerve terminal membrane, also known as the *presynaptic membrane*. These release sites are closely associated with membrane-bound voltage-gated calcium ion channels.

The postsynaptic portion of the NMJ (muscle end-plate) is characterized by a specialized, highly infolded muscle membrane holding the nicotinic ACh receptor (AChR) molecules (Figure 36-1A). Each AChR is a complex of multiple glycoprotein subunits configured to form an ion channel. New AChRs are constituted and replace old ones approximately every 8–11 days. When ACh molecules bind to the AChR a conformational change occurs, opening the ion channel and allowing sodium influx. AChRs are concentrated at the peaks of the junctional folds, directly opposite the active release sites of ACh vesicles on the presynaptic nerve terminals. After leaving the binding sites on AChRs, ACh molecules drift down into the troughs of the junctional folds, where the enzyme acetylcholinesterase (AChE) is concentrated. ACh is metabolized into choline and acetate for reuptake by the nerve terminal.

Neurophysiology of Neuromuscular Junction Transmission

When a propagated nerve action potential from a spinal motor neuron reaches the nerve terminal and depolarizes the nerve terminal membrane,

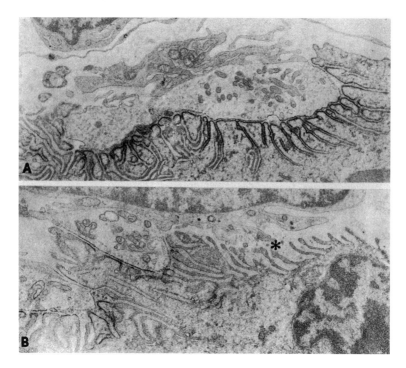

Figure 36-1. (A) Electron photomicrograph (magnification: ×11,000) of a normal-appearing neuromuscular junction showing a tightly apposed junction between the nerve terminal and the postsynaptic surface and highly infolded postsynaptic membrane folds. The specimen was treated to highlight acetylcholine receptors, visualized as dark outlining of the peaks of the membrane folds but not the troughs. (B) Electron photomicrograph (magnification: ×15,400) showing the pathologic features of myasthenia gravis. In the region of the asterisk there is widening of the synaptic cleft between the nerve terminal membrane and the postsynaptic membrane, simplification of the postsynaptic endplate folds, and absence of the dark outlining of the membrane peaks corresponding to loss of acetylcholine receptors. (Reprinted with permission from A Engel, JM Lindstrom, EH Lambert, et al. Ultrastructural localization of the acetylcholine receptor in myasthenia gravis and in its experimental autoimmune model. Neurology 1977;27:307.)

voltage-gated calcium channels open to admit calcium, facilitating the release of the ACh vesicles. With repetitive nerve terminal depolarization, the immediately releasable pool of ACh vesicles is depleted. In any train of stimuli to the nerve terminal, a characteristic reduction of ACh vesicle release occurs with each stimulus. The safety factor of NMJ transmission refers to the fact that as long as the frequency of nerve terminal depolarizations does not exceed approximately 5 per second, enough ACh is always released after each stimulus to produce a threshold depolarization of the muscle membrane, generating a propagated muscle fiber action potential and a muscle fiber contraction. The neurophysiologic features underlying presynaptic release of ACh are reviewed in Table 36-1.

When AChR ion channels open and an influx of sodium ions occurs, a small electrical depolarization of the muscle membrane occurs at that site. The measurable change in the resting membrane potential that occurs after the release of a single vesicle of ACh is termed a *miniature endplate potential* (MEPP) and reflects the steady-state leakage of ACh vesicles from the nerve terminal at rest, a phenomenon critical for maintaining the structural integrity of the endplate. With a full nerve terminal depolarization, a large number of ACh vesicles is released, producing a threshold depolarizing endplate potential (EPP), which in turn generates a propagated action potential along the length of the muscle fiber membrane. As the action potential is propagated along the muscle fiber membrane, electromechanical changes produce muscle fiber contraction.

Myasthenia Gravis

Pathophysiology

Autoimmune myasthenia gravis (MG), the most common postsynaptic defect of NMJ transmission, is the result of an antibody attack leveled against the AChR. The resulting disease is characterized by loss of AChRs, simplification and scarring of the postsynaptic junctional folds, and widening of the NMJ synaptic cleft (Figure 36-1B).

In MG, normal amounts of ACh are released from the nerve terminal, but because of the loss of AChRs, the safety factor of NMJ transmission is lost. As the amount of ACh release drops with successive stimuli to the nerve terminal, a point is reached when AChRs are underexposed to ACh, and insufficient ion channels are opened to produce a threshold EPP and a propagated action potential. In the absence of a propagated muscle fiber action potential, the muscle fiber will not contract, leading to the clinical observation of muscle weakness.

In a patient with MG, AChR antibody damage to AChRs is not evenly distributed over all muscle fibers and all muscle bellies. Some NMJs will have lost so many AChRs that not even the first release of ACh in a train of electrical stimuli to the nerve terminal will produce a threshold EPP, whereas other NMJs will be nearly normal. When measuring the effect in the whole muscle belly, an averaging of the effect of the AChR antibody damage in all individual muscle fibers takes place, producing a picture of progressive decline of muscle belly contraction during a train of depolarizations of the nerve terminals, mirroring the natural decline in ACh release during a train of depolarizations (Figure 36-2).

Clinical electrodiagnostic techniques have been developed to measure the degree to which patients suspected of having MG demonstrate loss of the safety factor of NMJ transmission. By applying a cutaneous electrical stimulus overlying a motor nerve trunk, one can repetitively depolarize the nerve terminals innervating a whole muscle belly. Electrodes applied over the muscle belly record an electrical signal integrated through a differential amplifier. The size of the resulting waveform is a summation of the propagated action potentials of all muscle fibers activated by the nerve trunk stimulus. In a normal individual, slow repetitive stimulation (2–5 per second) results in the recording of a compound muscle action potential (CMAP) for each stimulus, all of equal size. In MG, during a train of stimuli, a classic decrementing response is seen: There is progressive loss of the CMAP amplitude with each successive stimulus in the train, reflecting the result of progressive reduction of releasable ACh in the setting of a reduced number of available AChRs (Figure 36-3).

The role of the thymus in the etiology of MG remains uncertain. The thymus may serve as a source of antigenic stimulation of AChR antibody production, it may serve as a holding area for AChR antibody-secreting B cells, or it may in some other way promote a state of immune dysregulation that favors the perpetuation of MG.

Clinical Features

MG is a disorder of weakness and fatigability of skeletal muscle and is the most commonly occurring defect of NMJ transmission, with a prevalence of 1 per 10,000–20,000 population. A diagnostic cornerstone of the disease is the tendency for symptoms to be most prominent with physical activity and exercise and least noticeable after rest. Cranial muscles are often involved first, producing ptosis and diplopia as a result of weakness of the levator palpebrae and extraocular muscles, respectively. Weakness of mastication and swallowing often develops, and the natural facial expression may change, resulting in a loss of facial

Table 36-1. Physiologic Factors Governing Neuromuscular Junction Transmission

- Acetylcholine is released from the nerve terminal in vesicles.
- Only vesicles of acetylcholine at the active zones are available for immediate release.
- In any series of stimuli, later stimuli release progressively less acetylcholine.
- The largest decrease in acetylcholine release is between the first and second stimuli.
- Even after many stimuli at slow repetitive stimulation, enough acetylcholine is released to produce a threshold endplate potential and a propagated muscle fiber action potential.
- Calcium uptake into the nerve terminal potentiates release of acetylcholine.

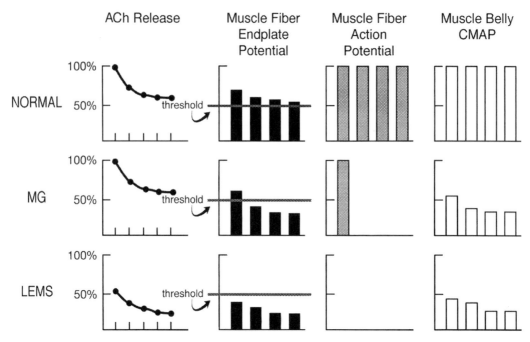

Figure 36-2. This figure compares acetylcholine (ACh) release and the electrophysiologic endplate response in a normal individual with two pathologic states: myasthenia gravis (MG) and the Lambert-Eaton syndrome (LEMS). The columns titled ACh Release, Muscle Fiber Endplate Potential, and Muscle Fiber Action Potential pertain to events at a single neuromuscular junction (NMJ), while the column titled Muscle Belly CMAP pertains to responses obtained from a whole muscle belly. At the muscle fiber endplate, if sufficient ion channels open and sufficient sodium influx occurs, the resulting endplate potential will be above the threshold required to generate a propagated muscle fiber action potential. The response recorded from a whole muscle belly (CMAP) after nerve trunk stimulation is a summation of all the individual muscle fiber action potentials generated after nerve trunk stimulation and represents an averaging of the responses from all NMJs in the muscle belly, some of which have severe impairment of transmission while others have little or no transmission defect. (CMAP = compound muscle action potential.) (Adapted from JE Desmedt. New Developments in Electromyography and Clinical Neurophysiology [Vol 1]. Basel: S. Karger, 1973;305.)

tone and a horizontal smile. Subsequently, weakness may develop in extremity muscles, and finally in muscles of respiration. Some patients have a pure ocular form of MG, demonstrating only ptosis and diplopia. Others may present only with extremity fatigability and weakness, or with fragmentary symptoms such as dysphagia or dysarthria. The clinical severity of MG has traditionally been classified into four categories, as listed in Table 36-2.

Early in the disease process, symptoms tend to vary remarkably from hour to hour and day to day, depending on the patient's activity level. Patients often have fewest symptoms on arising from rest,

and maximal symptoms late in the day. When symptoms are mild, no objective evidence of the disorder will be found on clinical examination. The patient's description of fluctuating symptoms of fatigue, blurred vision, and trouble swallowing can lead the physician into the erroneous diagnosis of a somatization disorder or depression.

Diagnosis

Aside from the patient's history, support for the diagnosis can come from the neurologic examination. In advanced cases, there is evidence of bifa-

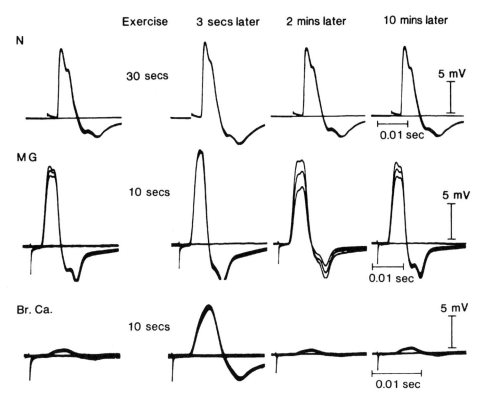

Figure 36-3. Effect of exercise on the action potential of the hypothenar muscles evoked by maximal stimulation of the ulnar nerve at the wrist. The response of the rested muscle (far left) is compared with responses 3 seconds, 2 minutes, and 10 minutes after the end of a maximal voluntary contraction of the muscle. Each record consists of three superimposed action potentials evoked at a rate of 3 per second. (N = responses of a normal subject; MG = responses of a patient with generalized myasthenia gravis.) In the rested muscle, a progressive decline of amplitude occurs during stimulation at a rate of 3 per second. Three seconds after exercise, this defect is repaired and there is some increase in the amplitude of response (post-tetanic facilitation). Two minutes after exercise, the defect is more marked than it was initially. At 10 minutes, the response is returning to its original level. (Br. Ca. = patient with the myasthenic syndrome associated with a small cell bronchogenic carcinoma.) The slight progressive decline in amplitude of response during stimulation at a rate of 3 per second that occurred in the rested muscle is not evident in the reproduced record. There is marked post-tetanic facilitation 3 seconds after exercise, but a depression of the response is seen 2 minutes after exercise. (Reprinted with permission from EH Lambert, ED Rooke, LM Eaton, et al. Myasthenic Syndrome Occasionally Associated with Bronchial Neoplasm: Neurophysiologic Studies. In HR Viets [ed], Myasthenia Gravis. The Second International Symposium Proceedings. Springfield, IL: Charles C. Thomas, 1961;364.)

cial weakness, ptosis, dysarthria, dysconjugate gaze, and extremity weakness. In subtle cases, there may be slight asymmetry of eyelid position, less than a full smile, and mild weakness of the orbicularis oculi muscles (tested by forcefully opening closed eyelids), the frontalis muscles (tested by forcefully lowering elevated eye brows), or the neck flexor muscles. Strong support for the diagnosis can come from observing fatigability of muscle strength. Sustained upgaze may produce progressive ptosis or dysconjugate gaze. During sustained upgaze, a classic finding is fleeting eyelid contractions known as *Cogan's eyelid twitches.* Fatigability can also be elicited in extremity muscles. Myasthenic weakness found on the examination can be distinguished from other causes of muscle weakness by intravenous administration of the acetylcholinesterase inhibitor drug edrophonium chloride, also known as the *Tensilon test.* Two milligrams are injected as a test dose to identify improvement of the weakness.

Table 36-2. Osserman Classification of Adult Myasthenia Gravis

I	Ocular myasthenia gravis
IIA	Mild generalized myasthenia gravis
IIB	Moderate generalized myasthenia gravis
III	Acute fulminating myasthenia gravis
IV	Late severe myasthenia gravis (i.e., onset of severe symptoms developing 2 or more years after onset of group I or II symptoms)

Table 36-3. Relative Value of Diagnostic Modalities in Myasthenia Gravis

Single-fiber electromyography: most sensitive test
   Abnormal in up to 80% of pure ocular myasthenia gravis patients
   Abnormal in more than 90% of generalized myasthenia gravis patients
Acetylcholine receptor antibody detection: most specific test
   Present in up to 70% of pure ocular myasthenia gravis patients
   Present in more than 90% of generalized myasthenia gravis patients
Repetitive stimulation tests: neither specific nor highly sensitive
   Abnormal in approximately 50% of patients with mild generalized myasthenia gravis
Tensilon test: test that is the easiest to perform but useful only in the presence of objective signs of weakness and not entirely specific for myasthenia gravis

In the absence of clear improvement, 8 mg is injected approximately 1 minute after the test dose. A clear change in the pattern of weakness should be apparent within 1–2 minutes. One milligram of injectable atropine should be available in case of symptomatic bradycardia from cholinergic excess.

Electrodiagnostic studies provide an extension of the clinical examination, offering quantitative support for the clinical diagnosis of MG. With repetitive electrical stimulation of a motor nerve trunk, such as the median nerve at the wrist, a classic finding is progressive reduction of the evoked motor amplitude when recording from a muscle belly, such as the abductor pollicis brevis. A maximal decremental response of greater than 10% signifies a defect of NMJ transmission. In the classic electromyographic picture of a postsynaptic defect of NMJ transmission, a three-stage pattern of the decremental response is seen: (1) more than 10% decrement in CMAP amplitude during a train of stimuli delivered to a rested muscle belly, (2) repair of the decremental response after a 10- to 20-second period of forceful exercise of the recorded muscle belly, and (3) exaggeration of the decremental response within 2–4 minutes of the exercise period (see Figure 36-3). In patients without a decremental response in rested muscle, a decremental response can sometimes be provoked by exhausting the muscle belly being recorded with 1 or more minutes of forceful isometric exercise. When repetitive stimulation studies are performed on proximal nerve trunks, such as the spinal accessory nerve (innervating the trapezius muscle), the sensitivity of this procedure increases, but in the absence of significant clinical fatigability of the muscle under study, repetitive stimulation studies are diagnostic in less than 50% of patients.

Single-fiber electromyography offers a diagnostic sensitivity of more than 90% in patients with generalized manifestations, and 75% in those with pure ocular symptoms. A thin needle electrode inserted in a muscle belly records the jitter, or variability, of NMJ transmission time defined as the delay between two muscle fiber action potentials propagated along two neighboring muscle fibers whose nerve terminals depolarize in a time-locked fashion (i.e., two muscle fibers innervated by the same nerve branch). Although extremely sensitive, single-fiber electromyographic abnormalities are not specific for NMJ disorders.

Identification of acetylcholine receptor antibody in the patient's serum can also confirm the diagnosis. By means of a series of immunoassays, antibody can be detected in the sera of 70–80% of patients with pure ocular MG and in 90–95% of those with generalized MG. False-positive antibody detection has been rarely encountered in patients exposed to the α-bungarotoxin in cobra venom or to certain intravenous NMJ blocking agents such as suxamethonium chloride or dimethyltubocurarine iodide. False-positive results have also been rarely reported in patients with amyotrophic lateral sclerosis (ALS) or pernicious anemia, and in patients taking the drug D-penicillamine. A summary of diagnostic modalities in MG and their relative value is listed in Table 36-3.

MG may occur in the setting of other autoimmune disorders, most commonly immune thyroid disease (antithyroglobulin antibodies) and pernicious anemia (anti–parietal cell antibody). Less common associations include rheumatoid arthritis, systemic lupus erythematosus, diabetes, and pemphigus. The serologic workup for MG should include thyroid function studies and the vitamin B_{12} concentration.

When the presentation of myasthenic symptoms occurs rapidly over weeks, the differential diagnosis is relatively narrow and includes brain stem disorders that are malignant (lymphoma, glioma, metastasis) or inflammatory (sarcoidosis, Lyme disease, chronic meningeal diseases) in etiology, botulism, and some forms of acute inflammatory demyelinating polyradiculoneuropathy (also known as *Guillain-Barré syndrome*).

When the onset of myasthenic symptoms is more slowly progressive and includes a prominence of ocular-bulbar manifestations, the differential diagnostic considerations include Graves' disease with extraocular involvement, ocular pharyngeal dystrophy, myotonic dystrophy, and mitochondrial myopathy. When the symptoms are primarily in the extremity muscles, disorders to be considered include Lambert-Eaton myasthenic syndrome (LEMS), polymyositis, chronic inflammatory demyelinating polyradiculoneuropathy (CIDP), and weakness associated with metabolic derangements (e.g., hypercalcemia, hypermagnesemia, hypophosphatemia, cortisol deficiency, Cushing's syndrome, hypothyroidism, or hyperthyroidism). The differential diagnosis of MG is summarized in Table 36-4.

Management of Myasthenia Gravis

After the diagnosis of MG has been established, structural abnormalities of the thymus gland must be sought. In patients younger than 50–60 years of age, thymectomy is an appropriate consideration whether or not there is evidence of thymic enlargement on computed tomographic (CT) scans of the chest. In 75% of patients undergoing thymectomy, there will be evidence of thymic hyperplasia. Approximately 15% of patients will have evidence of thymoma, a locally invasive malignancy for which surgery is indicated irrespective of the age of the patient. Many scientific reports have confirmed that, compared with those not having surgery, patients who undergo thymectomy are more likely

Table 36-4. Differential Diagnosis of Myasthenia Gravis

Brain stem mass lesions
Inflammatory/infectious diseases of the cranial nerves
Guillain-Barré syndrome (Miller-Fisher variant)
Graves' disease
Hypothyroidism/hyperthyroidism
Oculopharyngeal dystrophy
Myotonic dystrophy
Mitochondrial myopathy (progressive external ophthalmoplegia)
Lambert-Eaton syndrome
Polymyositis
Botulism
Organophosphate poisoning

to achieve remission or reduce their requirement for immunosuppressant medication.

For patients with mild, stable symptoms, an oral acetylcholinesterase inhibitor drug such as pyridostigmine may be sufficient treatment. The drug is usually started at a dosage of 30–60 mg every 6 hours and can be increased to up to 120 mg every 3–4 hours, but higher doses usually produce intolerable side effects of gastrointestinal upset and diarrhea. As a drug that merely increases the concentration of ACh in the neuromuscular synapse, pyridostigmine has no role in reversing the underlying immune destruction of the NMJ and should be replaced by more potent therapies if symptoms are progressive or life threatening.

For patients with progressive symptoms, corticosteroids have been the cornerstone of modern treatment. Treatment regimens vary widely and should be individualized to the patient's needs. In a stable patient, a slowly incrementing dosage, starting at 10 or 20 mg every other day, will minimize the risk of acute myasthenic worsening, which can occur in as many as 50% of marginally compensated patients during the first several weeks of therapy. In patients with rapidly progressive or severe symptoms, high-dose corticosteroids can be started along with plasmapheresis, during which 2–3 liters of the patient's plasma are removed and replaced by saline and albumin, thus rapidly decreasing the serum AChR antibody concentration. Clinical improvement from plasmapheresis is often apparent after 1 week of every-other-day treatment, while

Table 36-5. Agents Associated with Exacerbation of Myasthenia Gravis

Metabolic states	Hypermagnesemia, hypocalcemia
Neuromuscular blockers	Curare, succinylcholine
Cholinesterase inhibitors	Pyridostigmine (high dose), organophosphate compounds
Antibiotics	Aminoglycosides, polymyxins, clindamycin, lincomycin, tetracycline, erythromycin
Antiarrhythmics	Procaine-based drugs, quinine-based drugs, lidocaine, beta-adrenergic blockers
Miscellaneous	Lithium, calcium channel blockers, iodinated contrast agents, phenytoin, D-penicillamine, captopril

the benefits of corticosteroids are usually delayed by at least 2 weeks. Plasmapheresis should not be used as the sole immune modulating therapy in marginally compensated patients, as return or progression of the symptoms is not uncommon within several weeks of the last treatment, likely caused by rebound accumulation of antibody in the circulation. The risk of relapse is minimized by continuing with plasmapheresis until corticosteroid therapy begins to take effect. In patients requiring chronic immunosuppression, azathioprine can be added to reduce the long-term requirement of corticosteroids.

Myasthenic Crisis

Rapidly progressive myasthenic weakness is a potentially life-threatening event and is commonly described as *myasthenic crisis*. The patient with the new onset of the illness may present in crisis, although MG is usually slowly progressive. Patients with stable myasthenic symptoms may suddenly decompensate for a number of reasons. In some, the illness enters a progressive phase. In others, control may be lost as the result of intercurrent infection, drug interaction, pregnancy, or the postpartum state.

Many drugs adversely affect NMJ transmission, but the safety factor of NMJ transmission protects normal individuals in most cases. In a patient with MG or other disorders of NMJ transmission, drugs may have a profound effect (Table 36-5). Overdosage with acetylcholinesterase inhibitors is espe-

cially common in patients whose myasthenic weakness has markedly improved on immunosuppressant therapy. This paradoxic worsening in the controlled patient results from an excess concentration of ACh in the synapse, producing a state of constant depolarization of the motor endplate, failure of the endplate to repolarize, and eventual neuromuscular blockade and paralysis. Clinically, cholinergic crisis should be suspected in the presence of autonomic symptoms, including excessive abdominal cramping, diarrhea, increased bronchial secretions, sweating, salivation, bradycardia, and hypotension. Patients suspected of cholinergic crisis should be admitted to the hospital and withdrawn from acetylcholinesterase inhibitors under close supervision. Other drugs that can precipitate neuromuscular blockade include the many anesthetic muscle relaxants used intraoperatively, such as succinylcholine, as well as curare-like drugs and organophosphates. Antibiotics such as the polymyxins, lincomycin, and clindamycin can produce weakness by noncompetitive blockade of AChRs.

Some agents exert effects at the nerve terminal. Aminoglycoside antibiotics such as neomycin, gentamicin, and tobramycin are thought to interfere with calcium influx at presynaptic voltage-gated calcium channels. Iodinated contrast agents may produce similar effects as a result of the sodium citrate and sodium edetate used as sequestering agents in the compounds.

Other drugs have combined presynaptic and postsynaptic or undetermined mechanisms of NMJ transmission inhibition. Drugs in this category include antiarrhythmic and anesthetic agents containing procaine, lidocaine, and quinine. Drugs that have been occasionally reported to increase myasthenic weakness include calcium channel blocking agents, beta-adrenergic blocking agents (propranolol), lithium, phenytoin, phenothiazines, erythromycin, tetracycline, and phenytoin.

Neonatal Myasthenia Gravis

Neonatal myasthenia gravis occurs in up to 20% of the offspring of mothers with autoimmune MG. The likelihood of developing neonatal MG does not correlate with the severity of disease in the mother but does correlate to some extent with the maternal concentration of AChR antibody. In the newborn,

AChRs appear to be of the fetal type, differing in one of the five AChR subunits from adult AChRs. Mothers with a higher ratio of fetal AChR antibody to adult AChR antibody seem most likely to transfer the illness. It is not clear whether newborn AChR antibody is the result of transplacental transfer from the mother. Patients are symptomatic from birth, but usually show spontaneous resolution within 3 weeks, rarely as long as 7 weeks. Findings include facial weakness, ptosis, dysphagia, weak cry, and respiratory insufficiency. Rarely, ventilator assistance is required.

Congenital Myasthenia

A heterogeneous group of disorders is described as congenital myasthenia. They all share in common the absence of detectable AChR antibody and the presence of the defect at birth, although the clinical manifestations may not be apparent until childhood, adolescence, or adulthood. Each disorder represents a different genetic defect affecting some molecular component of NMJ transmission. A brief description of four separate entities follows.

Familial infantile myasthenia is an autosomal recessive disorder characterized by intermittent hypotonia and fatigable generalized weakness, ptosis, dysphagia, and respiratory insufficiency exacerbated by infection or excitement. The disorder responds to acetylcholinesterase inhibitors and is thought to arise from a defect in reuptake of the ACh precursor choline by the nerve terminal or some other step in ACh synthesis or release.

Congenital acetylcholinesterase deficiency is an autosomal recessive disorder that can result in severe generalized weakness and hypotonia, sometimes requiring ventilatory support. Older children and adults may show a characteristic exaggeration of scoliosis and lumbar lordosis after prolonged standing. This disorder does not respond to acetylcholinesterase inhibitors. A classic electrodiagnostic feature is the tendency to observe repetitive CMAPs after a single electrical stimulus to the motor nerve trunk.

The slow channel syndrome is so named because of the finding of prolongation of the open time of AChR ion channels. This disorder, inherited in an autosomal dominant fashion, shows characteristics very similar to those of MG except that there is relatively severe involvement of neck extensors and forearm extensor muscles. Patients fail to respond to acetylcholinesterase inhibitors.

A final group of congenital myasthenic disorders results from AChR deficiency, although a number of different pathophysiologic mechanisms have been identified in individual cases. These patients can present both clinically and electrodiagnostically in a fashion indistinguishable from autoimmune MG and respond to acetylcholinesterase inhibitors, but not to immunosuppressants.

Lambert-Eaton Myasthenic Syndrome

LEMS was first reported as a myasthenic disorder associated with bronchial carcinoma in 1953. Edward Lambert and colleagues first differentiated LEMS from MG in 1957 and subsequently discovered that it is caused by reduced release of ACh from the presynaptic nerve terminal membrane.

Pathophysiology

LEMS is the most common presynaptic disorder of NMJ transmission and is one of the classic paraneoplastic neurologic disorders, being associated with small cell carcinoma of the lung in more than 50% of cases. On freeze-fracture electron microscopic examination, the main pathologic feature can be seen as a disorganization of the normally linear arrays of active zone particles constituting the sites of immediate release of ACh vesicles. These pathologic changes can be produced by exposing normal presynaptic NMJs to the serum of patients with LEMS (Figure 36-4). These findings, as well as the ability to produce LEMS-like clinical features in mice receiving immunoglobulin from LEMS patients, demonstrated the immune-mediated nature of this illness.

The target to which LEMS immunoglobulin is directed appears to be the presynaptic nerve terminal membrane calcium channels. LEMS IgG crosslinks active zone particles on the nerve terminal membrane, the likely site of the voltage-gated calcium channels responsible for facilitating ACh release. Antibody directed against the P/Q subtype of calcium channel has been detected in the vast majority of LEMS patients both with and without small cell lung cancer. P/Q calcium channels are found on both the presynaptic membranes of NMJs and the

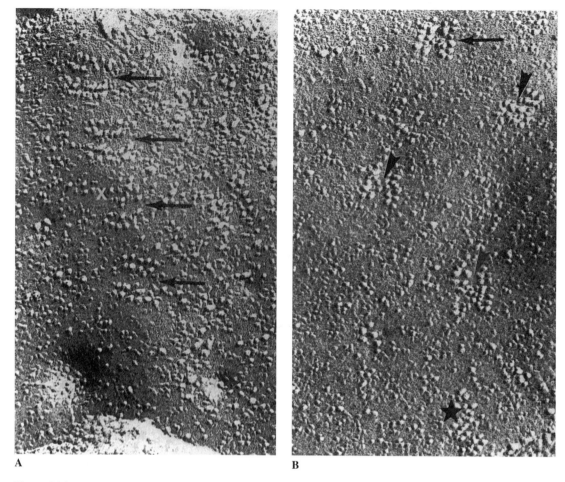

Figure 36-4. (A) Freeze-fracture electron photomicrograph of the presynaptic nerve terminal membrane, showing active zones identified by arrows, consisting of double parallel arrays of large membrane particles. Some of the active zones are incomplete (X). (B) Disorganization of active zones after treatment with IgG from patients with LEMS. The arrow indicates one normal array, the arrowheads abnormal active zones, and the star a particle cluster. (Reprinted with permission from T Fukuoka, AG Engel, B Lang, et al. Lambert-Eaton myasthenic syndrome: I. Early morphological effects of IgG on the presynaptic membrane active zones. Ann Neurol 1987;22:193.)

membranes of small cell carcinoma cells. The link between small cell lung carcinoma and LEMS is thought to involve antigenic determinants shared between this neuroectodermal tumor and the presynaptic nerve terminal membrane. Small cell lung cancer cells express voltage-gated calcium channels on their surface, and calcium influx through these channels is greatly reduced when exposed to LEMS IgG.

Patients with LEMS demonstrate other features of an autoimmune state. They have an especially increased incidence of autoimmune thyroid disease and pernicious anemia, but also vitiligo, celiac disease, type I diabetes, rheumatoid arthritis, psoriasis,

asthma, ulcerative colitis, scleroderma, and multiple sclerosis. Rarely, MG can be associated with LEMS. Finally, the clinical response of LEMS to plasmapheresis and other immunomodulating therapies lends support for an autoimmune etiology.

At the molecular level, the electrophysiologic hallmark of LEMS is a reduced number of MEPPs resulting from a decreased frequency of ACh vesicle release. The size of individual MEPPs remains normal. By contrast, in MG the number of MEPPs is normal while the size of MEPPs is reduced. With a single nerve terminal depolarization, the number of ACh vesicles released at the active release site of the nerve terminal is markedly reduced, resulting in generation of a smaller EPP at the muscle endplate. The release of ACh is diminished further in a train of depolarizations of the nerve terminal, at which point the safety factor of NMJ transmission fails and propagated muscle fiber action potentials are not produced because threshold EPPs are not generated. In this way the electrophysiologic appearance of a presynaptic disorder such as LEMS closely resembles that of MG (see Figure 36-2). When recording the electrophysiologic response to a single electrical stimulus to a nerve trunk from a whole muscle belly, the resulting CMAP is of low amplitude in LEMS, owing to insufficient EPP generation at many NMJs. By contrast, in MG, a single stimulus will usually result in a normal CMAP amplitude because the safety factor is not lost until the release of ACh diminishes in a train of stimuli.

Calcium transport into the nerve terminal membrane facilitates ACh release. Calcium influx can be transiently improved in LEMS by brief forceful voluntary exercise of the muscle or tetanic repetitive electrical nerve stimulation. Thus, LEMS is a disorder that is prominent at rest and somewhat improved by exercise, whereas MG symptoms are least prominent at rest and most apparent after exercise. However, the basic molecular physiology of NMJ transmission in these two disorders is very similar: The safety factor of NMJ transmission is lost, and slow repetitive electrical stimulation of the motor nerve trunk produces a decrementing train of CMAP amplitudes.

Clinical Features

LEMS is characterized primarily by progressive generalized weakness that is most prominent in the proximal leg muscles. Fatigability is less commonly described than in MG. In the later stages of disease craniobulbar involvement may occur, producing diplopia, ptosis, and dysphagia. Respiratory failure is an uncommon feature, although rarely it may be the presenting symptom of LEMS. Autonomic dysfunction such as dry mouth, dry eyes, constipation, and erectile dysfunction may be presenting symptoms in up to 6% of patients.

The neurologic examination often reveals a waddling gait. Weakness is more prominent in proximal muscles of the arms and legs, and there is a charac-

Table 36-6. Clinical manifestations of Lambert-Eaton Myasthenic Syndrome

Common
    Proximal more than distal extremity weakness
    Diminished or absent deep tendon reflexes
    Transient improvement with exercise of the muscle group
    Cholinergic autonomic failure
        Dry eyes, dry mouth
        Constipation
        Erectile dysfunction
Uncommon
    Craniobulbar dysfunction
        Diplopia, ptosis, dysphagia
    Respiratory insufficiency

teristic improvement in strength that occurs after a few seconds of full voluntary muscle contraction, corresponding to the facilitatory effect of calcium influx at the presynaptic site from tetanic repetitive stimulation. Muscle stretch reflexes are reduced or absent, and they may show improvement after brief, forceful exercise of the appropriate muscle group. Ptosis may be seen in some patients. The clinical manifestations of LEMS are summarized in Table 36-6.

Approximately 50% of patients with LEMS harbor a small cell lung carcinoma. Other malignancies have been associated with LEMS, including adenocarcinoma of the lung, mixed parotid tumor, systemic mastocytosis, lymphoma, and renal cell carcinoma. In many cases the neurologic symptoms antedate the diagnosis of the malignancy by as much as 2 years, often because the tumor mass responsible is initially extremely small. Sometimes the malignancy is found only at postmortem examination. Rarely, paraneoplastic LEMS may be accompanied by a second paraneoplastic neurologic disorder, usually a progressive cerebellar syndrome. Close to 50% of patients with LEMS have no associated malignancy and are thought to have a primary autoimmune disorder, sometimes accompanied by other autoimmune conditions.

Diagnosis

The clinical presentation of LEMS is rather stereotyped, but generalized weakness is a relatively nonspecific symptom. Often, such patients are first thought to have a myopathy, such as polymyositis, or a demyelinating peripheral polyneuropathy, such as CIDP. The combination of generalized weakness and areflexia of a duration of weeks to months should lead to a strong suspicion of the diagnosis. The electrodiagnostic features are almost always pathognomonic of the diagnosis of LEMS. The classic feature is a reduced amplitude CMAP recorded from a rested muscle evoked by a single electrical stimulus, followed by a marked increase in the CMAP amplitude when the electrical stimulus is preceded by a brief forceful voluntary contraction of the muscle of 10–20 seconds' duration (see Figure 36-3). The doubling of the CMAP amplitude at rest (100% facilitation) is said to be suggestive of the diagnosis of a presynaptic defect of NMJ transmission, whereas a 200% facilitation is said to be diagnostic. In some patients, the facilitation can exceed 1,000%. When patients are unable to deliver maximal voluntary contraction, a diagnostic incremental response can be seen with tetanic repetitive electrical stimulation at 30–50 Hz, but this is uncomfortable. Diagnostic incremental responses may not be seen in all muscles; in some cases proximal muscle responses must be recorded to confirm the diagnosis. With slow repetitive electrical stimulation (2–5 Hz), decremental responses like those in MG are typical.

Management

After the diagnosis of LEMS has been confirmed, a search for malignancy is indicated, including a CT scan of the chest, a blood screen, and a comprehensive physical examination. In the absence of an abnormality on the CT scan in a patient with a history of smoking, repeat scans every 6 months are indicated, especially in the face of progressive disease. In patients with a diagnosed malignancy, antineoplastic therapy is the most important treatment modality. However, in spite of optimum treatment, most patients with malignancy die within 2 years of diagnosis.

Specific treatment of the neurologic symptoms can begin by pharmacologically increasing the acetylcholine concentration in the synapse. Pyridostigmine in the same doses used for MG can relieve minor symptoms. 3,4-diaminopyridine has been shown to improve acetylcholine release by inhibiting presynaptic potassium channels. It can significantly improve symptoms at dosages of 5–25 mg three to four times per day. Minor side effects include perioral and acral paresthesias, epigastric distress, and insomnia. Seizures have been documented in a few patients and can be treated either with dosage reduction or addition of an anticonvulsant.

In patients with aggressive symptoms of LEMS, immunosuppressant treatment is appropriate. Corticosteroids such as prednisone are a reasonable first step, to which azathioprine can be added for additional immunosuppressant effect. Plasmapheresis, especially when administered long term in conjunction with corticosteroids, can be beneficial in aggressive cases, although its onset of action may be delayed compared with its effect in MG. The benefit of high-dose intravenous gamma-globulin is as yet unproven in more than anecdotal reports.

Drugs that adversely affect neuromuscular transmission in MG have similar effects in LEMS. Among the drugs considered potentially hazardous are aminoglycoside antibiotics, procainamide, quinidine, quinine, propranolol, calcium channel blockers, and iodinated radiocontrast agents.

Botulism

Botulism is a life-threatening presynaptic disorder of NMJ transmission produced by neurotoxins elaborated by the bacterium *Clostridium botulinum*. The disease occurs in three situations: by ingestion of toxin in food, by exposure to toxin produced in a traumatic wound infected by *C. botulinum,* and by exposure to toxin produced by *C. botulinum* colonizing the gastrointestinal tract of infants.

Pathophysiology

Botulinum toxin is an extremely potent blocker of ACh release from the presynaptic nerve terminal membrane. As few as 10 molecules of botulinum toxin can irreversibly stop ACh release. The result is complete failure of NMJ transmission across the NMJ, followed by degeneration of the motor endplate and functional denervation of the muscle fiber. Full recovery from botulism is delayed because nerve sprouts must be newly formed to reinnervate denervated muscle fibers, generating new NMJs to re-establish synaptic transmission.

There may be more than one mechanism by which botulinum toxin inhibits ACh release. A portion of the botulinum toxin molecule binds to the release site of ACh on the nerve terminal. The light chain of the toxin interacts with synaptobrevin-2, an integral protein component of the ACh vesicle membrane, leading to a failure of ACh vesicle fusion with the nerve terminal membrane.

The electrophysiologic manifestations of botulism are identical to those of LEMS, except that the damage to the ACh mobilization process is so complete that (1) no recordable muscle fiber action potential may be possible, (2) no recordable CMAP may be possible, (3) calcium influx into the nerve terminal may have little or no effect on the CMAP amplitude, and (4) if facilitation does occur, its duration can be prolonged.

Clinical Features

In those who ingest contaminated food, nausea and vomiting may occur within 12–36 hours. Neurologic symptoms may be delayed by up to 3 days. Cranial nerves are affected first: Diplopia occurs as a result of paralysis of extraocular muscles; blurred vision occurs because of fixed dilation of the pupils. Bulbar involvement results in dysphonia, dysarthria, and dysphagia. Later, weakness of extremity and respiratory muscles occurs. Failure of ACh transmission occurs across both nicotinic and muscarinic cholinergic synapses, producing autonomic dysfunction in the form of paralysis of pupillary function, loss of salivation (sometimes producing severe drying of the pharyngeal mucosa), ileus, constipation, urinary retention, and orthostatic hypotension.

Diagnosis

The diagnosis of botulism rests on clinical suspicion and confirmatory laboratory tests. Electrodiagnostic testing will show very low or absent evoked CMAPs. In mild to moderate disease, facilitation of the CMAP response may be achieved with tetanic repetitive stimulation. When the toxin load is not high, as when toxin is produced in the gut of infants, a clear facilitation with tetanic repetitive nerve stimulation is seen. The facilitation effect may last for 5 minutes or longer after tetanic stimulation, as opposed

to the situation in LEMS, where the effect lasts less than 1 minute. Toxin can be identified in the blood, stool, gastric contents, or food by means of a bioassay in mice. Culture of the organism anaerobically is difficult. Early on, botulism can be confused with disorders such as streptococcal pharyngitis (due to severe drying and redness of the oral mucosa) and intestinal obstruction producing ileus. The differential diagnosis also includes anticholinergic intoxication from drugs such as atropine, belladonna, and jimsonweed, or from mushroom poisoning. Some of the symptoms of botulism can also resemble those of Guillain-Barré syndrome.

Management

Antitoxin therapy has been recommended in adult cases and should be administered as soon as possible. Delayed use may still be beneficial; toxin has been found in the blood of some patients as long as 30 days after intoxication. Recent studies have not recommended antitoxin use in infantile botulism. All preparations of antitoxin are of equine origin, and up to 20% of patients have untoward reactions, so that hypersensitivity testing and desensitization may be necessary before use.

The use of penicillin to eradicate *C. botulinum* in the bowel of colonized patients is of uncertain value. Even in the case of wound infection by *C. botulinum*, use of antibiotics does not prevent intoxication.

Treatment with drugs that increase ACh release may yield some clinical benefit. Guanidine hydrochloride can improve general strength and respiratory function in as many as 50% of patients, but its use is severely limited by the potential complications of bone marrow suppression and renal toxicity. 3,4-diaminopyridine has been used successfully in the treatment of LEMS and may have a positive effect on the presynaptic release of ACh in patients with botulism.

Other Disorders of Neuromuscular Transmission

Organophosphate Poisoning

Exposure to organophosphates occurs primarily through the use of insecticides such as malathion and parathion. They act by irreversibly inhibiting acetylcholinesterase, producing weakness, muscle cramps and fasciculation, autonomic cholinergic hyperactivity, disorientation, and seizures. In mild cases, the electrodiagnostic findings can resemble pyridostigmine intoxication and congenital acetylcholinesterase deficiency, in that multiple CMAPs arise after a single electrical stimulus to the nerve trunk. The treatment of this condition includes pralidoxime and atropine.

Magnesium Intoxication

Magnesium acts as a calcium antagonist, competing for uptake at the voltage-gated calcium channels. In states of magnesium excess, such as renal failure or after magnesium sulfate treatment for eclampsia during pregnancy, calcium influx drops, ACh release is inhibited, and generalized weakness can develop. This effect can be reversed with calcium infusion.

Tick Bite Paralysis

The toxin produced by the pregnant female tick of several species has been shown to produce progressive generalized weakness over several days, sometimes affecting swallowing and respiratory muscles. In North America, the tick *Dermacentor andersoni* has been implicated in a number of cases. Deep tendon reflexes are lost and sensation is spared, giving rise to a clinical picture that resembles Guillain-Barré syndrome. CMAPs after nerve trunk stimulation are low in amplitude, but electrophysiologic defects of NMJ transmission have not been reported. Thus, the disorder has not been clearly demonstrated to be a defect of NMJ transmission. However, the rapid recovery of CMAP amplitude and clinical strength that occurs after tick removal (sometimes within 24 hours) leads to the speculation that some easily reversible blockade of NMJ transmission may be the cause.

Suggested Reading

Desmedt JE. The Neuromuscular Disorder in Myasthenia Gravis. II. Presynaptic Cholinergic Metabolism, Myasthenia-like Syndromes, and a Hypothesis. In JE Desmedt (ed), New Developments in Electromyography and Clinical Neurophysiology (Vol 1). Basel: S. Karger, 1973;305–342.

Drachman DB. Myasthenia gravis. N Engl J Med 1994;330:1797.

Eaton LM, Lambert EH. Electromyography and electric stimulation of nerves in diseases of motor unit: observations on myasthenic syndrome associated with malignant tumors. JAMA 1957;163:1117.

Gardnerova M, Eymard B, Morel E, et al. The fetal/adult acetylcholine receptor antibody ratio in mothers with myasthenia gravis as a marker for transfer of the disease to the newborn. Neurology 1997;48:50.

Harper CM Jr. Neuromuscular Transmission Disorders in Childhood. In HR Jones Jr, CF Bolton, CM Harper Jr (eds), Pediatric Clinical Electromyography. Philadelphia: Lippincott–Raven, 1996;353–385.

Lennon VA, Kryzer TJ, Griesmann GE, et al. Calcium-channel antibodies in the Lambert-Eaton syndrome and other paraneoplastic syndromes. N Engl J Med 1995;332:1467.

Levin KH. Paraneoplastic neuromuscular syndromes. Neurol Clin North Am 1997;15:597.

O'Neill JH, Murray NM, Newsom-Davis J. The Lambert-Eaton myasthenic syndrome. A review of 50 cases. Brain 1988;111:577.

Osserman KE, Genkins G. Studies in myasthenia gravis: review of twenty-year experience in over 1,200 patients. Mt Sinai J Med 1971;38:497.

Pickett JB. Neuromuscular Transmission. In AJ Sumner (ed), The Physiology of Peripheral Nerve Disease. Boston: Saunders, 1980;238–264.

Schaffner W. *Clostridium Botulinum* (Botulism). In RG Mandell, RG Douglas Jr, JE Bennett (eds), Principles and Practice of Infectious Diseases (3rd ed). New York: Churchill Livingstone, 1990.

Stalberg E, Trontelj JV. Single Fiber Electromyography (2nd ed). New York: Raven, 1994.

Swift TR. Disorders of neruomuscular transmission other than myasthenia gravis. Muscle Nerve 1981;4:334.

Chapter 37
Muscle Disorders

Terri Strassburger and John J. Kelly, Jr.

Chapter Plan

Approach to patients with muscle weakness
    (myopathy)
    Symptoms
    Signs and order of examination
    Laboratory tests
Myopathy syndromes
    Atrophic myopathies
    Inflammatory/necrotic myopathies
    Dystrophies
    Metabolic myopathies
    Congenital myopathies
Conclusion

Approach to Patients with Muscle Weakness (Myopathy)

Myopathies are intrinsic diseases of skeletal muscle. Anatomically, the muscle is a part of the motor unit, which is made up of the motor neuron, its axon, the neuromuscular junction, and the muscle. Because of the relative simplicity of the unit as well as the uniform structure and function of muscle, myopathies have somewhat similar clinical manifestations. Therefore, their differential diagnosis often depends on laboratory techniques, including electromyography (EMG), serum enzyme levels, and muscle biopsy.

Symptoms

The common symptoms of muscle disorders are weakness, cramps, stiffness, fatigue or exercise intolerance, pain, spasm, and twitching. Weakness, or an inability to generate force, is the most common symptom but can be difficult to differentiate from fatigability. In general, fatigue is more common in disorders of the neuromuscular junction, chronic systemic diseases, or psychiatric diseases and less commonly seen in intrinsic muscle disorders. However, true intolerance to exercise is a symptom of muscle disorders, in particular the glycogen storage diseases and mitochondrial disorders. In these patients, prolonged exercise leads to premature fatigue and muscle tenderness or myalgia. These patients usually complain of concomitant weakness.

In myopathies, weakness occurs predominantly in the proximal and bulbar muscles. The particular topography may give diagnostic clues to the underlying cause (Table 37-1). Patients may complain of difficulty arising from a chair, walking up stairs, raising the arms above shoulder level, truncal and limb weakness, drooping of the eyelids, double vision, and difficulty chewing or swallowing with bulbar weakness.

Muscle cramps, which are common in healthy individuals, can be seen in primary muscle disorders. Although nonspecific, they suggest certain metabolic disorders, tetanus, or dehydration.

Table 37-1. Major Clinical Neuromuscular Presentations

Syndrome	Weakness	Topography			Sensory
		Proximal	Distal	Bulbar	
Myopathy	Symmetric	+++	Rare	Occ	No
Polyneuropathy	Symmetric	Rare	+++	Rare	Yes
Motor neuron disease (ALS)	Asymmetric	Late	+++	++	No
Neuromuscular transmission	Symmetric	+++	Rare	+++	No

Rare = rarely involved; Occ = occasionally involved; ++ = often involved; +++ = almost always involved; Late = involved late in the course of the disease; ALS = amyotrophic lateral sclerosis.

In general, pain is not a common symptom of muscle disease. If prominent, there may be an accompanying peripheral neuropathy; radiculopathy; or primary blood vessel, bone, joint, or tendon disorder. Tenderness of muscles, however, can be seen in the inflammatory myopathies. In addition, physiologic contractures with muscle shortening and pain during activity occur in some metabolic myopathies. Historical information such as family history, symptom progression, and toxin exposure should be investigated in obscure cases.

Signs and Order of Examination

The clinical evaluation should be systematic and directed. Observation is invaluable especially in the case of a young child who has difficulty cooperating. Severe weakness may result in abnormal posture and gait. Excessive lumbar lordosis implies weak hip extensor muscles, waddling gait implies hip abductor weakness, and flaring of the shoulder blades implies shoulder girdle weakness. Difficulty in performing certain tasks, such as walking, hopping, or arising from a sitting position, implies true weakness as opposed to fatigability and can aid in the localization of the weakness. The results of this "functional muscle testing" can be abnormal when isometric strength testing may appear normal.

A rating scale of muscle testing should be used to quantitate the degree of weakness and localize the specific muscles involved. The Medical Research Council Scale is recommended, which recognizes five grades of muscle strength: 0, complete paralysis; 1, minimal contraction; 2, active movement with gravity eliminated; 3, weak contraction against gravity; 4, movement against gravity and resistance;

5, normal strength. The ocular, facial, pharyngeal, lingual, neck, shoulder, upper and lower limbs, truncal, and pelvic muscles should be tested. The powerful trunk and girdle muscles, the force of which can be difficult for the examiner to overcome, should be tested by asking the patient to squat then stand or walk on toes and heels. Patients who can squat and rise, walk on heels and toes, and hop on either foot have little or no weakness of lower limbs.

Muscles should be inspected for signs of wasting, fasciculations, or hypertrophy. Muscle hypertrophy, when confined to the calves, is seen in muscular dystrophy, most typically in Duchenne's and Becker's dystrophy. Generalized muscle hypertrophy can indicate a myotonic myopathy or storage myopathy.

The tendon reflexes are normally spared in most muscle diseases but can be reduced in muscular dystrophy or inflammatory myopathies when weakness is severe. In hypothyroid myopathy, the tendon reflexes are slow to relax. The sensory examination results are normal in pure myopathies.

The general physical examination can be extremely important in the evaluation of a patient with myopathy. Systemic features, such as frontal balding and cataracts (myotonic dystrophy [MD]), heart block, pigmentary retinopathy, sensorineural hearing loss (Kearns-Sayre mitochondrial myopathy) and skin rash (dermatomyositis) can give important diagnostic clues to the underlying etiology.

Laboratory Tests

Blood Studies

The findings on laboratory testing are summarized in Table 37-2. The serum concentration of creatine

Table 37-2. Laboratory Findings in Neuromuscular Diseases

Syndrome	CK	EMG	Nerve Biopsy	Muscle Biopsy	Other
Myopathy	+++	+++	–	+++	–
Polyneuropathy	–	+++	+++	–	–
Motor neuron disease	+	+++	–	Denerv	–
Neuromuscular transmission	–	+++	–	+/–	AChR

CK = creatine kinase; EMG = electromyography; – = normal or not helpful; + = mildly abnormal or helpful; +++ = abnormal and often diagnostic; Denerv = neurogenic denervation; AChR = acetylcholine receptor antibodies.

kinase (CK) is a reliable indicator of muscle damage or necrosis. The highest levels occur in patients with inflammatory myopathies, Duchenne's muscular dystrophy (DMD) and acute rhabdomyolysis. High concentrations occur in some metabolic myopathies but can also occur in patients without myopathies such as spinal muscular atrophy or motor neuron disease, in normal patients after strenuous exercise or viral illness, or with muscle trauma (EMG needle insertion). Serum CK levels are normal in most congenital myopathies, myotonic syndromes, and steroid myopathies. Specific diagnoses can be made using molecular genetics, which is available for some inherited muscle diseases and can lead to appropriate genetic counseling.

Electromyography

EMG is often essential to myopathy evaluation. It provides evidence of a primary myopathic process and allows it to be differentiated from a neurogenic disorder. Typically, the motor and sensory nerve conduction studies (NCSs) produced normal findings in myopathies. In certain conditions, however, a peripheral neuropathy may coexist with a myopathy, such as inflammatory myopathies associated with connective tissue diseases or mitochondrial myopathies. The needle examination in myopathies usually reveals short-duration, low-amplitude, polyphasic motor unit action potentials (MUAPs) (Figure 37-1). With voluntary contraction, there is early recruitment of MUAPs with a full interference pattern. Certain myopathies (i.e., inflammatory and toxic myopathies and DMD) show spontaneous fibrillation potentials and positive waves. The waxing and waning ("dive bomber") myotonic discharges are typical of the myotonic myopathies. The distribution of EMG changes

within the muscle indicates the extent and pattern of involvement and can be of diagnostic help. In addition, the EMG can aid in the determination of the site of muscle biopsy.

Muscle Biopsy

A muscle biopsy is often required to obtain a definitive diagnosis. Ideally, a moderately weak muscle that has not been the site of previous trauma (e.g., a previous EMG study) should be selected. If the muscle is severely affected, the muscle biopsy specimen is often difficult to interpret and may show only nonspecific (end-stage) changes. Muscle may be biopsied by needle or open methods. The needle biopsy requires only a minor incision and can be repeated at different sites, whereas the open biopsy requires a larger incision, but offers a larger tissue sample, which may be of benefit in myopathies that are patchy.

Myopathy Syndromes

Atrophic Myopathies

The atrophic myopathies are the most common muscle diseases encountered by the clinician. They are characterized by insidious onset of proximal muscle weakness, usually associated with an underlying medical problem, certain medications, or disuse of muscles. The most common causes are endocrine- (thyroid, parathyroid), medication- (steroids), and alcohol-related myopathies.

The most common endocrine myopathies are related to thyroid dysfunction, which can cause (1) a chronic thyrotoxic myopathy, (2) a hypothyroid myopathy, or (3) an infiltrative ophthalmoplegia. In

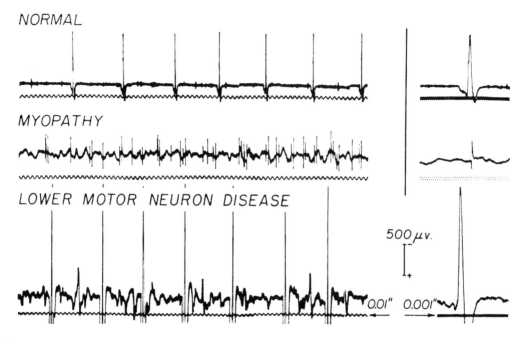

Figure 37-1. Motor unit action potentials during weak voluntary contraction (m. biceps brachii) in a normal person, in progressive muscular dystrophy (myopathy), and in amyotrophic lateral sclerosis (lower motor neuron disease). Action potentials on the left are recorded with a slow time base (time signal is 100 cycles per second). Action potentials on the right are recorded with a more rapid time base (time signal is 1,000 cycles per second). (Reprinted with permission from Mayo Clinic and Mayo Foundation. Clinical Examinations in Neurology [3rd ed]. Philadelphia: Saunders, 1971;285.)

chronic hyperthyroid myopathy, there is slowly progressive weakness and atrophy of muscles, particularly the thighs and shoulders. This may progress to a severe degree, suggesting the diagnosis of motor neuron disease; however, there are no fasciculations or spasticity. Myalgias may occur. The bulbar and sphincter muscles are spared. The deep tendon reflexes (DTRs) are generally normal, but may show a shortened relaxation time. Women are affected approximately three or four times more frequently than men. The serum CK level is usually normal (Table 37-3). Routine muscle biopsy specimens generally show nonspecific changes such as mild fatty infiltration and type I and II muscle fiber atrophy. The EMG findings are normal or only mildly abnormal. The results of NCSs are also normal, but the needle examination may show mild changes in MUAPs. An absence of muscle fiber membrane irritability (fibrillations and positive wave) is generally seen.

Hypothyroid myopathy is characterized by slowly progressive proximal weakness of the shoulder and pelvic girdle muscles. These patients complain of fatigability, myalgias, cramps, and "stiffness." Atrophy is generally not observed, and indeed, occasionally muscle hypertrophy occurs (Hoffman's syndrome). The reflexes may demonstrate delayed relaxation, but this is difficult to detect clinically. Myoedema, which is a painless and electrically silent mounding of muscle tissue when percussed, may be observed. The CK levels are generally mildly elevated. There is a 10 to 1 female-to-male ratio of patients with hypothyroid disease. Muscle biopsy shows atrophy of type I and II fibers with occasional muscle fiber necrosis. The EMG findings are usually normal. However, these patients often have associated entrapment neuropathies such as carpal tunnel syndrome. Needle examination occasionally can be myopathic. Symptoms and signs generally resolve rapidly when the patient reaches a euthyroid state.

A proximal myopathy with fatigability can be a complication of hyperparathyroidism, hypophosphatemia, acromegaly, or adrenal insufficiency. Typically, the serum CK level and EMG findings are normal. The muscle biopsy specimen appears normal or nonspecific with type II fiber atrophy.

Table 37-3. Myopathic Syndromes

Syndrome	CK	EMG	Biopsy	Other
Atrophic	Normal	+/–	Type II atrophy	–
Dystrophic	+/+++	++	Characteristic	Selective weakness
Inflammatory/necrotic	+++	+++	Inflammatory/necrotic	Rash in some
Metabolic	+/–	+/–	Characteristic	Cramps, myalgias, fatigue, CNS signs
Congenital	Normal	+/–	Characteristic	Static weakness

CK = creatine kinase; EMG = electromyography; CNS = central nervous system; – = normal or not helpful; + = mildly abnormal or helpful; ++ = moderately abnormal or helpful; +++ = abnormal and often diagnostic.

Alcoholic myopathy can be acute or chronic. In acute alcoholic myopathy, patients present with a rapid progression of muscle pain, cramping, swelling, and weakness during or immediately after an alcoholic binge. The location and degree of muscle involvement can be highly variable. If the alcohol consumption is great, rhabdomyolysis, myoglobinuria, and even renal failure can occur. Serum CK levels are markedly elevated during the attacks. Muscle biopsy specimens show widespread muscle fiber necrosis. Treatment requires supportive medical care and nutritional supplementation, and patients usually make a satisfactory recovery.

Patients with chronic alcoholic myopathy complain of an insidious onset of proximal limb girdle weakness over months. The degree of weakness is variable among patients. Muscle biopsy specimens show muscle fiber atrophy, necrosis, and regeneration.

Asymptomatic alcoholic myopathy is often found coincidentally when chronic alcoholic patients are evaluated for other medical reasons and elevated CK levels are found. There is no evidence of weakness clinically. These patients probably have a presymptomatic stage of acute or chronic alcoholic myopathy.

The EMG findings are similar in the above alcoholic myopathies. The motor and sensory NCSs may appear abnormal, indicating an axonal and demyelinating sensorimotor polyneuropathy caused by alcohol or nutritional deficiency. Occasionally, the proximal muscles show evidence of a myopathic process with some muscle membrane irritability, but this is highly variable and often absent. In acute alcoholic myopathy with rhabdomyolysis, dense fibrillation potentials and positive waves are seen.

Patients with iatrogenic steroid myopathy generally complain of proximal muscle weakness of the lower and upper extremities. The distal muscles, facial muscles, and sphincters are usually spared. Atrophy can be seen late in the course of the disease. Muscle pain may be a complaint, and the patient may develop a cushingoid appearance (increase of truncal adipose tissue and skin pigmentation). For reasons that are not clear, women are more prone to exogenous steroid-induced weakness than men are. Weakness may begin several weeks after initiation of steroids or may be observed within a few days after extremely high dosages. Not infrequently, the issue of steroid myopathy emerges when a patient is being treated for a myopathy with steroids and develops increasing weakness. It is often unclear whether the weakness is caused by increasing inflammatory myopathy or superimposed steroid myopathy. Serum CK levels may be helpful, as they are generally not elevated in steroid-induced myopathies. An improving EMG picture also suggests a steroid myopathy. Often a steroid taper is necessary to determine the cause. If the patient improves, the presumptive diagnosis is medication-induced weakness. The muscle biopsy shows type II fiber atrophy with a lack of necrosis. The EMG findings generally appear normal or show minimal myopathic changes without spontaneous activity (fibrillations and positive waves). Cushing's syndrome (endogenous excess of corticosteroids) is similar in its clinical and laboratory findings.

Inflammatory/Necrotic Myopathies

The inflammatory myopathies are characterized by proximal muscle weakness and inflammation on muscle biopsy. They are generally differentiated by the presence or absence of characteristic skin changes or their association with other connective tissue or autoimmune diseases. The three major subsets are polymyositis, dermatomyositis, and inclusion body myositis (IBM).

The clinical features of polymyositis and dermatomyositis are similar except for the characteristic rash in dermatomyositis. This is generally a erythematous flat rash on the face, upper trunk, elbows, knees, and metacarpophalangeal joints, with a violaceous discoloration of the upper eyelids (heliotrope), especially in children. Subcutaneous calcifications occur, more commonly in children, and can become large and even ulcerate through the skin. The weakness in both of these diseases is proximal and symmetric, primarily involving the shoulder and hip girdle musculature. In addition, the neck and pharyngeal muscles can be affected with dysphagia. The respiratory and external ocular muscles are generally spared. Patients may complain of muscle pain or tenderness, but this is actually uncommon. The rate of progression can be acute, subacute, or chronic. Other systemic complaints can accompany the disease, such as weight loss, fever, and, less commonly, cardiac conduction defects. A small percentage of patients with polymyositis and dermatomyositis display features of concomitant connective tissue disorders, such as systemic lupus erythematosus, rheumatoid arthritis, or scleroderma. Adult-onset dermatomyositis may be associated with an occult malignancy, especially in older patients. Toxic myopathies resulting from drug and toxin exposures can mimic inflammatory myopathies and must be excluded.

Typically, the serum CK level is greatly elevated in inflammatory myopathies (up to 50-fold) and often correlates roughly with the clinical severity and acuteness of the disease. Rarely, the CK level can be normal. The EMG findings typically appear myopathic, and additionally there are usually fibrillation potentials and positive sharp waves. Confirmation with muscle biopsy is advisable because other disorders can mimic inflammatory myopathies. Generally, an open biopsy is recommended because of the patchy nature of the disease. The biopsy specimen generally shows invasion of inflammatory cells, muscle fiber necrosis, and regeneration (Figure 37-2). If a patient possesses all four criteria (typical clinical, CK, EMG, and muscle biopsy findings) the patient is classified as having definite polymyositis or dermatomyositis. If three criteria are satisfied, the

patient is placed in the probable category; with two criteria the patient is placed in the possible category. Possible myositis patients are often given a course of high-dose prednisone as a therapeutic trial.

The treatment of choice for polymyositis and dermatomyositis is high-dose corticosteroids early in the course of the disease. Some patients may require immunosuppressive agents such as azathioprine and methotrexate for long-term therapy, especially if intolerant of steroid side effects. Physical therapy is important to prevent contractures.

IBM is characterized by a slowly progressive weakness over the course of years. The weakness generally begins in the proximal legs, but sometimes it begins distally or diffusely, later involving the arms and sometimes the pharynx (dysphagia). The muscles typically affected are the biceps brachii, triceps, iliopsoas, quadriceps, and tibialis anterior muscles. The deltoid, pectoralis major, forearm, and hand intrinsic muscles are also involved, but usually less than those noted above. The neck flexors, hip adductors, gluteal, hamstring, gastrocnemius, soleus, and toe flexors are relatively spared. Overall, approximately 50% of patients have some degree of distal weakness, but in only 35% of patients is the distal weakness the same or greater than that found proximally. Patients often have muscle atrophy and DTRs are often reduced or absent, especially in the lower extremities. IBM is more common in males (approximately 3 to 1).

Most patients with IBM will have a moderately elevated serum CK level, but generally not exceeding 10 times normal. The EMG findings are generally myopathic, and fibrillation potentials and positive sharp waves are usually seen in all muscles affected, which is an important distinguishing feature. A muscle biopsy is essential for diagnosis. Muscle fibers contain rimmed vacuoles (vacuoles lined by basophilic material) on light microscopic examination, and intranuclear and intracytoplasmic filamentous inclusions on electron microscopy studies. Typically, patients with IBM do not respond to corticosteroids or other immunosuppressive agents. Most are given a therapeutic trial, however, as there are occasional responders. The disease is slowly progressive but relentless. The patient often requires a wheelchair after 10 years of disease duration. Treatment is supportive.

Figure 37-2. (2) Polymyositis. The best known change in the biopsy specimens of patients with polymyositis is the inflammatory response. The routine hematoxylin and eosin stain demonstrates a perivascular inflammatory response in which the cells are gathered around a medium-sized blood vessel. This is a typical feature and strongly suggests the diagnosis. (3) In this patient the cellular response was apparently associated with necrotic fibers rather than with the blood vessels. Although this patient did indeed have polymyositis, interpretation of such a biopsy should be more cautious, since other genetic dystrophies may give rise to cellular responses associated with the fibers. (4) Another biopsy specimen shows a vacuolar change in many fibers. (Reprinted with permission from MH Brooke. A Clinician's View of Neuromuscular Diseases [2nd ed]. Baltimore: Williams & Wilkins, 1986;220.)

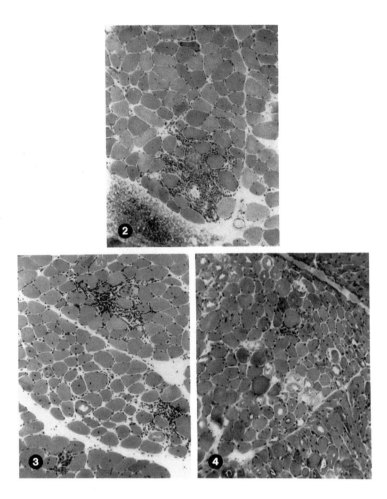

Dystrophies

The muscular dystrophies comprise a group of progressive muscle disorders that are usually inherited, although spontaneous mutations do occur. They are traditionally classified according to their mode of inheritance and clinical manifestation. Common features include symmetrical muscle weakness with atrophy, normal sensation, and hereditary transmission. Genetic testing using molecular markers has changed the classification of some of the dystrophies and aided in more accurate diagnosis.

The best known of the muscular dystrophies is DMD. Patients possess a defective gene causing absence of a membrane protein called *dystrophin*. DMD begins in early childhood, is relentlessly progressive, and leads to death in early adulthood. It is inherited as an X-linked recessive trait and is trans-

mitted to males from the mother, who is generally an asymptomatic carrier. Most male children have normal early motor development, but soon develop proximal muscle weakness manifested by difficulty arising from the floor (Gower's sign) or climbing stairs. The calf muscles and sometimes the quadriceps and deltoids become enlarged and firm yet weak (pseudohypertrophy), while the thigh and girdle muscles become atrophic and weak. The gait becomes waddling, there may be frequent falls, and there is a tendency for these children to walk on their toes to redistribute the center of gravity. The tendon reflexes are reduced in proportion to the muscle weakness; however, the Achilles tendon reflex may be spared. Weakness progresses to involve respiratory muscles; kyphoscoliosis ensues and contractures develop. Boys are wheelchair-bound by age 12 years. Cardiac involvement and mental impairment can occur, although death usually occurs as a result of respiratory insufficiency.

The serum CK levels are markedly elevated early in life in proportion to the tempo of muscle destruction and may drop to normal when muscle destruction is very advanced. Muscle biopsy specimens show fiber degeneration and regeneration and muscle replacement with fat and connective tissue. Immunohistochemical staining reveals complete absence of dystrophin. The EMG is myopathic with evidence of muscle fiber irritability. The dystrophin gene deletions can be detected by polymerase chain reaction (PCR) analysis of DNA from affected patients.

Becker's muscular dystrophy (BMD) is an X-linked recessive disorder allelic with DMD and is less common and less severe than DMD. It causes weakness and atrophy in the same topography as DMD as well as pseudohypertrophy of the calf muscles; however, maintenance of ambulation and life expectancy are considerably longer. Cardiac involvement and mental deficiency are absent or mild. Achilles tendon contractures are common and can occur early in the disease. The serum CK level is elevated, but not to the degree seen in DMD. In BMD, immunohistochemical staining of muscle biopsy specimens reveals a reduced amount of dystrophin, which can range from mild to severe. The severity of the disease correlates with the degree of dystrophin reduction.

There is no curative treatment for DMD or BMD. Supportive treatment such as pulmonary toilet, physical therapy, and orthopedic procedures such as spinal fusions can help symptomatically. Studies have shown high-dose steroids can slow deterioration slightly, but side effects are problematic.

The most frequently encountered dystrophy is MD, which is inherited in an autosomal dominant manner. Clinical symptoms may not present until adolescence or early adult life. Weakness is generally seen in the distal muscles as well as the neck and pharyngeal/laryngeal muscles. Myotonia is manifested by the slow relaxation of muscles after forceful contraction, such as eye or hand closure. The face typically appears thin and narrowed, with temporalis/masseter atrophy, ptosis, and frontal balding. Other organ systems are involved. Patients may present with cardiac arrhythmias, hypogonadism, endocrine abnormalities, mental deficien-

cies, and cataracts. Weakness can progress to involve the respiratory muscles. DTRs are depressed, whereas sensation is normal. Disease progression is slow. The defective gene has been localized to chromosome 19, with expansion of the CTG triplet repeat in the myotonin protein kinase gene. This DNA fragment increases in size in successive generations, causing increased disease severity (anticipation). Besides molecular testing, EMG can be very helpful in diagnosis. Trains of myotonic discharges are observed after needle insertion. These are sustained runs of single muscle fiber activity that outlast the inciting stimulus and sound like a dive-bomber. Myopathic changes are also observed. There is no specific treatment; however, the myotonia may respond to quinine or phenytoin. Other organ manifestations should be treated appropriately and a multispecialty approach is recommended for all dystrophies, most appropriately in a muscular dystrophy clinic.

Metabolic Myopathies

Metabolic myopathies constitute a heterogeneous group of diseases caused by a primary biochemical abnormality of the muscle cell. These abnormalities can range from mitochondrial disorders, defects in various enzymes in the metabolism of glucose/glycogen or lipids, or abnormalities of the muscle membrane ion channels.

Intramuscular glycogen provides energy for short-term strenuous exercise, whereas lipids or fatty acid metabolism provides energy for long-duration or endurance exercise. For these reasons, glycogen metabolic disorders often produce weakness, cramps, fatigue, or exercise intolerance early in strenuous exercise, whereas the lipid metabolic disorders produce poor endurance with prolonged exercise, especially after fasting.

The glycogen storage diseases are generally autosomal recessive. The muscle biopsy is either normal or shows evidence of abnormal accumulation of glycogen in vacuoles. The specific enzymatic defect (e.g., acid maltase, myophosphorylase, phosphofructokinase deficiency) can be detected by biochemical analysis of affected tissue (e.g., muscle, skin, or leukocytes). These diseases generally show a blunted or no rise of venous lactate levels after ischemic forearm exercise testing. EMG findings are varied but may show muscle membrane irritability (fibrillations and positive sharp waves) and myopathic changes. Other manifestations of the glycogen metabolic disorders may include myoglobinuria, systemic organ involvement such as the heart, liver, spleen, and central nervous system, and failure to thrive or hypotonia in infants.

The lipid storage diseases are heterogeneous and many are poorly defined. They are identified by the characteristic finding of lipid accumulation in myocytes. The two best characterized lipid disorders are carnitine deficiency myopathy and carnitine-palmitoyl transferase deficiency. Their deficiency prevents the transport of fatty acids into the muscle mitochondria where they are metabolized. Subtypes of carnitine deficiency may be restricted to muscle or may involve the liver, heart, and central nervous system. Some forms of carnitine deficiency are potentially treatable by the administration of oral carnitine. Thus, early diagnosis is important.

The clinical spectrum of the mitochondrial disorders is very diverse. They range from slowly progressive myopathies confined to a few muscles (chronic progressive external ophthalmoplegia) to severe, fatal infantile myopathies. In addition, they often involve extramuscular and extraneurologic tissues. The most well-described mitochondrial myopathies are the multisystem encephalomyopathies such as Kearns-Sayre, myoclonic epilepsy with ragged-red fibers, and mitochondrial encephalomyopathy with lactic acidosis and strokelike episodes. There may be overlap among these and other mitochondrial syndromes, and new phenotypes are still being identified. Common features include weakness, short stature, dementia, and sensorineural hearing loss. Many mitochondrial disorders have a maternal inheritance. Diagnosis is made based on clinical features, an elevated fasting venous lactate level, and muscle biopsy specimens that reveal ragged-red fibers (caused by proliferation of mitochondria) with modified Gomori's trichrome stain. The EMG findings may reveal evidence of a peripheral neuropathy or myopathy. The common mutations in the mitochondrial genome associated with some of the disorders can be identified with PCR.

The primary periodic paralyses present as episodic focal or generalized weakness associated with or without fluctuations in the serum potassium level. Three types are generally recognized—hypokalemic, hyperkalemic, and normokalemic—although some studies have shown that the normokalemic variety may be a variant of hyperkalemic periodic paralysis. They are inherited in an autosomal dominant manner with rare sporadic cases. The serum potassium level is usually normal between attacks of weakness and abnormal during an attack, which separates these from the secondary periodic paralyses caused by such disorders as renal failure or diuretic abuse. The weakness is caused by an abnormality in sodium or chloride channels resulting in failure of action potential propagation along the muscle membrane. The three primary periodic paralyses can be differentiated by the duration of the attacks, provocative features, and serum potassium levels during attacks. In hypokalemic periodic paralysis, the attacks are often precipitated by a high-carbohydrate meal and tend to be of long duration (many hours) whereas in hyperkalemic period paralysis, attacks can be precipitated by fasting or by rest after exercise and tend to be of short duration. The CK level may be moderately raised during and sometimes between attacks. When performed during an attack, the EMG findings may reveal myotonia (more often in hyperkalemic) or progressive reduction in motor unit recruitment. In addition, the compound muscle action potential shows a progressive reduction in amplitude. With disease progression, EMG findings may show myopathic changes even between attacks. Muscle biopsy specimens reveal vacuolar changes in muscle fibers with occasional necrosis. Provocative tests are also used for diagnosis. Hypokalemic periodic paralysis can be induced with oral glucose, whereas hyperkalemic periodic paralysis can be induced with oral potassium. Careful cardiac, blood pressure, and electrolyte monitoring is necessary if these provocative tests are performed. Treatment is aimed at correcting the potassium concentration. Oral potassium with a low-carbohydrate diet is used for hypokalemic periodic paralysis, and a potassium wasting diuretic such as hydrochlorothiazide is used for hyperkalemic periodic paralysis.

Secondary periodic paralyses are acquired disorders that result in serum potassium fluctuations, which in turn cause episodic weakness. They can be caused by endocrine abnormalities, toxins, medications (diuretics), or renal failure. Treatment is aimed at correcting the underlying disease state.

Congenital Myopathies

The congenital myopathies are a heterogeneous group of relatively nonprogressive muscle disorders that present at birth or shortly after with generalized weakness. The infant is hypotonic at birth and subsequently shows delayed motor milestones. There is usually a family history of muscle disease. As the infant grows, there is often some improvement in strength, but not to normal levels. Skeletal abnormalities and dysmorphic features are common. These disorders are classified by specific morphologic abnormalities of the myocyte, which can be detected by immunohistochemical staining or electron microscopic examination. The serum CK level is either normal or only mildly elevated, as muscle necrosis does not occur. The EMG findings, with a few exceptions, are also generally normal or mildly myopathic. Both parents should be studied since either may possess subtle clinical and laboratory findings. The three most common congenital myopathies are (1) central-core myopathy, (2) nemaline myopathy, and (3) centronuclear myopathy.

Infants with central core disease are hypotonic at birth or in infancy with symmetric proximal muscle weakness. There is little atrophy and the neck and facial muscles are spared. Rate of progression is highly variable. Skeletal deformities such as pes cavus and congenital hip dislocation are often present. The disease is transmitted in an autosomal dominant manner. Patients are susceptible to malignant hyperthermia and precautions should be taken when general anesthesia is considered. The muscle biopsy is diagnostic and specimens reveal cores in the center of muscle fibers with a lack of mitochondria within the cores. Histochemical stains are required to detect the central cores and may be missed if the stains are not performed. The findings on EMG are generally myopathic or normal.

Nemaline myopathy is a very heterogeneous disorder that can present at any time from birth through adulthood, with a variable degree of severity and progression. It is also autosomal dominant. The slowly progressive infantile form presents with hypotonia and proximal upper and lower extremity weakness. Cranial nerve musculature involvement can occur, with feeding difficulty and a weak cry. Skeletal deformities such as club feet, high arched palate, and facial dysmorphism are common. Spe-

cial staining techniques reveal the diagnostic "rod bodies" in muscle biopsy specimens. The findings on EMG can demonstrate a variety of changes, which are influenced partly by the age of the patient and the stage of the disease. In general, the EMG findings are myopathic without evidence of muscle fiber irritability.

Centronuclear myopathy, like nemaline myopathy, is also heterogeneous and can present at any time from birth through adulthood. The most common form is neonatal with autosomal recessive inheritance. These infants are born hypotonic, with proximal weakness and respiratory difficulties. Common findings include high arched palate, elongated face, ptosis, facial weakness, weak cry and suck, and dysphagia. Reflexes are often diminished or absent and sensation is normal. Motor milestones are delayed, and a wheelchair is often required by the second or third decade. The CK level is normal or slightly elevated. Muscle biopsy specimens show small type I hypotrophic muscle fibers with centrally located nuclei. Type II fibers appear normal in size. The EMG findings are variable and influenced by the severity of the disease. In general, although the EMG findings are myopathic, centronuclear myopathy differs from the other congenital myopathies by the presence of increased insertional activity with positive sharp waves and fibrillations.

Treatment of the congenital myopathies is supportive. The genetic basis for these disorders is currently unknown.

Conclusion

The clinical diagnosis of myopathies is aided by the use of blood laboratory tests, EMG, and muscle biopsy. The classification of myopathies is evolving with the use of molecular genetics. Ultimately, this will bring a better understanding of these diseases with better treatment options.

Suggested Reading

Adams RD, Victor M. Principles of Neurology. New York: McGraw-Hill, 1993;1184.

Beggs AH, Kunkel LM. Improved diagnosis of Duchenne/ Becker muscular dystrophy. J Clin Invest 1990;85:613.

Bohan A, Peter JB. Polymyositis and dermatomyositis. N Engl J Med 1975;292:344;403.

Buxton J, Shelbourne P, Davies J. Detection of an unstable fragment of DNA specific to individuals with myotonic dystrophy. Nature 1992;355:547.

Dalakas MC. Inflammatory Myopathies. In LP Rowland, S DiMauro (eds), Handbook of Clinical Neurology (Vol 18). Amsterdam: Elsevier, 1992;369–390.

Dumitru, D. Electrodiagnostic Medicine. Philadelphia: Hanley & Belfus, 1995;1031–1129.

Mastaglia FL, Laing NG. Investigation of muscle disease. J Neurol Neurosurg Psychiatry 1996;60:256.

Medical Research Council of the United Kingdom. Aids to the Examination of the Peripheral Nervous System. United Kingdom: Pendragon House, 1978.

Wallace DC. Mitochondrial DNA mutations and neuromuscular disease. Trends Genet 1989;5:9.

Zubrzycka-Gaarn EE, Bulman DE, Karpati G. The Duchenne muscular dystrophy gene product is localized in the sarcolemma of human skeletal muscle. Nature 1988;333:466.

Chapter 38
Infectious Disorders

A. Bacterial Infections

Patricia K. Coyle

Chapter Plan

Clinical syndromes
    Meningitis
    Abscess
    Subdural and epidural infections
    Toxin related
    Endocarditis
    Prosthetic device infection
Pathogens
    Acute pathogens
    Chronic pathogens
    Spirochetes
    Unusual pathogens
Pathogenesis
Diagnosis
Complications
Management
Sequelae
Future directions

Among the many classes of organisms that are able to invade and infect the nervous system, bacteria are second only to viruses as the most frequent pathogens. Bacteria are prokaryotes that lack a nucleus and other internal membrane structures. They contain a cytoplasmic membrane surrounded by a cell wall and a variety of other outer membrane structures, such as flagella, pili, and capsules. Bac-teria are haploid with a single chromosome, but with extrachromosomal plasmids that contain genes, which can contribute to properties such as virulence and antibiotic resistance. It is important to diagnose infections caused by bacteria because they are curable with appropriate antibiotics. If not treated promptly, they can cause death, and in survivors can result in permanent neurologic damage.

Clinical Syndromes

When bacteria infect the nervous system, they cause a variety of clinical syndromes. These reflect not only the anatomic structures involved, but also the functional systems and pathways that are disrupted (Table 38A-1). Although these syndromes differ in their presentation and features, they share in common the fact that unless they are appropriately treated, they will persist and worsen, leading to increasing complications. It is unusual for a bacterial infection to resolve spontaneously and without sequelae.

Meningitis

Meningitis is the most common bacterial neurologic infection. At least 25,000 cases occur each year in

Table 38A-1. Clinical Syndromes Associated with Bacterial Neurologic Infections

Syndrome	Target	Common Pathogens	Characteristic Features
Meningitis	Pia, arachnoid membranes, and subarachnoid space	*Streptococcus pneumoniae, Neisseria meningitidis, Mycobacterium tuberculosis, Listeria monocytogenes, Haemophilus influenzae*	Triad of fever, headache, stiff neck
Abscess	Parenchymal tissue	Streptococci (aerobic, anaerobic), gram-negative bacilli, *Staphylococcus aureus, Bacteroides* species; mixed	Predisposing factor; triad of fever, headache, focal deficit
Subdural empyema	Dura mater, subdural space	Streptococci (aerobic, anaerobic), staphylococci, gram-negative bacilli (aerobic), nonstreptococcal anaerobes	Predisposing factor; male predominance; fever, headache, neurologic deficits; intracranial more common than spinal
Epidural abscess	Epidural space	*S. aureus,* gram-negative bacilli (aerobic), streptococci (aerobic), anaerobes	Predisposing factor; spinal more common than intracranial; fever, localized pain, malaise
Toxin	Acetylcholine receptors, myelinated axons, presynaptic terminals	*Clostridium botulinum, Corynebacterium diphtheriae, Bordetella pertussis, Clostridium tetani*	Botulism: flaccid paralysis of cranial peripheral nerve Diphtheria: cranial and peripheral nerve demyelination Whooping cough: variety of neurologic complications Tetanus: trismus, opisthotonus, dysautonomia, paralysis
Endocarditis	Central nervous system, peripheral nervous system, blood vessels	Streptococci, *S. aureus,* other staphylococci, gram-negative bacilli	Variable neurologic syndromes; often multiple; often initial presentation; increased mortality
Shunt infection	Shunt device	Staphylococci, gram-negative bacilli, streptococci, diphtheroids; mixed	Variable

the United States, and many more cases occur in less-developed regions of the world. Meningitis is an infection of the subarachnoid space and its lining membranes, the pia and arachnoid membranes. Because this space contains cerebrospinal fluid (CSF), meningitis is typically associated with striking CSF changes. In the case of bacterial meningitis, which generally causes an acute septic picture, CSF changes include a high white cell count with neutrophil predominance, a very low glucose level, an elevated protein concentration, and increased opening pressure. Most bacterial meningitis cases (70%) occur in children younger than age 5 years. The classic clinical presentation is the triad of fever, headache, and meningismus (stiff neck). Patients may also experience photophobia, nausea, vomiting, pulmonary symptoms, and lethargy. This clinical picture changes somewhat at the extremes of age. Neonates are more likely to appear septic and to experience seizures as a complication of meningitis, whereas the elderly are more likely to present

with prominent mental status changes. They may have fever associated with confusion, stupor, or even coma, without manifesting classic features of headache and stiff neck. Bacterial meningitis is most often an acute or even fulminant process, and in extreme cases can lead to death in a matter of hours. The major bacteria associated with meningitis are discussed in the section on acute pathogens below. These agents must colonize the nasopharynx before their meningeal invasion. In contrast, mycobacteria cause chronic meningitis, defined as a meningitis lasting for 4 or more weeks. They are discussed in the section on chronic pathogens. In general, chronic meningitis patients are not as sick as those with acute meningitis. In unusual cases (individuals with underlying immune or anatomic defects that make them vulnerable to repeated infections), bacteria can even result in recurrent meningitis, involving repeated attacks of acute meningitis. Risk factors have been identified for bacterial meningitis based on the age of the host

(Table 38A-2). The presence of one or more of these risk factors should raise a suspicion of bacterial meningitis.

Abscess

Abscess is an infection of brain parenchyma. It consists of liquefied and necrotic brain tissue surrounded by a fibrotic capsule. An abscess is generally associated with marked surrounding edema. It can act as an expanding mass lesion, with risk of herniation. This is an uncommon problem, noted in only 0.2–1.3% of autopsy series. Men are more commonly affected than women, particularly adults ages 30–45 years. Only 25% of brain abscesses occur in children younger than age 15 years, with a peak in children ages 4–7 years. Infectious abscess results from direct spread of a contiguous infection (of the ear, mastoid, sinus, or dental region); hematogenous spread from a cardiac, pulmonary, or other distant site; or cranial trauma that breaches the skull barrier.

The frontal lobe is the most common site involved, followed by the temporal, frontoparietal, parietal, cerebellar, and occipital lobes. Unusual sites for location of a brain abscess include the pituitary gland within the sella turcica, the brain stem, the basal ganglia, and the thalamus. Generally abscess is a single large lesion. In 10–50% of cases, abscesses are multiple and can be very small, forming pellet-sized microabscesses. This reflects widespread hematogenous seeding of bacteria to the brain.

The classic clinical presentation of brain abscess is fever, hemicranial or generalized headache, and focal neurologic deficit. Unfortunately, this triad is present in less than one-half of patients. Fever occurs in 40–50% of patients, headache in up to 75%, and focal neurologic deficits (e.g., hemiplegia) in 50%. Most patients have mental status changes. Other features include seizures (25–45%), particularly with frontal lobe abscess, nausea/vomiting (22–50%), meningismus (25%), and papilledema (25%). Brain abscess is most often associated with a subacute course, with an average duration of symptoms of approximately 2 weeks.

A number of bacteria can cause brain abscess. Aerobic bacteria are isolated from approximately 60% of abscesses. The major pathogens are streptococci, gram-negative bacilli, and *Staphylococcus*

Table 38A-2. Risk Factors for Bacterial Meningitis

Neonates
  Low birth weight
  Labor and delivery complications
  Premature rupture of membranes
  Chorioamnionitis
  Maternal (gynecologic, peripartum infection, urologic)
  Underlying disease process
Adults
  Immune deficiency
    Type-specific anticapsular antibodies
    Bactericidal antibodies
    Complement
    Asplenia
    Primary/secondary immunodeficiency
  Infection focus
    Systemic
    Parameningeal
  Neuroanatomic barrier damage
    Head trauma
    Neurosurgery
    Cerebrospinal fluid leak
  Sickle cell disease
  Alcoholism

aureus. Anaerobes are isolated from over 30% of abscesses. Pathogens include *Bacteroides* species and anaerobic streptococci. Mixed infections occur in 30–60% of cases.

Subdural and Epidural Infections

Subdural empyema, which accounts for 15–25% of intracranial infections, is an infection of the space between the dura mater and arachnoid membranes. This compartment is a potential rather than an actual space. Most subdural empyemas (90%) are supratentorial, with occasional spinal cord empyemas. This infection occurs more commonly in men by a ratio of 3 to 1. Most patients (70%) are in the second or third decade of life.

Empyema generally presents with nonspecific symptoms over several days, followed by acute or subacute deterioration. More than 90% of patients have fever and headache, which is often localized. Headache worsens steadily and level of consciousness is ultimately affected. Focal deficits appear in 80–90% of patients. There may be chills,

Table 38A-3. Bacterial Neurologic Infections Caused by Toxins

Disease	Agent	Comments
Botulism	*Clostridium botulinum*	Four clinical types: food borne, wound, infant, infectious
Diphtheria	*Corynebacterium diphtheriae*	Noninflammatory demyelinating neuropathy: cranial nerves, peripheral nerves
Pertussis	*Bordetella pertussis*	Neurologic complications in >5%; toxin mechanism unclear: direct effect, adjuvant effect to enhance inflammation
Tetanus	*Clostridium tetani*	Four clinical types: generalized, localized, cephalic, neonatal

meningismus, vomiting, malaise, seizures, and papilledema. More than 10% of patients develop complications of venous sinus thrombosis or brain abscess. Infants with meningitis are at special risk for subdural empyema. Approximately 2% of neonates with bacterial meningitis develop empyema, presumably as a result of infection of a sterile subdural effusion. These effusions occur in 12–32% of neonatal meningitis cases. Risk factors for development of empyema in children and adults are infections of the head (sinuses, middle ear, face, scalp, cranial osteomyelitis), head trauma or surgery, and bacteremia from a distant infection site. In most cases a single organism is involved. Organisms include aerobic and anaerobic streptococci, staphylococci, aerobic gram-negative bacilli, and other anaerobes.

Spinal or intracranial epidural abscess is an infection of the epidural space. This infection is a medical and surgical emergency because it acts as a mass lesion to produce spinal cord compression or a variety of major cerebral complications. Spinal epidural abscess occurs most commonly in adults older than age 50 years. In contrast, intravenous drug users, who are at risk for this infection, are often younger. Spinal epidural abscess is generally posterior to the cord in the thoracic or lumbar region. It frequently involves several vertebral segments. Infection of the epidural space can occur as a result of spread from a contiguous infection site, secondary to penetrating trauma, or from hematogenous seeding, which is particularly common in children. In 20–40% of cases there is no obvious primary infection site. Patients present with fever, back pain, and generalized malaise. If not recognized and treated, they progress to radicular pain and finally cord compression. *S. aureus* is the major etiologic agent

of spinal epidural abscess, being responsible for 52–95% of cases.

Approximately 10% of epidural abscesses are intracranial. They complicate 2% of craniotomy procedures. They also occur as a result of contiguous infections involving head and skull structures. Patients present with fever, localized cranial tenderness, severe hemicranial headache, nausea, vomiting, and lethargy. As the abscess expands, focal deficits develop. Secondary complications include venous sinus thrombosis, subdural empyema, brain abscess, and meningitis. In patients with prior craniotomy the presentation may be quite subtle, suggesting a simple wound infection rather than a potentially deadly neurologic infection. Etiologic pathogens for intracranial epidural abscess are more diverse than for spinal abscess. They include streptococci, anaerobes, and staphylococci.

Toxin Related

Four bacterial infections cause neurologic disease not from direct infection effects but rather from indirect effects of released toxins (Table 38A-3). Botulism is a rare infection that involves seven distinct neurotoxins (A–G) elaborated by *Clostridium botulinum*, a diffuse cluster of agents organized into four distinct groups. These toxins are cytoplasmic proteins released by lysis. They bind to acetylcholine receptors at the neuromuscular junction, autonomic ganglia, and postganglionic parasympathetic fibers. Symptoms range from acute gastrointestinal (GI) problems to flaccid paralysis. Food-borne botulism is caused by ingestion of food contaminated with neurotoxin, most commonly A, B, or E. Low pH foods and canned foods are particular risks. The incubation period is short (18–36 hours). Patients present with GI symptoms (nausea, vomiting, diarrhea, constipation, cramps) accompanied or followed by flaccid weakness. The cranial nerves are involved first, with blurred vision, diplopia, dysarthria, dysphagia, ptosis, facial weakness, depressed gag response, and tongue weakness. Patients then go on to flaccid weakness of the arms and legs and in severe cases to respiratory paralysis. Parasympathetic involvement leads to dry mouth, sore throat, and paralytic ileus. Wound botulism (caused by toxin produced within an infected wound site) is the most unusual form of botulism, but can be seen in intravenous drug users. The incubation period is more prolonged (4–18 days), and there are no GI symptoms. Infant botulism, caused by ingestion of bacterial spores (often from contaminated honey) that produce toxins A or B, occurs up to age 6 months. It is the most common form of botulism. Constipation develops first, followed in 1–3 weeks by poor feeding and neurologic features. Infectious botulism is caused by ingestion of spores by adults or children, with intestinal colonization and subsequent production of toxin. The clinical manifestations are similar to food-borne infection.

Patients with botulism can have pupils that are normal or fixed and dilated, reflexes that are normal or decreased, and sensation that is normal or mildly diminished. Even profound deficits are potentially reversible, and full supportive care is critical. Patients should be admitted to an intensive care unit, with serial vital capacity monitoring to detect early respiratory failure. Botulinum antitoxin is given, and wounds are debrided. The mortality rate of patients hospitalized for botulism ranges from 1% to 10%. Symptoms may last months to several years, such as extended fatigue and shortness of breath.

Diphtheria is caused by respiratory tract infection with *Corynebacterium diphtheriae*. Bacteria that are infected with a lysogenic beta phage produce an exotoxin that inhibits protein synthesis. In severe infections, up to 75% of patients develop neurologic damage from the exotoxin. There is noninflammatory demyelination of cranial nerves and, to a lesser extent, peripheral nerves. Patients develop adjacent paralysis of the soft palate and posterior pharynx, the face, and even the oculomotor nerve. Within 10 days to 3 months there is peripheral motor weakness of the extremities, which begins proximally but goes on to involve distal muscles and footdrop. The mortality rate of diphtheria is 4–12%. Mortality is greatest at the extremes of age and generally occurs within the first few days of severe illness. Treatment involves rapid administration of diphtheria antitoxin, 14 days of antibiotics (erythromycins or penicillins), and full supportive care.

Bordetella pertussis also produces a localized infection of the respiratory tract—whooping cough. The bacterium produces a number of virulence factors, including pertussis toxin. Neurologic complications (e.g., confusion, seizures, vision and hearing loss, focal deficits, and even death) occur in more than 5% of infections. They develop during the so-called paroxysmal phase of whooping cough, which involves fits of coughing, whooping, gagging, and hypersalivation. Neurologic involvement is believed to reflect multifactorial mechanisms, including both direct effects of toxin as well as heightened inflammation caused by an adjuvant effect of toxin. The best treatment is prevention, with vaccine immunoprophylaxis. Erythromycins are used for symptomatic infection, along with optimal supportive care.

At least 1 million cases of tetanus occur each year, with 25% caused by occupational accidents. *Clostridium tetani* is an obligate anaerobe that requires a plasmid (extrachromosomal DNA) for toxin (tetanospasmin) production. Tetanus toxin inhibits release of neurotransmitter from presynaptic terminals. It can be transported by retrograde transmission to enter the central nervous system (CNS) and even cross transneuronal synapses. The result is a disruption of central motor control, autonomic function, and the neuromuscular junction. There are four recognized forms of tetanus. Generalized tetanus commonly presents with trismus (lockjaw) resulting from rigid masseter muscles. It is the most striking and easily recognized form of tetanus. Patients develop back and shoulder stiffness, risus sardonicus (sneering grin), abdominal rigidity, and generalized painful spasms (opisthotonus, fist clenching, flexor and extensor spasms) without loss of consciousness. Localized tetanus presents with fixed, rigid muscles at the site of an injury. The muscles are painful, and reflexes are increased. Patients with localized tetanus often go on to generalized tetanus. Cephalic tetanus is a form of localized disease that involves the lower cranial nerves. Patients develop facial weakness, dyspha-

Table 38A-4. Neurologic Complications
of Bacterial Endocarditis

Predisposing factors
  Cardiac
    Left-sided valvular disease
    Prosthetic heart valve
      Inappropriate anticoagulation
    Chronic rheumatic heart disease
    Congenital heart lesions
      Ventricular septal defect
      Bicuspid aortic valve
      Patent ductus arteriosus
      Tetralogy of Fallot
    Mitral valve prolapse
    Degenerative valvular disease
  Noncardiac
    Procedure-related valve injury
    Procedure-induced bacteremia
    Intravenous drug use
    Chronic hemodialysis
    Age >60 yrs
Frequent pathogens
  Native valves
    Streptococci (60%)
      Viridans group
      Streptococcus milleri
      Streptococcus bovis
    Staphylococcus aureus (20–30%)
      Intravenous drug use
    Brucella species (~10% in geographic region)
  Prosthetic valve
    Staphylococci, coagulase negative (30%)
    Streptococcus viridans (30%)
    S. aureus (10–14%)
    Gram-negative bacilli (10–20%)
Manifestations
  Stroke
    Embolic infarct
    Hemorrhage (subarachnoid, intracerebral, subdural)
  Encephalopathy
  Meningitis
  Abscess
  Seizure
  Headache
  Psychiatric
  Localized syndromes
    Brain stem
    Cranial neuropathy
    Spinal cord
    Peripheral nerve
Outcome
  Mortality 20–67%
  Morbidity ~34%

gia, and occasionally ophthalmoplegia. Chronic otitis may be an infection source, and these patients are frequently co-infected with *S. aureus*. The most common form of tetanus is neonatal tetanus, which accounts for approximately 50% of cases and has a mortality rate of 90%. It is caused by infection of the umbilical stump of an infant whose mother lacks immunity. The baby presents with weakness and inability to suck during the second week of life, followed by characteristic opisthotonus. Death may occur as a result of a hypersympathetic state. Overall, the mortality rate of tetanus is 15%. The most serious sequelae are respiratory compromise and autonomic dysfunction, which produces labile hypertension, tachycardia, arrhythmia, and fever. Treatment involves optimized intensive care, human tetanus immune globulin, tetanus toxoid, control of spasms/rigidity, and metronidazole.

Endocarditis

Some 20–40% of patients with infective endocarditis develop neurologic complications. Neurologic involvement is more common with increasing age. Up to 45% of patients older than age 60 years will experience neurologic difficulties such as mental confusion. Particular risk factors for neurologic involvement in endocarditis patients are left-sided valvular disease, prosthetic valve disease, insufficient anticoagulation in the setting of prosthetic valve endocarditis, and intravenous drug use in the setting of left-sided valve endocarditis (Table 38A-4). Neurologic involvement is the initial presentation in 16–23% of patients, but they generally have other signs pointing to an endocarditis. In these patients embolic stroke is often the first manifestation. Neurologic complications, which occur after treatment is started, tend to cluster within the first 2 weeks. In rare instances there may be late embolic events or rupture of a mycotic aneurysm months after presentation. Neurologic involvement in endocarditis is varied and includes encephalopathy, seizures, meningitis, abscess, headache, psychiatric syndromes, and a variety of focal syndromes. Meningitis (particularly when the pathogens are *S. aureus* or *Streptococcus pneumoniae*) now complicates less than 10% of endocarditis cases. Seizures are reported in 1.5–15.0% of cases. Confusion, a manifestation of encephalopathy, is particularly frequent in the elderly. Overall, the most common neurologic complication is stroke. This is generally embolic infarction of the cortex or cerebellum. There may be a single large embolus that occludes a major vessel, or multiple microemboli. The mortality rate in such patients ranges from 33% to 81%. Intracranial hemorrhage occurs in 3–6% of endocarditis cases. It may be caused by rupture of a mycotic aneurysm, erosion of a vessel wall, or hemorrhagic transformation of an ischemic infarction. Bleeding is a particular risk in anticoagulated endocarditis patients.

Prosthetic Device Infection

A number of devices are used to evaluate or treat neurologic patients. In effect, they are foreign bodies that are internal or external to the nervous system. They can become infected, with secondary involvement of the nervous system. Internalized devices include shunts used to divert CSF and reservoirs used for therapy access. Externalized devices include drainage systems and monitoring systems to track intracranial pressure or seizures. Infection complicates 2.8–14.0% of shunt surgeries. Some series suggest that the surgical complication rate should be less than 4%. Unfortunately, the presence of this foreign body provides an ongoing risk factor, and the actual case infection rate for implanted shunts is 8–40%. Infection has a bimodal time distribution. Most infections (70–85%) occur within 6 months of surgery, with a second cluster after 1 year. For implanted CSF reservoirs, the infection rate is 3–15%, and most cases develop within 1 month of placement. The major pathogens involved are *Staphylococcus epidermidis* (47–64%), followed by *S. aureus* (12–29%), gram-negative organisms such as *Escherichia coli, Klebsiella, Proteus,* and *Pseudomonas* (6–20%), streptococci (8–10%), diphtheroids (1–14%), and mixed flora (10–15%). The infection rate for externalized devices is 5–7% and increases with prolonged placement. Staphylococci account for approximately one-half of cases, and gram-negative organisms for approximately 25%. There are multiple ways for these foreign bodies to become infected, such as retrograde infection from the distal end, infection from wound or skin breakdown, hematogenous infection, and infection at the time of surgery. The clin-

ical presentation of prosthetic device infection is variable, and fever and pain are not always present. In the case of drainage devices, patients often present because of the associated shunt failure, with headache, nausea, drowsiness, and mental status changes. Some patients present because of associated wound, intracranial, blood, pleural, or peritoneal infection.

Pathogens

Acute Pathogens

Among the bacteria that cause acute/subacute neurologic infection, the major gram-positive pathogens are *S. pneumoniae*, group B streptococci, *Listeria monocytogenes*, and *S. aureus*. The major gram-negative pathogens are *Neisseria meningitidis*, *Haemophilus influenzae*, and a series of enteric agents (*E. coli*, *Klebsiella* species, *Pseudomonas aeruginosa*).

S. pneumoniae accounts for 30–50% of adult meningitis cases and 10–20% of childhood meningitis cases. It is the major cause of meningitis in adults, particularly older individuals. *S. pneumoniae* is divided into at least 84 different serotypes based on capsule polysaccharides, but within a given geographic region a few serotypes are responsible for most invasive infections. Concurrent pneumonia (15–25%), acute otitis media (30%), acute sinusitis, a history of head trauma (10%), sickle cell disease, asplenia, CSF fistula or leaks, and specific malignancies (chronic lymphocytic leukemia, multiple myeloma) are clues that neurologic infection may be caused by *S. pneumoniae*. Up to 25% of strains are now penicillin resistant because of altered penicillin-binding proteins, and 4–9% are resistant to cephalosporins. For this reason, recommended initial antibiotic coverage is vancomycin with ceftriaxone (cefotaxime in infants) to cover highly resistant strains. Once susceptibility is known, penicillin or ampicillin can be substituted as a more economical choice. It has been recommended that adult patients with meningitis who are being treated with adjunctive corticosteroids have rifampin substituted for vancomycin because of concerns about decreased CNS penetration of vancomycin with concurrent steroids. Patients should receive antibiotics for 10–14 days. A first-generation vaccine is currently available for *S. pneumoniae*, but it is used to prevent pneumonia. The vaccine is only 46–63% effective in preventing meningitis in immunocompetent individuals over age 2 years. Second-generation vaccines for *S. pneumoniae* are currently under study.

N. meningitidis accounts for 25–40% of meningitis in children and 10–35% of meningitis in adults, especially younger adults. Less than 10% of cases occur in patients older than age 45 years. Infection often occurs as part of an epidemic. Thirteen serogroups are recognized based on the capsule polysaccharide pattern. Serotypes within a group are further defined by outer membrane proteins. Petechiae or purpura are noted in 50–75% of *N. meningitidis* infections, which can be an important clinical clue. Fulminant infection produces adrenal failure, cardiovascular collapse, and disseminated intravascular coagulation. The preferred treatment for meningococcal infection is penicillin or ampicillin. Resistant strains are rare. Antibiotic susceptibility is tested only if there is a poor clinical response, in which case a cephalosporin is used. Patients are treated for 7 days. A first-generation vaccine for *N. meningitidis* is available, but it gives limited immunity and is poorly immunogenic in infants. A second-generation vaccine is currently under study. Chemoprophylaxis is recommended for people in close contact with infected patients. They are treated with rifampin for 2 days to eradicate nasopharyngeal colonization.

H. influenzae was once the major cause of childhood meningitis in the United States. With the advent of second-generation vaccines against serotype B, the critical pathogen, infections fell by 85–90%. The vaccine induces antibodies to the polyribosylribitol phosphate protein, which are highly protective. In areas of the world where vaccination is not carried out, however, this agent remains a major cause of meningitis. Up to 32% of *H. influenzae* strains are beta-lactamase producers, so that a third-generation cephalosporin (ceftriaxone or cefotaxime) is preferred over ampicillin as initial therapy. Patients are treated for 7 days. When there is a household contact younger than age 4 years, both the patient and household receive 4 days of chemoprophylaxis with rifampin to eliminate nasopharyngeal colonization.

Group B streptococci (*Streptococcus agalactiae*) are the major cause of neonatal meningitis. They are divided into six main serotypes. Most infants (80%) have concomitant pneumonia. *S. agalactiae* rarely causes neurologic infection in adults who have underlying disease processes. Recommended treatment in neonates is 14–21 days of ampicillin with gentamicin (they are synergistic). Adult infections are treated with penicillin G or ampicillin.

Listeria species, particularly *L. monocytogenes*, account for 5–10% of neonatal and 5% of adult meningitis cases. This is an intracellular pathogen. *L. monocytogenes* can also produce localized brain stem encephalitis. In neonates, infection results from subclinical maternal infection, or passage through an infected genital tract. In adults, infection is associated with diabetes, old age, alcohol abuse, and immunocompromise (defective cell-mediated immunity). Infection can also be food borne, which may account for up to 20% of sporadic *Listeria* infections. Meningitis caused by *L. monocytogenes* can produce focal deficits and seizures. Patients are treated with ampicillin or penicillin G combined with gentamicin for 14–21 days. The combination therapy shows enhanced bactericidal activity.

Among the staphylococci, *S. aureus* and *S. epidermidis* (a nonpathogenic skin contaminant) can on occasion produce neurologic infection. This is most common in the setting of indwelling catheter or shunt, endocarditis, or an event that breaches the CNS anatomic barriers (such as head trauma or neurosurgery). *S. aureus* is generally treated with nafcillin or oxacillin, whereas methicillin-resistant strains are treated with vancomycin. The CSF is monitored closely to determine whether local installation of intrathecal or intraventricular vancomycin is needed. *S. epidermidis* is generally treated with vancomycin plus an aminoglycoside.

Gram-negative enteric organisms such as *E. coli*, *Klebsiella-Enterobacter* species, and *P. aeruginosa* are occasional neurologic pathogens. They account for approximately 36–48% of neonatal meningitis cases and 1–10% of adult meningitis cases. They are likely CNS pathogens in the setting of head trauma; neurosurgery; or underlying conditions such as gram-negative sepsis, immunocompromise, ruptured brain abscess, or strongyloidiasis (a parasitic infection). Suspected gram-negative infections are generally treated with the third-generation cephalosporin ceftazidime (because it is effective against *Pseudomonas*), plus an aminoglycoside. These organisms can be difficult to treat. Antibiotic susceptibility should be tested, with consideration given to intrathecal or intraventricular therapy for patients who respond poorly.

Chronic Pathogens

Among the major bacteria that produce chronic neurologic infection are *Mycobacterium tuberculosis*, and *Brucella* species. *M. tuberculosis* is an obligate aerobe with a half-life of 15–20 hours. Humans are the only natural reservoir. Both immune and genetic factors in the host determine whether these bacteria are eliminated, contained, or go on to produce active tuberculosis (TB). TB has re-emerged as a significant infectious problem in the United States and continues to be a major problem worldwide. Infection with human immunodeficiency virus, the cause of acquired immunodeficiency syndrome, has been associated with increased risk of active TB. It is currently recommended that TB patients be tested for HIV positivity. CNS infection accounts for 5% of extrapulmonary TB. The vast majority of neurologic infections produce TB meningitis, although occasionally TB causes tuberculous epidural abscess, parenchymal tuberculoma or tuberculous abscess, or localized spinal cord disease (either as a space occupying lesion or an inflammatory arachnoiditis).

TB is the most frequent infectious cause of chronic meningitis. In children, TB meningitis commonly occurs in the setting of active infection. In adults, however, meningitis typically represents rupture of an old tubercle, so that signs of active systemic TB are absent. The CSF pattern is that of a chronic meningitis, with several hundred white cells (mainly mononuclear, although up to one-third of patients can show an initial neutrophil response), low glucose level, and high protein concentration. Approximately 50% of patients have an elevated CSF opening pressure. Acid-fast stain is reported to produce a positive result in 8–86% of cases, depending on the volume of CSF and number of samples sent. Clues to a diagnosis of TB meningitis include low sodium levels (25–92%), abnormal findings on brain neuroimaging (more than 75%), abnormal findings on chest x-ray films (25–50% of adults, 50–90% of children), positive findings on purified protein derivative tuberculin test, and positive extraneural cultures (morning urine, gastric washings, sputum, bone marrow). Specialized CSF studies, which can be diagnostic, include a positive finding on polymerase chain reaction (PCR) to detect *M. tuberculosis* DNA, detection of specific antigen or antibody, and detection of tuberculostearic acid. Unfortunately, culture requires weeks for *M. tuberculosis* to grow out. Treatment of TB meningitis involves chemotherapy for intracellular and extracellular organisms, combination drugs to avoid development of resistant strains, and use of drugs that penetrate the blood-brain barrier. Treatment is generally started using three first-line drugs and continued for months. The most commonly used agents are isoniazid, rifampin, and pyrazinamide, with occasional use of streptomycin and ethambutol. Multidrug-resistant (MDR) strains of *M. tuberculosis*, defined by resistance to two or more of the above first-line drugs, occurs in 9% of cases. The mortality rate of MDR TB is very high (62–92%). These patients require treatment with up to four or five drugs at a time, including a number of second-line agents, for 18–24 months.

Particularly common complications of TB meningitis are hydrocephalus, hyponatremia, seizures, and stroke resulting from thickened basilar meningeal exudate.

Approximately 5% of *Brucella* infections involve the nervous system. Neurobrucellosis is generally a subacute or chronic meningitis. It can result in an infectious vasculitis leading to infarction or mycotic aneurysm formation leading to hemorrhage. Unusual manifestations of neurologic *Brucella* infections include myelopathy, cerebellar syndrome, and radiculoneuropathy. Brucellosis is a zoonotic infection that is particularly endemic in the Mediterranean and Middle East regions. It is most commonly spread by infected milk from goats, sheep, or camels.

Spirochetes

Spirochetes are flexible and motile gram-negative bacteria that have a helical rod configuration, so that they coil. Motility is conveyed by endoflagella. Four spirochetal infections can involve the nervous system (Table 38A-5) and share in common several features. The bacterium enters the host through a skin or mucous membrane site. With the exception of syphilis, all of the diseases involve zoonotic or vector-borne transmission. Once inoculated,

Table 38A-5. Spirochete Bacterial Neurologic Infections

Infection	Bacterium	Comments
Syphilis	*Treponema pallidum*	Sexual transmission; neurosyphilis syndromes: asymptomatic, meningitis, meningovasculitis, parenchymatous (general paresis, tabes dorsalis), gumma
Lyme disease	*Borrelia burgdorferi*	Tick transmission; geographic restriction; neurologic Lyme disease syndromes: early stage disseminated infection (meningitis, cranial neuropathy, painful radiculoneuritis), late stage disseminated infection (encephalopathy, polyradiculoneuropathy, encephalomyelitis)
Leptospirosis	*Leptospira interrogans*	Animal contact transmission; biphasic illness; neurologic syndromes: meningitis (68–90%), vascular involvement, late uveitis
Relapsing fever	*Borrelia recurrentis;* other *Borrelia* species	Tick or louse transmission; recurrent febrile episodes; neurologic syndromes: meningitis, parenchymal lesions, cranial nerve palsy, hemorrhage

spirochetes disseminate throughout the body and spread to multiple organs, including the CNS. They can cause chronic CNS infection. Clinical disease activity in all these spirochetal diseases tends to be episodic, with periods of remission that range from days to years.

Syphilis has long been recognized to cause a wide array of neurologic syndromes associated with duration of infection. Up to 25% of patients develop silent CNS disease after initial infection with *Treponema pallidum*. Many clear the CNS infection spontaneously, but a few patients (<3%) develop clinical meningitis in the first 2 years after infection. Ten percent to 12% of patients with CNS involvement develop meningovascular syphilis, which typically presents as stroke in a young adult. Meningovascular syphilis occurs on the average 7 years into untreated infection. Generally these patients have nonspecific prodromal syndromes (involving headache, mood disturbance, dizziness, and behavioral changes) weeks to months before their acute stroke. A decade or more after infection, 5% of patients present with tertiary neurosyphilis, either a dementing syndrome (general paresis) or a spinal cord syndrome manifested by lightning pains and sensory ataxia of the legs (tabes dorsalis). Gummas are rare mass lesions that occur at any stage of infection. Neurosyphilis is treated with parenteral penicillin regimens.

Lyme disease is caused by a spirochete called *Borrelia burgdorferi*, which is transmitted by the bite of an infected ixodid (hard body) tick. Neurologic disease occurs in up to 40% of symptomatic infections. This infection is often heralded by an expanding, red, ringlike skin lesion (erythema migrans) at the tick bite site. Within 3 months of infection, patients may go on to develop a meningitis (generally quite mild, suggesting an aseptic viral rather than bacterial process); cranial nerve palsy (in most cases unilateral or bilateral facial nerve palsy); or an acute painful radiculoneuritis with localized muscle weakness, atrophy, and sensory deficits. The CSF is usually abnormal in these patients, with mononuclear pleocytosis, elevated protein level, and detectable antibodies to *B. burgdorferi*. Late neurologic syndromes (which can occur months to years after infection) include subtle encephalopathy, mild axonal neuropathy, and rare brain or spinal cord parenchymal syndromes. Treatment of neurologic Lyme disease syndromes generally involves parenteral third-generation cephalosporin (ceftriaxone or cefotaxime) given for several weeks.

Leptospirosis is a biphasic illness caused by *Leptospira interrogans*. Patients become infected through contact with urine or tissue from an infected animal. Some 5–10% of infections have severe hepatic and renal involvement (Weil's disease). Seven to 12 days after infection there is abrupt onset of fever, severe headache, conjunctivitis, severe myalgias, and other symptoms. Although spirochetes can be isolated from both blood and CSF at this point, patients spontaneously improve after several days. Several days later, 68–90% of patients develop a mild meningitis, with perhaps 7% of them developing a variety of additional neurologic syndromes. Treatment of leptospirosis involves either tetracyclines or penicillins, given for 1 week.

Relapsing fever is caused by a variety of *Borrelia* species distinct from the agent of Lyme disease.

Table 38A-6. Unusual Bacterial Neurologic Infections

Neurologic Infection	Bacterium	Manifestations	Therapy
Cat-scratch disease	*Bartonella henselae*	Encephalopathy (2–4%) (headache, seizures, transient neurologic deficient); neuroretinitis (unilateral vision loss); isolated neuropathies (cranial, peripheral); neuropsychiatric syndromes (in those positive for human immunodeficiency virus)	Oral doxycycline or erythromycin; possibly trimethoprim sulfamethoxazole, fluoroquinolone; temporary anticonvulsants (if needed)
Whipple's disease	*Tropheryma whippelii*	Dementia; ophthalmoplegia (supranuclear, vertical); myoclonus, hypothalamic dysfunction; oculomasticatory myorhythmia; headache; ocular disease (bilateral vision loss, uveitis, retinitis, optic neuropathy)	Penicillin + streptomycin for 2 wks, followed by trimethoprim sulfamethoxazole for 1 yr
Tularemia	*Francisella tularensis*	Severe headache; confusion; meningitis	Streptomycin; possibly gentamicin, chloramphenicol, tetracyclines

These spirochetes are transmitted by the bite of a tick or by an infected body louse. Illness is characterized by repeated bouts of spirochetemia associated with fever. Some 9% of patients develop neurologic infection (meningitis, encephalitis, hemorrhage, seizures, cranial and peripheral neuropathies). Infection is treated with any of several antibiotics (tetracyclines, penicillin, erythromycins, chloramphenicol) given for 5–10 days.

Unusual Pathogens

Other bacterial neurologic pathogens include *Bartonella henselae*, the agent of cat-scratch disease; *Tropheryma whippelii*, the agent of Whipple's disease; and *Francisella tularensis*, the agent of tularemia. These infections represent unusual but distinctive neurologic problems (Table 38A-6).

Pathogenesis

Both bacterial, host, and antimicrobial factors play a role in neurologic infection. Specific virulence factors can be identified for a given organism that help determine its ability to colonize, invade, and survive in tissues, including the CNS compartment. Outer surface adherence molecules, which vary for different types of bacteria, allow organisms to attach to and invade certain cells. In most neuro-

logic infections, bacteria must first colonize at an extraneural site, then spread to the nervous system. This generally involves hematogenous spread. If the organism encounters a host immune response that is able to neutralize it, neurologic infection is prevented. Thus, prior immunity through natural infection or vaccine-induced immunoprophylaxis offers the possibility of an effective prevention strategy. Once an organism penetrates the CNS compartment, however, the local immune system is inadequate to contain the infection. Meningitis occurs in the setting of normal CNS tissue. In contrast, abscess requires compromised brain tissue to serve as a nidus for initial infection. The abscess evolves through stages of parenchymal tissue infection involving cerebritis, central liquefaction, and, finally, capsule formation.

The host immune response to invading bacteria can be a double-edged sword. It has been recognized that immune and inflammatory mediators, which are part of the host defense response, contribute to damage. These mediators include reactive oxygen radicals, nitric oxide, excitatory amino acids, and cytokines. Bacterial cell wall components (e.g., peptidoglycan, teichoic acid, and lipopolysaccharide) are released by antibiotic-induced lysis of organisms. These components are potent inducers of proinflammatory cytokines (particularly tumor necrosis factor and interleukin-1β), which markedly enhance local inflammation. For a subarachnoid space infection such as meningitis, this magnified inflammatory response leads to a cascade of events: blood-brain barrier damage, brain edema, cerebral vasculitis, increased intracranial pressure, increased CSF outflow resistance, and altered cerebral blood flow. There is loss of brain autoregulation, cortical hypoxia, CSF acidosis, and neuronal injury.

The recognition that the host immune response participates in the damage produced by neurologic infection has led to the concept of adjuvant therapy (see the section on management). Finally, choice of antibiotics (whether they are bactericidal or bacteriostatic, whether they cause marked lysis, whether they are active intracellularly, and whether they penetrate the CNS compartment) will also play a role in the pathogenesis of bacterial neurologic infection.

Diagnosis

The diagnosis of bacterial neurologic infection begins with identification of the infection syndrome and then identification of the causal agent. The infection syndrome is generally suspected based on the clinical evaluation and confirmed by CSF evaluation, neuroimaging, biopsy, or occasionally other specific tests (Figure 38A-1).

Meningitis is diagnosed by CSF examination, which documents pleocytosis and other supportive abnormalities. Specific CSF studies that are most helpful in identifying the pathogen include culture (which generally takes 48 hours for acute agents), Gram's and acid-fast stains, and detection of bacterial antigens. Antigen assays are commercially available for the major acute pathogens. Supportive but nonspecific CSF findings for acute bacterial meningitis include elevated opening pressure, neutrophilic pleocytosis, very low glucose levels, elevated protein levels, elevated lactate levels, and elevated C reactive protein levels. Blood cultures may be positive for the causal agent. In suspected meningitis cases, neuroimaging (brain computed tomographic [CT] or magnetic resonance imaging [MRI] scan) is done before CSF examination when patients present in coma, with focal deficits, or with papilledema. Neuroimaging allows one to exclude other disease processes as well as to screen for meningitis complications (e.g., hydrocephalus,

stroke, subdural effusion, and subdural or intracranial infection).

In suspected brain abscess, a lumbar puncture is contraindicated because of the risk of herniation with a focal mass lesion. Neuroimaging is the diagnostic test of choice. CT scanning has a sensitivity of 95–99% beyond the cerebritis stage and is highly suggestive when there is ringlike enhancement of a mass lesion with surrounding edema. MRI is more sensitive than a CT scan and can detect cerebritis as well as provide better delineation of abnormal tissue. Neuroimaging is also the diagnostic test of choice for subdural empyema and epidural abscess. Again, MRI is preferred to CT scanning because it provides more information and better lesion delineation. In both these infections, which can be considered parameningeal masses, lumbar puncture is contraindicated. Organism identification for abscess, empyema, and epidural abscess generally occurs at the time of surgery or aspiration.

With regard to toxin-mediated infections, the diagnosis of botulism requires identification of toxin or isolation and staining of *C. botulinum*. Diphtheria is diagnosed based on the clinical picture and confirmed by positive throat culture. Special selective media must be used by the microbiology laboratory when *C. diphtheriae* is suspected. Pertussis (whooping cough) is diagnosed by culture, serologic study, or PCR. Tetanus can only be diagnosed clinically, although lack of immunity and supportive electromyographic studies are helpful clues.

The diagnosis of infective endocarditis is generally made on the basis of positive blood culture and abnormal echocardiography findings. Neurologic involvement is generally diagnosed through a combination of CSF analysis, neuroimaging, and sometimes angiography (MR angiography, conventional angiography). The most accurate way to diagnose hardware infection is direct culture of the device or fluid/tissue in contact with the device.

Complications

Bacterial neurologic infection can provoke marked inflammation within an enclosed compartment, with limited room for shifting of tissues and fluids (Table 38A-7). These infections can also disrupt vital neural tissue. Therefore compli-

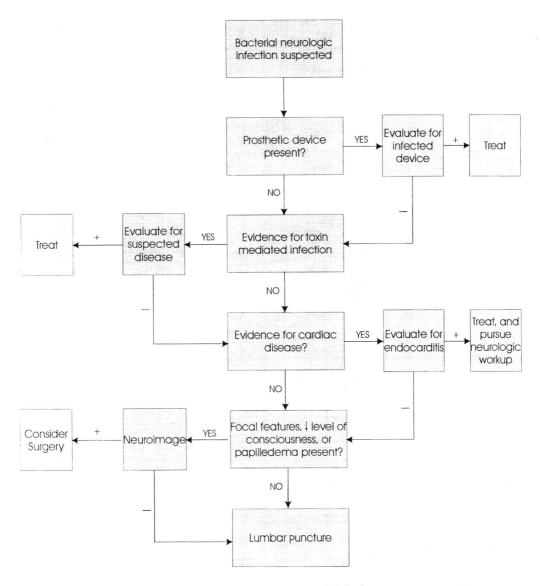

Figure 38A-1. Approach to the patient with suspected bacterial neurologic infection.

cations are often encountered and become life-threatening. They need to be recognized, monitored, and appropriately managed. For patients with significant intracranial pressure, externalized monitoring devices can be used to guide therapy. Increased pressure is treated with head elevation to 30 degrees, hyperventilation to a PCO_2 between 25 and 30 mm Hg, and bolus injections of mannitol. Pentobarbital coma is used if necessary.

Seizures can complicate neurologic infection and require aggressive therapy using appropriate doses of anticonvulsants.

Management

Management of bacterial neurologic infection is based on the syndrome, causal agent, and presence

Table 38A-7. Complications of Bacterial Neurologic Infections

Complication	Therapy
Intracranial pressure	Elevate head of bed 30 degrees
	Hyperventilate to P_{CO_2} of 25–30 mm Hg
	Consider intracranial monitor
	Administer mannitol: adults, 1.0-g bolus, then 0.25 g/kg every 2–3 hrs; children, 0.5–2.0 g/kg over 30 mins, then as needed
	Administer pentobarbital: initial 5–10 mg/kg at 1mg/kg/min, then 1–3 mg/kg/hr
Seizures	Anticonvulsants
	Reduce fever
Hyponatremia and syndrome of inappropriate antidiuretic hormone	Fluid restriction initially 75% maintenance (1,000–1,200 ml/m^2); 5% dextrose, 0.25–0.50% normal saline; 20–40 mEq/liter K$^+$
	Measure serum sodium, urine specific gravity every 6–12 hrs
	Gradual volume increase
Hydrocephalus	Ventricular tap or drain
	Acetazolamide
	Corticosteroids
Abscess	Antibiotic/surgery
Subdural effusion	Follow with serial imaging
	Occasional subdural taps
	Occasional drainage
Disseminated intravascular coagulation	Treat infection
	Replace platelets, coagulation factors
	Consider heparin
Cerebrovascular accident	Appropriate supportive therapy
	Consider reducing brain metabolism

of secondary complications. Antibiotic therapy is instituted based on the most likely causal agent (Table 38A-8). Treatment can then be adjusted once a pathogen is identified. Bactericidal intravenous antibiotics are preferred in most cases because they give high levels and CNS penetration. Antibiotics are given for 1–3 weeks for acute bacterial meningitis depending on the pathogen. In the case of abscess, parenteral antibiotics are given for 4–6 weeks, and they may be followed by prolonged oral agents (2–6 months) in appropriate cases. Empyemas and epidural abscesses are treated for 3–4 weeks, although epidural abscess associated with osteomyelitis requires more extended treatment (6–8 weeks). Endocarditis is also treated with appropriate antibiotics for 6–8 weeks. Duration of therapy for shunt infection depends on the organism, the extent of the infection, and CSF findings. Typically it ranges from 3 to 10 days.

Surgical management in combination with antibiotics is standard in the treatment of abscess, subdural and epidural infections, and prosthetic device infection. Surgery will also be required in 20–35% of endocarditis cases. Brain abscess is treated by excision or by CT-guided stereotaxic aspiration. In unusual circumstances (inoperable lesion, multiple abscesses, single small lesion, severely ill patient), surgery is withheld, while response to antibiotics is carefully monitored with serial neuroimaging. Subdural empyema is drained through multiple burr holes or craniotomy. Epidural abscess also requires surgical removal of the lesion. In the case of infected prosthetic devices such as shunts, removal of all infected hardware is done. Surgical treatment for endocarditis includes cardiac (valve replacement, vegetation debridement) procedures and excision of mycotic aneurysm.

Adjunctive therapy of bacterial infection to modulate an injurious host immune response is in its infancy. At the current time adjunctive therapy with corticosteroids is the only routinely available treat-

Table 38A-8. Suggested Empiric Antibiotic Treatment Protocols for Bacterial Neurologic Infections

Syndrome	Empiric Protocol
Meningitis	Start with third-generation cephalosporin (ceftriaxone, cefotaxime)
	Add ampicillin for infants, older adults (to cover *Streptococcus agalactiae, Listeria monocytogenes* infections)
	For immunosuppressed add ceftazidime (to cover *Pseudomonas*) and ampicillin
	For head trauma/neurosurgery use ceftazidime and vancomycin
Abscess	Start with penicillin G or third-generation cephalosporin, plus metronidazole or chloramphenicol (to cover anaerobes)
	Add nafcillin or vancomycin (for staphylococci)
	Use ceftazidime (for *Pseudomonas*)
	Use third-generation cephalosporin or trimethoprim-sulfamethoxazole (for *Enterobacteriaceae*)
Subdural empyema	Start with beta lactamase–stable penicillin or vancomycin, third-generation cephalosporin, and metronidazole
Epidural abscess	Start with nafcillin, cephalosporin, or vancomycin (to cover staphylococci)
	Consider third-generation cephalosporin plus aminoglycoside (to cover gram-negative organisms)
	Consider metronidazole (to cover anaerobes)
Hardware infection	Start with nafcillin or vancomycin plus rifampin (to cover staphylococci)
	Consider third-generation cephalosporin plus aminoglycoside (to cover gram-negative organisms)

ment. It is recommended only in limited circumstances: in children older than age 2 months who have acute bacterial meningitis; in adults with acute meningitis and positive Gram's stain CSF findings (indicating significant organism load) or increased intracranial pressure; and in TB meningitis when there is a depressed level of consciousness, increased intracranial pressure, or spinal block.

Finally, it is a given that management of any infectious syndrome involves appropriate supportive care. Cardiovascular and respiratory status must be stabilized. Ventilation, perfusion, temperature, and metabolic status are closely monitored and treated. Routine laboratory findings are assessed, with the clinician particularly looking for the development of hyponatremia or a syndrome of inappropriate antidiuretic hormone secretion.

Sequelae

Bacterial neurologic infections can result in death. In survivors such infections can also result in permanent neurologic damage. Factors that affect the likelihood of such sequelae include the causal agent itself, the age of the host, the presence of underlying disease in the host, and the interval before appropriate treatment is started. For acute bacterial

meningitis in adults, the overall mortality rate approximates 25%. For neonates, mortality ranges from 8% to 50%. Morbidity in survivors can include seizures, hearing or vision loss, cognitive deficits, focal neurologic abnormalities, hydrocephalus, neuroendocrine disturbance, and developmental disability. In one series of infants who survived gram-negative meningitis, 61% had neurologic damage.

For chronic TB meningitis, the mortality rate is also 20–30%. This rate is higher for patients who present with mental status changes or focal deficits. Morbidity ranges from 0% to 50% in adults and to 25–50% in children, and is identical to that seen with acute meningitis.

For brain abscess, mortality has ranged from 0% to 24%, and in the postantibiotic era has been less than 5%. Risk factors for death are a shorter duration and more rapid progression of symptoms before presentation, emphasizing the importance of a high index of suspicion in patients who are at risk for development of brain abscess. Neurologic sequelae in survivors occur in 30–55% of cases and are more likely when there are severe neurologic problems at the time of presentation and diagnosis. Up to 17% of survivors have incapacitating deficits. Children younger than age 5 years may show cognitive sequelae, whereas children older than age 5 years are more likely to show behavioral sequelae. The mortality rate of subdural empyema ranges from 0% to 41%, with a morbidity rate of 15–73%. Epidural abscess has had a mortality rate of 18–31%, although modern series report lower rates of 13–18%. The morbidity rate is as high as 55% and relates to delay in diagnosis as well as the extent of deficit at the time of diagnosis. Rapid diagnosis and treatment before significant deficits have occurred, or within 24 hours of deficits, can be associated with complete recovery.

In the case of bacterial endocarditis, patients with cerebral emboli have a 33–81% mortality rate, with hemorrhagic infarctions at particular risk. Mycotic aneurysms have a mortality rate of 46%, toxic encephalopathy a rate of 50%, and infection (meningitis or abscess) complications have a mortality rate of greater than 80%.

Future Directions

The ideal therapy for bacterial infection is prevention. Immunoprophylaxis, using an effective and safe vaccine, is theoretically feasible for any given pathogen. The second-generation vaccine for *H. influenzae*, although available for only a few years, has resulted in a dramatic reduction in infections in areas of the world where it is used. Future new and improved vaccines may ultimately lead to eradication of many of the above bacterial neurologic infections.

Until eradication becomes a reality, however, current treatments need to be improved. New and superior drugs, with excellent CNS penetration and minimal side effect profiles, are being developed to deal with changing sensitivity profiles of current pathogens. There has also been a rapid expansion of new information about the host's immune and inflammatory response as well as the ability to manipulate that response. This is leading to development of new modulatory adjunctive therapies in addition to corticosteroids. They include monoclonal antibodies that block adhesion molecules, anti-inflammatory cytokines, antioxidants, excitatory amino acid antagonists, and nitric oxide synthase inhibitors. In the future there is likely to be routine use of selected adjuvant therapy in addition to antibiotics to optimize treatment of bacterial neurologic infection. Symptomatic therapy needs to be optimized and to be widely available. Advances in neurologic therapeutics and critical care neurology are leading to improved management of sick patients with a positive impact on morbidity and mortality rates.

Finally, it is important to be able to diagnose infection quickly in order to start appropriate and effective antibiotic therapy and to manage infectious complications optimally. Molecular diagnostic techniques, such as PCR technology to detect organism-specific DNA, are being developed for bacterial agents that cannot be diagnosed through standard culture and stain techniques. Advances in both diagnosis and treatment will be needed to deal with the continuing challenge of emerging, re-emerging, and resistant neurologic bacterial pathogens.

Suggested Reading

Anderson BE, Neuman MA. *Bartonella* spp. as emerging human pathogens. Clin Microbiol Rev 1997;10:203.

Coxon RE, Fekade D, Knox K, et al. The effect of antibody against TNFα on cytokine response in Jarish-Herxheimer reactions of louse-borne relapsing fever. Q J Med 1997;90:213.

Coyle PK, Dattwyler R. Spirochetal infection of the central nervous system. Infect Dis Clin North Am 1990;4:731.

Coyle PK. Neurologic complications of lyme disease. Rheum Dis Clin North Am 1993;19:993.

Dill SR, Cobbs CG, McDonald CK. Subdural empyema: analysis of 32 cases and review. Clin Infect Dis 1995;20:372.

Farr RW. Leptospirosis. Clin Infect Dis 1995;21:1.

Heilpern KL, Lorber B. Focal intracranial infections. Infect Dis Clin North Am 1996;10:879.

Louis ED, Lynch T, Kaufmann P, et al. Diagnostic guidelines in central nervous system Whipple's disease. Ann Neurol 1996;40:561.

Pfister HW, Scheld WM. Brain injury in bacteria meningitis: therapeutic implications. Curr Opin Neurol 1997;10:254.

Porkert MT, Sotir M, Parrott-Moore P, Blumberg HM. Tuberculous meningitis at a large inner-city medical center. Am J Med Sci 1997;313:325.

Quagliarello VJ, Scheld WM. Treatment of bacterial meningitis. N Engl J Med 1997;336:708.

Roos KL. Central Nervous System Infectious Diseases and Therapy. New York: Marcel Dekker, 1997.

Scheld WM, Whitley RJ, Durack DT. Infections of the Central Nervous System (2nd ed). Philadelphia: Lippincott–Raven, 1997.

Segreti J, Harris AA. Acute bacterial meningitis. Infect Dis Clin North Am 1996;10:797.

Townsend GC, Scheld WM. The use of corticosteroids in the management of bacterial meningitis in adults. J Antimicrob Chemother 1996;37:1051.

Verdon R, Chevret S, Laissy JP, Wolff M. Tuberculous meningitis in adults: review of 48 cases. Clin Infect Dis 1996;22:982.

B. Viral Infections of the Nervous System

Nadir E. Bharucha and Roberta H. Raven

Chapter Plan

Viruses can affect the central nervous system (CNS), its coverings, and the peripheral nervous system. Most viral infections are benign and self-limiting systemic illnesses that rarely affect the nervous system. If the nervous system is involved, it is usually only the meninges, with meningitis resulting. Viruses affecting the brain produce an encephalitis. Infection of the spinal cord produces myelitis. When a clinical level is demonstrable, the term *transverse myelitis* is used. When the gray matter of the anterior horn cells is selectively affected by the poliovirus, the term *poliomyelitis* is used. If other viruses affect the anterior horn cells, the condition is termed a *poliolike illness*. The peripheral nervous system begins at the root. Root involvement only is radiculitis. Peripheral nerve involvement, usually a postviral phenomenon, is called *peripheral neuropathy*.

Pathogenesis of Viral Infections

Viruses affect the nervous system either directly, or indirectly by a postinfectious, immune-mediated mechanism. One indirectly caused condition is Reye's syndrome, in which there is an encephalopathy of unknown origin that occurs after a viral infection, usually varicella or influenza A or B, which has been treated with salicylates. When a virus has a direct effect, the virus itself enters the nervous system via the bloodstream or through the cranial or peripheral nerves. The virus enters the blood from the respiratory tract (e.g., influenza viruses, measles, mumps, varicella zoster), from the gut (enteroviruses, i.e., polio, coxsackie, echo), or from the skin through insect bites (arboviruses). Spread through nerves themselves occurs with rabies. In experiments, herpes simplex virus 1 (HSV-1) spreads through the olfactory nerve. In the case of varicella zoster, there is retrograde spread to the sensory ganglion at the time of primary infection, with anterograde spread through the nerve to skin at the time of the shingles. The immune-mediated, postviral, or postvaccinal clinical syndromes are postinfectious encephalomyelitis, transverse myelitis, and acute inflammatory demyelinating polyneuropathy or Guillain-Barré syndrome. Postinfectious encephalomyelitis usually occurs after a latent period of 2–12 days after a viral exanthem such as measles or a viral respiratory or gut infection. Sheep-brain antirabies vaccine produces a variety of central and peripheral nervous system complications. Transverse myelitis is more often immune-mediated than caused directly by the virus. The same viruses that produce postinfectious encephalomyelitis also cause immune-mediated transverse myelitis. The spinal cord is directly affected by varicella-zoster virus (VZV), which produces a transverse myelitis, by human T-cell leukemia/lymphotropic virus type I (HTLV-I), which produces tropical spastic paraplegia, by human immunodeficiency virus (HIV), which produces a myelopathy, and by dumb rabies, which causes an ascending myelitis. The poliovirus and enterovirus 71 directly and selectively affect anterior horn cells. Involvement of the peripheral nervous system directly by viruses, apart from VZV, HSV, and cytomegalovirus (CMV), is uncertain. Immune-mediated syndromes are far more common.

Meningitis

Epidemiology

The most common causes of viral meningitis are the enteroviruses, mumps, arboviruses, and HSV-2. Less common causes are lymphocytic choriomeningitis, the related Lassa virus, VZV, Epstein-Barr virus (EBV), and HIV. In Olmsted County, Minnesota, where Mayo Clinic's unique record linkage system provides community-based data, the age-adjusted incidence rate of presumed viral meningitis, polio excepted, was 10.9 per 100,000 population per annum between 1950 and 1981. A specific viral cause was identified in only 11% of these cases. Figures for developing countries are unavailable. Throughout the world, the illness mostly affects the young.

Enteroviral infections are spread by direct or indirect fecal-oral contact. An infected person can shed the virus in the feces for up to 4.5 months. Infection occurs principally in late summer and autumn in the developed countries, and in the rainy season in developing countries. Mumps, a paramyxovirus, starts as an upper respiratory infection. It then spreads in the blood to other target organs (salivary glands, testes, ovaries, breasts, brain, and meninges). Because of

vaccination with MMR (measles, mumps, rubella) vaccine, the incidence of mumps is declining. Lymphocytic choriomeningitis, an arenavirus, is also a respiratory tract infection that is spread after contact with rodents, their droppings or their urine. Lassa virus, too, is spread by the respiratory route but can spread directly.

Clinical Features

The clinical features are those of any meningitis, namely headache, neck stiffness, vomiting, photophobia, and fever. If there is an associated encephalitic component, there may also be altered sensorium and seizures. However, with a viral meningitis, the patient seems less ill than in pyogenic meningitis, and subsequently the progress is usually benign and self-limiting. In addition to the above, there may be associated neurologic or nonneurologic accompanying physical signs, which depend on the causative virus. Enteroviral infections can cause poliomyelitis or a poliolike illness. There may also be myocarditis or pericarditis, epidemic pleurodynia (Bornholm's disease), respiratory tract infection, herpangina, diarrhea, and skin rashes. Mumps causes an ependymitis with hydrocephalus in newborns. In the older age groups, parotitis is the major clinical feature. However, it should be remembered that parotitis is not specific for mumps, that it may never occur at all (40% of patients with CNS mumps do not have it), that it may follow aseptic meningitis, and that one-half of the patients with mumps have a pleocytosis in the cerebrospinal fluid (CSF) without any sign of meningitis. Lymphocytic choriomeningitis usually begins with a respiratory tract infection followed by meningitis. There may be associated parotitis, orchitis, arthritis, skin rash and alopecia.

Diagnosis

The CSF shows a lymphocytic pleocytosis that does not exceed 1,000 cells per μl. In one-third of patients with viral meningitis, there is a predominantly polymorphonuclear leukocytosis. In 13% of patients with pyogenic meningitis, there is a lymphocytosis. The greatest difficulty occurs in partially treated pyogenic meningitis and tuberculous meningitis, where the

Table 38B-1. Causes of Aseptic Meningitis

Infectious	
Viral	
Bacterial	Fastidious organisms—e.g., mycobacteria, spirochetes, *Mycoplasma, Brucella, Listeria, Rickettsia*, partially treated meningitis
Fungal	
Parasitic	
Parameningeal	Brain or craniospinal abscess, otitis, mastoiditis, sinusitis
Postinfectious	Rubeola, rubella, varicella
Postvaccine	Rabies, pertussis, influenza, yellow fever
Noninfectious	
Neoplastic	Primary, secondary, medulloblastoma, craniopharyngioma
Chemical	Contrast media, drugs, anesthetic agents
Immune-mediated	Vasculitis, hypersensitivity reactions, sera
Vascular	Subarachnoid hemorrhage
Toxic	Lead, mercury
Undefined	Sarcoidosis, Behçet's, Vogt-Koyanagi-Harada, Mollaret's, cat-scratch disease

Source: Reprinted with permission from WG Bradley, Daroff R, Fenichel G, Marsden CD (eds). Neurology in Clinical Practice (2nd ed). Boston: Butterworth–Heinemann, 1996;1260.

cells are predominantly lymphocytic. CSF protein is usually raised in viral meningitis, but typically not more than 130 mg per dl. Much of this extra protein is immunoglobulin (Ig)G, which diffuses across the blood-CSF barrier. Later, in convalescence and chronic infections, IgG is produced in the CSF itself by plasma cells. This IgG is usually specific. In mumps, oligoclonal bands can be found for up to a year after the illness. The CSF glucose level is usually normal, but it may be reduced. If reduced, the CSF-to–blood glucose ratio is between 0.3 and 0.5. Bacteria are absent in the CSF on staining and culture. Viral culture should be attempted from CSF and blood specimens and other body tissues. Serum antibody titers may show a fourfold rise during the acute stage, or specific IgM titers may be raised. It may be necessary to wait for the convalescence stage to demonstrate a rise in antibody titer, a situation that does not help the clinician. The typical CSF findings of lymphocytic pleocytosis with mildly elevated proteins, normal or slightly depressed glucose levels, and an absence of organisms are found in a host of infectious and noninfectious conditions termed *aseptic meningitis* (Table 38B-1).

Treatment

Basically, treatment is symptomatic, except if HSV or HIV is suspected. Inappropriate secretion of antidiuretic hormone (ADH) may occur and should be treated with fluid restriction.

Recurrent Aseptic Meningitis

Recurrent aseptic meningitis can be caused by several viruses. Bacteria can also cause the condition, particularly if there is an anatomic defect that allows the entry of organisms, if host defenses are impaired, or if there is a parameningeal focus of infection. Recurrent chemical meningitis occurs if a dermoid cyst periodically leaks its contents into the subarachnoid space.

Mollaret's meningitis is a condition of unknown etiology in which there are recurrent episodes of aseptic meningitis. The CSF shows the usual findings of aseptic meningitis as well as large, fragile "endothelial" cells called *Mollaret's cells*. There is accumulating evidence in the literature to the effect that HSV-2 DNA and, to a lesser extent, HSV-1 DNA are found in the CSF of patients with Mollaret's meningitis. Behçet's disease, Vogt-Koyanagi-Harada syndrome, and sarcoidosis all produce uveitis and meningoencephalitis. In Behçet's disease, there are also recurrent mouth and genital ulcers, arthritis, skin lesions, gastrointestinal tract symptoms, vasculitis, and epididymitis. Behçet's disease is common in the Mediterranean region, the Middle East, and parts

Table 38B-2. Viruses Causing Encephalitis

"Arboviruses"
Arenaviruses—cytomegalovirus, Lassa fever virus both cause epidemic encephalitis
Herpesviruses—herpes simplex virus 1 and 2, Epstein-Barr virus, cytomegalovirus, varicella-zoster virus
Paramyxoviruses—measles and mumps
Enteroviruses—polio, coxsackie, and echo
Miscellaneous—adenoviruses, influenzae, parainfluenzae, hepatitis, and rotavirus, rabies
Retroviruses—human immunodeficiency virus

of Asia. In Vogt-Koyanagi-Harada syndrome there is deafness, vitiligo, alopecia, and poliosis (patches of whitening of the hair of the scalp and eyebrows). All three conditions are treated with corticosteroids or immunosuppressants.

Encephalitis

Encephalitis means inflammation of the brain. The diagnosis is suspected when there is a combination of an encephalopathy and an acute febrile illness, usually in association with meningitis. Encephalopathy consists of altered sensorium of varying degrees, together with a variety of other focal disorders of the cerebrum, brain stem, or cerebellum. These include seizures, focal deficits of higher functions, usually of language and memory, hemiplegia, movement disorders, ocular palsies, nystagmus, and ataxia. Occasionally, the hypothalamic-pituitary axis is affected, causing hyponatremia as a result of inappropriate ADH secretion. Encephalitis can also cause diabetes insipidus or disturbances in temperature regulation. Encephalopathy is much more commonly caused by noninfectious than infectious causes. The noninfectious causes are trauma, metabolic disturbances, disorders of the cerebral circulation, toxic factors, and tumors. If fever is also present with these symptoms, the physician should suspect an infectious cause. The infectious causes may be either viral or nonviral. Nonviral causes are more common because of the high prevalence of malaria and tuberculosis in less developed parts of the world. Other bacteria, rickettsia, mycoplasma, fungi, and other parasites can also cause encephalitis. Diagnosis for all these is important because treatment is available.

Epidemiology

Encephalitis can be considered from several perspectives: (1) its time course, which may be acute or subacute/chronic; (2) its etiologic agent, which may be viral or nonviral; and (3) whether it is epidemic, as with arboviruses; endemic, as with dengue and measles; or sporadic, as with the herpesvirus group. The term *zoonotic encephalitis* is used when an animal reservoir is involved in its spread. Rabies is the most important example because it is widespread, dramatic, preventable, untreatable, and almost always fatal.

The term *subacute/chronic encephalitis* also includes slow infections of the CNS. They are caused by the conventional viruses, HIV, measles virus causing subacute sclerosing panencephalitis (SSPE), rubella, and JC papovavirus. The human prion diseases, kuru, Creutzfeldt-Jakob disease, Gerstmann-Straussler-Scheinker disease, and fatal familial insomnia also cause subacute/chronic encephalitis. Viral causes of encephalitis are listed in Table 38B-2.

In the United States, some idea of the different causes of the syndrome of infectious encephalitis can be obtained from a study done at the Walter Reed Army Institute, in which a specific cause was identified in 67% of patients. Most of these were viral infections: mumps (15%), arboviruses (11%), enterovirus (10%), lymphocytic choriomeningitis virus (9%), and herpes simplex (9%). A miscellaneous group of 7% included other viruses, rickettsia, leptospira, mycoplasma, and fungi. *Mycobacterium tuberculosis* was responsible for 6%.

Epidemic Encephalitis

Arboviral encephalitis is caused by viruses that use as their hosts blood-sucking insects (e.g., mosqui-

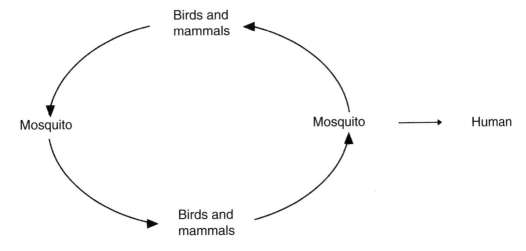

Figure 38B-1. Usual transmission cycle of arboviruses.

toes, ticks, sandflies). Humans are an inadvertent host in the cycle between these arthropods and their primary hosts, which are usually birds or other mammals (Figure 38B-1). There are exceptions, such as dengue, in which humans are the primary host. Also, in the urban epidemic form of St. Louis encephalitis, the cycle goes from a mosquito to a human to a mosquito (Figure 38B-2). The term "arbovirus" is not taxonomically correct.

The viruses in this group belong to the togaviral, flaviviral, rhabdoviral, filoviral, bunyaviral, and reoviral families. Mosquito-borne viruses cause eastern and western equine, Venezuelan equine, St. Louis, Murray Valley, California group (including La Crosse and California), West Nile, dengue fever, and Japanese encephalitides. Tick-borne viruses cause Kyasanur Forest disease complex, Russian spring-summer, Central European louping

Figure 38B-2. Transmission cycle of arboviruses with humans as primary host.

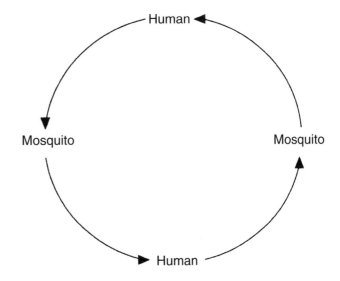

Table 38B-3. Etiology and Distribution of Arboviral Encephalitides

Name	Viral Family	Region
Eastern equine encephalitis	Togaviridae	North America
Western equine encephalitis	Togaviridae	North, Central, and South America
Venezuelan equine encephalitis	Togaviridae	Southern United States, Central America, northern South America
St. Louis encephalitis	Flaviviridae	North America, Caribbean
California group (except Tahyna)	Bunyaviridae	North America, Europe
Colorado tick fever	Reoviridae	North America
Powassan[a] encephalitis	Flaviviridae	North America
Japanese encephalitis	Flaviviridae	Asia
Kyasanur Forest disease complex	Flaviviridae	India
Murray Valley encephalitis	Flaviviridae	Australia, New Guinea
Dengue	Flaviviridae	Worldwide
Rift Valley fever encephalitis	Bunyaviridae	Africa
Russian spring-summer encephalitis	Flaviviridae	Western Siberia
Central European louping ill[b]	Flaviviridae	Europe, United Kingdom, Ireland

[a]Location in Ontario, Canada, where virus was first discovered.
[b]Named after leaping movements of infected sheep.

ill, Colorado tick fever, and Powassan encephalitides. Sandfly-borne viruses cause Rift Valley fever encephalitis.

Regional and seasonal factors are an important consideration when making the diagnosis (Table 38B-3). Restriction of these illnesses to definite areas at specific times of the year is the direct result of the breeding and feeding habits of the insect vector and the location of the host. Mosquito-borne diseases in temperate regions occur in late summer and early autumn. In the tropics, mosquito-borne disease occurs during the summer and monsoon months. The tick-borne encephalitides occur in spring and early summer.

The clinical features usually follow the pattern given in Figure 38B-3. The outcome ratio of inapparent-to-apparent infection, distribution, and important clinical features of various encephalitides are noted in Table 38B-4.

Sporadic Encephalitis

The herpes group of viruses, measles, mumps, and adenovirus are the most common causes of sporadic encephalitis. Several herpesviruses are capable of affecting the nervous system. Clinical disease usually follows a latent period, during which the virus is dormant. In HSV-1, the virus is dormant in the trigeminal sensory ganglion, in HSV-2 it is dormant in the sacral sensory ganglia, and in VZV it is in various sensory ganglia. In CMV, the site where the virus lies dormant is not known.

Herpes Simplex Encephalitis

Herpes simplex encephalitis is the most common sporadic, acute, focal encephalitis in the United States. It usually affects young people between the ages of 5 and 30 years and people older than 50 years of age. In children and adults, HSV-1 accounts for more than 95% of cases. In newborns, HSV-1 or -2 can cause encephalitis. In older age groups, HSV-2 causes genital herpes and meningitis but not encephalitis.

Pathogenesis

The virus probably enters the body through the mucous membrane of the mouth or eye. It travels through branches of the fifth nerve to the trigeminal ganglion, where it replicates and remains dormant. The mechanism of reactivation of the virus is unknown. The majority of people with herpes simplex encephalitis are not immunocompromised and indeed have anti–HSV-1 antibodies at the onset of clinical diagnosis.

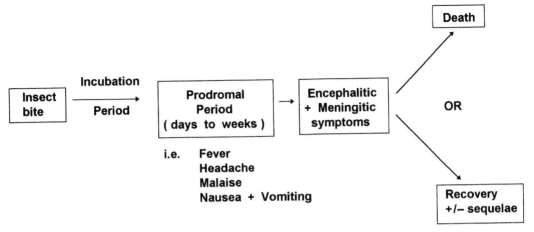

Figure 38B-3. Clinical course of arboviral encephalitis.

How the virus gets to the brain from the trigeminal ganglion is also unknown. It could be via branches of the fifth nerve to the meninges of the middle and anterior cranial fossae. Another proposed pathway is via the nose and olfactory pathways into the inferior temporofrontal regions.

Pathology

There is bilateral, asymmetric, anterior temporal and orbitofrontal inflammation. In newborns, the disease is more often disseminated in the brain. Gross changes consist of swelling, congestion, and hemorrhage. Deeper parts of the limbic system are also affected. Microscopically, there is evidence of inflammation and, in addition, there are homogeneous, eosinophilic, nuclear inclusions called *Cowdry Type A* inclusions. HSV antigen can be identified by immunologic tests, or DNA from HSV can be identified by polymerase chain reaction.

Clinical Features

As with any encephalitis, there is a prodromal phase, followed by the encephalitic syndrome. Features that suggest herpes simplex encephalitis are behavioral changes, olfactory or gustatory hallucinations, and prominent amnesia. However, it is impossible to make a diagnosis on clinical grounds alone.

Diagnosis

The CSF is abnormal in more than 95% of cases at some stage. It shows a picture similar to aseptic meningitis except that there is often an increased number of red cells. HSV-I antibodies and antigens can be identified in the CSF with a high degree of sensitivity and specificity. Unfortunately, the tests do not become positive until the second week of the illness. In newborn babies, the virus itself can be isolated from the CSF in approximately one-half of cases. This is not so in adults. Polymerase chain reaction is now being used more often to show HSV DNA in the CSF. Although this is a highly sensitive and specific method, false-positives and false-negatives do occur.

The electroencephalogram shows a predominantly frontotemporal abnormality, with periodic, lateralized, epileptiform discharges. Computed tomographic (CT) and magnetic resonance imaging (MRI) scans of the brain also show abnormalities in these regions. On CT scans, the lesions are hypointense with edema and enhancement. On MRI scans, the affected areas are hyperintense on T2-weighted images and, in addition, there are foci of hemorrhage with a parenchymal or gyral pattern of enhancement.

Brain biopsy still is the only available method for definitive diagnosis, but since the advent of acyclovir, this is usually not performed. When it was used regularly for diagnosing encephalitis, biopsy

Table 38B-4. Characteristics of Selected Arboviral Encephalitides

Name	Sequelae/Mortality	Inapparent: Apparent (I:A)	Distribution	Important Clinical Points
Eastern equine encephalitis	80% have sequelae	I:A low; children 2:1 to 8:1, adults 4:1 to 50:1; severe disease in children	Eastern Gulf Coast of United States, Caribbean, South America, least frequent in United States	Periorbital edema
Western equine encephalitis	Mortality 10%	I:A; children 8:1 to 50:1, adults 1,000:1	Western and Midwest United States	Problem worst in young children <2 yrs old
Venezuelan equine encephalitis	Mortality low		South and Central America	Neurologic complications uncommon; lymphadenopathy in one-third
St. Louis encephalitis		I:A 60:1; affects elderly, case fatality rate 5–10%	Central Western and Southern United States	Unusual features: (1) may be symptoms of urinary tract infection at onset, (2) may be muscle involvement with raised enzymes, (3) syndrome of inappropriate secretion of antidiuretic hormone
California group (except Tahyna)	Mortality 3%	I:A 26:1 or below; usually children 5–10 yrs old		Rapid evolution and resolution of symptoms; seizures prominent feature
Japanese encephalitis	5–50% fatal; 3–32% sequelae	I:A 25:1 to 1,000:1. In endemic areas common in children 3–15 yrs old. In epidemics all age groups affected.	In the north from east Russia to Japan; in the south from west coast of India to Indonesia	Animals: herons, egrets, pigs and cattle; focal motor weakness; arms > legs; UMN or LMN lesion; segmental sensory changes; features of parkinsonism; convulsions in children rather than adults
Dengue	Mortality nil	I >A	Worldwide	Endemic in tropics and subtropics; breakbone fever, usually in nonimmune adults and children; fever, arthralgias, and rash more like measles; spares palms and soles; associated with retro-orbital pain, headache, backache, limb pains; may be biphasic fever; recurs after 2 days ± bradycardia
Dengue hemorrhagic fever and dengue shock syndrome	Leading cause morbidity/mortality	Deadly; immune mediated	Tropical	Occurs in those exposed who have been pre-exposed to virus; bleeding very prominent; blood shows low platelets, leukopenia and hemoconcentration; lungs: bronchopneumonia; liver: mild dysfunction; electroencephalogram: diffuse changes; neurologic manifestations uncommon; encephalitis or peripheral mononeuritis leading to Bell's palsy, palatal palsy, ulnar nerve palsy, sciatic neuritis; Guillain-Barré syndrome
Rift Valley encephalitis	Mortality >50%	Affliction—usually benign	East Africa, Rift Valley, Kenya, Egypt, South Africa	Including encephalitis, retinopathy, hemorrhages, hepatitis

Russian spring-summer encephalitis	Mortality 20–30%; sequelae 20–30%	Far eastern Russia and China	Peak in May and June, hence the name; coma and seizures occur early; distinctive pattern: high cervical cord and low bulbar distribution; presents with LMN weakness and atrophy in the face, palate, neck, shoulders, and arms; chronic or late sequela is epilepsia partialis continua (Kozhevnikow's encephalitis)
Central European encephalitis	Less mortality and fewer sequelae than in Russian spring-summer encephalitis	Central Europe and western Russia	Clinical features similar to Russian spring-summer encephalitis

UMN = upper motor neuron; LMN = lower motor neuron.

confirmed the diagnosis in just under one-half of the cases and identified other treatable conditions in a number of patients. The false-negative rate was approximately 4%. The use of polymerase chain reaction to identify HSV DNA in the biopsy specimen improves the yield.

Complications of biopsy used to occur in approximately 2% of patients. Now, if the clinical picture, electroencephalography, and neuroimaging suggest HSV encephalitis, a trial of acyclovir is warranted.

Treatment

Acyclovir given intravenously in a dose of 10 mg per kg every 8 hours for 7–10 days should be started as soon as possible. Infected cells phosphorylate acyclovir to a triphosphate, which selectively inhibits viral DNA polymerase. This selectivity reduces side effects. Longer treatment with acyclovir and the use of steroids are still debatable. Symptomatic treatment of seizures and cerebral edema is required. Treatment with acyclovir reduces mortality from 80% to 20–30%. Major and minor sequelae are found in most of the survivors. If treatment is begun within 4 days of commencement of the illness, the survival at 18 months is increased from 72% to 92%. If the patient has a Glasgow Coma Scale score of 6 or less at the start of treatment, results are uniformly poor. Relapse occurs in 5% of cases. Acyclovir should be restarted at a dose of 15 mg per kg every 8 hours and continued for 3 weeks.

Varicella-Zoster Virus Infection

VZV causes varicella (chickenpox) in children and herpes zoster (HZ) in adults. Approximately 1 in 1,000 to 1 in 4,000 children with varicella experience neurologic complications, chiefly meningoencephalitis, but also Reye's syndrome, myelitis, or Guillain-Barré syndrome. Varicella in a pregnant woman in the third trimester results in an encephalitis in the baby. The meningoencephalitis that follows chicken pox usually occurs after a latent period but within 2 weeks of the onset of rash. It presents mainly as a cerebellar ataxia, sometimes with behavioral changes. The meningoencephalitis is believed to be an immune-mediated condition

and so is termed a *postinfectious encephalitis*. The distinction between infectious and postinfectious encephalitis is often unclear, as in some cases of post-varicella encephalitis, the organism or its genetic material has been identified in the CSF. The pathologic features include perivenous demyelination and intranuclear inclusion bodies.

HZ infection occurs in an unknown percentage of people who have had chickenpox. The reasons for reactivation of the virus, dormant in sensory ganglia, are unknown. The theories are that host immunity is impaired, that dormant virus is somehow reactivated by another exposure to VZV, or, rarely, that there is an underlying structural lesion of the nerve root. The rash, which occurs in the distribution of a dermatome, is first macular, then papular, then vesicular, pustular, and finally replaced by crusting. Before the rash, there is pain and itching. Sometimes, they occur for weeks or even months beforehand. The affected dermatomes are mostly thoracic or lumbar, but cranial nerves III, IV, V, VI, VII, IX, and X can also be affected. The first division of cranial nerve V and cranial nerve VII are the most commonly involved cranial nerves. These produce zoster ophthalmicus and Ramsay-Hunt syndrome, respectively. The most common complication of HZ is postherpetic neuralgia. Other, less common complications are segmental motor weakness, which may involve a cranial nerve; cerebral arteritis, which can affect the carotid artery, often on the same side and giving a contralateral hemiplegia; cerebral angiitis, affecting small cerebral vessels; encephalomyelitis; aseptic meningitis; progressive multifocal leukoencephalopathy; and the Guillain-Barré syndrome. In immunosuppressed people, infection is more severe, the rash is more likely to be generalized, and complications occur more frequently. Zoster sine herpete (zoster without a rash) is believed to be a definite clinical entity that may present with any of the other manifestations of HZ. VZV DNA has been identified in CSF using polymerase chain reaction 5–8 months after the onset of pain in some cases.

Treatment is with acyclovir, which should be started during the first week of the rash. In immunocompromised people it prevents progression of the rash, and in those with normal immune systems it might reduce the incidence and duration of postherpetic neuralgia. The usual adult dose of acyclovir is 800 mg five times a day for 7–10 days.

Longer courses are not of proven value, and corticosteroids may permit reactivation of the virus. The pain of postherpetic neuralgia is most effectively controlled by explanation to the patient and amitriptyline.

Epstein-Barr Virus Infection

The most common clinical presentation of EBV is infectious mononucleosis (IM), which presents with fever, sore throat, lymphadenopathy, atypical lymphocytosis, and heterophil antibodies. Less than 5% of patients with IM have neurologic complications, which develop 1–3 weeks after onset of the illness. Asymptomatic CSF abnormalities are found in patients with IM more often than neurologic manifestations. Occasionally, neurologic complications can be the presenting symptom of EBV infection, before other manifestations of IM develop. The neurologic manifestations are encephalitis, cranial nerve palsies, myelitis, and various patterns of peripheral nerve disease. Neurologic manifestations nearly always abate. There is no available definitive treatment. Diagnosis of EBV is made by identification of IgM antibodies to the viral capsid antigen.

Cytomegalovirus Infection

Infection with CMV in the developed nervous system is rare. It usually develops only in immunocompromised people. It presents as meningoencephalitis or as a Guillain-Barré–like syndrome. CMV infection in pregnancy affects the baby, producing encephalitis, microcephaly, intracerebral calcification, and mental retardation.

Paramyxoviruses

Mumps

Mumps is more commonly associated with meningoencephalitis than encephalitis and has been discussed in the section on meningitis. The encephalitis is unusual in children and adults, but can occur in utero, producing periaqueductal inflammation with hydrocephalus.

Measles

Measles does not usually acutely affect the CNS. On average, at 5 days after the onset of rash, in 1 in 1,000 patients with measles, it produces a postinfectious, immune-mediated encephalomyelitis. This results in death in 10% of patients and severe sequelae (seizures, mental regression, and focal deficit) in others. Measles can also produce a rare, fatal, inclusion body encephalitis, also known as *immunosuppressive measles encephalitis*, which occurs weeks to months after the primary infection in children with lymphatic malignancies or other immunosuppressive conditions. It presents with partial status epilepticus. The third encephalitic syndrome that can occur after measles infection is SSPE. This occurs years after primary measles infection, which took place usually within the first year of life. It is a problem seen mostly in developing countries where measles immunization is often not given. It consists of four stages: stage 1—behavioral changes and mental regression; stage 2—motor disability, seizures, and jerks with slow relaxation; stage 3—coma with decerebrate rigidity; stage 4—a flaccid, comatose state and death. Treatment is symptomatic, as there are no available definitive treatments.

Enteroviruses

Most cases of aseptic meningitis are caused by enteroviruses, which also cause between 10% and 20% of cases of viral encephalitis. Rarely, enteroviruses are responsible for a poliolike paralysis, cerebellar ataxia, epidemic myalgia, and polymyositis. Perinatal meningoencephalitis is caused by coxsackie and echoviruses. In an immunocompromised person, they can produce meningoencephalitis at any age and even progressive encephalitis or polymyositis.

Poliomyelitis

Polio is caused by a picornavirus by one of three serotypes: 1, 2, and 3. The term comes from the Greek word *polios*, meaning gray, and *myelos*, meaning spinal cord. Since the advent of mass immunization, paralytic poliomyelitis is a rare occurrence in developed countries. In the western hemisphere, there have been no new cases of wild-type polio since 1991 and in the United States, none since 1979. When it does occur, it does so in one of two groups: those who have not been immunized, as happened among the Amish community of the United States in 1979, and in recipients of live oral poliovirus vaccine (OPV) who are younger than 5 years of age and in their older contacts. Immunosuppressed people are more likely to get OPV-associated paralytic disease. In the general population, the incidence of OPV-associated paralytic poliomyelitis is 1 case per 2.6 million doses distributed.

In developing countries, paralytic poliomyelitis caused by the wild-type virus still occurs, but after the World Health Organization's intensive global elimination program, it is now found only in West and Central Africa and South Asia. The disease mostly affects children. Older children and adults are less often affected, but if they are, the disease is more severe. The virus enters via the gastrointestinal tract, where it spreads to the CNS via the blood. It is spread from person to person by the fecal-oral route. Poverty, poor or absent sanitation, and overcrowding coupled with lack of immunization make this possible. Incidence peaks in summer and during the monsoons. In a person incubating the disease, paralysis can be provoked by exercise, surgery (especially tonsillectomy), and intramuscular injections. These provocative factors are thought to produce reflex vasodilatation of capillaries supplying the relevant anterior horn cells, thereby permitting passage of the virus. Another possibility is that the virus enters the motor neuron at the neuromuscular junction with retrograde spread.

Pathology

In the acute stage of paralytic polio, neurons show dissolution of the Nissl granules. There are congested blood vessels with perivascular and perineuronal inflammatory cell infiltrates. In the chronic stage, there is loss of neurons with gliosis. Affected muscles show denervation atrophy. The neurons affected are usually the large motor neurons of the brain stem and spinal cord. Other structures that may be affected are the precentral motor cortex, thalamus, hypothalamus, other brain stem and cerebellar nuclei, and even sensory and autonomic neurons of the spinal cord.

Clinical Features

Ninety percent of infections are subclinical. Most of those with clinical disease manifest with a minor illness or abortive poliomyelitis, which consists of a brief, febrile illness affecting the upper respiratory or gastrointestinal tract. Neurologic involvement consists of a rapidly resolving aseptic meningitis and, more rarely, of paralytic poliomyelitis, which is the major illness. When neurologic involvement occurs in children, the sequence is usually that of a minor illness followed by resolution of symptoms, followed in 5–10 days by aseptic meningitis with fever, followed 2–5 days later by paralysis. In adults, the pre-paralytic phase may be much shorter. The earliest symptoms of paralysis are muscle tenderness, cramps, stiffness, and twitching. Maximal paralysis occurs within a few days of onset. Paralysis is asymmetric, affects the legs more than the arms and the proximal more than the distal muscles. Wasting of affected muscles begins a week after paralysis and progresses over several months. Sensory symptoms but not signs are common. Patients feel tingling and pain in the muscles. Autonomic manifestations, namely retention of urine, disturbances of sweating, and delay of gastric emptying with constipation also occur. Spinal poliomyelitis is much more common than the bulbar form.

Bulbar poliomyelitis presents with difficulty in swallowing and speaking resulting from involvement of cranial nerves IX and X, and difficulty in breathing, irregular heart rhythm, and poor blood pressure control resulting from involvement of the reticular formation in the medulla. There may be facial weakness (cranial nerve VII) but eye movements, chewing, and tongue movements are usually unimpaired.

Encephalitic poliomyelitis is uncommon. Autonomic manifestations are prominent. Hypoxia and hypercapnia are thought to produce an encephalopathy that is probably more common than an encephalitis per se.

Diagnosis and Differential Diagnosis

Diagnosis is clinical. Other paralytic disorders requiring exclusion are the Guillain-Barré syndrome and the syndrome of acute axonal neuropathy found in northern China. In both these conditions, there is no febrile illness at the time of paralysis. Weakness is more symmetric. Bifacial weakness is prominent and the CSF does not show lymphocytosis. Sensory nerve action potential studies are abnormal in Guillain-Barré syndrome but normal in polio and acute motor axonal neuropathy.

Several other viruses may also cause a poliolike illness. These are echoviruses, coxsackie A7, and enterovirus 71. They can be distinguished using serologic studies.

Acute hemorrhagic keratoconjunctivitis caused by enterovirus 70 occurs in epidemics. Conjunctivitis is followed by a poliolike illness with asymmetric lumbosacral radiculitis. It can also be diagnosed by serologic tests.

Treatment

There is no specific treatment for polio. Symptomatic and supportive treatment is the mainstay in the acute stage, followed by rehabilitation.

Prevention

The coat of the poliovirus contains four proteins, which determine antigenicity and the ability to attach to receptor sites in the gut. Immunity is determined by secretory IgA antibodies in the alimentary tract, which prevent colonization by poliovirus, and also by IgG antibodies in the blood, which neutralize virus as it enters the bloodstream. Infection with wild virus and OPV causes the formation of IgG and IgA antibodies. Inactivated poliovirus vaccine (IPV) causes formation of IgG antibodies only, and it is thus unable to prevent gut colonization. Therefore, the virus is shed in the stool and may infect other non-immunized people. However, IPV does reduce viral shedding from the oropharynx. An enhanced potency IPV has been produced. Sweden, Finland, and the Netherlands use IPV vaccine. Most other countries use OPV. The advantages of OPV are its ease of administration and that it prevents colonization of the gut by wild virus, therefore helping in the production of herd immunity. The vaccine virus is excreted in the stool and immunizes nonimmune contacts. Its disadvantage is that it requires refrigeration at 4°C in order to maintain its potency. Vaccine failures have been reported, usually from tropical countries. OPV is contra-indicated in immunocompromised people, and in normal people there is a very small risk of vaccine-associated poliomyelitis. IPV, besides being used routinely in certain countries, should be given to immunocompromised people who require immunity and to nonimmune adults.

Prognosis

Two to five percent of children and 15–30% of adults with acute paralytic poliomyelitis die. Of those who die, 26% have bulbar paralysis, 22% have respiratory paralysis, and 52% have both. Most recovery occurs within 6 months of onset.

Years or decades after the acute illness, some patients develop new symptoms of progressive muscle weakness, pain, fatigue, fasciculation, and even atrophy. This is believed to be caused by dysfunction and death of motor neurons that have taken over the function of those that died earlier.

Rabies

Rabies is caused by a bullet-shaped RNA virus belonging to the rhabdovirus group, which is part of the genus, Lyssavirus. Other members of the Lyssavirus genus such as Mohola, Duvenhage, and European bat Lyssa virus usually affect animals but rarely can cause a rabies-like illness in humans. Antirabies vaccine is ineffective against these viruses. Rabies can infect all mammals. It spreads to humans most often through the bite of an infected animal. Humans may rarely inhale the virus in a bat-infested cave or become infected by handling heavily contaminated material in the laboratory without first taking precautions. Human-to-human transmission has also been reported after corneal transplant and, very rarely, across the placenta and by breast feeding. Animal reservoirs vary in different parts of the world. The urban form of rabies is spread by dogs and cats. The sylvatic form spreads from raccoons, bats, foxes, skunks, wolves, and mongooses. Some parts of the world are free of rabies, namely Australia, the United Kingdom, and Antarctica. Some parts have a high incidence, particularly Asia, Africa, and South America. India has one of the highest rates in the world, 35.5 deaths per 1 million population in 1992.

Pathogenesis and Pathology

The virus starts to replicate at the site of the bite within cells of striated muscle, enters the peripheral nervous system at the neuromuscular junction, and spreads centrally along the axon. Most replication takes place within the gray matter of the CNS. Its effect on nerve cells is either direct or by interference with neurotransmitter function, probably via acetylcholine, 5-hydroxytryptamine, 8-aminobutyric acid, and N-methyl-D-aspartate, or else by interference with opiate receptors. It also induces an inflammatory response.

Typical features of encephalitis are seen in the limbic system and brain stem in furious rabies and in the spinal cord in dumb or paralytic rabies. Under the light microscope, typical intraneuronal inclusions called Negri bodies are seen. They contain virus particles. The virus spreads from the CNS through the autonomic nervous system to salivary glands, the gastrointestinal tract, heart, pancreas, and skin. The significance of this is that it is via salivary gland infection that the virus spreads and further that biopsy of hair follicles above the nuchal hair line may demonstrate the virus for diagnosis. There is no viremia. Degenerative changes are seen in the organs to which the virus has spread as well as in the peripheral nerves.

Clinical Manifestations

Rabies has an incubation period usually of 1–3 months but ranging from 4 days to many years. The length of the incubation period depends on the site of the bite, the critical factor being its distance from the CNS. The severity of the bite, the number of organisms introduced, and the state of the host defenses are also important determining factors. The prodromal period consists of the nonspecific symptoms of any encephalitic illness. Most important during the prodrome, because it gives the clue to the diagnosis, is the presence of pain, itching, or muscle twitching at the site of the bite, caused by proliferation of the virus either in the local dorsal root ganglion or in the anterior horn cell.

A few days after the onset of the prodrome, the next stage begins. In most cases, this is the encephalitic stage, which manifests as furious rabies, but in some, the spinal cord is predominantly affected (myelitic phase) producing paralytic or dumb rabies.

The Encephalitic Phase or Furious Rabies

The characteristic features of the encephalitic phase are alternating periods of agitation and lucidity. The agitation is associated with confusion, hallucinations, aggressiveness, and seizures. Hyperesthesia is prominent, and the patient is excessively sensitive to touch, light, breeze, and sound. There is autonomic instability with sweating, hypersalivation, and lacrimation. Hydrophobia is very characteristic. It consists of painful involuntary spasms of the pharynx, larynx, and respiratory muscles, including the diaphragm. Spasms are provoked by attempting to drink. Later, even the mention of water or the sight of it or the sound of running water can cause spasms. They can be provoked by blowing air on the face (aerophobia). Frothing of the mouth is caused by a combination of excessive salivation and hydrophobia. Other findings on examination include fever, ophthalmoplegia, facial palsies, impaired palatal and tongue movements, vocal cord paralysis, and upper motor neuron paralysis of the limbs with fasciculations. There are fluctuations of blood pressure, temperature, respiration, and urine output. Priapism also occurs. The patient dies either during a hydrophobic spasm or lapses into coma with flaccid paralysis. The patient almost always dies despite intensive care. There are, however, a very small number of well-documented cases of rabies in which the patient has survived.

The Myelitic Phase or Dumb Rabies

The myelitic phase is rare but is seen in patients bitten by vampire bats or in those who have had postexposure immunization to rabies. Patients have an ascending, flaccid paralysis to which they eventually succumb.

Diagnosis

Laboratory methods give little help in diagnosing rabies. The only available definitive test that will give a result early in the disease is skin biopsy from above the hairline at the back of the neck. Fluorescent antibody stain of the specimen shows viral antigen in the nerve twiglets around the hair follicles. Virus isolation from various sources in the first week and antibody estimation from the second week onward are confirmatory but take too long to be of use in the immediate management. Brain specimens can also be used to isolate virus or can be stained with fluorescent antibody stain or examined under a microscope for Negri bodies. Brain biopsy can be done while the patient is alive but is difficult because the structures affected are deep. Therefore, specimens are usually obtained at postmortem examination, either from the affected person or from a sick animal that has bitten a human and subsequently has been killed. If the animal is healthy at the time of the bite and if it remains healthy while under observation for 10 days, then it is unlikely to have rabies. For all these reasons, the diagnosis of rabies is usually made clinically. A history of a bite in a rabies-endemic country or travel to a country where rabies is endemic, together with an alternating state of agitation and lucidity accompanied by hydrophobia is pathognomonic. The differential diagnosis must include other forms of viral encephalitis, hysteria, tetanus (which can also be transmitted by a bite), and intoxication with datura. The differential diagnosis for dumb rabies includes the Guillain-Barré syndrome, poliomyelitis, and postvaccinal encephalomyelitis 2 weeks after inoculation with vaccines containing nervous tissue from other species.

Prevention and Treatment

Rabies is a preventable but not a treatable disease. Prevention can be achieved by vaccination with tissue-culture vaccine (human diploid cell or purified chick embryo cell vaccine). Pre-exposure prophylaxis should be given to those at risk of contact. Postexposure prophylaxis consists of local wound cleaning, passive immunization with human rabies immune globulin, and active immunization with a course of tissue culture vaccine. Definite criteria for different kinds of exposure to rabies virus (licking, scratching or biting; site of this; wild or domestic animal) have now been determined by the World Health Organization. As mentioned above, the suspected animal should be observed for 10 days. Unfortunately, nervous tissue vaccine and sheep brain vaccine are still widely used in Africa and Asia, as is suckling mouse brain vaccine in South America. They can cause various allergic reactions, such as myelitis, mononeuritis multiplex, meningoencephalitis, or a combination of these between 1 and 2 weeks after the first injection. Reactions to sheep brain vaccine occur in 1 in 220 courses, more often affect the CNS, and cause death in 3%. Reactions to mouse brain vaccine occur in 1 in 7,865 to 1 in 27,000 courses, more often affect the peripheral nervous system, and cause death in 22%.

Suggested Reading

Bale JF Jr. Viral encephalitis. Med Clin North Am 1993; 77:25.

Bhabha SK, Bharucha NE, Bharucha EP. Viral Infections. In WG Bradley, RB Daroff, GM Fenichel, CD Marsden (eds), Neurology in Clinical Practice—Principles of Diagnosis and Management (2nd ed). Boston: Butterworth–Heinemann, 1996;1259–1275.

Booss J, Esiry MM (eds). Viral Encephalitis—Pathology, Diagnosis and Management. Oxford, UK: Blackwell Scientific, 1986.

Connolly KJ, Hammer SM. The acute aseptic meningitis syndrome. Infect Dis Clin North Am 1990;4:599.

Davies LE. Acute Viral Meningitis and Encephalitis. In PGE Kennedy, RT Johnson (eds), Infections of the Nervous System. London: Butterworths, 1987;156–176.

Gourie-Devi M. Poliomyelitis and Other Anterior Horn Cell Disorders. In RA Shakir, PK Newmann, CM Poser (eds), Tropical Neurology. London: Saunders, 1996.

Griffin DG. Encephalitis, Myelitis, and Neuritis. In GL Mandell, JE Bennett, R Dolin (eds), Principles and Practice of Infectious Disease (4th ed). New York: Churchill Livingstone, 1995;874–887.

Ho DD, Hirsch MS. Acute viral encephalitis. Med Clin North Am 1985;69:415.

Jackson AC. Acute viral infections. Curr Opin Neurol 1995;8:170.

Johnson RT (ed). Viral Infections of the Nervous System. New York: Raven, 1982.

Johnson RT. The pathogenesis of acute viral encephalitis and postinfectious encephalitis. J Infect Dis 1987;155:359.

Nicolosi A, Hauser WA, Beghi E, Kurland LT. Epidemiology of central nervous system infections in Olmsted County, Minnesota, 1950–1981. J Infect Dis 1986;154;399.

Ratzan KR. Viral meningitis. Med Clin North Am 1985; 69:399.

Scheld WM, Whitley RT, Durack DT (eds). Infections of the CNS (2nd ed). Part I: Viral Infections and Related Disorders. Philadelphia: Lippincott–Raven, 1997;7–273.

The NIAID Collaborative Antiviral Study Group. Diseases that mimic herpes simplex encephalitis. Diagnosis, presentation and outcome. JAMA 1989;262:234.

Tsai TF. Arboviral infections in the United States. Infect Dis Clin North Am 1991;5:73.

Tunkel AR, Scheld WM. Acute Meningitis. In GL Mandell, JE Bennett, R Dolin (eds), Principles and Practice of Infectious Disease (4th ed). New York: Churchill Livingstone, 1995.

Viral Diseases. In GL Mandell, JE Bennett, R Dolin (eds), Principles and Practice of Infectious Disease (4th ed, Vol 2). New York: Churchill Livingstone, 1995.

Warrell DA, Warrell MJ. Rabies. In RA Shakir, PK Newmann, CM Poser (eds), Tropical Neurology. London: Saunders, 1996;51–76.

Whitley RJ. Viral Encephalitis. N Engl J Med 1990; 323:242.

C. Parasitic Infectious Disorders

Oscar H. Del Brutto

Chapter Plan

Protozoal infections
    Cerebral amebiasis
    Cerebral malaria
    Toxoplasmosis
    Trypanosomiasis
Cestode infections
    Coenurosis
    Cysticercosis
    Echinococcosis (hydatid disease)
    Sparganosis
Nematode infections
    Angiostrongyliasis
    Gnathostomiasis
    Strongyloidiasis
    Toxocariasis
    Trichinosis
Trematode infections
    Paragonimiasis
    Schistosomiasis

Parasitic diseases of the central nervous system (CNS) affect millions of people in Latin America, Asia, and Africa and represent a public health challenge for the developing world. In addition, increased tourism, refugee movements, massive immigration, and the acquired immunodeficiency syndrome (AIDS) epidemic have contributed to the diffusion of some formerly rare and geographically restricted parasitic diseases that are now widespread. Parasitic diseases of the CNS are pleomorphic and may produce subacute or chronic meningitis, acute or subacute encephalitis, space-occupying brain lesions, stroke, and myelopathy. Because these are nonspecific clinical manifestations, parasites are considered, in endemic areas, as "great imitators" because they may mimic almost any neurologic disease.

Protozoal Infections

Cerebral Amebiasis

Free-living amebae of the genus *Acanthamoeba* and *Naegleria*, as well as the intestinal parasite *Entamoeba histolytica*, may invade the CNS. *Acanthamoeba* invades the CNS by the hematogenous route from a primary infection of the skin or the respiratory tract; it is an opportunistic pathogen, affecting immunocompromised patients. In contrast, *Naegleria* infection occurs in normal hosts. *Naegleria* is acquired during swimming in warm fresh water; the parasites enter the nasal cavity and migrate through olfactory nerves to the CNS. *E. histolytica* migrates to the CNS from the colon or liver in patients with severe infections.

Pathology

CNS infection by *Acanthamoeba* results in the formation of hemorrhagic brain abscesses surrounded by a granulomatous inflammatory infiltrate. Invasion of arterial walls by trophozoites causes a necrotizing angiitis that may lead to cerebral infarcts. *Naegleria* induces purulent meningitis associated with diffuse hemorrhagic necrosis of the brain parenchyma; the involvement is more prominent in the frontal lobes and the olfactory bulbs, around the portal of entry of the microorganisms. *E. histolytica* infections present with multiple ill-defined brain abscesses formed by a central hemorrhagic area and a rim of necrotic tissue.

Clinical Manifestations and Diagnosis

Acanthamoeba produces a subacute disease called *granulomatous amebic encephalitis*, which is characterized by low-grade fever, focal signs, seizures, intracranial hypertension, and behavioral changes; the disease runs a progressive course over 2–8 weeks. *Naegleria* causes primary amebic meningoencephalitis, a fulminant disease carrying a grim prognosis that resembles acute bacterial meningitis. *E. histolytica* produces a multifocal encephalopathy that usually occurs in the setting of advanced systemic amebiasis. Examination of fresh cerebrospinal fluid (CSF) samples reveals mobile trophozoites in patients with *Naegleria* encephalitis. In contrast, the diagnosis of *Acanthamoeba* and *E. histolytica* infections usually rests on the demonstration of parasites in biopsy specimens.

Therapy

Amebic infections of the brain are highly fatal diseases. Amphotericin B and rifampin may be used in *Naegleria* infections, whereas surgery is advised for *Acanthamoeba* abscesses. Metronidazole and surgery are indicated for *E. histolytica* brain abscesses.

Cerebral Malaria

Up to 500 million people are infected by *Plasmodium* species every year, with approximately 1.5–3.0 million fatal cases, most of which occur in African children. From the four species of human malaria parasites, only *Plasmodium falciparum* invades the CNS and causes cerebral malaria. However, because all the species may cause high fever associated with delirium or seizures, the current definition of cerebral malaria requires all the following: (1) unarousable coma, (2) evidence of acute infection with *P. falciparum*, and (3) no other identifiable cause of coma.

Pathology

Autopsy studies have shown brain edema and small ring hemorrhages in the subcortical white matter in almost 80% of cases. Hemorrhages result from extravasation of erythrocytes due to endothelial damage. In addition, capillaries and venules are plugged by clumped, parasitized erythrocytes. Brains of patients who survived the acute phase of the disease have granulomatous lesions (Dürck nodules) at the site of ring hemorrhages.

Clinical Manifestations

Fever is the initial complaint. This is followed by progressive somnolence associated with seizures, extensor posturing, and disconjugate gaze. Retinal hemorrhages, when present, suggest a poor prognosis. Some patients, particularly children, present with focal signs related to cerebral infarcts or hemorrhages. Hypoglycemia, pulmonary edema, renal failure, bleeding diathesis, and hepatic dysfunction may complicate the course of the disease. Up to 25% of patients die despite medical care. Permanent sequelae, more common in children, include mental retardation, epilepsy, blindness, and motor deficits.

Diagnosis

P. falciparum may be seen by examining thin and thick blood smears prepared with Giemsa stain; repeated examinations may be needed because parasitemia is cyclical. The CSF is usually normal; however, routine CSF examination is mandatory to exclude other causes of encephalopathy. Computed tomographic (CT) and magnetic resonance imaging (MRI) scans may show brain swelling or small hemorrhages in severe cases.

Therapy

Because of chloroquine-resistant strains of *P. falciparum*, quinine is the drug of choice for cerebral malaria. After an initial loading dose (20 mg per kg), the maintenance dose of quinine should be adjusted according to plasma concentrations to prevent accumulation. Quinidine may be used when quinine is not available. Systemic complications must be recognized and treated. Symptomatic measures also include anticonvulsants, sedatives, and osmotic diuretics. Corticosteroids are harmful to comatose patients with cerebral malaria.

Toxoplasmosis

Toxoplasmosis has become a common parasitic disease of the CNS because it is a frequent opportunistic infection in AIDS patients. In these cases, the disease results from reactivation of a dormant infection with *Toxoplasma gondii*, a protozoa that is acquired by ingestion of contaminated cat feces or by eating undercooked meat. Immunocompetent hosts may also suffer from CNS toxoplasmosis during acute infections, and fetuses may be involved as a result of placental transmission of tachyzoites from women who acquire the disease during pregnancy.

Pathology

T. gondii may produce a focal or diffuse necrotizing encephalitis associated with perivascular inflammation. Focal lesions take the form of cerebral abscesses consisting of a necrotic center and a periphery in which multiple tachyzoites and cysts are seen together with patchy areas of necrosis and perivascular cuffing of lymphocytes. Glial nodules composed of astrocytes and microglial cells are common in the surrounding brain tissue.

Clinical Manifestations

Immunocompetent hosts rarely develop neurologic symptoms, although an acute encephalitis with fever, irritability, seizures, and drowsiness progressing to coma occurs in some cases. Immunocompromised hosts may also develop an acute encephalitic syndrome or, more frequently, a sub-acute disease characterized by focal signs associated with seizures and signs of intracranial hypertension. In AIDS patients, the clinical picture is usually complicated because of concurrent infection with other pathogens.

Diagnosis

In immunocompetent hosts, a fourfold rise in serum antibody titers is a sensitive indicator of acute infection. In contrast, immunosuppressed individuals usually have absent or low antibody titers despite severe disease. CT scans show ring-enhancing lesions surrounded by edema; lesions are usually multiple and may be located in the subcortical white matter, the basal ganglia, or the brain stem. MRI studies are better than CT scans for the detection of lesions (Figure 38C-1). Ring-enhancing lesions are not pathognomonic for cerebral toxoplasmosis because they may be observed in other diseases affecting AIDS patients; therefore, definitive diagnosis requires histologic demonstration of the parasite. Empiric therapy followed by repeated neuroimaging studies at 3 weeks has been proposed as an alternative to biopsy in AIDS patients.

Therapy

The combination of pyrimethamine (100–200 mg the first day followed by 50–75 mg per day for 6 weeks) and sulfadiazine (4–6 g per day for 6 weeks) is the therapy of choice for CNS toxoplasmosis. Clindamycin (600 mg every 6 hours) is an alternative drug in patients developing skin reactions to sulfadiazine. New drugs, including clarithromycin, trimetrexate, piritrexin, and atovaquone, have been used with promising results in AIDS patients with CNS toxoplasmosis. CNS toxoplasmosis tends to recur after discontinuation of therapy. In AIDS patients, permanent maintenance therapy with pyramethamine (25–50 mg per day) and sulfadiazine (2–4 g per day) is usually advised to decrease the risk of relapses.

Trypanosomiasis

Trypanosoma infections cause two different diseases in humans, sleeping sickness (African trypanosomiasis) and Chagas' disease (American

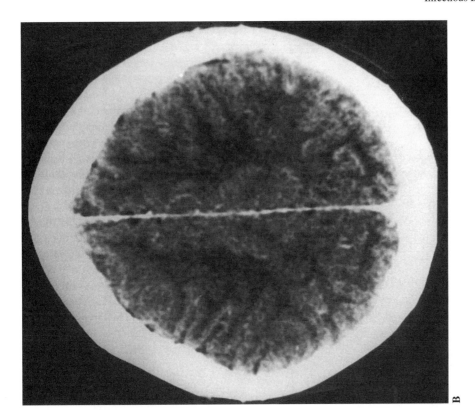

B

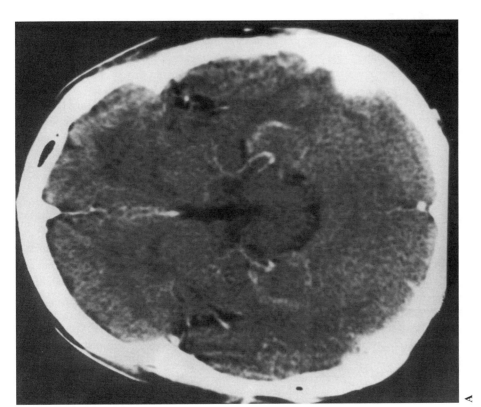

A

Figure 38C-1. Contrast-enhanced computed tomographic (CT) (A,B) and magnetic resonance imaging (MRI) (C,D) scans of a patient with acquired immunodeficiency syndrome with cerebral toxoplasmosis. The MRI study allows visualization of multiple brain abscesses that are not seen on the CT scan.

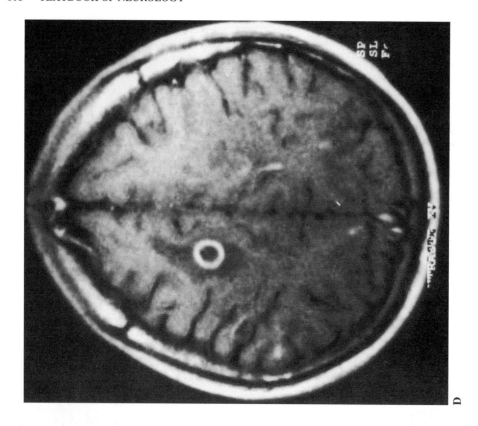

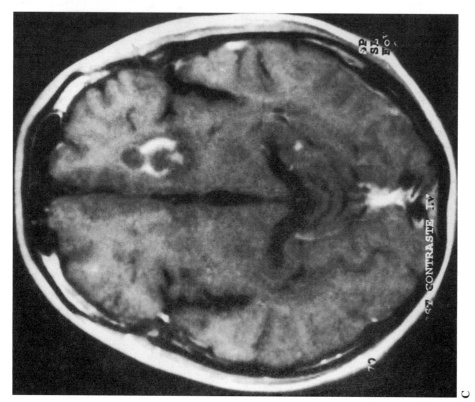

Figure 38C-1. *Continued.*

trypanosomiasis). The former is caused by *Trypanosoma brucei* and the latter by *Trypanosoma cruzi*. These parasites enter the human body by direct inoculation through a bite of their insect vector; the tsetse fly in the case of *T. brucei*, and bugs of the genus *Triatoma* in the case of *T. cruzi*. Blood transfusions still represent a frequent cause of *T. cruzi* infection in endemic areas.

American Trypanosomiasis (Chagas' Disease)

Acute Chagas' disease is characterized by unilateral orbital edema (Romaña's sign) and mild constitutional symptoms, although early invasion of the CNS by trypanosomes may cause irritability, stupor progressing to coma, seizures, focal signs, and CSF pleocytosis, particularly in infants and AIDS patients. The brains of these patients show multiple areas of hemorrhagic necrosis, glial proliferation, and perivascular infiltrates of inflammatory cells. Chronic disease is usually not associated with primary neurologic complications; however, some patients develop cardioembolic brain infarcts as the result of chagasic dilated cardiomyopathy. In addition, immunocompromised patients experience reactivation of chronic infections, resulting in a rapidly fatal meningoencephalitic syndrome similar to that observed in acute infections. During the acute phase, diagnosis is possible by demonstration of *T. cruzi* in blood smears, CSF samples, or xenodiagnosis. Chronic disease is confirmed by serologic testing. Nifurtimox and benznidazole may be used for acute disease and for acute reactivations of chronic disease. Chronic Chagas' disease has no specific treatment.

African Trypanosomiasis

Sleeping sickness may be caused by two subspecies of *T. brucei*: *T. gambiense* as the agent of West African trypanosomiasis and *T. rhodesiense* as that of East African trypanosomiasis. In both conditions, trypanosomes invade the CNS within the first days after inoculation and remain latent for long periods. Thereafter, the disease enters into a stage in which symptoms—fever, cervical lymphadenopathy (Winterbottom's sign), and hepatosplenomegaly—suggest reticuloendothelial activation. Then somnolence, apathy, involuntary movements and rigidity appear. Neurologic manifestations progress to dementia, stupor,

coma, and death. Although the West African and the East African forms of trypanosomiasis are similar, the former usually runs a more chronic course. Autopsy studies have shown diffuse gliosis; demyelination; and infiltrates of hypertrophied lymphocytes (Mott cells) involving the meninges, perivascular spaces, and brain parenchyma. During the initial stages, parasites may be isolated from blood, CSF, and lymph nodes. CSF examination may reveal moderate pleocytosis and the typical Mott cells. Chronic disease may be diagnosed by immune tests performed in serum or CSF. When CNS symptoms have appeared, therapy requires the use of melarsoprol, a toxic arsenical drug.

Cestode Infections

Coenurosis

Coenurosis is caused by *Coenurus cerebralis*, the larval stage of *Taenia multiceps*, the dog tapeworm. Its life cycle includes a canid as the definitive host and the sheep as the natural intermediate host. Humans who ingest dog feces contaminated with *T. multiceps* eggs become intermediate hosts of this cestode and acquire the disease. *C. cerebralis* is a cystic vesicle that includes a small larva with multiple scolices. Cysts are found in subcutaneous tissues, skeletal muscles, and the CNS. In the CNS, they are usually located at the base of the skull, where they induce arachnoiditis with obstruction of CSF transit and secondary hydrocephalus. Parenchymal brain involvement may also occur; these lesions are surrounded by an inflammatory infiltrate resulting from the host's reaction against the parasite. Seizures and focal signs occur in these cases. Focal signs may also be related to a brain infarct caused by inflammatory occlusion of leptomeningeal blood vessels. The CT findings include hydrocephalus and cystic or ring-enhancing lesions in the brain parenchyma or CSF cisterns. Diagnosis must be confirmed by biopsy of a brain lesion. There is no specific therapy for this condition.

Cysticercosis

Cysticercosis is caused by the larval stage of the tapeworm *Taenia solium*. Humans are the only definitive hosts of this cestode, whereas pigs are the natural intermediate hosts. The disease occurs when humans become intermediate hosts of *T. solium* by ingesting its eggs from contaminated food or through contact with feces of *T. solium* carriers. Cysticerci may invade almost every organ; however, the CNS is the most frequently affected.

Pathology

Cysticerci are liquid-filled vesicles consisting of two parts: a vesicular wall and a scolex. Parenchymal brain cysticerci are small and lodge in the cerebral cortex or the basal ganglia. Subarachnoid and ventricular cysticerci may attain a large size because of a mechanism of hydrophic degeneration. Spinal cysticerci may be found at both the cord parenchyma or the subarachnoid space. There are marked individual variations in the severity of the inflammatory reaction against cysticerci. Some parasites escape the host's immune detection, whereas others evoke an intense immune response causing both destruction of cysticerci and damage of the surrounding tissues. Common pathologic lesions related to cysticercosis are astrocytic gliosis, brain edema, arachnoiditis, hydrocephalus, and angiitis.

Clinical Manifestations

Seizures occur in up to 80% of patients with parenchymal brain cysts or calcifications; in endemic regions, the debut of seizures in otherwise healthy middle-aged individuals is suggestive of neurocysticercosis. Focal signs usually follow a subacute or chronic course, although they may occur abruptly in patients who develop a cerebral infarct as a complication of arachnoiditis. Intracranial hypertension occurs in up to 30% of patients; hydrocephalus and ventricular cysts are the most common causes of this syndrome. Intracranial hypertension usually has a subacute onset and a progressive course that may be punctuated by episodes of sudden loss of consciousness related to movements of the head (Bruns' syndrome) when the cause of hydrocephalus is a fourth ventricle cyst. Intracranial hypertension also occurs in patients with cysticercotic encephalitis, a severe form of the disease that occurs as the result of an intense immune response against massive cysticerci infection of the brain parenchyma. This condition is more frequent among children and young women. Clinical manifestations of spinal neurocysticercosis are nonspecific; spinal arachnoiditis is characterized by root pain and weakness of subacute onset, and cysts in the cord parenchyma usually course with motor and sensory deficits that vary according to the level of the lesion.

Diagnosis

CT scans provide objective evidence about the topography of cysticerci and the activity of the disease. Cystic lesions imaging the scolex (Figure 38C-2) and punctate calcifications are the most characteristic findings. Annular enhancing lesions, hydrocephalus, and abnormal enhancement of the leptomeninges are nonspecific and represent a diagnostic challenge. MRI is better than CT scanning for the recognition of brain stem, ventricular, and spinal cysts. A shortcoming of MRI, however, is its inability to detect small calcifications. Immunologic tests are a valuable complement to neuroimaging but should never be used alone to exclude or confirm the diagnosis. The most effective are the serum immunoblot and the CSF enzyme-linked immunosorbent assay (ELISA); however, some disappointing results have been reported with those tests because of cross-reactivity.

Therapy

Patients with parenchymal brain or subarachnoid cysts must be treated with albendazole (15 mg per kg per day for 8 days) or praziquantel (50 mg per kg per day for 15 days). These drugs result in disappearance of most cysts as well as in marked clinical improvement. Patients with calcifications should receive only symptomatic treatment. Ventricular cysts should be resected surgically. Cysticidal drugs may favor the occlusion of a blood vessel in patients with subarachnoid cysts or may worsen the brain edema accompanying cysticercotic encephalitis; administering corticosteroids is advised for the prevention of such complications. In addition, therapeutic priorities (shunts for hydrocephalus) must be considered before the use of cysticidal drugs.

Figure 38C-2. Contrast-enhanced computed tomographic scan showing characteristic cystic lesions of parenchymal brain cysticercosis. Hyperdense dots within the cysts represent the scolices.

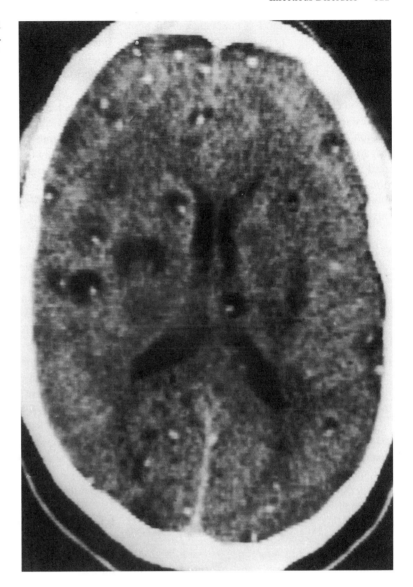

Echinococcosis (Hydatid Disease)

Hydatid disease is caused by larvae of cestodes of the genus *Echinococcus*. There are two different forms of hydatid disease: cystic hydatid disease, caused by *Echinococcus granulosus,* and alveolar hydatid disease, caused by *Echinococcus multilocularis*. Canids are the definitive hosts for *Echinococcus* species, and sheep or rodents are the intermediate hosts. Humans acquire the infection by ingesting food contaminated with eggs of these tapeworms. Echinococcal cysts can grow in the liver, the lungs, the heart, and the CNS. In the latter, the cysts may grow primarily or secondarily from metastatic dissemination of a developed visceral cyst.

Pathology

E. granulosus cysts are large, single, spherical, and well demarcated from the surrounding tissues, which do not show marked inflammation. In contrast, *E. multilocularis* cysts are small, tend to group in clusters, expand rapidly, elicit a severe immune reaction from the host, and tend to metastasize. In both species, the larvae may be found within the cysts.

Clinical Manifestations

Cystic and alveolar hydatid disease are characterized by seizures and progressive intracranial hypertension. Neurologic manifestations are more severe in patients with alveolar hydatid disease. Spinal cord involvement may be observed in both conditions; usual manifestations include root pain and motor or sensory deficits. Unilateral proptosis and diplopia occur in some patients with cystic hydatid disease of the orbit. In addition, primary hydatid cysts of the heart may embolize to the intracranial vascular bed and occlude a major cerebral artery with the subsequent development of a brain infarct.

Diagnosis

CT or MRI scans usually permit an accurate diagnosis of hydatid disease. Cystic hydatid disease is characterized by a large, spherical, nonenhancing, liquid-filled vesicle that is well demarcated from the surrounding brain parenchyma. Cysts are usually located within the brain parenchyma, although extradural cysts with bone erosion may occur. Lesions in alveolar hydatid disease are multiple and show abnormal contrast enhancement. Diagnosis by the Casoni's test or ELISA is not accurate because of cross-reactions with other parasites.

Therapy

Hydatid cysts were resected by surgery in the past. Reports suggest that albendazole (15 mg per kg per day for 28 days) destroys most of these cysts, obviating the hazards of transoperative rupture of a cyst. Albendazole is effective against both *E. granulosus* and *E. multilocularis* and may be used as the primary form of therapy, as prophylactic treatment before surgical resection of the cyst, or postoperatively to treat recurrent hydatid disease.

Sparganosis

Sparganosis is caused by the second-stage larvae of cestodes of the genus *Spirometra*. Dogs and cats are definitive hosts of this cestode, cyclops are the first intermediate hosts, and frogs and snakes are the second intermediate hosts. Humans acquire the infection by drinking water contaminated with cyclops harboring the larva or by eating infected frog or snake. After entering the body, the sparganum—a ribbon-shaped motile worm—migrates to skeletal muscles or subcutaneous tissue, where it produces slowly growing nodules. The larva also migrates through the foramina of the skull base and vertebral column to invade the brain parenchyma, the subarachnoid space, or the spinal canal. The tissue surrounding the parasite shows inflammatory changes. Focal necrosis along the tracks of migration of these larvae is a common finding. Cerebral sparganosis presents with seizures or focal signs of subacute onset. CT findings are usually confined to one cerebral hemisphere and include multifocal areas of low density within the subcortical white matter, focal cortical atrophy, ipsilateral ventricular enlargement, spotty calcifications, and enhancing nodules that may change in location on sequential scans. Diagnosis rests on the direct visualization of the parasite from a brain biopsy. Surgical resection of the parasite is the treatment of choice.

Nematode Infections

Angiostrongyliasis

Infection with *Angiostrongylus cantonensis*, the rat lung worm, is common in Southeast Asia and Oceania. Rats are the usual definitive hosts of this nematode and snails and slugs are intermediate hosts. Humans are infected by eating raw snails or vegetables contaminated with rat feces. Once ingested, the larva migrates to the CNS, where it induces an intense eosinophilic meningitis. Occasionally, migrating larvae induce hemorrhagic tracts within the brain parenchyma. Headache is usually the first and most prominent complaint of this condition, although cranial nerve palsies occur in some patients. CSF examination reveals pleocytosis (up to 2,000 cells per µl) with 20–70% eosinophils; protein levels are increased but glucose levels are normal. Neuroimaging studies usually appear normal. Angiostrongyliasis is a benign, self-limited condition. In some cases, CSF drainage results in relief of symptoms.

Gnathostomiasis

Gnathostomiasis primarily affects subcutaneous tissues. CNS involvement, albeit rare, is its most severe complication. Dogs and cats are definitive hosts of *Gnathostoma spinigerum*, cyclops are the first intermediate hosts, and many animal species are the second intermediate hosts. Humans become infected by eating undercooked fish or poultry contaminated with larvae of this nematode. This highly motile larva migrates to the spinal canal and then to the brain, leaving necrotic tracts along nerve roots, the spinal cord, the subarachnoid space, and the brain parenchyma. This explains the most common manifestations of gnathostomiasis, including radiculitis, transverse myelitis, meningitis, and subarachnoid or parenchymal brain hemorrhages. The latter occur in up to 30% of patients with cerebral gnathostomiasis and are the most lethal complication of the disease. Autopsy studies of some of these cases have shown the larvae at the end of long hemorrhagic tracts extending from the basal ganglia to the lower brain stem. Diagnosis should be suspected in patients who develop a progressive eosinophilic meningitis associated with focal signs and CT evidence of multiple parenchymal brain hemorrhages. Although albendazole is effective for the subcutaneous form of the disease, there are no studies on medical therapy for cerebral gnathostomiasis.

Strongyloidiasis

Strongyloides stercoralis inhabits the human intestinal tract. Under normal conditions, this nematode does not invade the CNS. However, disseminated disease may occur when the host's immune mechanisms fail to control the normal cycle of autoinfection (hyperinfection syndrome). CNS involvement is the most severe complication of such dissemination and may occur as the direct result of larval invasion of the CNS or may be secondary to recurrent bacteremias associated with migration of the larvae. Cerebral infarcts and brain abscesses have been reported in patients with disseminated strongyloidiasis. Definitive diagnosis of disseminated strongyloidiasis requires identification of the larvae in CSF or tissue specimens. However, the disease should be suspected in immunosuppressed patients who develop meningitis, focal neurologic signs, or acute encephalopathy. Mortality from disseminated strongyloidiasis is high, although some patients have improved with thiabendazole.

Toxocariasis

Toxocariasis is caused by nematodes of the genus *Toxocara*. Humans acquire the infection by ingesting soil contaminated with dog or cat feces containing *Toxocara* eggs. After ingestion, eggs mature into larvae that migrate to the tissues of the host, producing a disease called *visceral larva migrans*. The pathogenesis of brain damage in toxocariasis is related to the passage of migrating larvae through the brain parenchyma, leaving necrotic tracks or to the inflammatory response that develops around inert larvae. Usual manifestations include subacute encephalitis, parenchymal brain granulomas, or cerebral infarcts. Diagnosis may be suspected in patients with positive findings on toxocara ELISA or indirect hemagglutination assay. Therapy is symptomatic, although diethylcarbamazine (250 mg per day for 4 weeks) has been used with success in some cases.

Trichinosis

Trichinosis occurs after ingestion of undercooked pork meat contaminated with larvae of *Trichinella spiralis*. Larvae enter the bloodstream and encyst in skeletal muscle. Trichinosis is usually asymptomatic; however, severe forms with cardiac and neurologic manifestations may occur. CNS involvement is characterized by meningoencephalitis or stroke. Stroke subtypes include hemorrhagic infarcts related to venous thrombosis and subcortical infarcts caused by small artery disease. The pathogenesis of trichinosis-induced stroke is not well understood. Although it has been argued that migrating larval emboli are responsible for occlusion of cerebral vessels, recent studies suggest that hypereosinophilia is responsible for these vascular lesions. The latter is supported by the parallelism between the cardiac and neurologic manifestations of trichinosis and those of the idiopathic hypereosinophilic syndrome and by the fact that both cardiac and cerebral ischemic disease occur during the acute phase of trichinosis when eosinophilia is prominent. Eosinophils may directly induce vascular occlusion through a prothrombotic effect or may damage the vascular endothelium after being stimulated by cytokines produced in response to *T. spiralis* infection. Diagnosis of neurotrichinosis should be considered in patients who, besides a cerebral infarct, have fever, myalgia, periorbital edema, and peripheral eosinophilia. Support for the diagnosis is provided by the presence of anti-*Trichinella* antibodies or by the identification of the parasite in muscle tissue. Administering corticosteroids is advised in order to suppress the eosinophilic-induced vascular damage.

Trematode Infections

Paragonimiasis

Paragonimiasis is caused by lung flukes of the genus *Paragonimus* (*Paragonimus westermani, Paragonimus mexicanus, Paragonimus shrjabini*). Humans acquire the disease by ingesting larvae in contaminated raw or undercooked freshwater crabs or crayfish. Thereafter, these larvae enter the peritoneal cavity and migrate to the lungs. Further migration of the worms through the foramina of the skull base to the CNS may occur. CNS involvement is characterized by meningitis, granulomatous or calcified parenchymal brain lesions, and cerebral hemorrhages.

Clinical Manifestations

The meningitic form of the disease may be associated with focal signs of sudden onset related to small cerebral infarcts, which are caused by *Paragonimus*-induced endarteritis. Parenchymal brain lesions produce seizures, focal signs, and intracranial hypertension. Cerebral hemorrhages may occur along the track of a larva's migration or as the result of the necrotizing vasculitis that develops during early granuloma formation.

Diagnosis and Therapy

Diagnosis of CNS paragonimiasis is suggested by the presence of specific antibodies in the CSF or by CT findings of multiple calcifications located in the temporal and occipital lobes that resemble "soap bubbles." Support for the diagnosis is provided by demonstration of *Paragonimus* eggs in sputum because most patients have pulmonary disease. Therapy includes praziquantel (25 mg per kg per day for 1 week) and corticosteroids.

Schistosomiasis

Schistosomiasis is caused by trematodes of the species *Schistosoma* (*Schistosoma japonicum, Schistosoma mansoni, Schistosoma haematobium*). Humans are definitive hosts for these parasites, which enter the body through the skin after aquatic exposure to their larval forms. After maturation, the larvae migrate and settle, as adult worms, in the mesenteric veins. CNS schistosomiasis occurs when larvae migrate to the spinal cord or the cerebral vasculature. A diversity of neurologic manifestations may occur, mainly related to the *Schistosoma* species and the location of parasites; *S. japonicum* almost always affects the brain. In contrast, the other two species usually affect the spinal cord and occasionally the brain.

Schistosoma japonicum *Schistosomiasis*

Acute infection may produce diffuse meningoencephalitis with fever (Katayama fever), seizures, visual loss, neck stiffness, disorientation, and stupor. Chronic disease produces seizures, focal signs, and intracranial hypertension related to the development of parenchymal brain granulomas. Parenchymal brain and subarachnoid hemorrhages occur in some patients; they are related to segmental damage of small leptomeningeal or parenchymal blood vessels induced by the parasites.

Schistosoma mansoni *and* Schistosoma haematobium *Schistosomiasis*

Transverse myelitis related to inflammatory necrosis of the spinal cord is the most common manifestation of these forms of the disease and represents a common cause of paraplegia in endemic areas. Schistosomal transverse myelitis usually affects the lower cord and is characterized by flaccid paraplegia associated with sphincter dysfunction and sensory loss. In addition, granulomatous masses may involve the conus medullaris and cauda equina;

they cause pain in the lower back, saddle anesthesia, sphincter dysfunction, and weakness in the lower limbs. Occasionally, acute paraplegia has resulted from occlusion of the anterior spinal artery by the parasite.

Diagnosis and Therapy

CSF analysis usually shows mild mononuclear pleocytosis and increased protein contents. CT scans may show enhancing lesions in patients with *S. japonicum* schistosomiasis, and CT myelography or MRI scans reveal enlargement of the lower spinal cord in some patients with spinal schistosomiasis. Up to 75% of patients with spinal cord involvement have specific antibodies detected by ELISA. Examination of stool or urine specimens for schistosomal eggs is helpful when positive, but its absence does not exclude the diagnosis. Praziquantel (40–60 mg per kg in 3 doses for 1 day) is effective for patients with brain or spinal cord involvement. Corticosteroids are advised to ameliorate the process of endarteritis, which may cause further brain and spinal cord damage.

Suggested Reading

Cameron ML, Durack DT. Helminthic Infections. In WM Scheld, RJ Whitley, DT Durack (eds), Infections of the Central Nervous System (2nd ed). Philadelphia: Lippincott–Raven, 1997:845.

Chang KH, Chi JG, Cho SY, et al. Cerebral sparganosis: analysis of 34 cases with emphasis on CT features. Neuroradiology 1992;34:1.

Ciurea AV, Vasilescu G, Nuteanu L, Carp N. Cerebral hydatid disease in children. Experience of 27 cases. Childs Nerv Syst 1995;11:679.

Del Brutto OH, Sotelo J. Neurocysticercosis: an update. Rev Infect Dis 1988;10:1075.

Del Brutto OH, Sotelo J, Roman GC. Therapy for neurocysticercosis: a reappraisal. Clin Infect Dis 1993;17:730.

Fourestie V, Douceron H, Brugieres P, et al. Neurotrichinosis. A cerebrovascular disease associated with myocardial injury and hypereosinophilia. Brain 1993;116:603.

Haribhai HC, Bhigjee AI, Bill PLA, et al. Spinal cord schistosomiasis. A clinical, laboratory and radiological study, with a note on therapeutic aspects. Brain 1991;114:709.

Hung T-P, Chen E-R. Paragonimiasis of the central nervous system. Neurol Infect Epidemiol 1996;1:11.

Liu LX, Weller PF. Antiparasitic drugs. N Engl J Med 1996;334:1178.

Punyagupta S, Bunnag T, Juttijudata P, Rosen L. Eosinophilic meningitis in Thailand. Epidemiologic studies of 484 typical cases and the etiologic role of *Angiostrongylus cantonensis*. Am J Trop Med Hyg 1970;19:950.

Scrimgeour EM, Gajdusek DC. Involvement of the central nervous system in *Schistosoma mansoni* and *S. haematobium* infection. A review. Brain 1985;108:1023.

Simon MW, Wilson HD. The amebic meningoencephalitides. Pediatr Infect Dis 1986;5:562.

Villanueva MS. Trypanosomiasis of the central nervous system. Semin Neurol 1993;13:209.

Warrell DA. Cerebral Malaria. In RA Shakir, PK Newman, CM Poser (eds), Tropical Neurology. London: Saunders, 1996;213–245.

Weller PF, Liu LX. Eosinophilic meningitis. Semin Neurol 1993;13:161.

D. Acquired Immunodeficiency Syndrome and the Nervous System

Philippe Vuadens and Julien Bogousslavsky

Chapter Plan

Neuromuscular diseases
    Peripheral neuropathies
    Myopathies
Central nervous system diseases
    Spinal cord diseases
    Focal central nervous system disorders
    Meningitis
    Acquired immunodeficiency syndrome dementia
    complex
Antiretroviral agents and combination therapy

The nervous system is often involved in the course of human immunodeficiency virus (HIV) infection, not only by diseases that are related to immune dysfunction but also by direct effects of the retrovirus. The involvement of the nervous system may occur at each stage of HIV infection, from seroconversion to acquired immunodeficiency syndrome (AIDS), and various neurologic disorders can appear in the peripheral or central nervous system (CNS). The percentage of AIDS-related neurologic complications rises as immunocompetence decreases.

In this chapter, the main neurologic complications of HIV infection are discussed and divided in two sections according to their neuroanatomic location: central or peripheral lesions.

Neuromuscular Diseases

Neuromuscular diseases occur in 30–50% of HIV patients. Sometimes they can be masked by coexistent CNS disorders, such as focal brain lesions, myelopathy, or AIDS dementia complex (ADC). The prevalence of peripheral complications will probably increase as more appropriate medicaments for HIV and opportunistic infections lengthen survival (Table 38D-1).

Peripheral Neuropathies

Different forms of peripheral neuropathies occur during HIV disease. Their rate increases proportionately as immunosuppression increases. They can be the first manifestation of the disease (Figure 38D-1).

Inflammatory Demyelinating Polyneuropathy

Inflammatory demyelinating polyneuropathy is common in the early stages of HIV infection (seroconversion) and in patients who are seropositive but asymptomatic. The acute form is clinically similar to Guillain-Barré syndrome (GBS), which is characterized by rapidly ascending weakness of the limbs with areflexia and sometimes bilateral facial weakness. The sensory features are usually mild. The evolution is similar to that of typical GBS. Electrophysiologic studies confirm conduction blocks, prolonged F-wave latencies, and signs of demyelinization. Cerebrospinal fluid (CSF) analysis reveals a lymphocytic pleocytosis of 15–50 cells per μl, with an elevated protein level (50–250 mg per dl).

The subacute or chronic forms are more frequent and are distinguished by a slower course that may be monophasic or relapsing, predominantly producing motor weakness. They generally occur with the decline in the CD4 cell count. The motor deficit is diffuse or patchy with minor sensory deficits.

The prognosis for HIV patients with acute or chronic demyelinating polyneuropathies is similar to that for seronegative patients. It is usually excellent in 1–6 months, even without specific treatment, in patients with the acute form. Specific treatments include steroids, plasmapheresis, or intravenous immunoglobulin.

Mononeuropathy Multiplex

Mononeuropathy multiplex is characterized by asymmetric or proximal lesions of the peripheral nerves that occur in association with a CD4 cell count of more than 200 per μl. In advanced immunosuppression with a CD4 cell count of less than 50 per μl, a more extensive form of mononeuropathy multiplex may develop that involves several peripheral nerves and numerous cranial nerves.

Among the cranial nerves, the facial nerve is the most frequently involved, and in all stages of HIV disease the result is similar to that seen in Bell's palsy. In the upper limb, the ulnar nerve is usually

Table 38D-1. Timing of Peripheral Neuropathies

Syndrome	Asymptomatic	AIDS Stage
AIDP	++	+
CIDP	++	+
Mononeuropathy multiplex	–	+
Distal symmetrical polyneuropathy	Sometimes	++
Autonomic neuropathy	–	++
Toxic neuropathy	+	+
Polyradiculopathy	–	++

AIDS = acquired immunodeficiency syndrome; AIDP = acute inflammatory demyelinating neuropathy; CIDP = chronic inflammatory neuropathy; + = present; – = absent; ++ = more frequent.

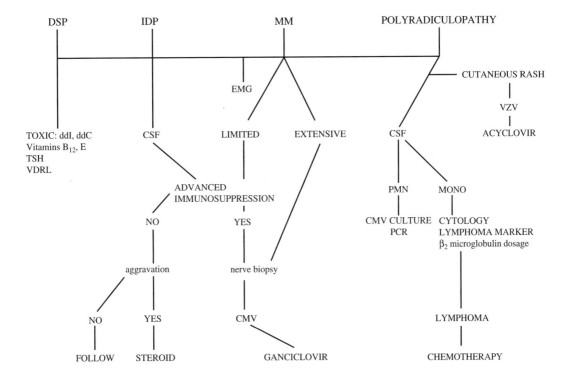

Figure 38D-1. Algorithm for the management of human immunodeficiency virus-related neuropathy. (DSP = distal sensory neuropathy; IDP = inflammatory demyelinating polyneuropathy; MM = mononeuritis multiplex; CMV = cytomegalovirus; VZV = varicella-zoster virus; PMN = polymorphonuclear cell; MONO = mononuclear cell; PCR = polymerase chain reaction; CSF = cerebrospinal fluid; EMG = electromyography; TSH = thyroid-stimulating hormone; ddI = didanosine; ddC = zalcitabine. (Adapted from D Simpson, RK Olmey. Peripheral Neuropathies Associated with Human Immunodeficiency Virus Infection. In PJ Dick [ed], Peripheral Neuropathies: New Concepts and Treatments. Philadelphia: Saunders, 1992;685–711.)

the first nerve to be injured; in the lower limb it is the femoral or sciatic nerve.

The diagnosis is not always easy when the symptoms begin, but the asymmetric presentation of the lesions is a good criterion for diagnosis. CSF analysis reveals a lymphocytic pleocytosis with a high protein level. Electrophysiologic studies show focal or multifocal axonal lesions that are usually asymmetric. Sometimes there is an overlap with a distal symmetric polyneuropathy. Different patterns of nerve biopsy abnormalities are described. An axonal degeneration is present with polymorphonuclear infiltrates. Necrotizing arteritis is less common.

The evolution varies, but usually spontaneous remission occurs, especially if the CD4 cell count is higher than 50 per μl. When recovery is incomplete, steroids, plasmapheresis, or immunoglobulin may be warranted.

In every case of mononeuropathy multiplex, cytomegalovirus (CMV) or varicella zoster infections must be excluded. Patients with systemic CMV infection (retinitis, gastroenteritis, or pulmonary disease) are more susceptible to mononeuropathy multiplex. A few authors recommend empiric therapy for CMV even in the absence of proof of CMV infection in severely immunosuppressed patients.

Distal Symmetric Polyneuropathy

Distal symmetric polyneuropathy is the most frequent neuropathy seen in HIV disease. Usually, it is subclinical and becomes symptomatic during the stages of AIDS-related complex or AIDS. It is usually a painful sensorimotor polyneuropathy. The major symptoms are paresthesias and dysesthesias in the lower extremities. The upper limbs are usually affected later. Diminution or abolition of tendon reflexes is an invariable sign. Sensation is always affected more than motor function in the distal segments of the limbs, more in the legs than in the arms. Vibratory sense is involved more than position and tactile senses. Pinprick and temperature sensation are disturbed in a stocking-and-glove distribution. Weakness is generally limited to the foot muscles.

The electrophysiologic features of this type of polyneuropathy are similar to those of other axonal forms of distal polyneuropathies. Small or absent sural nerve potentials are the most frequent abnormalities. Sural nerve biopsy specimens demonstrate axonal degeneration and vasculitis. HIV has never

been isolated from sural nerve by culture. The etiology remains uncertain. Spreading from the dorsal root ganglia to distal nerves by HIV seems plausible, but vasculitic components in the nerves suggest an immunoallergic reaction. Nutritional and toxic factors also play important roles.

Treatment is only limited to modifying the pain level with amitriptyline or carbamazepine. Specific antiviral agents such as zidovudine (AZT) do not seem to improve the polyneuropathy.

Autonomic Neuropathy

Symptomatic autonomic neuropathy is infrequent, although subclinical abnormalities are common in HIV disease. Parasympathetic disturbances include tachycardia, urinary dysfunction, and impotence. Sympathetic failure accounts for orthostatic hypotension, faintness, diarrhea, and anhidrosis. The risk for symptomatic autonomic abnormalities occurs late in HIV disease.

Many factors contribute to the autonomic disturbances: malnutrition and dehydration, drugs used in the treatment of HIV-associated complications, and both peripheral and CNS abnormalities. Treatment is limited to the relief of symptoms by the management of the fluid and electrolyte imbalance and antiarrhythmic agents.

Toxic Neuropathy

Toxic neuropathies are frequently associated with antiretroviral treatment. 2',3'-Dideoxycytidine (ddC) and dideoxyinosine (ddI) induce a painful polyneuropathy with sensory deficit, usually after several weeks of treatment and especially with high doses. Symptoms typically begin with paresthesias, dysesthesias, and pain in the feet with crescent intensity. The clinical picture is very similar to that of HIV-associated distal polyneuropathy, but the fingers are more often involved. Toxic polyneuropathy related to stavudine therapy has also been reported. Vitamin deficiencies, especially of vitamins B_{12} and E, may also induce a polyneuropathy, as can antimicrobial agents such as isoniazid, metronidazole, dapsone, or nitrofurantoin.

Polyradiculopathy and Myeloradiculopathy

The clinical features of polyradiculopathy and myeloradiculopathy are characterized by radicular pain and paresthesias in a cauda equina distribution associated with rapidly progressive paraparesis and sphincter disturbances. Sometimes the upper limbs or cranial nerves can be involved.

Electrodiagnostic studies demonstrate proximal axonal disease in lumbar nerve roots with widespread denervation in the lower limbs and paraspinal muscles. These features allow polyradiculopathy to be differentiated from distal polyneuropathy or mononeuropathy multiplex. On magnetic resonance imaging (MRI) scans, the inflammation of lumbar nerve roots can sometimes be visualized. The CSF analysis is characterized by elevated protein levels, marked polymorphonuclear pleocytosis (15–2,000 cells per µl), and often hypoglycorrhachia. Pathologic findings are inflammation and necrosis of ventral and dorsal nerve roots. The necrosis spreads progressively and focal myelitis may appear.

The diagnosis of polyradiculopathy must be prompt. This type of neurologic complication occurs when CD4 cell counts are very low, usually in the AIDS stage when opportunistic diseases have already occurred. Considerable evidence suggests that that many polyradiculopathies result from CMV infection. Therefore, 50% of CSF culture results are positive for CMV. Even if these results are negative, all patients must be promptly treated with ganciclovir or foscarnet because of high mortality. This is especially important when CSF results reveal marked polymorphonuclear pleocytosis. Other conditions can also induce AIDS-associated polyradiculopathy: neurosyphilis, lymphomatous meningitis, toxoplasmosis, and herpes group and varicella zoster infections.

Myopathies

Myopathies can occur in all stages of HIV disease and can be the first manifestation of the disease. HIV infection and its treatment are sometimes associated with myopathies and there are many causes.

Human Immunodeficiency Virus–Associated Polymyositis

The predominant clinical feature in HIV-associated polymyositis is a progressive proximal muscle weakness associated with myalgia in 25–50% of cases. Typically, patients have difficulty in rising from a chair or climbing stairs. The neurologic examination reveals symmetric proximal paresis with prominent involvement of hip flexors and the neck.

The serum creatine kinase (CK) level is high in more than 90% of cases. The level does not correlate with weakness but with myonecrosis. Myopathic electromyographic results are characterized by brief, small, and polyphasic motor unit potentials with fibrillation potentials. The most common histopathologic finding is scattered myofiber degeneration with occasional inflammatory infiltrates but without vasculitis. In a few cases, rod bodies myopathy is discovered, which is characterized by atrophy of type I fibers with intracytoplasmic rod bodies of nemaline without inflammatory infiltrates.

The pathogenesis is unknown, but immune mechanisms have been evoked because antigens have been demonstrated in macrophages invading muscle. HIV itself has never been detected in muscle biopsy specimens. HIV-associated myopathy may be treated with corticosteroids, like idiopathic polymyositis, but this treatment should be used cautiously because of the risk of further immunosuppression.

Rarely, other opportunistic infections can be detected in muscles of HIV patients. These include toxoplasmosis, CMV, microsporidia, *Cryptococcus neoformans, Mycobacterium avium,* and *Staphylococcus aureus.* Often the clinical features are those of focal myositis.

Myopathy Related to Zidovudine Treatment

Since 1987, with the introduction of zidovudine, many authors have reported cases of myopathy caused by zidovudine toxicity. This type of manifestation occurs in 10% of treated patients, the rate increasing with the length of treatment. The clinical features are characterized by proximal weakness, myalgia, and elevated serum CK levels. Muscle biopsy specimens reveal mitochondrial dysfunction with ragged-red fibers and cytochrome *c* oxidase deficiency, but the significance of these histologic abnormalities is unclear, because zidovudine-treated patients can be asymptomatic with ragged-red fibers in muscle biopsy specimens.

The management of patients with zidovudine toxicity is dose reduction or withdrawal. The percentage of improvement after zidovudine withdrawal varies from 20% to 100% in different studies. If no amelioration is gained, a diagnosis of polymyositis must be sought through muscle biopsy, and corticosteroid treatment must be initiated.

Muscle Wasting Syndrome

Diffuse wasting of muscles may occur in HIV-infected patients with weight loss and chronic muscle weakness, without systemic or nutritional factors. According to the Centers for Disease Control and Prevention, the clinical criteria of this syndrome must associate weight loss (more than 10%) plus chronic diarrhea (more than 30 days) or chronic weakness and fever (more than 30 days). High cytokine levels may play a role in this muscular wasting. In every case, an opportunistic infection must be ruled out (CMV, cryptosporidiosis, microsporidiosis, *Pneumocystis carinii*). When the weight loss involves the lipid mass, nutritive supplements are proposed. In the presence of predominant muscle wasting, testosterone is recommended and a substitution introduced in case of a low level. If the testosterone level is normal, therapy with growth hormone or anti–tumor necrosis factor agents may be useful.

Myopathy Associated with Vasculitis

Various vasculitides can occur in HIV-infected patients, including necrotizing vasculitis, rheumatoid purpura of Henoch-Schönlein, and hypersensitivity vasculitis.

Myasthenia Gravis

A few cases of myasthenia gravis have been reported in HIV patients, although this association may be fortuitous.

Central Nervous System Diseases

Spinal Cord Diseases

Spinal cord disease is frequently found at autopsy in AIDS patients. Several causes must be considered, either related to HIV or to other infections.

Vacuolar Myelopathy

Typically, vacuolar myelopathy occurs in the AIDS stage, involving clinically 5–10% of AIDS patients. However, at autopsy it is present in up 50% of patients. Symptomatic patients develop a slowly progressive spastic paraparesis, gait ataxia, and impaired sensation, sometimes with urinary incontinence. The ataxia is related to loss of joint position sense. There is no sensory level, but a sensory neuropathy is frequently associated.

The diagnosis is one of exclusion. The CSF is nondiagnostic, and MRI scans usually appear normal. The pathologic modifications include a degeneration of the lateral and posterior columns of the spinal cord with spongy degeneration and intramyelin vacuolation. The vacuoles contain lipid-laden macrophages. The pathogenesis remains uncertain. The direct role of HIV has not been proved. Moreover, the pattern of vacuolar myelopathy resembles the subacute degeneration of the spinal cord resulting from vitamin B_{12} deficiency, but the vitamin level is normal. Antiretroviral therapy has little efficacy against this myelopathy.

Herpes Group–Associated Myelitis

The herpesvirus group (herpes zoster, herpes simplex, CMV) may produce a spinal cord syndrome. Varicella-zoster virus typically induces dermatomal vesicular rash, followed 1–3 weeks later by a myelitis. Patients rapidly develop paraplegia with sensory loss. The pathologic features include inflammation and ischemic infarction, which can evolve to hemorrhagic and necrotic lesions. The diagnosis is established by identification of skin lesions, demonstration of virus in CSF cultures, or serologic or polymerase chain reaction (PCR) findings.

At the spinal level, CMV infection produces a progressive polyradiculomyelopathy, initially characterized by lower extremity and sacral paresthesias and followed by a progressive and ascending paraparesis with sensory loss and bowel and urinary dysfunctions. It generally occurs in patients with advanced HIV infection (CD4 cell count of less than 50 cells per μl). The CSF reveals a polymorphonuclear pleocytosis and positive CMV cultures. MRI scans may show enhancement of nerve roots or spinal cord hyperintensities. Herpes simplex virus may also cause myelitis, and it is often associated with CMV infection.

Compressive lesions of the spinal cord include lymphomas; toxoplasmosis; and abscesses caused by bacteria, fungi, or mycobacteria. Rare cases of syphilitic myelitis are reported and cord infarction may occur in patients with vasculitis.

Focal Central Nervous System Disorders

The most frequent focal affliction of the brain in HIV-infected patients is toxoplasmosis, followed by primary cerebral lymphoma and progressive multifocal leukoencephalopathy (PML). Often these afflictions are indistinguishable on clinical examination (Table 38D-2). Less common causes of focal lesions include *Candida* abscess, *Nocardia* abscess, syphilitic gumma, cryptococcoma, fungal or parasitic abscess, and vascular lesions.

Toxoplasmosis

Toxoplasmosis is the most common focal neurologic complication in HIV disease, occurring in about 30% of patients when immunosuppression is lower than 50 CD4 cells per μl. It is also the most frequent cause of intracerebral mass lesions occurring in association with HIV disease. It occurs as a consequence of infection with *Toxoplasma gondii*, a protozoan. In almost all cases, *Toxoplasma* encephalitis results in a recrudescence of infection rather than a new infection.

The neurologic symptoms are generally focal and associated with a global encephalopathy. They depend on the location of the lesions. The first signs are headache, fever, malaise, and confusion, arising over the course of 1–2 weeks. Focal signs of CNS involvement are hemiparesis, brain stem or cerebellar features, epileptic seizures, chorea, lethargy, and rarely myelitis or medullary cona syndrome. The course of the illness is subacute, ranging from 1 to 2 weeks. A prodrome and malaise for several days before the onset of the neurologic signs are not always observed, and focal signs can represent the first manifestation of toxoplasmosis.

CT or MRI scans usually reveal multiple nodular lesions, sometimes ring enhanced with edema and mass effect (Figure 38D-2). The lesions are very often localized in the basal ganglia or the frontoparietal lobes. Although not specific, MRI is more sensitive than CT scanning in demonstrating focal lesions.

CSF results are also nonspecific but often abnormal. An elevation of the CSF protein level is seen in the majority of cases, and a mononuclear pleocytosis (fewer than 100 cells per μl) occurs in one-third of cases. Rarely, mild hypoglycorrhachia is noted. Serologic examination and CSF antibodies are rarely diagnostic. These tests fail to distinguish between acute and chronic infection. The probability of demonstrating seronegative *Toxoplasma* infection is probably more important in patients with advanced immunosuppression. It therefore is very useful to evaluate the *Toxoplasma* serostatus of HIV patients early in their course. Prophylaxis is recommended for *Toxoplasma*-seropositive patients with CD4 cell counts of fewer than 200 per μl. Buffy coat or PCR examination of the CSF can help to detect *T. gondii*, but the sensitivity is still poor.

When doubt remains, brain biopsy is the best means for confirming the diagnosis of cerebral toxoplasmosis. Before a surgical procedure is used, the algorithm that has been developed to help manage these patients should be applied (Figure 38D-3). A 2-week trial of antitoxoplasmosis therapy is recommended. If clinical improvement is obtained, toxoplasmosis is confirmed and the treatment is continued. If there is no clinical and radiologic improvement, brain biopsy should be performed.

The therapy is oral pyrimethamine, 150 mg as an initial dose followed by 75 mg per day, and sulfadiazine, 6–8 g per day divided into four doses, associated with 5 mg folinic acid. Clindamycin (600 mg four times a day) and pyrimethamine are an effective alternative treatment. Other therapeutic possibilities include azithromycin, clarithromycin, doxycycline, and atovaquone. After 6 weeks of this initial treatment, maintenance therapy must be continued life-long with trimethoprim-sulfamethoxazole (three tablets per week). The dose must be adapted to the severity of immunosuppression. The prognosis is usually poor, with mean survivals ranging from 120 to 265 days. It is correlated with mental function at the time therapy is introduced.

Table 38D-2. Clinical and Radiologic Differentiation of Central Nervous System Diseases in Human Immunodeficiency Virus Infection

	Clinical Findings				Radiologic Findings			
	Presentation	Consciousness	Fever/Headache	Focal Signs	Number of Lesions	Pattern	Enhancement	Location
AIDS dementia complex	Weeks/months	Normal	–	–	Diffuse	Ill-defined	–	White matter
Toxoplasmosis	<2 weeks	Decreased	+	+++	One to many	Ring mass	++	Basal ganglia
Lymphoma	2–8 weeks	Decreased or normal	–	+	One to many	Solid mass	+++	Periventricular
PML	Weeks/months	Normal	–	++	One to many	No mass	–	White matter
Cryptococcus	<2 weeks	Decreased	+++	–	One to many	Punctuate	–	Basal ganglia
Cytomegalovirus	<2 weeks	Decreased or normal	+	–	One to many	Confluent	++	Periventricular

– = absent; + = mild; ++ = moderate; +++ = severe; AIDS = acquired immunodeficiency syndrome; PML = progressive multifocal leukoencephalopathy.

Source: Modified from JC McArthur. HIV-Associated Dementia. In Annual Course of the American Academy of Neurology (Vol 5). Boston: American Academy of Neurology, 1995:228-9–228-25.

Figure 38D-2. Two nodular enhancing focal lesions caused by toxoplasmosis.

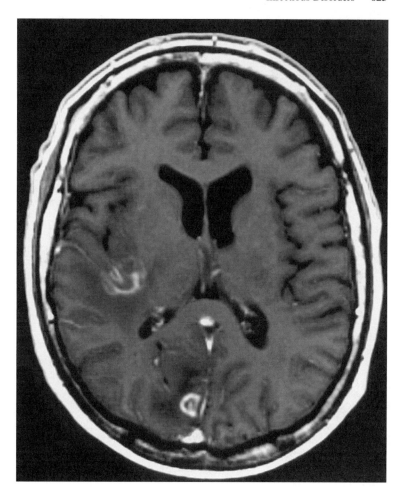

Primary Central Nervous System Lymphoma

Lymphoma usually develops late in HIV patients when CD4 cell counts are fewer than 100 cells per μl. The presence of Epstein-Barr virus is very often detected in tissue. The clinical presentation is mainly characterized by headache, mental changes, seizures, or focal deficits. Patients are sometimes confused and lethargic and have memory loss.

Radiologic studies show single or multiple homogeneous, contrast-enhancing lesions (Figure 38D-4). The lesions are multiple in 60–80% of cases. It is often difficult to differentiate between lymphoma or toxoplasmosis. Thallium-201 single-photon emission computed tomography scanning or fluorodeoxyglucose positron emission tomography scanning can help in distinguishing between them because the radioisotope is taken up by lymphoma-

tous cells. Stereotactic biopsy helps to definitively confirm the diagnosis definitively.

The prognosis is poor, with a median survival of less than 1 month for untreated patients. Radiation therapy may prolong life by 4–6 months. The possibility of using chemotherapy depends on the underlying immunodeficiency status and the risk of opportunistic infections.

Other CNS tumors can occur in HIV patients, but their incidence does not increase in HIV populations as compared with non-HIV populations. Kaposi's sarcoma rarely involves the nervous system, but metastatic lesions can develop in the brain.

Progressive Multifocal Leukoencephalopathy

PML results from JC virus, a human papillomavirus, and occurs in 2–3% of AIDS patients. It is

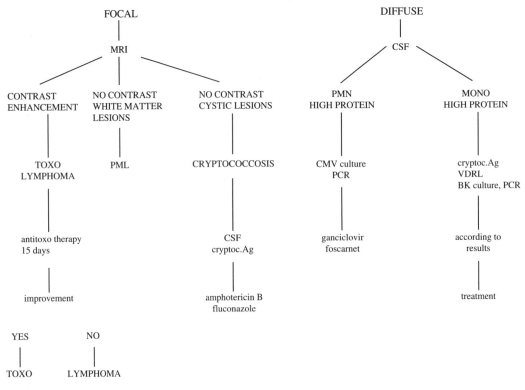

Figure 38D-3. Algorithm for management of human immunodeficiency virus patients with focal or diffuse features. This algorithm is not exhaustive. (MRI = magnetic resonance imaging; CSF = cerebrospinal fluid; PMN = polymorphonuclear cell; PCR = polymerase chain reaction; TOXO = toxoplasmosis; PML = progressive multifocal leukoencephalopathy; cryptoc = cryptococcosis; CMV = cytomegalovirus; MONO = mononuclear cell; BK = mycobacterium; antitoxo = antitoxoplasmosis.)

a subacute, progressive, demyelinating disease that can be the presenting manifestation of AIDS. The clinical picture is progressive over weeks and generally begins with limb weakness. Cognitive dysfunction or visual field defects are also very common, followed by gait disturbance, limb incoordination, speech disorders, and headache. Although focal presentations are the rule, a subacute dementia characterizes the course of illness in occasional cases.

The CSF is usually normal, but mild abnormalities have been described. CT scans typically reveal nonenhancing, hypodense lesions in the white matter, predominantly in the parieto-occipital region and the cerebellum; these lesions are without mass effect. An MRI scan is more sensitive in demonstrating these lesions (Figure 38D-5). The specificity and sensitivity of PCR in detecting virus in the CSF are not optimal in all laboratories; however,

generally the clinical and radiologic features are characteristic enough to confirm the diagnosis, and biopsy is not necessary in most cases.

There is no effective treatment for PML and the survival varies between 1 and 4 months after diagnosis. A few cases have a prolonged survival (more than 1 year). Different treatments, such as cytosine arabinoside, adenosine arabinoside, interferon-alpha, and DNA intercalators, have been proposed, but their efficacy remains to be proved.

Meningitis

Aseptic Meningitis

Retrospective studies suggest an incidence of aseptic meningitis in HIV patients of between 5% and 10% of cases. It especially occurs during the

Figure 38D-4. Enhancing focal mass lesion prominently surrounded by edema caused by cerebral lymphoma.

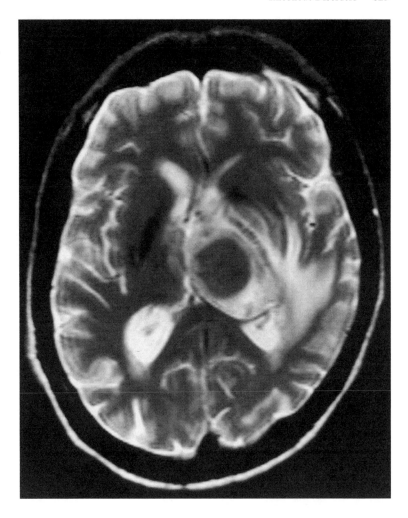

asymptomatic phase of HIV infection. It often is the manifestation of seroconversion (30–40% of cases), associated with a mononucleosis-like syndrome. The clinical picture includes headache, fever, malaise, and moderate meningismus. Involvement of the cranial nerves may sometimes be present. The CSF reveals a moderate pleocytosis, with the white blood cell count ranging between 20 and 80 cells per µl and a discrete elevation of the protein level. The symptoms decrease in a few days, but may take up to 4 weeks to resolve. More common is a chronic HIV meningitis characterized by a persistent pleocytosis. It is usually asymptomatic, but in most individuals, headache may be a chronic manifestation. Moreover, CSF abnormalities, especially mild pleocy-

tosis, are very common in asymptomatic HIV individuals. They are not predictive of the subsequent development of neurologic diseases.

Cryptococcosis

The incidence of cryptococcosis in HIV patients is estimated at approximately 7%. It is infrequent in children with HIV, and it can be the first manifestation of HIV infection. The main clinical manifestation is cryptococcal meningitis in patients with AIDS. Mass lesions of the brain, cryptococcomas, may also develop.

The usual clinical manifestations are fever, headache, a stiff neck, and photophobia. The appearance of these signs ranges between a few

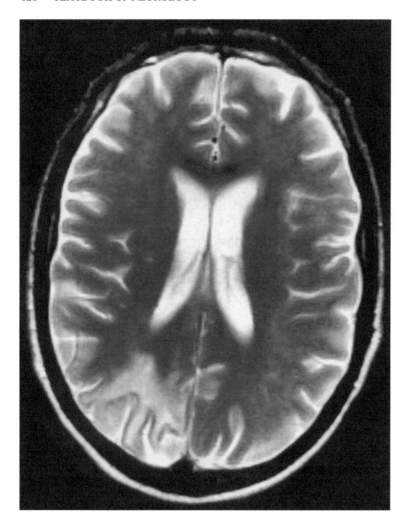

Figure 38D-5. A white matter lesion caused by progressive multifocal leukoencephalopathy that spares the cortex. The lesion is hyperintense, without mass effect, and does not enhance.

days to 3 weeks. Signs of increased intracranial pressure or cranial nerve involvement may occur and portend a poor prognosis. If the diagnosis is not recognized, a fulminant form of meningitis develops, with altered mentation and elevated intracranial pressure with brain swelling or hydrocephaly. In advanced cases, the yeasts invade the brain parenchyma along the Virchow-Robin spaces and may coalesce to develop cryptococcomas, especially in the basal ganglia. These mass lesions can produce hemiparesis or epileptic seizures.

The typical CSF findings in cryptococcal meningitis are an elevated opening pressure in more than two-thirds of patients, with a high protein level, pleocytosis, and low sugar level. The main diagnostic test is the detection of cryptococcal antigen. This assay is very specific and sensitive, more so than fungal cultures or CSF India ink staining. It should be performed on all patients with meningitis, especially if the CD4 cell count is fewer than 200 cells per μl. MRI scans show meningeal enhancement or multiple small hyperintensities on T2-weighted sequences. Nonenhancing mass lesions, cryptococcomas, are rarely demonstrated.

Treatment must be promptly begun with amphotericin B or fluconazole for a period of 2–3 weeks, until the symptoms resolve and CSF cultures produce negative results. Because of relapses, a maintenance regimen is continued with fluconazole for life.

Neurosyphilis in Human Immunodeficiency Virus Infection

In the AIDS era, the neurologic manifestations of syphilis have changed. The incidence of tabes has decreased, and the meningovascular complications have increased. The clinical features of neurosyphilis are observed during the secondary or tertiary stages, characterized by diverse groups of neurologic syndromes.

The presentation of syphilitic meningitis is similar to many forms of meningitis, with fever, headache, photophobia, and a stiff neck. Cranial nerves VII and VIII, with facial paresis and hearing loss, are typically affected. This form of neurologic manifestation occurs during secondary syphilis or the first 12 months of infection. At the spinal level, the main complication is a meningomyelitis, the manifestations of which are paraparesis at the thoracic level, sensory loss, and sphincter disturbances. Meningovascular syphilis is caused by an endarteritis of small and medium-sized vessels, the consequences of which are brain or spinal strokes. This is a tardive complication occurring 2–10 years after infection. Tabes dorsalis and general paresis are rare in AIDS patients.

There are no strict criteria for CSF abnormalities in the diagnosis of neurosyphilis. The presence of pleocytosis or increased total protein indicates inflammation but confirms nothing about etiology, especially in HIV patients, because HIV infection impairs cellular immunity, which is important in the response to *Treponema pallidum*. The diagnosis of symptomatic neurosyphilis is then based on clinical features and serologic tests. Nontreponemal tests include the VDRL or RPR (rapid plasma reagin). Although the specificity of the VDRL test is high, its sensitivity is between 30% and 70%. Thus, a nonreactive test does not exclude the diagnosis of neurosyphilis. On the contrary, a reactive CSF VDRL test establishes the diagnosis and the patient must be treated. The specific treponemal tests are the FTA-ABS (fluorescent treponemal antibody absorption) and the MHA-TP (microhemagglutination assay). They are reactive with active neurosyphilis. A negative CSF serology excludes neurosyphilis.

Therefore, in suspected neurosyphilis, if the serum FTA and MHA test results are positive, the VDRL test must be performed on CSF obtained by a lumbar puncture. In case of reactive test results, patients will be treated. When the CSF-VDRL test result is negative, the treatment depends on reactive CSF FTA and MHA test results. When the serum FTA or MHA test results are reactive but the VDRL, FTA, and MHA test results are nonreactive in the CSF, therapy is proposed if the CSF cell count is higher than 20 per ml.

The treatment of neurosyphilis includes intravenous penicillin G, 2–4 million units every 4 hours for 10–14 days, or intramuscular procaine penicillin, 2.4 million units daily for 10–14 days with probenecid. Alternatives are ceftriaxone or doxycycline.

Patients must be followed regularly after therapy with serum nontreponemal titers at 3-month intervals and CSF analysis every 6 months until the cell count is normal. Retreatment is indicated if serum VDRL or RPR findings are higher than two or more dilutions, if pleocytosis persists at 6 months or later, or if CSF-VDRL results have increased or new neurologic features have appeared.

Cytomegalovirus

In HIV-infected patients, signs of CMV infection in the brain are very frequent, but often the diagnosis is proved at autopsy. In the CNS, CMV causes a subacute encephalitis or ventriculitis. The symptoms are often not specific and may be very similar to those of ADC. Patients complain of headache, stiff neck, and cognitive changes. The clinical picture of lethargy, confusion, dementia, cranial nerve palsies, or other focal deficits develops in approximately 3 weeks. Other locations or involvement of other organs are frequent: retinitis, interstitial pneumopathy, hepatitis, and adrenalitis with hyponatremia. The CSF sample may be normal, or it may reveal a mild pleocytosis or a discrete elevation of the protein level. Cultures are generally negative, and the sensitivity and specificity of CSF CMV serologic studies are not known because the seropositive tests do not always correlate with the clinical signs. A PCR study for CMV RNA and DNA is sensitive and specific, but they may be also detected in asymptomatic patients. Quantification of viral DNA will be more useful in evaluating patients. Neuroimaging may be normal or may reveal meningeal or ventricular enhancement or an increased periventricular T2 signal. Treatment with ganciclovir or foscarnet may be beneficial.

Table 38D-3. Definitional Criteria for Human Immunodeficiency Virus–Associated Dementia Complex

---

Probable (each of the following)
1. Abnormality present for at least 1 month in two or more cognitive fields and impairing daily life
2. Abnormality in motor function or performance or decline in motivation or emotional control
3. Absence of altered consciousness
4. Absence of another cause

Possible (one of the following)
1. Another cause is present and the cause of criterion 1 is uncertain
2. Etiology of criterion 1 is uncertain related to incomplete evaluation

---

Source: Adapted from RS Janssen, DR Cornblath, LG Epstein, et al. Nomenclature and research case definitions for neurological manifestations of human immunodeficiency virus type-1 (HIV-1) infection. Report of a Working Group of the American Academy of Neurology AIDS Task Force. Neurology 1991;41:778.

Mycobacterial Infections

The infection of the CNS by mycobacterial agents is infrequent. It is almost always caused by *Mycobacterium tuberculosis,* although other atypical mycobacteria are also observed. The risk of CNS infections is higher among Haitians, black Americans, and intravenous drug abusers.

The neurologic findings of CNS tuberculosis are meningitis, cerebral or spinal abscesses, and tuberculoma. The presenting symptoms and signs of tuberculous meningitis in HIV patients include fever, headache, altered level of consciousness, malaise, nausea, and vomiting. Intracerebral lesions are frequent with tuberculous meningitis.

Acquired Immunodeficiency Syndrome Dementia Complex

ADC is one of the most serious complications of HIV infection. Navia and others described the clinical features of this syndrome in 1986. This term associates the progressive appearance of cognitive and behavioral dysfunctions and motor deficits with AIDS. It is actually recognized that HIV-1 produces this clinical syndrome. This neurologic syndrome is variously named, and the terms *AIDS dementia complex, HIV dementia, HIV encephalopathy, HIV-associated*
dementia complex, and *HIV-1–associated cognitive/motor complex* are synonymous. The term *ADC* has been favored for several years and remains the most commonly used term. The prevalence of ADC varies from 7% to 60%, depending on the population studied. It increases with immunosuppression, especially in severely immunosuppressed patients (CD4 cell count of less than 200 cells per µl).

Initial symptoms include forgetfulness, difficulty with concentration, apathy, inertia, and loss of interest in daily activities. It is common for patients to recognize these difficulties while reading or during discussions. This progressively results in social withdrawal. Confusion or disorientation may also develop. Behavioral modifications consist of loss of libido, emotional lability, depression, and loss of emotional responsiveness. Agitation, anxiety, mania, or psychosis can sometimes be the first manifestations of this syndrome. Typically, patients complain of taking a longer time to perform daily tasks, think, follow conversations, or read. Motor dysfunctions include difficulty in walking and writing, a tendency to drop things, weakness, and hand tremor.

The clinical progression of ADC follows the deterioration of immune function. As the immune functions deteriorate, patients find it more and more difficult to perform complex tasks. These clinical features suggest a subcortical involvement characterized by a general slowing of thought processes and motor activities. Later, they evolve into dementia with global cognitive dysfunctions, primitive reflexes, sphincteral disturbances, and paraparesis.

Definitional criteria proposed by the American Academy of Neurology separate patients with cognitive dysfunctions interfering with daily life (HIV-1–associated dementia complex) from patients with mild cognitive dysfunction or motor abnormalities (HIV-1–associated minor cognitive/motor disorder) (Table 38D-3). The Centers for Disease Control and Prevention defines ADC as a cognitive or motor dysfunction that progresses over weeks or months in the absence of opportunistic infections or CNS tumor. To these criteria of diagnosis, Price and Brew have joined a severity scale, combining the functional repercussions on daily activities of both cerebral and spinal cord dysfunction. This scale is very useful for following the evolution or response to treatment (Table 38D-4).

Because of the subcortical nature of ADC, the most useful neuropsychological tests are those that focus on psychomotor speed and performance, for exam-

Table 38D-4. Staging of Acquired Immunodeficiency Syndrome Dementia Complex

Stage	Description
Stage 0 (normal)	Normal mental and motor function
Stage 0.5 (equivocal/subclinical)	Mild symptoms without impairing daily life
	Mild signs (snout response, slowed ocular or limb movements)
Stage 1 (mild)	Able to perform activities of daily life but with unequivocal evidence of intellectual or motor impairment
Stage 2 (moderate)	Able to perform activities of self-care but cannot work or maintain the more demanding activities of daily life
Stage 3 (severe)	Major intellectual deficit or motor disability
Stage 4 (end stage)	Nearly vegetative

Source: Adapted from RW Price, BJ Brew. The AIDS dementia complex. J Infect Dis 1988;158:1079.

ple, the trail-making test, the digit symbol test, the grooved pegboard test, and the finger tapping test.

Although there is no definitive diagnostic test for the diagnosis of ADC, various paraclinical techniques can help to support or refute the clinical diagnosis. CSF abnormalities are frequent in the majority of patients with ADC, but such changes can also be demonstrated in asymptomatic HIV patients. An increase in total protein occurs frequently (70% of cases), but pleocytosis is uncommon. Eight percent of patients with HIV dementia show an increase of the immunoglobulin (Ig)G index, with oligoclonal bands in 35% of cases. If these abnormalities are not specific, normal CSF protein levels in HIV-demented patients exclude the diagnosis of ADC. HIV-1 isolation from the CSF or the detection of HIV-specific antibodies or antigens are not specific to HIV dementia. However, p24 antigen levels in the CSF should be correlated with the severity of ADC. Beta$_2$-microglobulin is the most useful CSF marker because its level is correlated with the extent of neuropsychological impairment and the stage of ADC. When the beta$_2$-microglobulin level is above 3.8 mg per liter, the positive predictive value for HIV dementia is 88%. Levels of other CSF markers, such as neopterin, quinolinic acid, cytokines, and prostaglandins, are also increased, but these abnormalities are not specific. CT scans allow other diagnoses to be excluded and generally reveal atrophy or hypodensity in the white matter. MRI scans are more sensitive in detecting modifications in the white matter. On T2-weighted sequences, these are characterized by hyperintensities of a patchy, ill-defined nature that involve the deep white matter

symmetrically and confluently. Sometimes punctate lesions of less than 1 cm in diameter can be seen on MRI scans and involve the basal ganglia. The electroencephalogram has little diagnostic value. Stereotyped biphasic complexes have been reported in asymptomatic HIV patients, but the EEG findings can be normal in mildly or moderately demented patients. According to a consensus of neuropathologists, three main pathologic changes are described in ADC: HIV encephalitis, HIV leukoencephalopathy, and diffuse poliodystrophy. HIV encephalitis involves mainly the deep white matter, the basal ganglia, and the brain stem. It is characterized by multiple disseminated perivascular foci of microglia, macrophages, and multinucleated giant cells. The presence of multinucleated giant cells is necessary to fulfill the pathologic criteria. If they are absent, HIV antigen or nucleic acids must be demonstrated by immunocytochemical analysis or in situ hybridization. The presence of HIV-1 is an excellent criterion of HIV encephalitis because the microglia and macrophages are the main reservoir of HIV-1 in the brain.

HIV leukoencephalopathy is the main and the most frequent neuropathologic abnormality in AIDS. It is characterized by diffuse myelin pallor and gliosis. There is microglial proliferation with astrocytosis and activated macrophages, but rarely multinucleated giant cells. There are few inflammatory infiltrates and viral antigens. In approximately 40% of cases, neuropathologic modifications of gray matter are also present, termed *poliodystrophy*. They show reactive astrogliosis with microglial proliferation and astrocytosis, inducing cerebral atro-

Table 38D-5. Primary Antiretroviral Agents

Reverse Transcriptase Inhibitors	Proteinase Inhibitors
Zidovudine (AZT)	Saquinavir
Zalcitabine (ddC)	Indinavir
Didanosine (ddI)	Ritonavir
Lamivudine (3TC)	
Stavudine (d4T)	
Nevirapine	
Delavirdine	
Loviride	

phy and neuronal loss. The pathogenesis of ADC is not limited to infection of macrophages and microglia by HIV-1. Direct and indirect mechanisms contribute to the pathogenesis of HIV dementia, involving interactions between HIV-1, the CNS, and the immune system. Price has proposed cell models of ADC pathogenesis that explain the interactions of these three "elements." Direct damage is caused by various viral products, such as cytokines, arachidonic acid, and viral proteins, which are neurotoxic. Indirect damage is related to macrophages and microglia invasion, resulting in release of different toxic products, which act on neural cells to cause their dysfunction, proliferation, and death.

Since the introduction of zidovudine, the prevalence of ADC has decreased, suggesting a beneficial effect of this substance. Several studies have confirmed that HIV dementia is uncommon with zidovudine treatment. The same treatment also results in clinical and neuropsychological improvement of demented patients. In the brain the number of multinucleated giant cells is dramatically decreased while patients are taking zidovudine. No therapeutic effect has been noted with stavudine, 3TC, zalcitabine, or didanosine.

Antiretroviral Agents and Combination Therapy

Several antiretroviral agents that target different sites of viral replication are available. Two main groups of drugs are particularly useful: the reverse transcriptase inhibitors and the proteinase inhibitors (Table 38D-5).

Zidovudine (AZT), a nucleoside reverse transcriptase inhibitor, was the first drug to be used against HIV and several studies revealed that AZT slowed the progression of disease in symptomatic patients, but this beneficial effect is not sustained over the long term. However, because of its ability to penetrate the CNS, it is effective against ADC (no such effects have been reported with ddI or ddC).

More recently, many data have provided evidence that a combination of antiretroviral agents are more effective than monotherapy and especially for patients who had never received nucleoside reverse transcriptase inhibitors. At first the combination of AZT and ddI or ddC was studied, but the association of AZT and stavudine or lamivudine has also demonstrated a superior effect in reducing viral load and delaying the occurrence of viral resistance. In addition, nucleosides combined with non-nucleoside inhibitors or proteinase inhibitors show greater effects than monotherapy.

Most recent studies even recommend triple combinations, including a proteinase inhibitor. Because a high turnover of virions and CD4 cells is present early in the HIV infection, the therapy should be initiated as early as possible (at the time of primary infection when it is symptomatic). The therapeutic regimen is maintained for at least 1 year. In asymptomatic patients, therapy is proposed or reintroduced when the CD4 cell count is lower than 55 per µl and the viral load is higher than 5,000 copies per milliliter of plasma.

Other types of treatment or combinations of drugs are under consideration, but many questions remain, especially the identification of the most appropriate combination and the timing of antiretroviral therapy. The limiting factor of these different therapeutic possibilities is, for most countries, the potential cost, not forgetting patient compliance and adverse effects.

Suggested Reading

Barohn RJ, Gronseth GS, LeForce BR, McVey AL, et al. Peripheral nervous system involvement in a large cohort of human immunodeficiency virus-infected individuals. Arch Neurol 1993;50:167.

Berenguer J, Moreno S, Laguna F, Vicente T, et al. Tuberculous meningitis in patients infected with the human immunodeficiency virus. N Engl J Med 1992;326:668.

Janssen RS, Cornblath DR, Epstein LG, et al. Nomenclature and research case definitions for neurological manifestations of human immunodeficiency virus type-1 (HIV-1) infection. Report of a Working Group of the American Academy of Neurology AIDS Task Force. Neurology 1991;41:778.

Katz D, Berger JR. Neurosyphilis in AIDS. Arch Neurol 1989;46:895.

Marshall DW, Brey RL, Cahill WT, Houk RW, et al. Spectrum of cerebrospinal fluid findings in various stages of human immunodeficiency virus infection. Arch Neurol 1988;45:954.

McArthur JC. Neurologic manifestations of AIDS. Medicine 1987;66:407.

McArthur JC. HIV-Associated Dementia. In Annual Course of the American Academy of Neurology (Vol 5). Boston: American Academy of Neurology, 1995;228-9–228-25.

McArthur JC, Selnes OA, Glass JD, Hoover DR, et al. HIV Dementia: Incidence and Risk Factors. In RW Price, SW Perry (eds), HIV, AIDS and the Brain. New York: Raven, 1994;251–272.

McCutchan JA. Cytomegalovirus infections of the nervous system in patients with AIDS. Clin Infect Dis 1995; 20:747.

Navia BA, Jordan BD, Price RW. The AIDS dementia complex. I. Clinical features. Ann Neurol 1986;19:517.

Petito CK, Navia BA, Cho ES, Jordan BD, et al. Vacuolar myelopathy pathologically resembling subacute combined degeneration in patients with acquired immune deficiency syndrome. N Engl J Med 1985;312:874.

Porter SB, Sande MA. Toxoplasmosis of the central nervous system in the acquired immunodeficiency syndrome. N Engl J Med 1992;327:1643.

Price RW, Brew BJ. The AIDS dementia complex. J Infect Dis 1988;158:1079.

Price RW, Brew B, Sidtis JJ, Rosenblum M, et al. The brain in AIDS: central nervous system HIV-1 infection and the AIDS dementia complex. Science 1988;239:586.

Remick SC, Diamond C, Migliozzi JA, Solis O, et al. Primary central nervous system lymphoma in patients with and without the acquired immune deficiency syndrome. A retrospective analysis and review of the literature. Medicine 1990;69:345.

Simpson D, Olney RK. Peripheral Neuropathies Associated with Human Immunodeficiency Virus Infection. In PJ Dick (ed), Peripheral Neuropathies: New Concepts and Treatments. Philadelphia: Saunders, 1992;685–711.

Simpson DM, Citak KA, Godfrey E, Godbold J, et al. Myopathies associated with human immunodeficiency virus and zidovudine: can their effects be distinguished? Neurology 1993;43:971.

So YT, Olney RK. Acute lumbosacral polyradiculopathy in acquired immunodeficiency syndrome: experience in 23 patients. Ann Neurol 1994;35:53.

White MH, Armstrong D. Cryptococcosis. Infect Dis Clin North Am 1994;8:383.

Whiteman ML, Post MJ, Berger JR, Tate LG, et al. Progressive multifocal leukoencephalopathy in 47 HIV-seropositive patients: neuroimaging with clinical and pathologic correlation. Radiology 1993;187:233.

Chapter 39
Tumors of the Central Nervous System

N. Scott Litofsky and Lawrence D. Recht

Chapter Plan

Classification
Epidemiology
Symptoms and signs
Differential diagnosis
Evaluation
Therapeutic modalities
    Symptomatic therapies
    Surgery
    Radiation therapy
    Pharmacologic therapies
Brief survey of central nervous system neoplasms
    Central nervous system metastases
    High-grade (malignant) gliomas
    Low-grade (benign) gliomas
    Primary central nervous system lymphomas
    Medulloblastomas
    Meningiomas
    Pituitary adenomas
    Craniopharyngiomas
    Vestibular schwannomas
    Pineal region germ cell tumors

Classification

Tumors of the central nervous system (CNS) are classified according to whether they are *metastatic* or *primary* in origin (Table 39-1). Metastatic tumors are those which spread into CNS either via hematogenous spread from systemic sites (especially the lung and breast) or through direct extension from adjacent structures such as bone.

Primary tumors themselves can be subdivided into those that arise from intrinsic neural tissues and those that arise from surrounding structures such as leptomeninges. Tumors may assume the appearance of any of the intrinsic neural cell types—astrocytes, oligodendrocytes, ependymal cells, and even neurons—and they are classified on this basis (although this does not necessarily mean that these tumors arise from these cells).

Frequently, intrinsic tumors are labeled either "benign" or "malignant." Although it is true that certain tumors such as meningiomas and pituitary adenomas are indolent and not likely to invade surrounding neural tissues, there is some hazard in using these labels to describe CNS tumors because, in the special case of the CNS, even slow-growing tumors can be located in unfavorable locations. For example, they may involve eloquent neural regions or may be attached to neural or vascular structures that limit their ability for complete resectability. Patients with these "benign" tumors that cannot be completely removed surgically often eventually have neurologic deterioration and death from progression of recurrent tumor. As such, a tumor that may be regarded as "benign," such as a meningioma, may eventually behave in a "malignant" fashion.

Table 39-1. Types of Central Nervous System Tumors

Metastatic
    Common sites
        Lung
        Breast
        Kidney
        Colon
        Melanoma
        Other
Primary
    Gliomas
        Glioblastoma
        Anaplastic astrocytoma
        Astrocytoma
        Oligodendroglioma
        Ependymoma
        Juvenile pilocytic astrocytoma
        Ganglioglioma
    Primary central nervous system lymphoma
    Medulloblastoma
    Meningioma
    Craniopharyngioma
    Hemangioblastoma
    Pituitary adenoma
    Schwannoma
    Germ-cell tumor

Epidemiology

Brain tumors represent an important category of cancers as well as CNS diseases. They are not rare events; yearly incidence rates in the United States range from 17 to 20 per 100,000. Brain tumors are the most common solid neoplasm in children, and numerous studies suggest that their incidence is increasing, especially in elderly patients. Approximately one-half of these tumors are metastatic, which numerically represent the most common CNS neoplasm. The rest are composed of primary tumors, of which malignant gliomas are the most frequent, comprising another one-fourth (see Table 39-1).

A number of potentially causative agents have been proposed as underlying the development of particular primary brain tumors. For example, there are a number of familial syndromes, including the neurofibromatoses and the Li-Fraumeni syndrome, in which congenital lack of tumor suppressor oncogenes leads to a higher incidence of cancers in general and primary brain tumors in particular. Infectious agents such as Epstein-Barr virus can also be detected in a high percentage of patients with primary CNS lymphomas (PCNSLs) associated with immunocompromise. Moreover, when epidemiologic studies are conducted, patients with brain tumors are found more frequently to be exposed to a number of environmental toxins such as organic solvents. Although numerous potential associations and correlations exist, exactly why a particular brain tumor develops remains unknown.

Symptoms and Signs

Tumors of the CNS can cause a wide variety of symptoms depending on their location and rapidity of growth. One of the most common symptoms is *headache,* which occurs in approximately one-half of patients at some time in the course of the tumor. Headache occurs as a result of elevated intracranial pressure (ICP), which stretches the nociceptors, or pain receptors, in the dura and on the blood vessels of the brain. Nighttime recumbency increases the intravascular volume within the brain, which subsequently increases ICP. Similarly, the hypoventilation that occurs with sleep also will cause hypercarbia and subsequent cerebral vasodilatation, which will increase intravascular volume within the head. The typical headache thus occurs in the morning when the patient arises. Patients may describe it as a sensation of pressure or of a band constricting the head. The headache tends to improve as the day progresses because hypercarbia improves and venous drainage increases. Occasionally, the headache may be more localized, such as is seen with meningiomas, which can cause headache at the points of their dural attachments.

In children especially, morning headaches may be accompanied by vomiting that is often projectile in nature and occurs without associated nausea. Pressure on the area postrema from elevated ICP probably accounts for this. The importance of morning headache associated with vomiting in a child cannot be overemphasized: Any child with these symptoms should be considered as harboring an intracranial mass lesion until proven otherwise. Immediate neuroimaging is thus warranted.

Seizure is often the first symptom of a brain tumor, occurring in approximately 25% of patients at the time of presentation. Tumors adjacent to the cerebral cortex are more likely to cause seizures than those associated with deeper structures or those located in the posterior fossa. Similarly, tumors in relatively epileptogenic areas such as the frontal or temporal lobes or those adjacent to the motor and sensory cortex are more likely to produce seizures. Seizures may be either partial or generalized in type; frequently patients with temporal lobe tumors will complain of a characteristic aura associated with a bad taste or smell, the so-called *uncinate* fit.

Signs suggestive of elevated ICP should also be sought. The hallmark finding is papilledema. As ICP exceeds central venous pressure, the normal venous pulsations of the retina cease. Further elevations of ICP occlude the central vein of the retina, leading to engorgement of the optic cup with subsequent blurring of its margins. Cognition can be also affected by elevated ICP. Patients may have decreased concentration or attention, problems maintaining a cognitive set, difficulties with orientation, or a decrement in their level of consciousness.

More helpful in localization are a number of location-specific neurologic deficits related to compression or invasion of neural or vascular structures by tumor. Lesions adjacent to the motor strip in the cerebral cortex, deeper tumors compressing the internal capsule, or lesions adjacent to or in the brain stem may all produce motor deficits as a result of compression of the corticospinal tract. Hemispheric cerebellar lesions as well as lesions of the basal ganglia or thalamus can be associated with loss of coordination and ataxia. Vision may be affected by tumors of the anterior skull base (e.g., meningiomas), which result in monocular visual loss; of the optic chiasm, which result in bitemporal field loss; or of the optic tract, which produce homonymous hemianopia. Tumors of the occipital cortex itself are usually distinguished from tract lesions by the presence of central (macular) sparing.

Tumors of the pineal region can produce a dorsal midbrain or Parinaud's syndrome, which is characterized by light-near dissociation, mydriasis, loss of convergence movements, and paralysis of upgaze. Pressure from the third ventricle on the tectum will preferentially compress the retinotectal tract, leading to diminution of the light reflex. Pupillary constriction from accommodation, which is transmitted through the optic tract, the lateral geniculate body, the optic radiation, the occipital cortex, and then the midbrain, is not affected. Upgaze is also affected by pressure on the tectum in the third ventricle when elevated ICP is present.

Lesions of the skull base also present with characteristic location-dependent syndromes. For example, tumors of the cerebellopontine angle, such as vestibular schwannomas, present with characteristic hearing decrement or tinnitus, whereas tumors involving the cavernous sinus will cause ophthalmoplegia.

Patients with spinal tumors frequently experience localized back pain that tends to be worse at night. Nerve roots being compressed by spinal lesions may cause arm pain, thoracic pain, or leg pain, depending on the level of the tumor. Unilateral spinal lesions may cause Brown-Sequard–type syndromes with ipsilateral loss of proprioception, light touch, and vibration sense and contralateral motor dysfunction and loss of pain and temperature sensation.

Symptoms related to endocrinopathy are also location specific. Lesions adjacent to the sella may compress pituitary tissue, leading to endocrine hypofunction. Symptoms may include fatigue, nausea, cold intolerance, weight gain or loss, amenorrhea, and decreased libido. Similarly, functional pituitary tumors secreting growth hormone, corticotropin, prolactin, or thyroid-stimulating hormone may be associated with endocrine hyperfunction. Last, craniopharyngioma and germinoma of the suprasellar area may be associated with diabetes insipidus as a result of suppression of antidiuretic hormone (ADH) secretion or precocious puberty, especially in children.

Differential Diagnosis

Because of their protean manifestations, neoplasms should be part of the differential diagnosis of virtually every symptom and sign that suggests CNS dysfunction. Tumors may be initially mistaken at the time of presentation for meningitis, encephalitis, and multiple sclerosis. Brain tumors can present acutely, especially in the elderly, suggesting stroke as the cause. This underscores why obtaining radiologic images of patients with suspected stroke is imperative.

Conversely, many diseases can mimic tumor and only a high index of suspicion leads the clinician to the correct diagnosis. Infectious diseases are probably the most common mimickers of brain tumor worldwide. Frequently, historical details can help.

For example, the most frequent cause of mass lesions in India is tuberculosis; in Central America it is cysticercosis. Therefore, travel histories are crucial. In acquired immunodeficiency syndrome (AIDS) patients, single mass lesions are at least as frequently infectious in cause as neoplastic. Bacterial abscesses can be mistaken for brain tumors in a nonimmunocompromised host; useful clues favoring abscess are the presence of systemic symptoms such as fever and imaging studies revealing symmetric ring enhancement and an inordinate amount of edema.

Other neurologic conditions can also initially manifest themselves as tumor. For example, in young patients, demyelinating lesions can present as single enhancing lesions; although frequently only biopsy will cinch the diagnosis, questioning these patients about prior episodes consistent with demyelination can suggest the correct cause. Giant aneurysms and vascular malformations can also be mistaken for tumor, especially in a patient with seizures or headache rather than CNS bleeding. Structural spinal disorders that must be differentiated from tumor include spondylosis, herniated nucleus pulposus, and syringomyelia.

Evaluation

Computed tomographic (CT) scans provide a reasonable imaging study with which to characterize brain masses. If the patient presents in extremis with a precarious neurologic or systemic condition, a CT scan of the head is probably the optimal first study because it can be performed fairly rapidly under closely monitored conditions. Intravenous iodinated contrast should be administered if the non–contrast-enhanced scan is suggestive of an intracranial mass. A CT scan is superior to magnetic resonance imaging (MRI) for examination of bone and it has particular importance for neoplasms that involve the skull base. Its shortcomings include a uniplanar view, as most scans are performed with only axial slices of the brain. This provides less anatomic detail than MRI scans.

MRI allows superior visualization of the relationships of lesions to neural and vascular structures. Because multiplanar axial, coronal, and sagittal views are routinely obtained, better visualization of neoplasms is possible. Gadolinium enhancement helps define lesions further. Not infrequently, lesions that are either not visible or only very subtle on CT scans are obvious when MRI is performed. This feature is particularly helpful in the workup of patients with CNS metastases in which the presence of multiple metastatic lesions profoundly affects management choices. MRI scans with and without gadolinium are also the preferred study for spinal neoplasms. Both axial and sagittal views can be obtained to determine whether the lesion is extradural, intradural extramedullary, or intramedullary in location. Definition of this relationship may focus diagnostic possibilities more precisely.

MRI and CT scans have superseded numerous older techniques that previously were routinely used in the management of these patients. Nevertheless, these tests still may yield additional information and aid workup in many cases. A lumbar puncture is frequently the only way in which carcinomatous meningitis can be documented. Furthermore, because several neural tumors, such as primitive neuroectodermal tumors, germ cell tumors, and glioblastoma, may seed CSF pathways with drop metastases, lumbar puncture is an important diagnostic procedure in the workup and evaluation of patients with these neoplasms.

Although MR angiography is rapidly becoming widely used, there are still occasional instances in which a conventional cerebral angiography is helpful in defining the vascular anatomy of a lesion preoperatively. Because of its nonspecificity, electroencephalography is of limited usefulness in the workup of patients with neoplastic lesions; on the other hand, it can be very helpful in the management of tumor-associated epilepsies. Although more invasive than MRI scanning, myelography with CT scanning can sometimes provide additional information about spinal neoplasms.

Single-photon emission computed tomography scanning can also prove useful in distinguishing highly anaplastic tumors from inflammatory lesions. Because [201]Th, the tracer routinely used, is absorbed only by viable tissue, a ratio can be generated comparing uptake in abnormal brain areas with radiographically normal ones. This test can also be particularly helpful in distinguishing the effects of treatment (e.g., radiation, chemotherapy) of recurrent tumors when imaging studies reveal enhancing lesions after therapy.

Therapeutic Modalities

Brain tumor treatments can be subdivided into symptomatic, surgical, radiotherapeutic, and pharmacologic categories (Table 39-2).

Symptomatic Therapies

Irrespective of tumor type, certain treatments are routinely administered to patients with CNS neoplasms to provide palliative relief of symptoms arising from either increased ICP, seizures, or focal neurologic deficits. Because they are directed more toward stabilization of normal function rather than specifically being directed at reducing or eradicating tumor, they are frequently termed *nonspecific* or *symptomatic treatments*.

Raised ICP can manifest itself as headache, depressed mental status, or focal neurologic deficits. When ICP becomes extremely high, cerebral herniation may result, representing a true neurologic emergency. Symptoms of raised ICP can be treated in a variety of ways (Table 39-3). Elevating the head of the bed will increase venous drainage and reduce the intracranial vascular volume. Fluid restriction can also reduce intravascular volume and reduce symptoms of mass effect. In the nonemergent situation, glucocorticoids can improve both headache and neurologic deficits by reducing vasogenic edema. Typically, dexamethasone (4–10 mg intravenously or orally every 6 hours) is administered because of its minimal mineralocorticoid actions, and improvement may be seen within 24 hours. Mild narcotics, such as codeine, 30 mg every 4 hours, can help alleviate headache. Respiratory depression and resulting hypercarbia that can result from sedation may produce cerebral vasodilatation, so use of these agents must be judicious.

In the setting of herniation, intubation with mechanical hyperventilation can reduce cerebral volume by causing vasoconstriction with quick (within minutes) but temporary reversal of signs. Because its actions are only temporary, further treatments should be concurrently administered. Mannitol, an osmotic diuretic, can reduce total body water content and reduce brain volume, improving symptoms related to mass effect. The typical dose is 0.25 g per kg intravenously every 6 hours. In the case of associated hydrocephalus, placement of a ventriculostomy can also be used to divert CSF to reduce intracranial volume.

Effective treatment of seizures is an important way in which the physician can improve the quality of life for a patient with a CNS neoplasm. Guidelines for administration and follow-up of these patients are similar to those for patients with epilepsy. After a seizure has occurred, patients are usually treated with phenytoin, carbamazepine, or

Table 39-2. Brain Tumor Therapies

Non–tumor directed (symptomatic)
    Corticosteroids
    Osmotic agents
    Ventriculostomy/shunting procedures
Surgery
    Stereotactic biopsy
    Craniotomy
Radiation therapy
    External beam irradiation
    Stereotactic focused irradiation
Pharmacologic
    Chemotherapy
    Immunotherapy

Table 39-3. Management of Elevated Intracranial Pressure

Emergent (Clinical Herniation)	**Nonemergent Inpatient**	**Nonemergent Outpatient**
Mechanical hyperventilation	Mannitol	Decadron
Mannitol	Decadron	Fluid restriction
Decadron	Fluid restriction, head elevation	Osmoglyn, head elevation
Tumor resection	Tumor resection	Tumor resection
If hydrocephalus: ventriculostomy	If hydrocephalus: ventriculostomy or cerebrospinal fluid shunt placement	If hydrocephalus: cerebrospinal fluid shunt placement

phenobarbital. In the setting of frequent seizures or status epilepticus, intravenous loading is indicated. Otherwise, medications can be administered orally. Recurrent seizures commonly occur, especially in patients with hemispheric gliomas, and can be quite refractory to treatment. Newer second-line agents are rarely effective in these cases but sometimes tumor-specific treatment such as surgical removal or even tumor irradiation will effectively decrease seizures.

Interestingly, anticonvulsants do not effectively prevent a first seizure from occurring. Therefore, some workers would recommend that these agents not be administered prophylactically in most patients because of these drug's frequent pharmacologic interactions and side effects.

Surgery

Surgery provides an opportunity to both definitively diagnose and treat CNS neoplasms. As such, it is performed in the vast majority of cases, with the major exceptions being patients with known cancers and multiple mass lesions. In addition, surgery can also serve as an effective symptomatic therapy by decompressing the brain and other neural structures. The type of surgical intervention is based on the clinical status of the patient and imaging studies.

In cases in which there are multiple lesions of the brain (and not sufficient evidence of a known primary focus), there are smaller lesions without mass effect, or surgical cure is not thought possible, stereotactic brain biopsy is the recommended modality for establishing a tissue diagnosis. In centers in which the procedure is well performed, the diagnostic accuracy of this maneuver approaches 95%, and morbidity is very low.

A more extensive resection is indicated in those patients with large single lesions causing mass effect or those in whom the differential diagnosis suggests pathologic entities that are amenable to surgical cure such as pituitary adenomas, meningiomas, juvenile pilocytic astrocytomas (JPAs), gangliogliomas, vestibular schwannomas, and benign teratomas. Patients with metastatic disease to the brain have a better outcome if a solitary brain lesion is surgically resected, so a patient with an accessible lesion should also be considered for craniotomy.

Radiation Therapy

Although a major component of the adjuvant therapy for most types of CNS neoplasms, CNS irradiation is not without serious long-term morbidities, which are both volume and dose fraction dependent. Therefore, most radiation therapists will tailor treatment so that as little brain is irradiated as gently as possible. In cases of advanced metastatic disease in which survival is very limited, a short course of whole brain irradiation consisting of ten fractions of 300 cGy is still indicated; in all other cases, lower fractions and reduced volumes are generally used.

In general, radiation therapy prolongs the survival of patients with many different tumor types. However, both the normal oligodendroglial and endothelial cells are vulnerable to its effects, which over the long term can produce bothersome toxicities. Radiation necrosis can occur secondary to endothelial cell injury; it represents a coagulative necrosis of brain tissue. Its presentation is usually indistinguishable from tumor recurrence—that is, an enlarging enhancing lesion at the tumor site with clinical deterioration. Although it may respond to high-dose steroids, resection of the necrotic mass is often necessary. A number of syndromes also may develop because of damage to white matter (leukoencephalopathy). Optic neuropathy and endocrinopathies frequently occur because of the proximity of the optic apparatus and hypothalamus to lesions within the suprasellar area. More generalized leukoencephalopathies manifesting as a global deterioration in neurologic function can develop within months after the completion of radiation therapy; this complication is particularly frequent in elderly patients.

Newer radiotherapeutic techniques such as stereotactic radiosurgery, interstitial brachytherapy, gamma knife therapy, and boron neutron capture therapy are all being assessed as ways in which to focus radiation exclusively into tumor, thus improving the therapeutic index of radiation therapy. Currently, however, none has proved superior to conventional external beam irradiation techniques.

Pharmacologic Therapies

Most CNS neoplasms respond poorly if at all to conventional chemotherapies for a number of reasons, including an inability of drugs to broach the blood-brain barrier and tumor cell heterogeneity, which causes marked intratumoral differences in chemosensitivity. Nevertheless, chemotherapy is frequently used in the more aggressive CNS neoplasms and a number of studies suggest at least some benefit. In the glioma subgroup of CNS neoplasms, the addition of a single agent, nitrosourea, to radiation therapy modestly improves survival in patients with glioblastoma and anaplastic astrocytomas. Anaplastic oligodendroglioma seems particularly chemosensitive. Certain less common neoplasms, such as PCNSLs and germ cell neoplasms, may be treatable with chemotherapy alone. Unfortunately, although a number of agents are being actively investigated, no chemotherapeutic or biologic agent currently seems likely to become the preeminent brain tumor therapy.

Brief Survey of Central Nervous System Neoplasms

Central Nervous System Metastases

CNS metastases represent the most common CNS neoplasm. The most common primary sources are lung, breast, kidney, melanoma, and gastrointestinal tract. When extrapulmonary cancers are responsible, there is frequently but not invariably concurrent lung metastasis.

CNS metastases are usually located at the gray-white matter junctions. On imaging studies, they appear as single or multiple, homogeneously or ring-enhancing masses. They can occur at any time during the clinical oncologic course; often, especially in lung cancers, they may herald the diagnosis. In these patients, chest and abdominal CT scans, a careful examination of the skin, rectal examination and stool guaiac testing, and a mammogram in women constitute an adequate initial metastatic workup. If these tests are nonconfirmatory, stereotactic biopsy can be used to establish a diagnosis.

Similar to the situation in systemic metastatic disease, CNS metastases are generally associated with a very poor prognosis, measurable in months; sometimes, however, especially in those patients with metastatic breast cancer, longer survivals are noted. Management depends on the clinical status of the patient and the location and multiplicity of the lesions. Patients who have a solitary brain metastasis have better outcomes if their tumors are surgically resected in addition to being irradiated; if a solitary lesion is noted in the setting of stable or quiescent systemic disease, surgical resection is indicated. In patients with advanced systemic disease or multiple lesions, whole brain radiation therapy is generally recommended.

Metastatic disease to the spine frequency causes neurologic symptoms by compression of the spinal cord or cauda equina. As with cranial disease, dexamethasone can improve neurologic symptoms and pain. For patients with known cancer, radiation therapy can palliate symptoms. Surgical decompression may be necessary for patients in whom a cancer diagnosis has not yet been established, in patients who have failed radiation therapy, or in those with spinal instability resulting from bone destruction by tumor.

High-Grade (Malignant) Gliomas

High-grade gliomas are the most commonly encountered primary brain tumors. They occur most frequently in middle-aged or older adults. The most aggressive tumor of this group is the glioblastoma multiforme, which is characterized pathologically by endothelial proliferation, a high degree of hypercellularity, anaplasia, and tissue necrosis. Anaplastic astrocytomas occur less commonly than glioblastomas; they are distinguished pathologically from glioblastoma multiforme primarily by the absence of necrosis. Because there is marked overlap between their clinical and imaging characteristics, these tumors are usually considered as representing a spectrum of the same pathologic process.

High-grade gliomas can arise anywhere within the CNS. They grow rapidly and are resistant to therapy. Although they appear most often as single enhancing lesions on imaging studies, they are highly invasive within the CNS and are not surgically curable. Even with intensive aggressive multimodality therapies, recurrence either at the local site or distantly within the CNS is the rule. Perhaps 10% of patients with glioblastoma multiforme survive longer than 2 years. Median survival for anaplastic astrocytomas is slightly better, being in the range of 3 years, although anaplastic astrocytomas will often degenerate into glioblastoma multiforme in their terminal phases.

Low-Grade (Benign) Gliomas

A number of diverse CNS neoplasms have cellular characteristics reminiscent of CNS supporting cells and behave in a less aggressive fashion than their high-grade counterparts. Compared with the malignant gliomas, they occur in younger patients. They occur approximately one-fourth as often as malignant gliomas.

Although they are often referred to as benign, most low-grade gliomas are better thought of as low-grade malignancies; although their course can extend longer than 10 years, cures are infrequent and they still eventually prove fatal, usually in the setting of histologic transformation into a more malignant subtype.

A number of subtypes constitute this class. Astrocytomas appear to be composed of well-differentiated astrocytic cells; patients often present with seizures when tumors are cortically based. On imaging studies, tumors appear as either hypodense (on CT scans) or hypointense (on T1-weighted MRI scans) and are usually nonenhancing. When they are polar and located near the surface, extensive resection alone can be associated with prolonged survival; this is not possible in most cases, however, because tumors tend to be located either in deeper locations or in eloquent cortex. Many workers advocate a less extensive resection followed by radiation therapy in these cases.

Oligodendrogliomas are another class of low-grade glioma that behaves similarly to astrocytoma. Pathologically, cells resemble oligodendrocytes; frequently, areas of astrocytoma are admixed with areas of oligodendroglioma (oligoastrocytoma). Intratumoral calcification is frequently noted, which provides a diagnostic clue on CT scans or even plain radiographs. These tumors have the highest frequency of hemorrhage among glioma subtypes. Median survival is comparable with that of diffuse low-grade astrocytoma.

Two special cases of truly benign gliomas—that is, tumors that are often associated with very prolonged survivals, even cure—are the JPA and the ganglioglioma. The JPA occurs most frequently in older children and adolescents and tends to be located in the cerebellum or optic pathways. It is distinguished pathologically by the appearance of Rosenthal fibers and microcystic changes; it is this latter characteristic that accounts for the propensity of these tumors to enhance on imaging studies (rather than blood-brain barrier breakdown, which underlies enhancement of more malignant gliomas). These tumors are circumscribed and well delineated from the surrounding brain. This lack of infiltration allows frequent surgical resection of the entire lesion. Radiation therapy is almost never indicated. Gangliogliomas are composed of well-differentiated astrocytic cells admixed with neoplastic neurons. They also frequently occur in children, most often arising in the temporal lobe. They are frequently found serendipitously when temporal lobectomy is performed for seizure control. Long-term survival is very common in patients with gangliogliomas, although recurrence can occur.

Primary Central Nervous System Lymphomas

Once considered a rare disease, PCNSLs are being encountered more frequently by clinicians. PCNSLs can be subdivided into those that occur in an immunocompromised patient (most frequently in patients with AIDS) and those who are immunocompetent. Incidence is probably increasing in both groups.

Lymphomas tend to arise in the periventricular area. They are most often composed of B cells. Only 20% will have systemic disease and even in these patients, systemic symptoms are infrequent. CSF and ocular involvement are more commonly encountered. In the AIDS population, lesions on imaging studies may have a central low density with peripheral enhancement or have relatively homogeneous enhancement. In the non-AIDS population, enhancement is typically homogeneous. Tissue diagnosis usually via stereotactic biopsy is essential for beginning specifically directed therapy. Because these tumors are responsive to both chemotherapy and radiation therapy, surgical extirpation usually is not necessary. Radiation therapy may provide long-term palliation, and a number of studies have shown that chemotherapy is also effective in an immunocompetent host. Long-term survival in these patients, although not common, occurs much more frequently than with malignant gliomas and justifies intensive treatment.

In patients with AIDS, radiation therapy can alter the natural history of the disease; thus, patients who are treated tend to die of other AIDS complications at somewhat later intervals and after a better quality of life than those in whom treatment is withheld.

Medulloblastomas

Medulloblastoma is the most common of the primitive neuroectodermal tumors—a family of small blue cell tumors with immunohistochemical markers of both glial and neuronal tissues. Medulloblastomas occur mostly in the pediatric age group, arise from the cerebellar vermis, are highly proliferative, and often will seed the spinal fluid pathways. They are one of the few types of CNS tumors that frequently give rise to systemic metastases, with bone and bone marrow being common metastatic sites. Outcome is dependent on the extent of disease, the presence of hydrocephalus, the extent of surgical resection, and patient age (patients younger than 4 years fare less well). In addition to surgery, craniospinal radiation and chemotherapy are often used. Five-year survival is approximately 50%, and long-term survival is frequently seen in good-risk patients (no dissemination, tumor not invading brain stem, tumor undifferentiated, patient age older than 4 years, and total resection).

Meningiomas

Approximately 10% of primary tumors are meningiomas—durally based neoplasms that arise from arachnoidal cap cells. Although histologically malignant meningiomas are encountered, for the most part, these neoplasms are slow growing and potentially curable if totally resected. Patients with meningiomas can have symptoms of headache, neurologic deficit, or seizure. Occasionally, these tumors are found incidentally when patients undergo imaging for other reasons. Unfortunately, meningiomas often cannot be completely resected because they have a tendency to invest themselves into and around neural and vascular structures as well as to invade the skull and dural sinuses. Incidentally discovered meningiomas may not require specific therapy; in other patients, complete resection is the goal. For those tumors in which total resection is not possible, radiation therapy can occasionally control disease.

Pituitary Adenomas

Arising in the adenohypophysis, pituitary adenomas can produce symptoms either from hypersecretion of one of the pituitary hormones or hypopituitarism resulting from compression of the normal gland. The most common subtypes are prolactin-secreting tumors followed by nonfunctional tumors, corticotropin-secreting tumors, and growth hormone-secreting tumors. Besides endocrine dysfunction, visual loss from compression of the optic chiasm or headache and loss of consciousness from hemorrhage into the tumor (pituitary apoplexy) can occur.

Tumors that secrete prolactin (prolactinomas) are usually responsive to the dopamine agonist bromocriptine, which may shrink even large macroadenomas and improve both endocrine dysfunction and symptomatic visual loss. In cases that are unresponsive, transsphenoidal surgery can be performed, with complete tumor removal being possible even if the tumor extends into the suprasellar cistern. In patients who have hypopituitarism, hypothyroidism and hypocortisolemia should be corrected before surgical intervention is attempted. Radiation therapy is sometimes used when tumor removal is not possible, such as when the cavernous sinus is involved.

Craniopharyngiomas

Craniopharyngiomas are suprasellar tumors that develop from residua of the hypophyseal duct. Although these tumors are slow growing, they should also be considered low-grade malignancies. Additionally, they tend to invest themselves and become firmly adherent to vital neural and vascular structures, which limits surgical excision. There are two peaks in incidence: in the second and fifth decades.

Patients frequently present with visual or endocrine dysfunction; occasionally a calcified, cystic suprasellar mass is noted on imaging studies. Treatment options include radical excision, which may produce significant morbidity, or partial resection with subsequent radiation therapy in the early postoperative period. Patients who are younger than 6 years of age, patients who have had total or near total resection, or patients who are in poor neurologic condition might best be observed for a time before treatment with external beam radiation therapy.

Vestibular Schwannomas

Vestibular schwannomas arise in the internal auditory canal in the cerebellopontine angle. They arise from the Schwann cells of the vestibular branch of the eighth cranial nerve. There is a tendency for bilateral occurrence in patients with type II neurofibromatosis. Patients with small tumors may present only with tinnitus or hearing loss, whereas larger tumors may cause coordination deficits, motor deficits, or symptoms related to hydrocephalus.

The exact surgical approach depends on the clinical signs and the size of the tumor. For tumors less than 1 cm in which the patient has adequate hearing in that ear, a suboccipital approach can be performed in an attempt to preserve both hearing and facial nerve function. For tumors greater than 1.5 cm, it is very difficult to preserve hearing; the goal of surgery is to remove the tumor and preserve facial nerve function.

Pineal Region Germ Cell Tumors

Pineal region tumors are an uncommon, complicated group of tumors. The differential diagnosis of these tumors includes gliomas, meningiomas, primitive neuroectodermal tumors, and benign cysts, but numerous different types of germ cell tumors must also be considered. Management of these lesions is directed by making a definitive diagnosis, which always requires neurodiagnostic imaging and CSF markers, and often tissue sampling. Germinomas and mature teratomas usually have negative markers, although germinomas may have a slightly elevated beta human chorionic gonadotropin (βHCG). Choriocarcinomas have highly elevated βHCG levels, and endodermal sinus tumors produce α-fetoprotein, as do some embryonal carcinomas. Immature teratomas express both markers. Management of these lesions is controversial. Some believe that all lesions should be surgically excised, although mature teratoma is really the only lesion that is surgically curable. An alternative mode of management is to obtain CSF for markers and plan to perform a stereotactic biopsy. If markers are absent and the pathologic condition is germinoma, then treatment with chemotherapy and radiation therapy is appropriate. If CSF markers are present, then therapy can proceed without tissue sampling. If patients have hydrocephalus, surgical decompression can open CSF pathways and prevent the need for a ventriculoperitoneal shunt. Alternatively, patients can be treated with a shunt if necessary. Hydrocephalus, if mild, may respond to tumor shrinkage by adjuvant therapy alone.

Suggested Reading

Apuzzo MLJ, Chandrasoma P, Cohen D, et al. Computed imaging stereotaxy: experience and perspective related to 500 procedures applied to brain masses. Neurosurgery 1987;20:930.

Baskin DS, Wilson CB. Surgical management of craniopharyngiomas. J Neurosurg 1986;65:22.

Black PMcL. Meningiomas. Neurosurgery 1993;32:643.

Cairncross JG, Macdonald DR, Ramsay DS. Aggressive oligodendroglioma: a chemosensitive tumor. Neurosurgery 1992;31:78.

Evans AE, Jenkin DT, Sposto R, et al. The treatment of medulloblastoma. Results of a prospective randomized trial of radiation therapy with and without CCNU, vincristine, and prednisone. J Neurosurg 1990;72:572.

Hardy J. Transsphenoidal microsurgery of the normal and pathological pituitary. Clin Neurosurg 1969;16:185.

Kaye AH, Laws ER (eds). Brain Tumors. New York: Churchill Livingstone, 1995.

Lunsford LD, Kondziolka D, Flickinger JC. Stereotactic radiosurgery: current spectrum and results. Clin Neurosurg 1992;38:405.

McKeran RO, Thomas DGT. The Clinical Study of Gliomas. In DGT Thomas, DL Graham (eds), Brain Tumors: Scientific Basis, Clinical Investigation, and Current Therapy. Baltimore: Butterworth, 1980;194–230.

Ojemann RG. Management of acoustic neuromas (vestibular schwannomas). Clin Neurosurg 1993;40:498.

Patchell RA, Tibbs PA, Walsh JW, et al. A randomized trial of surgery in the treatment of single metastasis to the brain. N Engl J Med 1990;322:494.

Recht LD, Bernstein M. Low-grade gliomas. Neurol Clin 1995;13:847.

Rorke LB, Gilles FH, Davis RL, et al. Revision of the World Health Organization classification of childhood brain tumors. Cancer 1985;56:1869.

Salcman M. Malignant glioma management. Neurosurg Clin North Am 1990;1:49.

Tomlinson FH, Kurtin PJ, Suman VJ, et al. Primary intracerebral malignant lymphoma: a clinicopathological study of 89 patients. J Neurosurg 1995;82:558.

Chapter 40
Paraneoplastic Neurologic Syndromes

Ramón Reñé and Francesc Graus

Chapter Plan

Paraneoplastic neurologic syndromes (PNSs) are a group of disorders of unknown etiology that occur exclusively, or with increased frequency, in the setting of cancer. PNSs may involve any structure of the central or peripheral nervous system (Table 40-1). PNSs represent less than 1% of the neurologic complications of cancer, but they are important in clinical practice because they are associated with specific types of tumors and usually antedate the diagnosis of the cancer, which almost always is in a localized stage when the chance to cure the tumor is highest.

Several antineuronal antibodies have been described in the serum and cerebrospinal fluid (CSF) of patients with some PNSs (Tables 40-2 and 40-3), which supports the hypothesis that PNSs could be the result of an immunologic response triggered against tumoral antigens and misdirected to similar antigens expressed in the nervous system. However, this model of immuno-mediated disease has been unambiguously proved only in Lambert-Eaton myasthenic syndrome (LEMS). Although the pathogenic role of the other autoantibodies remains unclear, they are of clinical relevance because (1) they represent excellent diagnostic markers of some PNSs and related tumors; its detection confirms the paraneoplastic character of the neurologic dysfunction and directs the search of the underlying cancer to a few organs; (2) they may identify patients with clinical features that are unusual for a given PNS; and (3) they support a theoretical ground for the use of immunosuppressor therapies.

In this chapter we describe the most frequent PNSs, the methodologic approach to patients with a suspected PNS, and the current status of the treatment of these neurologic disorders.

Table 40-1. Paraneoplastic Neurologic Syndromes

Paraneoplastic syndromes of the central nervous system
    Encephalomyelitis
    Limbic encephalitis
    Bulbar encephalitis
    Myelitis
    Cerebellar degeneration
    Retinopathy
    Opsoclonus-myoclonus
    Stiff-person syndrome
    Necrotizing myelopathy
Paraneoplastic syndromes of the peripheral nervous system
    Subacute motor neuronopathy
    Subacute sensory neuronopathy
    Sensorimotor neuropathies
    Multineuritis and vasculitis
    Autonomic neuropathies
    Neuromyotonia
Paraneoplastic syndromes of the neuromuscular junction
    and muscle
    Lambert-Eaton myasthenic syndrome
    Dermatomyositis
    Acute necrotizing myopathy
    Carcinomatous neuromyopathy

Paraneoplastic Syndromes of the Central Nervous System

Paraneoplastic Encephalomyelitis/ Subacute Sensory Neuronopathy

Paraneoplastic encephalomyelitis/subacute sensory neuronopathy (PEM/SSN) includes several neurologic syndromes characterized by pathologic changes of neuronal loss, microglial proliferation, and inflammatory infiltrates in the nervous system. The areas more frequently involved are the hippocampus, the lower brain stem, the spinal cord, and the dorsal root ganglia. The clinical picture reflects the variable anatomic involvement and includes encephalopathy (limbic encephalitis), brain stem syndromes (bulbar encephalitis), autonomic dysfunction, myelitis, and SSN. Although some patients may have a clinical involvement of only one of these areas through the entire clinical course, 75% of them present with a multifocal disorder.

In 75% of PEM/SSN patients, the underlying neoplasm is a small-cell lung cancer (SCLC). SSN is the most common clinical syndrome and in 20% of the patients, SSN is the only clinical evidence of disease. (For teaching purposes, SSN is described within the section Paraneoplastic Syndromes of the Peripheral Nervous System; see below.) The second most common clinical syndrome that may remain isolated throughout the clinical course is limbic encephalitis. Symptoms include severe impairment of recent memory, neuropsychiatric manifestations (anxiety, depression, confusion, inadequate behavior, hallucinations), and seizures. The electroencephalogram shows generalized slow waves or focal abnormal discharges over the temporal areas. Computed tomographic (CT) scans of the head usually appear normal but magnetic resonance imaging (MRI) may demonstrate early in the course of the disease an increased signal in one hippocampus (or both) on T2-weighted images (Figure 40-1). The abnormal signal disappears over time and subsequent MRI scans only show atrophy of the medial part of one or both temporal lobes.

Other common manifestations of PEM/SSN are brain stem encephalitis, cerebellar symptoms,

Table 40-2. Antineuronal Antibodies in Paraneoplastic Neurologic Syndromes

Antibody	Syndrome	Tumor
Anti-VGCC	Lambert-Eaton myasthenic syndrome	SCLC
Anti-Hu	Encephalomyelitis/sensory neuropathy	SCLC
Anti-recoverin	Cancer-associated retinopathy	SCLC
Anti-Yo	Cerebellar degeneration	Ovary/breast
Anti-Ri	Brain stem encephalitis	Breast
Anti-128 kd	Stiff-person syndrome	Breast
Anti-Tr	Cerebellar degeneration	Hodgkin's

SCLC = small-cell lung cancer.

Table 40-3. Characteristics of Antineuronal Antibodies

Antibody	Antigen(s)	Location	Function
Anti-VGCC	P-type VGCC	NM junction	Neurotransmitter release
Anti-Hu	HuD, HuC, HelN1	Nuclear[a]	RNA-binding proteins
Anti-recoverin	Recoverin	Photoreceptor	cGMP-gated signal transduction
Anti-Yo	CDR62/CDR34	Purkinje	Unknown
Anti-Ri	NOVA	Nuclear[b]	RNA-binding proteins
Anti-128 kd	Amphiphysin	Synapsis	Vesicle-associated
anti-Tr	Unknown	Purkinje	Unknown

NM = neuromuscular; VGCC = voltage-gated calcium channels; GMP = guanosine monophosphate.
[a]Present in all neurons.
[b]Absent in neurons of the peripheral nervous system.

motor weakness, and autonomic dysfunction. Clinical symptoms reflecting impairment of these areas may remain isolated at the onset of the disease, but unlike SSN and limbic encephalitis, evidence of multifocal involvement rapidly appears over time in almost all of these patients. The symptoms of brain stem encephalitis reflect the predominant involvement of the floor of the fourth ventricle and the inferior olives and include vertigo, nystagmus, oscillopsia, ataxia, diplopia, dysarthria, and dysphagia. Motor weakness caused by damage of the motor neurons in the spinal cord is observed in 20% of PEM/SSN patients. In a few of them, the predominant muscle weakness may suggest an initial diagnosis of amyotrophic lateral sclerosis (ALS) or even Guillain-Barré syndrome.

The autonomic nervous system is affected in 30% of patients; the most common symptoms are orthostatic hypotension, urinary retention, pupillary abnormalities, impotence, and dry mouth. A few patients develop a chronic intestinal pseudo-obstruction as a result of damage of the neurons of the myenteric plexus. Patients complain of nausea and vomiting, constipation, abdominal pain, and weight loss. Radiologic studies disclose a marked distension of the gastrointestinal tract (Figure 40-2). Like SSN, the intestinal pseudo-obstruction may be isolated or associated with other features of the PEM/SSN syndrome.

Most patients with PEM/SSN have anti-Hu antibodies. An exception would be patients with an isolated limbic encephalitis throughout the complete clinical course. In this setting, anti-Hu antibodies usually are not present.

Paraneoplastic Cerebellar Degeneration

Paraneoplastic cerebellar degeneration (PCD) is characterized by a rapidly evolving severe pancerebellar syndrome caused by a widespread loss of cerebellar Purkinje cells. PCD is mostly associated with gynecologic and breast tumors, SCLC, and Hodgkin's disease.

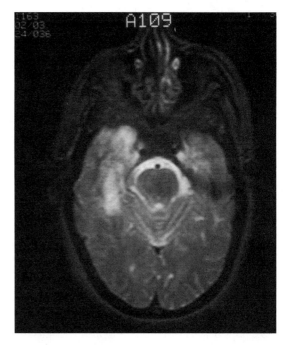

Figure 40-1. A T2-weighted magnetic resonance imaging scan demonstrates a high-intensity lesion in the medial aspect of the left temporal lobe.

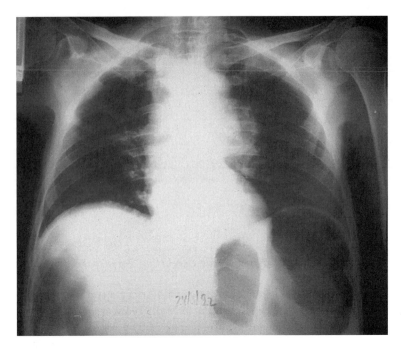

Figure 40-2. A chest x-ray film showing the tumor in the left hilus and severe dilatation of the left colon that displaces the stomach.

Patients with PCD and ovarian or breast cancer almost always have anti-Yo antibodies. Approximately 60% of anti-Yo–positive patients do not have a known cancer when they develop the PCD. The onset of symptoms is subacute with gait ataxia that progresses to severe truncal and appendicular ataxia with dysarthria, downbeat nystagmus, and oscillopsia. Clinical dysfunction may stabilize after a few months but by then the patient is often severely disabled. CT and MRI scans initially appear normal but later cerebellar atrophy is noted. Exceptionally, anti-Yo antibodies have been reported in male patients with PCD and lung cancer or in women with PCD and cancer other than of the ovary or breast.

Patients with PCD associated with Hodgkin's disease are usually men, and the cerebellar dysfunction may occur in the setting of prolonged remission of the neoplasm. Improvement, either spontaneous or after corticosteroid treatment, is reported in 10% of the patients. Up to 25% of these patients have antineuronal antibodies. These antibodies are not characterized well enough to indicate they are associated with Hodgkin's disease. We have described an antibody, called anti-Tr, that immunoreacts with a characteristic pattern in rat cerebellum and is restricted to patients with PCD and Hodgkin's disease. Until the cloning of the Tr antigens, which will allow the definitive identification of the antibody, the immunohistochemical pattern may be used to identify the anti-Tr antibodies and direct the search for the underlying tumor to Hodgkin's disease (Figure 40-3).

Patients who present to the neurologist with a cerebellar syndrome and finally develop a SCLC may develop extracerebellar symptoms typical of PEM/SSN or remain with an isolated cerebellar syndrome throughout the clinical course. In the latter case, anti-Hu antibodies are usually absent. In both clinical situations, up to 16% of patients also have clinical features of LEMS.

Paraneoplastic Opsoclonus Myoclonus Syndrome

Opsoclonus is a disorder of ocular motility characterized by irregular, continuous, large amplitude conjugate saccades in all directions of gaze. Opsoclonus occurs with a wide variety of conditions including viral encephalitis, metabolic encephalopathies, brain stem gliomas, thalamic hemorrhages, multiple sclerosis, and drug intoxications. The anatomic site responsible for opsoclonus is unknown.

Figure 40-3. Immunohistochemical study of rat cerebellum. Anti-Tr antibodies (A) produce a dotted pattern in the molecular cell layer (upper part of the figure) not seen with anti-Yo antibodies (B). Both antibodies immunoreact with the cytoplasm of the Purkinje cells.

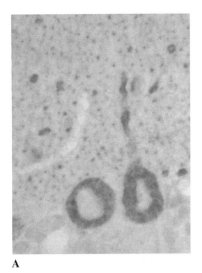

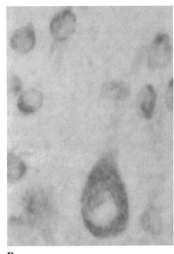

A   B

Paraneoplastic opsoclonus myoclonus may be the presenting symptom in approximately 2–5% of children with neuroblastoma, and 50% of children who develop opsoclonus have neuroblastoma. The patients also present myoclonus of the limbs and trunk, hypotonia, and irritability. The symptoms run a fluctuating course with occasional spontaneous remissions and good response to corticosteroids and treatment of the underlying tumor.

Paraneoplastic opsoclonus in adults is mainly associated with two different types of tumors. Women with breast or fallopian cancer develop a clinical picture of subacute onset characterized by opsoclonus, truncal and gait ataxia, dizziness, dysphagia, dysarthria, oscillopsia, and diplopia. The serum and CSF contain an antibody called anti-Ri that recognizes a family of neuronal RNA-binding proteins (NOVA antigens) preferentially expressed in the brain stem neurons. Although the first cases with anti-Ri antibodies had opsoclonus, some patients never develop this sign, but all present evidence of brain stem dysfunction. In the two autopsy cases reported, the main finding was neuronal loss and inflammatory infiltrates in the brain stem. These data suggest anti-Ri antibody identifies a particular type of brain stem encephalitis.

The second tumor most commonly associated with opsoclonus is SCLC; these patients present a myoclonus-opsoclonus syndrome similar to that observed in children with neuroblastoma. Rarely, opsoclonus has also been reported with other neo-

plasms including carcinoma of the uterus, urinary bladder, breast, thyroid, thymus, and lung and Hodgkin's disease.

Retinopathy

Paraneoplastic retinopathy is usually associated with SCLC or melanoma. The retinopathy that occurs in SCLC, called *cancer-associated retinopathy* (CAR), usually antedates the diagnosis of the tumor and has a subacute onset with episodic visual obscurations, light-induced glare, photosensitivity, and night blindness followed by progressive painless visual loss. Ophthalmologic examination shows ring-like scotomata and a narrowed retinal arteriolar caliber. The electroretinogram discloses absent or attenuated responses but latencies of visual evoked potentials are within the normal range. The most important pathologic change is severe loss of photoreceptors. Patients with CAR and SCLC harbor antibodies that recognize a 26-kd calcium binding protein, named *recoverin*, present in the photoreceptors.

In contrast, the paraneoplastic retinopathy associated with melanoma usually appears months to years after diagnosis of metastatic melanoma. The retinopathy presents clinical features similar to those of CAR, but the electroretinogram demonstrates a pattern more consistent with damage of bipolar cells of the retina rather than the photoreceptors. The serum of these patients does not have anti-recoverin antibodies but immunoreacts with a subset of bipolar retinal cells.

Paraneoplastic Stiff-Person Syndrome

Stiff-person syndrome is characterized by stiffness of axial muscles with superimposed painful muscle spasms and typical electromyographic findings of continuous muscle activity abolished by intravenous or oral diazepam. Approximately 1% of cases of stiff-person syndrome are paraneoplastic, associated with Hodgkin's disease, thymoma, or breast or lung cancer. Patients with paraneoplastic stiff-person syndrome and breast cancer harbor in their serum and CSF an antibody that reacts against a synaptic protein of 128-kd molecular mass called *amphiphysin*. Anti-amphiphysin antibodies were recently also reported in three patients with PEM/SSN and SCLC.

Necrotizing Myelopathy

A few cases of necrotizing myelopathy have been described in association with cancer, mostly lymphomas and lung cancer. Necrotizing myelopathy has an acute or subacute clinical course characterized by a rapid development of ascending paraplegia. Postmortem studies show widespread necrosis of the spinal cord, even beyond the clinically affected segment. Pathologic changes involve all components of the spinal cord, the dorsal columns usually being more affected than the ventral cord. Inflammation is markedly absent. The CSF is normal or shows moderate protein elevations. Myelograms appear normal or demonstrate nonspecific swelling of the spinal cord. MRI studies of pathologically confirmed necrotizing myelopathy are lacking.

Paraneoplastic Syndromes of the Peripheral Nervous System

Motor Neuron Syndromes

Epidemiologic studies have ruled out a possible link between ALS and cancer. However, some paraneo-

plastic syndromes present clinical features resembling those of ALS. Three syndromes must be considered. First, a few patients with PEM/SSN may present with isolated motor weakness, but in only exceptional patients does the motor deficit remain isolated to raise a diagnostic problem with ALS. Second, a few patients with cancer, usually lymphoma, macroglobulinemia, or kidney adenocarcinoma, develop a clinical picture similar to that of ALS, but they improve with treatment of the tumor. Patients with lymphoma and motor neuron syndromes often show serum paraprotein and elevated protein levels in the CSF. A third type of paraneoplastic motor neuron disorder is subacute motor neuronopathy, which is associated with Hodgkin's disease or lymphoma and characterized by subacute, painless, proximal, asymmetric muscle weakness with predominant involvement of the lower extremities and sparing of the bulbar muscles. Pain and fasciculations are absent and tendon reflexes are decreased or abolished. Motor and sensory nerve conduction studies are normal and electromyographic studies are suggestive of lower motor dysfunction. The CSF may show a high protein concentration. The syndrome usually appears after the treatment of the lymphoma and runs an independent and usually benign clinical course and sometimes may spontaneously improve.

Subacute Sensory Neuronopathy

SSN is caused by damage to sensory neurons in the dorsal root ganglia. The main clinical complaints at the onset are pain and paresthesias with asymmetric distribution that involve arms rather than the legs. Later, pain is replaced by numbness, limb ataxia, and pseudoathetotic movements of the hands. The neurologic examination shows abolition of the deep tendon reflexes and involvement of all modalities of sensation but with clear predominance of the joint position and vibratory senses. Thirty percent of the patients complain of unilateral or bilateral numbness on the face resulting from trigeminal ganglia damage. Sensorineural deafness and sensory deficits in the trunk are less usual. The typical SSN has a subacute onset and progresses rapidly to involve the four limbs and then may stabilize, although by the time it does so (6–9 months), the patient may be confined to bed or chair because of ataxia. In 10% of patients, the neuropathy runs a mild, very slow clinical evolu-

Table 40-4. Sensorimotor Neuropathies Associated with Plasma Cell Dyscrasias

Dyscrasia	Onset	Incidence	Pathologic Features	Response to Treatment	Antibody
Waldenstrom's	Early	<5%	Demyelinating	Partial	MAG
	Late	<5%	Axonal	No	Vimentin
Myeloma					
Osteosclerotic	Early	40%	Axonal atrophy	Yes	None
Osteolytic	Early*	<1%	Axonal	No	None
With amyloidosis	Late	<5%	Amyloid deposits	No	None

MAG = myelin-associated glycoprotein.
*The incidence of mild neuropathies late in the course of the myeloma is higher, 10–15%, and 20% of them are caused by amyloidosis.

tion. These patients may remain ambulatory and with an independent life for years in absence of any anti-tumoral or immunosuppressive treatment.

The CSF may show mild lymphocytic pleocytosis. Electromyographic studies disclose abolished sensory nerve action potentials. Motor nerve conductions are usually normal, although signs of denervation such as fibrillation or increased amplitude of motor unit potentials may be present when motor neurons are involved in the setting of PEM/SSN. Sural nerve biopsy specimens show fiber loss without features of regeneration or demyelination. Perivascular inflammatory infiltrates without necrosis of the vessel walls may be observed in the epineural vessels.

Sensorimotor Neuropathies

Severe sensorimotor neuropathies antedating the diagnosis of cancer occur in less than 1% of patients with cancer and may be associated with any tumor, but are usually seen in patients with lung cancer. The clinical features do not differ from those seen in sensorimotor neuropathies from other causes or in chronic inflammatory demyelinating polyneuropathy.

Paraneoplastic neuropathies associated with plasma cell dyscrasias are clinically heterogeneous and their incidence varies depending on the underlying disease. Because these neuropathies are described elsewhere in the book, the most relevant features are summarized in Table 40-4.

An acute polyradiculoneuropathy with clinical, electromyographic, and CSF features identical to those of typical Guillain-Barré syndrome has been

reported in patients with Hodgkin's disease. In patients with subacute sensorimotor neuropathy associated with lymphoma and leukemia, the clinical picture may be caused by direct infiltration of the peripheral nerves. The neoplastic origin of the neuropathy may be overlooked when the neuropathy is the first manifestation of the lymphoma or in patients who improve with corticosteroids. Diagnosis is confirmed when malignant cells are present in peripheral nerve biopsy specimens.

Mononeuritis Multiplex and Vasculitis

In a few patients with cancer, sensorimotor neuropathy is caused by vasculitis. The neuropathy is painful, rapidly progressive, and usually asymmetric. Patients may also have proximal muscle weakness caused by a coincident muscle vasculitis. Neurologic symptoms usually precede the diagnosis of the tumor, because the most common underlying neoplasms are prostate and kidney adenocarcinomas, lymphomas, and lung cancers. Diagnosis is confirmed by the demonstration of epineural microvasculitis in the nerve biopsy specimen. A muscle biopsy is indicated because it may increase the chances of finding the vasculitis.

Neuromyotonia

The term *neuromyotonia* describes the association of myokymia, cramps, impaired muscle relaxation, hyperhidrosis, and an elevated creatine kinase level with electromyographic evidence of prolonged bursts of motor unit potentials firing at a frequency of 40–200 Hz. These discharges arise from ectopic generation in peripheral nerve. A few patients with neuromyotonia have an underlying thymoma or SCLC. The autoimmune pathogenesis of acquired neuromyotonia is supported by the presence of antibodies directed against voltage-gated potassium channels and successful passive transfer studies.

Paraneoplastic Syndromes of the Neuromuscular Junction and Muscle

Lambert-Eaton Myasthenic Syndrome

LEMS is characterized by a defect in the presynaptic quanta release of acetylcholine. Cancer, usually an SCLC, develops in up to 55% of patients with LEMS. The clinical, electrophysiologic, and immunologic features are identical in LEMS patients with or without SCLC. The presenting symptoms are proximal leg muscle weakness and fatigability with a high incidence of autonomic problems, including blurred vision, sexual impotence, dry mouth, sluggish pupillary responses, and reduced lacrimation and sweating. Symptoms of cranial nerve dysfunction, such as diplopia, eyelid ptosis, and difficult swallowing, are mild or transitory. Distal unexplained paresthesias are frequent. The neurologic examination discloses proximal weakness and decreased deep tendon reflexes. Typically, a sustained voluntary contraction for a few seconds may result in an increase in muscle strength and potentiation of the reflexes.

The diagnosis of LEMS is confirmed by electromyographic studies. There is a reduced amplitude of the compound muscle action potentials, which increase more than 100% during repetitive supramaximal nerve stimulation or after a short period of maximum voluntary contraction. Antibodies against the P-type voltage-gated calcium channels are found in the serum of 85% of patients with paraneoplastic or nonparaneoplastic LEMS. P-type voltage-gated calcium channels are present in some SCLC lines and at the neuromuscular junction. LEMS is transferred to animals injected with immunoglobulin G (IgG) from LEMS patients, which suggests the antibodies are responsible for the syndrome.

Polymyositis and Dermatomyositis

Polymyositis and dermatomyositis are associated with cancer in 9% of adult patients. The clinical, electromyographic, and biopsy features are not different in patients with or without cancer. The relative risk of cancer is higher with dermatomyositis than without, 2.4 versus 1.8, particularly in women. Besides, dermatomyositis patients are more likely to develop the cancer in the year before or after the diagnosis of the myositis. The most commonly associated tumors are breast, ovarian, lung, and gastrointestinal malignancies. The paraneoplastic disorder runs an independent course from the associated cancer, but in some patients there may be clinical improvement when the tumor is treated.

Acute Necrotizing Myopathy

Acute necrotizing myopathy presents as a painful, proximal, rapidly progressive muscle weakness that involves respiratory muscles and usually causes the death of the patient in weeks or months. The syndrome has been reported in a few patients with lung, gastrointestinal, bladder, and breast carcinomas. The electromyogram discloses myopathic changes, and serum levels of creatine kinase are elevated. The syndrome differs from paraneoplastic polymyositis by having a more aggressive clinical course and the presence in the muscle biopsy specimens of extensive necrosis with absent or sparse inflammatory infiltrates.

Diagnostic Approach to Patients with Suspected Paraneoplastic Neurologic Syndromes

The clinical evaluation of patients with suspected PNS is difficult because similar syndromes may occur in the absence of cancer, and the tumor is not usually evident at the onset of the neurologic disorder in the majority of patients.

In patients not known to have cancer there are several neurologic syndromes that strongly suggest a paraneoplastic etiology and indicate the search of an underlying cancer (Table 40-5). The diagnosis of sensorimotor neuropathy, neuromyotonia, or dermatomyositis is not an indication for an aggressive search for an underlying neoplasm unless there are clues in clinical or laboratory examination findings. In PNS patients with clinical features or with anti-neuronal antibodies highly associated with a given cancer, studies to discover the cancer should be repeated every 3 months the first year and every 6 months the second and third years. If a tumor is not evident after 3 years, the syndrome may not be a PNS, and the subsequent diagnosis of a neoplasm probably is coincidental. When the same syndromes appear in the setting of a previously known cancer, a number of nonparaneoplastic disorders must be excluded (Table 40-6).

The most helpful test that suggests the parane-oplastic etiology of the syndrome is the detection of well-defined antineuronal antibodies (see Table 40-1). When the diagnosis of PCD is suspected, the detection of antineuronal antibodies will be helpful in ordering the appropriate tests. The diagnostic approach to anti-Yo–positive women should include a breast and pelvic examination, mammogram, and pelvic CT scan. If malignancy is not found, repeat mammography, pelvic examination under anesthesia, and uterine dilation and curettage are recommended. Surgical exploration and

Table 40-5. Neurologic Syndromes that Strongly Suggest a Paraneoplastic Neurologic Syndrome

Limbic encephalopathy
Subacute lower brain stem dysfunction
Multifocal involvement of the nervous system with sensory
  neuropathy
Subacute pancerebellar syndrome
Opsoclonus
Subacute retinopathy
Subacute motor neuronopathy
Subacute sensory neuronopathy
Lambert-Eaton myasthenic syndrome
Dermatomyositis in older patients

removal of pelvic organs may be considered, particularly in postmenopausal women. The detection of the anti-Hu antibody confirms that the cerebellar dysfunction is a component of PEM/SSN syndrome, and the tumor search should be directed to the lung. Because LEMS may coexist in patients with PCD and SCLC, an electromyogram is indicated in all patients with PCD with anti-Hu antibodies or without detectable antibodies. If anti-Tr

Table 40-6. Paraneoplastic Neurologic Syndrome in Patients with Known Cancer

Paraneoplastic Syndrome	Differential Diagnosis
Encephalomyelitis/limbic encephalitis	Brain/leptomeningeal metastasis
	Herpetic encephalitis
	Wernicke-Korsakoff syndrome
	Side effects of cancer treatment
Brain stem encephalitis	Brain/leptomeningeal metastasis
	Cerebrovascular disease
	Listeria rhomboencephalitis
Cerebellar degeneration	Brain/leptomeningeal metastasis
	Ara-C neurotoxicity
Opsoclonus	Cerebrovascular disease
	Drug neurotoxicity
Retinopathy	Leptomeningeal metastasis
	Side effect of chemotherapy
Subacute motor neuronopathy	Postradiotherapy motor neuropathy
Subacute sensory neuronopathy	Cisplatin/taxol neuropathy
Lambert-Eaton myasthenic syndrome	Cancer cachexia
Neuromyotonia	Metastasis to nerve roots of plexus
	Radiation-induced plexopathy
	Chemotherapy neurotoxicity
	Hypomagnesemia

antibody is present, a search for Hodgkin's disease is indicated.

In patients with suspected SSN, limbic or bulbar encephalitis, or multifocal CNS involvement suggestive of PEM/SSN, the most important diagnostic test is the search for the anti-Hu antibody. The detection of the antibody in patients with no known cancer should prompt the search for an SCLC. When a tumor other than an SCLC is discovered, the tumor must be tested for the presence of Hu antigens, and if results are negative, the search for an SCLC should continue. It is important remember that in some patients with limbic encephalitis as the only clinical evidence of the PEM/SSN syndrome, the anti-Hu antibody may be absent even when the underlying cancer is an SCLC.

Treatment of Paraneoplastic Neurologic Syndromes

The clinical course of PNS is not always uniform. Spontaneous improvement is reported in a few patients with PEM/SSN and SCLC, opsoclonus-myoclonus syndrome associated with neuroblastoma, PCD in Hodgkin's disease, acute or chronic sensorimotor neuropathies, and subacute motor neuronopathies. Furthermore, some patients with sensory neuronopathy and anti-Hu antibodies may present with a slowly indolent clinical course over years in the absence of any treatment.

Cancer treatment does not improve the PNS in many patients. However, the efficacy of antineoplastic therapy is difficult to assess because (1) PNSs are rare and multicenter therapeutical trials are lacking; (2) there is no successful treatment for some tumors; (3) PNS frequently appears before the tumor is diagnosed; and (4) some PNSs are characterized by neuronal loss and a beneficial treatment may arrest the progression but not lead to clinical improvement. In spite of these problems, aggressive treatment of the underlying cancer is recommended in all patients with PNS because, at least in a few patients, neurologic improvement or stabilization is reported in almost all types of PNS after the treatment of the tumor. In patients with LEMS, treatment of the associated SCLC is important to control the neurologic syndrome; when a patient with LEMS does not respond to immunotherapy, an occult SCLC must be sought.

Several immunosuppressive therapies, including corticosteroids, plasmapheresis, and intravenous high-dose immunoglobulins, have been used in the treatment of PNS. Corticosteroids are useful in the opsoclonus-myoclonus syndrome associated with neuroblastoma, LEMS, multineuritis with vasculitis, dermatomyositis, and in a few patients with limbic encephalitis. In most of these disorders, the damage to the nervous system is functional more than structural and the target neurons of the autoimmune attack may regenerate, so clinical improvement may be expected after treatment.

In PNS with neuronal degeneration such as PEM/SSN or PCD, immunosuppressive therapies have not been successful with the exception of isolated cases of PCD that improved with intravenous immunoglobulins. Plasmapheresis and intravenous immunoglobulin therapies also have been effective in LEMS and dermatomyositis refractory to corticosteroid treatment.

Suggested Reading

Anderson NE, Budde-Steffen C, Rosenblum MK, et al. Opsoclonus, myoclonus, ataxia, and encephalopathy in adults with cancer: a distinct paraneoplastic syndrome. Medicine 1988;67:100.

Brownell B, Hughes JT. Degeneration of muscle in association with carcinoma of the bronchus. J Neurol Neurosurg Psychiatry 1975;38:363.

Dalmau J, Graus F, Rosenblum MK, Posner JB. Anti-Hu-associated paraneoplastic encephalomyelitis/sensory neuronopathy. A clinical study of 71 patients. Medicine 1992;71:59.

Folli F, Solimena M, Cofiell R, et al. Autoantibodies to a 128-kd synaptic protein in three women with the stiff-man syndrome and breast cancer. N Engl J Med 1993;328:546.

Graus F, Dalmau J, Valldeoriola F, et al. Immunological characterization of a neuronal antibody (anti-Tr) associated with paraneoplastic cerebellar degeneration and Hodgkin's disease. J Neuroimmunol 1997;74:55.

Graus F, Delattre JY. Immune modulation of paraneoplastic neurologic disorders. Clin Neurol Neurosurg 1995;97:113.

Graus F, Reñe R. Paraneoplastic neuropathies. Eur Neurol 1993;33:279.

Jacobson DM, Thirkill ChE, Tipping SJ. A clinical triad to diagnose paraneoplastic retinopathy. Ann Neurol 1990;28:162.

Luque A, Furneaux HM, Ferziger R, et al. Anti-Ri: an antibody associated with paraneoplastic opsoclonus and breast cancer. Ann Neurol 1991;29:241.

Mancall EL, Rosales RK. Necrotizing myelopathy associated with visceral carcinoma. Brain 1964;87:639.

Newsom-Davis J, Mills KR. Immunological associations of acquired neuromyotonia (Isaacs' syndrome). Brain 1993;116:453.

O'Neill JH, Murray NMF, Newsom-Davis J. The Lambert-Eaton myasthenic syndrome. Brain 1988;111:577.

Peterson K, Rosenblum MK, Kotanides H, Posner JB. Paraneoplastic cerebellar degeneration. I. A clinical analysis of 55 anti-Yo antibody-positive patients. Neurology 1992; 42:1931.

Schold SC, Cho ES, Somasundaram M, Posner JB. Subacute motor neuronopathy: a remote effect of lymphoma. Ann Neurol 1979;5:271.

Sigurgeirsson B, Lindelöf B, Edhag O, Allander E. Risk of cancer in patients with dermatomyositis or polymyositis. N Engl J Med 1992;326:363.

Chapter 41

Hydrocephalus and Other Disorders of Cerebrospinal Fluid Circulation

Flemming Gjerris

Chapter Plan

Many studies of disorders of cerebrospinal fluid (CSF) circulation such as hydrocephalus and idiopathic intracranial hypertension (IIH) have been conducted in the last decade. New investigative methods such as magnetic resonance imaging (MRI) and MR spectroscopy have resulted in a better understanding of the pathogenesis and pathophysiology of these diseases regarding distinguishing between active hydrocephalus and degenerative brain disorders. The CSF dynamics can be investigated either by intrathecal invasive methods or by different MRI techniques. Values of resistance to CSF outflow (R_{out}) evaluated in some neurosurgical research centers are used as predictors for CSF shunting procedures. The most well-known disorders of CSF circulation are shown in Table 41-1.

Cerebrospinal Fluid Circulation

A better understanding of dynamic disorders of the CSF circulation is attained by a thorough knowledge of the anatomy and physiology of the CSF pathways. CSF dynamics are defined as all factors contributing to the formation, circulation, and absorption of the CSF. Only a short review of these dynamics is given here; for details see Chapter 11.

Anatomy and Physiology of the Cerebrospinal Fluid Pathways

The different compartments of the CSF are shown in Figure 41-1, and the various CSF volumes and other variables are given in Table 41-2. The interstitial fluid compartment is a very narrow space (150 Å),

Table 41-1. Diseases with Disturbances of Cerebrospinal Fluid Circulation

Hydrocephalus
Idiopathic intracranial hypertension
Subarachnoid hemorrhage
Meningitis
Meningeal carcinomatosis
Chronic meningoencephalitis
Head injuries
Spinal tumors
Surgery of the posterior fossa
Other pathologic conditions

separated from the small intracerebral vessels by a highly impermeable capillary double-layer cell membrane (the blood-brain barrier). The inside of the ventricular system is covered by the ependyma.

The main site of origin of CSF, a clear, colorless fluid, is the intensely vascularized choroid plexus.

CSF is created partly as a filtration process and partly as an active secretion. Other sources of CSF are interstitial fluid seeping away from the brain, either transependymal or transpial, to the subarachnoid space. The CSF formation rate (F_r) differs remarkably in various species and is approximately 0.35 ml per minute in humans, a total of 500 ml per day. The size of the CSF volume is closely correlated with F_r, R_{out}, and intracranial pressure (ICP). The normal CSF volume in an adult is 150 ml, thus requiring a turnover of three times a day. F_r can be inhibited by low temperature, by changes in CSF osmolality, and by some drugs, and it decreases slightly during increased ICP. CSF flows caudally in the ventricular system, compelled by movements of the ependymal cilia, by respiratory and arterial pulsations, and by small pressure gradients between the ventricular system and the sinuses. It moves into the spinal space, the cisterns, and sulci of the brain to the arachnoid villi, which act as one-way valves, carrying CSF to

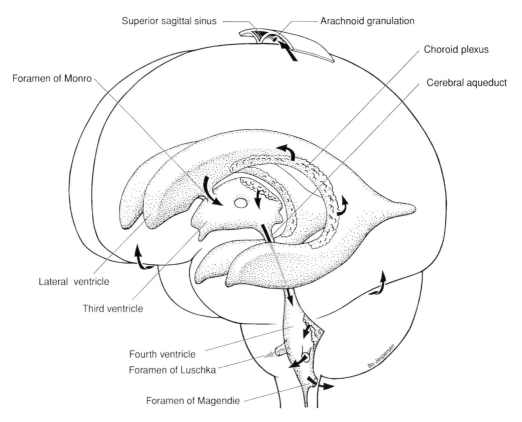

Superior sagittal sinus — Arachnoid granulation
Choroid plexus
Foramen of Monro
Cerebral aqueduct
Lateral ventricle
Third ventricle
Fourth ventricle
Foramen of Luschka
Foramen of Magendie

Bo Jespersen

Figure 41-1. The ventricular system of the brain. Arrows indicate the circulation of cerebrospinal fluid from the site of formation in the choroid plexus to the site of absorption in the villi of the sagittal sinus.

the venous outflow system. However, new MRI investigations together with isotope cisternography studies have questioned the well-known theory of a bulk flow in the CSF circulation. The length and diameter of the aqueduct influence CSF flow. Humans have the lowest R_{out} of all species. The main part of CSF absorption takes place through the villi into the sinuses, but new findings suggest a fairly large absorption into the brain itself. The relationship between CSF absorption and ICP is linear, and absorption begins at an ICP of 5 mm Hg.

The concentrations of single solutes (e.g., protein, transmitter) differ widely in the various parts of the CSF compartment. The differences in rostral-caudal concentration gradients for many transmitters make it difficult to interpret peptide or transmitter concentrations measured at the lumbar level.

Intracranial Pressure and Cerebrospinal Fluid Outflow

ICP is measured and monitored either by the epidural, subdural, intraventricular, or lumbar routes. Intraventricular monitoring by a frontal burr-hole is the gold standard and has many advantages. ICP is kept constant by different outflow resistance factors, which also are the major protective mechanisms against excessively high elevations of ICP. CSF vasopressin probably regulates some absorptive mechanism of intracranial water, and a linear correlation between ICP and the concentration of CSF vasopressin has been found (Figure 41-2).

Resistance to Cerebrospinal Fluid Outflow: Measurement and Reproducibility

R_{out} is in clinical practice measured by three different CSF manipulation methods: infusion (perfusion), bolus injection, and isotope dilution.

The infusion and perfusion methods monitor ICP during intrathecal infusion of lactated Ringer's solution at either a constant rate or a constant pressure. The absorbed flow values are plotted against the different ICP levels measured; the slope of the regression line is conductance to CSF outflow and the reciprocal value is R_{out} (Figure 41-3). The advantages of the method are CSF analysis and long-term ICP monitoring, but the risks of complications limit

Table 41-2. Normal Volumes of Intracranial and Intraspinal Spaces and Other Variables

Brain and spinal cord	1,250–1,500 g
Cerebral blood volume	50–100 ml (20–30 ml)
Cerebral blood flow	50–60 ml/100 g brain/min
Cerebrospinal fluid volume	100–150 ml (40–80 ml)
Ventricular system	15–25 ml
Interstitial fluid volume	100–150 ml
Intracranial pressure (steady state)	<15 mm Hg = <2 kPa
Resistance to cerebrospinal fluid outflow (R_{out})	<10 mm Hg/ml/min

Note: Numbers in parentheses are the intracranial reserve capacity.

general use. R_{out} values obtained by the computed infusion test correlate with values assessed from lumboventricular perfusions. They are reproducible and reliable. One measurement of R_{out} is sufficient, gives trustworthy information about disturbances in the CSF circulation, and is easy to perform.

The bolus injection method is fast and simple. A rapid intrathecal injection of a small bolus results in an instant ICP increase followed by a pressure decline. R_{out} is calculated from the changes in ICP. Comparisons between the injection method and other methods on estimation of R_{out} show that bolus values are lower than perfusion values.

CSF flow can also be estimated by isotopes introduced intrathecally by either the lumbar or the ventricular route. The tracer is followed by a gamma camera both in space and time up to 48 hours, and the findings are described morphologically or dynamically.

The majority of normal R_{out} values in humans (Table 41-3) have been obtained from patients. It has been found that the normal R_{out} is less than 10 mm Hg per milliliter per minute as determined by a lumbar computed infusion method in both healthy subjects and patients with spinal degenerative disorders (see Table 41-3).

Hydrocephalus

History, Definition, and Classification

Hydrocephalus is an increased CSF volume or a dilated ventricular system. There is no consensus on

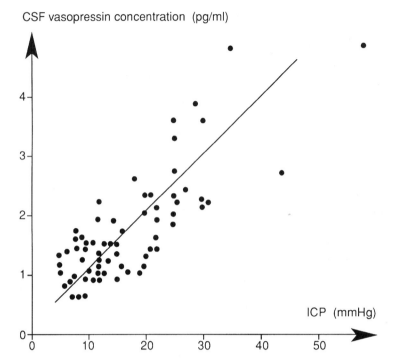

Figure 41-2. Relationship between intracranial pressure and cerebrospinal fluid (CSF) vasopressin concentration in patients with normal or raised intracranial pressure (ICP). (Modified from PS Sørensen, F Gjerris, M Hammer. Cerebrospinal fluid vasopressin and increased intracranial pressure. Ann Neurol 1984;15:435.)

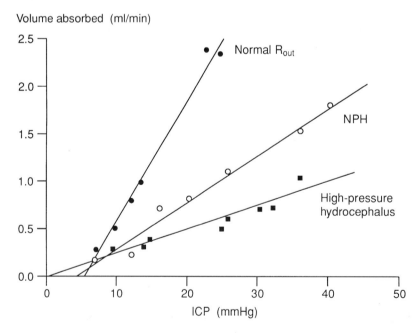

Figure 41-3. Cerebrospinal fluid outflow resistance (R_{out}) values obtained from three persons: one patient with normal R_{out}, one patient with normal-pressure hydrocephalus (NPH) and a high R_{out}, and one patient with high-pressure hydrocephalus and a very high R_{out}.

Table 41-3. Normal Cerebrospinal Fluid Outflow Resistance (R_{out}) Values

Authors (year)	Materials	Resistance to Cerebrospinal Fluid Outflow (mm Hg/ml/min)
Ekstedt (1978)	Patients	<8.33
Sklar et al. (1979)	Patients	<10.00
Børgesen et al. (1989)	Patients	<12.00
Tans and Poortvliet (1983)	Patients	<13.00
Albeck et al. (1991)	Normal individuals	<9.10
Albeck et al. (1998)	Patients (spinal diseases)	<10.00

these definitions. The modern concept of the pathophysiology of hydrocephalus dates back to the sixteenth century, when Stensen (Steno) in his postmortem examination of a hydrocephalic calf was the first to give a pathophysiologic explanation of hydrocephalus.

The incidence in infants is approximately 1 per 1,000 live births; when combined with myelomeningocele the incidence is approximately 3 per 1,000 live births. In adults it occurs in 15% of patients after subarachnoid hemorrhage and in 1% after meningitis.

Hydrocephalus can be classified in many ways, depending on the age of the patient (i.e., infantile, juvenile, or adult), on the pathologic or clinical findings (i.e., obstructive or nonobstructive, acute or chronic, active or arrested), and on the results of different investigations (i.e., communicating or noncommunicating hydrocephalus). None of these divisions is mutually exclusive. A classification by ICP and R_{out} values provided by intrathecal invasive methods divides patients into those with high-pressure hydrocephalus (HPH) or those with normal-pressure hydrocephalus (NPH) and into those with hydrocephalus with a high R_{out} or a normal R_{out}, respectively. The

last group also includes so-called atrophic hydrocephalus, or brain atrophy, a condition in which ICP is normal, there is passive enlargement of the ventricular system, and the R_{out} is normal. Many of these patients suffer from Alzheimer's disease or other degenerative disorders of the brain.

Etiology and Pathogenesis

The causes of hydrocephalus are manifold and complex (Table 41-4) and differ depending on the age of the patient at the time of diagnosis.

Hydrocephalus is basically caused by disturbances in secretion, circulation, or absorption of the CSF or obstruction of the venous outflow system. Increased CSF secretion is described only in children with plexus papillomas, in which the volume of the plexus is so large that the CSF formation rate exceeds absorption capacity. The CSF circulation can be restricted in the ventricular system (e.g., by tumors) (Figure 41-4), in the subarachnoid space (e.g., by subarachnoid hemorrhage), or by hyperosmolality in the CSF (e.g., by a spinal tumor leaking protein). Problems with CSF absorption are seen in

Table 41-4. The Most Common Causes of Hydrocephalus

Infants	Children and Adults
Chiari type II malformation	Aqueductal stenosis
Aqueductal occlusion	Arachnoid or intraventricular cysts
Dandy-Walker syndrome	Midline brain neoplasms (posterior fossa)
Malformations of the brain	Subarachnoid hemorrhage
Tumors of the brain	Meningitis and other infections
Arteriovenous malformations (vein of Galen)	Head injuries
Arachnoid cysts and idiopathic causes	Idiopathic causes

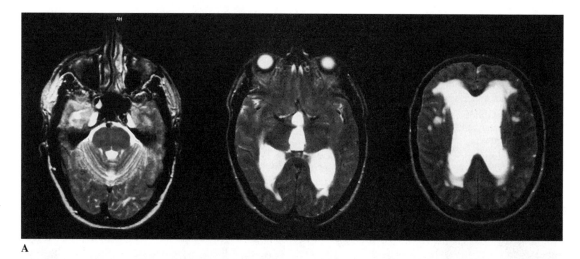

A

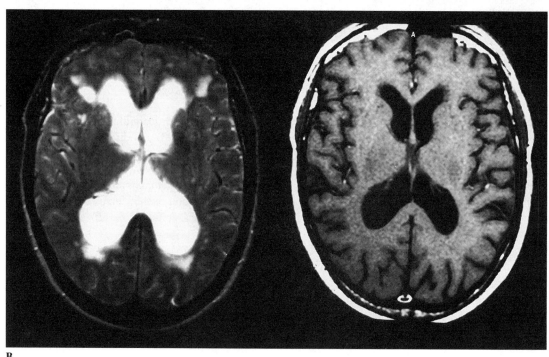

B

Figure 41-4. Hydrocephalus and a pineal tumor are demonstrated on these magnetic resonance imaging scans before and after an endoscopic third ventriculostomy. The tumor blocks the aqueduct and gives rise to hydrocephalus with severe periventricular edema (A and left side of B), which disappeared 3 months after the ventriculostomy (right side of B). Biopsy of the tumor by a supratentorial occipital approach showed it to be a benign cyst.

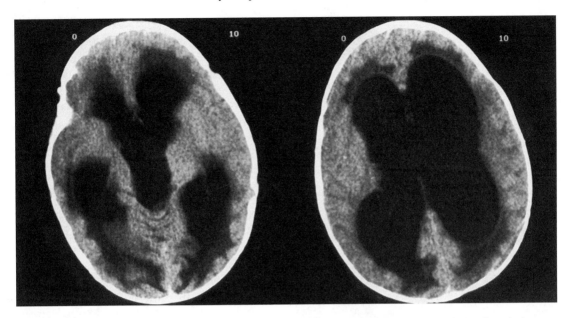

Figure 41-5. Severe hydrocephalus shown on a computed tomographic scan, demonstrating the typical periventricular lucency of the white matter around the anterior part of the frontal horns and the posterior part of the occipital horns.

conditions in which debris, high numbers of abnormal cells, high protein content, or scar tissue block the resorption channels in the arachnoid villi. Blockage of the cerebral venous drainage caused by systemic venous hypertension or thrombosis of the sinuses is not an important factor in the pathogenesis of hydrocephalus.

Pathophysiology

Complete or incomplete obstruction in any of the CSF pathways causes an increase in R_{out} and ICP followed by a dilation of the ventricular system cranial to the hindrance (see Figure 41-4). In kaolin-induced hydrocephalus in animals, a markedly elevated ICP and reduced production of CSF are found during the first week, with a decline in ICP toward the end of the next 4 weeks, as is seen in humans, in whom R_{out} and ICP increase after subarachnoid hemorrhage. As the size of the ventricles increases, the intraventricular pressure decreases. This paradoxical phenomenon is the result of a reversible variation in the extracellular fluid volume of the brain and mechanical stress on the ventricular walls. Many other factors influence the dilation and shape of the ventricles, especially after a prolonged

increase in ICP. The elevation of the cerebral venous pressure also plays a role in the maintenance of the hydrocephalic state.

Depending on the site of obstruction, the lateral ventricles are the first to dilate, followed caudally by the third ventricle, the aqueduct, and the fourth ventricle. Progressing hydrocephalus causes cytologic changes in both the cortex and especially the periventricular white matter. The ependymal lining is flattened and the subependymal layer is torn and stretched. The subependymal white matter degenerates and becomes edematous with decreased cell function. The periventricular lucency or edema is mainly confined to the white matter (Figure 41-5); this so-called hydrocephalic edema is hardly ever seen in the central gray matter. Very often a sharp demarcation between the edematous white matter and the intact gray matter is seen. CSF is presumably pressed through the ependyma into the subependymal area, and some CSF absorption takes place into the blood through the pial vessels. This periventricular edema has been explained as a transependymal absorption of CSF, but theoretically it is not easy to explain water absorption through the capillaries or the small veins of the subependymal layer. Hydrocephalic edema has also been explained as stasis of the

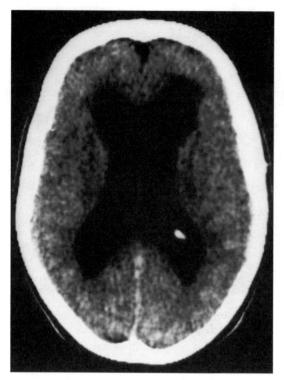

Figure 41-6. Severe hydrocephalus on a computed tomographic scan demonstrating absence of sulci or small sulci.

interstitial fluid. It correlates with a high R_{out} and thus indicates a low absorption of CSF. Hydrocephalic edema is demonstrated in Figure 41-5; the exhausted reserve capacity of the venous and CSF spaces in the disappearance or diminishing of sulci and cisterns can be seen on the computed tomography (CT) or MRI scans in Figures 41-5 and 41-6.

Diagnostics and Imaging Investigations

In infants, ultrasonography, transillumination of the thin skull, measurement of head circumference, and CT or MRI studies are among the most valuable studies. High-resolution cranial ultrasonography via the anterior fontanel or open sutures is particularly useful in premature infants, especially in the follow-up after intraventricular hemorrhage. It requires no anesthesia, is easy to use in serial investigations, and is the first choice in the initial evaluation. A flow diagram for management of hydrocephalus in infants is shown in Figure 41-7.

In older children and adults, CT or MRI scans are the investigations of first choice (Figure 41-8). They reveal many of the causes of hydrocephalus and are efficient means of follow-up before and after treatment. MRI visualizes the structures in all planes (axial, coronal, and sagittal) and gives an exact location and extent of the pathologic process. CT and MRI scans illustrate the dilated ventricular

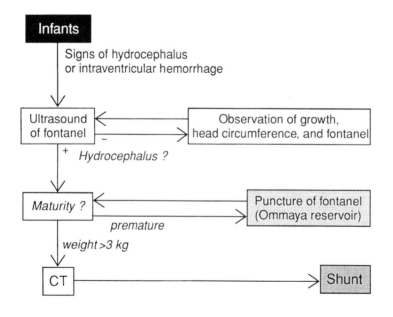

Figure 41-7. Flow diagram of diagnostics and treatment in hydrocephalic infants after intraventricular hemorrhage and with hydrocephalus of unknown cause. (CT = computed tomography.)

Figure 41-8. Flow diagram of diagnostics and treatment in older children and adults with suggestions of active hydrocephalus. (CT = computed tomography; MRI = magnetic resonance imaging; ICP = intracranial pressure; NPH = normal-pressure hydrocephalus; R_{out} = resistance to cerebrospinal fluid outflow.) (Modified from F Gjerris, SE Børgesen, PS Sørensen [eds]. Outflow of Cerebrospinal Fluid. Copenhagen: Munksgaard, 1989.)

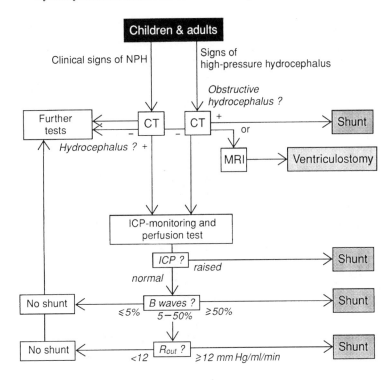

system, the size of the sulci, and periventricular edema, which is reversible after CSF shunting (see Figure 41-4B). In many patients these investigations also show the anatomic site of blockage of the CSF pathways (see Figures 41-4 and 41-9). CSF dynamics and blood flow in the sagittal sinus can be investigated by different MRI techniques—for example, flow void and two-dimensional cine phase-contrast MRI. From some of these MRI investigations it is possible to determine CSF flow in the cerebral aqueduct itself (see Figure 41-9). Some of these MRI methods are relatively new and the mathematics behind them complex, and evidence for their routine use still must be evaluated.

Various intrathecal infusion or perfusion methods are useful, partly for scientific reasons and partly because of assumptions about the effect of shunting (see Table 41-3 and Figure 41-3). The CSF tap test by the lumbar route has been described as a useful predictive investigation, but scientific evidence and a comparison with CSF dynamic tests is still needed. Many other investigations have been used for selection of NPH patients for CSF shunt-

ing; however, until now, the most useful single predictive test in our hands is measurement of R_{out} (see Figure 41-3), and it should be used as the gold standard in comparison with new predictive methods such as different MRI techniques. It is very useful and has a high predictive value in many studies. The flow diagram (see Figure 41-8) can be used as a guide for diagnostic investigations and treatment of a hydrocephalic child or adult.

High-Pressure Hydrocephalus

HPH is defined as a hydrocephalic state with increased ICP. Many of these patients have papilledema. The recent onset of bilateral papilledema always signifies an ICP of at least 20 mm Hg. If ICP is monitored, the lower level of ICP used in the definition of HPH should be 15 mm Hg. Even a moderate elevation of ICP should be defined as HPH and not NPH, especially because it is well known that the prognosis after CSF shunting is much better in HPH than in NPH. The different causes are outlined in Table 41-4.

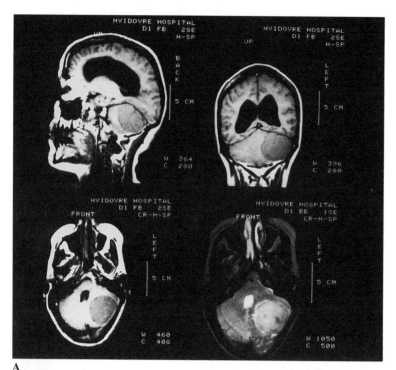

A

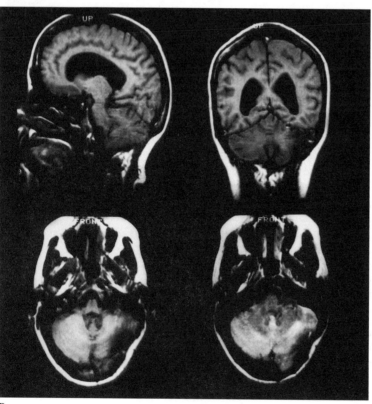

B

Figure 41-9. Magnetic resonance imaging scan before and after surgery for a huge meningioma in the posterior fossa. The severe hydrocephalus before the operation (A) disappeared quickly after the operation (B). Cerebrospinal fluid flow was close to zero, measured in the aqueduct by magnetic resonance spectroscopy before the operation and normal at follow-up examination of the patient 3 months after the operation.

Symptoms and Signs

Symptoms and signs are dependent on the age of the patient at the time of diagnosis, the different causes, and the location of the pathologic process. In infants, acute symptoms include irritability and attacks of screaming, drowsiness, and episodes of vomiting, rarely projectile. The most common signs are increasing head circumference, a bulging fontanel (investigated with the child in an upright position), dilated scalp veins, separated sutures, sixth nerve palsy, sunset phenomenon with downward deviation of the eyes and sclera visible above the iris, and neck stiffness and intermittent opisthotonic position of the head and back.

The symptoms in older children are headache and vomiting, which in typical cases occur in the morning, often with improvement after vomiting. There are complaints of blurred or double vision. Behavioral disturbances and declining school performance are well-described symptoms, which are often uncovered late in the clinical course as being the result of increased ICP. In children with midline tumors, the initial symptoms can be alterations in stance and gait, either caused by hydrocephalus and the subsequent pressure on the long nerve tracts passing close to the dilated frontal horns or by the cerebellar vermian process itself. Sixth nerve palsy, which is a nonlocalizing sign, papilledema, a "cracked pot sound," visual defects (increased blind spot), and a discrete, slight paraplegia are among the more common signs. Severe chronic papilledema accompanied by optic atrophy, progressing coma, and brain herniation are uncommon today, possibly because of better and faster diagnosis, both clinically and from CT or MRI scans. Similar symptoms and signs are described in adults in whom a slow-growing HPH (see Figure 41-6) also can result in severe headache, epileptic fits, progressing dementia, and gait disturbances.

Intracranial Pressure, Cerebrospinal Fluid Outflow, Cerebral Blood Flow, and Brain Metabolism

In HPH the ICP is elevated, very often with abnormal pressure waves and B waves. R_{out} may be more than 40 mm Hg per ml per minute in active HPH, and high ICP and R_{out} should be suspected when CT or MRI scans in addition to hydrocephalus show small or absent cortical sulci and fissures.

Cerebral blood flow studies and positron emission tomography (PET) characteristically show a regional reduction in flow and metabolism and only a global decrease in cerebral blood flow if the patient is very severely demented or unconscious.

Treatment and Complications

Treatment depends on the age of the patient at the time of diagnosis, the causes, and the examination findings. Even though both acetazolamide and furosemide lower ICP, treatment with these drugs does not cause the hydrocephalic state to diminish or resolve, neither clinically nor on CT or MRI scans. Patients with rapidly progressing signs of brain herniation should be treated with mannitol (0.5–1.0 g/kg body weight) intravenously and steroids until the obstructing process is removed, if possible (see Figure 41-9).

In infants with obstructive (both nontumoral and neoplastic) hydrocephalus, third ventriculostomy should be considered, because these children might have normal CSF resorption over the hemispheres or into the villi. Hydrocephalus after intraventricular hemorrhage in infants (see Figures 41-5 and 41-7) should be treated with serial punctures by the lumbar route or via an Ommaya catheter placed in the frontal region. They should be tapped regularly until the CSF clears up and should only be treated with a shunt when their body weight is more than 3 kg.

In older children and adults, endoscopic ventriculostomy should be considered. This operation is in many cases successful (see Figure 41-4). The success rate of the operation seems to depend on the cause of the hydrocephalic state and is much lower after meningitis or other hydrocephalus courses, where CSF circulation in the subarachnoid spaces and villous absorption may be impaired by the primary pathologic process. Ventriculostomy may be performed either as a first-choice treatment for hydrocephalus or secondarily after previous shunting—that is, for aqueductal stenosis. CSF shunting is necessary in many cases, and the flow diagram in Figure 41-8 can be followed. The main principle in the shunt is a ventricular catheter (mostly frontal), a pressure-resistant one-way valve, and a distal catheter, either to the peritoneum (first choice) or to the right atrium. The main configurations are the spring-ball, diaphragm, or slit-valve types. Some programmable types can have the opening pressure regulated from outside the skull. The different types open at different pressures or are

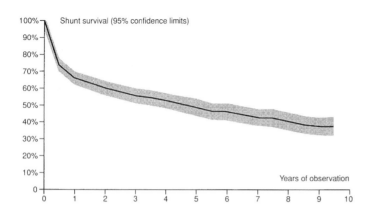

Figure 41-10. Shunt survival with 95% confidence limits. (Modified from F Gjerris, SE Børgesen. Current concepts of measurement of cerebrospinal fluid absorption and biomechanics of hydrocephalus. Adv Tech Stand Neurosurg 1992;19:145.)

pressure/flow regulated. There is not much evidence and nearly no consensus on the effect of prophylactic antibiotics, although most neurosurgical departments employ this treatment.

Complications are well known, numerous, and described in up to 40% of the shunted patients. Shunt failure is more often seen in infants than adults, and the most common are infection, obstruction, disconnection, or overdrainage. Chronic overdrainage (shunt dependency) is well known and can result in secondary aqueductal stenosis, which can make future treatment even more difficult. Fifty percent of the shunts are revised or not functioning after 5 years (Figure 41-10). An appalling late complication after atrial shunting is pulmonary thrombosis.

Prognosis

In infants, the prognosis very often depends on associated factors, such as congenital defects of the brain or spinal cord (e.g., myelomeningoceles or Dandy-Walker syndrome). Five-year survival in children treated for congenital hydrocephalus is 80%, but normal brain development or function is described in only approximately 50%. Adults treated by third ventriculostomy or a shunt have a good prognosis, depending on the cause of hydrocephalus, but even in obstructive brain metastases a long survival period without headache and other disabling symptoms is described.

Normal-Pressure Hydrocephalus

NPH is clinically an entity of progressing dementia, gait disturbances, and urinary disturbances, with hydrocephalus on CT or MRI scans, a normal ICP, and an abnormal R_{out}. In the definition of NPH, a sharp upper limit of ICP is necessary—that is, 15 mm Hg—to distinguish it from HPH. The disorder has many eponyms—for example, chronic adult hydrocephalus, low-pressure hydrocephalus, or occult hydrocephalus—and no consensus in the classification has been reached until now.

NPH is seen after subarachnoid hemorrhage, meningitis, head injury, and intracranial surgery. Sixty percent of NPH patients have an unknown cause to the hydrocephalic state, and in typical cases it is a disease of adulthood. Cases of NPH in children, especially after intraventricular bleeding or surgery for brain tumors, are well known but uncommon.

Symptoms and Signs

The classic clinical triad is insidious progressing dementia, gait disturbances, and urinary disturbances. The disease begins in many patients as walking difficulties, dizziness, balance problems, and small steps. Gait ataxia or apraxia is described by many patients as unsteadiness or uncertainty and is best demonstrated on special force-plate equipment. Difficulties with fine finger movements, tremor, and impairment of handwriting are not uncommon.

Intracranial Pressure, Cerebrospinal Fluid Outflow, Cerebral Blood Flow, Brain Metabolism, and Brain Biopsy

Twenty-four-hour (or overnight) ICP monitoring followed by measurement of R_{out} is helpful and reveals a high number of episodes of B waves, which correlate well with the values of R_{out}. The higher the R_{out},

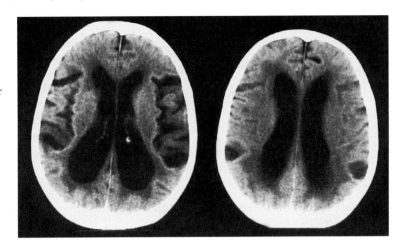

Figure 41-11. A computed tomographic scan of the brain of a patient with the triad of progressing dementia, gait disturbances, and urinary incontinence, demonstrating great fissures and sulci (for evaluation, see text).

the more frequent the B waves. The high percentage of B waves in NPH patients is probably caused by oscillations in cerebrovascular volume. There is a considerable variation of R_{out} from normal to very high values in NPH, but decreased CSF bulk flow—expressed as increased R_{out}—is well described in many studies.

The hydrocephalic edema seen on CT and MRI scans (see Figures 41-4, 41-5, and 41-6) is reversible even in NPH. In the evaluation of patients with signs of NPH, care should be taken in interpreting the findings on CT or MRI scans alone. Large fissures and sulci (Figure 41-11) do not speak against a treatable NPH condition, and these patients should be evaluated carefully—that is, by CSF dynamics (see Figure 41-3). MRI scans are better than CT scans in showing diffuse white matter disorders of the brain—for example, Binswanger's disease. The pathophysiology of NPH has been discussed earlier and is easier to understand in patients with subarachnoid hemorrhage and meningitis than in patients with an unknown cause.

Global cerebral blood flow is most often normal in NPH patients, and regional cerebral blood flow is significantly reduced, very often with enlarged subcortical low-flow regions and enhanced side-to-side asymmetry in central white matter and the inferior and midtemporal cortex. PET investigations using glucose markers have shown hypometabolism in different areas in patients with Alzheimer's disease and NPH.

In the group with NPH of unknown causes, a brain biopsy may be considered, especially because

the histologic findings can provide an explanation of either the failure rate or the brief clinical improvement after CSF shunting in elderly demented patients, even in NPH patients with an elevated R_{out}. In studies of NPH patients, brain biopsy demonstrated arachnoid fibrosis, Alzheimer's disease, or arteriosclerosis in more than one-half of patients.

Treatment and Complications

It is not easy to decide the best diagnostic procedure or the correct treatment in NPH patients, but an algorithm (see Figure 41-8) can be followed. Reliable predictive factors of improvement are (1) the triad of progressing dementia, gait disturbances, and urinary incontinence; (2) absent or small sulci, enlarged temporal horns or third ventricle, and periventricular lucency on imaging studies; (3) on single photon emission computed tomography (SPECT) or PET, low flow areas in the brain; (4) an R_{out} of more than 20 mm Hg per ml per minute; and finally (5) more than 50% B waves on ICP monitoring. If shunting is needed, a ventriculoperitoneal or ventriculoatrial medium-pressure shunt is the treatment of choice. Some authors recommend low-pressure shunts, but the data show no better results than with the use of a medium-pressure shunt, and the rate of complications, especially subdural effusions, is much higher. One should be careful in placing a shunt in severely demented patients with an unknown cause to their NPH unless they have an R_{out} of more than 20 mm Hg per ml per minute. Complications after CSF shunting are found in

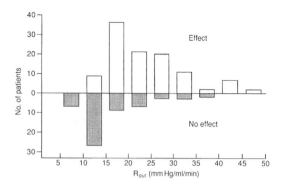

Figure 41-12. Resistance to cerebrospinal fluid outflow (R_{out}) values in patients with normal-pressure hydrocephalus before cerebrospinal fluid shunting. Patients who improved had higher R_{out} values than unimproved patients. (Modified from F Gjerris, SE Børgesen. Current concepts of measurement of cerebrospinal fluid absorption and biomechanics of hydrocephalus. Adv Tech Stand Neurosurg 1992;19:145.)

more than 30% of NPH patients, mostly infections or subdural effusions.

Prognosis

The outcome for NPH patients after CSF shunting is best when the cause of the NPH is known. It is much more difficult to predict the prognosis in patients with unknown cause. Strong selection criteria for improvement are necessary. Patients should be considered improved only if there is either amelioration in one or more functional grades or if there is recovery in dementia, gait disturbances, and urinary incontinence or if the family's estimation is good or excellent. One of the best predictive factors is the value of R_{out}. No patients with an R_{out} of less than 10 mm Hg per ml per minute should be given a shunt, because there is no improvement after shunting (Figure 41-12). Between 70% and 80% of patients with a high R_{out} improve clinically after shunting, and the mean R_{out} in NPH patients improving after CSF shunting is higher than in unimproved patients (see Figure 41-12). Many so-called NPH patients with an unknown cause have normal R_{out} values or do not improve after CSF shunting. Approximately one-half of these patients have brain abnormalities such as meningeal fibrosis, Alzheimer's disease, or ischemic changes on brain biopsy specimens at the time of CSF shunting, but no correlation is found between these findings and the clinical condition or the CSF dynamic values.

No single imaging method can identify responders and nonresponders after CSF shunting in patients with NPH. The improvement rate is higher when the third ventricle and temporal horns are enlarged and when sulci and fissures have normal sizes or when sulci are absent. The best prognosis in dementia alone in NPH patients, evaluated neuropsychologically before and after shunting, is found in patients with a combination of a known cause, a short history, high R_{out}, and small sulci or hydrocephalic edema on imaging studies. The same predictive value of R_{out} is demonstrated in NPH patients when gait disturbances are evaluated alone (Figure 41-13). Serious predictive prognostic signs are vascular episodes in the history, chronically systemic hypertension, and concomitant signs of arteriosclerotic brain disease.

Regional studies of cerebral blood flow (CBF) and PET investigations before and after CSF shunting in NPH patients show an increase in CBF and metabolism with a normalization or reduction in the area of the subcortical low-flow region in most of the patients, but so far the results are not clear enough to provide a certain indicative guide for CSF shunt operations.

Idiopathic Intracranial Hypertension

The clinical syndrome of IIH was described 100 years ago by Quincke, but in other terms—that is, *meningitis serosa*. It was later described in detail by many authors, who settled on the term *benign intracranial hypertension*. Because the prognosis for the visual impairment is not as excellent as previously believed, the term *IIH* is preferable. The diagnosis of IIH is one of exclusion.

Definition and Classification

IIH is a syndrome characterized by papilledema, no focal cerebral signs, normal findings on CT or MRI scans, and normal composition of the CSF. The presence of a space-occupying lesion or hydrocephalus on imaging investigations and signs of infection in the CSF exclude the diagnosis of IIH. An identical clinical picture is seen in chronic meningoencephalitis, cerebral sinus thrombosis, intrathoracic lesions, polyradiculitis, and spinal cord

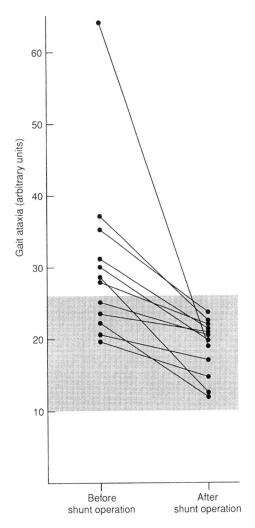

Figure 41-13. Stance and gait ataxia in patients with normal pressure hydrocephalus before and after shunting. (Modified from PS Sørensen, EC Jansen, F Gjerris. Motor disturbances in normal-pressure hydrocephalus. Arch Neurol 1986;43:34.)

Table 41-5. Causes of Idiopathic Intracranial Hypertension

Primary Causes	Secondary Causes
Idiopathic	Thrombosis of the sinuses
Metabolic diseases	Polycythemia
Endocrine diseases	Infections
A number of drugs	Spinal tumors

especially in obese females between 25 and 35 years of age. In the other age groups, the sex ratio is nearly equal. Many causes (see Table 41-5) have been described, often associated with endocrine disorders or the use of different drugs, but only a few cases are well documented. The different disorders that can produce a similar clinical picture must be excluded by the findings on CT, MRI, angiography, MR angiography, or lumbar puncture before it is safe to conclude the diagnosis of IIH.

Pathophysiology

Intracellular and extracellular brain swelling or edema is suggested, and an increase in brain water is also a possibility in patients with IIH. A slightly increased cerebral blood volume is described. CBF is normal, even in patients with an ICP of more than 40 mm Hg. Reduced CSF absorption resulting from increased R_{out} is a constant finding in many studies. Increased brain water self-diffusion is also demonstrated on MRI scans. The CSF dynamics and flow in the sagittal sinus measured by phase-contrast cine-MRI scanning are normal in patients with IIH.

It has been suggested that IIH could develop because of an increase of R_{out} at the level of the villi, caused by some of the proposed precipitating factors leading to an intracellular and interstitial accumulation of brain water and a "stiffer brain" or caused by agents or noxious events that might interfere with membrane function and brain water permeability. The elevated pressure in the subarachnoid space and on the cerebral veins causes cerebral vasodilatation and increased cerebral blood volume, resulting in a further elevation in ICP and R_{out} until the CSF absorptive level is in equilibrium. Patients with CSF absorption block who develop IIH probably have pre-existing

tumors (Table 41-5). If an etiologic diagnosis is suspected, it may be necessary to add a proper modifier to the term *IIH*—for example, cerebral sinus thrombosis or withdrawal of steroids.

Etiology and Pathogenesis

The incidence of IIH is close to 1 per 100,000, with an increase to 3 per 100,000 in women in the age group 15–44 years. It is found in all age groups,

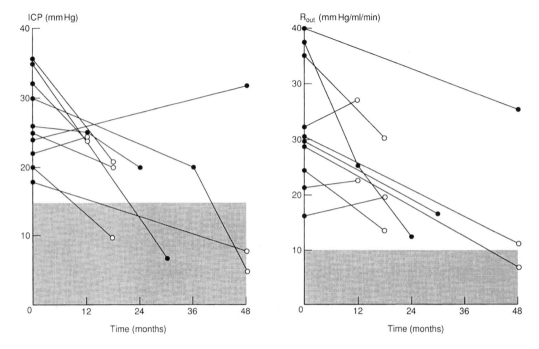

Figure 41-14. Intracranial pressure (ICP) and resistance to cerebrospinal fluid outflow (R_{out}) in patients treated for idiopathic intracranial hypertension. Closed circles denote clinical symptoms of increased ICP, open circles symptom-free patients. (Modified from PS Sørensen, F Gjerris, J Schmidt. Resistance to CSF Outflow in Benign Intracranial Hypertension. In F Gjerris, SE Børgesen, PS Sørensen [eds], Outflow of the Cerebrospinal Fluid. Copenhagen: Munksgaard, 1989;343–352.)

cerebral edema and do not generate hydrocephalus because the noncompliant edematous brain resists distension. No new findings contradict this hypothesis.

Diagnostics and Imaging Investigations

The ventricular system is normal or diminished on CT or MRI scans. An empty sella on plain x-ray films or CT scans of the skull is described in approximately 10%, and 25% of patients with IIH have changes of chronically elevated ICP. ICP investigation, most often by the lumbar route and R_{out} measurements, is recommended and is also a tool for follow-up.

Intracranial Pressure, Cerebrospinal Fluid Outflow, Cerebral Blood Flow, and Brain Metabolism

Nearly all patients have signs of increased ICP in the initial period of their disease. Lumbar puncture should be performed after normal brain imaging and is of no risk in patients with IIH. The composition of the CSF should be completely normal. Thirty to 120 minutes of lumbar pressure monitoring, which corresponds closely to ICP, is necessary and sufficient to reveal an increased steady-state ICP and abnormal pressure waves. Measurement of R_{out} by a lumbar computed infusion method is of considerable diagnostic value and an important variable in the surveillance of patients with IIH. It is reliable and can be repeated several times during the course of the disease, with a minimum of inconvenience to the patient (Figure 41-14). Increased R_{out} is initially found in most patients with IIH.

Symptoms and Signs

The symptoms of IIH are headache, visual obscurations, and double vision. Nearly 90% of patients have headache. Many of the patients have had symptoms for less than 3 months at the time of diagnosis. No focal neurologic signs except for those attributable to increased ICP—that is, papilledema, sixth nerve palsy, and enlarged blind spots, are found at the time of admission. Obesity is a consistent finding together with a significant weight gain 6–12 months before the symptoms of increased ICP have been noticed. Uncommon are dizziness, vomiting, and paresthesias. Visual obscurations or blurring of vision are ominous symptoms, which indicate that visual acuity is jeopardized. In rare cases blindness may occur rapidly, within one day, which is why vision should be monitored carefully when the diagnosis of IIH is established.

Treatment and Complications

Standard treatment is acetazolamide, 500–1,500 mg daily, and furosemide, 80 mg daily, for 6–24 months. Only a few patients do not respond to the medical treatment. If the eye symptoms do not improve quickly, patients should have the vision monitored by visual evoked potentials. A shunt operation, most often a lumboperitoneal shunt (easiest to perform with a small ventricular system) to avoid permanent visual defects may be necessary. Another possibility is optic nerve sheath decompression. The symptoms and signs of increased ICP disappear in the majority of IIH patients despite a sustained elevated ICP in some patients, who apparently also have a long-standing increase in R_{out}. Some patients develop chronic changes of the optic discs with gliosis, mimicking chronic papilledema.

Prognosis

IIH is usually a self-limiting disorder with a high spontaneous remission rate, and in many patients it carries a good long-term prognosis. Permanent visual loss is seen in a minority, and recurrence, even 5–15 years after the first attack, is described in up to 10%. Blindness can develop very quickly, within a few days, which is why patients should be monitored carefully during the treatment. In most patients monitored long term, both ICP and R_{out} decrease or normalize (see Figure 41-14), and the prognosis is good or excellent.

Other Cerebrospinal Fluid Circulation Disorders

Intracranial Hypertension

Subarachnoid hemorrhage, meningitis, meningeal carcinomatosis, and protein-producing spinal tumors may give rise to increased viscosity of the CSF, resulting in increased resistance to CSF circulation and outflow. This has been demonstrated in various clinical and experimental pathologic conditions. Functional or structural obstruction to CSF outflow in the above-mentioned diseases usually results in hydrocephalus, but in rare cases a condition similar to IIH is described. HPH and NPH with increased R_{out} are found after subarachnoid hemorrhage and meningitis, but it has been found in some cases that even ICP and R_{out} normalize over time; the ventricular system does not always diminish. Hydrocephalus is also found in pituitary apoplexy with blood in the CSF, in meningeal carcinomatosis, and after chronic meningoencephalitis with an increased number of abnormal CSF cells. When CT or MRI scans exclude a space-occupying lesion or severe hydrocephalus, a diagnostic lumbar puncture can be carried out without danger of brain herniation in most of these patients. Hydrocephalus or IIH is also seen after head injuries, in protein- or cell-producing spinal tumors, and in hydrocephalus after surgery of the posterior fossa.

Intracranial Hypotension

Low levels of CSF pressure have been characterized under the term *CSF hypotension syndrome* or *intracranial hypotension syndrome*, which secondarily may be caused by a variety of different disorders—for example, dehydration in infants, CSF fistulas after dural puncture, or CSF shunting. It is also described with an unknown etiology, the so-called spontaneous (primary) intracranial hypotension syndrome.

Definition and Incidence

Intracranial hypotension is present when the CSF pressure is 60 mm H_2O (4.5 mm Hg) or lower and is more often found in women (especially during pregnancy) than in men (3 to 1). The incidence varies with age, predominantly between 15 to 49 years of age. The disorder is very infrequent above the age of 65 years. Intracranial hypotension is most commonly seen in connection with lumbar puncture, often caused by an inexpedient technique.

Primary Intracranial Hypotension

Spontaneous, or idiopathic, intracranial hypotension is a rare but well-known clinical entity first described by Schaltenbrand in 1938. In some cases of spontaneous intracranial hypotension characterized by severe postural headache, modern investigations such as MRI scanning have disclosed CSF leaks, mostly in the spinal canal.

Symptoms and Signs.   The cardinal symptom is severe postural headache, which in many patients is partly or completely reduced by a recumbent position. The headache is aggravated by coughing or sneezing. Nausea or emesis, dizziness, neck pain, horizontal diplopia, changes in hearing, photophobia, upper limb pains or paresthesias, visual blurring, or dysgeusia are described in many patients. Positive clinical findings are visual field defects and sixth nerve palsy.

Investigations and Study Findings.   Patients with a postural headache should undergo neuroimaging, preferably MRI scanning with gadolinium, of both the brain and spine before a lumbar puncture. Lumbar puncture with pressure monitoring of at least 30 minutes is obligatory, including estimation of protein, blood cells, and malignant cells, especially if the MRI scan shows meningeal enhancement. CSF opening pressure is low in approximately one-half of patients and may be normal. A variable pleocytosis of 5 or more cells per cubic ml is also found in one-half of patients, as is a variable, mostly slight increase in CSF protein level.

The syndrome of low-pressure headache and pachymeningeal gadolinium enhancement on MRI scans is recognized with increasing frequency. One of the principal MRI features is diffuse pachymeningeal gadolinium enhancement, which in some of the literature is found in nearly all the patients. In some patients with spontaneous intracranial hypotension, MRI scans also reveal displacement of the optic chiasm, flattening of the pons, and downward displacement of the cerebellar tonsils. MRI

scans with gadolinium and MR spectroscopy with diffusion and perfusion studies may show a characteristic picture in patients with metastases or dural enhancement secondary to CSF leak. Dural enhancement is most frequently associated with metastatic malignancies. Other imaging studies in intracranial hypotension patients have shown that the diffuse enhancement of the pachymeninx often is associated with subdural fluid collections. Biopsy specimens of the meninges in patients with intracranial hypotension have either shown a thin subdural zone of fibroblasts and thin-walled vessels in an amorphous matrix or normal findings. Diffuse benign arachnoidal cell proliferation is also noted, probably a reaction triggered by long-standing changes. Usually there is no evidence of inflammation, infection, or metastatic neoplasia. Radioisotope cisternography demonstrates in some of these intracranial hypotension patients a fast accumulation of isotope in the bladder and early disappearance of radioactivity from the intracranial CSF space and is described as useful in illustrating a CSF fistula.

Pathophysiology and Pathology.   The findings on MRI scans, radioisotope cisternography, and dural biopsies suggest that the meningeal abnormalities found in intracranial hypotension patients probably represent reactive secondary phenomena, possibly related to the decreased CSF volume and hydrostatic CSF pressure changes, and not a primary meningeal process. Low blood concentration of vitamin A, which is thought to diminish the production of CSF, has been mentioned as a factor predisposing individuals to intracranial hypotension. Abnormal radioisotope cisternography with rapid absorption of the isotope from the CSF space suggests that an undetected CSF leakage or hyperabsorption could be a pathophysiologic factor in intracranial hypotension. The diffuse meningeal enhancement may also be explained by the dural venous dilatation that accompanies a reduced CSF volume.

Diagnosis.   Idiopathic intracranial hypotension is a diagnosis of exclusion and no evidence of underlying systemic or neoplastic diseases should be found. The dural enhancement found on MRI scans in patients with spontaneous intracranial hypotension should be kept in mind in hypertrophic pachymeningitis of unknown etiology. All secondary causes of intracranial hypotension should be eliminated, which in spontaneous intracranial hypotension means a vigorous attempt to diagnose and localize unknown CSF fistulas, especially in the spinal canal.

Differential Diagnosis.   The meningeal enhancement with gadolinium shown by MRI in patients with spontaneous intracranial hypotension should be differentiated from diseases associated with infectious or neoplastic pachymeningitis, but in spontaneous intracranial hypotension it is not always necessary to do an extensive workup for carcinomatosis or infection. It is important to remember that a low CSF pressure or a so-called dry tap can be caused by a spinal subarachnoid blockage provoked by an intradural tumor.

Treatment and Prognosis.   Severe, intractable headache associated with spontaneous intracranial hypotension may respond to intravenous or oral caffeine and bedrest. Intrathecal infusion of saline is recommended in the treatment of severe cases of intracranial hypotension. The prognosis in typical cases is good, and usually the symptoms gradually improve without any treatment. The intense meningeal enhancement on MRI scans resolves once the intracranial hypotension improves. The abnormal findings on isotope cisternography become normal spontaneously or after treatment.

Secondary Intracranial Hypotension

Secondary intracranial hypotension may be seen as a consequence of disorders that include dural puncture (e.g., spinal anesthesia or myelography), or operations in which CSF is lost (e.g., surgery including the dura or skull base). Hearing loss and dizziness, most often transitory, have been explained by the low CSF pressure, which affects the endolymphatic space. Experimental craniotomy studies demonstrate that the cochlear aqueduct provides a pathway between the CSF and the perilymphatic space. In prospective studies of the effect of neurosurgery or spinal anesthesia on hearing, it is suggested that the mechanism of demonstrated hearing loss is a direct result of the decrease in pressure or volume of the CSF reflected within the perilymphatic fluid and comparable with transitory endolymphatic hydrops.

Lumbar Puncture.   The characteristic clinical presentation of severe postural headaches with a low CSF pressure on subsequent lumbar puncture and a history of prior dural puncture should draw attention to the diagnosis of secondary intracranial hypotension. Intracranial hypotension results from the leakage of CSF via the dural hole, which produces hypotension in the subarachnoid space. The diameter of the lumbar puncture cannula is the main factor and the use of a small-diameter (25-gauge and less) cannula reduces the frequency of intracranial hypotension. Specially designed cannulas are recommended. No specific treatment is required in the beginning, as the symptoms spontaneously resolve in 80% of patients. After 1 week an epidural blood patch or intrathecal infusion of saline allows a 90% success rate. Prevention of intracranial hypotension after lumbar puncture is important and depends of the diameter of the cannula and the spinal puncture technique.

Cerebrospinal Fluid Fistulas and Hyperdrainage after Cerebrospinal Fluid Shunting.   CSF fistulas might be found spontaneously or as sequelae after intracranial or spinal operations. They can be classified based on the location of the CSF fistula—that is, skull base, spine, and CSF shunt overdrainage.

Symptoms and Signs.   The general symptoms and signs are the same as in spontaneous intracranial hypotension and focal symptoms and signs depend of the exact sign of the fistula. Many patients complain of rhinorrhea or a salty taste with a CSF fistula in a paranasal sinus, of otorrhea or a hearing loss with a CSF fistula in the petrous bone, and of neck or dorsal pain with a CSF fistula in the spinal canal.

Investigations and Study Findings.   The investigations are the same as for spontaneous intracranial hypotension. Spinal and skull base CSF leaks are often difficult to demonstrate radiographically or surgically, but isotope cisternography, CT-myelography, and brain and spinal MRI studies often do disclose a CSF fistula, especially in the cervical or upper thoracic spinal canal. Often these are seen as meningeal diverticula. They are uncommon but increasingly recognized as a cause of "spontaneous" intracranial hypotension. MRI scans show the same dural enhancement and downward displacement of the optic chiasm and cerebellar tonsils, resembling a Chiari I malformation as in spontaneous intracranial hypotension.

In CSF shunt overdrainage or hyperdrainage, many patients complain of severe headache and some develop subdural effusions together with a small ventricular system on CT or MRI scans. The patients may have caudal displacement of the brain on midsagittal images, and if the subdural effusions in intracranial hypotension patients are operated on, they are never under pressure.

Treatment and Prognosis.   Surgery on CSF fistulas and correction of CSF shunts are often necessary. The meningeal enhancement or the subdural effusions on MRI scans or the abnormal cisternographic findings are reversible when the CSF fistula is ligated or closed by an epidural blood patch or saline infusion or after a shunt is revised.

Suggested Reading

Albeck MJ, Børgesen SE, Gjerris F, et al. Intracranial pressure and cerebrospinal fluid outflow conductance in healthy subjects. J Neurosurg 1991;74:597.

Albeck MJ, Skak C, Nielsen PR, et al. Age-dependency of resistance to cerebrospinal fluid outflow. J Neurosurg 1998 (in press).

Bech RA, Juhler M, Waldemar G, et al. Correlation between frontal brain and leptomeningeal biopsy specimens to CSF outflow resistance and B-wave activity in patients suspected of normal-pressure hydrocephalus. Neurosurgery 1997;40:497.

Borgbjerg BM, Gjerris F, Albeck M, et al. A comparison between ventriculo-peritoneal and ventriculo-atrial cerebrospinal fluid shunts in relation to rate of revision and durability. Acta Neurochir (Wien) 1998 (in press).

Børgesen SE, Gjerris F, Schmidt J. Measurement of Resistance to CSF Outflow by Subarachnoid Perfusion. In F Gjerris, SE Børgesen, PS Sørensen (eds), Outflow of Cerebrospinal Fluid. Copenhagen: Munksgaard, 1989;121–129.

Czosnyka M, Gjerris F, Maksymowicz W, et al. Computerised Lumbar Infusion Test—Multicentre Experience in Clinical Studies in Hydrocephalus. In H Nagai, K Kamiya, S Ishii (eds), Intracranial Pressure IX. New York: Springer-Verlag, 1995;494–495.

Ekstedt J. CSF hydrodynamic studies in man. J Neurol Neurosurg Psychiatry 1978;41:345.

Gideon P, Sørensen PS, Thomsen C, et al. Measurement of blood flow in the superior sagittal sinus in healthy volunteers and in patients with normal-pressure hydrocephalus and idiopathic intracranial hypertension with phase-contrast cine MR imaging. Acta Radiol 1996;37:171.

Gjerris F, Børgesen SE. Current concepts of measurement of cerebrospinal fluid absorption and biomechanics of hydrocephalus. Adv Tech Stand Neurosurg 1992;19:145.

Gjerris F, Børgesen SE. Pathophysiology of the CSF Circulation. In A Crockard, R Hayward, JT Hoff (eds), Neurosurgery—The Scientific Basis of Clinical Practice (3rd ed). Boston: Blackwell, 1998 (in press).

Gjerris F, Børgesen SE, Sørensen PS (eds). Outflow of Cerebrospinal Fluid. Copenhagen: Munksgaard, 1989.

Mokri B, Piepgras DG, Miller GM. Syndrome of orthostatic headaches and diffuse pachymeningeal gadolinium enhancement. Mayo Clin Proc 1997;72:400.

Raimondi AJ. A unifying theory for the definition and classification of hydrocephalus. Child Nerv Syst 1994;10:2.

Schievink WI, Meyer FB, Atkinson JL, Mokri B. Spontaneous spinal cerebrospinal fluid leaks and intracranial hypotension. J Neurosurg 1996;84:598.

Sklar FH, Beyer CW, Ramanathan M, et al. Cerebrospinal fluid dynamics in patients with pseudotumor cerebri. Neurosurgery 1979;5:208.

Sørensen PS, Gjerris F, Hammer M. Cerebrospinal fluid vasopressin and increased intracranial pressure. Ann Neurol 1984;15:435.

Sørensen PS, Jansen EC, Gjerris F. Motor disturbances in normal-pressure hydrocephalus. Arch Neurol 1986;43:34.

Tans TJ, Poortvliet DCJ. Steady-State and Bolus Infusions in Hydrocephalus. In S Ishii, H Nagai, M Brock (eds), Intracranial Pressure V. Berlin: Springer-Verlag, 1983;636–640.

Tedeschi E, Hasselbalch SG, Waldemar G, et al. Heterogeneous cerebral glucose metabolism in normal-pressure hydrocephalus. J Neurol Neurosurg Psychiatry 1995;59:608.

Waldemar G, Schmidt JF, Delecluse F, et al. High resolution SPECT with [99mTc]-d,l-HMPAO in normal-pressure hydrocephalus before and after shunt operation. J Neurol Neurosurg Psychiatry 1993;56:655.

Chapter 42
Epilepsy

Christine J. Kilpatrick and Stephen M. Davis

Chapter Plan

With an estimated prevalence of at least 1%, epilepsy is one of the most common neurologic disorders. In addition, it is estimated that approximately 1 in 50 people have a single seizure at some stage in their lives.

An epileptic *seizure* results from abnormal discharge of cortical neurons. This electrical discharge may result in a disturbance of sensory, motor or psychic function, or conscious state with or without convulsive movements. Hence, the clinical features of seizures vary. *Epilepsy* refers to a chronic condition characterized by recurrent seizures.

Classification

The International Classification of Epileptic Seizures (ICES), published in 1970 and revised in 1981, is well accepted throughout the world. More recently the International Classification of Epilepsies and Epileptic Syndromes (ICE) has gained increasing acceptance as a useful characterization of the epilepsies. It is important to distinguish between the classification of seizures and the classification of epilepsies and epileptic syndromes. Seizures are best considered as symptoms, whereas the epilepsies and epileptic syndromes may include several seizure types and are characterized by a number of clinical features, including age of onset, etiology, family history, prognosis, and response to treatment.

Classification of Seizures

The ICES is based on seizure semiology and the site of electroencephalographic (EEG) activity. There are two main seizure types (Table 42-1): partial seizure and generalized seizure.

Table 42-1. A Classification of Epileptic Seizures Based on the International League Against Epilepsy Classification of Epileptic Seizures (1981)

Partial seizures
    Simple partial seizure
    Complex partial seizure
    Secondarily generalized tonic-clonic seizure
Generalized seizures
    Tonic-clonic seizure
    Absence seizure
    Myoclonic seizure
    Tonic seizure
    Atonic seizure
Unclassified epileptic seizures

In partial seizures, the EEG activity begins in a focus of the cerebral cortex. There are three types of partial seizures: simple partial seizures, complex partial seizures, and partial seizures that secondarily generalize to tonic-clonic seizures.

In simple partial seizures, the conscious state is preserved. The nature of the simple partial seizure depends on the site of the electrical activity. Involvement of the frontal lobe may present as jerking of the contralateral limb, involvement of the parietal lobe as sensory disturbance, and involvement of the temporal lobe as psychic phenomena.

In complex partial seizures, the most common type of partial seizure, the conscious state is impaired. The majority of complex partial seizures arise in the temporal lobe, the frontal lobe being another common site of origin. A complex partial seizure often begins with an aura, which is a warning of the onset of the seizure that in isolation is a simple partial seizure. If the seizure arises in the temporal lobe, the aura may take the form of déjà vu, intense fear, or an epigastric rising sensation. The patient then loses awareness and may stare and have a blank expression. This is often associated with automatisms, automatisms being defined as a confusional state during which nonpurposeful movements occur. Oral automatisms such as lip-smacking, chewing, and swallowing and limb automatisms such as rubbing and fiddling of a limb are common. Unilateral dystonic posturing of the upper limb is commonly seen in complex partial seizures of temporal lobe origin and is a reliable lateralizing feature indicating contralateral seizure activity.

A simple partial seizure may occur in isolation or progress to a complex partial seizure. If the focal electrical discharge generalizes, both a simple partial seizure and a complex partial seizure may evolve into a secondarily generalized tonic-clonic seizure.

In generalized seizures, the electrical discharges are bilateral, synchronous, and symmetric, involving both cerebral hemispheres from the onset. Despite this common electrophysiologic basis, the clinical features of generalized seizures vary significantly. The common generalized seizures include the following:

- Tonic-clonic seizure
- Absence seizure
- Myoclonic seizure
- Tonic seizure
- Atonic seizure

Tonic-clonic seizure is the most common type of generalized seizure and may have some or all of the following features:

- Loss of consciousness
- Tonic phase with stiffening of the body
- Tongue biting, incontinence, apnea
- Clonic phase with rhythmic jerking of limbs
- Postictal phase with drowsiness and confusion

The same clinical event may be initiated by a simple or complex partial seizure, in which case it is a secondarily generalized tonic-clonic seizure.

Absence seizures are characterized by brief loss of consciousness and awareness, during which the patient, usually a child, may stare blankly. The onset and recovery are abrupt without postictal confusion. Minor motor features such as eye blinking may occur, but there is no loss of postural control. During the seizure, the EEG recording shows bilateral synchronous 3-Hz spike-wave activity. The seizure and EEG changes can often be provoked by hyperventilation.

Myoclonic seizures are characterized by brief muscle jerks. These are usually single but may be multiple. Consciousness is usually preserved. The jerks usually involve the limbs and trunk, but on occasions may cause the patient to fall.

Atonic and tonic seizures often occur in the presence of diffuse cerebral damage and are frequently associated with intellectual disability. In atonic seizures, there is a sudden loss of postural tone and the patient falls to the ground, whereas with tonic seizures, there is a sudden increase in tone of the limbs, often with tonic extension of the upper limbs and associated brief loss of consciousness.

Classification of Epilepsies and Epileptic Syndromes

The epilepsies are divided into four subgroups (Table 42-2):

- Partial, focal, or localization-related epilepsies
- Generalized epilepsies
- Epilepsies and syndromes undetermined whether focal or generalized
- Special syndromes

The partial, focal, or localization-related epilepsies are divided into idiopathic and symptomatic or cryptogenic categories.

In idiopathic partial epilepsy, there is no structural basis for the focal, clinical, and electrical features. Benign childhood epilepsy with centrotemporal spikes (rolandic epilepsy) is a common form of idiopathic partial epilepsy. The condition occurs in otherwise normal children and usually remits in adolescence. Seizures are often sleep related and characterized by orofacial or oropharyngeal involvement, which frequently evolve into secondarily generalized tonic-clonic seizures. Genetic predisposition is frequent and there is a male predominance. The interictal EEG recording demonstrates a spike focus in the centrotemporal region that may shift from side to side. The seizures are usually responsive to carbamazepine.

In symptomatic partial epilepsy, there is an underlying structural cause such as hippocampal sclerosis or glioma. The most common symptomatic partial epilepsy is temporal lobe epilepsy caused by hippocampal sclerosis. Cryptogenic partial epilepsies are presumed to be symptomatic, but the cause is unknown.

The generalized epilepsies are divided into two groups: idiopathic (primary) generalized epilepsies, and symptomatic or cryptogenic (secondary) generalized epilepsies. Idiopathic (primary) generalized epilepsy, in its pure form, constitutes a condition in which there is no underlying pathologic abnormality, all seizures are initially generalized, onset is usually in childhood or early adult life, intellect is usually normal, and in many cases there is a genetic

Table 42-2. A Classification of Epilepsies Based on the Revised Classification of Epilepsies and Epileptic Syndromes (1989)

Partial, focal, or localization-related epilepsies
   Idiopathic partial epilepsies
      Benign childhood epilepsy with centrotemporal spikes
      Childhood epilepsy with occipital paroxysms
         Symptomatic partial epilepsies
      Temporal lobe epilepsies
      Frontal lobe epilepsies
      Parietal lobe epilepsies
      Occipital lobe epilepsies
         Cryptogenic partial epilepsies
Generalized epilepsies
   Idiopathic (primary) generalized epilepsies
      Benign neonatal familial convulsions
      Benign neonatal convulsions
      Benign myoclonic epilepsy in infancy
      Childhood absence epilepsy
      Juvenile absence epilepsy
      Juvenile myoclonic epilepsy
      Epilepsy with tonic-clonic seizures on awakening
         Symptomatic or cryptogenic generalized epilepsies
      West syndrome
      Lennox-Gastaut syndrome
      Epilepsy with myoclonic-astatic seizures
      Epilepsy with myoclonic absences
         Specific syndrome—seizures complicating disease state
Epilepsies and syndromes undetermined whether focal or generalized
   Neonatal seizures
   Epilepsy with continuous spike wave during slow wave sleep
   Tonic-clonic seizures in which clinical and EEG findings do not permit classification as generalized or partial onset
Special syndromes
   Febrile convulsions
   Isolated seizures or status epilepticus
   Metabolic and toxic-induced seizures

basis. The idiopathic generalized epilepsies usually have a good prognosis and in most cases, an excellent response to valproate.

Idiopathic generalized epilepsy is subdivided into a number of clinical syndromes. The most common are benign neonatal convulsions, childhood absence epilepsy, juvenile absence epilepsy, and juvenile myoclonic epilepsy. Benign neonatal convulsions occur in the first week of life and are very frequent repeated clonic or apneic seizures. Seizures do not recur and there is no associated psychomotor deficit. Childhood absence epilepsy begins in childhood and is characterized by frequent absence seizures. There is a genetic predisposition in otherwise normal children. Approximately 50% of patients have occasional generalized tonic-clonic seizures occurring in adolescence. Characteristically, the seizures are responsive to treatment and the condition often remits in adult life.

Juvenile absence epilepsy begins in adolescence with absence seizures being less frequent and tonic-clonic seizures more frequent than in childhood absence epilepsy. Response to therapy is good. Juvenile myoclonic epilepsy is now recognized as a common type of epilepsy beginning in adolescence. Characteristically, patients present after a generalized tonic-clonic seizure, but a preceding history of myoclonic jerks is usually obtained. Seizures are often precipitated by sleep deprivation and alcohol excess. Absence seizures may occasionally occur and genetic predisposition is common. Seizures are well controlled with valproate but have a high chance of recurrence after drug withdrawal.

Symptomatic or cryptogenic (secondary) generalized epilepsies, in their pure form, constitute a diffuse gray matter disease, often acquired. The condition usually has a poor prognosis. The most common symptomatic or cryptogenic epilepsies are West syndrome and Lennox-Gastaut syndrome. West syndrome is characterized by infantile spasms, arrest of psychomotor development, and a hypsarrhythmic EEG pattern. Onset peaks between age 4 and 7 months and prognosis is generally poor. Lennox-Gastaut syndrome presents in childhood and is usually associated with intellectual disability, which is often progressive. The syndrome is associated with multiple seizure types, predominantly atonic, tonic, and absence seizures. The EEG typically has a slow background rhythm with less than 3-Hz spike-waves and often multifocal abnormalities. Response to antiepileptic drugs is poor, although the best results are achieved with valproate, clonazepam, and lamotrigine.

Although in some patients with seizures one cannot make a syndromal diagnosis, an attempt at diagnosis should be made in all patients, particularly those with generalized seizures, in order to provide a more informed prognosis to the patient and appropriate advice with respect to antiepileptic drug treatment and duration of therapy.

Etiology

The etiology of epilepsy is variable and strongly related to age, seizure type, and epilepsy type. In many patients, it is probably multifactorial. In childhood, genetic factors and congenital disorders, such as cortical dysplasias, are common, whereas in adolescence with idiopathic generalized epilepsy, genetic factors are dominant. In older patients, tumor and cerebrovascular disease are more prominent. Partial epilepsies are more likely to be associated with an underlying structural cause, whereas generalized epilepsies more often have a genetic basis.

There is considerable evidence to suggest a genetic contribution to the etiology of epilepsy. This is particularly true of the idiopathic generalized epilepsies and benign focal epilepsies of childhood (idiopathic partial epilepsies). It is likely there is also a genetically transmitted susceptibility in the symptomatic partial epilepsies. In recent years, linkage studies have identified a single gene locus in several epilepsy syndromes.

Hippocampal sclerosis accounts for approximately 70% of cases with intractable temporal lobe epilepsy being considered for surgery. The etiology of hippocampal sclerosis is uncertain and there is a strong association with febrile seizures of infancy. The condition can be detected on magnetic resonance imaging (MRI) scans as atrophy of the hippocampus best seen on T1-weighted coronal images, increased signal on T2-weighted coronal images, and signal loss in inversion recovery (Figure 42-1). The technique of volumetric MRI has increased its ability to detect hippocampal atrophy.

Temporal lobe epilepsy secondary to hippocampal sclerosis is a well-recognized symptomatic partial epilepsy syndrome, often referred to as *mesial temporal lobe epilepsy*. The characteristic clinical features include the following:

- Onset in late childhood or adolescence
- Frequent complex partial seizures
- Rare secondarily generalized seizures
- Often intractable to antiepileptic drugs
- Past history of febrile seizures of infancy
- Responsiveness to temporal lobe surgery

Cerebrovascular disease is a common cause of epilepsy, particularly in the elderly. Early seizures

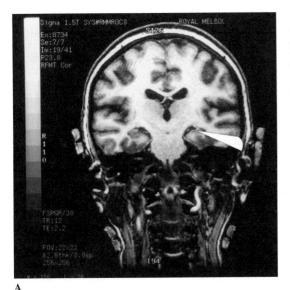

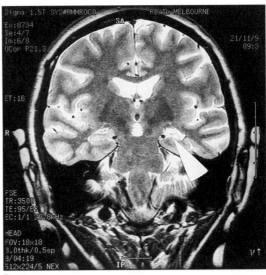

A

B

Figure 42-1. (A) A coronal T1-weighted magnetic resonance imaging (MRI) scan showing atrophy of the left hippocampus. (B) A coronal T2-weighted image showing atrophy and increased signal of the left hippocampus. (C) A coronal MRI inversion recovery image demonstrating atrophy and signal loss in the left hippocampus.

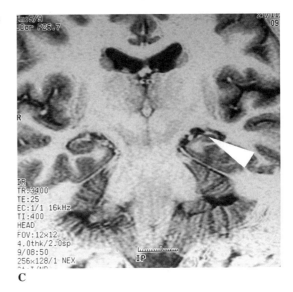

C

(seizures within 2 weeks of stroke onset) are a common complication of cortical infarcts and lobar hemorrhages, and in studies assessing the etiology of late-onset epilepsy, cerebrovascular disease is identified as the cause in approximately 20% of cases. Other types of cerebrovascular disease, such as cavernomas, arteriovenous malformations, venous infarcts, and subarachnoid hemorrhage, are also common causes of seizures, with cavernomas being a common cause of intractable partial epilepsy.

Cerebral tumor accounts for approximately 10% of patients with newly diagnosed, late-onset epilepsy,

the incidence being higher in patients with partial seizures. Epilepsy is more commonly seen in patients with low-grade gliomas than high-grade gliomas and is more common in frontal and temporal lobe tumors. Dysembryoplastic neuroepithelial tumor (DNET), a benign tumor, is a common cause of intractable partial epilepsy and is often surgically resectable.

Cortical dysplasias, which represent abnormalities of neuronal migration in fetal development, are common causes of chronic epilepsy. These lesions can often be detected on MRI scans and, when localized, are resectable.

Table 42-3. Features Differentiating Absence Seizures from Complex Partial Seizures

Features	Absence	Complex Partial Seizure
Age at onset	Childhood/adolescence	Any age
Etiology	Idiopathic	Focal lesion cerebral cortex
Electroencephalogram, ictal	3-Hz spike-wave	Lateralized anterior temporal rhythmic theta activity
Duration	Brief (seconds)	Longer (minutes)
Number of seizures per day	Multiple	Rarely more than 1–2
Aura	Nil	Common
Associated features	Minimal	Automatisms—oral or limb
		Dystonic posturing
Postictal state	Nil	Confused

Trauma is a common cause of chronic epilepsy in all age groups. Seizures that occur within minutes of a head injury tend not to recur, whereas early seizures—that is, seizures within 1 week of a head injury—have a high chance of recurrence. Late seizures may occur up to several years after a head injury and are usually recurrent.

Investigations

The assessment of a patient with an epileptic seizure aims to achieve the following:

- Confirm the diagnosis of a seizure
- Identify the seizure type
- Identify, if possible, the epilepsy syndrome
- Establish the etiology of the seizure
- Determine the prognosis
- Establish the need for antiepileptic drug treatment

Assessment and investigations that aim to establish the etiology of a seizure include the following:

- History and examination
- Interictal EEG recording
- Neuroimaging (computed tomographic [CT] scan, MRI scan)

The clinical history may provide important clues to the cause of the seizure disorder. A history of myoclonic jerks in an adolescent with a tonic-clonic seizure after sleep deprivation strongly suggests a diagnosis of juvenile myoclonic epilepsy. A history of complex partial seizures in a patient with a history of febrile seizures of infancy is suggestive of mesial temporal lobe epilepsy secondary to hippocampal sclerosis. In many patients, however, a definitive diagnosis of seizure type and etiology cannot be made and further investigations are indicated. For example, a history of blank spells may suggest both absence seizures and complex partial seizures, and in a patient with a tonic-clonic seizure, it is often unclear whether or not the seizure was a primarily or a secondarily generalized tonic-clonic seizure (Table 42-3).

Interictal EEG recording with surface electrodes may appear normal, which does not exclude the diagnosis of epilepsy, may show focal abnormalities, which may be regional excess slow waves (Figure 42-2), or may show focal epileptiform activity (Figure 42-3), suggesting the seizure is partial in type. It may show generalized spike-wave activity (Figure 42-4), which is suggestive of an idiopathic (primary) generalized epilepsy.

Neuroimaging is essential to establish the cause of the seizure. MRI is the investigation of choice, providing a reliable diagnosis of hippocampal sclerosis, cortical dysplasia, and small foreign tissue lesions such as cavernomas, low-grade glioma, and DNET, which are frequently not detected on CT scans. Current MRI methods include consecutive thin slice (<1.5 mm) volumetric T1-weighted imaging, T2-weighted imaging, and inversion recovery scanning, using a 1.5-Tesla machine. More advanced MRI methods, such as FLAIR (fluid attenuated inversion recovery) are likely to increase the diagnostic yield. Using current MRI methods, a causal lesion is found in the majority of patients with a partial epilepsy.

Other tests, such as cerebrospinal fluid (CSF) examination, biochemical and hematologic estimations, and functional neuroimaging with single photon emission computed tomography (SPECT)

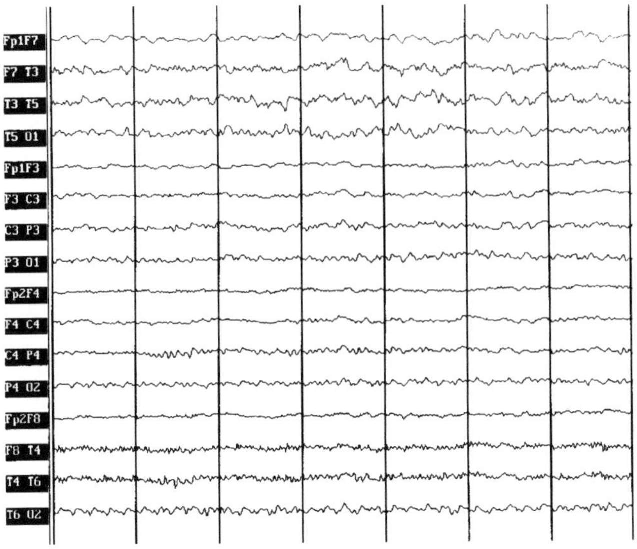

Figure 42-2. An interictal electroencephalographic recording with surface electrodes demonstrating excess theta activity over the left temporal region.

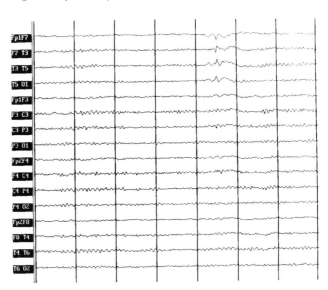

Figure 42-3. An interictal electroencephalographic recording with surface electrodes demonstrating sharp wave focus in the left temporal region.

and positron emission tomography (PET) are sometimes required.

Prolonged video-EEG monitoring is useful when there is diagnostic uncertainty as to the nature of the events, in determining seizure type, and in localizing the seizure focus before surgery.

Differential Diagnosis

The diagnosis of a seizure is a clinical one. There are a number of conditions that can be confused with and misdiagnosed as epileptic seizures:

- Psychogenic seizures
- Syncope (vasovagal and cardiac arrhythmias)
- Aggressive outbursts
- Transient ischemic attacks
- Episodic phenomena during sleep
- Transient global amnesia

Prognosis of a Single Seizure

When assessing a patient after an epileptic seizure, of major concern is an estimate of the risk of seizure recurrence and hence the need for treatment.

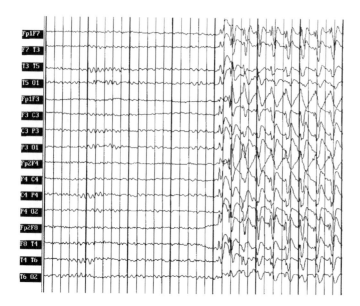

The risk of seizure recurrence is influenced by the following:

- Seizure type
- A finding of generalized spike-wave activity on interictal EEG recordings
- Neurologic examination findings
- Results of neuroimaging

Partial seizures, spike-wave discharges on EEG recordings, abnormal neurologic examination findings, and a lesion on MRI scans all increase the risk of seizure recurrence. If neuroimaging results are negative, the interictal EEG recording normal, and the seizure unprovoked, the risk of recurrence is approximately 50% over a 3-year follow-up period. Some syndromes such as juvenile myoclonic epilepsy are associated with a high risk of seizure recurrence without appropriate treatment.

Table 42-4. Seizure Types and Antiepileptic Drug of Choice

Seizure Type	Drug of Choice
Absence	Ethosuximide
Myoclonic	Valproate
Tonic-clonic	Valproate
Simple partial seizure	Carbamazepine
Complex partial seizure	Carbamazepine
Secondarily generalized tonic-clonic	Carbamazepine

Treatment

Medical Treatment

It is essential that the diagnosis of an epileptic seizure be definite before commencing antiepileptic drug therapy. In recent years, there has been a tendency to commence treatment after a single unprovoked seizure, provided the diagnosis is certain. Because certain drugs are more effective for one seizure type and epilepsy syndrome than another, accurate diagnosis is essential. Treatment appropriate to the seizure type and epilepsy syndrome should commence with one of the first-line antiepileptic drugs. If this fails—that is, the drug is either ineffective at a maximum tolerated dose or the patient develops intolerable side effects—then a second agent should be tried, either another first-line drug or one of the newer antiepileptic drugs. Although one aims to achieve monotherapy, in some patients combination therapy is more effective. Currently, the newer antiepileptic drugs are used as second-line agents, but it is likely in the future they will be used earlier in the treatment of epilepsy.

In current management, carbamazepine is the drug of choice for complex and simple partial seizures and secondarily generalized tonic-clonic seizures (Tables 42-4 and 42-5). Valproate is the first-line drug for primarily generalized tonic-clonic

Table 42-5. Established Antiepileptic Drugs

Drug	Indications: Seizure Type	Indications: Epilepsy Syndrome	Disadvantages	Value of Plasma Concentrations

Carbamazepine	SPS, CPS
	Secondarily generalized
	   tonic-clonic
	Generalized tonic-clonic
		Symptomatic and idiopathic
		  partial epilepsies
			Sedation
			Rash
			Leukopenia
			Hepatic induction
			Teratogenic
			SB (0.5–1.0%)
				Moderate

Valproate	Myoclonic Absence Generalized tonic-clonic	Idiopathic and symptomatic generalized epilepsies	Gastrointestinal upset Weight gain Hair loss Hepatotoxicity Teratogenic SB (1–2%)	Minimal

Ethosuximide	Absence	Childhood absence epilepsy
		  (absence seizures only)
			Gastrointestinal upset
			Ineffective against
			   other seizure types
				Moderate

Phenytoin	SPS, CPS
	Secondarily generalized
	   tonic-clonic
	Generalized tonic-clonic
		Partial epilepsies
		Post-traumatic epilepsy
			Sedation
			Cosmetic effects
			Nonlinear kinetics
			Hepatic induction
			Rash
			Teratogenic
			  cleft lip/palate, CHD
				Useful

Phenobarbitone	SPS, CPS Secondarily generalized tonic-clonic Generalized tonic-clonic	Partial epilepsies	Sedation Hepatic induction	Moderate

SPS = single partial seizure; CPS = complex partial seizure; SB = spina bifida; CHD = congenital heart disease.

seizures and myoclonic seizures. Ethosuximide is often the initial agent in children with absence seizures alone, but if there are associated tonic-clonic seizures, valproate is the drug of choice. Phenytoin is usually preferred in the management of patients with post-traumatic epilepsy and postoperative seizures.

In general, idiopathic generalized epilepsies respond best to valproate, with lamotrigine being a useful alternative. Symptomatic generalized epilepsies, such as West syndrome, respond to corticotropin or vigabatrin, and Lennox-Gastaut syndrome is best treated with valproate or lamotrigine. Idiopathic and symptomatic partial epilepsies respond best to carbamazepine.

The three new antiepileptic drugs—lamotrigine, vigabatrin, and gabapentin—have each been shown to be effective as add-on therapy in the treatment of partial seizures, with vigabatrin probably being the most effective in this patient population (Table 42-6).

Clinical experience and subsequent trials have shown lamotrigine to have a broad spectrum of activity with particular use in the generalized seizures, whereas vigabatrin may exacerbate generalized seizures, particularly absence and myoclonic seizures, and should be avoided in these patients. To reduce the risk of rash associated with lamotrigine, the drug should be introduced slowly, particularly in patients comedicated with valproate, which prolongs the half-life of this drug. Given the potential side effects of aggression and depression with vigabatrin, this drug should be avoided in patients with a past psychiatric history. Gabapentin does not interact with other drugs and is associated with relatively few side effects. Felbamate, a promising new antiepileptic drug particularly for the treatment of Lennox-Gastaut syndrome, has now a limited role in the management of epilepsy because of the adverse effect of aplastic anemia.

Table 42-6. Newer Antiepileptic Drugs

Drug	Seizure Type	Value of Plasma Concentrations	Advantages	Disadvantages
Lamotrigine	Partial and generalized	Uncertain, probably useful	Alerting effect Less sedative effect than most other anti-epileptic drugs	Rash Nausea, dizziness Valproate increases half-life Slow introduction required, particularly when comedicated with valproate
Vigabatrin	Partial Infantile spasms	Nil	Effective drug Sedation less than some first-line drugs	Depression, aggression Rarely psychosis May exacerbate myoclonic and absence seizures Avoid use in idiopathic generalized epilepsies
Gabapentin	Partial	Uncertain	Minimal side effects No drug interactions	Occasional sedation

Therapeutic Monitoring

Plasma concentrations of all the established and some of the newer antiepileptic drugs can be measured. Measuring plasma levels of antiepileptic drugs can aid in choosing the appropriate dose to minimize side effects and maximize antiepileptic effects. Phenytoin plasma levels are particularly valuable, with a good correlation between plasma concentration, therapeutic effect, and toxicity. Plasma concentrations of carbamazepine and barbiturates are of modest benefit, but the correlation between plasma concentrations of valproate and therapeutic effect and toxicity is poor. The value of lamotrigine plasma levels is uncertain and given the mechanism of action of vigabatrin, plasma levels of this drug are not used (see Tables 42-5 and 42-6).

Surgical Treatment

Although surgery for epilepsy has been performed for over a century, it is following the introduction of MRI that the concept of surgically remediable epilepsy syndromes has been recognized and epilepsy surgery has become relatively common.

Epilepsy surgery is indicated in patients who are unresponsive to available antiepileptic drugs, and in whom seizures are shown to arise from a single focus that can be excised. The most successful outcome is in patients with a focal lesion on MRI scans. The most common surgical procedure is temporal lobectomy.

Temporal Lobectomy

The most common surgically remediable epilepsy syndrome is temporal lobe epilepsy secondary to hippocampal sclerosis—that is, mesial temporal lobe epilepsy. Other surgically resectable epileptogenic lesions of the temporal lobe include DNET, low-grade glioma, cavernoma, and focal cortical dysplasia.

Assessment of patients for temporal lobe surgery includes the following:

- Clinical history
- Video-EEG monitoring with surface and sphenoidal electrodes and, if required, intracranial recording
- MRI scan
- Interictal and ictal SPECT
- Interictal PET
- Neuropsychology assessment
- Intracranial carotid Sodium Amytal test (Wada's)

Success of epilepsy surgery is dependent on accurate localization of the seizure focus. A detailed history of seizures from the patient and observers is essential to establish seizure type and frequency. A past history of febrile seizures of infancy suggests hippocampal sclerosis as the underlying cause.

Video-EEG monitoring, recording at least three habitual seizures, is essential to confirm the diagnosis of complex partial seizures and to localize and lateralize seizure onset, based on both the clinical features and electrophysiologic recordings.

MRI studies, preferably using volumetric acquisition of images, is essential in assessing the cause of the epilepsy. Functional imaging with interictal and ictal SPECT using hexamethyl-propyleneamineoxime showing hypoperfusion and hyperperfusion of the seizure focus, respectively, is helpful confirmatory evidence of the seizure focus (Figure 42-5). Interictal PET, demonstrating hypometabolism of the seizure focus, also provides further evidence of the site of seizure activity. These imaging techniques, both structural and functional, have circumvented the need for intracranial monitoring in most patients.

All patients should undergo a detailed neuropsychological assessment. This allows assessment of overall intellectual function, detection of verbal or nonverbal memory deficits suggestive of left or right hippocampal dysfunction, respectively, and an assessment of whether or not the contralateral temporal lobe is able to sustain memory function after a temporal lobectomy.

The intracarotid Sodium Amytal test is performed in patients in whom the neuropsychological deficits are not concordant with the proposed side of temporal lobectomy; there is evidence of bilateral hippocampal dysfunction; or there is a need to be certain of language dominance. In some epilepsy surgery centers, the intracarotid Sodium Amytal is performed routinely. The procedure involves unilateral intracarotid injection of Sodium Amytal to temporarily ablate the function of the ipsilateral temporal lobe. If the investigations are concordant for seizure localization and lateralization, an excellent outcome from surgery can be expected in 70–80% of cases.

Prognosis of Epilepsy

Approximately 70% of patients with newly diagnosed epilepsy treated with a single antiepileptic drug are seizure free. Only an additional 10–15% of patients, however, will become seizure free with

the addition of a second agent. Some epilepsy syndromes, such as juvenile myoclonic epilepsy, have an excellent response to treatment, with approximately 80% seizure free, whereas other syndromes such as Lennox-Gastaut syndrome have a poor prognosis despite multiple antiepileptic drugs.

Withdrawal of Antiepileptic Drugs

When a patient is seizure free for several years, the issue of drug withdrawal is usually raised. Factors that caution against drug withdrawal because of anticipated seizure recurrence are the following:

- Frequent seizures before the seizure-free period
- A history of partial seizures
- Multiple drugs required to achieve seizure-free status
- Epileptiform activity on interictal EEG recordings
- Lesion on MRI scan
- Intellectual disability
- Syndromal diagnosis of juvenile myoclonic epilepsy

If antiepileptic drugs are withdrawn, it should be done slowly over several months.

Status Epilepticus

Status epilepticus is defined as recurrent seizures without recovery of consciousness between attacks. It occurs in a minority of patients with chronic epilepsy and is rarely the first presentation of epilepsy. *Convulsive status epilepticus* is a medical emergency. Seizures that are multiple, although not continuous, may herald status epilepticus and should be treated in the same manner. Status epilepticus may be precipitated by the abrupt withdrawal of antiepileptic drugs, intercurrent infection, alcohol withdrawal, and new intracranial disease. Nonconvulsive status epilepticus accounts for approximately 25% of all cases of status epilepticus. It may in fact be more common, as cases are often not identified. There are two types of nonconvulsive status: generalized (absence status) and partial (complex partial status).

Absence status is the more common type and is characterized by a prolonged confusional state with

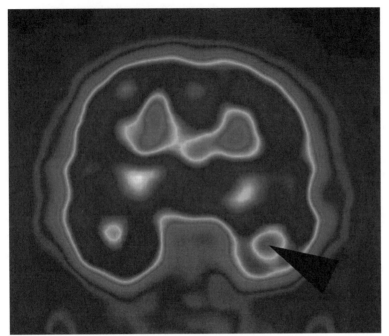

A

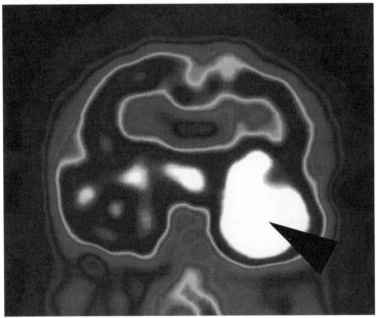

B

Figure 42-5. (A) An interictal ^{99}Tc-HMPAO single-photon emission computed tomographic (SPECT) study in a patient with mesial temporal lobe epilepsy showing hypoperfusion (*arrow*) of the left temporal lobe. (B) An ictal ^{99}Tc-HMPAO SPECT study showing marked hyperperfusion (*arrow*) of the left temporal lobe.

generalized epileptiform discharges on the EEG recording. The condition is not life-threatening and treatment depends on available facilities. The condition usually responds to intravenous diazepam or clonazepam. Complex partial status should be treated in a similar manner.

The principles of management of convulsive status epilepticus are the following:

- Stop the seizures (intravenous diazepam, intravenous clonazepam, or intravenous phenytoin)
- Protect the airway
- Establish the cause
  Consider psychogenic seizures
  CT scan
  Consider CSF examination

Women and Epilepsy

When managing women of childbearing age with epilepsy, a number of specific issues need to be considered.

Contraception

Enzyme-inducing drugs such as carbamazepine, phenytoin, or phenobarbitone may reduce the efficacy of the oral contraceptive pill. Women taking these drugs should use a combined high-dose oral contraceptive preparation, but the risk of pill failure remains.

Teratogenicity

The risk of congenital malformations in children born to women with epilepsy is higher than in the nonepileptic population and is higher again in women taking antiepileptic drugs. The risk appears to be greater with multiple antiepileptic drugs and to be dose- and plasma concentration–related. It is estimated the risk is 2- to 3-fold that for nonepileptic women. Probably all antiepileptic drugs are potentially teratogenic; some, however, have specific risks. Valproate is associated with a 1–2% risk of spina bifida; carbamazepine with a 0.5–1.0% risk of spina bifida; and phenytoin with congenital heart disease, cleft lip, and cleft palate. Folate supplements reduce the risk of spina bifida in the offspring at risk for this condition;

women treated with antiepileptic drugs, in particular valproate or carbamazepine, should take folate supplements (5 mg per day) before conception and during the first 3 months of the pregnancy. The safety of the newer antiepileptic drugs is unknown. If the epilepsy is well controlled, patients may wish to withdraw antiepileptic therapy before pregnancy. The risk of further seizures and the associated potential harm to both mother and baby, however, needs to be balanced against the risk of teratogenicity. The goal should be to control the epilepsy.

Seizure Frequency During Pregnancy

Most studies report an increase in seizure frequency in approximately 30% of patients during pregnancy. This may be in part the result of increased metabolism of the antiepileptic drugs and poor compliance with lowering of plasma concentrations or it may the result of withdrawal of therapy in order to reduce the risk of teratogenicity. Doses of antiepileptic drugs may need to be adjusted as the pregnancy progresses.

Breast-Feeding

Although all the antiepileptic drugs are excreted to varying amounts in breast milk, breast-feeding is usually not contraindicated, except when treatment includes sedative antiepileptic drugs such as benzodiazepines or barbiturates.

Driving

Every country has its own specific guidelines with respect to driving and epilepsy. In many countries, the different seizure types and epilepsy syndromes and their respective prognoses are taken into consideration. In general, patients with established epilepsy, particularly partial epilepsy, should be seizure free for 2 years before driving. After a single seizure, abstaining from driving for a period of 3–6 months is recommended.

Conclusion

In recent years, there have been significant advances in the management of patients with epilepsy. These include a recognition of the importance of accurate diagnosis of seizure type and epilepsy syndrome, leading to improved medical management, an increase in available antiepileptic drugs, and a shift away from invasive monitoring with more emphasis on neuroimaging, in particular MRI, in the selection of patients for epilepsy surgery. It is anticipated development of MRI techniques will result in a better understanding of the etiology of many epilepsy syndromes and lead to earlier referral for and greater access to epilepsy surgery.

Suggested Reading

Berg AT, Shinnar S. The risk of seizure recurrence following a first unprovoked seizure: a quantitative review. Neurology 1991;4:965.

Berger MS, Keles E. Epilepsy Associated with Brain Tumors. In AH Kaye, ER Laws (eds), Brain Tumors. New York: Churchill Livingstone, 1995;239–246.

Commission of Classification and Terminology of the International League Against Epilepsy. Proposal for revised clinical and electroencephalographic classification of epileptic seizures. Epilepsia 1981;22:489.

Commission of Classification and Terminology of the International League Against Epilepsy. Proposal for revised classification of epilepsies and epileptic syndromes. Epilepsia 1989;30:389.

Cook MJ, Kilpatrick CJ. Imaging in epilepsy. Curr Opin Neurol 1994;7:123.

Delgado-Escueta AV, Janz D. Consensus guidelines: preconception counselling, management and care of the pregnant woman with epilepsy. Neurology 1992;42(Suppl 5):149.

Delgado-Escueta A, Serratosa J, Liu A, et al. Progress in mapping human epilepsy genes. Epilepsia 1994;35(Suppl 1):529.

Kilpatrick CJ, Davis SM, Tress BM, et al. Epileptic seizures in acute stroke. Arch Neurol 1990;47:157.

Levy RH, Mattson RH, Meldrum BS (eds). Antiepileptic Drugs (4th ed). New York: Raven, 1995.

MRC Vitamin Study Research Group. Prevention of neural tube defects: results of the Medical Research Council Vitamin study. Lancet 1991;338:131.

Shorvon S. Status Epilepticus: Its Clinical Features and Treatment in Children and Adults. Cambridge, UK: Cambridge University Press, 1994.

Wieser H-G, Engel J Jr, Williamson PD, et al. Surgically Remediable Temporal Lobe Syndromes. In J Engel Jr (ed), Surgical Treatment of the Epilepsies (2nd ed). New York: Raven, 1993;49–63.

Wolf P. Treatment of the Idiopathic (Primary) Generalised Epilepsies. In S Shorvon, F Dreifuss, D Fish, D Thomas (eds), The Treatment of Epilepsy. Cambridge, UK: Blackwell Science, 1996;238–246.

Chapter 43
Neurologic Disorders of Systemic Illness

Annelise Dewarrat and Julien Bogousslavsky

Chapter Plan

Electrolytic Disorders

General Considerations

The clinical expressions of electrolytic disorders are diffuse encephalopathy and neuromuscular disorders. In general, neurologic manifestations correlate with both the degree and the acuteness of the metabolic disorder. Metabolic encephalopathy of all causes is characterized by behavioral changes, apathy, attentional disorders, disorientation, confusion, and various degrees of decreased consciousness evolving to coma in severe cases. Brain stem reflexes are preserved. Tremor, asterixis, multifocal myoclonus, and seizures are frequent. Focal neurologic deficits such as hemiparesis or extensor plantar responses are sometimes found in diffuse encephalopathies. In these conditions, a computed tomographic (CT) scan must be obtained to exclude a focal lesion such as a stroke or a subdural hematoma. An electroencephalographic (EEG) recording often shows nonspecific and diffuse slowing of the cerebral activity. An antecedent history and general examination may be helpful, but biologic tests are the key to the diagnosis.

Osmolality Disturbances

Sodium is the major cation of the extracellular fluid compartment and the principal determinant of serum osmolality. Hyponatremia reflects, with rare exceptions, a hypo-osmolar state. The two principal causes of hyperosmolar states are hypernatremia and severe nonketotic hyperglycemia. Osmolality disturbances almost exclusively induce central nervous system (CNS) disturbances. A slowly developing osmolality disturbance is better tolerated than an acute one because brain tissue is able to regulate its intracellular volume by increasing or decreasing intracellular osmolality via an increment or a decrement of organic osmolytes.

Hypo-Osmolar State: Hyponatremia

Clinical Manifestations.   Hyponatremia is one of the most common electrolytic disturbances seen in hospitalized patients. Acute hyponatremia (less than 24 hours' duration) is more dangerous and has a higher morbidity and mortality than more chronic hyponatremia. Patients with a serum sodium concentration below 125 mmol per liter may develop a diffuse encephalopathy and seizures if the serum sodium level falls below 115 mmol per liter. Anorexia, nausea, and vomiting can precede these manifestations. Neuromuscular symptoms such as cramps, fasciculations, and muscle weakness are rarely of clinical importance.

Pathophysiology.   A hypo-osmolar state results in a shift of water from the extracellular fluid down an osmotic gradient into cells. Brain edema, altered excitability of the neural membrane, and transient increased local brain extracellular fluid concentrations of organic osmolytes, namely glutamate, explain the clinical manifestations.

Neuromuscular irritability is possibly related to an increased concentration of cytosol calcium because of inactivation of the sodium-calcium carrier system. The elevation of the cytosolic calcium concentration lowers the excitation-contraction threshold and results in cramps.

Central Pontine Myelinolysis.   Central pontine myelinolysis (CPM) is a well-known complication of rapid correction of hyponatremia. The rate and magnitude of correction of chronic hyponatremia and probably the initial sodium concentration are the known risk factors of CPM. Ion-induced injury without adequate protection from organic osmolytes and disruption of the blood-brain barrier are the pathogenic mechanisms currently suggested by animal experiments. CPM is frequently associated with severe debilitating diseases such as cancer, chronic alcoholism and malnutrition, severe burns with major osmolality fluctuations, and liver transplantation. Delayed appearance of an acute spastic quadriparesis with pseudobulbar palsy is the classical manifestation. Oculomotor palsies may be associated rarely. Behavioral changes are prominent and decreased consciousness is common. Atypical associated features such as cerebellar ataxia and extrapyramidal signs and various delayed-onset movement disorders such as parkinsonism and dystonia are reported. Magnetic resonance imaging (MRI) shows areas of increased signal intensity on T2-weighted and decreased signal intensity on T1-weighted sequences in the central pons (Figure 43-1) and frequently associated bilateral extrapontine lesions, mainly in the neostriatum, lateral thalamus, internal capsule, and sometimes subcortical white matter. The outcome prognosis varies widely, from death to complete recovery, but most survivors have significant residual disability.

Treatment of Symptomatic Hyponatremia.   There is no consensus on the management of hyponatremia. In acute symptomatic hyponatremia of less than 24-hours' duration, rapid correction carries few dangers and can be life saving. Symptomatic hyponatremia of unknown duration should not be corrected at a rate greater than 8–12 mmol per liter per day.

Figure 43-1. Magnetic resonance imaging scan of the brain from a 52-year-old alcoholic man who developed, 3 days after correction of a severe hyponatremia, acute quadriparesis, bulbar palsy, and disturbances of consciousness. A T2-weighted sequence confirmed a pontine hyperintense signal suggestive of central pontine myelinolysis.

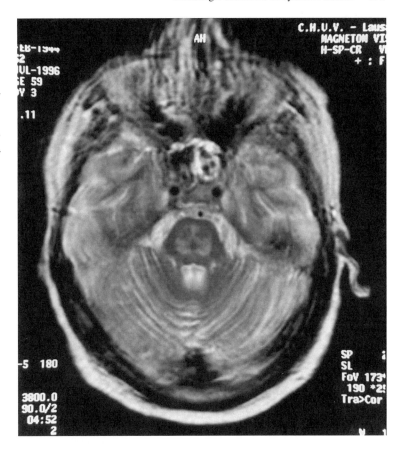

Hyperosmolar States

Hypernatremia

CLINICAL MANIFESTATIONS. Most symptoms of hypernatremia relate to the CNS. Symptoms of encephalopathy usually accompany serum sodium levels in excess of approximately 160 mEq per liter or total osmolalities of 340 or more mOsm per kg. Hemorrhagic encephalopathy can be a complication of hypernatremia. Rapid shrinkage in brain volume could lead to increased stress on the veins with subdural, subarachnoid, or intracerebral hemorrhages. In a few cases, a hypernatremic myopathy with proximal weakness and cramps and moderate rhabdomyolysis may be observed.

PATHOPHYSIOLOGY. Hypernatremia-induced hyperosmolality of the extracellular fluid results in brain cell dehydration and probably in modification of neurotransmitter release and brain energy metabolism. Disruption of the blood-brain barrier may also occur. In hypernatremic myopathy, an Na-K pump that is overworking to correct the intracellular electrolyte imbalance could be responsible for a depletion of the intramuscular energy stores.

TREATMENT. There is no consensus about the optimal rate of fluid administration in patients with hypernatremia. Seizures, fatal cases of cerebral edema, and permanent brain damage have occurred as complications of a too-rapid correction of hypernatremia. The rate of correction of chronic hypernatremia (defined as hypernatremia of >2 days' duration) should not exceed 0.7 mmol per liter per hour or approximately 10% of the serum concentration per day. Hyperacute hypernatremia (<12 hours' duration) may be treated rapidly.

Nonketotic Hyperosmolar Hyperglycemia. Nonketotic hyperosmolar hyperglycemia is a frequent cause of alterations of consciousness in elderly subjects with known mild non–insulin-requiring diabetes or in nondiabetics. An associated acute illness (infection, gastrointestinal bleeding, myocardial infarction, or surgery) precipitates the hyperglycemia in most of them. Mortality remains high.

CLINICAL MANIFESTATIONS.   A variable altered state of consciousness ranging to coma is always present in this condition and strongly correlates with a hyperosmolar state induced by osmotic diuresis. The blood sugar level usually ranges from 45 to 65 mmol per liter and plasma osmolality is always greater than 350 mOsm per kg. An absence of or very low levels of ketonemia differentiate this condition from diabetic ketoacidosis (DKA). Severe dehydration and moderate renal insufficiency are associated. Focal neurologic deficits, such as hemiparesis or Babinski's sign, mimicking acute stroke, are common in hyperglycemic nonketotic coma. Partial motor or generalized seizures occur in approximately 10–15% of patients. Rarely hemichorea or ballism may be caused by nonketotic hyperglycemia.

TREATMENT.   Correction of severe hyperosmolar hypovolemia by administration of relatively hypotonic fluids along with insulin to reduce the hyperglycemia must be done carefully to avoid a fall in osmolality that is too rapid and cerebral edema.

Potassium Disorders

Potassium is the principal intracellular cation. The transmembrane concentration gradient of potassium is maintained by selective permeability and active (Na/K/ATPase) and passive transport processes, and determines the resting transmembrane electrical potential of nerves and muscles cells. Potassium disturbances exclusively induce neuromuscular symptoms.

Hypokalemia

Clinical Manifestations.   At a serum potassium concentration of less than 3.5 mmol per liter, mild weakness, fatigability, and myalgia can occur. Trunk, neck, and proximal limb weakness evolving to areflexic flaccid quadriplegia with respiratory insufficiency is a threat when the concentration falls to less than 2 mmol per liter. Rhabdomyolysis and myoglobinuria may be seen and correlate with a segmental necrosis of the muscle fibers on muscle

biopsy specimens. Electrocardiographic modifications of the repolarization are well known but ordinarily without serious cardiac consequences.

Pathophysiology.   Pathophysiologic mechanisms underlying hypokalemic myopathy are modifications of membrane potentials (initial hyperpolarization and subsequent hypopolarization), blood flow, and energy metabolism.

Hyperkalemia

Clinical Manifestations.   The most important clinical manifestations of hyperkalemia are related to potentially life-threatening alterations in cardiac excitability. Peaked T waves, prolongation of the PR interval, loss of P waves, widening of the QRS complex, and then asystolia occur when the potassium concentration exceeds 7–8 mmol per liter. Hyperkalemia may produce muscle weakness but not structural muscle damage. When the serum potassium level is greater than 6.5 mmol per liter, paresthesias, fatigue, and weakness with reduced tone and reflexes are manifested. With severe hyperkalemia, higher than 8 mmol per liter, ascending muscle paralysis may occur and progress to flaccid quadriplegia with respiratory impairment.

Pathophysiology.   Initial membrane hyperexcitability from reduction of the resting membrane potentials is followed by diminution of the rate of rise and amplitude of the action potential. This slows conduction, may produce block, and is responsible for muscle weakness and cardiac conduction defects.

Calcium Disorders

Calcium plays a critical role in a variety of cellular and organ functions, including neuromuscular activity and modulation of membrane permeability.

Hypocalcemia

The prominent feature of hypocalcemia is neuromuscular irritability leading to tetany; tingling paresthesias involving the extremities and circumoral region are followed by carpopedal spasm and, in more severe situations, by laryngeal stridor, dys-

Figure 43-2. Computed tomographic scan of the brain of a young woman with hypoparathyroidism after surgical thyroidectomy. Note the asymptomatic calcifications involving deep gray nuclei.

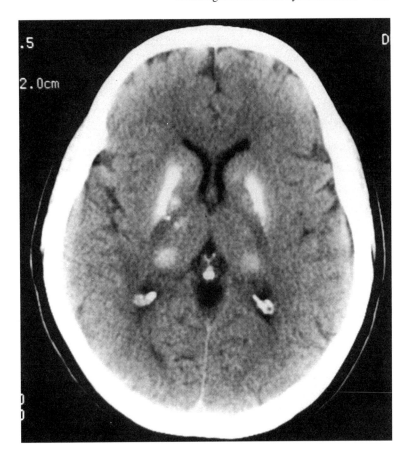

pnea, and generalized spasms. Mild diffuse encephalopathy and psychiatric disturbances are reported in up to one-half of patients with hypocalcemia related to hypoparathyroidism. Dementia may occur. Convulsions are common, especially in children. Severe encephalopathy with coma is exceptional. Brain calcifications, involving mainly the basal ganglia and sometimes the dentate nucleus and white matter, can be found almost exclusively in chronic idiopathic hypoparathyroidism (Figure 43-2). Pseudotumor cerebri with papilledema and increased intracranial pressure has been reported.

Hypercalcemia

Hypercalcemia induces both central and peripheral nervous system manifestations. Hypercalcemic encephalopathy may be severely confining or range to coma. Generalized or focal seizures occur rarely. Hyperparathyroidism is a classic cause of treatable dementia. Headaches and depression are other common symptoms. Hypertension and related cerebrovascular events are frequent complications. Brown tumors of the skeleton may develop in exceptional cases, and involvement of vertebral bodies with progressive myelopathy or radiculopathies have been reported. Myopathy is one of the prominent effects of hypercalcemia. In the long-lasting hypercalcemia of primary hyperparathyroidism, severe muscle weakness may be associated with amyotrophy and could mimic amyotrophic lateral sclerosis. Serum creatine phosphokinase levels are usually normal.

Phosphorus Disorders

Phosphate is the dominant intracellular anion and plays a critical role in many aspects of cell structure (component of phospholipid cell membranes, nucleic acids) and function (adenosine triphosphate [ATP] synthesis mainly, but also enzyme cofactor in glycolysis and 2,3-DPG synthesis).

In hypophosphatemia, neuromuscular symptoms are prevalent, but CNS manifestations are reported. Profound muscular weakness may occur. Acute reversible respiratory failure and failure to wean have been described in intensive care patients. Acute rhabdomyolysis is reported during treatment of alcoholic withdrawal, refeeding after starvation, and treatment of DKA. Pre-existing muscle cell injury related to nutritional derangements is a contributing factor, as are other associated electrolyte disorders. Paresthesias and weakness have been attributed to peripheral nerve conduction dysfunction. Perioral dysesthesias, ataxia and dysarthria, confusion, and in severe cases, seizures and coma are reported.

Magnesium Disorders

Magnesium is the second most abundant intracellular cation. The kidney is the major regulator of the serum magnesium concentration. Magnesium is an enzymatic cofactor in both carbohydrate and protein metabolism. It has an action similar to calcium on muscle and nerve membranes and an opposite action on neuromuscular function.

Hypermagnesemia

Hypermagnesemia is usually iatrogenic, most commonly in renal failure, particularly after exogenous magnesium administration (antacids, enemas, parenteral alimentation) or parenteral therapy. Depression of neuromuscular function occurs along with a reduction in deep tendon reflexes when serum magnesium levels are higher than 4 mmol per liter. At levels of more than 10 mmol per liter, flaccid quadriplegia or respiratory failure and apnea may occur. Stupor and coma develop at higher levels as life-threatening cardiac conduction defects.

Hypomagnesemia

Hypomagnesemia is caused by reduced intake, impaired absorption from excessive gastrointestinal losses (diarrhea, laxatives), or renal losses, mostly from use of diuretics. It is frequently associated with hypocalcemia and hypokalemia. At serum levels of less than 0.6 mmol per liter, increased neuromuscular excitability occurs, with muscle twitching, cramps, carpopedal spasm, paresthesias, muscle weakness, mild encephalopathy, and cardiac arrhythmias.

Metabolic and Endocrine Disorders

Diabetic Ketoacidosis

DKA is caused by insulin deficiency and precipitated by a failure of the patient to take insulin, infection, intercurrent illness, or emotional stress. CNS manifestations are more frequent in hyperosmolar nonketotic decompensation of diabetes than in DKA. Coma occurs in only approximately 10% of the patients with DKA, but a majority of them have moderate degrees of altered consciousness. Two causes of worsening altered consciousness during initial therapy are a rapid fall in the serum glucose level and osmolality with associated cerebral edema and excessive bicarbonate replacement resulting in rebound CNS acidosis. The latter occurs because carbon dioxide is more readily diffusible across the blood-brain barrier than is bicarbonate ion, causing the CNS pH to fall at a time when the peripheral pH is rising.

Nonketotic Hyperosmolar Hyperglycemia

Nonketotic hyperosmolar hyperglycemia is discussed under "Hyperosmolar States."

Hypoglycemia

Clinical Manifestations

Hypoglycemic encephalopathy occurs when the serum glucose level falls below 2.5 mmol per liter, but sometimes it occurs at higher glucose levels. Low blood glucose levels and a rapid regression of symptoms after administration of a hypertonic glucose solution are the hallmarks of the disease. Bizarre behaviors, sometimes mimicking psychiatric disturbances, confusion, and altered consciousness ranging from stupor to coma are signs of hypoglycemic encephalopathy. Although the depth of coma generally correlates with blood glucose levels, considerable overlap is described. Profound coma with mydriasis, bradycardia, irregular respiration, and hypotonia develops when glycemia falls to less than 0.5 mmol per liter. Focal or generalized seizures may occur. Transient episodes of reversible hemiplegia are classically reported. Paroxysmal choreoathetosis caused by hypoglycemia can occur. The duration of the hypoglycemia seems to be the principal determinant of death and neurologic and cognitive sequelae.

Pathophysiology

The brain has a particular metabolic dependence on glucose, the essential energetic substrate. Daily glucose consumption of the brain is 100–150 g and the few stores, principally glycogen, would maintain the brain's normal function for no more than 2–3 minutes if the blood supply is abruptly cut off.

Neuropathology

Selective neuronal vulnerability has been described in autopsy cases. If laminar necrosis of cortical ribbon is similar to the damage caused by cerebral hypoxia, involvement of Ammon's horn is particularly conspicuous. The putamen and the caudate nucleus are greatly altered, but the Purkinje cells of the cerebellum are less often involved than in hypoxia.

Diabetic Neuropathies

Diabetes is the primary cause of peripheral neuropathy. The duration of diabetes, age, genetic predisposition, and poor control of diabetes are known risk factors. Many distinct clinical types of diabetic neuropathies are defined and must be recognized for proper management (Table 43-1). The clinical types are not mutually exclusive. For example, radiculoplexopathy coexists generally with distal sensory neuropathy.

Symmetric Neuropathies

Distal sensory and sensorimotor neuropathy is the most common type of diabetic neuropathy, often being mildly symptomatic or asymptomatic. Both

Table 43-1. Clinical Classification of Diabetic Neuropathy

Symmetric neuropathies
Distal sensory and sensorimotor neuropathy
Large fiber–type neuropathy
Small fiber–type neuropathy
Acute painful neuropathy
Autonomic neuropathy
"Insulin" neuropathy
Asymmetric neuropathies
Mononeuropathy (cranial and limb)
Radiculopathy
Lumbar plexopathy or radiculoplexopathy
Chronic inflammatory polyradiculoneuropathy

Source: Adapted from PA Low, GA Suarez. Diabetic Neuropathies. In HP Hartung (ed), Peripheral Neuropathies: Part I. London: Baillère's Tindall, 1995;401–426.

small and large myelinated fibers are commonly affected, but a predominantly large fiber-type neuropathy with severe sensory ataxia or a small fiber-type neuropathy with distal burning pain, loss of pain and temperature sensation, and autonomic dysfunction are recognized. An acute painful diabetic neuropathy, often related to poor diabetes control, with associated profound weight loss is described. A good evolution is expected after adequate diabetic control is achieved. It is important to recognize autonomic neuropathy because it carries an increased risk of death from severe arrhythmias, silent myocardial infarction, and unrecognized hypoglycemia. Many organs and functions are involved as a result of disturbances of both the sympathetic and parasympathetic systems, mainly the cardiovascular system, the genitourinary and digestive tracts, the thermoregulatory system and pupillary function, and because of unawareness of hypoglycemia.

Asymmetric Neuropathies

The most common mononeuropathy is an isolated third nerve cranial neuropathy. Pain behind or above the eye is present in approximately one-half of cases. Pupillomotor function is generally spared. In decreased order of frequency, the sixth, the fourth, and the seventh nerves may be affected. The limb nerves most commonly involved are the ulnar, median, radial, femoral, lateral cutaneous of the thigh, and common peroneal nerves. Lesions occur at the common sites of external pressure palsies. Plexopathies and radiculoplexopathies are invariably associated with a distal sensory neuropathy. Weight loss and deep pain, localized in the thigh but also in the buttock or the lumbar region, are followed by proximal weakness and amyotrophy. The muscles affected are the iliopsoas, quadriceps, and adductors. The knee reflex is typically reduced or absent. The hip flexors and hamstrings are most commonly spared. Not infrequently both sides can be involved subsequently in an asymmetric fashion.

Thyroid Diseases

Thyroid dysfunction must be considered in the differential diagnosis of many central and peripheral nervous system disorders, because neurologic signs may often precede the other systemic manifestations, especially in the elderly.

Hyperthyroidism

Hyperthyroidism has many causes (e.g., Grave's disease, toxic multinodular goiter, toxic adenoma) and affects many organs. Neurologic manifestations are divided into neuromuscular and central nervous system disorders.

Neuromuscular Disorders.   Myopathy is the most frequent neuromuscular manifestation of hyperthyroidism, with an incidence of approximately 60%. Clinical examination reveals a predominantly proximal weakness and usually only mild muscle atrophy. Deep tendon reflexes may be normal or have a shortened relaxation time. Bulbar muscles and the esophagus may rarely be involved. Rarely, the clinical picture resembles anterior horn cell disease, with fasciculations and myokymia. Serum levels of muscular enzymes are usually normal. There have been several reports of acute thyrotoxic myopathy with severe generalized weakness and bulbar palsy. Some of these are probably cases of acute myasthenia gravis coincident with thyrotoxicosis (common autoimmune mechanisms). Thyrotoxic periodic paralysis has been reported on rare occasions in hyperthyroidism. The symptoms are quite similar to those of familial hypokalemic periodic paralysis. Grave's ophthalmopathy is an organ-specific autoimmune process strongly linked to Grave's hyperthyroidism. Clinical manifestations are painful bilateral or sometimes unilateral exophthalmos and diplopia. An orbital inflammatory process involves muscles and soft tissues and results in eyelid retraction, proptosis, periorbital edema, chemosis, and disturbances in ocular motility with early involvement of the inferior rectus muscles. Threatening complications are visual loss by keratitis, corneal ulceration, and compressive optic neuropathy.

Central Nervous System Disorders.   Neuropsychiatric manifestations such as emotional lability, irritability, hyperactivity, and insomnia are common. Psychosis is reported in 2% of cases. Thyroid storm, a life-threatening decompensation of the hyperthyroid state often precipitated by infection or surgery, always includes CNS dysfunction (restlessness, confusion, and delirium sometimes progressing to coma). Seizures and status epilepticus may occur. Essential systemic signs are fever, tachyarrhythmias, and high-output cardiac failure. Vomiting, diarrhea, and jaundice may be associated. Elderly patients often present with a misleading picture known as "apathetic hyperthyroidism," with lethargy, depression, and dementia.

More than 90% of patients have an exaggerated physiologic tremor of the hands and fingers. Chorea have been reported in 2% of patients, although its relationship to hyperthyroidism remains controversial. Focal motor or generalized seizures have been sometimes reported. Myelopathy with hyperreflexia, Babinski's sign, and spasticity have been described, and are reversible with the treatment of hyperthyroidism.

Hypothyroidism

The most common causes of hypothyroidism are acquired thyroid gland malfunction, mainly destruction related to Hashimoto's thyroiditis, or iatrogenic malfunction (from surgery or medical treatment). Neurologic manifestations are divided in neuromuscular and CNS disorders.

Neuromuscular Disorders.   Slight signs and symptoms of myopathy are reported in the majority of patients and may be the only manifestation of the disease. Fatigue, stiffness, myalgia, and rarely cramps are reported. Slight proximal weakness may be associated with slowed relaxation of the reflexes. Serum creatine kinase (CK) levels are elevated in most hypothyroid patients. The carpal tunnel syndrome, commonly bilateral, is the most frequent peripheral nerve disorder in hypothyroidism. Mechanical compression of the median nerve is caused by deposition of acid mucopolysaccharide protein complexes beneath the flexor retinaculum carpi. Rarely, tarsal tunnel syndrome or compression of the cubital nerve at the canal of Guyon have been reported. Complete resolution with thyroid hormone replacement is the rule. Sensorineural deafness has been reported. Ptosis of the upper lids occurs in relation to diminished sympathetic tone. Dysarthria and hoarseness occur in many patients, most probably from local myxedematous infiltration of the tongue and vocal cords. Diffuse sensorimotor axonomyelinic polyneuropathy is a classic complication of hypothyroidism. Sensory symptoms are prominent, with paresthesias, painful dysesthesias in the hands and feet, and sometimes lancinating pain, but objective sensory loss in a distal glove-and-stocking uncommonly are inconstantly found. Distal weakness and wasting may occur.

Central Nervous System Disorders.   Neuropsychiatric manifestations are encountered in more than one-half of patients, particularly in elderly individuals. The occurrence of dementia or sometimes psychosis early in the course of hypothyroidism and in the absence of other myxedematous features may delay the diagnosis. Associated reduced consciousness should always point to hypothyroidism. In myxedema coma, the marked impairment of CNS function is associated with hypothermia, hypoventilation, bradycardia, hyponatremia, hypoglycemia, and rhabdomyolysis and often precipitated by cold exposure and infection. Cerebellar ataxia is reported in 5–30% of cases. Seizures are rare in hypothyroid patients but have been noted in up to 25% of those in myxedema coma. Obstructive sleep apnea is related to obesity, infiltration of the tongue and upper airways by myxedematous tissue, and abnormalities in respiratory drive.

Hashimoto's Encephalopathy

A diffuse encephalopathy associated with Hashimoto's thyroiditis and elevated antithyroglobulin antibody titers but normal thyroid function has been reported. The clinical presentation includes stroke-like repetitive onset of confusion and focal deficits followed by myoclonic encephalopathy and partial complex or generalized tonic-clonic seizures, often with progressive neuropsychological impairment. Improvement with steroid treatment may support an autoimmune etiologic mechanism.

Parathyroid Diseases

The neurologic manifestations of hyperparathyroidism and hypoparathyroidism are described under "Hypercalcemia" and "Hypocalcemia."

Adrenal Diseases

Adrenal diseases are rare but iatrogenic. Cushing's syndrome is a frequent complication of chronic steroid treatment.

Cushing's Syndrome

Neurologic manifestations of glucocorticoid excess are related to CNS and muscle dysfunctions. In Cushing's disease, a pituitary tumor may be responsible for visual symptoms by local invasion of the chiasma or cavernous sinus and also for insufficiency of other endocrine glands.

Neuropsychiatric manifestations are reported, including depression, impaired concentration, and poor recent memory, as well as severe confusion, hallucinations, and psychosis. Hypertension and diabetes are frequent complications of Cushing's syndrome and are major risk factors for cerebrovascular complications. Symptomatic myopathy is present in 50–80% of cases. In steroid-induced myopathy, weakness, and atrophy are dose dependent, and fluorinated glucocorticoids produce a more severe myopathy. Proximal weakness develops insidiously and involves the legs more severely than the arms. Myalgias are not frequent. CK levels are usually normal. In the intensive care unit, an acute myopathy can develop within a few days of administration of large doses of glucocorticoids in patients with asthma who require mechanical ventilation with or without concomitant administration of curare agents. In this situation, muscle necrosis correlates with a marked increase of CK levels. The prognosis is usually good.

Addison's Disease

Addison's disease, an autoimmune destruction of the adrenals, accounts for most of a primary adrenocortical insufficiency and can be part of a polyglandular failure syndrome. Tuberculosis is the second most frequent cause. Other causes are acquired immunodeficiency syndrome, hemorrhage, infection, and tumors. Secondary adrenocortical insufficiency results from inadequate corticotropin production, mostly consecutive with hypothalamic or pituitary tumors or withdrawal of chronic administration of glucocorticoids. Neuropsychiatric manifestations ranging from depression to psychosis are other features. Apart from a lack of glucocorticoid, other metabolic disturbances (hyponatremia, hyperkalemia, and hypoglycemia) may induce a diffuse encephalopathy. In addisonian crises, stupor and coma may supervene, associated with flaccid weakness of the four limbs. Generalized convulsions related to hyponatremia and papilledema are reported. Severe myopathy with generalized weakness and cramps is reported in 25–50% of patients. Respiratory muscle weakness can occur. CK levels are normal.

Pituitary Disorders

Acromegaly

Growth hormone hypersecretion is caused mostly by a pituitary somatotrophic tumor or rarely hyperplasia. Neuromuscular complications are common. Myopathy with initial increased muscle bulk and strength progresses insidiously to proximal weakness and fatigability in 50% of acromegalic patients. Muscle wasting is minimal. CK levels may be slightly elevated. Approximately 35% of acromegalic patients have bilateral carpal tunnel syndrome. Local changes are synovial edema, hyperplasia of ligaments and tendons, and proliferation of cartilage and bone. Resolution is the rule with correction of growth hormone excess. A sensorimotor axonomyelinic polyneuropathy is a complication of acromegaly. Most often, pain and paresthesias of the hands and feet are reported, but weakness may be severe. Hypertrophy of the peripheral nerves should be sought.

Pituitary Apoplexy

Pituitary apoplexy is a rare complication of a pituitary tumor related to sudden intratumoral infarction or hemorrhage. The neurologic picture is often dramatic, with severe headache of sudden onset, visual loss from compression of the optic chiasma, diplopia from compression of the ocular nerves in the cavernous sinus, stupor or coma, stiff neck, and sometimes focal neurologic signs (Figure 43-3).

Cardiorespiratory Failure and Respiratory Diseases

Postanoxic Ischemic Encephalopathy

Postanoxic ischemic encephalopathy remains a frequent cause of persistent brain damage or death after effective cardiopulmonary resuscitation.

Pathophysiology

Brain energy metabolism is highly dependent on oxygen supply. Postanoxic ischemic encephalopathy is caused by a rapid reduction of the oxygen content of the blood or a sudden reduction of the cerebral blood flow. Complete arrest of cerebral blood flow induces loss of consciousness within 6–8 seconds, with convulsions, pupillary dilation, and bilateral extensor responses. With rapid cardiopulmonary resuscitation, coma is reversible without sequelae. After more than 5 minutes under normothermic conditions, irreversible neuronal damage is observed.

Neuropathology

The neuropathologic picture is characterized by cortical laminar necrosis, neuronal losses in the hippocampus, loss of Purkinje cells in the cerebellum, and, in severe cases, damage to the thalamus and basal ganglia. Watershed infarcts can be found, especially when carotid artery stenosis is present.

Prognostic Factors

Circulatory arrest of long duration, advanced age, and underlying disease (cardiogenic shock, recurrent arrhythmias, or cardiac arrest from myocardial infarction, or multiorgan failure) are factors indica-

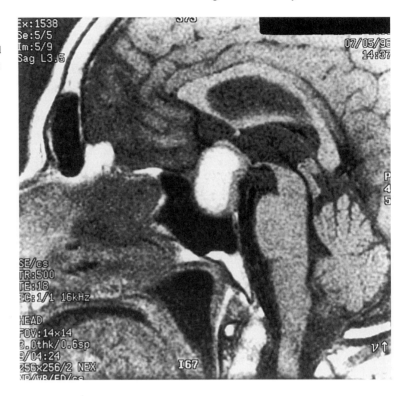

Figure 43-3. Magnetic resonance imaging scan of the brain from a 63-year-old woman who developed headaches and a sudden worsening of progressive visual disturbances characterized by a superior bitemporal quadrantanopia and right optic neuropathy. A sagittal T1-weighted image revealed hemorrhage in a macroadenoma of the pituitary gland.

tive of a poor prognosis. Repeated neurologic examinations and EEG studies during the first few days are often needed to determine outcome. In one study, the best predictor of poor outcome was an absence of motor response to painful stimuli after 3 days of intensive care. All these patients remained in a permanent vegetative state and not one survived at 1 year follow-up. Myoclonus status, defined as generalized intermittent, spontaneous, and stimulus-sensitive myoclonus of the face and limbs that persists for more than 30 minutes, is another predictor of poor outcome.

Laboratory Investigations

CT scans often appear normal. Sometimes diffuse edema, bilateral watershed infarctions, thalamic hypodensities, cerebellar infarctions, and contrast-enhanced laminar necrosis occur. MRI scans may appear normal and have no prognostic value. An EEG is part of the initial neurologic evaluation and evolution at 48 or 72 hours may be helpful. Some EEG patterns (alpha coma, burst suppression pattern) are strong predictors of poor out-

come. Short-latency sensory evoked potential studies are now considered an early reliable prognostic investigation. Bilateral loss of short latency sensory evoked potentials is associated with a mortality rate of 100% in adult nontraumatic comatose patients.

Delayed Postanoxic Encephalopathy

Delayed postanoxic encephalopathy is a rare complication of carbon monoxide poisoning, drug overdose, or anoxia from cardiac arrest. One to 4 weeks after an apparent full recovery from the initial anoxic coma, the patient develops behavioral changes with apathy, confusion, and irritability, often mistaken for a psychiatric disease but associated with gait difficulties and incontinence. Frontal release signs, pseudobulbar palsy, increased deep tendon reflexes with bilateral extensor plantar responses, rigidity, and reduced consciousness, sometimes progressing to coma and death are observed. Slow recovery may occur in 50–70% of cases. Neuropathologic studies reveal diffuse, severe, bilateral hemispheric demyelination sparing the subcortical arcuate fibers and brain stem. Lipid-laden macrophages and reactive astrocytes are present. Pallidal necrosis is sometimes found. The pathophysiology is unknown.

Respiratory Failure

Clinical Manifestations

Ventilation failure, characterized by hypoxemia and hypercapnia with consequent respiratory acidosis, may lead to a progressive diffuse encephalopathy and coma. Abrupt worsening may be induced by sedative drugs. Asterixis and tremor are common. Postural and action tremor may be partly caused by beta-adrenergic drugs. Unlike the situation in other metabolic encephalopathies, hemiparesis or seizures are rare. Headache of a generalized, frontal, or occipital localization, sometimes occurring nocturnally or early in the morning, is reported in chronic respiratory failure. Papilledema may be present. In advanced chronic obstructive pulmonary disease, often with severe weight loss and malnutrition, a subclinical axonal polyneuropathy has been described. Mild distal sensory changes and an absence of deep tendon reflexes without weakness are found on clinical examination.

Pathophysiology

The pathophysiologic mechanisms of respiratory encephalopathy are not fully understood. The degree of carbon dioxide retention is probably the main determinant of neurologic manifestations. At the cellular level, acidosis of the brain induced by hypercapnia interferes with energy metabolism. Thus, the rate and duration of carbon dioxide accumulation and the buffering capacity of the brain may be critical.

Etiology

Pulmonary diseases are the most frequent causes. Narcotics or sedatives depress the brain stem respiratory drive. Neuromuscular disorders such as Guillain-Barré syndrome, myasthenia gravis, critical illness neuropathy, amyotrophic lateral sclerosis, poliomyelitis, and rarely polymyositis or some types of muscular dystrophy may induce respiratory failure. CNS lesions, such as spinal cord injury at or above C3 and unilateral caudal brain stem infarction, are other potential causes of ventilatory failure.

Cardiac Disease

General Considerations

Many cardiac diseases may be complicated by stroke, and cardioembolism accounts for approximately 15–20% of all ischemic strokes. Establishing a firm diagnosis of cardioembolic stroke may be difficult, and nearly one-fourth of patients with a potential cardiac source of embolism may have a coexisting potential arterial cause of stroke. A nonprogressive onset of stroke, hemianopia without hemiparesis or hemisensory disturbances, Wernicke's aphasia, ideomotor apraxia, involvement of specific territories (posterior division of the middle cerebral artery, anterior cerebral artery, cerebellum, multiple territories), and a hemorrhagic component are associated with the presence of a potential cardiac source of embolism. The advent of transesophageal echocardiography (TEE) allowed reliable identification of more potential cardioembolic sources, mainly interatrial septal abnormalities (patent foramen ovale [PFO] and atrial septal aneurysm [ASA]). The main causes of cardioembolic stroke are atrial fibrillation (45%), left ventricular segmental akinesia after myocardial infarct (25%), prosthetic heart valve (10%), and rheumatic valve disease (10%). PFO with or without an ASA may be a frequent cause in young patients. Other rarer causes are dilated cardiomyopathy, endocarditis, and atrial myxomas.

Atrial Fibrillation

Nonvalvular atrial fibrillation (NVAF) is the most common source of cardioembolism. The prevalence increases with age. Patients with NVAF have a fivefold increased risk of stroke compared with age-matched controls. Stroke risk is 4–5% per year. Clinical and echocardiographic risk factors that increase stroke risk are age, hypertension, recent cardiac failure or thromboembolism, left atrial enlargement, left ventricular dysfunction, and spontaneous intra-auricular contrast. Five randomized trials established the benefit of oral anticoagulation (international normalized ratio [INR] between 2 and 4) in primary and secondary prevention of stroke in NVAF. The stroke risk reduction is approximately 65%. Although warfarin (Coumadin) is superior to aspirin in NVAF, aspirin is an efficient alternative when an anticoagulant is contraindicated.

Myocardial Infarction

Approximately 2.5% of patients with acute myocardial infarction (AMI) experience a stroke within 2–4 weeks, mostly in the first week. Early stroke is most commonly cardioembolic from left ventricular thrombi, and the stroke risk is higher in anterior myocardial infarction. At the moment, there is no consensus for stroke prevention in the acute phase of myocardial infarction. Both heparin and aspirin alone may reduce by half the risk of stroke. However, for high-risk patients with anterior transmural myocardial infarction, prevailing opinion may favor early anticoagulation followed by selection for further anticoagulation guided by echocardiography. The pathogenesis of late stroke may be unrelated to myocardial infarction. Other potential cardiac causes of stroke—mostly atrial fibrillation, severe internal carotid artery disease, and lacunar stroke—may be found.

Cerebrovascular Complications of Thrombolytic Therapy for Acute Myocardial Infarction

The clinical benefit of thrombolytic therapy in AMI has been clearly established and it is now given routinely. Although an increased rate of stroke, especially hemorrhages, is reported during the first 24 hours after thrombolysis, this seems to be balanced by late cerebrovascular events in control patients. The overall stroke incidence in the recent large coronary thrombolysis trials was approximately 1%. Age, poor hemodynamics, and anterior myocardial infarction were associated with an increased risk of stroke. Stroke subtypes are difficult to ascertain because clinical and radiologic evaluation were not always complete. Strokes were divided among one-third each for intracerebral hemorrhages, ischemic cerebral infarctions, and undefined events. Most hematomas are localized in the subcortical white matter, and additional hematomas

may develop in previously infarcted areas. Multiple parenchymal hemorrhages and hemorrhages in multiple intracranial compartments, including the intraventricular, subdural, and subarachnoid spaces, are more prevalent in fibrinolysis-associated hemorrhages. Outcome is often poor. A major risk factor for hemorrhage is an age of 70 years or more. Hypertension, combined fibrinolytic and antithrombotic treatment, cerebrovascular diseases such as arteriovenous malformation, cerebral amyloid angiopathy, and microvascular lesions are potential causes.

Rheumatic Mitral Valve Disease

The incidence of systemic embolism is greater in rheumatic mitral valve disease than in any other common form of heart disease, varying from 1.5% to 4.7% per year, and it increases sevenfold with the development of atrial fibrillation. Age, decreased cardiac function, and left atrial size are independent risk factors for thromboembolism. Risk of recurrence is high. Thus, long-term oral anticoagulation (INR of 2–3) is recommended for rheumatic mitral valve disease complicated by chronic or paroxysmal atrial fibrillation or with a history of systemic embolism. If recurrent systemic embolism occurs despite adequate oral anticoagulation, low-dose aspirin may be added.

Prosthetic Heart Valves

Mechanical valves and bioprosthetic valves have different levels of thrombogenicity. Mechanical valves require long-term anticoagulation with a recommended INR of between 3.0 and 4.5. Nevertheless, the rate of embolism in anticoagulated patients with mechanical valves is still 3% per year for the mitral valve and 1.5% per year for the aortic valve. Bioprosthetic valves, which have a lower inherent thrombogenicity, do not require long-term anticoagulation in the absence of atrial fibrillation, a history of systemic embolism, or a finding of left atrial thrombus at the time of surgery. For patients with a bioprosthetic valve in the mitral position, oral anticoagulation (INR of 2–3) is indicated for 3 months after mitral valve replacement and is optional for a bioprosthetic valve in the aortic position. After 3 months, antithrombotic therapy is not indicated unless the embolic risk factors mentioned above are present.

Patent Foramen Ovale and Atrial Septal Aneurysm

TEE with contrast can reliably detect PFO and ASA. Although the foramen ovale remains patent throughout life in approximately 30% of persons, many studies have demonstrated a higher prevalence of PFO in young patients with unexplained ischemic stroke than in control subjects. Paradoxical embolism from a venous source through a right-to-left shunt is usually incriminated, but direct evidence for paradoxical embolism is commonly lacking, and systematic screening for deep venous thrombosis in the lower limb or pelvis has led to extremely variable estimates. Despite these ongoing controversies, the possibility of paradoxical embolism should be considered in young patients with ischemic stroke and PFO, provided other causes are excluded. ASA may contribute to an increased risk of paradoxical embolism in patients with PFO and may even act as a direct source of embolism. There is no consensus about secondary prevention. Antithrombotics are commonly given. A subgroup of patients may benefit from surgical closure of the PFO.

Infective Endocarditis

Approximately one-third of patients with infective endocarditis have neurologic complications, most often with *Staphylococcus aureus*. Approximately 20% of them have ischemic stroke. The clustering of embolic events during uncontrolled infection is constantly found. Of all emboli, almost two-thirds may occur on presentation and an additional 11% during the subsequent 48 hours. Symptomatic intracranial hemorrhage occurs early, with an incidence of approximately 5%. Three mechanisms may be involved: The most frequent may be septic emboli during uncontrolled infection (particularly with virulent organisms), which may be responsible for acute erosive arteritis with rupture. Sterile emboli can cause infarcts that undergo secondary hemorrhagic transformation, usually

mild and asymptomatic in the absence of anticoagulation therapy. The true incidence of mycotic aneurysm is not known, because cerebral angiography is not routinely performed and because aneurysms may heal with antibiotic treatment. Mycotic aneurysm may be an uncommon cause of intracranial hemorrhage, accounting for only 0.8–2.8% of cases. Diffuse encephalopathy with stupor or coma may be found in 20% of cases. Multiple small cerebral emboli have been found in autopsy cases. Meningitis may be present in 4%. Brain abscesses are rare, less than 1% of those with infective endocarditis have brain abscesses. Persistent headaches without neurologic signs and vertebral osteomyelitis are reported in 3%.

Nonbacterial Thrombotic Endocarditis

Nonbacterial thrombotic endocarditis (NBTE) is characterized by uninfected fibrin vegetations of one or more heart valves. Overall incidence at autopsy is approximately 1%. The condition is associated most commonly with cancer (more than 50% with adenocarcinoma, 20% with leukemias and lymphomas, and 20% with diverse solid tumors) but also with other chronic debilitating disorders and acute fulminant diseases such as septicemia or burns. Most patients suffering from cancer-associated NBTE have identifiable coagulation abnormalities. Deep-vein thrombosis and disseminated intravascular coagulation (DIC) may be found. The brain is a common site of embolization, and infarctions are often multiple. Transthoracic echocardiography results are often negative; TEE may be more rewarding. Heparin seems to be the most effective treatment.

Atrial Myxoma

Atrial myxoma is an exceptional cardiac tumor. Cardiac symptoms such as dyspnea and syncopes usually dominate the picture. Emboli of myxomatous tissue or thrombus from the surface of the mass occur in 25–45% of cases and half of them in the brain and retina, often multiple. Aneurysms may develop on peripheral branches of the intracranial arteries from invasion of the arterial walls by myxomatous embolic tissue. Intracranial metastases from myxomatous proliferation, mostly arising from the choroid plexus, are rarely reported. Non-specific systemic complaints of fever, fatigue, weight loss, anemia, elevation of the erythrocyte sedimentation rate, and hypergammaglobulinemia can occur.

Gastrointestinal Disorders

Hepatic Diseases

Hepatic Encephalopathy

The reversible neuropsychiatric syndrome of hepatic encephalopathy (HE) occurs in the evolution of chronic progressive liver failure of all types or in surgical portosystemic shunts.

Clinical Manifestations.   Four clinical stages are commonly described and are useful for their prognostic significance. The first stage is characterized by early psychiatric changes such as apathy or euphoria, anxiety, restlessness, and inverted sleep patterns. Neurologic examination reveals short attention span, dyscalculia, impaired handwriting, tremor, and slowed coordination. In the second stage, an altered level of consciousness may alternate with agitation, reduced attention, and disorientation. Asterixis, ataxia, dysarthria, and altered limb tone are obvious. The third stage is characterized by increasing drowsiness, disorientation for place, delirium, and paranoia. In the fourth stage, coma with abnormal flexion or extension responses, brisk oculocephalic reflexes, and sluggish pupillary reactions are present. In the last stages, seizures, hyperreflexia, Babinski's sign, and myoclonus are reported. Focal neurologic signs can appear in patients with deep coma. A constant and characteristic finding of HE is hyperventilation with respiratory alkalosis, most likely from increased respiratory drive triggered by accumulated toxins. Signs of hepatic liver disease are often obvious on general examination and laboratory analysis.

Pathophysiology.   Recent data suggest that neurotransmission failure rather than decreased brain energy metabolism is the cause of HE. Ammonia neurotoxicity, false neurotransmitter synthesis from decarboxylation of various amino acids in the large intestine, increased transport of blood-borne gamma-aminobutyric acid (GABA) or endogenous benzodiazepines, and other toxins are the presumed pathogenetic mechanisms of HE.

Laboratory Tests.   Blood ammonia levels are frequently elevated but do not always correlate with the severity of neurologic impairment. EEG recordings show nonspecific slow waves and triphasic wave patterns. The predictive value of evoked potentials for outcome in HE is unresolved. A CT scan is useful to exclude a hemorrhagic complication such as subdural hematoma. In fulminant hepatic failure, radiologic signs of brain swelling are demonstrated. Hyperintense globus pallidus on T1-weighted MRI scans was demonstrated in cirrhotic patients, which correlated with the severity of the liver failure and was reversible with liver transplantation.

Portocaval Encephalomyelopathy

Portocaval encephalomyelopathy is a rare complication of surgical or spontaneous portosystemic anastomosis in hepatic cirrhosis. A progressive, irreversible, pure spastic paraplegia develops, always after one or more episodes of reversible HE. Signs of posterior column involvement and sphincteric disturbances are rarely present. Neuropathologic studies have shown the cerebral lesions of HE (Alzheimer's type II gliosis in the cortex, the basal ganglia, and more rarely in the cerebellum). In the medulla, there is demyelination and axonal loss involving selectively the dorsolumbar crossed corticospinal tracts and rarely the direct corticospinal tracts, the spinocerebellar tracts, and the posterior columns. The pathophysiologic mechanism of this complication is unknown.

Inflammatory Bowel Diseases

Ulcerative colitis (UC) and Crohn's disease (CD) may be complicated during their course by extraintestinal manifestations affecting various organ systems. Neurologic involvement has been reported in 3% of a large series of patients. The neurologic disorder may precede the onset of intestinal symptoms in one-fourth of patients. Neurologic complications were as frequent in UC as in CD, but involvement of the peripheral nervous system occurred mostly in UC, whereas myopathy and myelopathy characterized CD. The pathogenesis of neurologic complications in inflammatory bowel disease is unknown. A dysimmune mechanism, commonly presumed in inflammatory bowel disease, could be the pathophysiologic basis of some of the neurologic complications.

Peripheral nervous system involvement was the most frequent neurologic complication in a series (31.5%). Acute inflammatory demyelinating polyradiculoneuropathy was most common. Mononeuritis multiplex, bibrachial plexopathy, and a recurrent facial nerve palsy were rare manifestations. Inflammatory myopathy (mostly dermatomyositis) was also reported (16%). Myasthenia gravis preceded CD presentation in one patient.

Chronic progressive myelopathy of unknown cause was the second most frequent neurologic manifestation (26%) in inflammatory bowel disease and was most common in patients with CD. An inflammatory demyelinating origin could be suspected in two of them (intrathecal oligoclonal band synthesis or T2-weighted hyperintense periventricular lesions on brain MRI scans).

Cerebrovascular disorders, manifested as sinus venous thrombosis and recurrent ischemic strokes, were reported as a frequent neurologic complication (21%). In other studies, cerebrovascular diseases were documented in 0.12–4.00% of inflammatory bowel disease patients, constituting the most commonly described neurologic manifestation. The cerebral and retinal arterial and venous circulations may be affected by a hypercoagulability-related thrombosis, a vasculitis, and a consumption coagulopathy leading to hemorrhagic events. Bacterial meningitis by direct extension of inflammatory masses has been reported in CD.

Whipple's Disease

Whipple's disease is a rare, chronic, multisystem granulomatous infectious disease caused by *Tropheryma whippelii* and involving preferentially the small intestine. Onset is usually in middle age, with a male predominance. Presenting symptoms are weight loss, diarrhea with steatorrhea, arthral-

gias, abdominal pain, cardiac involvement, lymphadenopathy, and hyperpigmentation. CNS involvement is an infrequent complication, occurring in 6–16% of cases. Less than 5% of all cases of Whipple's disease may present as isolated CNS Whipple's disease without other systemic involvement. The clinical presentation of progressive dementia, myoclonus, and supranuclear ophthalmoparesis is highly suggestive. A peculiar pathognomonic movement disorder named *oculomasticatory myorhythmia* has been described. Pendular vergence oscillations of the eyes occur with synchronous rhythmic contractions of masticatory muscles. Hypothalamic dysfunction, seizures, cerebellar ataxia, pyramidal signs, and parkinsonism have been reported. Peripheral neuropathy and myopathy are rare and perhaps related to nutritional deficiency. CSF analysis may reveal normal results or may reveal increased protein content, inflammatory cells, and rarely periodic acid-Schiff (PAS)–positive macrophages. MRI scans show hyperintense lesions in the brain stem, hypothalamus, medial temporal lobes, or hemispheres. New tests using the polymerase chain reaction technique could be helpful in the diagnosis in cases without the pathognomonic PAS-positive macrophages on intestinal biopsy specimens. Long-term treatment with trimethoprim-sulfamethoxazole is recommended.

Celiac Disease

Although most commonly diagnosed in childhood, celiac disease or gluten-sensitive enteropathy may occur at any age. Gastrointestinal symptoms and signs of malabsorption are often discrete. Jejunal biopsy specimens demonstrating villous atrophy of the small bowel mucosa are required for diagnosis. Anti-gliadin and anti-endomysial antibodies may be highly sensitive and specific depending on the severity of the disease. Neurologic complications occur in approximately 10% of cases. A progressive and variable combination of cerebellar ataxia, combined posterior and lateral column spinal cord dysfunction, and dementia has been described. Malabsorption may be responsible for multiple nutrient and vitamin deficiencies. Vitamin E deficiency is probably one cause of nervous system dysfunction in celiac disease. Other toxic, genetic, and immunologic factors are also involved. Bilateral parieto-occipital calcifications associated with celiac disease, folate deficiency, and epilepsy are a recently recognized entity in children. Basilar impression of the skull from localized bone disease at a critical period of skeletal development is rarely symptomatic. Peripheral nervous system disorders are other complications of celiac disease. Both axonal or predominantly demyelinating neuropathies, metabolic myopathy related to hypokalemia or calcium and vitamin D deficiencies, and polymyositis have been reported. Neurologic manifestations are not always reversible with vitamin supplementation and a gluten-free diet.

Renal Disease: Renal Failure

Uremic Encephalopathy

The uremic syndrome is the consequence of any form of severe acute or chronic renal failure, involves many organs, and is reversible with dialysis. In systemic diseases (vasculitis, amyloidosis), specific nervous system involvement is related to the underlying process.

Clinical Manifestations

The clinical features of uremic encephalopathy consist of a continuum of nonspecific signs of CNS dysfunction and appear to be related to the rate of development of renal failure. Altered alertness and awareness of the environment, apathy, slurring of speech, and impaired concentration with diminished attention span are the earliest signs. Sometimes florid delirium with agitation, misidentifications, or visual hallucinations are reported. Sensorial clouding progresses to stupor and coma in the advanced stage. Motor signs, such as asterixis and tremor, occur in the early stage of uremic encephalopathy. Multifocal myoclonus is observed, usually in patients with advanced metabolic disturbances and severe clouding of consciousness. Motor abnormalities are characterized in the early stage by clumsiness of the hands, unsteadiness of gait, abnormal release of frontal signs, and altered limb tone. In the late stages, decorticate attitudes appear more commonly than

decerebrate ones. Focal motor signs, sometimes alternating from one side to the other and reversible after hemodialysis, are reported. Hyperkalemia may induce flaccid quadriparesis. Convulsions, either generalized or focal motor, are most often late manifestations. Meningeal signs, pleocytosis, and increased protein content of the cerebrospinal fluid have been reported. Among general signs, hyperventilation—compensatory to metabolic acidosis—cannot be omitted.

Pathophysiology

It is commonly suggested that many symptoms of uremia result from accumulation of products of protein metabolism, but the true identity of the uremic toxins remains unknown. Some of the metabolic consequences are decreased intermediary metabolism, cellular ion transport abnormalities, decreased pentose phosphate shunt, disturbed neurotransmitter function (namely GABA), and increased brain calcium content. It must be mentioned that other metabolic disorders secondary to renal failure, such as acidosis, hyponatremia, hyperkalemia, hypocalcemia, hypermagnesemia, dehydration or hyperhydration, and drugs, participate in the brain dysfunction. Hypertensive encephalopathy may be a complication of severe acute or chronic renal failure.

Laboratory Tests

EEG recordings often show nonspecific slow background activity and an excess of theta and delta waves, as in others metabolic encephalopathies, but they could be useful in excluding seizures or nonconvulsive status in stuporous patients. CT scans exclude a complication such as subdural hematoma.

Uremic Polyneuropathy

Uremic neuropathy is a distal, symmetric, mixed sensorimotor polyneuropathy that is mostly subclinical. The incidence among patients with chronic renal failure is approximately 60%. Cramps in the lower extremities and restless legs and moving toes are reported early. Distal sensory symptoms are frequent. The earliest neurologic signs are loss of ankle reflexes and reduced vibratory sensation in the distal lower limbs. Touch and joint position sense may be reduced. Slight distal paresis of the toe extensors may be present. A few patients can develop a severe and rapidly evolving sensorimotor polyneuropathy; additional factors are toxic drugs, sepsis, and diabetes. The differential diagnosis must include other metabolic neuropathies and systemic illnesses responsible for both renal failure and neuropathy, such as polyarteritis nodosa, systemic lupus erythematosus, primary systemic amyloidosis, multiple myeloma, and diabetes. Carpal tunnel syndrome is the most common mononeuropathy in chronic renal failure. Vascular shunts could be responsible for ischemic neuropathies (median and ulnar nerves), but a more frequent cause is amyloid deposits composed of beta-2-microglobulin. Other features of dialysis-associated amyloidosis are arthropathy and pathologic fractures. Rarely, cranial nerves can be affected, most commonly the eighth nerve.

Myopathy

Patients with chronic renal failure frequently complain of proximal lower limb weakness. Impaired vitamin D metabolism and secondary hyperparathyroidism are responsible for calcium metabolism dysfunction in muscles. Partial removal of hyperfunctioning parathyroid glands, vitamin D supplementation, or renal transplant improve the weakness.

Hematologic Disorders

Red Blood Cell Disorders

Iron Deficiency Anemia

Nonspecific neurologic symptoms of headache, poor concentration, dizziness, tinnitus, and fatigue are common in iron deficiency anemia. Benign intracranial hypertension with headache, papilledema, and progressive visual loss in severe cases has been reported rarely. Severe iron deficiency anemia, sometimes associated with thrombocytosis, may aggravate focal cerebrovascular symptoms related to large vessel occlusive atherosclerosis.

Megaloblastic Anemia

Megaloblastic anemia is discussed in Chapter 6.

Sickle Cell Anemia

Stroke is a frequent complication of sickle cell anemia, occurring in 5–17%, with a maximum incidence in the first two decades of life and particularly in homozygous individuals. Strokes are more commonly ischemic, and the predominant mechanism is a large vessel occlusive vasculopathy of the distal internal carotid artery and proximal middle and anterior cerebral arteries. Intimal hyperplasia and fibrosis of proximal intracranial blood vessels may result from primary endothelial damage complicated by mural thrombosis. Moyamoya syndrome, intracranial hemorrhage, and cerebral thrombophlebitis may occur. Seizures are common.

Polycythemias

Polycythemia vera is associated with an increased incidence of both ischemic stroke and cerebral hemorrhage. In this myeloproliferative disorder, the incidence of ischemic stroke is approximately 10–20% and is related to hematocrit level, associated thrombocytosis, and platelet function disorders. The hyperviscosity syndrome and cerebral venous thrombosis are other complications. Spurious and secondary polycythemias are risk factors for ischemic stroke.

White Blood Cell Disorders

Neurologic complications of leukemias, lymphomas, and cancer, in general, may be directly related to the disease or follow CNS infections or neurotoxicity of drugs. Only direct complications are discussed here. Paraneoplastic syndromes are discussed in Chapter 15.

Leukemias

Acute lymphocytic leukemia, which is most common in children, has a high propensity for CNS involvement. In acute nonlymphocytic leukemia, space-occupying lesions—granulocytic sarcomas near the periosteum and in the dura, orbit, and brain—are more likely to develop than meningeal infiltration. CNS infiltration in chronic leukemia is unusual except in the late phase of blastic transformation. Meningeal leukemia is by far the most common complication of leukemia. Confusion, cranial nerve palsies, and painful radicular deficits may coexist. Positive CSF cytology are diagnostic but may be found only after repeated lumbar puncture. CT or MRI scans with gadolinium may demonstrate leptomeningeal deposits or enhancement. A high incidence of intracerebral hemorrhage exists when acute leukemia (most commonly nonlymphocytic) and blast crisis when a leukocyte count of greater than 300,000 per μl are present. Leukostasis, DIC, or other coagulopathies are causes of intracranial hemorrhage. A hyperviscosity syndrome must be recognized and treated rapidly. It is characterized by dizziness, tinnitus, blurred vision, and impairment of consciousness. Distention of retinal veins, papilledema, and focal neurologic signs may be found. Ischemic stroke, related to leukostasis or DIC, is less common than hemorrhage. Cerebral venous thromboses are reported.

Lymphomas

CNS infiltration is frequent in non-Hodgkin's lymphoma (NHL) but exceptional in Hodgkin's disease (HD). In NHL, the less differentiated the cell type, the more likely the occurrence of CNS infiltration. Leptomeningeal infiltration, occuring almost exclusively in NHL, and epidural spinal cord or nerve root compressions, in both NHL and HD, are the most common neurologic complications. Intravascular lymphoma or neoplastic angioendotheliomatosis are very rare systemic disorders involving the brain, spinal cord, and peripheral nervous system. Symptoms may include a subacute developing dementia with or without focal neurologic signs. Neurolymphomatosis is a rapidly progressive and fatal painful neuropathy caused by exclusive infiltration by lymphoma. Cerebrovascular complications of lymphoma occur most commonly at the time of relapse or in progressive disease. Ischemic strokes related to DIC, NBTE, and septic embolism and cerebral venous thrombosis from coagulopathy are more common than hemorrhages.

Plasma Cell Dyscrasias

The incidence of spinal cord compression from an isolated plasmacytoma or multiple myeloma is approximately 10%. Vertebral body collapse or epidural extension is found. Nerve root compression occurs by the same mechanism. Leptomeningeal myelomatosis and orbital myeloma are exceptional. A hyperviscosity syndrome is a more common complication of Waldenström's macroglobulinemia than multiple myeloma. The symptoms consist of a triad of skin and mucosal bleeding, diminished visual acuity with dilation of retinal veins, retinal hemorrhages or papilledema, and neurologic manifestations characterized by headache, vertigo, decreased consciousness, and seizures. The overall incidence of polyneuropathy in plasma cell dyscrasias approximates 10%, most commonly associated with IgM gammopathies (monoclonal gammopathies of undetermined significance [MGUS] or Waldenström's macroglobulinemia). MGUS-associated polyneuropathy is generally a chronic, symmetric, predominantly sensory and ataxic polyneuropathy with tremor. IgM paraprotein may act as an antibody to myelin-associated glycoprotein. In Waldenström's macroglobulinemia, polyneuropathies are more heterogeneous, most commonly sensorimotor, and axonomyelinic. A symmetric axonal, sensory, or sensorimotor or rarely a demyelinating predominantly motor polyneuropathy may complicate IgG or IgA gammopathies (MGUS or myeloma). The proportion of IgG and IgA paraproteins in which reactivity with defined neural antigens has been identified is lower than for IgM paraproteins. In solitary plasmacytoma or osteosclerotic myeloma (sometimes part of the POEMS syndrome), a chronic inflammatory demyelinating polyneuropathy with predominantly motor signs is found. Amyloid neuropathy is another complication of gammopathies. Amyloid deposits come from the variable portion of the Ig light chain of the monoclonal protein. Painful sensory and autonomic neuropathy is one of the systemic manifestations. Weakness develops later. Prognosis is poor from cardiac and renal infiltration. Cryoglobulinemic neuropathy may be associated with lymphoproliferative disorders. Cryoglobulins are serum immunoglobulins that precipitate on cooling and dissolve when heated.

Clinical manifestations are Raynaud's phenomenon, purpura, arthralgias, glomerulonephritis, polyneuropathy, and stroke.

Platelet Disorders and Coagulopathies

Thrombocytopenia

Many diseases and drugs may cause thrombocytopenia. Intracranial hemorrhage may occur when thrombocytes fall to less than 20,000 per μl. Bleeding tendency may also result from abnormal platelet function, either secondary to a congenital defect or acquired from drugs, especially aspirin, or paraproteinemia or uremia.

Thrombocytosis

In essential thrombocythemia, a myeloproliferative disorder, both the number and function of the platelets are abnormal. Ischemic stroke, more commonly transient ischemic attacks, may occur in 30% of cases. Stroke is a rare complication of thrombocytosis secondary to splenectomy or iron deficiency anemia.

Thrombotic Thrombocytopenic Purpura

Thrombotic thrombocytopenic purpura is characterized by prominent neurologic symptoms, microangiopathic hemolytic anemia, thrombocytopenia, fever, and renal disease. Biopsy specimens show widespread hyaline occlusion of terminal arterioles and capillaries in many organs. A diffuse encephalopathy with altered mental status, confusion, decreased consciousness, and generalized seizures may be associated with focal neurologic deficits. Usually deep lacunar and small cortical infarcts are found, but major artery branch occlusion may also occur.

Disseminated Intravascular Coagulation

DIC is a relatively common acquired hemorrhagic thrombotic syndrome that occurs as a result of thrombin formation in the systemic circulation. Widespread clotting results in depletion of coagulation factors and platelet and secondary fibrinolysis with resultant hemorrhages. Detection of fibrin degradation products is a strong indicator of DIC. Sepsis, burns, cancer, and head injury are the most common causes of DIC. Patients with DIC have clinical symptoms of both hemorrhages and thrombosis. Neurologic complications are intracerebral hemorrhage, ischemic stroke, and probably more common venous sinus thrombosis.

Hemophilias

Intracranial hemorrhage is the most severe complication of hemophilia, which is an inherited hemorrhagic diathesis. Epidural spinal cord bleeding is rare. Peripheral nerve lesions caused by intramuscular hematoma are the most common neurologic complications of hemophilia. Many nerve trunks may be involved, most frequently the femoral nerve.

Hypercoagulable States

A deficiency of natural anticoagulants, such as antithrombin III, protein C or activated protein C resistance, and protein S are hereditary. Some of them may be acquired (hepatic insufficiency, nephrotic syndrome, DIC, pregnancy, and anticoagulation). In hereditary deficiencies, the risk of lower limb venous thrombosis is clearly increased. Cerebral venous thrombosis and stroke are rare. The antiphospholipid antibody syndrome may result in arterial and venous thrombosis, recurrent fetal loss, thrombocytopenia, livedo reticularis, chorea, and migraine.

Suggested Reading

Bogousslavsky J, Cachin C, Regli F, et al. Cardiac sources of embolism and cerebral infarction—clinical consequences and vascular concomitants: the Lausanne stroke registry. Neurology 1991;41:855.

Bogousslavsky J, Garazi S, Jeanrenaud X, et al., for the Lausanne Stroke with Paradoxical Embolism Study Group. Stroke recurrence in patients with patent foramen ovale: the Lausanne Study. Neurology 1996;46;1301.

Dyck PJ, Thomas PK, et al. (eds). Peripheral Neuropathy. Philadelphia: Saunders, 1993;1219–1274.

Ghika-Schmid F, Ghika J, Regli F, et al. Hashimoto's myoclonic encephalopthy: an underdiagnosed treatable condition? Mov Disord 1996;11:555.

Illowsky Karp B, Laureno R. Pontine and extrapontine myelinolysis: a neurologic disorder following rapid correction of hyponatremia. Medicine 1993;72:359.

Kaminski HJ, Ruff RL. Endocrine Myopathies. In AG Engel, C Franzini-Armstrong (eds), Myology. New York: McGraw–Hill, 1994;1726–1753.

Kanter MC, Hart RG. Neurologic complications of infective endocarditis. Neurology 1991;41:1015.

Knochel JP. Neuromuscular manifestations of electrolyte disorders. Am J Med 1982;72:521.

Lossos A, River Y, Eliakim A, Steiner I. Neurologic aspects of inflammatory bowel disease. Neurology 1995;45:416.

Louis ED, Lynch T, Kaufmann P, et al. Diagnostic guidelines in central nervous system Whipple's disease. Ann Neurol 1996;40:561.

Low PA, Suarez GA. Diabetic Neuropathies. In HP Hartung (ed), Peripheral Neuropathies: Part I. London: Baillère's Tindall, 1995;401–426.

Martin R, Bogousslavsky J, for the Lausanne Stroke Registry Group. Mechanisms of late stroke after myocardial infarct: the Lausanne Stroke Registry. J Neurol Neurosurg Psychiatry 1993;56:760.

Posner JB. Neurologic Complications of Cancer. Philadelphia: Davis, 1995.

Tonner DR, Schlechte JA. Neurologic complications of thyroid and parathyroid disease. Med Clin North Am 1993;77:251.

Uldry PA, Regli F, Berger JP. Complications neurologiques en Médecine interne. Paris: Masson, 1991.

Wijdicks EFM. Neurology of Critical Illness. Philadelphia: Davis, 1995.

Young GB, Ropper AH, Bolton CF. Coma and impaired consciousness. A clinical perspective. New York: McGraw–Hill, 1998.

Chapter 44
Head Injury

Christopher S. Ogilvy and Frederick G. Barker II

Chapter Plan

Pathophysiology of head injury
    Mechanisms
    Types of head injury
Evaluation of patients with head injury
    History
    Physical examination
    Laboratory investigations
    Radiologic investigations
Management of patients with various severities of
        head injury
    Mild head injury (Glasgow Coma Scale score of
        13–15)
    Moderate head injury (Glasgow Coma Scale
        score of 8–12)
    Severe head injury (Glasgow Coma Scale score
        of less than 8)
    Pediatric head injuries
    Penetrating head injury

The correct initial diagnosis and management of head injury are based on a firm understanding of pathophysiology coupled with anatomy. Head injury can be deceptive in that apparent mild injury can initially produce a clinical picture that hides the true severity of the underlying cranial or brain injury. A pertinent history and physical findings may be crucial in deciding how to proceed with radiologic evaluation or clinical observation of head-injured patients. Moderate and severe head injuries present one of many areas in medicine where evaluation and treatment often proceed simultaneously. A review of the pathophysiologic events that occur after varying degrees of head injury is provided followed by specific recommendations for treating mild, moderate, and severe head injury. Special conditions that are commonly seen by emergency room personnel are also discussed along with the management of head injuries in pediatric patients.

Pathophysiology of Head Injury

One way to consider the topic of head injury is to divide head injury into two basic types of insults: primary insults and secondary insults. A *primary insult* is defined as the transfer of kinetic energy to the scalp, skull, and brain tissue. At times this has been referred to as the *impact injury*. Secondary injury is caused by complications of direct injury to the brain or its coverings or to the extracranial organ systems that support the brain. The most significant of these secondary injuries cause further damage to cerebral structures.

Secondary insults can occur as a consequence of brain swelling, brain ischemia, frank infarction, or intracranial hemorrhage. In addition, systemic abnormalities may induce secondary insults. Hypoxemia and hypercapnia resulting from pulmonary problems may result in extensive cerebral injury or worsening of primary brain injuries. Cerebral hypoperfusion caused by blood loss or cardiac failure also may result in a secondary insult to the brain. Septicemia may induce severe secondary insults to cerebral parenchyma. Primary injuries to the brain can be considered in terms of their effect on the skin and scalp, injury to the skull or coverings of the brain, and injury to the brain tissue itself.

Mechanisms

The mechanism of primary head injuries is usually the result of transfer of kinetic energy into cranial structures. The two major mechanisms of energy transfer involve *contact phenomena* and *inertial effects*. Contact phenomena are caused by collisions of the head with other objects. In the usual course of events the head is moving and strikes a fixed object such as a windshield or support structures of an automobile. Moving objects can cause the same effect by striking a stationary skull, such as blunt objects struck against the head. This mechanism often causes clinically significant focal injury to the portion of the brain directly beneath the impact site and results in a *coup* type of injury. Dissipation of energy as the skull is struck can result in effects remote from the impact site. This dissipation of energy through skull and brain can account for skull fractures at sites distant from the focus of impact. Injuries to the skull and brain tissue at sites diametrically opposed to the site of impact result in *contrecoup* injuries. Deep hemorrhages in brain tissue can also occur.

Inertial effects are caused by sudden movement of the head in an acceleration or deceleration force. These types of injuries are almost always confined to the brain, supporting structures, and blood vessels. This type of injury is often responsible for the development of acute subdural hematomas in the absence of any obvious evidence of head trauma. This type of injury can also cause diffuse axonal injury within the brain tissue. Although the division of injuries between contact and inertial effects is convenient in separating types of injuries in the laboratory setting or for purposes of discussion, these injuries usually occur in conjunction. For instance, one rarely sees inertial effects without some type of contact phenomenon occurring as a cause of the inertial change.

Types of Head Injury

Skull Fractures

Skull fractures are a result of significant head trauma, usually of the direct type. A simple classification of skull fractures into open, closed, linear, or depressed followed by descriptive comments about the size, location, degree of bony fragmentation, and displacement helps in the discussion of these injuries with other physicians as well as in planning management.

A linear fracture of the skull is the type most commonly seen. This injury is caused by an out-bending of the bone at a distance from the impact site as a result of general skull deformation during impact. These fractures typically point toward the site of impact yet may not reach the impact area. These fractures may enter the calvarial sutures and cause disruption of the involved sutures. When this occurs, the term *diastasis* is used to describe suture separations greater than 3 mm. This term is also used to describe the width of a fracture not involving a suture line. These fractures occur more frequently in children because of the increased pliability of the pediatric skull. In the pediatric population, the force of impact needed to produce a fracture is less than in adults. The radiologic evaluation of these injuries and clinical management will be discussed below.

A depressed fracture is caused by more localized forces. These fractures may be stellate or comminuted with complex fragments depending on the type of injury incurred. In adults, these fractures tend to be comminuted. In children the depressed fracture may occur as a fragmentation, or a *greenstick fracture*. There is more likely to be injury to the brain parenchyma in depressed fractures than in nondepressed fractures. Often these are coup type injuries with underlying cerebral contusions. Focal deficits may occur, such as monoplegia or hemiplegia. We have seen several cases in which direct blows to the dominant temporal parietal region or frontal region will produce a classic Wernicke's type (receptive) or Broca's type (expressive) aphasia.

Although a skull fracture is often the result of significant cranial impact, the fracture alone does not represent a serious head injury. Most skull

Figure 44-1. A computed tomographic scan of a 14-year-old boy who presented with worsening headache several hours after hitting his head while playing basketball. There is a right temporal epidural hematoma present. Although there is no mass effect on the perimesencephalic cistern, the patient was taken to the operating room for removal of the clot because of his worsening headache. At surgery, a fracture through a branch of the middle meningeal artery was identified.

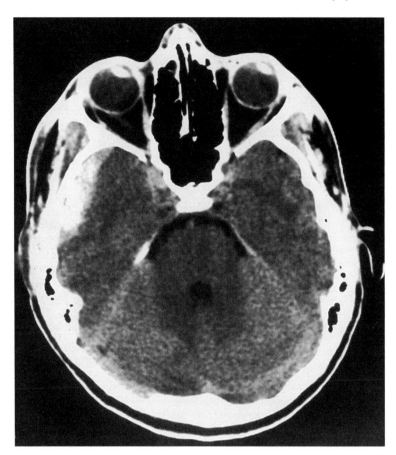

fractures have no lasting significance. It is the facial or brain injuries that occur in conjunction with the fracture that cause major morbidity and mortality.

Brain Injuries

Focal Hemorrhages.   There are four major categories of intracranial hemorrhage that may occur as a result of head trauma. Bleeding between the skull and dura results in the development of an epidural hematoma. Bleeding between the dura and arachnoid gives rise to a subdural hematoma, whereas bleeding into the subarachnoid space produces a typical subarachnoid hemorrhage. The fourth type of hemorrhage is intraparenchymal hematoma. Of these various types, subarachnoid hemorrhage is by far the most common in patients who sustain a closed head injury.

Epidural Hematomas.   Epidural hematomas are almost exclusively caused by trauma and usually are acute lesions. Rarely, a patient will present with a subacute or chronic epidural hematoma. The classic locations for epidural hematomas are the temporal and frontal regions associated with an overlying skull fracture (Figure 44-1). Skull fractures occur in 75–90% of patients with epidural hematomas. These collections of blood typically occur as a result of lacerations of branches from the meningeal artery by fractured bone edges. The typical elliptical of these lesions seen on CT scans is shown in Figure 44-2. In this case, the cause was a posterior parietal skull fracture that severed a posterior branch of the middle meningeal artery. The clot may not cross suture lines because of the adherence of the dura to the suture. The size of these lesions is dependent on several factors, including the tightness of adherence of the dura to the inner

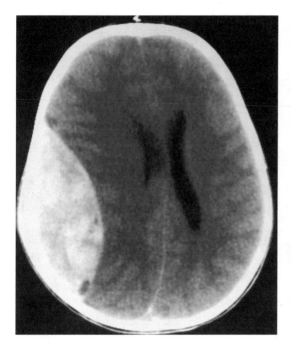

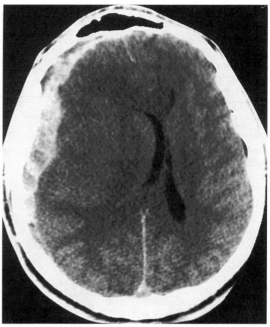

Figure 44-2. This 4-year-old child became comatose while being examined by his pediatrician after a fall from a chair 3 hours earlier. The large ellipse-shaped collection of blood is consistent with an epidural hematoma. At surgery, a posterior branch of the middle meningeal artery was found to be torn by a linear, minimally displaced skull fracture. The child made an uneventful recovery and was discharged 6 days after surgery.

Figure 44-3. A large amount (more than 1.5 cm) of midline shift is present on this computed tomographic scan of a 25-year-old man involved in a motor vehicle crash. The subdural collection of blood over the right hemisphere follows the gyri and produces an irregular margin instead of the elliptical pattern seen in epidural hematomas. At surgery, the source of this particular hematoma proved to be a torn cortical vein.

table of the skull and degree of laceration into the meningeal artery. As is discussed below, the management of these lesions represents a true neurosurgical emergency.

Subdural Hematomas.   Subdural hematomas can present as chronic, subacute, or acute collections of blood in the subdural space. Acute subdural hematomas have been defined as lesions with symptoms present for up to 7 days. Acute subdural hematomas are hyperdense collections on CT scans and usually more diffuse than epidural hematomas. The inner margin of these lesions often follows the gyri and sulci over the cortex of the brain surface, producing an irregular margin instead of the elliptical pattern seen in epidural hematomas (Figure 44-3). Subdural hematomas can be present on the side of a direct blow to the head or may be present contrecoup to a skull frac-

ture or impact site. Acute subdural hematomas may result from tears in the venous system over the cortex or injury to cortical arteries.

The management of these lesions should be emergent surgical evacuation. The patient's preoperative neurologic status correlates with the postoperative survival. Reducing the time between impact and lesion evacuation improves the likelihood of a favorable neurologic outcome. Patient age is another factor related to outcome, with older patients having a higher mortality than younger patients. At times, a small subdural hematoma may be present with a large amount of midline shift on the CT scan. The degree of parenchymal injury associated with an acute subdural hematoma is one of the factors that correlates with decreased survival. This phenomenon is produced by a contusion with diffuse swelling of brain underlying the hematoma and not the collection of blood itself. In these cases often the only neurosurgical procedure indicated is insertion of an intracranial pressure (ICP) monitor. Tiny acute subdural hematomas (3–5 mm) can be managed conservatively with close observation. These lesions may resolve on their own.

Subacute subdural hematomas have been defined as lesions in which patients have had associated symptoms for 7 days to 14–22 days. These lesions were isodense to brain tissue on CT scans in three-fourths of the cases looked at in one series. Symptoms may include headache, confusion, or mild focal neurologic dysfunction such as pronator drift and hemineglect. Surgical management of subacute hematomas usually involves a craniotomy to remove the partially liquefied clot material.

Chronic subdural hematomas represent a further evolution of the sequence of events that occurs when blood is present in the subdural space. These lesions usually are produced by relatively minor head injuries. Patients prone to develop this type of lesion include the elderly, where cortical atrophy leads to an enlarged subdural space. With minor low velocity impacts to the cranial vault, veins and arteries in the subdural space are more apt to tear. Other patients at risk include those on long-term anticoagulation for cardiac or vascular disease. The lesions most certainly begin as small collections of blood in the subdural space. With the passage of time, subdural blood liquefies and membranes form over both sides of the collections. There is a process of neovascularization that occurs within the membranes. Chronic subdural hematomas often present in patients with progressive weakness, hemineglect, or worsening headaches weeks to months after the initial head injury. These progressive symptoms are thought to relate to the gradual enlargement of these collections with time. Increase in size is thought to occur through a process of fluid production by the vessels present on the membranes forming around the collection of blood.

Once a chronic subdural hematoma is identified, it can be removed surgically or followed expectantly. The exact surgical technique used is a matter of some controversy. Loculations of the subdural fluid may be visible on CT scans, requiring a craniotomy to fully drain the lesion. In many lesions, two burr holes will suffice to adequately drain the chronic collections. Some surgeons favor placement of a tube in the subdural space and use this to drain the collection either percutaneously or with an external drainage system. Before any surgical procedure, the risk of stopping oral anticoagulants and reversing the prolonged clotting studies must be balanced by the benefit of the procedure. If safe, we favor administration of fresh frozen plasma and vitamin K to reverse warfarin-induced prolongation of the prothrombin time before proceeding to the operating room.

Focal Parenchymal Injuries.   Focal brain injuries secondary to trauma take the form of intra-parenchymal hematomas, contusions, or infarctions. A cerebral contusion represents brain tissue with small areas of hemorrhage. The areas of hemorrhage are separated by areas of edema. The initial CT appearance of contusions is often a nonhomogeneous area of high density (Figure 44-4A). Over the first 3–5 days, there is a gradual increase in the edema in the area of a contusion (Figure 44-4B). This can produce a mass effect necessitating surgical decompression.

In the case of traumatic cerebral hematomas, the common locations are in the anterior poles of the temporal or frontal lobes. It is these areas that are subjected to the greatest force as the brain decelerates against the skull in the anterior-posterior plane. In most cases, these hematomas occur at the time of injury; however, delayed intraparenchymal hemorrhages have been described.

Post-traumatic infarction should be considered in patients with focal neurologic deficits yet with no obvious findings on the scan to suggest a cause of the deficit. Areas of acute ischemia may not be visible on CT scans for 24–72 hours after the event. After this interval, the areas become hypodense on CT scans and have surrounding areas of enhancement when intravenous contrast is administered. After trauma, focal ischemic deficits are usually caused by arterial dissection of the carotid or vertebral system. In alert patients, neck pain with transient or lasting focal deficits should alert the physician to the possibility of a dissection. In obtunded patients, an angiogram should be considered when patients develop a focal finding in the neurologic examination without an obvious explanation visible on the CT scan.

A final form of focal parenchymal injury are those lesions caused by penetrating injuries to the brain. These can be piercing-type injuries caused by knives, nails, screwdrivers, sticks, and other sharp

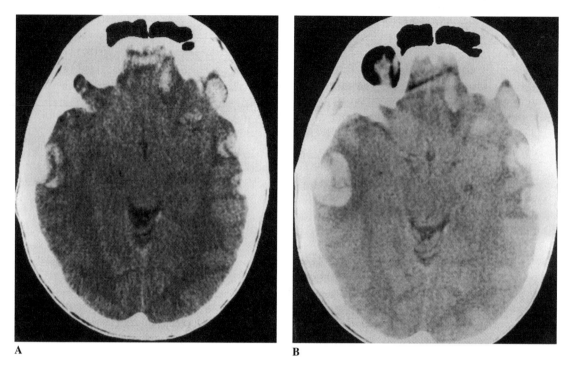

Figure 44-4. (A) A computed tomographic (CT) scan of a college athlete who fell while pole vaulting and sustained a concussion. There are multiple contusions present around the periphery of the temporal and frontal lobes. (B) A CT scan obtained 5 days after the incident demonstrates enlargement of the high-density regions of the contusions, with surrounding low density (edema).

objects driven into the cranial vault by another human or by a machine. These types of objects can penetrate the thinner regions of the skull (temporal bone) or enter through an existing foramen (e.g., the orbit, foramen magnum, ethmoidal plate). When a sharp object is driven inside the skull, it usually produces a focal hemorrhage with a surrounding contusion. Small epidural or subdural hematomas may also occur. Parenchymal lesions are also caused by missiles penetrating the cranial vault.

When power-driven missiles (usually bullets or shell fragments) injure the brain, the initial abnormality seen on CT scans may not represent the entire extent of the lesion. Missiles transmit kinetic energy to brain tissue. The amount of energy (E) a missile has as it enters the brain is predicted by the formula $E = (\frac{1}{2}M) \times V^2$, where M is the mass of the missile, and V is the difference between the velocity of the missile entering the skull and the velocity of the missile leaving the skull.

It should be clear that velocity has a much larger effect on the amount of energy delivered to brain tissue than does bullet size. Therefore, the injury from high-velocity (often military) weapons is more extensive than a comparably placed lesion from a low-velocity (civilian) weapon. If a patient with a gunshot wound survives, tissue infarction can be seen to develop in the area adjacent to the bullet track on CT scans obtained several hours or days after the insult.

Diffuse Parenchymal Injuries.   As a result of head injury, diffuse subarachnoid hemorrhage can occur. This type of hemorrhage is often mild and does not by itself produce symptoms. Occasionally subarachnoid hemorrhage can be focal and severe, which carries with it the same risk of vasospasm as does subarachnoid hemorrhage from ruptured intracranial aneurysms. Although the most common cause of subarachnoid hemorrhage is trauma, the details of the trauma should be considered carefully. If a patient has been involved in an unexplained single vehicle crash or an unwitnessed fall, the possibility of a ruptured intracranial aneurysm should be entertained. In addition, traumatic aneurysms are known to occur. These lesions are usually the result of penetrating injuries, yet can occur with closed head injuries on intracranial vessels in close proximity to the falx, the tentorium, or a skull fracture.

A second cause of diffuse parenchymal damage is shearing injuries (Figure 44-5). In this situation, a significant axial rotation of the cerebral contents has occurred, producing disruption of axonal pathways (white matter tracts). This can be visualized on CT scans as areas of multiple small hemorrhages into the deep white matter. One common location for these hemorrhages to be visualized is in the corpus callosum.

Evaluation of Patients with Head Injury

Correct diagnosis is a prerequisite to proper treatment, and head injury is no exception. As with other disorders of the nervous system, the most expeditious diagnosis is based on history, physical examination findings, laboratory evaluations, and radiographic studies.

History

The historical features of the workup are often minimized or ignored by a physician confronted by severe head trauma, but it generally offers the quickest and most reliable guide to the severity of the injury. In a conscious patient, symptoms of headache, nausea, drowsiness, or vertigo may be elicited. The patient's recall of the accident should be recorded accurately, as this may serve as an indicator of the severity of a concussion. Neurologic injuries antedating the current injury are particularly important. In short, a complete history should be obtained.

When the patient is unconscious, the tendency is to immediately proceed to the physical examination. While the initial stabilization is proceeding, however, crucial questions may be posed to the team transporting the patient: Was the patient ever conscious? Were there others injured, and if so, how severely? What was the mechanism of the injury? Was the patient wearing a seat belt? How fast was the vehicle traveling? Was the patient breathing when initially found? These questions assume addi-

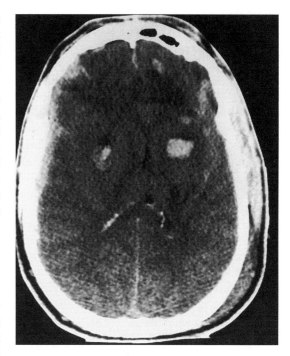

Figure 44-5. A severe head injury in a pedestrian struck by a car and thrown 30 feet. There is diffuse shear injury of sufficient force to cause focal intraparenchymal hematomas in the region of the basal ganglia bilaterally. A small right-sided subdural hematoma is also present. Despite lack of midline shift, the patient had a Glasgow Coma Scale score of 3 as a result of the bilateral (diffuse) nature of the injury.

tional importance when the patient's condition has been iatrogenically altered—by pharmacologic paralysis to assist management or by a change in position in a patient with a cervical spine injury.

Physical Examination

There are two parts to the physical examination: general and neurologic. The general examination focuses on the patient's head. This should be carefully examined both visually and with palpation. Cushing stated that the physical examination was not complete until the head is shaved, and in some instances this still holds true, particularly when the entry or exit point is sought in a gunshot wound. The skull is carefully palpated to check for a fracture. The face is similarly inspected and palpated for penetrating trauma or fracture. The fundi are examined for retinal hemorrhage (particularly in a child) and gross ocular damage is excluded. Where papilledema is present in the setting of an acute injury, the possibility that it may have preceded the injury should be strongly suspected, because this sign generally takes at least 24 hours to develop. Foreign bodies in the eyes should be noted for proper extraction. Any penetrating wound of the orbit deserves special attention in view of the common intracranial nature of this injury. The eardrums should be examined bilaterally and the presence or absence of hemotympanum or Battle's sign noted.

The neurologic examination of a conscious patient with head injury is not different from the standard neurologic examination and should evaluate mental status; the cranial nerves; motor, sensory, and cerebellar functions; gait; and reflexes. For a patient in coma the examination is, perforce, less complete, but the basic framework is the same. The three basic components of the Glasgow Coma Scale (GCS), initially defined in 1974 and widely used to gauge the severity of severe head injury, are "best" verbal and motor responses and the ability to open the eyes in response to verbal or painful stimuli (see Chapter 13, Table 13-1). The scale has some obvious shortcomings: for instance, unilateral posturing is ignored if the contralateral side has good motor function.

The complete coma examination documents mental status as the patient's response to either questions and commands or to a painful stimulus. The degree of confusion or disorientation should be noted. The patient's recall of events surrounding the injury should be noted and always compared with descriptions of other witnesses (when available). The cranial nerve examination includes cranial nerves II (blink to threat, pupillary response), III, IV, VI (pupillary reaction, direct and consensual, ciliospinal response, and eye movement—either voluntary or in response to a vestibular stimulus such as ice water irrigation of the ear), V (corneal reflex), VII (corneals, and grimace to pain), VIII (vestibular response, as above), and IX/X (gag). Motor examination records the response to noxious stimuli in the limbs and trunk. Sensory examination is limited to the presence or absence of motor responses in the limbs. Cerebellar and gait testing is obviously impossible. The reflexes, particularly the Babinski, are of clear importance.

Laboratory Investigations

Standard investigations should include an evaluation of hematocrit, platelets, and coagulation variables; blood and possibly urine screens for toxic substances such as alcohol or cocaine; and routine blood chemistry analysis. A blood sample should be sent to the blood bank for typing. Other tests should be guided by the patient's overall condition. For instance, blood gas analysis is only relevant (from a strictly neurosurgical standpoint) when consciousness is impaired. However, thrombocytopenia or the coagulopathy of chronic liver failure may be important even in seemingly trivial head injuries.

Radiologic Investigations

Cervical spine injuries are not covered in detail. We re-emphasize the importance of plain cervical spine films in the immediate evaluation of all injuries in the head, and particularly in those patients who are comatose or in whom an operation is planned. Complete cervical spine radiologic evaluation requires adequate anteroposterior, lateral, odontoid, and oblique views. Our policy is to immobilize the neck in a hard cervical collar until these studies are completed.

Skull Films

There are few more controversial subjects than the value of skull radiographs. Our preference is to forgo skull films except in certain circumstances. To a large extent, their use has decreased in importance because computed tomographic (CT) scanning has become more widespread in availability. However, if skull films have already been obtained by another physician, they should be carefully reviewed for evidence of skull fractures (particularly in the plane parallel to the CT scan cuts) as well as facial fractures, pneumocephalus, or intracranial foreign bodies. Every CT scan includes a scout view, which functions to some extent as a lateral skull view and which must be carefully examined for the same features.

Computed Tomographic Scanning

Perhaps more than any other issue, the question of which patients should rapidly undergo a CT scan involves medicolegal considerations. The following guidelines should not be interpreted as hard-and-fast rules, yet they do provide a general framework in deciding who to scan. The CT scan is occasionally referred to as the "neurosurgeon's chest x-ray," but it must be remembered that the number of patients who will have an abnormality of clinical importance on the scan becomes vanishingly small if a careful and complete neurologic examination produces entirely normal findings. The true magnitude of this number has not been subjected to rigorous study. When the criterion for "normal" is a GCS score of 15, however, one study found 13% of patients had an abnormality on the CT scan, and 3% of patients were submitted to immediate surgery. The authors of this study did not report the presence or absence of subtle neurologic signs in these patients. The GCS, however, loses sensitivity when nearly-normal patients are considered: Unilateral motor deficits, subtle aphasias, blindness, drowsiness, or even a fixed dilated pupil are all consistent with a GCS score of 15.

In general, we believe a CT scan is indicated whenever a head injury is followed by a new neurologic deficit or one that cannot be conclusively demonstrated to be old, whenever a patient with a concussion will be removed from reliable observation (e.g., by general anesthesia for surgery on an abdominal injury), or whenever a penetrating wound of the brain is suspected. Opinions vary about whether the patient with an uncomplicated closed and undepressed skull fracture (demonstrated by skull films) and normal findings on neurologic examination requires a CT scan, but when the fracture crosses the area of the middle meningeal artery, a venous sinus, or an air-containing sinus, a scan should certainly be obtained. The presence of a skull fracture is a reliable indicator of a more severe intracranial injury, and these patients are 20 times more likely to require craniotomy; certainly a CT scan in this situation is reassuring.

Pediatric head injuries pose a separate problem. A young child is to a large extent unexaminable, in that large portions of the brain have not yet fully developed their specific functions and hence cannot be evaluated. We are much more liberal with the use of skull films in the toddler and infant age groups, and the presence or absence of a skull fracture is more frequently a factor in the decision regarding CT scanning. Our threshold to mildly sedate a child

to obtain a CT scan is low. One study found abnormalities on CT scans in 31% of children with GCS scores of greater than 12.

Management of Patients with Various Severities of Head Injury

Once the initial neurologic evaluation is complete and the GCS score is known, the physician must proceed with general medical and neurologic stabilization of the patient and management of the neurologic injury. The management in these injuries will be discussed by dividing the severity into three major groups as described by others, namely, mild (GCS score of 13–15), moderate (GCS score of 8–12), and severe (GCS score of less than 8). Management of any serious or potentially serious head injury should proceed with neurosurgical back-up available. Often the neurosurgeon will be present during much of the evaluation and treatment. In other settings, the neurosurgeon is only involved if surgery is needed. The lines of communication between the emergency room physician and neurosurgeon should be open at all times in order to provide rapid, appropriate care for patients with head injuries.

Mild Head Injury (Glasgow Coma Scale Score of 13–15)

As described above, the value of the GCS diminishes as the patient more nearly approximates normal, and the simple determination that the GCS score is 15 can leave significant neurologic injury undetected.

Head Injury Without Concussion

The patient who has hit his or her head and has not suffered a concussion is unlikely to harbor a significant intracranial injury; however, there are exceptions. For instance, a concussion is not a prerequisite for the development of an epidural hematoma. Such patients will, however, complain of severe headache, and neurologic deficits usually quickly follow. The most trivial blow to the head in an elderly person or the anticoagulated patient can cause a subdural hematoma. This is usually a more insidious problem. In general, the physician should consider a CT scan more seriously in these patients, even in the presence of normal examination findings.

The vast majority of patients with these injuries can, after a thorough history and examination in the emergency department, simply be reassured and discharged. A sheet of instructions listing the various signs of developing trouble after a head injury should be given in the emergency department to all patients who are to be discharged after a head injury (Figure 44-6). The importance of observation by a reliable companion for 24 hours after the injury is emphasized.

Head Injury with Concussion

Cerebral concussion is defined as an immediate and transient impairment (not necessarily loss) of consciousness. Thus, a football player who is struck in the head and continues to play yet later cannot remember the game has sustained a concussion. A classic concussion usually involves amnesia for the events surrounding the injury, either preceding the blow (retrograde amnesia) or after the return of awareness (anterograde amnesia). Thus, the history given by such a patient should, wherever possible, be confirmed by a witness to the event. A surprising proportion of patients will be uncertain whether they have been "knocked out."

Inherent in these definitions is a rapid return to normal consciousness, and thus the syndrome of concussion generally has a good prognosis, with few lasting sequelae. However, a well-defined post-concussion syndrome, including headaches, difficulty concentrating or reading, dizziness, patchy numbness, and a variety of other nondescript phenomena, soon becomes familiar to any physician who sees these patients in follow-up. The management of these patients, which can at times be difficult, falls outside the scope of this chapter. In general, the concussion is not followed by serious sequelae and no specific treatment is prescribed. The patient may be discharged home with observation provided that he or she has returned to a normal state.

The concussion, however, may be a marker of more severe injury to the brain, and more caution is enjoined on the physician treating these patients. Some hospitals have policies regarding admission of all patients who have lost consciousness for a certain period of time. In our experience, the witnesses of such an accident are almost never present or reliable, and when they are, they usually have not taken care to note the precise length of time that the patient was unconscious. We prefer to regard such information as only one factor in the treatment decision.

All patients who have suffered a concussion should, if possible, be under reliable observation for 24 hours. This need not be on an inpatient basis. As the physician's impression of the severity of injury increases (guided by the patient's symptoms, the presence of drowsiness or "fogginess," and the duration of unconsciousness), either CT scanning, inpatient observation, or both should be more seriously considered.

Moderate Head Injury (Glasgow Coma Scale Score of 8–12)

The group of patients with GCS scores from 8 to 12 warrants expeditious evaluation and treatment. It is often patients in this group who can follow simple commands yet have intracranial lesions (parenchymal contusions, epidural or subdural hematomas) that can be treated effectively with surgery if recognized early. For patients with moderate head injuries, the overall outcome from head injury has been shown to be related to the severity of the injury. Interestingly, 42% of patients with moderate injury had a history of previous head injury.

The initial goal of the physician managing a patient with moderate head injury is to decide whether the patient is a candidate for emergent craniotomy. The gathering of information on which to base this decision proceeds as outlined above. The results of the CT scan play a major role in deciding whether a particular patient warrants surgical intervention as well as help the surgeon plan the details (location, size) of a craniotomy. A commonly used indicator for deciding to operate is the degree of midline shift on the CT scan. If the shift is 5 mm or greater, serious consideration should be given to proceeding to the operating room. In the case of focal extra-axial collections in younger patients, the rule often holds true, especially for temporal lobe lesions. Great care should be taken in trying to generalize this rule to all injuries. If a hemisphere is diffusely swollen, with 5 mm to 1 cm

---

Aftercare Instruction Sheet: Head Injury

You have suffered a head injury, and even though you are being allowed to go home, a relative or friend should stay with you, **and you both should read the following patient instructions:**

During the first 24 hours:
1. Eat and drink very little. Clear liquids are best if your stomach is upset.
2. Drink **no** alcoholic beverages.
3. Relax in bed if possible—no school or work. Do not exert yourself in any way.
4. Do not take sedatives or sleeping pills.
5. Do not drive a car or operate tools or instruments that could harm you if you were not alert.
6. Try to nap or sleep with the head elevated on at least one or two pillows. Do not sleep flat.
7. If you previously lost consciousness ("passed-out") after injury, we advise that you not sleep for periods of more than 2 hours without being awakened. You should not be left alone.
8. Avoid aspirin or compounds containing aspirin. Use acetaminophen (Tylenol) instead.

If any of the following symptoms appear, call your doctor or return to the emergency department immediately:
1. Persistent nausea or vomiting (more than twice)
2. Confusion, unusual drowsiness, or loss of memory
3. Dizziness, trouble walking, or staggering gait
4. Convulsions or seizures ("fits") (These are twitching or jerking movements of either the eyes, arms, legs, or body.)
5. Pupils of unequal size (The pupil is the dark center portion of the eye.)
6. A severe headache or a headache that is worsening or persistent
7. Personality changes
8. Weakness or trouble with the use of arms or legs; or areas of skin numbness
9. Unconsciousness or fainting
10. Stiff neck or fever
11. Visual disturbances including blurring of vision and double vision
12. Unusual sounds in the ear(s), such as ringing
13. Bleeding or clear liquid drainage from the ears or nose
14. Difficulty speaking or slurred speech
15. Excessive shortness of breath or difficulty breathing
16. Any unusual or abnormal symptoms

It is important that you report to your follow-up doctor for any new or remaining problems after your head injury. It is not uncommon for patients to have persistent or recurring headaches after their head injury; however, these patients and patients who have remaining difficulties should be followed either by their own physician or a follow-up doctor.

Should you have any questions or difficulties, do not hesitate to contact your own physician or return to the emergency department.

Figure 44-6. Standard instructions given to patients discharged after minor head injury.

of midline shift, the decision to place an ICP monitor and manage the patient medically can avoid undue morbidity incurred by surgery as a result of brain tissue herniating through the craniotomy site. Although this type of injury often occurs in more severe injuries, it has been encountered in patients with moderate head injury.

If a parenchymal abnormality or extra-axial abnormality is identified on the CT scan, the decision to operate is also guided by the patient's overall medical condition. These patients are often stable enough neurologically that one can proceed with the evaluation (diagnostic radiographs) of potential major injuries involving other organ systems. However, it should be remembered that the window of time in which to evaluate these other injuries may be truncated at any time by neurologic deterioration, and therefore serial neurologic examination is mandatory.

Once the decision not to operate on a patient with a moderate head injury has been made, medical management of the injury should begin. Anticonvulsant therapy is usually initiated at this time unless there is some contraindication (e.g., hypotension, drug allergy, intoxication). Anticonvulsants are continued at therapeutic blood levels for 2 weeks. Careful neurologic observation over time (hours) and the results of a toxic screen of blood and urine often provide the answer to whether a patient has generalized mental status impairment as a result of intoxication, their head injury, or a combination of the two neurologic insults.

Severe Head Injury (Glasgow Coma Scale Score of Less Than 8)

The majority of the literature regarding head injury consists of studies on the most severely injured patients. In general, patients with severe head injuries have a significantly worse outcome compared with patients with moderate or mild injuries despite aggressive medical and surgical management. It is in these patients in whom associated injuries of other major organ systems result in systemic conditions (hypotension, hypoxia) that induce secondary neurologic injuries. The appearance of diffuse hemispheric swelling on the initial CT scan has been found to be associated with an early episode of either hypoxia or hypotension. Rapid assessment of these problems is critical in maximizing potential neurologic recovery. Similar to patients with moderate head injury, rapid evaluation of the severity of neurologic injury must proceed at the same time as evaluation of other major organ systems and treatment. As noted above, after initial systemic stabilization, the next step is to decide whether intracranial surgery is needed and, if so, what type of procedure should be performed.

After initial neurologic examination of a patient with a severe head injury (a process that should take 3–5 minutes), the patient should be immediately intubated endotracheally if this has not already been accomplished by emergency medical technologists at the scene of the accident. Care must be taken to avoid manipulation of the neck. Nasotracheal intubation should be avoided in the event that the patient has a basilar skull fracture of the anterior cranial fossa of sufficient size to allow the nasotracheal tube to enter the cranial fossa (the same rule applies to placement of an orogastric tube as opposed to a nasogastric tube). Hyperventilation should proceed by setting the ventilator at a rate of 12–13 per minute and using a tidal volume of 15 ml per kg of body weight (usually 750–1,000 ml in an adult). Arterial blood gases should be checked to avoid overzealous hyperventilation (P_{CO_2} should not be allowed to be less than 25–30 mm Hg). Once adequate ventilation is established and the patient has been stabilized from a cardiovascular standpoint, a cranial CT scan should be obtained (this can realistically be accomplished approximately 15–20 minutes after the patient has arrived in the emergency department, assuming the blood pressure and heart rate are stable).

Should signs of herniation or a mass lesion appear before CT scanning, intravenous mannitol therapy should be initiated, and obtaining the scan should be expedited. The usual dose of mannitol in this setting is 1–2 g per kg of body weight (intravenous bags or bottles come in a volume of 100 g and therefore 1 bag is adequate). Intravenous fluids should be isotonic (0.9% normal saline or lactated Ringer's solution), and infusion should be kept to a low rate to minimize aggravation of cerebral edema.

Once the CT scan is obtained, the decision to operate is usually based on the location of the lesion as well as the degree of midline shift. Even in the setting of apparent medical contraindications (e.g., heart disease, lung disease, other major injuries), a patient with a significant collection of epidural or subdural blood or one with a sizable intraparenchymal hematoma should be taken directly from the CT scanner to the operating room. The need for exploratory burr holes in an emergency ward equipped with a CT scanner is rare. However, in patients unable to tolerate a CT scan, exploratory burr holes remain the only method for ruling out acute subdural or epidural hematomas. The most important characteristics of scans predictive of elevated ICP and death are midline shift, compression or obliteration of the mesencephalic cisterns, and the presence of subarachnoid blood.

Intracranial Pressure Monitoring

Continuous measurement of ICP provides a means of deciding when to institute certain medical therapies or of deciding when to proceed with surgery in patients not operated on initially. ICP also gives an indication of the effectiveness of a given medical therapy. Subarachnoid, subdural, intraparenchymal, or intraventricular devices are all available for measuring ICP, and the use of each type has pros and cons.

Although not a substitute for an adequate neurologic examination, the ICP can rise before clinical neurologic deterioration. Measurement of ICP and systemic blood pressure (SBP) allows a constant monitoring of cerebral perfusion pressure (CPP) (CPP = SBP – ICP). Indeed, one of the main detrimental effects of elevated ICP is the reduction of cerebral perfusion. Prompt recognition of increased ICP (ICP of more than 15 mm Hg) can increase survival and potentially improve neurologic outcome. Usually, insertion of an ICP monitor is done once the patient is in an intensive care unit or postoperatively.

Medical Management

The acute medical management of patients with severe head injury is the same in patients after craniotomy and in patients managed without surgery. In the emergency room, the patient is hyperventilated and given mannitol osmotherapy as described earlier. The use of steroids in the setting of head injury remains controversial. Despite some basic laboratory evidence suggesting a role for steroids in the control of edema associated with head injury, the majority of clinical studies using steroids in patients with head injuries have failed to demonstrate any beneficial effect. Although there are theoretical disadvantages to using steroids, in the form of increased complications from impaired wound healing, decreased resistance from infection, or hyperglycemia, these do not appear to be statistically significant. The other form of medical therapy used at some institutions is intravenous barbiturates.

The use of barbiturates in the therapy of severe head injury is based on the fact that barbiturates reduce cerebral blood flow and the metabolic rate of normal brain. In retrospective clinical studies using high-dose barbiturates, mortality was reported to be reduced and ICP better controlled in certain patients with severe head injury. However, in a prospective, randomized study of barbiturate coma in head injury, no difference in ICP levels, mortality, or neurologic outcome was established for patients treated with barbiturates compared with the control group. Given the potential side effect of hypotension, the use of barbiturates in the emergency ward in the management of head injury is not indicated.

Pediatric Head Injuries

In general, the evaluation of children with head injury should proceed as outlined for adults. There are certain differences, however, in the pediatric population regarding head injury of which the emergency room physician should be aware. The most important fact to bear in mind is that child abuse may present with head injury. The shaken baby can develop a tentorial or interhemispheric subdural hematoma as a result of torn cerebral veins. The presence of retinal hemorrhages, particularly in children under 2 years of age, is extremely suggestive of child abuse. The neurologic examination and the use of skull films in children have been discussed earlier.

Initial fluid management of a comatose child should involve the use of 5% dextrose in one-half normal or normal saline, run at one-half to two-thirds the normal maintenance volume. Seemingly small volumes of blood loss or intravenous fluid replacement can cause large changes in blood pressure in infants and toddlers. These volume changes can be made smoother by the insertion of an ICP monitor to avoid large changes in ICP.

Surgical intervention most commonly involves management of a depressed skull fracture with or without an acute epidural hematoma. Rapid recognition of this problem in a comatose child can lead to complete recovery after surgery. Scalp lacerations must be attended to promptly in children to avoid significant blood loss. Children will develop hypotensive shock in a matter of 30–60 minutes if scalp lacerations, which appear trivial by adult standards, are not closed.

Another form of intervention in infants with an open fontanel (usually younger than 1 year of age) is the fontanel, or subdural, tap. This procedure can be done electively in children with chronic subdural hematomas. The technique of fontanel taps should be performed emergently in infants with a bulging fontanel and retinal hemorrhages suggestive of severe head injury (usually caused by child abuse). The indications for tapping these children, such as apnea, decerebrate posturing, or unreactive dilated pupils, have been described by others. We have used these indications with adequate results if the procedure can be done soon after injury.

Penetrating Head Injury

In cases in which the injury has been caused by a sharp object driven into the head (e.g., screwdriver, ice pick, knife), the initial evaluation and management proceed as outlined above. If the object remains in the brain or protrudes from the skull, it should be left in place until adequate radiologic evaluation has been obtained. The majority of these patients require surgery even if the penetrating object has been removed (assuming they arrive at the emergency department with some evidence of neurologic function). The possibility of arterial injury with traumatic aneurysm formation or arterial transection must be kept in mind when managing these patients, and the emergency room physician should confer early with the neurosurgeon and radiologist to decide if an angiogram is indicated.

Civilian gunshot wounds to the head are associated with a high morbidity and mortality. In 100 patients managed aggressively, only 13% had a good outcome and 20% had moderate disability. In patients with GCS scores after resuscitation of 3–5 and no operable hematomas on CT scan, further aggressive medical or surgical therapy was of no benefit.

Suggested Reading

Barnett GH, Chapman PH. Insertion and Care of Intracranial Pressure Monitoring Devices. In AH Ropper, SF Kennedy (eds), Neurological and Neurosurgical Intensive Care (2nd ed). Rockville, MD: Aspen,1988;43–55.

Bruce DA, Schut L, Sutton LN. Pediatric Head Injury. In RH Wilkins, SS Rengachary (eds), Neurosurgery. New York: McGraw-Hill, 1985;1600–1604.

Clifton GL. Controversies in medical management of head injury. Clin Neurosurg 1988;34:587.

Cooper PR. Resuscitation of the Multiply Injured Patient. In RH Wilkins, SS Rengachary (eds), Neurosurgery. New York: McGraw-Hill, 1985;1587–1592.

Dacey RG, Alves WM, Rimel RW, et al. Neurosurgical complications after apparently minor head injury—assessment of risk in a series of 610 patients. J Neurosurg 1986;65:203.

Eisenberg HM, Cayard C, Papanicolaou AC, et al. The Effects of Three Potentially Preventable Complications on Outcome After Severe Closed Head Injury. In The Vth International Symposium on Intracranial Pressure. Berlin: Springer–Verlag, 1983;549–553.

Eisinberg HM, Gary HE, Aldrich EF, et al. Initial CT findings in 753 patients with severe head injury. A report from the NIH traumatic coma data bank. J Neurosurg 1990;73:688.

Grahm TW, Williams FC, Harrington T, Spetzler RF. Civilian gunshot wounds to the head: a prospective study. Neurosurgery 1990;27:696.

Harsh GR III, Harsh GR IV. Penetrating Wounds of the Head. In RH Wilkins, SS Rengachary (eds), Neurosurgery. New York: McGraw–Hill, 1985;1670–1678.

Marshall LF, Bowers SA. Outcome Prediction on Severe Head Injury. In RH Wilkins, SS Rengachary (eds), Neurosurgery. New York: McGraw–Hill, 1985;1605–1608.

Narayan RK. Emergency Room Management of the Head-injured Patient. In DP Becker, SK Gudeman (eds), Textbook of Head Injury. Philadelphia: Saunders, 1989;23–66.

Rimel RW, Giordani B, Barth JT, et al. Disability caused by minor head injury. Neurosurgery 1981;9:221.

Rimel RW, Giordani B, Barth JT, Jane JA. Moderate head injury: completing the clinical spectrum of brain trauma. Neurosurgery 1982;11:344.

Rivara F, Tanaguchi D, Parish RA, et al. Poor prediction of positive computed tomographic scans by clinical criteria in symptomatic pediatric head trauma. Pediatrics 1987;80:579.

Rockoff MA, Kennedy SK. Physiology and Clinical Aspects of Raised Intracranial Pressure. In AH Ropper, SF Kennedy (eds), Neurological and Neurosurgical Intensive Care (2nd ed). Rockville, MD: Aspen, 1988;9–22.

Saul TG. Is ICP monitoring worthwhile? Clin Neurosurg 1988;34:560.

Selig JM, Becker DP, Miller JD, et al. Traumatic acute subdural hematoma: major mortality reduction in comatose patients treated within 4 hours. N Engl J Med 1981; 304:1511.

Stein SC, Ross SE. The value of computed tomographic scans in patients with low-risk head injuries. Neurosurgery 1990;26:638.

Temkin NR, Dikmen SS, Wilensky AJ, et al. A randomized, double-blind study of phenytoin for the prevention of post-traumatic seizures. N Engl J Med 1990; 323:497.

Ward JD, Becker DP, Miller JD, et al. Failure of prophylactic barbiturate coma in the treatment of severe head injury. J Neurosurg 1985;62:383.

Chapter 45
Sleep Disorders

Ursula E. Anwer

Chapter Plan

Normal sleep
    Sleep testing
    Sleep cycles
    Circadian rhythms
Sleep disorders
    Dyssomnias
    Parasomnias
    Sleep disorders in association with medical illness,
        neurologic disease, or psychiatric conditions

Normal Sleep

Sleep is a period of rest. It is seen throughout the animal world, and we human beings are well aware that sleep is a daily requirement. If we do not sleep enough and soundly, we do not feel well and may have a substandard performance during our daytime activities.

The purpose of sleep is still not known, although there are various theories. Two theories are most prevalent. The first is the restoration theory that hypothesizes that sleep is necessary to mend the daily wear and tear and reconstitute body energy. The second theory focuses more on the brain, stating that sleep might be required to sort out the experiences of the day and consolidate memories.

Newborns spend most of their time sleeping. Young babies sleep several times during a 24-hour cycle. By the age of 3–5 months, sleep consolidates to a longer nighttime period with a few daytime sleep periods, which gradually changes in the toddler stage to sleeping mostly at night and napping only once or twice. Adults usually have only one sleep period at night, although with age, there seems to be a shift back to polyphasic sleep.

The amount of sleep in adults varies. The average time required to feel well during the following day is 7–8 hours. Some people only require 4 hours, whereas others require 11 hours of sleep. It is not only important to sleep the individually required amount, but also the quality of sleep needs to be normal to feel vigorous and rested the following day.

Sleep Testing

Polysomnography evolved in the 1950s and revolutionized sleep research and sleep medicine. Five sleep stages are characterized by polysomnography. We differentiate rapid eye movement (REM) sleep from non-REM sleep. Sleep stages are usually scored according to rules proposed by Kalen and Rechtschaffen. The rules are based on electroencephalographic (EEG), electro-oculographic (EOG), and electromyographic (EMG) findings. EEG leads are usually placed according to the standard EEG rules over the occipital and vertex areas (Figure 45-1). The occipital lead is important in differentiating the awake alpha rhythm and its disappearance into stage 1 of sleep. The vertex electrode is important for the rest of the sleep stages,

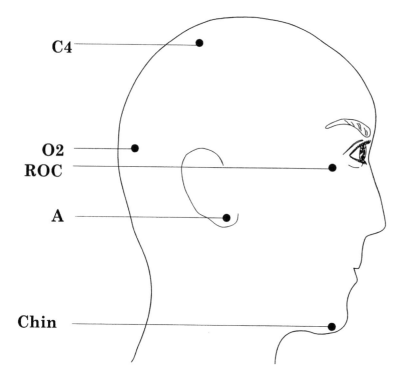

Figure 45-1. Basic lead placement in polysomnography: C4 = EEG, right vertex; O2 = EEG, right occiput; ROC = EEG lead, right outer canthus (left outer canthus not shown); EMG = chin. (EEG = electroencephalographic; EMG = electromyographic; A = inert electrode ear.)

because vertex sharp waves, K complexes, and sleep spindles are best seen there. The electro-oculogram demonstrates the rapid eye movements of REM sleep; the chin lead demonstrates changes in muscle tone, which vary according to sleep stages and should be absent in REM sleep. Nasal airflow, respiratory movements, oximetry, and leg movements are also monitored in most patients who are evaluated at a sleep laboratory (Figure 45-2).

A similar monitoring setup is used for the multiple sleep latency test (MSLT). The MSLT was developed to measure the extent of a patient's daytime hypersomnolence. The patient takes four naps in the sleep laboratory. The mean sleep latency should be more than 10 minutes.

Stage one of non-REM sleep (Figure 45-3A) indicates sleep onset. It is marked by slowing of the EEG background into a mixed frequency, mostly theta waves (4–7 Hz). The eye monitors show roving eye movements. Stage two (Figure 45-3B) is characterized by sleep spindles and K complexes with less than 20% high-voltage delta waves (less than 4 Hz). Stage three consists of 20–50% high-voltage (at least 75 μV) delta waves, leading to stage 4, which by definition requires at least 50% high-voltage delta waves (Figure 45-3C). Stages three and four, slow-wave sleep, decrease with advanced age. REM sleep itself (Figure 45-3D) is characterized by a desynchronized EEG recording. There are rapid eye movements but otherwise a total suppression of muscle activity except for the diaphragm. When humans awake during REM sleep, they usually report vivid dreaming. The percentage of REM sleep is approximately 20–25% per night, which is very constant, starting at around age 2 years and continuing for the rest of life.

Sleep Cycles

Polysomnographic studies have shown that sleep is organized into four to five cycles. Each cycle lasts approximately 90 minutes and consists of the sleeper going into stage 1 of sleep, then stage 2, then stages 3 and 4 to return to lower sleep stages and then REM sleep (Figure 45-4). The percentage of stages 3 and 4 is at its highest during the first cycle of sleep and diminishes during the following cycles. REM sleep, on the other hand, is

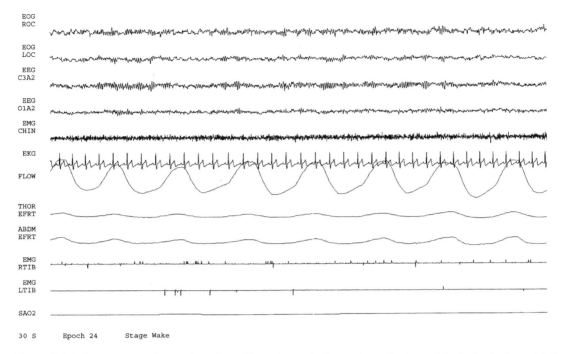

EOG ROC
EOG LOC
EEG C3A2
EEG O1A2
EMG CHIN
EKG
FLOW
THOR EFRT
ABDM EFRT
EMG RTIB
EMG LTIB
SAO2

30 S   Epoch 24   Stage Wake

Figure 45-2. Polysomnogram of an awake patient with regular respirations and a predominant alpha rhythm in the occipital lead. (EOG ROC and EOG LOC = electro-oculogram, right and left outer canthus; EEG C3A2 = vertex electroencephalic [EEG] electrode; EEG O1A2 = occipital electrode; EMG chin = electromyogram at chin; ECG = electrocardiogram; flow = nasal air flow measured by thermistor; THOR EFRT and ABDM EFRT = thoracic and abdominal belts measuring respiratory effort; EMG RTIB and EMG LTIB = electromyography from right and left anterior tibialis muscles to determine leg movements; SAO2 = oxygen saturation measured by oximetry is usually at the fingerberry or ear lobe.)

very brief during the first sleep cycle and becomes longer during subsequent cycles.

Circadian Rhythms

The beginning of sleep, the time of drowsiness, is regulated by an intrinsic circadian rhythm. The mammalian brain has a circadian pacemaker in the hypothalamus, the suprachiasmatic nucleus (SCN). Without external *zeitgebers,* clues about the time of the day, humans have a free-running circadian sleep-wake cycle of slightly more than 24 hours. The visual system, the daily light period, synchronizes the circadian clock. Other *zeitgebers* influence this rhythm, as for example the level of activity, meals, and probably auditory and other stimuli.

The circadian rhythm not only regulates the sleep-wake cycle, but it also regulates other physiologic rhythms as well. Some of them are not only linked to the sleep cycle, but also to specific stages of sleep.

Melatonin is secreted by the pineal gland, most likely as a sleep facilitator. Its secretion starts in the dark period and is inhibited by light. Cortisol secretion increases during the night, peaks in the early morning hours, and reaches its lowest level shortly before bedtime. Growth hormone secretion peaks during slow-wave sleep, usually during the first sleep cycle. Core temperature starts to fall in the evening and is at its lowest in the early morning hours. Temperature regulation is virtually absent during REM sleep, similar to the condition of poikilothermia. In summary, good sleeping requires sleep at the right time during the circadian rhythm, a sufficient amount of time spent sleeping, and good quality sleep.

Sleep Disorders

Some patients with sleep disorders complain about daytime sleepiness, others about the inability to sleep. In other cases, there may be an abnormal

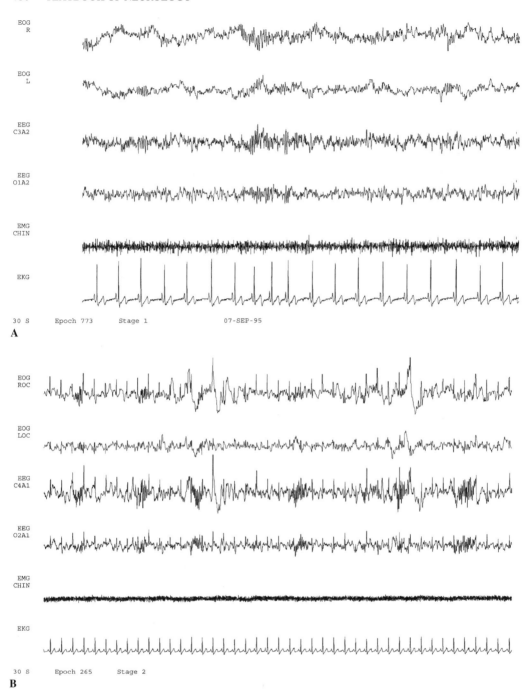

Figure 45-3. Polysomnogram of a patient in stages 1, 2, 4, and REM sleep. (A) Stage 1. The alpha rhythm in the occipital electroencephalographic (EEG) lead disappears and changes into a relative low frequency, low-voltage EEG activity with mixed frequency. The electro-oculographic (EOG) leads demonstrate roving eye movements. (B) Stage 2. The EEG, especially over the vertex, demonstrates K complexes and sleep spindles in a setting of a mixed-frequency, low-voltage EEG activity. (C) Stage 4. More than 50% of the EEG activity consists of high-voltage delta waves. (D) REM sleep. The EEG activity is desynchronized. Saw-toothing is seen over the vertex. The patient has eye movements recorded in both eye channels. The chin EMG is of relatively low voltage, indicative of atonia. (ROC = right outer canthus; LOC = left outer canthus.)

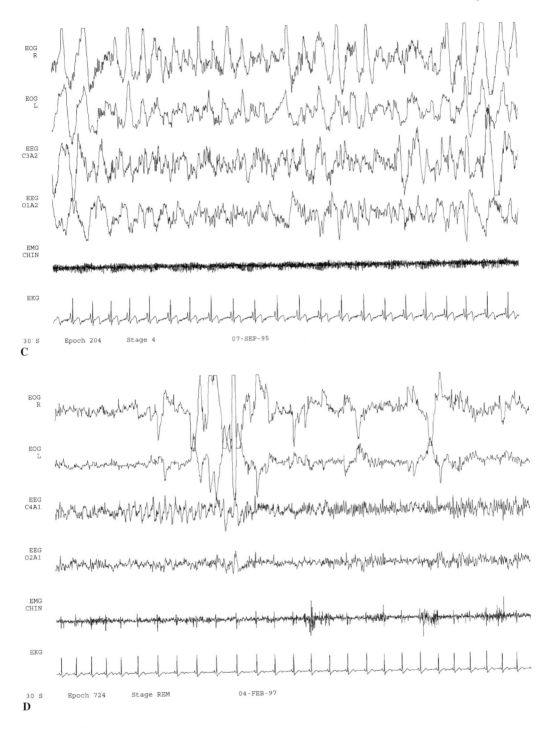

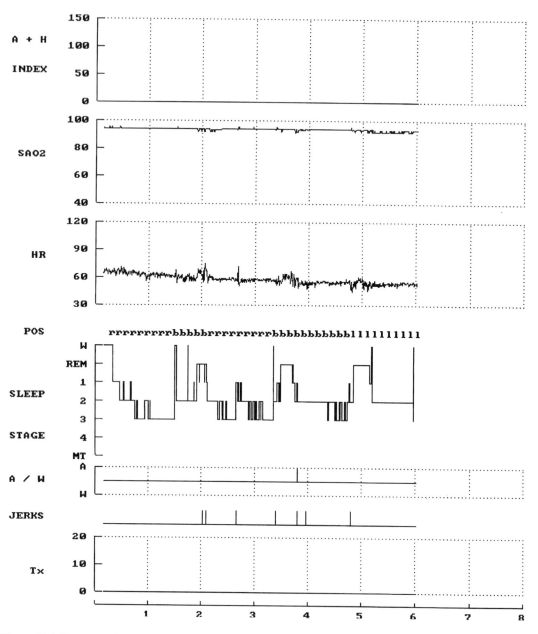

Figure 45-4. Histogram of a normal 30-year-old patient based on continuous overnight monitoring of the electroencephalographic, electro-oculographic, and chin electromyographic activity, as explained in Figures 45-1 and 45-2. The
patient does not have any respiratory disturbances. His oxygen saturation is within normal limits, and his heart rate varies
only slightly. He has a relatively higher amount of stage 3 of sleep toward the beginning of the night, with progressively
longer REM periods toward the end of the night. Rare leg movements are seen. (A+H index [apnea plus hypopnea index] =
the numbers of apneas and hypopneas per hour of sleep; SAO2 = arterial oxygen saturation monitored by oximetry over the
fingerberry; HR = heart rate; POS = position at night; MT = movements; A/W = awakenings; jerks = leg movements; Tx =
therapy with nasal continuous positive airway pressure; REM = rapid eye movement.)

sleep behavior at night making the sleeper and the bed partner concerned. The *International Classification of Sleep Disorders* categorized sleep disorders into three broad categories—dyssomnias, parasomnias, and medical-psychiatric sleep disorders—and added a fourth for patients with less-well-defined problems. Only a few of these disorders, the most prevalent ones, are discussed.

Dyssomnias

Dyssomnias are subdivided into intrinsic, extrinsic, and circadian sleep disorders. Intrinsic sleep disorders originate from within the body and extrinsic disorders are usually caused by external factors, mostly environmental disturbances. Circadian rhythm sleep disorders may occur because of an internal rhythm abnormality or a mismatch of the internal versus environmental *zeitgebers.*

Patients complaining about sleepiness during the daytime must be taken seriously. Most of them have a dyssomnia that should be treated to prevent serious mishappenings during the wakeful period, such as motor vehicle crashes, accidents at work, or simply embarrassment of the patient in his or her social environment.

Intrinsic Sleep Disorders

Narcolepsy.   Narcolepsy is characterized by excessive daytime hypersomnolence. Patients have an irresistible urge to sleep and may have sleep attacks, which usually happen in a relatively monotonous environment or with monotonous activity. The mean MSLT score is usually less than 5 minutes. Short naps are refreshing and can be associated with dreaming. Narcolepsy is a REM-dissociative disorder. Features of REM sleep occur at inappropriate times in the sleep-wake cycle. One is cataplexy, which is the equivalent of the paralysis during REM sleep. It is the second hallmark of narcolepsy. It is not always present at the onset of the disorder, but if present along with these sleep attacks, it is almost pathognomonic. Cataplexy is usually induced by an emotional event, be it sadness or happiness. The patient feels a sudden loss of segmental or total muscle control that usually lasts for a few minutes, and in extreme cases it can result in falls. Sleep paralysis and hypnagogic hallucinations as well as nocturnal sleep disruption are also associated features of narcolepsy. Patients may awaken from sleep being paralyzed, which can be extremely frightening. Hypnagogic hallucinations are vivid, usually visual perceptions at sleep onset of unreal objects, most likely presenting sleep-onset dreaming in the still-awake state.

REM suppressants are widely used to limit REM sleep and REM fragments during the daytime. The most frequently used medications are antidepressants, either tricyclics or selective serotonin reuptake inhibitors. Central nervous system (CNS) stimulants are prescribed to combat the excessive daytime sleepiness.

Obstructive Sleep Apnea.   The obstructive sleep apnea syndrome is characterized by repetitive episodes of upper airway obstruction during sleep lasting at least 10 seconds. There is complete cessation of air movement around the mouth or nose in spite of continuous inspiratory and expiratory efforts, which are detected by abdominal and thoracic movements (Figure 45-5A). Hypopneas, by definition, are characterized by a 50% reduction of airflow. Both apneas and hypopneas can result in a drop of oxygen saturation, which is usually monitored by oximetry. Hypoxia and also hypercapnia are both respiratory stimulators and can cause an arousal and renewed respiratory movements. The repetitive arousals cause disruption of the nocturnal sleep pattern (Figures 45-5B, 45-6A). The patient awakens in the morning not feeling refreshed and experiences excessive daytime hypersomnolence. The prevalence of obstructive sleep apnea is probably 1–2% in the general population. It is associated with obesity and the male sex, but it increases in incidence in postmenopausal women. It is also seen more frequently with certain anatomic features, for example, a small upper airway, as seen with large tonsils or with an enlarged tongue, or with retrognathia. Treatment of moderate to severe obstructive sleep apnea is imperative not only because it can cause sleep disruptions, but it may also cause cardiac problems and has been associated with an increased risk for stroke.

The treatment should be individualized. In some patients it is sufficient to change the sleeping position away from supine. A tonsillectomy might cure the syndrome in children. Tricyclic antidepressants can be prescribed in mild cases, especially if they are REM-related. The gold standard for moderate to

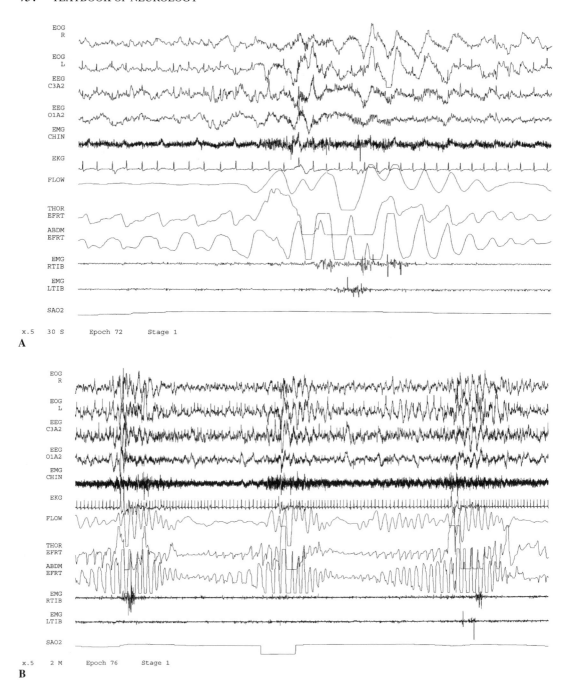

Figure 45-5. Polysomnogram showing obstructive sleep apnea. (A) In spite of respiratory efforts proven by respiratory movements in the thoracic and abdominal belts, there is no air flow at the nose and mouth. An arousal with increased respiratory effort leads to return of nasal air flow. (B) Obstructive sleep apnea compressed in time. A 2-minute epoch shows repeated arousals with cyclic increases in respiratory effort and fluctuations in oxygen saturation. (EOG R and EOG L = electro-oculogram, right and left outer canthus; EEG C3A2 = vertex electroencephalic [EEG] electrode; EEG O1A2 = occipital electrode; EMG chin = electromyogram at chin; ECG = electrocardiogram; flow = nasal air flow measured by thermistor; THOR EFRT and ABDM EFRT = thoracic and abdominal belts measuring respiratory effort; EMG RTIB and EMG LTIB = electromyography from right and left anterior tibialis muscles to determine leg movements; SAO2 = oxygen saturation measured by oximetry is usually at the fingerberry or ear lobe.)

severe obstructive sleep apnea is continuous positive airway pressure (CPAP), which keeps the airway open with a pneumatic splint (see Figure 45-6). For patients who do not tolerate nasal CPAP, there is the option of using a dental appliance or surgery. Dental appliances are worn at night to displace the mandible and tongue forward, creating a larger upper airway. Surgical procedures range from laser uvulopalatoplasty, to soft palate resection via uvulopalatopharyngoplasty, to geniotubercle advancement, and in extreme cases midface advancement, which is performed in only a few centers.

Periodic Limb Movement Disorder.   Periodic limb movement disorder (PLMS) is characterized by periodic episodes of repetitive, mostly leg movements during sleep. The movement usually consists of hip, knee, and ankle flexion with extension of the big toe occurring every 20–40 seconds either unilaterally or in alternating legs or both legs (Figure 45-7). The movement is rarely seen in the upper extremities. The generator for these movements remains to be determined. It is thought to be either in the spinal cord or in the brain stem. If PLMS is associated with frequent arousals and causes daytime hypersomnolence, it needs to be treated. The first line of therapy is usually benzodiazepines and then most of the medications prescribed for the restless leg syndrome (RLS).

Restless Leg Syndrome.   Patients with RLS have an uncomfortable sensation in their legs, usually before sleep onset, that is relieved by movement. The patients describe it as a tingling, like an insect crawling or a stinging sensation with at times an irresistible urge to move. Because it occurs in a relaxed atmosphere before sleep onset, it prevents sleep. Unfortunately, the patient may suffer the same situation if he or she wakes up during the night. In some patients the presleep RLS is carried over to the daytime and disturbs relaxed restful moments. Listening to a concert or sitting quietly in an airplane can become torture for these patients. Frequently, patients with RLS also have PLMS. RLS is associated with a variety of illnesses. Frequent associations are with peripheral neuropathy, uremia, and anemia. Therapy should include an attempt to treat the underlying condition. If no underlying condition is detected, the medication of choice is usually a benzodiazepine.

Some physicians prefer dopaminergic agents. Opioids can be useful as well.

Extrinsic Sleep Disorders

Extrinsic sleep disorders are primarily a reaction to an environmental stimulus, either resulting in the inability to initiate sleep or the inability to maintain sleep. An unusual sensory stimulus can disrupt sleep onset or maintenance—for example, sleeping in a hotel, a loud noise, a bed partner with a sleep problem, light, or unusual temperatures. Intense mental work as well as vigorous exercise just before bedtime can delay sleep onset. Alcohol consumption or caffeine intake in the evening hours can disrupt sleep. It is important to get a complete psychosocial history from every patient with a sleep complaint. Extrinsic sleep disorders are at times easily treatable, simply by avoidance of the responsible stimulus.

Circadian Rhythm Sleep Disorders

Modern life has changed our natural light/dark cycle, enabling us to live in brightly illuminated spaces, creating the illusion of daytime and enabling shift work. Modern traveling has created the problem of jet lag. Some people adapt more easily to shift work than others. Adaptation to a new circadian rhythm is more difficult with age. In general, people are able to change their circadian rhythm by about 1–2 hours a day. Phase delay is easier than phase advance. Traveling west is easier than going east. People who work stable night shifts usually do better than those working rotating shifts because they adapt their circadian rhythm, including their temperature and other physiologic rhythms, to the new time frame. Bright light will delay sleep onset; darkness is conducive to sleep. Bright light late at night will delay sleep onset and awakening; bright light in the early morning hours can advance sleep onset. This technique can be used to help adjust people with shift work, as well as jet lag.

Parasomnias

Parasomnias are phenomena appearing during sleep, rarely resulting in a complaint of daytime hypersomnolence or insomnia. They can be sub-

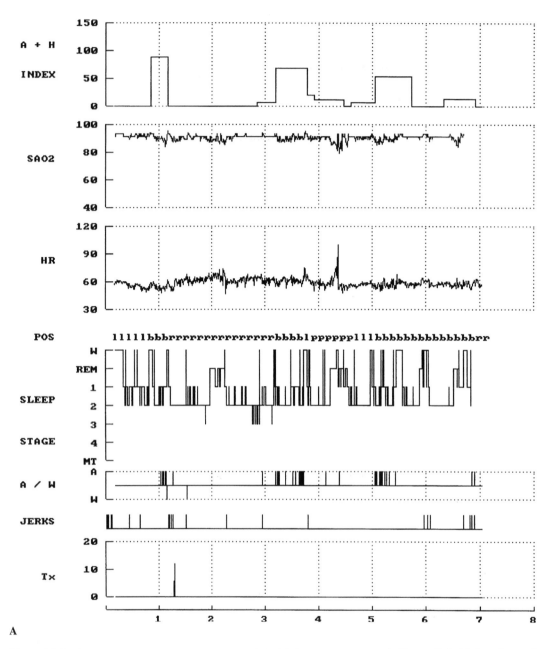

A

Figure 45-6. Histograms of a sleep apnea patient recorded with the same montage as in Figure 45-2. (A) Baseline study. The patient has fragmented sleep with almost no stage 3 and stage 4 of sleep as well as a low amount of REM sleep. The apnea and hypopnea index is well above the accepted index of 5. The oxygen saturation fluctuates into the low 80% range. (B) Study with treatment. Histogram of the same sleep apnea patient but with nasal continuous positive airway pressure. Sleep is less fragmented. The patient has stage 3 of sleep and a larger amount of REM sleep. There are only minor fluctuations of his oxygen saturation. (A+H index [apnea plus hypopnea index] = the numbers of apneas and hypopneas per hour of sleep; SAO2 = arterial oxygen saturation monitored by oximetry over the fingerberry; HR = heart rate; POS = position at night; MT = movements; A/W = awakenings; jerks = leg movements; Tx = therapy with nasal continuous positive airway pressure; REM = rapid eye movement.)

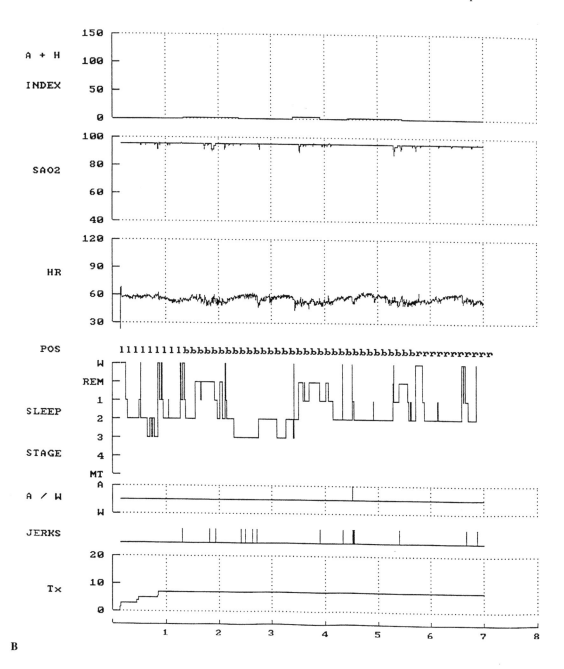

B

classified as disorders of arousal, partial arousal, sleep stage transition, and REM. These disorders are generally more prevalent in childhood.

Arousal Disorders

An altered waking mechanism seems to be responsible for arousal disorders. This can result in sleep "drunkenness," sleep walking, and, especially in children, night terrors.

Sleep Drunkenness.   In sleep drunkenness, a person is awakened but is not completely awake. The person is disoriented to time and space. There may be retrograde and anterograde memory impairment. There may be misperception of reality

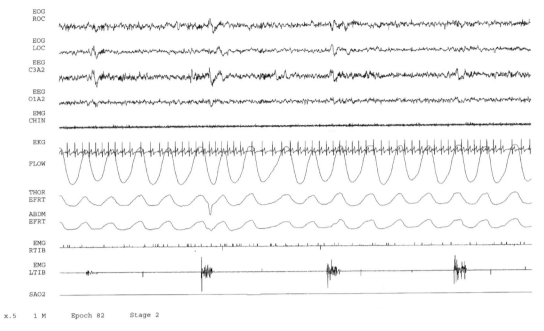

EOG ROC
EOG LOC
EEG C3A2
EEG O1A2
EMG CHIN
EKG
FLOW
THOR EFRT
ABDM EFRT
EMG RTIB
EMG LTIB
SAO2

x.5   1 M   Epoch 82   Stage 2

Figure 45-7. Polysomnogram of a patient with periodic limb movement disorder. Three leg movements are recorded at the left leg, each resulting in a minor arousal (K complex). The patient has regular respirations and is in stage 2 of sleep. (EOG ROC and EOG LOC = electro-oculogram, right and left outer canthus; EEG C3A2 = vertex electroencephalic [EEG] electrode; EEG O1A2 = occipital electrode; EMG chin = electromyogram at chin; ECG = electrocardiogram; flow = nasal air flow measured by thermistor; THOR EFRT and ABDM EFRT = thoracic and abdominal belts measuring respiratory effort; EMG RTIB and EMG LTIB = electromyography from right and left anterior tibialis muscles to determine leg movements; SAO2 = oxygen saturation measured by oximetry is usually at the fingerberry or ear lobe.)

with a fully functioning motor system. The person is able to walk, dress, and even drive a car. This state can last for minutes up to a few hours. Planning and premeditation of actions is not possible during this state. Confusional arousals can be precipitated by an arousal out of stages 3 and 4 of sleep, which is more prevalent during the first third of the night. It can be precipitated by sleep deprivation, by alcohol, or by CNS depressant drugs, which should be avoided in persons prone to this disorder.

Sleep Walking.   Sleep walking is common in young children. It tends to disappear in adolescence but can still occur in adulthood. It also happens out of stages 3 and 4 of sleep. The person may just sit up and mumble or get up and get fully or partially dressed and walk. There may be inappropriate behavior, which can result in falls and injury. The episode is usually terminated by the sleeper returning to bed to continue sleeping. There is usually complete amnesia about the event. Sleep walking occurs mostly during the first third of the night and can also be precipitated by sleep deprivation, fever, and certain medications that induce slow-wave sleep.

Night Terrors.   Night terrors are characterized by a sudden arousal from slow-wave sleep with a horrifying scream; behavior expressing intense fear; and, with the fear, associated autonomic expressions of tachycardia, mydriasis, diaphoresis, and increased muscle tone. Like sleep walking, night terrors occur predominately in children and mostly disappear in adolescence. They are not associated with psychopathologic conditions, although if they happen in older children and adults there may be a psychologically stressful event along with sleep deprivation precipitating the event.

Sleep-Wake Transition Disorders

Sleep-wake transition disorders are usually of benign character. They include rhythmic movements at sleep onset, such as head banging, head rolling, or body rocking and rolling. This occurs mostly in children up to the age of 4 years during drowsiness and into light sleep. Sleep starts and hypnic jerks are a normal occurrence at sleep onset and can be recalled in 60–70% of the population. They consist of asymmetric, nonrhythmic body jerks. No EEG abnormality is seen with them. RLS technically is also a sleep-wake transition disorder, but it is considered a dyssomnia because it results in an insomnia.

Parasomnias Associated with Rapid Eye Movement Sleep

Nightmares.   In contrast to night terrors, nightmares are usually experienced during the second part of the night, when the relative percentage of REM sleep is the highest. They are vivid, frightening dreams from which the sleeper usually wakes up sweaty and tachycardic. In contrast to night terrors, the sleeper does not wake up confused and is able to retell at least part of the horrifying dream. Psychologically stressful events can precipitate nightmares, as occurs in war veterans. Psychotherapy may be helpful to prevent them. Antidepressants, such as REM suppressants, can be useful, but their rapid withdrawal can in turn precipitate nightmares. Patients taking betablockers or dopaminergic medications are also at higher risk for nightmares.

Rapid Eye Movement Sleep Behavior Disorder. Patients with REM sleep behavior disorder lack the atonia of REM sleep, but otherwise experience REM sleep at the same frequency and density. Patients act out their dreams, which can be dangerous for the patient and bed partner. A loving bed partner's arm may be interwoven into the patient's dream as a dangerous horrifying snake that needs to be killed. The sleeper's movements may vary from arm and leg movements to punching and getting up and fighting with an object or a person mistaken as being part of the dream content. These episodes can occur every 90–100 minutes during each returning REM cycle but are not stereotypi-cal. Polysomnography shows typical REM sleep but no atonia.

The prevalence of REM sleep behavior disorder increases with age. Patients with structural lesions in the pontine tegmentum are at increased risk for this disorder (e.g., patients with multiple sclerosis, lacunar strokes, or, for some reason, early Parkinson's disease patients). It is thought that the perinucleus ceruleus area in the pontine tegmentum is the generator for the muscle atonia, creating an inhibition of the anterior horn cells during REM sleep. Clonazepam at bedtime is usually sufficient to suppress this disorder.

Sleep Disorders in Association with Medical Illness, Neurologic Disease, or Psychiatric Conditions

Many disorders that can affect basic neurologic function or sleep coordination can alter sleep. These can be electrolyte abnormalities in medical disease or alterations in the brain anatomy or physiology with neurologic and psychiatric diseases. These disorders might result in complaints of insomnia or daytime hypersomnolence.

Sleep Disorders with Medical Illness

Most medical problems affect sleep. A simple common cold or a febrile illness can result in drowsiness. Respiratory problems can lead to nocturnal hypoxemia or hypercapnia with frequent arousals and a disruption of sleep architecture. Esophageal reflux or peptic ulcer disease can awaken the patient at night. Any pain severe enough to arouse the patient can cause fragmented sleep. Diabetes mellitus, hypertension, and hypothyroidism are associated with obstructive sleep apnea. This brief list of medical conditions is only a small sample of disorders demonstrating potential sleep-wake alterations. Not only do these conditions change sleep, but also sleep itself can cause or worsen medical problems. For example, patients with obstructive sleep apnea can have arrhythmias at night.

One should not overlook the effect of various medications on sleep and its architecture. Steroids and methylxanthines, which are used for asthma patients, can precipitate insomnia. Beta-blockers may trigger nightmares. Anticholinergic medications can alter REM sleep.

Sleep Disorders with Neurologic Disease

Sleep is not a passive phenomenon during which the brain simply enters into a low functioning mode. Sleep seems to be orchestrated by different regions and nuclei in the brain, mostly the brain stem and hypothalamus. Any anatomic lesion or CNS dysfunction may bring this orchestra out of fine tune, resulting in a sleep disturbance. A hypothalamic lesion, for example, a stroke in the posterior hypothalamus, can result in somnolence, whereas a lesion in the anterior hypothalamus can result in insomnia. A lesion in the pons around the nucleus ceruleus can cause loss of atonia during REM sleep, as seen in REM behavior disorder.

Neurodegenerative Diseases. Neurodegenerative diseases are associated with sleep problems. In Alzheimer's disease there is a profound involvement of the central cholinergic nuclei, which may be responsible for some of the sleep disturbances. Patients with advanced Alzheimer's disease often experience fragmented sleep with increased daytime sleep and less sleep at night. The well-known "sundowning" might be a result of this. Fragmented sleep is also seen in patients with Parkinson's disease. Their tremor can be carried into light sleep. The relative immobility in advanced cases causes sleep problems. Dopaminergic medications can help this, but on the other hand, they can also be the culprit of nocturnal insomnia, nightmares, and hallucinations. Fatal familial insomnia is a prion disease causing destruction of mainly the anterior and dorsal medial thalamus. These patients develop progressive insomnia and autonomic dysfunction and eventually do not sleep at all. The disease results in coma and death after only a few months.

Seizure Disorders. Twenty percent to 30% of seizures are predominantly nocturnal. Sleep deprivation is a known activator of seizures. Most nocturnal seizures occur in stages 1 and 2, whereas REM sleep is a seizure suppressant. In general, nocturnal seizures seem to suppress REM sleep, cause fragmentation of sleep, and increase the percentage of stages 1 and 2 of sleep. At times it is difficult to determine whether the anticonvulsants or seizures are responsible for a change in sleep architecture, although it is thought that anticonvulsants have a stabilizing effect on the sleep EEG findings. At times, only polysomnography is able to tell whether a patient's sleep disturbance is caused by seizures or a different phenomenon, for example, a parasomnia.

Neuromuscular Disorders. Neuromuscular disorders have their main impact on sleep by impairing respiration. Any change in diaphragmatic function or function of the intercostal and accessory respiratory muscles can alter respiratory function by potentially being responsible for alveolar hypoventilation. The resulting hypoxemia and hypercapnia will lead to fragmented sleep and daytime hypersomnolence. Treatment of the underlying disorder will result in normal sleep—for example, successfully treating a patient with Guillain-Barré syndrome with plasmaphereses. If the neuromuscular disorder cannot be resolved, for example, in patients with motor neuron disease, the patients need to have respiratory support at night such as bilevel positive airway pressure or eventually even the assistance of a respirator.

Sleep Disorders with Psychiatric Conditions

Most patients with a psychiatric disorder also suffer from sleep disturbances. Insomnia is the most frequent complaint with problems initiating sleep, or there can be disruption of nocturnal sleep resulting in daytime hypersomnolence. Often it is difficult to determine whether the sleep disturbance is caused by the psychiatric problem or whether it is a side effect of a medication. In these cases a careful evaluation by the sleep specialist together with a psychiatrist is required.

The most prevalent sleep problem in depression is early awakening and not being able to return to sleep. Polysomnography shows early REM onset with increased REM density and poor sleep efficiency with early awakening. Successful antidepressant therapy has been judged by its ability to shift REM sleep to a later, more normal time of the sleep cycle. Manic patients have less total sleep time with less stage 3 and stage 4 of sleep. There is no consistent effect on REM sleep.

Some patients with panic attacks experience them predominantly at night. Polysomnography may be needed to differentiate these attacks from nocturnal seizures or obstructive sleep apnea. Patients with panic disorder often have difficulties falling asleep.

Nocturnal panic attacks can occur at any stage of sleep, but mostly occur in non-REM sleep.

Successful treatment of the psychiatric condition usually eradicates the sleep disorder as well. On the other hand, a sleep complaint may herald the occurrence or recurrence of a psychopathologic condition.

Patients complaining of a sleep disorder need a complete evaluation of their lifestyle, their sleep habits, nocturnal events witnessed by a bed partner, and a complete medical and psychiatric history. Only such a global assessment will enable the sleep specialist to formulate the right diagnosis and treatment plan.

Suggested Reading

Aldrich MS. The neurobiology of narcolepsy-cataplexy. Prog Neurobiol 1993;41:533.

Becker PB, Jamieson AO, Brown WD. Dopaminergic agents in restless leg syndrome and periodic limb movements of sleep: response and complications of extended treatment in 49 cases. Sleep 1993;16:713.

Bliwise DL, Caroll JS, Lee KA, Nekich JC, et al. Sleep and sundowning in nursing home patients with dementia. Psychiatry Res 1993;48:277.

Brzezinski A. Mechanisms of disease: melatonin in humans. N Engl J Med 1997;336:186.

Carskadon MA, Dement WC. Normal Human Sleep: An Overview. In MH Kruyger, T Roth, WC Dement (eds), Principles and Practice of Sleep Medicine. Philadelphia: Saunders, 1994;16–25.

Carskadon MA, Dement WC, Mitler MM, et al. Guidelines for the multiple sleep latency test (MSLT). A standard measure of sleepiness. Sleep 1986;9:519.

Coccagna G. Restless Leg Syndrome/Periodic Leg Movements in Sleep. In MJ Thorpy (ed), Handbook of Sleep Disorders. New York: Marcel Dekker, 1990;457–478.

Dyken ME, Rodnitzky RL. Periodic, aperiodic, and rhythmic motor disorders of sleep. Neurology 1992;42:S68.

Guilleminault C, Stoohs R, Quera-Salva MA. Sleep-related obstructive and nonobstructive apneas and neurologic disorders. Neurology 1992;42:S53.

Kaplan PW, Allen RP, Buchholz DW, Walters JK. A double-blind, placebo-controlled study of the treatment of periodic limb movements in sleep using carbidopa/levodopa and propoxyphene. Sleep 1993;16:717.

Keefauver SP, Guilleminault C. Sleep Terrors and Sleepwalking. In MH Kruyger, T Roth, WC Dement (eds), Principles and Practice of Sleep Medicine. Philadelphia: Saunders, 1994;567–573.

Kimoff RJ. Sleep fragmentation in obstructive sleep apnea. Sleep 1996;19:S61.

Levy P, Pepin JL, Mayer P, Wuyam B, et al. Management of simple snoring, upper airway resistance syndrome, and moderate sleep apnea syndrome. Sleep 1996;19:S101.

Mahowald MW, Schenck CH. REM-Sleep Behavior Disorder. In MJ Thorpy (ed), Handbook of Sleep Disorders. New York: Marcel Dekker, 1990;567–594.

Miller JD, Morin LP, Schwartz WJ, Moore RY. New insights into the mammalian circadian clock. Sleep 1996;19:641.

Pepin JL, Veale D, Mayer P, Bettega G, et al. Critical analysis of the results of surgery in the treatment of snoring, upper airway resistance syndrome (UARS), and obstructive sleep apnea (OSA). Sleep 1996;19:S90.

Rechtschaffen A, Kales A. A Manual of Standardized Techniques and Scoring System for Sleep Stages of Human Sleep. Los Angeles: Brain Information Service/Brain Research Institute, University of California at Los Angeles, 1968.

Thorpy MJ. Disorders of Arousal. In MJ Thorpy (ed), Handbook of Sleep Disorders. New York: Marcel Dekker, 1990;531–549.

Chapter 46
Tropical Neurologic Disorders

Gustavo C. Román

Chapter Plan

Tropical neurology
    Definition
    Basic neuroepidemiologic concepts
    History of travel and migration
Diagnostic guidelines according to clinical syndromes
    Seizures
    Encephalopathy, stupor, and coma
    Meningitis
    Encephalopathy with focal signs (intracranial
        space-occupying lesions)
    Acute-onset flaccid paralysis
    Tropical spastic paraparesis
    Peripheral neuropathies

Tropical Neurology

Definition

Tropical neurology is the study of nervous system disorders that occur with high prevalence in tropical and subtropical zones of the world (i.e., regions situated along the equator, extending to 30 degrees latitude north and south). The tropical climate is characterized by high temperatures, abundant sunlight, days and nights of equal length, and an absence of four seasons. Three-fourths of the population of the world or 3 billion people live in developing countries of the tropics; these countries produce only 15% of the world's net revenue and consume a meager 6% of the worldwide food production. This explains in part the tropical problems of illiteracy; malnutrition; deficient environmental sanitation; neurotoxicity; and water-borne and arthropod-transmitted infections of viral, bacterial, and parasitic origin. The principal determinants of neurologic diseases in underdeveloped countries are the socioeconomic conditions.

Basic Neuroepidemiologic Concepts

The pattern of occurrence of neurologic diseases changes in different geographic regions. Disease frequency is measured by epidemiologic indices such as incidence (number of new cases), mortality (number of fatal cases), and prevalence (total number of cases, new and old, present at a given time in a defined population). Environmental, climatic, racial, cultural, and dietary factors, among others, result in variations in disease frequency. Very few conditions are exclusively "tropical" because their vectors require a particular warm climate or a peculiar ecologic niche. In fact, "tropical diseases" such as malaria, leprosy, and cysticercosis occurred in Europe and North America in the late 1800s in conditions of poor environmental sanitation.

History of Travel and Migration

It is often remarked that air travel and modern communications have reduced the world to a global village. This change is also evident in the patterns of disease occurrence. As a result of international

743

Table 46-1. Etiologic Factors in Epilepsy in the Tropics

Perinatal factors
    Maternal infections during pregnancy, labor, and delivery
        Low birth weight
        Maternal malnutrition
        Maternal anemia (malaria, iron-deficient diet, hook-
            worms)
        Preterm deliveries
        Aged multiparous mothers
    Cerebral palsy: kernicterus (G6PD deficiency, umbilical
        cord sepsis)
Febrile seizures
    Malaria
Head injuries
    Traffic accidents
    Violence
Parasitic infections
    Metazoan infections
        Cysticercosis (*Taenia solium*)
        Schistosomiasis (bilharziasis)
            Schistosoma japonicum (Southeast Asia)
        Paragonimiasis (*Paragonimus westermani*)
        Sparganosis
        Hydatid disease
        Larva migrans (*Toxocara canis, Toxocara cati, Ascaris*)
    Protozoan infections
        Toxoplasmosis (*Toxoplasma gondii*)
        African trypanosomiasis (*Trypanosoma brucei*)
        American trypanosomiasis: Chagas' disease (*Try-
            panosoma cruzi*)
	Malaria (*Plasmodium falciparum*)
	    Cerebral malaria
	    Febrile seizures
	Amoebiasis (*Entamoeba histolytica, Naegleria,*
	    Acanthamoeba)
	Bacterial infections
	    Tuberculosis
	        Tuberculous meningitis
	        Tuberculous encephalopathy
	        Tuberculomas
	    Pyogenic meningitis
	        Meningococcal meningitis, other pyogenic bacteria,
	            Streptococcus suis (Asia)
	        Bacillus anthracis (India)
	Viral infections
	    Herpes encephalitis, mumps, respiratory viruses, entero-
	        viruses, rabies, rubella, arenaviruses, arboviruses
	        (flaviviruses)
	    Japanese encephalitis virus
	    Postinfectious encephalitides: measles, mumps, rubella
	    Subacute sclerosing panencephalitis
	    Creutzfeldt-Jakob disease
	Toxic agents
	    Alcohol
	    Lead
	    Benzahexachloride
	    Chloroquine
	Heredity

G6PD = glucose 6 phosphate dehydrogenase.
Source: Reprinted with permission from N Senananyake, GC Román. Aetiological factors of epilepsy in the tropics. J Trop Geogr Neurol 1991;1:69.

travel, tourism, and migration, physicians practicing in temperate regions often diagnose and treat patients with tropical diseases. Therefore, a history of travel or migration should be elicited when evaluating seemingly common neurologic disorders. For instance, headache, fever, and chills in a tourist may be the prodromata of cerebral malaria. Lower limb spasticity in a migrant may signal tropical spastic paraparesis caused by human T-cell lymphotrophic virus type I (HTLV-I) infection. A typical ulnar neuropathy may be caused by leprosy. Focal seizures may be the result of neurocysticercosis. Embolic stroke in a South American migrant may be caused by chagasic cardiomyopathy. The following section provides a diagnostic approach to the most common neurologic problems observed in tropical regions of the world, including Latin America, Africa, the Indian subcontinent, Asia, and the Pacific Islands.

Diagnostic Guidelines According to Clinical Syndromes

Seizures

The age-adjusted prevalence of active epilepsy in tropical countries ranges between 10 and 15 per 1,000 inhabitants. This is almost twice the prevalence in Western countries and represents an enormous health expenditure for the developing world. In contrast to industrialized countries, partial seizures with secondary generalization predominate in the tropics, probably indicating a higher proportion of patients with symptomatic epilepsy resulting from infections, perinatal brain injury, head trauma, and neurotoxins such as lead, chloroquine, or pesticides. Table 46-1 summarizes the main etiologic factors of epilepsy in the tropics; most of these causes of epilepsy are preventable. Prenatal and perinatal control, alcohol-use education, and mandatory enforcement of strict traffic regulations to prevent head injuries from accidents and drunk driving are required to decrease the high frequency of symptomatic epilepsy in the tropics. Neurocysticercosis, tuberculosis, malaria, epidemic meningococcal meningitis, Japanese encephalitis, and most parasitic and bacterial intracranial infections can be prevented by vaccination or controlled with appropriate treatment and public health measures.

Neurocysticercosis (*Taenia solium*) is the main cause of epilepsy in the tropics, causing up to 25% of cases. Neurocysticercosis results when human hosts ingest fertilized *T. solium* eggs passed in the stools of human tapeworm carriers. Thus, this is a human-to-human infection acquired by the fecal-enteric route in areas with deficient environmental sanitation. *T. solium* carriers are extremely contagious and are usually found in the patient's close environment (home, restaurant). Contrary to common belief, humans who ingest poorly cooked pork meat infested with larvae of the tapeworm *Taenia solium* develop intestinal taeniasis, *not* neurocysticercosis. Treatment with praziquantel or albendazole is effective.

Table 46-2. Etiologic Factors in Stupor and Coma in the Tropics

Infections
Cerebral malaria
Trypanosomiasis
Typhoid fever
Meningitis
Encephalitis
Drugs
Multiple agents, including alcohol
Metabolic disturbances
Hypoglycemia
Hyperglycemia
Uremia
Trauma
Traffic accidents
Violence
Epilepsy
Postictal state
Hyperthermia
Heat stroke
Sickle cell disease
Brain abscess
Tumors, including tuberculomas
Cerebrovascular accidents

Source: Reprinted with permission from World Health Organization Malaria Action Programme. Severe and complicated malaria. Trans R Soc Trop Med Hyg 1986;80(Suppl):1.

Encephalopathy, Stupor, and Coma

In contrast to factors that cause coma in Western countries, infection is the most common cause of coma in the tropics (Table 46-2). For diagnostic purposes, separation can be made between febrile and afebrile patients with encephalopathy in the tropics.

Febrile patients in the tropics who are acutely ill and present with signs of severe encephalopathy and decreased responsiveness must be considered to have cerebral malaria (*Plasmodium falciparum*) until proved otherwise. Seizures may occur, particularly in children. Focal signs such as hemiparesis or cranial nerve palsies are not prominent. Cerebrospinal fluid (CSF) examination is mandatory to eliminate other infections; in cerebral malaria the CSF is usually normal, except for increased pressure. Asexual forms of the parasite are usually demonstrated in thick peripheral blood smears. Urgent treatment with intravenous quinine or artemisin derivatives is required because of the high mortality.

Malaria is the most frequent parasitic disease in the tropics, with almost one-half of the population of the globe at risk for infection and more than 300 million persons infected. Africa alone has approximately 200 million cases of malaria, and more than 1 million children die every year in sub-Saharan Africa from complicated malaria. Malaria is endemic in tropical regions of the Americas, Africa, Asia, and subtropical areas of the Eastern Mediterranean. Malaria may even be acquired by mosquito bites during brief stops in airports ("runway malaria"). Malaria prophylaxis is mandatory for travelers and tourists to endemic areas. Arthropod-borne inoculation of viruses (dengue, yellow fever, Japanese encephalitis) or parasites (malaria, trypanosomiasis) is favored in the tropics by poor housing conditions and lack of control of the vector population.

Afebrile patients in the tropics with confusion, delirium, decreased level of consciousness (stupor or coma), and without focal neurologic findings may be suffering from drug effects (including alcohol), neurotoxins (suicide attempts), head trauma, seizures in the postictal state, metabolic disturbances (diabetes, uremia), stroke, or hyperthermia.

Human rabies, usually transmitted by animal bites (most commonly dogs) must be included in the differential diagnosis. Typical features include prodromata of paresthesias in the limb where the bite occurred leading to excoriation by scratching as well as nonspecific systemic signs such as fatigue, headache, myalgias, chills, and sometimes fever. Furious rabies is characterized by hysterical or psychotic behavior, psychomotor agitation, panic attacks, hydrophobia, and aerophobia leading to laryngopharyngeal and inspiratory spasms followed by coma and death. In paralytic rabies (usually resulting from contact with infected bats), signs suggestive of ascending myeloneuropathy or Guillain-Barré syndrome may be present.

African trypanosomiasis (sleeping sickness), caused by *Trypanosoma brucei,* is widely distributed in sub-Saharan Africa, where approximately 40 million people are at risk of infection. In the chronic stage African trypanosomiasis is characterized by progressive neurologic dysfunction with behavioral changes; pyramidal, extrapyramidal and cerebellar signs; cranial nerve involvement; cerebellar ataxia; and generalized and partial seizures.

American trypanosomiasis (Chagas' disease), caused by *Trypanosoma cruzi,* is a zoonotic disease prevalent in rural areas of Central and South America. Most cases of acute Chagas' disease occur in children and may be accompanied by manifestations of meningoencephalitis with drowsiness, irritability, focal neurologic signs, and seizures. The chronic form is primarily a cardiac and gastrointestinal disease producing cardiac dilatation and arrhythmias. Brain involvement is usually the result of embolism, often accompanied by focal or generalized seizures.

Meningitis

Patients with meningitis have severe headache and are delirious and febrile; examination discloses the presence of neck stiffness and meningeal signs (Kernig's and Brudzinski's). A high degree of suspicion is mandatory for the early diagnosis of meningitis by means of spinal tap. In sub-Saharan Africa epidemics of meningitis caused by meningococcus are common. Effective vaccination is available. Other forms include pneumococcal infection in patients with sickle cell disease, *Haemophilus influenzae* meningitis, other bacterial meningitides, and tuberculous meningitis. Swimming in freshwater ponds may result in amebic meningitis as a result of invasion via the cribriform plate of organisms of the genus *Naegleria*. Meningitis may occur with larva migrans, caused by infection with intestinal parasites of dogs (*Toxocara canis*) or cats (*Toxocara cati*). Seizures and rare focal neurologic signs may occur. Distomatosis, caused by *Fasciola hepatica* infection resulting from consumption of contaminated watercress, may produce meningitis. Eosinophilic meningitis is endemic in Southeast Asia (Thailand, Indonesia, Taiwan), the South Pacific islands, and Hawaii. Infection is caused by consumption of snails, slugs, and freshwater prawns contaminated with the larvae of *Angiostrongylus cantonensis*. Meningitis, with radicular symptoms and cranial nerve involvement, is frequent. In the same geographic areas, consumption of fish contaminated with *Gnathostoma spinigerum* may lead to a similar syndrome with extreme pain produced by the migrating larvae.

Encephalopathy with Focal Signs (Intracranial Space-Occupying Lesions)

Other than tumors, trauma, and intracranial hemorrhage, a number of neurologic infections commonly observed in the tropics present with symptoms suggestive of an intracranial tumor. These include tuberculoma, brain abscess (bacterial, fungal, and amebic), herpes simplex encephalitis, and several parasitic infections. Migration of adult or larval parasites into the nervous system produces signs of encephalopathy, increased intracranial pressure, and focal neurologic signs, including seizures. Parasites may invade the human host by oral ingestion of larvae or eggs, such as in the case of the tapeworms, some filariae such as dracunculosis (*Dracunculus medinensis*), and most intestinal parasites.

Computed tomographic (CT) images of the brain provide important etiologic information regarding parasitic infections: a single voluminous cyst is most likely caused by hydatidosis (*Taenia echinococcus*); multiple small cysts usually are caused by neurocysticercosis (although giant cysts or intraventricular cysts are not rare); thin-walled cysts resembling a soap-bubble are usually caused by paragonimiasis (*Paragonimus westermani, Paragonimus ringeri*). Multiple contrast-enhancing lesions may be caused by bilharziasis (*Schistosoma japonicum*), filariasis, or toxoplasmosis (*Toxoplasma gondii*). Toxoplasmosis has become one of the most common opportunistic infections of the nervous system in patients with acquired immunodeficiency syndrome.

Schistosoma japonicum in Southeast Asia is responsible for most cases of cerebral schistosomiasis and usually presents with seizures. Acute schistosomiasis (Katayama's fever) may produce an encephalopathy with coma, papilledema, focal neurologic signs, and seizures. A chronic form may be caused by embolization of schistosoma eggs to the brain, most commonly manifested by partial seizures.

Paragonimiasis is one of the most common parasitoses in the Far East (China, Korea), Southeast Asia, and some parts of Africa and South America. Human infection occurs by eating contaminated raw or undercooked crabs or crayfish. Primary lesions occur in the lungs, leading to hemoptysis. Sputum examination reveals typical parasite eggs. Worms penetrate through the foramina at the base of the skull and continue to migrate inside the brain.

Cerebral sparganosis, caused by the migrating larvae of various cestodes (*Diphyllobothrium, Spirometra*) is also manifested frequently by focal motor seizures. Sparganosis is endemic in Asia (China, Japan, Korea, and Southeast Asia), where it is acquired by drinking water contaminated with cyclops harboring larvae; by eating infected fish, frogs, or snakes; and by the local practice of applying poultices of frog flesh to a wound or to the eye.

Acute-Onset Flaccid Paralysis

When spinal cord compression or myelitis is suspected, urgent magnetic resonance imaging (MRI) of the spinal cord should be performed. In places where this is not available, a contrast myelogram should be done. The differential diagnosis of acute myelopathy includes a number of inflammatory and vascular conditions, but in adults in the tropics the most common cause is bilharziasis resulting from spinal cord involvement by *Schistosoma haematobium* in Africa and the Middle East, or by *Schistosoma mansoni* in the Caribbean, Venezuela, and Brazil. Bilharziasis or schistosomiasis is a major health problem in the tropics. Some 600 million people in 79 endemic countries are estimated to be at risk. MRI scans confirm the presence of hyperintense lesions caused by the presence of the parasite in the region of the conus medullaris. Bilharzial infection occurs when the host is swimming and there is active perforation of the skin by the parasites and invasion of the bloodstream.

In children with evidence of spinal cord transection evolving over a period of hours or days, usually with back pain, the most common cause is *acute transverse myelitis,* often occurring after a viral infection or vaccination. The diagnosis remains one of exclusion. Corticosteroid treatment is recommended. Bat bites may cause rabies, usually presenting as a transverse myelitis

Multiple sclerosis is considered a rare disease in the tropics. However, a number of documented cases have been reported from Africa and Latin America. Devic's disease (neuromyelitis optica), which is characterized by the simultaneous occurrence of bilateral optic neuritis and transverse myelitis, is considered a form of multiple sclerosis observed more commonly in Asia (India, Japan) and the Caribbean. The clinical similarity with subacute myelo-optic neuropathy caused by clioquinol, led to the possible association of this clinical form with the use of herbal teas in the Caribbean, probably because of toxic effects from halogenated quinolines present in plants of the Annonaceae family.

With the decline of poliomyelitis as a cause of acute flaccid paralysis, the Guillain-Barré syndrome (GBS) is rapidly becoming the most frequent cause of acute paralysis in children in the tropics. The incidence of GBS in the tropics appears to be higher than in industrialized countries. In Central America, poisoning with *Karwinskia calderoni* and *Karwinskia humboldtiana* resembles GBS. Clusters of GBS cases have occurred in association with swine-flu vaccination, poliomyelitis vaccination, and after postexposure rabies vaccination in Latin America, India, and Thailand. Causal agents invoked in GBS include cytomegalovirus, Epstein-Barr virus, the human immunodeficiency virus, dengue virus, varicella-zoster, measles virus, and *Mycoplasma pneumoniae*. In the tropics, rabies may present as an ascending or descending paralysis and the typical hydrophobia and aerophobia may be mistaken for bulbar and respiratory paralysis. A seasonal syndrome resembling GBS has been observed in China. Clinically this is a pure motor axonopathy, probably associated with infection with *Campylobacter* organisms. Changes similar to those observed neuropathologically in China have also been noted in patients from Mexico, Colombia, and Cuba.

Other conditions include botulism, elapid snake envenoming, and epidemic paralysis from consumption of gossypol, a phenolic compound present in cottonseed oil causing renal loss of potassium. Licorice (*Glycyrrhiza glabra*) may produce a similar picture.

Tropical Spastic Paraparesis

The most common cause of late-onset spastic paraplegia in the tropics is infection with HTLV-I. Onset is insidious, with leg stiffness and cramps. Increased urinary frequency, severe constipation, impotence in males, proximal weakness of the legs and problem walking occur. The spinal fluid is usually normal, with monoclonal bands caused by high-titers of anti-HTLV-I antibodies. Clinical forms resembling amyotrophic lateral sclerosis (pseudo-ALS) have been observed in patients infected with HTLV-I. Muscle wasting and fasciculations are present, involving distal muscles of the hands, shoulders, and tongue. These cases occur in areas of HTLV-I endemia in Japan and the Caribbean. Konzo, a form of acute-onset spastic paraplegia occurring in African children who survive on a diet of cassava, appears to be caused by excessive cyanide consumption and poor dietary intake of sulfur-containing amino acids.

Peripheral Neuropathies

Peripheral neuropathies are relatively common in the tropics and include a number of inflammatory and postinfectious conditions as well as toxic conditions, diabetes, genetic forms, alcoholism, and a common group of nutritional neuropathies caused by deficiencies of micronutrients (Table 46-3).

Leprosy is one of the most frequent causes of neuropathy in the world. Leprosy occurs throughout the tropics and subtropics, including Southeast Asia, Africa, Central and South America, the western

Pacific, the eastern Mediterranean, Japan, Korea, China, Hawaii, and the southern United States (Florida and Louisiana).

The group of nutritional neuropathies includes axonal neuropathies such as beriberi, caused by a thiamine deficiency, and subacute combined degeneration, caused by a cyanocobalamin deficiency. Specific vitamin deficits seldom occur, since most instances of human malnutrition are usually the result of an overall dietary deficiency. Tropical malabsorption plays a significant role by decreasing the availability of vitamins. Nutritional neuropathies may occur as epidemic outbreaks or as problems endemic to a particular geographic area. Precipitating factors include pregnancy and lactation, infections such as malaria and diarrhea, and increased metabolic requirements for thiamine resulting from increased carbohydrate intake and intense physical activity under hot and humid weather conditions. A toxic-nutritional component is present in alcoholic neuropathy, in tobacco-alcohol amblyopia, and in association with consumption of cyanide-producing tropical foodstuffs such as cassava.

Neurologic signs occur relatively late, when the combination of factors finally leads to deficiency of essential nutrients severe enough to injure the nervous system or when protective nutrients, such as sulfur-containing amino acids and antioxidant carotenoids (e.g., lycopene), become unavailable. The most sensitive elements (dorsal root ganglia, large myelinated distal axons, bipolar retinal neurons, cochlear neurons) are the first to suffer damage and manifest symptoms earliest. In various combinations this results in Strachan's syndrome, which is characterized by orogenital dermatitis, painful sensory neuropathy, amblyopia, and deafness. Strachan's syndrome was first reported in Jamaica, in malnourished populations in Africa, and among prisoners of war in tropical camps during World War II under conditions of dietary restriction, and it has been observed in Cuba in more than 50,000 patients. Clinical manifestations included retrobulbar optic neuropathy, sensorineural deafness, predominantly sensory and autonomic neuropathy, and dorsolateral myelopathy. Neurologic symptoms were preceded by weight loss, anorexia, chronic fatigue, lack of energy, irritability, sleep disturbances, and difficulties with concentration and memory. Political and economic conditions leading

Table 46-3. Peripheral Neuropathies and Myopathies in the Tropics

Inflammatory and postinfectious neuropathies	Amyloidosis
Leprosy	Uremia
Guillain-Barré syndrome	Sarcoidosis
Acute demyelinating neuropathy	Myxedema
Acute motor axonal neuropathy (Chinese paralytic	Connective tissue diseases
syndrome)	Acute intermittent porphyria
Post-rabies vaccine paralysis	Critical illness neuropathy
Other postinfectious neuropathies	Nutritional neuropathy
Neuropathies of infectious diseases	Beriberi and other B-group vitamin deficiencies
Campylobacter jejuni	Strachan's syndrome
Rabies	Tropical malabsorption-malnutrition
Diphtheria	Alcoholic neuropathy
Mycoplasma	Other causes
Lyme borreliosis (Bannwarth's syndrome)	Trauma, neoplasia, genetic neuropathies
Human immunodeficiency virus (acquired immuno-	Disorders of neuromuscular transmission
deficiency syndrome)	Myasthenia gravis
Human T-cell lymphotrophic virus types I/II	Botulism
Toxic neuropathies	Animal poisons
Heavy metals	Neurotoxic snake bite
Arsenic	Marine neurotoxins
Lead	Dart-poison frogs (South America)
Thallium	Tick-bite paralysis
Insecticides	Plant poisons
Organophosphorous esters	Curare
Plant poisons	Insecticide intoxication (intermediate syndrome)
Manihot (cassava)	Disorders of muscle
Karwinskia humboldtiana	Polymyositis (idiopathic inflammatory myopathy)
Gloriosa superba	Human T-cell lymphotrophic virus type I-associated
Podophyllum peltatum	polymyositis and myopathies
Animal poisons	Trichinosis
Ciguatoxin	Familial hypokalemic and hyperkalemic periodic
Paralytic shellfish poisoning (saxitoxin)	paralyses
Tick-bite paralysis	Cottonseed oil (epidemic hypokalemic paralysis),
Systemic diseases	licorice
Diabetes mellitus	

Source: Reprinted with permission from GC Román. Tropical Neuropathies. Baillières Clin Neurol 1995;4:469.

to severe limitations of food availability resulted in the epidemic in Cuba.

Toxic neuropathies are caused by a large number of products used in industry, agriculture, and medicine that selectively affect the peripheral nerves. In the tropics, widespread and indiscriminate use of toxic pesticides (including those that are banned in industrial countries); lack of education on their proper handling and storage; and predisposing factors such as malnutrition, infection, and genetic susceptibility increase the problem. Furthermore, in the tropics a large number of natural neurotoxins of plant or animal origin may induce toxic neuropathies or induce alterations of the neuromuscular transmission.

Among the heavy metal compounds causing peripheral neuropathy, the most common are arsenic, lead, and thallium. The most common pharmacologic products responsible for peripheral neuropathies in the tropics include isoniazid and ethambutol, sulfonamides, nitrofurantoin, chloramphenicol, metronidazole, chloroquine, clioquinol, dapsone, and aromatic diamines used for the treatment of leishmaniasis and trypanosomiasis. Neurotoxic industrial agents include n-hexane, methyl-n-butyl ketone, carbon disulfide, acrylamide, and trichloroethylene. Tri-ortho-cresyl phosphate (TOCP) intoxication was the cause of the Jamaica ginger paralysis. Epidemics also occurred in

Morocco, Durban, Bombay, and Sri Lanka as a result of contamination or adulteration of food or cooking oils with mineral oil containing TOCP. The clinical picture is characterized by symmetric weakness and wasting of distal muscles of the upper extremities with claw-hand and wrist-drop, minimal sensory abnormalities, and pyramidal signs late in the course. Organophosphorous pesticides may produce a delayed, distal, central as well as peripheral axonopathy known as organophosphate-induced delayed neuropathy. Delayed neurotoxicity should be differentiated from the intermediate syndrome, a postsynaptic neuromuscular junction lesion occurring 2–3 days after poisoning. Ocular toxicity (Saku disease) has been reported with fenthion, dichlorovos, fenitrothion, malathion, parathion, and methyl-parathion.

Suggested Reading

Caparros-Lefebre D, Charpentier D, Joseph H, Strobel M, et al. High prevalence of SMON after use of tropical herbal medicine. Neurology 1997;48(Suppl 2):A95.

Commission on Tropical Diseases of the International League Against Epilepsy. Relationship between epilepsy and tropical diseases. Epilepsia 1994;35:89.

de Bittencourt PRM, Adamolekum B, Bharucha N, et al. Epilepsy in the tropics: I. Epidemiology, socioeconomic risk factors, and etiology. Epilepsia 1996;37:1121.

Del Brutto O, Sotelo J, Román GC. Therapy for neurocysticercosis: a reappraisal. Clin Infect Dis 1993;17:730.

Del Brutto O, Sotelo J, Román GC. Neurocysticercosis: A Clinical Handbook. Heereweg, The Netherlands: Swetz & Zeitlinger, 1998.

Román GC. An epidemic in Cuba of optic neuropathy, sensorineural deafness, peripheral neuropathy and dorsolateral myelopathy. J Neurol Sci 1994;127:11.

Román GC. Epidemic neuropathy in Cuba: a plea to end the United States economic embargo on a humanitarian basis. Neurology 1994;44:1784.

Román GC. Tropical Neurology. In WG Bradley, RB Daroff, GM Fenichel, CD Marsden (eds), Neurology in Clinical Practice (2nd ed). Boston: Butterworth–Heinemann, 1996;2103–2128.

Román GC. Neurology in Public Health. In R Detels, WW Holland, J McEwen, GS Omenn (eds), Oxford Textbook of Public Health (3rd ed). Oxford, UK: Oxford University Press, 1997;1195–1223.

Román GC. Tropical neuropathies. Baillière's Clin Neurol 1995;4:469.

Román GC, Spencer PS, Schoenberg BS. Tropical myeloneuropathies: the hidden endemias. Neurology 1985;35:1158.

Román GC, Vernant JC, Osame M. HTLV-I and the Nervous System. New York: Liss, 1989.

Senananyake N, Román GC. Aetiological factors of epilepsy in the tropics. J Trop Geogr Neurol 1991;1:69.

Shakir RA, Newman PK, Poser CM (eds). Tropical Neurology. London: Saunders, 1996.

Toro G, Román GC, Navarro de Román LI. Neurologia Tropical. Bogota: Printer, 1983.

World Health Organization Malaria Action Programme. Severe and complicated malaria. Trans R Soc Trop Med Hyg 1986;80(Suppl):1.

Chapter 47

Psychogenic and Conversion Disorders

Patrice Guex and Friedrich Stiefel

Chapter Plan

Interfaces between neurology and psychiatry
Psychogenic disorders
Conversion disorder
    Etiology
    Diagnosis
    Clinical presentation and differential diagnosis
    Predisposing factors
    Epidemiology
    Therapeutic approaches
    Outcome

Neurology and psychiatry have common grounds: They share a part of their history, a part of their clinical and scientific interests, and a part of their patients. In this chapter, the common grounds are briefly discussed, the clinical disorders that implicate the efforts of both disciplines are summarized, and psychogenic and conversion disorders are emphasized.

Interfaces Between Neurology and Psychiatry

Historically there was little distinction between psychiatry and neurology, and the overlapping clinical fields of the two disciplines have led in many countries of the Western world to mandatory training or examinations that cover topics of both disciplines. Recent achievements in the neurosciences and in biological psychiatry have again augmented the interfaces between the two disciplines, and there is an increased awareness that a number of disorders, even somatoform disorders, may have a common cause and present clinical features observed in both disciplines. Although there is common ground, the clinical and scientific interests and the diagnostic and therapeutic tools of neurologists and psychiatrists do differ. It is therefore consistent that frontiers between the two disciplines are delineated and that disorders such as conversion disorders are part of the psychiatric expertise.

A variety of neurologic disorders are associated with psychiatric symptoms. Frontal and temporal lobe tumors; systemic lupus erythematosus; temporal lobe epilepsy; hydrocephalus; and focal lesions from stroke, abscess, or infection can all demonstrate the clinical features of standard psychiatric disease. Many other neurologic diseases, such as multiple sclerosis, seizure disorder, Parkinson's disease, or Huntington's chorea, are often associated with psychiatric symptoms resulting from structural changes in the brain or the psychosocial impact these diseases have for the patient. In addition, there are many standard treatments in neurology, such as the use of corticosteroids, which may induce psychiatric symptoms. Any psychiatric symptom therefore must be followed by a careful medical and neurologic examination to rule out an organic disease.

Psychiatric disorders may also be associated with neurologic symptoms. Some psychiatric disor-

Table 47-1. Psychiatric Disorders That May
Resemble Neurologic Disorders

Somatoform disorders
    Undifferentiated somatoform disorder
    Conversion disorder
    Pain disorder
Factitious disorders
Dissociative disorders
    Dissociative amnesia
    Dissociative fugue
    Dissociative identity disorder
    Depersonalization disorder
Substance-related disorders
Medication-induced movement disorders
Acute stress disorder
Mood disorders

---

ders manifest with minor nonlocalizing neurologic abnormalities (e.g., schizophrenia) or with cognitive and neuropsychologic symptoms (e.g., depression). A few psychiatric disorders mimic neurologic disease and a considerable amount of testing may be needed before the diagnosis is established. These disorders are the topic of this chapter.

Although a single diagnosis sometimes explains the clinical observations, there are situations in which a psychiatric and a neurologic condition coexist. Patients with seizures may have intermittent psychogenic seizures, strokes occur in patients with anxiety disorders, and patients with a pre-existing personality disorder also develop brain tumors. It is understandable that in such situations, the psychological factors affect the medical condition and the medical factors affect the psychological condition. These combined disorders are certainly the most frequent situations seen in daily work and sometimes also demand the clinical efforts of both disciplines.

Psychogenic Disorders

Table 47-1 illustrates a selection of psychiatric disorders that may at times mimic a neurologic symptomatology. We have summarized and classified these disorders as "psychogenic disorders," although such a classification is not an official one. In contrast to conversion disorder, which often closely resembles a neurologic disorder, the psychiatric disorders listed in Table 47-1 rarely present as a pure

neurologic disorder. Some clinical features of psychogenic disorders are briefly reviewed in the following sections. It must be remembered that most of the disorders listed in Table 47-1 have not attracted much attention in the past; psychiatric patients with physical symptoms address their complaints to the wrong physicians, and it is therefore not astonishing that only recent developments, such as the high costs and inefficient care of this patient population, have helped to focus clinical and scientific interest on this borderline between medicine and psychiatry.

The clinical picture of an undifferentiated somatoform consists of one or more physical complaints of at least 6 months' duration that cannot be fully explained by a known medical or mental disorder and that cause significant distress or social or occupational impairments. In pain disorder, pain is the predominant focus of the clinical presentation. These two disorders may sometimes express a neurologic symptom or resemble pain of neurologic origin. The diagnosis of pain as an expression of pain disorder is very difficult to establish, and usually doubts about the accuracy of the diagnosis remain. Pain is never just a pure nociceptive, physical experience, but involves different dimensions of a person, such as personality, affect, cognition, behavior, and social relations, and is therefore best conceptualized within a complex, multidimensional model. This clinical experience has been supported over the last decades by many neuroanatomic and neurotransmitter studies showing direct relations between affect and pain perception. In factitious disorder, the symptoms are caused by an intentional production or feigning. The motivation for this behavior is to assume the sick role; some of these patients feign neurologic symptoms and are therefore admitted to neurology wards. Patients with factitious disorder do not have external incentives for the behavior. Dissociative amnesia is an inability to recall important personal information, usually of a traumatic or stressful nature. The disturbance is not caused by another psychiatric disturbance, the side effects of a substance, or a general medical condition. Such states of amnesia can mimic amnesia of neurologic origin. The same holds true for dissociative fugue (unexpected travel away with inability to recall one's past and a confusion about personal identity), dissociative identity disorder (at least two identities or personality states recurrently take control of the person's behavior), or depersonalization disorder, which may be mistaken for a neurologic disorder such as temporal lobe epilepsy or complex partial seizures. Substance-related disorders and medication-induced movement disorders may resemble gait and coordination problems, vertigo, Parkinson's disease, and other conditions of neurologic origin. Acute stress disorder and anxiety may mimic neurologic symptoms such as amnesia or tremor, and depression may be associated with cognitive deficits seen in neurologic diseases or dementia.

Although it is beyond the scope of this chapter to discuss each of these disorders, a few general remarks may be helpful to differentiate psychogenic from neurologic disease. As indicated in Table 47-2, we classify indicators in favor of a psychogenic origin of a disorder into factors from the patient's history and factors resulting from observation, examination, and investigation. A symptomatology that is physiologically not possible is usually regarded as a strong indicator of a psychogenic disorder or a psychogenic aggravation of a neurologic disease. However, a study found at least one feature of a nonphysiologic sensory examination in 29 of 30 neurology patients with documented central nervous system (CNS) injury, 25 of whom had acute strokes. It is our clinical experience that psychogenic disorders often coincide with neurologic illness. All the other factors listed in Table 47-2 may be of help in diagnosing psychogenic disorders, but they are less important and also observed in disorders with an organic origin.

The history of the patient may already contain some valuable clues in favor of a psychogenic disorder. If a psychiatric history is present, any of the disorders listed in Table 47-1 may be present, explaining the symptomatology, especially if the history reveals a coincidence between symptom occurrence and severe psychosocial stress. Patients with abrupt changes in behavior or personality, on the other hand, are more likely to suffer from organic disease. If the symptom has permitted the patient to avoid unpleasant situations or to receive increased attention or affection by the environment (secondary gain), a psychogenic disorder also may be considered. However, many patients with somatic diseases also have secondary gains, which cannot always be interpreted as pathologic phenomena. Whereas one single factor listed in Table 47-2 is not helpful in differentiation, an accumu-

Table 47-2. Clues That Suggest Psychogenic Disorders

Patient's history
    History of psychiatric illness or symptoms
    Temporal coincidences between symptom and psychosocial stressors
    Absence of abrupt changes in behavior or personality
    Secondary gain of the symptom
Observations, examination, and investigations
    Symptom is physiologically not possible
    Appropriate investigation fails to find an organic origin
    Inconsistencies in symptom expression
    Excessive attention seeking through symptom expression
    Unresponsiveness or aggravation under adequate and usually successful treatment

lation of different factors may suggest a psychogenic disorder and psychiatric consultation should be considered.

The failure of an appropriate investigation to find an organic origin of the symptomatology is in itself not a proof for but may complement the other indicators of psychogenic disorders. It has to be remembered that in some of the follow-up studies of patients with somatoform disorders, up to 30% suffered a serious medical illness a few years later. Unfortunately such studies were carried out decades ago, and the diagnostic tools and the likelihood for correctly diagnosing a puzzling neurologic disorder have increased since then. The observation of the patient when he or she is unaware or when he or she is concentrating on tasks during clinical examination sometimes reveals inconsistencies with symptoms presented at the beginning of the consultation. This may be another clue for differentiating psychogenic from organic disorders. In this context, it is important to remember that malingerers cannot be considered to be suffering from psychogenic disorders. These persons intentionally produce false or exaggerated symptoms and are motivated by external incentives such as duties or financial compensations. Malingering is suspected in cases of noncooperation during diagnostic evaluation and if symptoms subside completely when the patient obtains his or her goals. Patients with psychogenic disorders may also show an intentional production of symptoms (e.g., patients with factitious disorders), but external incentives for their behavior as mentioned above are absent. Malingering is in our personal experience extremely rare and such a suspicion is more often an expression of a negative attitude on the part of the treating physician toward patients with unexplained symptoms or disorders of psychogenic origin. Patients with psychogenic disorder often quite obviously seek attention through symptom expression; such a behavior can be very irritating for the treating physician and staff and explains the occurrence of negative attitudes toward the patient. Unresponsiveness or aggravation under adequate and usually successful treatment often occur in patients with psychogenic disorders. These patients often consciously or unconsciously "reject" a medication aimed at ameliorating the physical symptom. To repeat, such clues must be considered with great caution and they do not prove the presence of a psychogenic disorder.

Conversion Disorder

The name *conversion disorder* indicates the clinical observation that "inner" psychic conflicts are converted into bodily phenomena. In ancient medicine, hysterical phenomena were thought to be a consequence of the uterus migrating within the body; later these patients were thought to be possessed by the devil (medieval medicine) or suffering from a gynecologic (eighteenth century) or neurologic disease (nineteenth century). It was Freud and Breuer who first unmasked these phenomena as psychogenic. Conversion disorder was formerly named *hysteria, conversion syndrome,* or *conversion neurosis;* the word "hysteric/hysteria" now denominates patients with a specific personality disorder called *histrionic personality disorder.* These patients show a pattern of excessive emotionality and attention seeking and were thought to produce conversion symptoms. Meanwhile, it is well established that conversion disorder can be associated with histrionic personality disorder, but also with other concomitant psychiatric disorders and that patients with histrionic personality disorder do not necessarily have a conversion disorder.

Etiology

The etiology of conversion disorder is thought to be a consequence of a special way of dealing with psychologically conflictual situations. This development is always an unconscious process, but the patient may to some extent modulate the severity without having voluntary control over the symptom. A classic example to illustrate the mechanisms of conversion disorder is the case of a young man with a fluctuating weakness in the right arm without demonstrable organic causes and without a known physiologic mechanism. In subsequent psychotherapeutic sessions, the young man indicates that he recently married and that since then, a growing number of situations have resulted in arguments with his wife. In one such situation he reports that he nearly lost control and stopped short before hitting his wife. Later he recognizes that at that moment the weakness in his right arm occurred, and the weakness was later aggravated in situations when the patient felt intense anger toward his wife. The symptom of the conversion disorder illustrates the conflictual situation of the patient who would like to hit his wife and who simultaneously would like to resist his aggressive impulses. The context and the development of this symptom were first hidden from consciousness and the notion of a relationship between the psychic experiences and the bodily phenomenon was only slowly accessible and acceptable to the patient. A resolution of the symptom followed these insights, and therapy for the couple permitted the partners to verbalize their thoughts and feelings without resorting to bodily expressions.

Diagnosis

As discussed for the other psychogenic disorders, it is not possible to diagnose a conversion disorder with absolute certainty. The suspicion of a conversion disorder relies on the observation that a symptom is physiologically not possible; other factors in favor of a conversion disorder were discussed above and listed in Table 47-2. In addition to these factors, some specific factors may arise in the context of a conversion disorder. The observed symptom illustrates the conflictual situation; the patient may have observed other people with similar symptoms ("identification") and he or she is not too worried about the bodily condition ("la belle indifférence"). The symptom allows the patient to obtain a primary gain (unable to hit in the example above) and a secondary gain (decreased aggressiveness and increased affection by his wife). The symptom thus lessens intrapsychic anguish, called *primary gain*, and enables the patient to avoid difficult situations and obtain additional support, called *secondary gain*. These factors are sometimes difficult to establish or appear retrospectively during psychotherapy, and their absence does not exclude a conversion disorder. In such situations, amobarbital sodium infusion as a diagnostic test is advocated in the medical literature. Amobarbital is infused intravenously (100–500 mg over 10–30 minutes) while the physician tests the neurologic symptoms, noting their change or disappearance under the infusion. Although we have observed the emergence of interesting psychological material under amobarbital, we advocate such a procedure only in exceptional situations. Because the diagnosis per se of a psychogenic disorder is often not a matter of urgency and can usually be established without amobarbital infusion, the administration of amobarbital can be perceived by the patient as a sign of distrust and as a humiliating procedure that deteriorates the therapeutic relationship.

Clinical Presentation and Differential Diagnosis

Conversion disorder may mimic a variety of neurologic symptoms and diseases such as paralysis, aphonia, blindness, gait and coordination disturbances, vertigo, seizures, anesthesia, and others. Table 47-3 contains the diagnostic criteria of the *Diagnostic and Statistical Manual of Mental Disorders* (DSM-IV) for conversion disorder. These criteria illustrate that pain has been eliminated as a conversion symptom and is now classified as pain disorder and that conversion disorder has to be differentiated from other psychogenic disorders mentioned above. The criteria also illustrate that symptom expression is culturally bounded and a consequence of a learning experience. This fact explains that a rather vivid symptom expression can be within the range of normal behavior.

Predisposing Factors

Predisposing factors for the development of conversion disorders include a prior medical illness as the

Table 47-3. Diagnostic Criteria for Conversion Disorder

A. One or more symptoms or deficits affecting voluntary motor or sensory function that suggest a neurologic or other general medical condition.
B. Psychological factors are judged to be associated with the symptom or deficit because the initiation or exacerbation of the symptom or deficit is preceded by conflicts or other stressors.
C. The symptom or deficit is not intentionally produced or feigned (as in factitious disorder or malingering).
D. The symptom or deficit cannot, after appropriate investigation, be fully explained by a general medical condition or by the direct effects of a substance or as a culturally sanctioned behavior or experience.
E. The symptom or deficit causes clinically significant distress or impairment in social, occupational, or other important areas of functioning or warrants medical evaluation.
F. The symptom or deficit is not limited to pain or sexual dysfunction, does not occur exclusively during the course of somatization disorder, and is not better accounted for by another mental disorder.

source of the symptom, exposure to other patients with conversion disorders (identification), a preexisting psychopathologic state such as a personality disorder (histrionic, passive-dependent, and passive-aggressive) or depression and schizophrenia, and the presence of a psychosocial stressor. Conversion disorder is also frequently observed in patients with CNS organicity, intellectual deficits, and mental retardation. In general, conversion is a rather immature mode of facing psychosocial stress.

Epidemiology

Although conversion disorder is a rare diagnosis in neurology, it is the source of frequent requests for psychiatric consultation in the general hospital. It has been noted that between 5% and 14% of patients who undergo a psychiatric consultation in a general hospital have experienced a conversion. Conversion disorder is observed two to five times more often in women than in men and is more frequent in adolescents and young adults, persons in lower socioeconomic groups and rural populations, and persons with lower educational levels. It is important to stress that the incidence of conversion disorder is also influenced by social and cultural factors. The incidence has decreased in patients from western Europe over the last decades, although it is still frequently observed in patients from Mediterranean countries and from southern Europe. It is suspected that an increased knowledge about these phenomena in the general population and an increased intellectualization of the society is responsible for this development. Patients with a disposition for conversion disorder in these societies probably now regress to lower levels of defense, such as somatization disorder or pain disorder, or they show more subtle manifestations, such as complex and slowly responding medical conditions, which are not diagnosed as conversion disorder and are "accepted" within medicine and the general population and therefore not the object of disrespect.

Therapeutic Approaches

Spontaneous remission of conversion disorder is common and many patients are never hospitalized or evaluated by a specialist. For some of the hospitalized patients, the change in environment and the supportive setting of a medical unit is sufficient for the resolution of the symptom. For others, a psychiatric consultation is indicated. It is important to stress that the way a psychiatric consultation is introduced to the patient is crucial for the further development of the disorder. It is counterproductive to let the patient know that "it's all in your head" and that he or she should therefore accept psychiatric help. Such an approach usually induces an aggravation of the symptom and a refusal of the patients to comply with the psychiatrist. A more beneficial way of introducing psychiatric help is to tell the patient that a physical symptom is always associated with and aggravated by psychosocial stress and that a mental health specialist can possibly help to find a more comprehensive way of treating the condition. Continuation of physical therapy during psychotherapy is often commendable to help the patient to find an "honorable way out of the symptom." If frustration and anger about patients "who are faking their symptoms" arises in the staff, psychiatric liaison and instruction of the team is beneficial before negative reactions toward the patient occur. A psychiatrist can inform the team on how conversion disorder is understood and how these patients differ from

malingerers. This is also an occasion to instruct the team that support, attention, and care should be given to the patient regularly and not only in moments when the symptoms are accentuated.

Outcome

Studies assessing patients with conversion disorder other than pseudoseizures have found that the outcome was favorable in patients younger than age 40 years who already improved during hospitalization. It is also known that favorable outcome is related to an acute onset of conversion disorder, the presence of a stressful but resolvable conflict, a good premorbid level of psychological functioning, and the absence of concomitant somatic or psychiatric disorders. In almost one-half of the patients who were followed, positive reassurance and exercises alone were beneficial for improvement, and only a few patients suffered from an organic deficit that may have been related to the initial episode. The incidence of false-positive diagnoses for conversion disorder is much lower than in prior reports indicating up to 30%; this may be because of the improvement of diagnostic possibilities over the last decades and the exclusion of patients with pseudoseizures and known organic disease.

Although the resolution of the conversion symptom may occur quite commonly during hospitalization, less is known about the long-term outcome. Psychiatrists are often confronted with patients with chronification, recurrence of symptoms during stressful life events, and changes to other forms of somatization. It is obvious that the outcome depends on the selection of the population that is followed, and general remarks such as "spontaneous remission is common and outcome usually favorable" do not take into account the existence of those patients who end up with a disability or with another form of psychogenic disorder. It may therefore be wise to request a psychiatric consultation before discharging a patient who has only slightly improved during hospitalization.

Suggested Reading

Cassem NH, Barsky AJ. Functional Somatic Symptoms and Somatoform Disorders. In NH Cassem (ed), Handbook of General Hospital Psychiatry (3rd ed). St. Louis: Mosby-Year Book, 1991;131–157.

Couprie W, Wijdicks EFM, Rooijmans HGM, et al. Outcome in conversion disorder: a follow up study. J Neurol Neurosurg Psychiatry 1995;58:750.

Cumston CG. An Introduction to the History of Medicine. New York: Dorset, 1987;299–302.

Diagnostic and Statistical Manual of Mental Disorders (4th ed). Washington, DC: American Psychiatric Association 1994;221–222.

Ford CV, Folks DG. Conversion disorders: an overview. Psychosomatics 1985;26:371.

Freud S. Hysterie und Angst. Studienausgabe, Band IV. Frankfurt: Fischer Verlag Taschenbuchverlag, 1982.

Fricchione G, Weilburg JB, Murray GB. Neurology and Neurosurgery. In JR Rundell, G Wise (eds), Textbook of Consultation-Liaison Psychiatry. Washington, DC: American Psychiatric Press, 1996;697–719.

Gould R, Miller BL, Goldberg MA, et al. The validity of hysterical signs and symptoms. J Nerv Ment Dis 1986; 174:593.

Hollander E, Neville D, Frenkel M, et al. Dysmorphic disorder—diagnostic issues and related disorders. Psychosomatics 1992;33:156.

James L, Singer A, Zurynski Y, et al. Evoked response potentials and regional cerebral blood flow in somatization disorder. Psychother Psychosom 1987;47:190.

Lazare A. Conversion symptoms. N Engl J Med 1981; 305:745.

Lipowski ZJ. Somatization: a borderland between medicine and psychiatry. Can Med Assoc J 1986;135:609.

Penman MF. When neurological symptoms are not what they appear: the challenge of caring for patients with conversion disorders. Axon 1993;15:19.

Perry CP, Jacobs D. Clinical applications of the amytal interview in psychiatric emergency settings. Am J Psychiatry 1982;109:889.

Rochford JM, Detre T, Tucker GJ, Harrow M, et al. Neuropsychological impairments in functional psychiatric disease. Arch Gen Psychiatry 1970;22:114.

Slater ETO, Glithero E. A follow-up of patients diagnosed as suffering from "hysteria." J Psychosom Res 1965;9:9.

Stiefel F. Psychosocial aspects of cancer pain. Support Care Cancer 1993;1:130.

Strub RL, Black FW. Other Neurobehavioral Syndromes and Neurologic Aspects of Psychiatric Disease. In RL Straub, FW Black (eds), Neurobehavioral Disorders—A Clinical Approach. Philadelphia: Davis, 1988; 469–471.

Tucker GJ, Neppe VM. Neurology and psychiatry. Gen Hosp Psychiatry 1988;10:24.

Wise MG, Rundell JR. Consultation Psychiatry. Washington DC: American Psychiatric Association, 1994;101.

Chapter 48
Neurologic Disorders of Pregnancy

Catherine Lamy and Jean-Louis Mas

Chapter Plan

It is not uncommon to encounter a variety of neurologic diseases in patients during their reproductive years. Many neurologic disorders, such as stroke or peripheral neuropathies, can develop in a pregnant patient. In addition, the pregnant state can affect numerous pre-existing neurologic conditions, including epilepsy, multiple sclerosis (MS), myasthenia gravis, muscle diseases, headaches, and brain tumors. Diseases of the nervous system can also have adverse effects on the mother, fetus, and newborn. The extent to which each disease may affect the course of pregnancy and the degree to which a given pregnancy may affect the relative stability of the disorder are concerns shared by every prospective mother and the physicians (obstetrician and neurologist) who care for her. This chapter presents a selective review of the most common neurologic problems that may be seen during pregnancy.

Stroke

Although it accounts for 4–11% of all maternal deaths, cerebral vascular disease in pregnancy and the puerperium remains poorly understood.

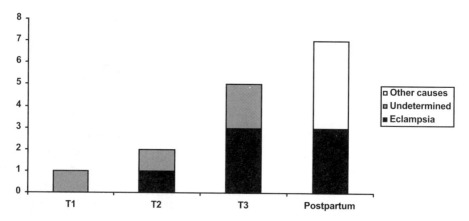

Figure 48-1. "Ile de France" study. Gestational age at the time of arterial ischemic stroke according to the main etiologic subgroups. T1: first trimester of pregnancy; T2: second trimester of pregnancy; T3: third trimester of pregnancy. Other causes were protein S deficiency, confirmed after pregnancy ($n = 1$), extracranial vertebral artery dissection ($n = 1$), postpartum angiopathy ($n = 1$), amniotic fluid embolism associated with disseminated intravascular coagulation ($n = 1$).

Arterial Ischemic Stroke

The incidence of arterial cerebral ischemic strokes varies from 3.8 to 11 per 100,000 deliveries. Figure 48-1 shows that ischemic strokes do not occur evenly throughout gestation; most of them occur during postpartum or the third trimester of pregnancy. In one study, the postpartum state (relative risk: 8.7; 95% confidence interval, 4.6–16.7) but not pregnancy itself (relative risk: 0.7; 95% confidence interval, 0.3–1.6), was associated with an increased risk of cerebral infarction.

The causes of ischemic strokes can be divided into pregnancy-specific causes and non–pregnancy-specific causes. Their relative frequency is poorly known. Only three conditions are actually specific for pregnancy: eclampsia, amniotic fluid embolism, and choriocarcinoma. The classic neurologic features of the pre-eclamptic–eclamptic syndrome include headaches, visual abnormalities, impairment of consciousness, and seizures. In addition, some patients have focal deficits of sudden onset consistent with a clinical diagnosis of stroke. The precise pathogenesis of these strokelike focal deficits is not fully understood. A minority of women have persisting neurologic deficits and neuroradiologic abnormalities suggesting brain infarction. In some of these patients, vasospasm has been demonstrated on angiograms, and one proposed mechanism for cerebral infarction is hypertension-induced vaso-

constriction causing ischemia. In most cases, however, the reversibility of the neurologic clinical signs and neuroradiologic lesions (Figure 48-2) within a few days or weeks strongly argues against the existence of true cerebral ischemic necrosis. The clinical and neuroimaging findings are more consistent with cerebral vasogenic edema, which is thought to result from the vasomotor disturbances of hypertension. According to the prevailing theory, the rapid increase in blood pressure induces a loss of autoregulation, which leads to arteriolar dilation, opening of tight junctions, and vasogenic edema. The precise mechanism, however, remains uncertain and other causes of altered vascular reactivity, such as sympathetic overactivity and endothelial cell dysfunction, have been reported in eclampsia.

The two other pregnancy-specific causes, *choriocarcinoma* and *amniotic fluid embolism*, are rarely responsible for focal cerebral ischemia. *Postpartum angiopathy* is characterized by the rapid occurrence of severe headaches, nausea or vomiting, seizures, and, less often, neurologic signs shortly after a normal pregnancy. This picture may suggest the diagnosis of subarachnoid hemorrhage, but computed tomographic (CT) scans and the cerebrospinal fluid usually appear normal. Cerebral angiography shows multiple segmental narrowings of the arteries arising from the circle of Willis, which resolve within a few weeks. Rapid spontaneous clinical recovery occurs in the vast majority of cases. The etiology is unknown,

Figure 48-2. Postpartum eclampsia. Left upper limb paresis of sudden onset (at 72 hours postpartum) disappearing within 48 hours. (A) Magnetic resonance imaging (MRI) scan, axial T2-weighted sequences (TR 2,000, TE 100). High-intensity signal in the cortex and white matter.

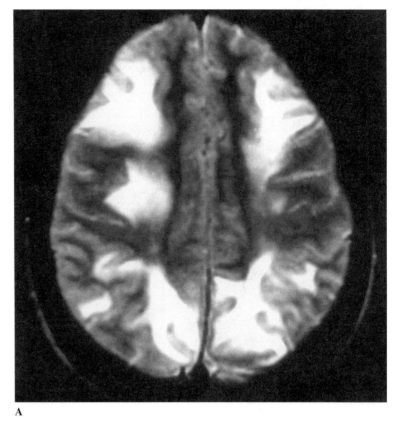

A

but a vasomotor response secondary to various stimuli has been suggested. Several cases have been associated with use of ergot alkaloids during labor. A similar syndrome has been reported outside of pregnancy under various nosologies. *Peripartum cardiomyopathy* refers to a rare dilated cardiomyopathy presenting with signs of cardiac failure in the last month of pregnancy or within a few months after delivery in the absence of pre-existing heart disease. Stroke occurs in approximately 5% of the cases and may be the initial manifestation of the disease. It usually results from cardioembolism and more rarely from cerebral hypoperfusion secondary to cardiac failure. Heart size returns to normal in more than one-half of the patients, but recurrences may arise with subsequent pregnancies. It is unclear whether this syndrome is pregnancy-specific or merely unmasked by gestational physiologic stresses. Most of the known causes of ischemic stroke in the young have been reported during pregnancy (Table 48-1). In most of these conditions, it is uncertain whether pregnancy is coincidental or plays a role in the occurrence of stroke.

In approximately 25% of patients, the cause of the stroke remains undetermined despite an extensive etiologic workup. The high relative risk of stroke during the postpartum period suggests a causal role for the rapid changes in hormonal status that follow a live birth or a stillbirth, perhaps by means of hemodynamic, coagulative, or vessel-wall changes.

Overall, the management of an acute ischemic stroke should not differ between pregnant and nonpregnant women. Usual symptomatic measures are needed when the stroke is severe. They include low-dose heparin therapy to prevent venous thromboembolic phenomena, hemodynamic monitoring with avoidance of any acute blood pressure change that could have adverse maternal and fetal effects, and prevention of secondary complications of stroke such as bronchopneumonia. Mannitol may be used postpartum to lower intracranial pressure but should be avoided antepartum because of the change in fetal plasma osmolality and subsequent dehydration.

When anticoagulation is indicated during pregnancy, standard or low-molecular weight heparin is

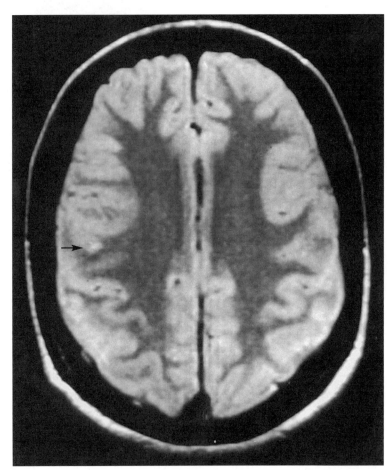

Figure 48-2. *Continued.* (B) Disappearance of the diffuse abnormalities on the control MRI scan (3 months later). Persistence of a nodular hypersignal at the junction of the cortex and white matter (*arrow*).

B

the preferred anticoagulant because, as a large molecule, it does not cross the placenta and its short half-life makes dose adjustment easier in case of overdose, bleeding, or premature delivery. Oral anticoagulation should be avoided between 7 and 12 weeks of gestation because of the risk of warfarin embryopathy and after 36 weeks because of the risk of serious perinatal bleeding caused by the trauma of delivery to the anticoagulated fetus.

Low-dose aspirin (60–150 mg per day) has been largely administered by obstetricians during the second and third trimesters of pregnancy in women at risk for pregnancy-induced hypertension without evidence of fetal or maternal adverse effects. Based on this evidence, low doses of aspirin can be used safely during the second and third trimesters of pregnancy; however, its safety during the first trimester remains controversial.

The risk of stroke recurrence in subsequent pregnancies is unknown but appears to be low, as judged by the paucity of reports. The occurrence of a pregnancy-related stroke does not contraindicate a subsequent pregnancy. The decision depends on the cause of the stroke, the residual deficit, and the desire for pregnancy. Subsequent use of oral contraception should probably be avoided in the majority of cases.

Cerebral Venous Thrombosis

The incidence of cerebral venous thrombosis (CVT) during pregnancy or the puerperium remains uncertain. Epidemiologic studies are difficult to perform because CVT may have a misleading presentation and a definite diagnosis requires angiography, magnetic resonance imaging (MRI), or autopsy. In Western Europe and North America, incidence rates ranging from 2 to 60 per 100,000 deliveries have been reported. In these countries, the pregnant and puerperal states account for 5–20% of all CVTs. In contrast, in India, the incidence of CVT is estimated at 200 to 500 per 100,000 deliveries, and in a recent Mexican study, the puerperal state accounted for 60% of all CVTs.

A clear relationship between CVT and the puerperium has long been recognized, with the majority of cases occurring in the second week postpartum. Traumatic damage to the endothelial lining of cerebral sinuses and veins during labor, a hypercoagulable state, and blood stasis are the most likely explanations for the occurrence of most CVTs in the puerperium. Puerperal infections and dehydration may contribute to the high frequency of CVTs in developing countries. CVTs in pregnancy or the puerperium have also been related to various causes (see Table 48-1), stressing the need for an etiologic workup, particularly when a CVT occurs during pregnancy.

The current mortality rate in Western countries with modern methods of diagnosis and the spreading use of anticoagulation is unknown but may be less than 5%. Recurrence of CVT in a subsequent pregnancy has been reported. The exact risk is unknown but is probably low as judged by the paucity of reports. Prophylactic treatment with low-dose heparin beginning after delivery and lasting for the first postpartum weeks can be recommended in subsequent pregnancies. This attitude could be extended to women who had a CVT outside of pregnancy or other risk factors for venous thrombosis.

Nontraumatic Subarachnoid Hemorrhage

Nontraumatic subarachnoid hemorrhages may account for 5–10% of all maternal deaths in pregnancy. As in the nonpregnant state, the most common cause is rupture of a vascular malformation. Other causes include eclampsia and various rare conditions (see Table 48-1).

The classic notion that rupture of an arterial aneurysm occurs more frequently during labor has not been confirmed. In a retrospective review of 114 patients with verified ruptured arterial aneurysms, only two sustained a hemorrhage during labor or

Table 48-1. Main Causes of Stroke Reported During Pregnancy or the Puerperium

Arterial ischemic strokes
  Cardioembolic disorders
    Rheumatic heart disease, prosthetic heart valves
    Atrial fibrillation
    Bacterial and nonbacterial endocarditis
    Peripartum cardiomyopathy
    Mitral valve prolapse
    Paradoxical embolus
  Cerebral angiopathies
    Atherosclerosis
    Arterial dissection
    Fibromuscular dysplasia
    Cerebral vasculitis: systemic lupus erythematosus, Takayasu's disease, periarteritis nodosa, isolated angiitis of the brain
    Postpartum cerebral angiopathy
  Hematologic disorders
    Sickle cell anemia
    Sneddon's syndrome
    Antiphospholipid antibodies
    Thrombotic thrombocythemic purpura
    Homocystinuria
    Antithrombin III, protein C, protein S deficiencies
    Disseminated intravascular coagulation
  Other causes
    Eclampsia
    Choriocarcinoma
    Amniotic fluid embolism, air embolism, fat embolism
    Drug abuse
    Sheehan's syndrome
Cerebral venous thrombosis
  Antithrombin III, protein S, protein C deficiencies
  Eclampsia
  Sickle cell disease
  Paroxysmal nocturnal hemoglobinuria
  Homocystinuria
Intracranial hemorrhages
  Arterial aneurysm
  Arteriovenous malformation
  Eclampsia
  Cerebral venous thrombosis
  Choriocarcinoma
  Bacterial endocarditis
  Drug abuse
  Disseminated intravascular coagulation
  Moyamoya disease
  Hematologic disorders
  Tumor
  Ruptured spinal cord vascular malformation
  Arterial hypertension

delivery. Although this is a controversial issue, the increased tendency of an aneurysm to bleed with advancing gestational age suggests that hemodynamic, hormonal, or other physiologic changes of pregnancy may play a role in aneurysmal rupture.

Most authors agree that surgical management after subarachnoid hemorrhage in pregnancy should be the same as that for the nonpregnant state. Clipping has been successfully achieved during all stages of pregnancy. In the review of Dias and Sekhar, surgical management was associated with lower maternal and fetal mortality. No data are available concerning endovascular treatments during pregnancy. The method of delivery should be based on obstetrical considerations.

Intracerebral Hemorrhage

The risk of intracerebral hemorrhage during pregnancy varies from 4.6 to 9.0 per 100,000 deliveries and may be five to six times higher than in nonpregnant women. As with cerebral infarctions, the postpartum state but not pregnancy itself seems to be associated with an increased risk of intracerebral hemorrhage.

Ruptured vascular malformations and eclampsia are the most common causes of intracerebral hemorrhage. These causes accounted for 40–80% of all intracerebral hemorrhages in two studies. Cerebral hemorrhage is a common finding in women dying of eclampsia, and it is generally agreed that hemorrhage is a result of severe hypertension, although coagulation disorders associated with eclampsia may also play a role. Hemorrhages range from multiple cortical petechiae or small hemorrhagic lesions, particularly at the junction between the cortex and the white matter, to massive hematomas, which may rupture into the ventricular system or the subarachnoid space.

In the past, arteriovenous malformations have been thought to be particularly prone to rupture during pregnancy, but recent studies do not support this common belief. In a retrospective study of 451 women with arteriovenous malformations and no previous hemorrhage, the rate of first cerebral bleeding was identical in the pregnant and nonpregnant states. For women with a history of previous hemorrhage, the risk of a second hemorrhage occurring during pregnancy is not known with accuracy. The importance of hemodynamic

changes associated with labor and delivery in promoting intracerebral hemorrhage is also uncertain. In this study, there were 375 vaginal deliveries, none of which was complicated by cerebral hemorrhage. The hemorrhages occurred evenly throughout gestation and the postpartum period. As with ruptured aneurysms, the decision to operate after angiomatous hemorrhage should be based on neurosurgical principles. No data are available regarding embolization of arteriovenous malformations in pregnancy. Stereotactic radiotherapy is not used in pregnant women. When an arteriovenous malformation is discovered in a nonpregnant woman, pregnancy should be deferred until treatment is concluded. Other causes of intracerebral hemorrhage (see Table 48-1) include hypertension, hematologic disorders, and other rare conditions such as choriocarcinoma (see "Brain Tumors").

Diagnostic Approach

Except for the problem of strokelike deficits in the setting of eclampsia, the diagnosis of arterial ischemic stroke does not pose any particular problem. CVT presents with a wide spectrum of symptoms and signs and can be confused with other diseases, in particular with eclampsia, encephalitis, intracerebral hemorrhage, and even with post–lumbar puncture headache. The differential diagnosis of hemorrhagic stroke includes eclampsia, pituitary necrosis, and CVT. It is noteworthy that hypertension and albuminuria, two main features of eclampsia, have been observed in approximately one-third of intracranial hemorrhages resulting from a ruptured vascular malformation during pregnancy.

As far as the etiology of stroke is concerned, one must not only consider the few pregnancy-specific causes of strokes such as eclampsia, but also any of the known causes of stroke in the young because some of these may need specific management. Pregnancy does not contraindicate radiologic procedures. The teratogenic risk linked to radiation exposure is limited to the embryogenesis period, which runs from the second to the fourteenth week of gestation. A CT scan done with abdominal shielding limits fetal exposure to a trivial amount (approximately 2 mrad). Cerebral angiography results in approximately the same amount of fetal exposure plus whatever results from fluoroscopy during catheter insertion before abdominal

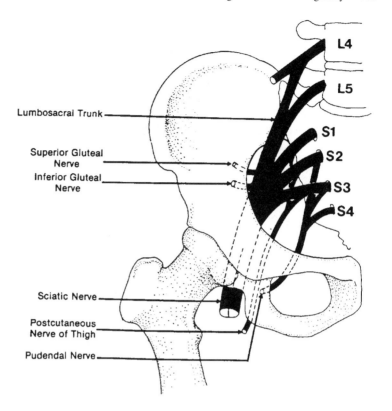

Figure 48-3. The lumbosacral plexus and the lumbosacral trunk. (Reprinted with permission from The Sciatic Nerve, the Gluteal and Pudenda Nerves, and the Posterior Cutaneous Nerve of the Thigh. In JD Steward [ed], Focal Peripheral Neuropathies. New York: Raven, 1993;322.)

shielding begins, which can be limited in skilled hands. After 6 months, iodine injection may induce fetal hypothyroidism which can be diagnosed and treated at birth with an excellent prognosis. MRI scanning does not appear to produce any short-term effect on the fetus, but any long-term risk remains to be determined. Gadolinium injection should not be used. Pregnancy does not appear to add any special problem to performing transesophageal echocardiography.

The etiologic evaluation should proceed as in the nonpregnant state. Too frequently, the stroke is considered a complication of pregnancy, and another underlying cause may be missed. Only a better definition of the causes and pathophysiologic mechanisms of strokes related to pregnancy and the puerperium will allow a better approach to diagnosis and treatment.

Peripheral Neuropathies

This section discusses obstetric paralysis and neuropathies that may have a higher incidence during

pregnancy or that require special precautions during pregnancy and delivery.

Maternal Obstetric Paralysis

Compression of a peripheral nerve may occur during labor and delivery. The injury may be caused by the fetal head, the application of forceps, trauma or hematoma during cesarean section, or improper positioning of the legs in the holders. Disproportion of the size of the fetal head to the pelvis, speed of delivery, dystocia, and primiparity are common features of deliveries resulting in postpartum neuropathies. Other possible causes of obstetric paralysis are lumbar intervertebral disc herniations and damage to lumbosacral roots from an epidural anesthetic catheter, although they are uncommon.

Postpartum Footdrop

The lumbosacral plexus (Figure 48-3) is formed from the L4–S2 roots. The L4 and L5 roots form

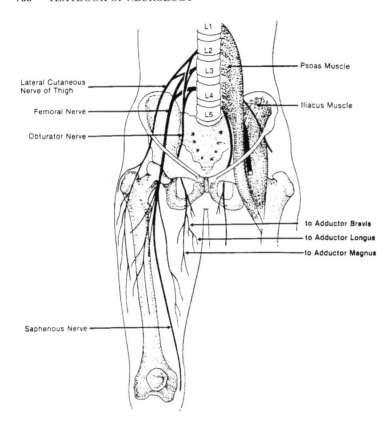

Figure 48-4. The femoral nerve, obturator nerve, and lateral cutaneous nerve of the thigh. (Reprinted with permission from The Femoral and Saphenous Nerves. In JD Steward [ed], Focal Peripheral Neuropathies, New York: Raven, 1993;388.)

the lumbosacral trunk that enters the true pelvis to join the sacral roots. This is the point at which the lumbosacral trunk can be easily compressed by the descending fetal head. Patients present with postpartum footdrop, often accompanied by a variable sensory deficit in the peroneal nerve distribution. The footdrop is almost always unilateral. A similar clinical presentation can result when the legholders compress the peroneal nerve where it crosses the fibular head. Nerve conduction study can distinguish between these two situations, which may have different outcomes. If the footdrop persists, electromyography is recommended to assess the extent and amount of axonal damage. Paresis with minimal axonal damage has a good prognosis. Physical therapy may be necessary. Subsequent pregnancies should be monitored for craniopelvic disproportion and difficult delivery.

Femoral Neuropathy

Femoral neuropathy after vaginal delivery is now rare. It is usually a painless condition that becomes

obvious when the patient walks for the first time after delivery. Anterior thigh paresthesia is common. There is some hip flexion weakness and more profound knee extension weakness. Walking up stairs is difficult. The condition can be unilateral or bilateral. Direct injury of the nerve trunks within the pelvis by either the fetal head or instruments is the cause of most cases of postpartum femoral neuropathy. Prolonged labor and cephalopelvic disproportion certainly contribute. Another possible mechanism is compression of the femoral nerve (Figure 48-4) against the inguinal ligament as a result of flexion of the thighs on the abdomen with abduction and outward rotation of the hips. However, in almost all postpartum cases, iliopsoas muscle weakness implies a more proximal lesion within the pelvis. Most lesions have a good prognosis, and no specific therapy is necessary.

Obturator Neuropathy

Postpartum obturator neuropathy is usually unilateral and combined with femoral neuropathy,

Figure 48-5. The median nerve in the carpal tunnel. (Reprinted with permission from The Median Nerve. In JD Steward [ed], Focal Peripheral Neuropathies. New York: Raven, 1993;158.)

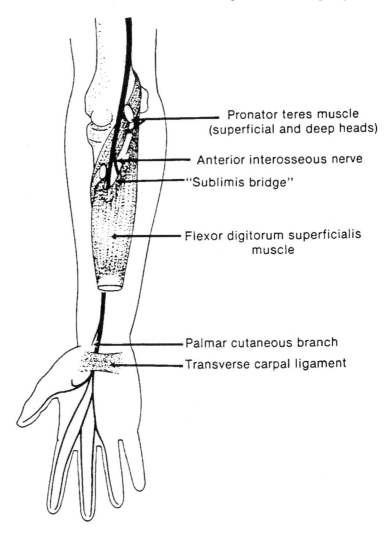

Pronator teres muscle (superficial and deep heads)

Anterior interosseous nerve

"Sublimis bridge"

Flexor digitorum superficialis muscle

Palmar cutaneous branch

Transverse carpal ligament

but bilateral cases have occurred. The obturator nerve, composed of fibers from the third and fourth lumbar roots, runs along the pelvic wall underneath the psoas major muscle (see Figure 48-4). It emerges near the pelvic brim where it can be exposed to the fetal head or highly placed forceps. At the time of compression, the woman may complain of a sharp pain in the groin and upper thigh. Later, weakness of hip adduction and rotation will be found, usually accompanied by diminished perception of light touch and pinprick over the upper inner thigh. Clinical examination is sufficient for early diagnosis. The lesion is usually incomplete, and functional recovery is typically good.

Other Mononeuropathies During Pregnancy

Carpal Tunnel Syndrome

Carpal tunnel syndrome is the most frequent neuropathy seen during pregnancy. It typically begins in the later half of pregnancy and usually involves the thumb and index and middle fingers with symptoms of numbness, tingling, and needles. Patients shake their hands in an attempt to alleviate symptoms, which are usually worse during the night or morning, and frequently awaken patients. The cause of carpal tunnel syndrome is compression of the median nerve in the carpal tunnel (Figure 48-5). Excessive weight gain and fluid retention are risk

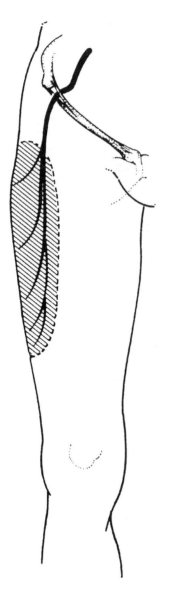

Figure 48-6. Lateral femoral cutaneous nerve. Shaded area represents skin distribution of the nerve. (Reprinted with permission from The Lateral Cutaneous Nerve of the Thigh. In JD Steward [ed], Focal Peripheral Neuropathies. New York: Raven, 1993;402.)

factors for development of this syndrome. The diagnosis can be confirmed by neurophysiologic testing, which should include a transcarpal orthodromic nerve conduction study. The first line of therapy consists of nocturnal splinting of the wrist. The most effective second-stage treatment is local injection of steroids into the carpal tunnel.

Meralgia Paresthetica

Meralgia paresthetica is a minor but bothersome disorder. The symptoms usually begin approximately the thirteenth week of gestation. Typically, numbness, tingling, and stinging pain occur in the middle third of the lateral thigh (Figure 48-6); symptoms worsen with standing or walking. Mild sensory loss to light touch and pinprick may be mapped out in the central area of hypesthesia. There is no associated weakness or reflex changes. The condition may be bilateral. A rapid weight gain is common. Because resolution of symptoms can be expected within the 3 months after delivery, treatment consists of explaining the symptoms to the patient and reassuring her of their transient course. Excessive weight gain should also be avoided. Temporary relief may be afforded by infiltrating local anesthetics into the nerve as it passes the inguinal ligament. Recurrent episodes may occur with subsequent pregnancies.

Facial Mononeuropathy (Bell's Palsy)

The idiopathic form of facial palsy seems to appear with slightly higher incidence in pregnancy. The majority of cases occur during the third trimester and the first 2 weeks postpartum. The prognosis is good if the initial paralysis is partial; only a minority of women are left with persistent facial nerve dysfunction as a result of severe axonal damage. When the paralysis is severe, many authors favor a 10-day course of prednisone treatment, starting at 40–60 mg daily and tapering rapidly, despite the possibility of steroid side effects on the mother or child. Oculoprotective treatment is always indicated.

Neuralgic Amyotrophy

Neuralgic amyotrophy is a condition characterized by acute and generally severe pain in and around the girdle followed by weakness and atrophy of single (especially serratus anterior) or multiple upper extremity muscles. The relation between pregnancy and neuralgic amyotrophy was first recognized in the rare familial variety of the condition, transmitted as an autosomal-dominant trait. In some of these families, affected women are prone to experience single or recurrent attacks during pregnancy or shortly postpartum. This syndrome appears to be clinically, electrophysiologically, and genetically distinct from the hereditary neuropathy with liability to pressure palsies, in which episodes of neuralgic amyotrophy can occur during and after pregnancy. Nonfamilial cases associated with postpartum have also been reported. The predominating pathogenetic mechanism in most cases of neuralgic amyotrophy is axonal injury rather than focal demyelination. The course and prognosis for neuralgic amyotrophy are similar for the sporadic, familial, or gestational form. The prognosis is good in most cases, but recovery may be quite delayed. No special therapy is of proven value.

Polyneuropathies During Pregnancy

There are no specific polyneuropathies of pregnancy. Malnutrition and vitamin deficiency are not significant causes of polyneuropathy in pregnancy in developed countries. Pregnancy has not been shown to trigger or aggravate diabetic neuropathy. Neuropathies associated with underlying diseases such as collagen disease may appear or relapse during pregnancy. Acute attacks of porphyrias, including an acute neuropathy, may be precipitated by pregnancy, anesthesia, surgery, and administration of drugs (porphyrinogenic drugs). We focus on Guillain-Barré syndrome, which is a frequent disease of the young, and on chronic inflammatory polyneuropathy, which seems to have a higher frequency in pregnancy.

Guillain-Barré Syndrome

Guillain-Barré syndrome, an acute inflammatory polyneuropathy, occurs randomly during pregnancy and the puerperium with no greater incidence than expected in nonpregnant women of childbearing age. The course of the disease does not differ from that in nonpregnant patients. The treatment should be the same as in the nonpregnant state, including early and, if necessary, repeated plasmapheresis or repeated administration of gamma globulins. Prevention of complications is a constant worry. Even if she is not bedridden, the chances of a pregnant woman developing peripheral thrombophlebitis and pul-

monary emboli are increased. Pregnant women have mildly restricted respiration depending on the size of the gravid uterus and thus may need assisted ventilation sooner and longer than would be otherwise expected. Even with weakness advancing to tetraplegia, a pregnant woman can be assured that her fetus is not affected. Pregnancy, labor, and delivery proceed normally for most women with Guillain-Barré syndrome. Premature birth may be associated with severe cases in the third trimester. Tocolytics should be avoided if autonomic instability exists. Uterine contractions are normally strong, but an inability to bear down increases the likelihood that forceps will be needed.

Chronic Inflammatory Demyelinating Polyneuropathy

Chronic inflammatory demyelinating polyneuropathy is a relatively rare, autoimmune peripheral nerve myelin disorder. The relapse rate during a pregnancy year is approximately three times greater than expected. Most of the exacerbations occur in the third trimester and the postpartum period, but worsening has been reported throughout pregnancy and while taking contraceptive pills. The cause is unknown. Treatment includes corticosteroids, plasmapheresis, or both; these treatments can be used during pregnancy if necessary. Obstetric aspects of these cases have been sparsely described, but no particular difficulty has been reported. The infants of affected mothers are normal.

Epilepsy

Epilepsy is one of the most common neurologic disorders, affecting approximately 1% of the population. Approximately 1 million women with epilepsy in the United States are of childbearing age, and most of them receive antiepileptic drugs. It is estimated that 1 in every 200 pregnancies takes place in a woman with epilepsy, making this condition one of the most common serious neurologic disorders encountered by obstetricians.

In the past, women with epilepsy were strongly encouraged not to have children simply because they had epilepsy, or they were told that they must stop all antiepileptic drugs if they wanted to be

Table 48-2. Relative Timing of Major Congenital Malformations Observed in Offspring of Women Treated with Antiepileptic Drugs

Organs	Malformations	Approximate Interval in Days or Weeks (After First Day of Last Menstrual Period)
Central nervous sytem	Meningomyelocele	28 days
Heart	Ventricular defect	6 weeks
Face	Cleft lip	36 days
	Cleft maxillary palate	10 weeks

pregnant, regardless of their seizures history. With modern antiepileptic drugs, seizures are controlled in approximately 75% of persons with epilepsy, allowing the majority of women with epilepsy to become pregnant if they wish. However, pregnancies in women with epilepsy remain high risk because of an increased frequency of maternal seizures; complications of pregnancy, labor, and delivery; and the fact that their children have higher rates of adverse pregnancy outcomes. In spite of this, more than 90% of women with epilepsy can expect to experience normal pregnancies and have normal babies.

Effects of Pregnancy on Epilepsy and Antiepileptic Drugs

The relationship between seizure frequency and pregnancy has been reported in a number of studies. Approximately 25% of women have an increased seizure frequency during pregnancy. The best predictor of the effect of pregnancy on seizures may be the prepregnancy seizure frequency. Increased seizure frequency may be caused by hormonal and metabolic changes, sleep deprivation, noncompliance, and a pharmacokinetically caused decrease in antiepileptic drug levels. Compliance is often a problem during pregnancy because the message that any drugs taken during pregnancy can be dangerous to the fetus has been imprinted in the mind of the public. Therefore, women should be told about the risks of antiepileptic drugs but also about the risks of seizures both to the mother and the fetus. The risk of major congenital malformations is largely limited to the first trimester (Table 48-2). Therefore, increased dosages of antiepileptic drugs in the later

trimesters, if necessary, are not associated with an increased risk of malformations. Total serum antiepileptic drug levels and, if possible, free antiepileptic drug fractions, should be measured before pregnancy and at regular intervals throughout pregnancy and the dosage adjusted as necessary. However, a decrease in serum antiepileptic drug levels does not in itself justify an increase in dosage. The overall clinical state should be assessed.

Effects of Epilepsy and Antiepileptic Drugs on Pregnancy

The risk of major malformations, minor anomalies, and dysmorphic features is approximately twofold to threefold higher in infants of mothers with epilepsy who received treatment with antiepileptic drugs compared with the infants of mothers without epilepsy (Table 48-3). Major congenital malformations include cleft lip and palate, cardiac defects, neural tube defects, and urogenital defects. Higher rates of congenital malformations are observed in infants of mothers with epilepsy who received multiple antiepileptic drugs rather than monotherapy. All antiepileptic drugs currently marketed cross the placenta and have been implicated in increasing the risk of congenital malformations (this does not include felbamate, gabapentin, and vigabatrin, for which there are insufficient data in humans). No congenital malformations are specific to one antiepileptic drug. Orofacial clefts are the most commonly reported malformations in infants of mothers with epilepsy, followed by midline heart defect. The prevalence of spina bifida is approximately 1–2% with valproate exposure and 0.5% with carbamazepine. If valproate or carbamazepine

Table 48-3. Guidelines: Preconception Counseling and Management of Pregnant Women with Epilepsy

1. The risk of major malformations, minor abnormalities, and dysmorphic features is twofold to threefold higher in infants of women with epilepsy taking antiepileptic drugs compared with the risk in infants of mothers without epilepsy.
2. Possibilities for prenatal diagnosis of major malformations should be discussed. If valproate or carbamazepine is the necessary antiepileptic drug, high-resolution ultrasonography should be done at 16–19 weeks, looking for neural tube defects. Amniocentesis for alpha-fetoprotein dosage should be offered if ultrasound examination is inconclusive. Ultrasonography at 22–24 weeks can detect oral clefts and heart abnormalities.
3. Effects of tonic-clonic seizures on the fetus are not well established. However, tonic-clonic seizures might be deleterious for the fetus, injure the mother, and lead to miscarriage.
4. The diet before conception should contain adequate amounts of folate. Folate daily supplement should be continued during the period of organogenesis.
5. If the patient is seizure-free for at least 2 years, withdrawal of antiepileptic drugs should be considered before conception.
6. The first-choice drug for seizure type and epilepsy syndrome should be used.
7. The lowest effective dose should be used and polytherapy should be avoided.
8. Valproate and carbamazepine should be avoided when there is a family history of neural tube defects.
9. Plasma antiepileptic drug levels and, if possible, free plasma antiepileptic drugs levels should be monitored regularly.
10. In cases of valproate treatment, high plasma levels should be avoided and doses should be divided over the day.
11. Vitamin K should be administered prophylactically to mothers taking antiepileptic drugs during the last month of pregnancy.
12. Antiepileptic drugs levels should be checked during the first weeks of the puerperium.

is to be used, high-resolution ultrasonography should be done at 16–19 weeks, looking for neural tube defects. Amniocentesis should be offered if ultrasound examination is inconclusive with amniotic fluid analysis of alfa fetoprotein. Ultrasonography at 22–24 weeks can detect oral clefts and heart abnormalities. In the detection of neural tube defects, high-resolution ultrasound has approximate resolutions of 95%. Various syndromes of minor malformations and dysmorphic features, especially facial and distal digital anomalies, have been described with antiepileptic drugs (trimethadione, hydantoin, primidone, phenobarbital, valproate, and carbamazepine). The long-term impact on the growth and psychomotor development of infants exposed prenatally to antiepileptic drugs remains uncertain at this time. The effects of tonic seizures on the fetus during pregnancy are not well established. However, tonic-clonic convulsions might be deleterious to the fetus, injure the mother, and lead to miscarriage.

Vitamin K_1 should be administered beginning 3 weeks before expected delivery until birth to prevent neonatal hemorrhage. Antiepileptic drug levels should be followed during the first weeks of the puerperium because they can rise and cause toxicity. Most women with epilepsy have a normal vaginal delivery. There is approximately a twofold

increased risk of vaginal hemorrhage, eclampsia, premature labor, and cesarean section in women with epilepsy. Tonic-clonic seizures occur during labor in 1–2% of women with epilepsy, and 24 hours after delivery in another 1–2%. Maintenance of plasma levels known to protect against seizures during the third trimester of pregnancy is a preventive measure against the occurrence of seizures during labor. Taking antiepileptic drugs during labor to ensure adequate plasma levels is also important, and the patient must be cautioned against missing doses as labor continues. All of the commonly used antiepileptic drugs are measurable in varying concentrations in breast milk. However, taking antiepileptic drugs for epilepsy does not constitute a contraindication to breast feeding. The exceptions are sedative drugs such as phenobarbital or benzodiazepines. After delivery, phenobarbital, primidone, and benzodiazepines will remain in neonatal plasma for several days, causing sedative effects and possibly a neonatal withdrawal syndrome.

Before Conception

All women of childbearing age with epilepsy should be advised, preferably before conception, about the risks associated with pregnancy and the ways to minimize those risks. First, the diagnosis of epilepsy should be based on firm data. Nonepileptic seizures; syncope; and other neurologic, medical, and psychiatric syndromes may be misdiagnosed as epilepsy, promoting the use of unnecessary and potentially harmful antiepileptic drugs. Second, the need for continued antiepileptic drug therapy should also be re-evaluated before conception. Antiepileptic drug withdrawal in patients planning pregnancy who have been free of seizures for at last 2 years may be considered. When withdrawal of antiepileptic drug treatment is not possible, crossover from multiple drugs to monotherapy should be considered and gradually attempted before conception. Monotherapy and use of the lowest effective dose reduces the risk of adverse outcomes. In many cases, a balance must be achieved between the risks to the fetus and the degree of seizure control. The use of a single daily dose is not advisable. Valproate and carbamazepine should be avoided when there is a personal or family history of neural tube defects. Third, growing evidence suggests that the preconceptual use of multivitamins with folate may reduce the risk of neural tube defects. Because women with epilepsy were not specifically studied, it remains to be definitively shown whether folate supplements given before and early in pregnancy prevent neural tube defects in the offspring of mothers with epilepsy. Based on available data, it seems reasonable to provide such supplements to each prospective mother. Whether the optimal dose in this population is 4 mg per day, or approximately 1 mg per day, or some other value remains to be demonstrated. What is crucial to remember is that the neural tube closes caudally at approximately day 28 after conception. Because many women do not realize they are pregnant until 3–4 weeks into the pregnancy, it is important to advise women who wish to be pregnant to consider taking a vitamin supplement for at least one month before attempting to conceive.

Risk of Epilepsy to Offspring

The overall risk of epilepsy in the offspring of epileptic parents is 3–4%. The higher risk for epilepsy is in offspring of parents with absence seizures and the lowest risk is associated with parents who have simple focal seizures.

Multiple Sclerosis

MS is the most common acquired inflammatory demyelinating disorder of the central nervous system, affecting approximately 250,000 people in the United States. MS primarily affects young adults, with a female-to-male ratio of 3 to 2. Consequently, women of childbearing age are a major target group for the disease. Women with MS are increasingly asking about the advisability of pregnancy. Specific concerns are (1) the effects of pregnancy on maternal MS; (2) the overall outcome of pregnancy; and (3) the risk that the child will also develop MS.

Effects of Pregnancy on Multiple Sclerosis

Although there are conflicting data, the risk of relapses appears to be decreased during pregnancy itself and increased in the puerperium. The risk of a progressive course may also be decreased in women who are pregnant after MS onset. Suppression of disease activity during the second half of pregnancy has also been observed in several immunologically mediated diseases, such as rheumatoid arthritis and systemic lupus erythematosus. This favorable effect may relate to immunologic or hormonal changes that occur during this period. Numerous studies have noted that an exacerbation of MS occurs in 20–40% of patients in the postpartum period. A meta-analysis calculated a mean relative risk of relapse in the postpartum period of 3.9 compared with the same patients when not pregnant and 5.4 compared with all nonpregnant patients. Multicenter, longitudinal prospective studies comparing the number of relapses, disability status, and MRI scans of lesions before and throughout pregnancy are needed to address the effect of pregnancy on MS more definitively.

Several retrospective studies have addressed the important issue of long-term disability consequent to pregnancy. They have failed to indicate an adverse effect of pregnancy on the prognosis for long-term disability in MS, even in patients who had experienced pregnancy-related relapses. In clinical practice, although the course of MS is unpredictable, only 33% of patients will be severely impaired 10 years after onset. Younger women with mild MS should be encouraged to make decisions about childbearing independent of MS factors, whereas older women with more severe disabilities may appropriately decide to avoid pregnancy.

Effects of Multiple Sclerosis on Pregnancy

Uncomplicated MS seems to have no effect on pregnancy, labor, or delivery. Before becoming pregnant, women with MS should stop immunosuppressive drugs and all nonessential drugs. Diazepam, phenytoin, and carbamazepine should be avoided during the first trimester because they are linked to an increased risk of malformations. Prednisone use, although nonteratogenic in humans, may result in neonatal adrenal suppression. Adrenocorticotropic hormones pose an increased risk for virilization of female fetuses during the first trimester. When MS symptoms provoke major impairments in function, corticosteroids can be used briefly during pregnancy. Some MS patients are more likely to experience constipation or urinary tract infections than normal patients because of the pressure of a gravid uterus on a neurogenic bowel or bladder.

The mode of delivery should be decided strictly on obstetric criteria. The rate of spontaneous abortions, congenital malformations, or stillbirths among women with MS is not increased. Epidural anesthesia may be used. During labor, fatigue related to MS may favor the use of forceps to shorten delivery.

The postpartum period is often a physically and emotionally stressful period. Because of functional impairment, some patients may have difficulty caring for their babies. There is no contraindication to breast feeding unless patients require drugs deemed toxic to the baby. No measures to decrease the risk of postpartum exacerbations are known; adequate rest and help with infant care duties are desirable.

Risk of Multiple Sclerosis to Offspring

MS is more common in kindred and there is an increased risk of MS in offspring. The lifetime risk of MS developing in the child of an affected parent is approximately 0.5–3.0%, compared with a general population risk in temperate zones of approximately 0.1%.

Myasthenia Gravis

Myasthenia gravis is an autoimmune disorder that results in failure of neuromuscular transmission. The disease is characterized by fluctuating weakness and fatigability. Myasthenia is primarily a disease of young women of childbearing age.

Effects of Pregnancy on Myasthenia Gravis

Pregnancy may have an important influence on myasthenia, although the effect is unpredictable. Overall, one-third of the women worsen, one-third improve, and one-third are unchanged by pregnancy. The changes may occur in any trimester. Exacerbations tend to be most sudden and most dangerous in the postpartum period. Many drugs given during pregnancy may worsen known myasthenia symptoms or precipitate the first presentation (Table 48-4).

Preconception counseling is the ideal, with the goal of achieving optimal management of myasthenia before pregnancy. A woman with generalized myasthenia gravis who is considering pregnancy should have a thymectomy before becoming pregnant. If performed before pregnancy, thymectomy can decrease the incidence of disease exacerbation during pregnancy and also favorably influence the incidence of neonatal myasthenia. Treatment of myasthenia gravis during pregnancy can include anticholinesterases. Corticosteroids are preferred over the other immune suppressants in pregnant patients. Plasmapheresis rapidly lowers acetylcholine antibody titers and may be indicated when high maternal titers threaten fetal development of neonatal myasthenia.

Effects of Myasthenia Gravis on Pregnancy

The risk of congenital abnormalities or abortion is not increased in women with myasthenia gravis, but the incidence of premature labor may be increased. Myasthenia does not affect the uterine muscles; therefore, vaginal delivery is possible. Nonetheless, progress late in delivery may be slow because of maternal exhaustion, and forceps-assisted delivery may be necessary. Cesarean section is not justified solely because the mother is myasthenic. Regional

Table 48-4. Drugs to Be Avoided in Myasthenia

Antibiotics	Neuromuscular Blocking Agents	Cardiovascular	Antirheumatics	Antiepileptic Drugs	Psychotropics	Others
Aminoglycosides	Curare	Procainamide	Chloroquine	Phenytoin	Lithium carbonate	Magnesium sulfate
Polymyxin A,B	Pancuronium	Quinidine	D-Penicillamine	Trimethadione	Chlorpromazine	Corticosteroids
Clindamycin	Succinylcholine	Quinine			Promazine	Thyroid replacement
Tetracyclines		Lidocaine			Phenelzine	Corticotropin
Colistin		Beta-blockers			Sedatives	Anticholinesterases
Lincomycin		Ca^{2+} channel blockers			Narcotics	
		Trimethaphan				

anesthesia is preferred over other anesthetic methods; neuromuscular blocking agents such as curare must be avoided. During labor, the need for anticholinesterase medication is increased; women taking corticosteroids should have an additional dose because of the fatigue of labor. Support services may help to eliminate or to reduce potent stressors during the postpartum period. Medication dosages may need to be adjusted as the mother's body returns to its prepregnant state.

Unlike most other neurologic diseases, maternal myasthenia can directly affect the fetus. The perinatal death rate is increased because of antenatal and perinatal myasthenia. Both conditions are presumed secondary to transplacental transfer of maternal acetylcholine receptor antibodies. Antenatal effects derive from inhibited skeletal muscle movements and development, resulting in pulmonary hypoplasia, arthrogryposis multiplex, and polyhydramnios. Offspring of mothers with previously affected infants or with especially high titers of acetylcholine receptor antibodies are at higher risk. Ultrasound monitoring of fetal movements and assessment of acetylcholine receptor antibody titers may identify those at-risk women.

Neonatal myasthenia is less severe but more common. It occurs in 15–20% of the offspring of mothers with myasthenia. No relationship exists between the maternal disease and the neonatal disease. The newborn with myasthenia gravis is characterized clinically by hypotonia, weak suck, feeding difficulties, feeble crying, and respiratory distress. The diagnosis is usually obvious and can be confirmed by a Tensilon test. Neonatal myasthenia often occurs in the first day or two of life and generally remits spontaneously within 2 or 4 weeks. Treatment is supportive but can be supplemented by cholinesterase inhibitors. Careful attention to secretions is imperative. Recovery is eventually complete and no further therapy is necessary. Neonatal myasthenia does not represent a risk to the infant of later myasthenia gravis.

Muscle Diseases

This section addresses those muscle diseases for which a relationship to pregnancy has been described or for which prenatal genetic counseling and testing are important.

Myotonic Dystrophy

Myotonic dystrophy (Steinert's disease) is a multisystem disorder inherited as an autosomal dominant trait that is characterized by variable expression of progressive, predominantly distal, skeletal muscle weakness with clinical and electrical myotonia. Other symptoms include cataracts; frontal balding; cardiac conduction defects; smooth-muscle weakness of the esophagus, stomach, bowel, and uterus; and various endocrine dysfunctions. Onset is usually in the second to third decade. Large sibships are not uncommon in families with myotonic dystrophy, and fertility is usually moderately reduced.

Effects of Pregnancy on Myotonic Dystrophy

The course of myotonic dystrophy may worsen during pregnancy, usually during the last trimester. Clinical worsening may be temporary, with a return to baseline values after delivery. Myotonia, muscle wasting, and weakness can also first become apparent during pregnancy.

Effects of Myotonic Dystrophy on Pregnancy

Myotonic dystrophy has a potentially devastating impact on the pregnancy itself. Numerous obstetric complications may be observed: spontaneous abortion, abnormal presentation, premature labor, prolonged labor in both the first and second stages as a result of poor uterine contractions and an inability to bear down, retained placenta, placenta previa, and postpartum hemorrhage from failure of uterine contraction after delivery. Response to oxytocin is variable. Cesarean section may be necessary, but anesthesia and surgery also carry special risks. Local anesthesia is preferable. Depolarizing neuromuscular blockade has been reported to cause myotonic spasm. Thiopental can cause marked respiratory depression. Optimal management for the parturient requires a preoperative clinical assessment of cardiac and respiratory function and careful postoperative monitoring of ventilation and cardiac rhythm.

Congenital Myotonic Dystrophy

Myotonic dystrophy can present intrauterine, at birth, or in early childhood. For reasons still unclear, congenital myotonic dystrophy occurs only when the mother is affected. The risk of an affected woman having a congenitally affected child is 10%. The risk increases to nearly 40% if she has already had congenitally affected offspring. Even asymptomatic women may have congenitally affected children. The severity of congenital myotonic dystrophy is variable. It can manifest in utero as polyhydramnios and reduced fetal movements. Neonatal onset of myotonic dystrophy is frequently fatal because of respiratory failure. Symptoms at birth in survivors are hypotonia, diffuse weakness, arthrogryposis, developmental delay, poor feeding, and mental retardation. A less severe disease with talipes, facial diplegia, hypotonia, mental retardation, and temporary respiratory and feeding troubles is also possible. The symptoms may improve for some years, but the congenitally affected patients invariably present with the classic form of the disease in late adolescence or early adult life.

Genetic Counseling

The finding of the gene responsible for myotonic dystrophy on chromosome 19 means carrier and prenatal detection can be performed with near 100% accuracy, allowing better genetic counseling. It is also important to develop an understanding of the disease, determine the risk for congenital myotonic dystrophy, and offer options for dealing with these risks.

Duchenne and Becker Type Muscular Dystrophies

The Duchenne and Becker type muscular dystrophies are allelic X-linked recessive disorders arising from defects in a gene coding for a large structural protein called *dystrophin*. Females are at risk for being carriers for the dystrophy. Because of its severe and inexorable clinical course and the lack of a cure, prepregnancy genetic counseling for women with affected offspring, siblings, or other relatives is important. Unfortunately, the dystrophin region is quite large, and up to one-third of cases of Duchenne and Becker type dystrophies are new mutations. In families with known dystrophies, carrier detec-

tion and prenatal diagnosis of an affected fetus is available.

Several other inherited muscle diseases (e.g., fascioscapulohumeral dystrophy, hyperkalemic periodic paralysis, paramyotonia congenita, mitochondrial myopathies, Emery-Dreifuss muscular dystrophy, X-linked centronuclear myopathy) are amenable to carrier detection and prenatal diagnosis by DNA analysis.

Headaches

Migraine and tension headaches often occur in women of childbearing age. It is not surprising, therefore, that headache is also the most common neurologic symptom in pregnancy, but pregnancy complicates the usual clinical picture. It modifies the course of several headache symptoms, and its presence raises special concerns about diagnosis and treatment.

Evaluation of the Pregnant Headache Patient

The best screening tests for evaluating patients with headache in general are a careful history and thorough general physical and neurologic examinations. When headaches are long-standing and the examination findings are normal, further tests are seldom necessary. Laboratory and radiologic tests are usually indicated if the headaches are of recent onset (particularly if the headaches are atypical), if there has been a recent change in a previously stable headache pattern, or if the neurologic examination findings are not normal. The same guidelines apply in evaluating the pregnant patient.

The onset of headaches during pregnancy or the puerperium can raise concerns about serious underlying illness: pre-eclampsia/eclampsia, pseudotumor cerebri, CVT (particularly during the puerperal period), intracranial hemorrhage, *Listeria* meningitis, and rapid expansion of a brain tumor, among others. New-onset headaches accompanied by neurologic abnormalities or headaches not conforming to standard headache syndromes should be investigated. When investigation is necessary, an MRI scan (without gadolinium injection) provides the most information with the least risk. If the MRI study shows no mass and if it is clinically warranted, pregnancy poses no special contraindication to lumbar puncture.

Behavior of Established Headache Syndromes in Pregnancy

Migraine

Approximately 70% of migrainous women improve or remit completely during pregnancy. In most studies, improvement is observed mainly during the last two trimesters of pregnancy. Improvement is more likely in women whose episodes of migraine are mainly menstrual. Of the remaining 30%, approximately two-thirds are unchanged, and one-third worsen, especially in the case of migraine with aura. Migraine may also appear for the first time during pregnancy, attacks with aura being the most commonly reported. However, migraine with aura should not be diagnosed for the first time in pregnant women unless thorough consideration has been given to other possibilities. When migraine begins during pregnancy, it does so most often in the first trimester.

Migraine never represents a threat for pregnancy, the fetus, or the delivery. It is therefore important that the treatment of migraine should not be noxious for the pregnancy. Few data are available about the risks of many antimigrainous drugs during pregnancy, delivery, and breast feeding. For the acute treatment of migraine attacks, paracetamol with or without metoclopramide is considered during pregnancy and breast feeding as the drug of first choice. The safety of aspirin during the first trimester of pregnancy is still a subject of debate, particularly for daily use. Several prospective studies concerning a large number of women taking aspirin episodically during the first 4 months of pregnancy have not shown a teratogenic risk. The potential adverse effects of aspirin or other non-steroidal anti-inflammatory drugs late in pregnancy are maternal and fetal hemorrhage, premature closure of the ductus arteriosus, prolongation of labor, and a delay in the onset of labor. The risks are probably low when the drug is taken episodically, but it is better to avoid them during the last trimester of pregnancy. Ergotamine tartrate and parenteral dihydroergotamine are classically contraindicated during pregnancy because of their uterotonic effect. Ergotamine tartrate is embryotoxic in animals, but there is no evidence of a teratogenic effect in humans when it is used at the normal dose. Ergotamine is contraindicated during breast feeding. Sumatriptan causes fetal malformations in rabbits. Prophylactic treatment of migraine is rarely indicated during pregnancy. If considered, preventive measures should first include nondrug treatments such as biofeedback, relaxation, or acupuncture and avoiding trigger factors. Possible drugs include dihydroergotamine, beta-blockers, amitriptyline, pizotifen, and flunarizine. It must be emphasized that for the last two drugs, only small series are available. Propranolol has been used safely during pregnancy to treat hypertension, and there is no evidence that it is teratogenic. Amitriptyline should be stopped at least 2 weeks before delivery. Special caution is required during pregnancy when prophylactic and acute treatments are associated.

Tension Headache

Certain changes in posture and psychological stress may contribute to tension headaches during pregnancy; female hormones seem to be of less causal importance compared to migraine. The tension-type headache pattern seems to be unchanged during pregnancy in the majority of women. The focus of treatment should be nondrug therapy such as behavioral and postural modification. Mild analgesics such as acetaminophen can be used periodically. The daily use of analgesics can itself perpetuate the headaches, and discontinuing their use can lead to improvement.

Postpartum Headache

Postnatal headaches are common. Migraine is particularly common in the postpartum period, especially in women with a previous personal or family history of migraine. Thrombosis of the superior sagittal or lateral sinuses may present as a progressively severe headache without neurologic symptoms or signs. Low-pressure headache may occur as a result of spinal procedures related to delivery. Diagnosis should be based on a careful history and examination as outlined above. A brain MRI scan is the test of choice to assess the patency of the dural sinuses.

Brain Tumors

Pregnancy does not increase the risk of brain tumors, and the types of brain tumors seen in pregnant women are identical to those seen in nonpregnant women of the same age, except for choriocarcinoma, which is specifically associated with pregnancy. By contrast, physiologic changes induced by pregnancy affect the biologic behavior of glial tumors, meningiomas, and pituitary adenomas. First, tumors may enlarge as a result of increased blood volume and fluid retention. Second, sex hormones may stimulate the growth of brain tumors. Brain tumors may also be more difficult to diagnose in pregnant women because nonfocal symptoms such as headaches, nausea and malaise overlap those of pregnancy. Generalized seizures occurring during the latter half of pregnancy can be confused with eclampsia. MRI and CT scans are the most useful modalities for diagnosis. Finally, brain tumors pose specific therapeutic problems in pregnant women.

Gliomas

Gliomas are the most common primary brain tumors in the general population and in pregnant patients as well. They arise from astrocytes or oligodendrocytes and give rise to tumors of varying malignancy. In the management of glial tumors during pregnancy, one should consider the benign or suspected malignant nature of the tumor, the stage of pregnancy during which the tumor is detected, the neurologic stability of the patient, the maternal and fetal outcomes with medical versus surgical management, the efficacy of vaginal versus cesarean delivery, and fetal viability. If possible, symptoms may be controlled by medical management until after delivery. Measures can include rest and corticosteroids. Urgent treatment of a low-grade glioma is almost never necessary. By contrast, if the mother is early in pregnancy and is suspected of having a high-grade tumor or is neurologically deteriorating, surgical treatment should not be postponed. Premature delivery can be considered when the fetus weighs more than 1,500 g.

Meningiomas

Meningiomas arise from dural tissue and are extra-axial. A rapid and occasionally temporary enlarge-ment of a meningioma may be observed during pregnancy, which may be facilitated by the presence of sex steroid receptors in most meningiomas. Surgical resection of a meningioma can be safely performed in a pregnant patient but should be postponed until after delivery if possible.

Pituitary Adenomas

Pituitary tumors are classified according to size as macroadenomas and microadenomas, and by the secreted hormone, which can be prolactin, growth hormone, corticotropin, thyrotropin, or gonadotropin, or the tumor can be nonsecretory. A previously asymptomatic pituitary adenoma may become symptomatic during pregnancy as a result of physiologic growth of the pituitary gland or growth of the tumor. Known tumors may also cause more problems during pregnancy. The most common symptoms of pituitary growth during pregnancy are headaches and visual field impairment. Most symptoms are mild and progress subacutely, allowing the physician time to intervene before the onset of irreversible neurologic deficits. Pregnancy-related pituitary apoplexy seems to be very rare. The diagnosis and serial evaluation of pituitary tumors have been greatly facilitated by MRI.

Prolactinoma is the most frequent of secreting pituitary adenomas. It is often discovered among women of childbearing age. Complications of microprolactinomas during pregnancy seem to be rare. Macroprolactinomas produce complications more often, particularly visual field loss, and require good tumor control before pregnancy and a rigorous follow-up throughout pregnancy. Treatment may be surgical, medical, or a combination. The use of dopaminergic drugs, which allow tumoral control and recovery of fertility in the majority of women with prolactinomas, have reduced the indications for surgery. Bromocriptine is usually stopped during pregnancy but may be safely reinstituted and maintained throughout gestation if symptoms reappear. This is usually sufficient to resolve neurologic symptoms. There has been no report of adverse effects of bromocriptine on the fetus when used throughout pregnancy.

Lymphocytic adenohypophysitis can cause pituitary expansion and hypopituitarism closely mimicking the features of a pituitary adenoma. It occurs exclusively in young women in relation to pregnancy. There is a preference for destruction of corticotropin and thyrotropin secreting cells. The presence of diffuse homogeneous contrast enhancement on CT or MRI scans may be a diagnostic feature of this disease when contrast injection may be performed. There is, at yet, no proven specific treatment. There are anecdotal reports of a beneficial effect of steroids but there is also evidence that spontaneous resolution may occur.

Brain Metastases: Choriocarcinoma

Systemic cancer is unusual in young women and is rarely present during pregnancy. No particular systemic neoplasm is associated with pregnancy except choriocarcinoma. Choriocarcinoma is a tumor caused by malignant transformation of the trophoblast. This disease is uncommon in Western countries (1 in 40,000 pregnancies in the United States), whereas its incidence ranges from 1 in 4,000 to 1 in 250 in Asia, Africa, and the Middle East. Most choriocarcinomas follow molar pregnancy, but the cancer may also follow term delivery, abortion, and ectopic pregnancy. Malignant transformation occurs most frequently within a year of pregnancy, but delays of up to several years have been reported. Brain metastases complicate approximately 20% of choriocarcinomas. In the brain, trophoblasts may invade blood vessels, just as they would in the uterus. The damaged vessels may thrombose and lead to single or multiple cerebral infarctions, or the embolus may fail to lodge and pass distally, leading to transient ischemic attacks. Other vessels may develop neoplastic aneurysms or varicosities. These vessels may bleed into the tumor mass, the brain parenchyma surrounding the tumor mass, or the subarachnoid space. With recent advances in chemotherapy and radiation, many patients can be cured.

Suggested Reading

Berie A. Peripheral Nerve Disorders in Pregnancy. In O Devinsky, E Feldmann, B Hainline (eds), Neurological Complications of Pregnancy. New York: Raven, 1994;179–192.

Bousser MG, Massiou H. Migraine in the Reproductive Cycle. In J Olesen, P Tfelt-Hansen, KMA Welch (eds), The Headaches. New York: Raven, 1993;413–419.

Cook SD, Troiano R, Bansil S, Dowling P. Multiple Sclerosis and Pregnancy. In O Devinsky, E Feldmann, B Hainline (eds), Neurological Complications of Pregnancy. New York: Raven, 1994;83–95.

DeAngelis. Central Nervous System Neoplasms in Pregnancy. In O Devinsky, E Feldmann, B Hainline (eds), Neurological Complications of Pregnancy. New York: Raven, 1994;139–152.

Delgado-Escueta AV, Janz D. Consensus guidelines: preconception counseling, management and care of the pregnant woman with epilepsy. Neurology 1992;42(Suppl 5):149.

Dias MS, Sekhar LN. Intracranial hemorrhage from aneurysms and arteriovenous malformations during pregnancy and the puerperium. Neurosurgery 1990;27:855.

Gilchrist JM. Muscle Disease in the Pregnant Woman. In O Devinsky, E Feldmann, B Hainline (eds), Neurological Complications of Pregnancy. New York: Raven, 1994; 193–208.

Horton JC, Chambers WA, Lyons SL, Adams RD, et al. Pregnancy and the risk of hemorrhage from cerebral arteriovenous malformations. Neurosurgery 1990;27:867.

Kittner SJ, Stern BJ, Feeser BR, et al. Pregnancy and the risk of stroke. N Engl J Med 1996;335:768.

Lindhout D, Omtzigt JGC. Pregnancy and the risk of teratogenicity. Epilepsia 1992;33(Suppl 4):41.

Mas JL, Lamy C. Stroke in Pregnancy and Post-partum. In M Ginsberg, J Bogousslavsky (eds), Cerebrovascular Disease. Cambridge, UK: Blackwell Scientific, 1998; 1684–1697

Rosenbaum RB, Donaldson. Peripheral nerve and neuromuscular disorders. Neurol Clin 1994;12:461.

Sadovnick AD, Eisen K, Hashimoto SA, et al. Pregnancy and multiple sclerosis. A prospective study. Arch Neurol 1994;51:1120.

Sharshar T, Lamy C, Mas JL. Incidence and causes of strokes associated with pregnancy and puerperium. A study in public hospitals of Ile de France. Stroke 1995;26:930.

Yerby MS, Devinsky O. Epilepsy and Pregnancy. In O Devinsky, E Feldmann, B Hainline (eds), Neurological Complications of Pregnancy. New York: Raven, 1994;45–63.

Chapter 49

Congenital Abnormalities of the Central Nervous System Presenting in Adulthood

N. Scott Litofsky and Robin I. Davidson

Chapter Plan

Most congenital malformations are identified in childhood. Some patients, however, will remain asymptomatic until later in life. In fact, occasionally patients' malformations are first identified after the onset of symptoms in adulthood.

It is not clear why particular patients remain asymptomatic until adulthood. In some cases, the growth of the patient in young adulthood can change anatomic relationships of the malformation enough to cause symptoms. In others, ligamentous laxity associated with the malformation can progress over time to the point of the abnormality becoming symptomatic. Last, trauma can cause a precipitous presentation of the malformation.

This chapter discusses a variety of congenital malformations that may first appear in adulthood. The pathologic features, presenting signs and symptoms, diagnostic evaluation, and treatment of the various malformations are included.

Chiari I Malformation

Chiari I malformation is a congenital abnormality of the hindbrain in which some or all of the cerebellar tonsils are positioned inferior to the foramen magnum. Although the tonsils may extend inferiorly several cervical segments, they usually do not extend more than a few centimeters or much below the level of C1. Typically, significant arachnoidal adhesions occur between the cerebellar tonsils and the medulla and spinal cord; banding around the upper cervical cord related to these adhesions may be present. The posterior inferior cerebellar arteries course inferiorly with the tonsillar herniation. Other structures in the hindbrain and upper cervical cord are normal—that is, the fourth ventricle, cerebellum, and spinal cord are in the normal position with normal anatomic relations to the surrounding structures.

Although the rest of the hindbrain may be normal, patients with Chiari I malformation may have one of several other central nervous system (CNS) malformations in association. Approximately 10% of patients will have hydrocephalus. Patients may also develop syringomyelia (cavitation within the spinal cord), which is thought to originate as the result of abnormal flow of cerebrospinal fluid (CSF) through the foramen magnum with a resulting pressure differential between the subarachnoid space and the internal spinal cord. In some patients the syrinx may be small, extending only several centimeters, whereas in others it may extend as far as the length of the spinal cord. It is important to recognize these associated CNS malformations as they may influence the treatment required.

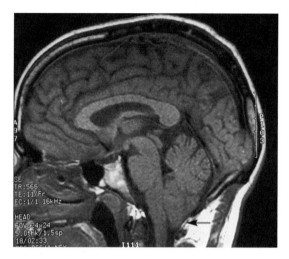

Figure 49-1. This sagittal magnetic resonance imaging scan shows the Chiari I malformation in a patient presenting with neck and arm pain. Note the position of the cerebellar tonsils relative to the foramen magnum (*arrow*).

Patient Presentation

The presentation of patients with Chiari I malformation will depend in part on the severity of the malformation as well as associated hydrocephalus or syringomyelia. One of the most common presenting symptoms is that of occipital headache. This symptom is probably caused by the distortion of the leptomeningeal structures at the site of the Chiari I malformation. The pain may radiate superiorly or inferiorly from the posterior skull base, often involving the neck or shoulder. Frequently it is associated with a decreased range of motion of the neck as the patient guards against movement that exacerbates the pain. Nuchal spasm may be evident as well. In those instances in which hydrocephalus is also present, patients may have a more global headache. Long tract findings may be present as well. Patients may have weakness in one or more extremities. They may also have sensory loss, either in the extremities or in the capelike distribution seen in patients with syringomyelia. Patients may be hyperreflexic or occasionally (in patients with syringomyelia) hyporeflexic.

Lower cranial neuropathy may occur with patients experiencing swallowing difficulties, weakness of shoulder shrug or neck rotation, poor gag, hoarseness, or stridor. These deficits may lead to frequent aspiration with resulting pneumonia. Vertigo with nystagmus may also occur. Apnea may rarely be a problem. These deficits can result from either compression of the medulla or from a syrinx extending into the bulbar area.

Differential Diagnosis

The differential diagnosis for Chiari I malformation includes many of the other abnormalities of the craniovertebral junction. These include basilar invagination, os odontoideum, or atlantoaxial degeneration (from a variety of causes). Cervical spondylosis should also be included in the differential diagnosis, as should syringomyelia from its other causes. Tumors of the foramen magnum may present similarly as well. Last, one must consider neurologic disorders such as multiple sclerosis.

Evaluation

Magnetic resonance imaging (MRI) scans provide the best characterization of the neural elements at the craniovertebral junction and thus MRI is the preferred study for evaluating a Chiari I malformation (Figure 49-1). Often the Chiari malformation is identified on cervical spine MRI scans when evaluating a patient for symptoms that are thought to be related to cervical spondylosis. The extent of the cerebellar tonsillar descent can be established

Figure 49-2. This sagittal magnetic resonance imaging scan shows a Chiari I malformation, syringomyelia, and hydrocephalus. Note the enlarged fourth ventricle on this view. The patient presented with headache, blurry vision, and gait difficulty. Symptoms resolved solely with a ventriculoperitoneal shunt.

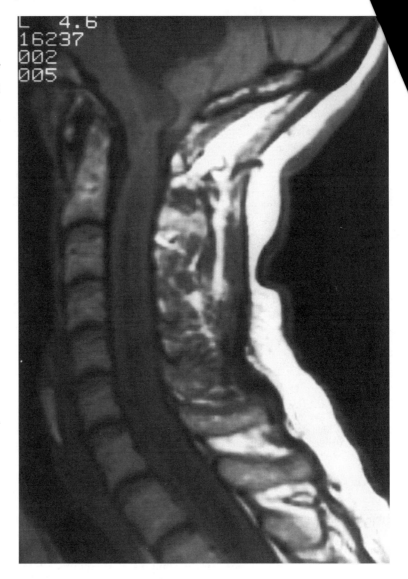

quite readily on MRI scans. However, this study alone is insufficient for evaluating the patient; one must pay attention to any associated structural abnormalities by ruling out hydrocephalus and syringomyelia, as these other abnormalities may influence treatment. MRI scans of the brain or computed tomographic (CT) scanning are sufficient for evaluating the presence of hydrocephalus. MRI scans of the spine are preferred for evaluating syringomyelia (Figure 49-2). In those patients in whom MRI is not feasible, CT cisternography with myelographic techniques can demonstrate the cerebellar tonsillar herniation.

Treatment

Treatment of Chiari I malformation is surgical. The treatment depends on which associated abnormalities, if any, are identified (Figure 49-3). If hydrocephalus is identified, the first step in treatment should be placement of a ventriculoperitoneal shunt. Reduction of intracranial pressure may reduce the displacement of the cerebellar tonsils and improve the patient's symptoms significantly. If other bony abnormalities such as basilar invagination coexist with the Chiari malformation, then initial treatment to address the anterior brain

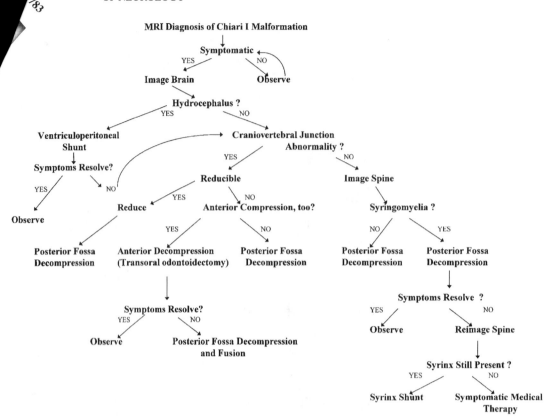

Figure 49-3. Management of Chiari I malformation. (MRI = magnetic resonance imaging.) (Portions adapted from JG Piper, AH Menezes. Chiari Malformation in the Adult. In AH Menezes, VKH Sonntag [eds], Principles of Spinal Surgery. New York: McGraw–Hill, 1996;379–394.)

stem compression may be required before decompression of the tonsillar herniation posteriorly. A transoral odontoidectomy is usually necessary in these cases, followed by a posterior decompression and fusion.

If hydrocephalus is not present or if the patient continues to have symptoms related to the Chiari malformation after a ventriculoperitoneal shunt is placed, treatment should then proceed to a posterior fossa decompression. This consists of cervical laminectomies extending the span of the tonsillar herniation with removal of the occipital bone in the area of the foramen magnum. A duraplasty is also performed to enlarge the cisterna magna. This involves opening the dura and grafting the dura with pericranium, fascia, or a dural substitute. Any identified arachnoidal adhesions or banding should be lysed microscopically before the grafting is performed.

Results of treatment depend on the degree as well as the duration of the symptoms. Good results are often encountered in patients who have mild symptoms or in patients who have symptoms involving only cerebellar dysfunction or headache. Patients diagnosed late in their course or who have developed lower cranial neuropathy tend to do less well. Therefore, it is important to establish the diagnosis early in the patient's course when symptoms are at their mildest.

Skeletal Abnormalities Involving the Craniovertebral Junction

A variety of malformations involving the bony components of the craniovertebral junction can present in adulthood. These abnormalities involve relationships of the foramen magnum, the axis, the atlas

Figure 49-4. This sagittal magnetic resonance imaging scan shows an abnormality at the craniovertebral junction. Although difficult to classify, it seems most consistent with assimilation of the atlas. Note the severe posterior compression at the foramen magnum, which caused a progressive myelopathy.

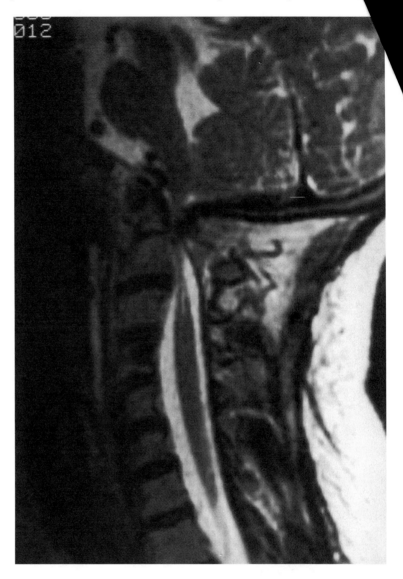

and odontoid process, the clivus, and the squamosal portion of the occipital bone. Occasionally these bony abnormalities may also be associated with Chiari I malformation.

Basilar invagination, also known as platybasia, usually is associated with a shortened clivus, which is also oriented more horizontally than normal. This abnormality causes the odontoid process to protrude into the posterior fossa. The pons or medulla is compressed or kinked, causing the neurologic symptoms associated with the malformation. Approximately 30% of these patients will also have an associated Chiari I malformation.

Assimilation of the atlas occurs when the ring of C1 fails to develop segmentally separate from the foramen magnum (Figure 49-4). This abnormality can lead to an irreducible basilar invagination or ligamentous instability of the atlantoaxial joint. Again, an associated Chiari malformation is prevalent, occurring in more than 40% of these patients.

The odontoid process may also develop abnormally. The dens may be hypoplastic, causing associated ligamentous maldevelopment with atlantoaxial instability. An os odontoideum, in which the odontoid tip does not fuse with the main body of the

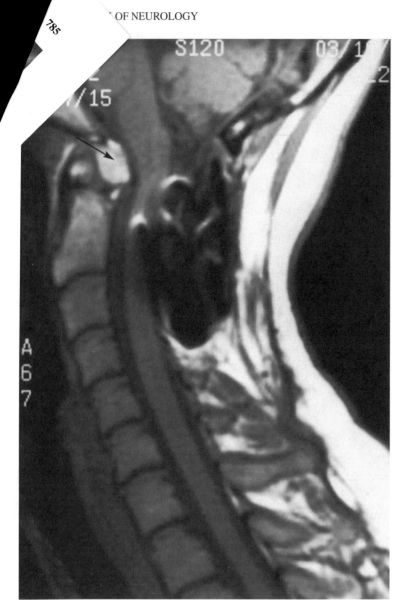

Figure 49-5. This sagittal magnetic resonance imaging scan shows an os odontoideum, with the superior portion of the dens (*arrow*) clearly separated from the rest of the odontoid process. Because of the instability at the craniovertebral junction, the patient presented with myelopathy. The artifact posterior to the spinal cord is related to a previous fusion.

dens, can lead to development of cruciate ligament incompetence, which is also associated with atlantoaxial instability (Figure 49-5).

A number of inherited disorders are associated with abnormalities of the craniovertebral junction. Atlantoaxial instability may be present in up to 25% of patients with Down syndrome (trisomy 21), although less than 1% are actually symptomatic (Figure 49-6). Atlantoaxial instability also occurs frequently in achondroplasia, although the presentation is typically in childhood. Patients with osteogenesis imperfecta, an inherited disor-

der of excessive bone fragility, often develop basilar impression, which becomes progressive over time. A number of other skeletal dysplasias are associated with symptomatic abnormalities of the craniovertebral junction.

Patient Presentation

Patients with abnormalities of the craniovertebral junction may present with a number of different signs and symptoms. The most common presenta-

Figure 49-6. This lateral x-ray film of the cervical spine in a 35-year-old Down syndrome patient shows widening of the atlanto-odontoid joint (*arrows*). She presented with neck pain and urinary incontinence.

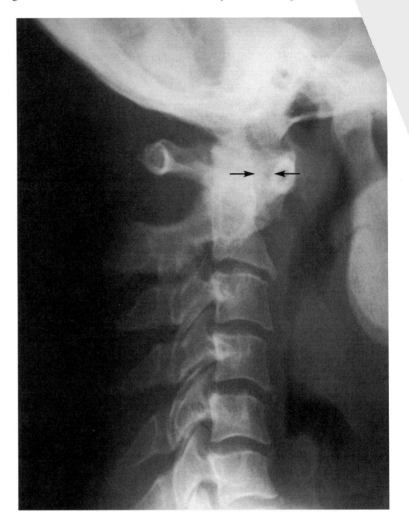

tion is myelopathy, which almost all symptomatic patients experience. Motor and sensory deficits may be present. Motor deficits can occur as a hemiparesis or a paraparesis, either involving the upper extremities or the lower extremities. Quadriparesis is also possible, as is a central cord-type syndrome. Not infrequently, patients may experience bulbar signs with lower cranial nerve deficits. Almost one in four patients experiences tinnitus or decreased hearing. Patients may also suffer from vertebrobasilar insufficiency with syncope, a change in consciousness, or transient visual loss. These symptoms relate to instability causing intermittent compression of the vertebral arteries. Pain is a frequent symptom. Usually patients complain of occipital headache or neck discomfort.

Of note, many previous asymptomatic patients begin to show evidence of their abnormality after minor trauma. The traumatic event may exacerbate the condition by further weakening fatiguing ligamentous structures, creating more instability. Alternatively, the trauma can directly injure neural structures at the site of compression by causing microvascular compromise or contusion.

Differential Diagnosis

The differential diagnosis must include the Chiari I malformation. As one might expect, the other considerations are the same as those discussed previously for Chiari I malformation.

...tients with craniovertebral junction ... must address several issues. First the ...normality must be clearly identified. The ...and location of the neural compression must ...etermined. Any associated CNS abnormalities ...ust also be identified. Last, skeletal stability must be assessed. MRI scans, especially sagittal images, demonstrate well the relationship of the bony and soft tissue abnormalities to the neural structures. MRI is also helpful for identifying whether a Chiari I malformation is present. Plain x-ray films and occasionally CT scans are helpful for defining the specific bony abnormalities present. Flexion/extension views on plain x-ray films can demonstrate gross instability.

Treatment

Treatment depends on the complete nature of the abnormality identified. Patients who have an unstable but reducible abnormality usually require closed reduction followed by immobilization in a halo vest or other orthotic device. A posterior operative fusion, usually from the occiput to at least C2, will definitively address the lesion. If the abnormality is irreducible, then the approach will depend on the site of neural compression. If, as in most patients with basilar invagination, the compression is anterior, then a transoral odontoidectomy is often necessary. For posterior compression, the removal of the posteriorly compressing elements is appropriate. If instability is present, a posterior fusion may also be necessary. Patients who have both anterior compression and instability may require a multi-staged approach consisting of a transoral odontoidectomy, then placement into a halo vest, followed by a posterior fusion.

Spinal Dysraphism with Tethering

Spinal dysraphic lesions may cause adults to develop slow dissolution in spinal cord or cauda equina function in two clinical settings. In the first instance, an infant or child who has undergone a prior repair of a myelomeningocele, meningocele, myeloschisis, lipomyelomeningocele, or filar fibrolipoma may require re-exploration at a later date. The patient may have achieved a neurologic plateau for a period of time; however, progressive dysfunction may surface again in adolescence or adulthood, during which motor and sensory root involvement of bowel, bladder, and lower extremities may again require surgical intervention.

In the second setting, the one that is addressed in this section, a more occult or subtle form of spinal dysraphism may slowly or, rarely, more rapidly present for the first time in adulthood. These problems include previously untreated small lipomyelomeningoceles, epidermoid cysts, diastematomyelia, and the fibrolipomas of the filum terminale. The lesion may occur with or without a concomitant cutaneous landmark such as a dimple, sinus tract, skin tag, hairy nevus, or midline "birthmark" or hemangioma. These abnormalities are often associated with the radiographic appearance of a low-lying conus medullaris, known as "tethering."

In a lipomyelomeningocele, a lipoma attached to a myeloschisis placode grows through dural and spina bifida defects into the subcutaneous tissues. A palpable mass is usually present. The spinal cord often is herniated out of the intravertebral canal with the neural tissue covered by fat (Figure 49-7).

Fibrolipoma of the filum terminale appears as a thickened filum that tethers the conus. It is usually more than 2 mm in diameter. A significant number of asymptomatic adults will also have this abnormality.

A diastematomyelia consists of a splitting of the spinal cord. This split spinal cord is often tethered by a bony, cartilaginous, or fibrous septum, which prevents free upward movement of the cord. Each hemicord usually has its own set of nerve roots.

Epidermoid cysts of the spinal cord consist of an epithelial membrane with central deposits of keratinized material (Figure 49-8). They are often associated with a dermal sinus and spina bifida.

Patient Presentation

Adult patients with spinal dysraphism usually present clinically with a spectrum of symptoms and findings that reflect a variegated, partial, or incomplete cauda equina syndrome or polyradiculopathy. A myelopathic or upper motor neuron pattern can

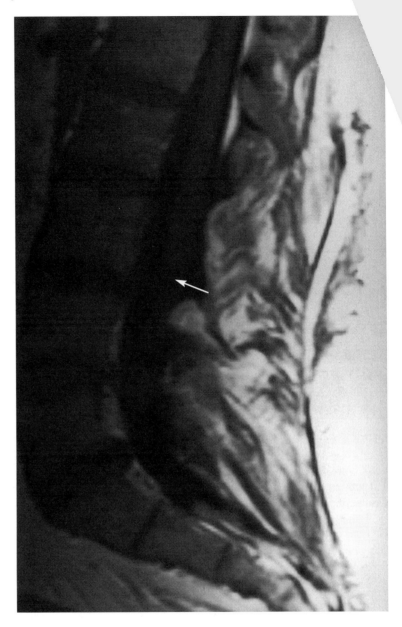

Figure 49-7. This sagittal magnetic resonance imaging scan shows the low-lying conus (*arrow*) tethered by a lipomyelomeningocele. The fat, hyperintense on this T1-weighted image, is attached to the cord.

also occur with a diastema situated above the conus. Symptoms can include back and leg pain, paresthesias and hypesthesia, progressive scoliosis, pes cavus deformity, muscle weakness, and urinary retention or incontinence. Pathophysiologic features have been ascribed to slowly progressive tension, torsion, and vascular compromise of the conus and nerve roots. Occasionally patients will present because of the cosmetic nature of the subcutaneous mass or the associated skin lesion. Although many of these patients had no previous symptoms, a portion of this population represents individuals whose symptoms were also present early on in life and were overlooked or static or patients who were believed by an earlier generation of neurosurgeons not to be operative candidates.

In our series of 85 patients with symptoms and signs of spinal dysraphism, 34 were infants with a clinically obvious diagnosis of myeloschisis, 38 were children, and 13 were adults. This adult popu-

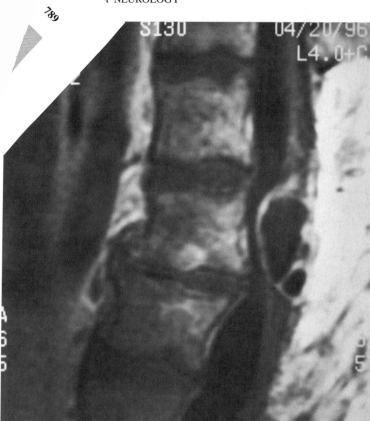

Figure 49-8. This sagittal magnetic resonance imaging scan shows an intraspinal lesion with lipomatous and epidermoid components tethering the cord.

lation consisted of eight women and five men. Clinical presentation occurred between the late teens through the early 50s. The primary diagnosis covered the spectrum of dysraphic diseases and included five patients with lipomyelomeningocele, two with diastematomyelia, two with intradural epidermoid, three with fibrolipoma of the filum terminale, and one with myelomeningocele. Symptoms and signs in this group included a unilateral mixed (motor/sensory) radiculopathy in eight patients, back and leg pain in nine patients (the root distribution was always L5 or S1), a bilateral mixed radiculopathy (again involving L5 and S1 roots) in four patients, a fatty subcutaneous mass in five patients, and deteriorating bladder function in three patients.

Evaluation

The diagnosis of a dysraphic lesion should be suspected clinically in a patient with back or leg pain, urinary symptoms, or radicular symptoms in association with any midline cutaneous anomaly of the thoracolumbosacral spine. A plain film evaluation will often reveal an occult spina bifida, but anterior or posterior fusion anomalies, hemivertebrae, kyphoscoliosis, and a diastema can also be revealed. MRI provides detailed structural information. It should be directed at the level of a normally placed conus as well as the clinically warranted levels below and above. The level of the conus and the lesion itself is well defined on sagittal, coronal, and axial views. A postoperative study should also be carried out to establish a baseline with which to compare any future studies obtained in the face of progressive or recurrent symptoms and signs. Urodynamic studies and urologic and orthopedic consultations are also mandated.

Treatment

Definitive treatment consists only of surgical intervention, the objective of which is to halt progression of neurologic decompensation and, it is hoped, to improve or eliminate pain. Surgical adjuncts include the use of an operating microscope, laser or ultrasonically driven dissection, and neurophysiologic monitoring.

In lipomyelomeningoceles, the fatty mass is usually resected. Separating the myeloschisis plate from the spinal cord will allow the cord to retract superiorly. Similarly, cutting the fibrolipoma of the filum frees the tethering of the cord. The septum of the diastematomyelia must be resected to de-tether the abnormality. In epidermoid cysts, the dermal sinus must also be excised, if present.

In our series of 13 patients, 17 operations were performed, with 14 utilizing intraoperative electromyography. Two patients had had prior procedures. One patient had a cosmetic reduction of her lesion to the level of the fascia; four underwent complete and four underwent partial resection of a fibrolipoma or epidermoid; two underwent excision and adhesiolysis; and two operations were resections of a diastema.

The natural history of patients with these lesions is one of slow progression. Surgical intervention may not halt this process, but it usually does. Pain is usually relieved by surgery as well. Re-operation, not uncommon in children and infants, appears to be justified in an adult with progressive neurologic dysfunction or pain. In our series, four patients received cosmetic improvement, and eight noted relief of pain. Four patients noted improvement in strength and four in sensation. One patient's genitourinary function was improved. No patients were made worse by the procedures utilized. There were no occurrences of meningitis. One superficial wound infection was treated with local care, and one CSF leak required a superficial repair. Four patients required a second operative procedure within a year of their initial operation for symptom recurrence.

Arachnoid Cyst

Arachnoid cysts are congenital abnormalities adjacent to the subarachnoid space. They consist of a membrane formed from arachnoid cells and laminated collagen bundles containing CSF. Occasionally there may be clusters and whorls of mesothelial cells. The underlying brain is normal. Although they may occur almost anywhere within the neural axis, the most common site is within the sylvian fis-

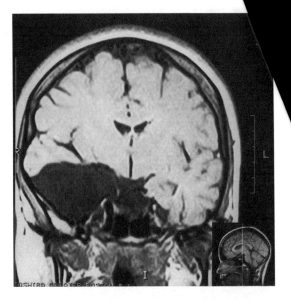

Figure 49-9. This coronal magnetic resonance imaging scan shows a middle fossa arachnoid cyst in a young woman presenting with headache. The lesion, compressing the temporal lobe, has the same intensity as cerebrospinal fluid.

sure/middle fossa (Figure 49-9). They can also be found on the cerebral convexity, in the suprasellar cistern, the cerebellopontine cistern, the interhemispheric fissure, the pineal area, the posterior fossa midline (Figure 49-10), and within the ventricles.

The congenital nature of arachnoid cysts has been proposed based on their usual presentation in children. Other features indicative of a congenital development include the often bilateral nature of sylvian fissure cysts, their occurrence in siblings, the splitting of the arachnoid membrane at the margin of the cyst, the failure of the cyst cavity to collapse completely after evacuation of the cyst, the absence of periopercular development in patients with sylvian fissure cysts, normal gyral and sulcal formation beneath the cysts, and focal expansion of the skull adjacent to the cyst even if there is no evidence of a shift or elevated intracranial pressure.

Patient Presentation

Patients may present with a variety of symptoms depending on the location of the cyst. In those instances in which intracranial pressure is elevated,

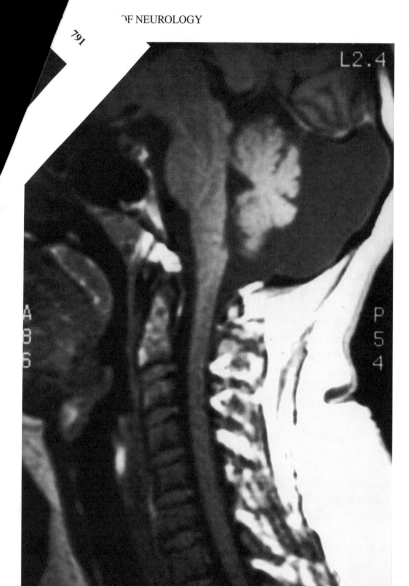

Figure 49-10. This sagittal magnetic resonance imaging scan shows a midline posterior fossa arachnoid cyst compressing the cerebellum. The patient presented with headache and neck spasm.

patients may present with headache. Cysts adjacent to epileptogenic areas may be associated with seizures. Suprasellar cysts can be associated with endocrinopathy, symptoms of hydrocephalus, or visual compromise (such as bitemporal hemianopia). Other cranial nerves can be affected, such as hearing loss or vestibular dysfunction caused by cysts in the cerebellopontine angle. Cerebellopontine angle cysts may also cause incoordination if the cerebellar hemisphere is compressed. Hemiparesis may occur from very large sylvian fissure cysts or convexity cysts. Cysts in the pineal region may be associated with Parinaud's syndrome. Although patients may have signs of intracranial pressure or focal neurologic deficits, often the only abnormality will be an expanded, deformed skull.

Usually, symptomatic arachnoid cysts are identified during childhood. Presentation in adulthood is often but not always related to an episode of head trauma. Hemorrhage may occur into the cyst, which leads to acute elevation in intracranial pressure and symptoms. Alternatively, trauma may lead to a tear in the cyst wall with development of a chronic subdural fluid collection and symptoms related to compression of the brain. It is also not uncommon for a patient to be diagnosed with an arachnoid cyst discovered incidentally after minor head trauma.

Differential Diagnosis

The differential diagnosis for arachnoid cysts includes the gamut of intracranial masses that can cause the patient's specific symptoms and signs. Among the entities to consider are epidermoid cysts, tumors (either primary or metastatic), large vascular malformations, cerebral abscesses, hydrocephalus, or chronic subdural fluid collections. Radiography usually differentiates the various considerations.

Evaluation

As with most CNS abnormalities, MRI has become the diagnostic modality of choice for the evaluation of arachnoid cysts. Typically the lesions have the same intensity characteristics as CSF. They are hypointense on T1-weighted images (see Figures 49-9 and 49-10) and hyperintense on T2-weighted images. They tend to have smooth borders, which is particularly helpful in differentiating arachnoid cysts from epidermoids. Compression of the surrounding brain is often noted, but the degree of compression is usually less than one would expect given the size of the mass. On CT scans, one can see thinning and distortion of the adjacent bone with focal expansion of the skull. The lesion does not enhance with gadolinium on MRI scans or intravenous contrast on CT scans.

Treatment

Treatment of an arachnoid cyst depends on the clinical status of the patient. For those patients in whom an arachnoid cyst is identified incidentally or those who present solely with seizures, observation of the cyst may be most appropriate. The patient can undergo imaging at sequential intervals to see if the cyst enlarges, which it typically will not do. For a symptomatic cyst, two options can be considered. One option is placement of a cyst shunt, usually with diversion of the cyst fluid to the peritoneal cav-

ity. Alternatively, craniotomy with fenestration the cyst into surrounding CSF cisterns can be formed. The value of craniotomy is that it can obviate the need for permanent placement of a foreign body. On the other hand, surgical risks are higher than for placement of a shunt and the cyst can recur on occasion.

Symptoms of elevated intracranial pressure related to the arachnoid cyst usually resolve after treatment. However, the brain often will not completely re-expand to fill the volume previously occupied by the cyst. The issues regarding seizure resolution are unknown. Seizures may be related to the developmental dysgenesis of the adjacent cerebral cortex and may continue even after treatment of the cyst.

Hydrocephalus Secondary to Aqueductal Stenosis

Although most congenital causes of hydrocephalus present in infancy and childhood, occasionally patients with congenital aqueductal stenosis will not become symptomatic until adulthood. In aqueductal stenosis, the cerebral aqueduct of Sylvius is significantly narrowed. This narrowing can recur as the result of surrounding gliosis, forking of the aqueduct, true narrowing of the aqueduct, or formation of a septum within the aqueduct. Not uncommonly, this malformation is hereditary.

Patient Presentation

Patients may present acutely or chronically with the signs and symptoms of elevated intracranial pressure. These symptoms can include headache, with or without papilledema or loss of retinal venous pulsations. Patients may have changes in their mental status consisting of a decrease in their level of consciousness or difficulties with their cognitive skills. Double vision from paresis of cranial nerve VI may be present. Other ocular findings include light-near dissociation and decreased upgaze. Last, patients may have gait difficulties from a spastic paraparesis. None of these symptoms is specific for either aqueductal stenosis or hydrocephalus from any cause, but they do suggest that the diagnosis of hydrocephalus should be considered.

ate imaging study for confirm-
is depends on the status of the
ts who present acutely with a severe
decrement in their level of conscious-
uld be evaluated emergently with a CT
which can identify the hydrocephalus. MRI
vides better anatomic detail. The sagittal view
can be particularly helpful, showing the narrowing
of the cerebral aqueduct. The lateral ventricles are
enlarged, as is the third ventricle, but the fourth
ventricle is quite small. The aqueduct can either be
seen to be narrowed or occasionally a septum can
be identified within it.

Treatment

The most definitive treatment option is placement
of a ventricular shunt, usually to the peritoneum.
The procedure is relatively straightforward and well
tolerated by most patients. However, the permanent
piece of indwelling hardware is required for the
remainder of the life of the patient, and shunts may
malfunction with recurrence of symptoms. An alternative available because of the noncommunicating
nature of the hydrocephalus of aqueductal stenosis
is a third ventriculostomy. This procedure consists
of either a stereotactic or endoscopic perforation of
the thinned floor of the third ventricle, which can
be performed with relatively minimal complications. It allows the CSF to bypass the aqueductal
stenosis and to circulate around the cerebral convexities from the opening in the floor of the third
ventricle to be absorbed by the arachnoid granulations. Third ventriculostomy can be effective for
many patients. However, a significant number of
patients with congenital aqueductal stenosis will
also have poor absorption of CSF by the arachnoid
granulations. Therefore, despite having the third
ventriculostomy, they may continue to have symptoms related to hydrocephalus and require a subsequent shunting procedure.

Suggested Reading

Alvarez N, Rubin L. Atlantoaxial instability in adults with
    Down syndrome: a clinical and radiological survey.
    Applied Res Mental Retardation 1986;7:67.
Baldwin H, Rekate H, Sontag V. Diagnosis, surgical man-
    agement and outcome of the adult tethered cord syn-
    drome. BNI Q 1991;7:16.
Baerji NK, Millar JHD. Chiari malformation presenting in
    adult life. Its relationship to syringomyelia. Brain 1974;
    97:157.
Di Lorenzo N, Fortuna A, Guidetti B. Craniovertebral junc-
    tion malformations. Clinicoradiographic findings, long-
    term results, and surgical indications in 63 cases. J
    Neurosurg 1982;57:603.
Harkey HL, Crockard HA, Stevens JM, et al. The operative
    management of basilar impression in osteogenesis imper-
    fecta. Neurosurgery 1990;27:782.
Menezes AH, Ryken TC: Abnormalities of the Craniocervi-
    cal Junction. In WR Cheek (ed), Pediatric Neurosurgery
    (3rd ed). Philadelphia: Saunders, 1994;139–158.
Menezes AH, VanGilder JC, Graf CJ, et al. Craniocervical
    abnormalities. A comprehensive approach. J Neurosurg
    1980;53:444.
Milhorat TH. Hydrocephalus: Pathophysiology and Clinical
    Features. In RH Wilkins, SS Rengachary (eds), Neuro-
    surgery. New York: McGraw–Hill, 1985;2135–2139.
Pang D, Wilberger J. Tethered cord syndrome in adults. J
    Neurosurg 1982;57:32.
Piper JG, Menezes AH. Chiari Malformation in the Adult. In
    AH Menezes, VKH Sonntag (eds), Principles of Spinal
    Surgery. New York: McGraw–Hill, 1996;379–394.
Pueschel SM, Herndon JH, Gelch MM, et al. Symptomatic
    atlandoaxial subluxation in persons with Down syn-
    drome. J Pediatr Orthop 1984;4:682.
Raffel C, McComb JG. Arachnoid Cysts. In WR Cheek (ed),
    Pediatric Neurosurgery (3rd ed). Philadelphia: Saunders,
    1994;104–110.
Reigel DH, McClone DG. Tethered Spinal Cord. In WR
    Cheek (ed), Pediatric Neurosurgery (3rd ed). Philadel-
    phia: Saunders, 1994;77–95.
VanGilder JC, Menezes AH. Craniovertebral junction abnor-
    malities. Clin Neurosurg 1983;30:514.

Chapter 50

Rare Hereditary Storage Disorders in Adults

Jean-Jacques Martin and Chantal Ceuterick

Chapter Plan

Inborn errors of metabolism are well known in children. Strategies of investigations have been well explored and advanced with molecular biology techniques. It has become apparent that similar disorders may exist in adults but are seldom recognized. Some lysosomal diseases are caused by the same enzymatic deficiencies that cause diseases in children. It is therefore difficult to explain why a molecular defect present since conception becomes expressed many years later. Other disorders such as the adult type of neuronal ceroid lipofuscinosis belong to a group of conditions that have infantile, late infantile, or juvenile variants. Although they share some common clinical and anatomic-pathologic features, they are in fact different in terms of molecular genetics, gene products, and pathogenetic mechanisms.

With the exception of some specific clinical patterns, most of the adult patients present with various symptoms such as dementia, psychosis, pyramidal signs, dystonia, ataxia, epilepsy, and peripheral neuropathy. In many of the adult-onset storage disorders, the accent is often first on psychiatric symptoms, followed by the emergence of neurologic signs. On neurology wards, such patients may receive a diagnosis of neurodegenerative disorder. More common causes should be considered before one realizes that one could be dealing with a storage disease.

This chapter addresses some rare metabolic conditions occurring in adults. Sometimes the disease starts in adolescence and has a protracted course, which

Table 50-1. Adult Forms (Late-Onset) Metabolic Disorders Affecting the Gray Matter

Disease	Histopathologic Features	Neurologic Features
Adult type of neuronal ceroid lipofuscinosis (Kufs' disease)	Intraneuronal storage of osmiophilic inclusions with fingerprint, curvilinear, and rectilinear profiles; storage in smooth muscle cells, eccrine sweat glands, skeletal muscle fibers	Progressive myoclonus epilepsy, dementia, ataxia, pyramidal and extrapyramidal signs, no blindness, no pigmentary retinal degeneration
Niemann-Pick disease type C	Intraneuronal storage of pleomorphic cytoplasmic bodies; sea-blue histiocytes in the bone marrow	Cerebellar syndrome, dementia, down-gaze palsy
GM$_2$ gangliosidosis	Membranous cytoplasmic bodies	Motor neuron disease
GM$_1$ gangliosidosis	Neurovisceral storage of membranous cytoplasmic bodies and of vacuoles with electron-lucent contents	Extrapyramidal signs such as dystonia, dysarthria, facial grimacing and parkinsonism, mild intellectual impairment
Fabry's disease	Dense myelinlike bodies in endothelial cells, smooth muscle cells, perithelial cells	Cerebrovascular complications, mainly in the vertebrobasilar circulation; peripheral neuropathy; autonomous neuropathy; bouts of excruciating pains
Mucopolysaccharidoses (many different types, including Scheie's, Hunter's, Sanfilippo, and Morquio's syndromes)	Zebra-like inclusions	Mental retardation, behavioral abnormalities, cervical myelopathy resulting from a spinal stenosis
Oligosaccharidoses (many different conditions, including sialidoses, galactosialidosis, and mannosidosis)	Membrane-bound inclusions with electron-lucent contents and/or lamellar profiles	Ataxia, psychomotor retardation, epilepsy, deafness
Mucolipidosis IV	Polymorphous lamellar inclusions and membranous cytoplasmic bodies	Severe psychomotor retardation
Gaucher's disease type 1	Tubular inclusions in Gaucher cells	Cerebral embolism, spinal cord compression, neuropathies, plexopathies, or spontaneous hematomyelia

does not prevent the patients from reaching adulthood. Gray matter diseases are discussed first, or at least those with a prevalence toward lesions in the neurons (Table 50-1), then the white matter diseases (Table 50-2), and finally less easily classifiable conditions.

Methods of Investigation

Many of the modern advances in the management of hereditary disorders affecting the nervous system are the result of gene mapping of the disease locus using molecular biology techniques, defining the presence of mutations, and assessing the nature of the gene product. Enzymatic assays of leukocytes or cultured fibroblasts preceded the positional cloning of the gene abnormalities and remain useful in the diagnosis (Table 50-3).

Morphology still has a role to play, but with changing indications, and this applies also to adult patients affected by rare storage disorders. Because late-onset neurometabolic disorders are much less frequent, the diagnosis will be more difficult to make and pathologic examinations of brain and extraneural tissues have been less frequently reported. Diagnostic morphologic investigations using electron microscopic (EM) examination of tissue biopsy specimens and to some extent light microscopy remain useful. EM studies are necessary when the basic biochemical defect remains unknown, and at the present time, the diagnosis of several diseases still depends entirely on ultrastructural elements. Less invasive biopsy procedures should be used. Biopsies are mandatory for older patients whose condition may be misdiagnosed or undiagnosed because of an unusual clinical course,

Table 50-2. Adult Forms (Late-Onset) Metabolic Disorders Affecting the White Matter

Disease	Histopathologic Features	Clinical Features
Schilder's disease (myelinoclastic type)	Giant multiple sclerosislike lesions	(1) Dementia, spastic paraplegia, optic atrophy; (2) in bursts; (3) pseudotumoral form; (4) psychiatric symptoms
Adrenoleukodystrophy	Demyelination with caudorostral or rostrocaudal progression; free spicular inclusions in glial cells, Schwann cells, and adrenal cells	Psychosis, intellectual decline, visual problems, cerebellar ataxia, quadriplegia
Adrenomyeloneuropathy	Focal demyelination in posterior columns and lateral spinal tracts; free spicular inclusions in Schwann cells	Spastic paraparesis, peripheral neuropathy, sphincter disturbances, disturbances of the proprioception
Metachromatic leukodystrophy	Demyelination, brown metachromatic deposits, lysosomal tuffstone bodies and priomatic inclusions in neurons, oligoglia, macrophages, and Schwann cells	Variegated psychiatric manifestations, ataxia, paraparesis, pyramidal signs, and polyneuropathy
Globoid cell leuko-dystrophy (Krabbe's disease)	Demyelination with globoid cells in the white matter, curved spicular inclusions in central and peripheral nervous system	Progressive tetraparesis, pseudobulbar palsy, optic atrophy, ataxia, dementia
Alexander's disease	Rosenthal's fibers in the astrocytes; large amounts of tightly packed material merging with aggregates of osmiophilic material	Intermittent signs resembling bouts of multiple sclerosis with ataxia, pyramidal signs, and bulbar dysfunction
Orthochromatic or sudanophilic leuko-dystrophies	Pallor of the myelin, isomorphic fibrillary gliosis, variable amounts of neutral fats in macro- and microglia, islands of better-preserved myelin in the Löwenberg-Hill type	Progressive mild or pronounced cognitive deterioration, pyramidal features
Cerebrotendinous xanthomatosis	Deposition of cholestanol in variable places of the central nervous system with macrophages and glial reaction	Behavioral problems, epilepsy, psychomotor retardation, dementia, pyramidal, extrapyramidal, cerebellar, spinal, and peripheral nerve signs

nonspecific neurologic manifestations, or normal enzyme activities. The definitive diagnosis relies on a combination of clinical, biochemical, genetic, and morphologic data.

Skin and Conjunctival Biopsies

The utility of skin and conjunctiva has been well documented, and diagnostic morphologic criteria have been established in a large number of neurometabolic disorders. To get maximal diagnostic morphologic information in late-onset disorders, one must keep in mind that ultrastructural lesions are less severe or less easy to find than in young patients. Additional biopsy tissue may sometimes be necessary when the skin biopsy specimen is not informative. Skin is more suitable than conjunctiva because more diversified structures may be examined, such as eccrine sweat glands and smooth muscle cells as well as numerous terminal axonal endings close to eccrine sweat glands or lying between smooth muscle cells. Skin biopsy remains a valuable noninvasive diagnostic procedure even in adult-onset neurometabolic disorders with a still-unknown biochemical defect such as in the neuronal ceroid lipofuscinoses (NCLFs), Niemann-Pick type C disease, and Lafora's disease. Each major subtype of NCLF is characterized by granular osmiophilic deposits, membrane-bound curvilinear profiles (CPs), rectilinear profiles (RPs), and fingerprint profiles (FPs). In the adult form, or Kufs' disease, mixed CPs, RPs, and FPs are only present in eccrine sweat glands. Because FPs are occasionally found in eccrine sweat glands from non-NCLF adult patients, however, other tissues must be examined to confirm the diagnosis.

Peripheral Nerve Biopsy

Although peripheral nerves may be damaged in many lysosomal and nonlysosomal disorders, their

Table 50-3. Methods of Investigation

Clinical
    Clinical features
    Inheritance
    Neurologic examination
    Neuroradiology
    Neurophysiology
        Electromyography and conduction velocities
        Somatosensory evoked potentials
        Brain stem evoked potentials
        Central motor conduction
        Electroretinography
        Visual evoked potentials
        Electroencephalography
    Neuropsychology
Clinical laboratory
    Urine
        Oligosaccharides
        Mucopolysaccharides
        Amino acids
        Organic acids
    Serum
        Pyruvate and lactate
        Carnitine
        Very long chain fatty acids
        Amino acids
        Phytanic acid
Morphologic studies
    Skin and conjunctival biopsies
        Lysosomal storage disorders, neuronal ceroid lipofus-
          cinoses, neuroaxonal dystrophy, Lafora's disease
    Peripheral nerve biopsy
        Essentially the same disorders with a better quanti-
          tative evaluation of the lesions
    Skeletal muscle biopsy
        The same plus mitochondrial diseases in combination
          with study of respiratory chain complexes and of
          mitochondrial DNA
    Bone marrow biopsy
        Sea-blue histiocytes in Niemann-Pick disease type C
          and Gaucher cells in Gaucher's disease
    Rectal biopsy
        When neurons must be examined (e.g., in adult
          neuronal ceroid lipofuscinosis)
    Brain biopsy
        When other methods have failed (e.g., for Alexander's
          disease)
    Liver biopsy
        Peroxisomal diseases
Enzyme studies
    Urine, leukocytes, cultured fibroblasts
Molecular genetic analysis
    Leukocytes, muscle biopsy

biopsy constitutes a more invasive diagnostic procedure. Schwann cells of myelinated and unmyelinated axons, axonal structures, and endoneurial endothelial cells and fibroblasts are screened. Peripheral nerve biopsies are more frequently used for patients with a late-onset and slower course of disease, such as in adult forms of metachromatic leukodystrophy (MLD), Krabbe's globoid cell leukodystrophy (GLD), and adrenomyeloneuropathy (AMN). If cutaneous myelinated nerve twigs are missing or do not show spicular inclusions, such as may be the case in AMN, a peripheral nerve biopsy specimen must be obtained to demonstrate the characteristic electron-lucent spicular clefts in Schwann cells. The evaluation of the storage density and accompanying lesions such as demyelination and remyelination are better quantified and evaluated on a nerve biopsy specimen.

Skeletal Muscle Biopsy

Skeletal muscle may also be affected in many neurometabolic disorders. Apart from muscle fibers, other cells, such as satellite cells, endomysial endothelial cells, fibroblasts, and intramuscular nerve fascicles, may be examined. Combined skin and skeletal muscle biopsies are useful for a diagnosis of Kufs' disease. Muscle biopsy is also necessary to discover ragged-red fibers with altered mitochondria showing abnormal cristae configuration and paracrystalline inclusions in mitochondrial encephalomyopathies.

Bone Marrow Biopsy

Numerous Gaucher cells with characteristic bundles of twisted tubular inclusions are found in the adult (type 1) non-neuronopathic form of Gaucher's disease. Sea-blue histiocytes and foam cells are found in patients and in heterozygotes with Niemann-Pick disease type A and C or juvenile dystonic lipidosis.

Rectal Biopsy

A full-thickness rectal wall biopsy procedure is required to obtain myenteric plexuses with autonomic neurons when neurons are best examined, such as in Kufs' disease. Other cells, such as Schwann cells and smooth muscle cells, can be simultaneously examined.

Brain Biopsy

Alexander's disease can be only confirmed by a brain biopsy, in which Rosenthal fibers will be found in astrocytic processes. A brain biopsy is the last resort when other alternative biopsy methods have failed, such as in Kufs' disease.

Liver Biopsy

Less frequently used is liver biopsy, which may be important in some peroxisomal diseases in which peroxisomes are visualized by cytochemical and immunocytochemical analysis.

Adult Forms of Gray Matter Disorders

Neuronal Ceroid Lipofuscinosis

Adult neuronal ceroid lipofuscinosis (ANCLF), or Kufs' disease, is clinically distinct from the other neuronal ceroid lipofuscinoses (NCLFs). The storage of lipopigments has been predominantly reported in neurons as opposed to the other forms of NCLFs, in which the storage affects the nervous system, visceral organs, conjunctiva, and skin. ANCLF is a rare condition that is difficult to diagnose. In fact, more than 50% of the reported cases of Kufs' disease are not ANCLF and very likely correspond to a heterogeneous spectrum of lipidoses. Many other diseases, such as late-onset lipidoses, may indeed mimic the adult NCLF phenotype.

In ANCLF, as in the other forms of NCLFs, an accumulation of autofluorescent lipopigments in neuronal perikarya and in axonal hillocks is observed in the isocortex and allocortex, the basal ganglia, the thalamus, the brain stem nuclei, the cerebellar dentate nucleus, and the neurons of the anterior horns in the spinal cord. Cerebellar atrophy is present. Storage pigments in neurons of NCLF brains have been shown to be immunoreactive with monoclonal antibodies directed against the 17–24 amino acid residues of amyloid β-protein, as in aging neuronal lipofuscin and Alzheimer's disease (AD). This was confirmed by the ultrastructural localization of the immunoreactivity on CPs, and to a lesser extent on FPs, suggesting that the processing of amyloid β-protein precursor could be defective in NCLF brains as well as in AD and perhaps also in the aging brain. EM examination of the lipopigments reveals membrane-bound inclusions with a combination of FPs, CPs, and RPs, creating a variegated spectrum in neurons, while CPs are found in skeletal muscle and CPs and FPs in eccrine sweat glands.

Various clinical and genetic phenotypes of ANCLF may be recognized:

1. Clinical phenotype A includes progressive myoclonus epilepsy with dementia, ataxia, and late-occurring pyramidal and extrapyramidal features. The vision is normal. No pigmentary retinal degeneration is noted. Marked photosensitivity is observed in some patients.
2. Clinical phenotype B is characterized by behavioral changes and dementia associated with motor disturbances such as cerebellar or extrapyramidal signs. Again, the vision is normal without pigmentary retinal degeneration. Facial dyskinesias are common. Some examples of the type B include epilepsy of a nonprogressive nature.

The disease starts mostly around the age of 30 years, but an onset during adolescence has been reported. Cases of late adult onset with clinical symptoms at age 60–65 years have also been described.

ANCLF is most often an autosomal recessive condition, but a few families have an autosomal dominant inheritance. It is important to stress that in contradistinction to the juvenile and protracted juvenile NCLFs, which can overlap with ANCLF because of prolonged survival, there is no pigmentary degeneration of the retina in ANCLF.

The diagnosis of ANCLF may be suggested by a careful evaluation of the ultrastructure of skin, muscle, and rectal biopsy specimens, but the diagnosis is fraught with many hazards. A brain biopsy might prove necessary to ascertain the diagnosis. The purpose of the biopsies is to detect osmiophilic inclusions containing varying patterns of CPs, RPs, and FPs. Factors complicating the interpretation are the ultrastructural heterogeneity of neuronal lipofuscin in the normal human cerebral cortex and the ultrastructural diversity of residual bodies in NCLFs.

Niemann-Pick Disease

The adult type B of the sphingomyelinase-deficient disease category is characterized by visceral manifestations such as hepatosplenomegaly, foam cells in the bone marrow, and diffuse infiltration of the lungs. There are no neurologic changes. In some cases, secondary complications occur, such as portal hypertension, respiratory problems, or generalized amyloidosis. An intermediate subacute form has also been described that satisfies the criteria for Niemann-Pick disease type B but with additional signs of neuronal involvement, such as retinal storage, peripheral neuropathy, mild neurologic signs, or psychiatric disorders.

Niemann-Pick disease type C (NPC, or dystonic juvenile lipidosis) is an entity distinct from Niemann-Pick disease types A and B. In contradistinction to Niemann-Pick types A and B, sphingomyelinase levels may be perfectly normal or secondarily decreased while visceral storage of sphingomyelin and cholesterol only increases to two or three times the normal values. Bis(monoacylglycero)phosphate accumulates moderately, whereas there is only a limited elevation of glucosylceramide or glucocerebroside levels. There is neuronal storage of neutral glycosphingolipids such as glucocerebroside and lactosylceramide. The primary defect is still unknown. It could be caused by defects in the intracellular transfer of endocytosed cholesterol from lysosomes. This could lead to a delayed induction of cellular cholesterol homeostatic regulations, to the accumulation of unesterified cholesterol in lysosomes, and to secondary alterations, such as a decrease in sphingomyelinase activity. Although many of the cases of NPC appear in late infancy, some patients may reach adult age; the progression is slower and the visceromegaly can remain inapparent. Among the main clinical signs, besides a cerebellar syndrome and a dementia, there is a supranuclear ophthalmoplegia affecting initially vertical eye movements and convergence and extending later on to all directions of gaze. Adult patients with NPC may present with features of chronic psychosis years before neurologic features occur. Progressive gait disturbances and supranuclear gaze dysfunction then appear. The most common initial signs are dysarthria (44%), dementia (31%), psychosis (25%), limb ataxia (25%), and gait ataxia (25%). The spleen is enlarged because of the storage of complex lipids such as sphingomyelin. One of the main laboratory features is the discovery of sea-blue histiocytes in the bone marrow. There is a deficiency of the stimulation of the biosynthesis of cholesterol esters from exogenous cholesterol in patients' fibroblasts.

NPC has also been described as DAF syndrome (*d*own-gaze, *a*taxia-athetosis, *f*oam cells). Niemann-Pick type D has been described only in people originating from Nova Scotia and resembles NPC.

Gangliosidoses

Clinical heterogeneity has been documented in patients with GM_2 gangliosidosis caused by hexosaminidase deficiency. The clinical presentation differs in function of the age at onset. The most classic forms are the infantile ones such as Tay-Sachs disease and Sandhoff's disease with megalencephaly, blindness, seizures, quadriparesis, and death in early childhood. An adult phenotype has been described that is characterized by a motor neuron disease. One can, for example, find adult GM_2 gangliosidosis presenting as a juvenile amyotrophic lateral sclerosis associated with a clinical picture of mild dementia or as a cerebellar ataxia and axonal motor-sensory peripheral neuropathy, while others are characterized by a spinal muscular atrophy. The neurologic involvement may increase with age. In general, most of the patients show evidence of multisystem degeneration in addition to motor neuron disease. Signs of intraneuronal storage are mainly found in the subcortical nuclei, the cerebellum, the brain stem, and the anterior horns of the spinal cord. Because of the main clinical symptoms, the differential diagnosis should include amyotrophic lateral sclerosis, Kugelberg-Welander spinal muscular atrophy, olivopontocerebellar atrophy, progressive supranuclear paralysis, spasmodic paraplegia, dystonia, psychoses, and dementias.

Sandhoff's disease is biochemically characterized by decreased activity of the two isoenzymes, hexosaminidase A, composed of α and β subunits, and hexosaminidase B, composed of β subunits only. It is caused by a mutation of a gene coding for the β subunits. The severity of the disease is correlated with the decrease in enzyme activity. In the classic infantile form, the activity of the isoenzymes of β-hexosaminidase is virtually zero, whereas residual activity has been detected in juvenile and adult forms. The latter can be expressed as a clinical picture of spinocerebellar degeneration with an autosomal recessive mode of inheritance.

GM$_1$ gangliosidosis is a hereditary neurovisceral disorder caused by a deficiency of the lysosomal acid β-galactosidase. Gene mutations causing different residual enzyme activities are related to the severity of the manifestations. Besides the infantile and late infantile/juvenile forms, there is an adult/chronic form. This rare form is clinically different from the infantile and late juvenile forms of the disorder. It is characterized by a protracted clinical course and extrapyramidal signs such as dystonia, dysarthria, gait and speech disturbances, facial grimacing, and parkinsonism. Intellectual impairment is mild if present. Histologically, the basal ganglia are predominantly involved, whereas the other areas of the central nervous system (CNS) are relatively unaffected. There is no cherry red spot, dysmorphism, or visceromegaly. There is no severe intellectual impairment. Some patients were followed with a diagnosis of cerebral palsy, torsion dystonia, parkinsonism, or striatonigral degeneration before the final diagnosis was established. Neuroimaging demonstrates abnormalities in the basal ganglia in most patients. Rare compound-heterozygous patients show more severe neurologic manifestations and a more rapid clinical course than those of homozygotes.

Fabry's Disease

Fabry's disease, or angiokeratoma corporis diffusum, is a sex-linked disorder resulting from an α-galactosidase deficiency. This deficiency leads to the progressive accumulation of glycosphingolipids, predominantly ceramide trihexoside, in lysosomes of the vascular endothelium. This storage in endothelial cells, smooth muscle cells, and perithelial cells of blood vessels produces a dolichoectasia of intracranial cerebral arteries and an occlusion of small vessels. It results in tissue ischemia and infarction, producing cardiac (myocardial failure or infarction, hypertrophic obstructive cardiomyopathy, dilated cardiomyopathy), renal, or cerebrovascular complications at a relatively young age. The average age at onset of cerebrovascular symptoms is 33.8 years for hemizygous individuals and 40.3 years for heterozygotes. The most frequent symp-

toms in decreasing order of frequency are hemiparesis, vertigo, diplopia, dysarthria, nystagmus, nausea and vomiting, headache, hemiataxia, and gait ataxia. The cerebrovascular manifestations of Fabry's disease are mainly caused by dilatative arteriopathy of the vertebrobasilar circulation. They recur frequently and carry a poor prognosis. Indeed the vertebrobasilar circulation is symptomatic in 67% of the hemizygotes and 60% of the heterozygotes, but the reason for this predilection is not clear. Intracerebral hemorrhage is sometimes found. Neuroimaging shows either a large infarct or multiple small infarcts. Angiography reveals elongated, ectatic, tortuous vertebral and basilar arteries, which could cause a reduction of blood flow or become obstructed, resulting in brain stem or cerebellar ischemia. Fabry's disease should be considered in the differential diagnosis of ischemic stroke in the young, especially if there are accompanying radiologic findings of dolichoectatic intracranial vessels.

Peripheral neuropathy and autonomous neuropathy are also part of the neurologic features. Characteristic skin lesions, anhidrosis associated with sweat gland failure, acroparesthesias, episodic crises of excruciating pains, and corneal and lenticular opacities are present in hemizygote males. Heterozygote females are either asymptomatic or express fewer signs of the disease, but sometimes they may exhibit symptoms similar to those of male patients. Intraneuronal storage of globotriaosylceramide or ceramide trihexoside has also been demonstrated by immunocytochemistry analysis in spinal cord, spinal ganglia, brain stem, amygdala, hypothalamus, substantia nigra, and cortex. This deposition could perhaps explain the lancinating limb pains because of dorsal root ganglia neuronopathy, primary small fiber peripheral neuropathy, and involvement of substantia gelatinosa neurons. The clinical expression of this highly selective neuronal involvement is not clear. Skin lesions, slit-lamp examination for corneal dystrophy, and enzymatic assay of α-galactosidase on leukocytes should support the diagnosis of Fabry's disease.

Mucopolysaccharidoses

The α-L-iduronidase deficiency diseases cover a spectrum of clinical severity ranging from the very severe Hurler's syndrome to the relatively mild

Scheie's syndrome through an intermediate Hurler-Scheie syndrome. The mildest Scheie's syndrome is compatible with normal intelligence, stature, and lifespan. The disease progresses slowly with cloudy corneas, joint stiffness, and aortic valve disease. In the intermediate Hurler-Scheie form, the patient may survive until early adulthood.

Hunter's syndrome is a hereditary X-linked recessive disease characterized by the accumulation of dermatan and heparan sulfate in the tissues as a result of a deficiency in iduronate sulfatase. Besides the severe form in infancy, a milder form can be diagnosed in adolescence or adulthood. A spinal stenosis with cervical myelopathy has been described in children but also in affected adults. The large head and coarse facies of the patient together with short, broad, and webbed hands and feet will help to make the diagnosis, and morphologic ultrastructural studies, biochemical analysis of urinary glycosaminoglycans, and assay of activity of iduronate sulfatase activity in cultured skin fibroblasts will contribute to the exact diagnosis.

There are four types of Sanfilippo mucopolysaccharidoses caused by deficiencies of specific enzymes that cause excessive degradation and therefore excessive excretion of heparan sulfate. There are rather mild somatic effects, significant mental deficiency, and dramatic behavioral abnormalities with aggressiveness, hyperkinesis, and insomnia. Because of a lack of recognition of the condition, adult patients can be discovered either as the propositus or as the affected sibling of a known patient. Anamnestic data will reveal the existence of abnormal psychomotor development, delay of speech, and disturbed behavior. The somatic features may be mild and not attract peculiar attention.

Mucopolysaccharidosis type IVA results from a deficiency of galactose-6-sulfatase and produces either the classic Morquio's disease or a milder form of the disease. Mucopolysaccharidosis type VII or β-glucuronidase deficiency may also be described in young adults with pectus carinatum, gross thoracic kyphoscoliosis, hip dysplasia, and signs of storage in skin, gingival biopsy specimens, and leukocytes.

Oligosaccharidoses

Sialidoses are genetic neurologic conditions with autosomal-recessive inheritance in which sialidase or α-L-N-acetylneuraminidase is primarily deficient. A first normomorphic group (I) without somatic changes is the so-called cherry red spot–myoclonus syndrome. The patients present with cherry red spots, myoclonus, cerebellar ataxia, and grand mal epilepsy. A second dysmorphic (II) group includes somatic changes. The main storage substances are sialic acid–rich oligosaccharides (SOS) and SOS-containing proteins. A formerly related condition, galactosialidosis in which sialidase and β-galactosidase are both deficient, is caused by gene mutations in a protective protein and has been separated from sialidosis type II, in which it was formerly included. The symptoms are the same plus skeletal dysplasia, mild gargoyle features, inguinal hernia, and angiokeratoma. Adult onset has been described.

Mannosidosis type II, which is characterized by the storage of oligosaccharides rich in mannose, is caused by a deficiency of the lysosomal enzyme α-D-mannosidase. Type I, with psychomotor retardation, deafness, facial dysmorphism, thickening of the skull, oxycephaly, diffuse abnormalities of the bones, hepatosplenomegaly, and severe recurrent infections leads to early death. Type II corresponds to a less severe form and allows survival into adulthood.

Mucolipidosis Type IV

Mucolipidosis type IV is a lysosomal storage disorder characterized by the lysosomal accumulation of mono- and polysialogangliosides and phospholipids. Most of the patients are Ashkenazi Jews. The disease is characterized by severe psychomotor retardation, corneal opacities, retinal degeneration, and strabismus. Skin and conjunctival biopsy specimens show very suggestive patterns. The disease has an early age of onset, but onset can be prolonged at least during the first three decades of life. Rare examples of a milder course with less severe clinical manifestations and onset in the second decade of life have been reported.

Gaucher's Disease

Excessive quantities of glucocerebroside accumulate in the organs of patients with Gaucher's disease because of a deficiency of the enzyme glucocerebrosidase. It has been subdivided into three clinical phenotypes:

1. Patients with type 1 disease (formerly classified as the adult form) are free of primary neurologic involvement, and any neurologic symptoms observed in such patients are the result of secondary complications of the illness. They may exhibit hepatosplenomegaly, anemia, thrombocytopenia, and skeletal, pulmonary, and renal involvement. In the category of the secondary complications, cerebral and pulmonary fat emboli secondary to severe skeletal involvement have been noted. Spinal cord compression may result from vertebral body collapse. Neuropathy, spontaneous hematomyelia, and plexopathies secondary to coagulopathies have also been reported.

2. Type 2 Gaucher's disease is referred to as the infantile form and produces extensive CNS damage.

3. Type 3 Gaucher's disease, or the juvenile form, shows progressive neurologic involvement beginning in adolescence or early adulthood and consisting of myoclonic and generalized tonic-clonic seizures, horizontal supranuclear gaze palsy, dementia, spasticity, and ataxia.

Adult Forms of White Matter Disorders

Schilder's Disease

Schilder's disease represents three different conditions: (1) an acute form of multiple sclerosis further subdivided into a bilocular type A with symmetric areas of demyelination, or a diffuse-disseminated B type (Schilder 1912); (2) a familial leukodystrophy (Schilder 1913); (3) a subacute sclerosing panencephalitis (Schilder 1924). It is different from the so-called Schilder's "sclérose intra-cérébrale centrolobaire symétrique," which concerns focal vascular or anoxic lesions in the white matter. It is therefore better to avoid using the term *Schilder's disease* unless one is able to specify whether it is a myelinoclastic disorder (Schilder, 1912), a dysmyelinating disease (Schilder, 1913), or an inflammatory condition (Schilder, 1924) analogous to subacute sclerosing panencephalitis. Even so, it is wiser to use a more specific denomination to avoid confusing the issue. The myelinoclastic multiple sclerosislike form includes different clinical pictures: (1) a progressive dementia with spastic paraplegia and optic atrophy; (2) a polysclerotic form with successive bursts; (3) a pseudotumoral form with increased intracranial pressure; and (4) a form in which psychiatric symptoms predominate.

Adrenoleukodystrophy (Adult Form)

Adrenoleukodystrophy (ALD) belongs to the group of peroxisomal diseases with impairment of the β-oxidation system. It is an X-linked disorder with as its main clinical features adrenal cortical insufficiency and demyelination in the CNS. Diagnosis can be made by the assay of very long chain fatty acids (VLCFAs) in plasma or cultured skin fibroblasts, supported by the discovery of spicular and lamellar inclusions in the Schwann cells of cutaneous nerve twigs, and confirmed by DNA examination. The childhood form represents approximately 40% of all cases, the second most important group being AMN (±25%), which is characterized by spasticity and gait disturbances in adolescents and adults. There are also rarer examples of adult cerebral ALD. Adult female carriers may present with mild pyramidal features and deep sensory disturbances. The onset of the symptoms of adult ALD is after the age of 21 years, but the disorder can even be diagnosed later, between the ages of 27 and 57 years. Psychiatric symptoms such as a schizophrenialike psychosis may be the only manifestation at the time of diagnosis (17%) or may represent part of the clinical picture. Other features are a progressive intellectual decline, dementia, Balint's syndrome (psychic paralysis of visual fixation, optic ataxia, disturbance of visual attention with relatively intact vision), an acute confusional state with short-term memory loss, and even a Klüver-Bucy syndrome or a progressive cerebellar ataxia. A mixed sensory-motor neuropathy may be present. The course of the disease tends to have a milder and more protracted course than the childhood form. Adult ALD is difficult to recognize, the more so because clinical or laboratory evidence of adrenocortical dysfunction may be absent. The assay of VLCFAs in serum should be included in the diagnostic work-up if magnetic resonance imaging (MRI) scans show evidence of demyelination in an adult patient.

Adrenomyeloneuropathy

AMN is typically found in an older age group than classic ALD and affects preferentially the spinal cord and peripheral nerves. It presents with a spastic paraparesis, peripheral neuropathy, sphincter disturbances, sensory abnormalities, psychiatric disturbances, and hypogonadism. The levels of VLCFAs in plasma, MRI findings showing spinal cord atrophy, and an X-linked mode of inheritance allow a differential diagnosis with the pure hereditary spastic paraparesis of Strümpell-Lorain, which can be transmitted as a dominant, an autosomal recessive, or an X-linked recessive trait.

Metachromatic Leukodystrophy

MLD is a storage disorder caused by a deficiency of arylsulfatase A, which produces an intralysosomal storage of cerebroside sulfate in oligoglia, macrophages, some neurons (e.g., those of the cerebellar dentate nuclei), and also in Schwann cells in the peripheral nerves. Other tissues may be affected, such as the kidneys or the gallbladder. The responsible gene is approximately 3 kb long and consists of 8 exons. A correlation exists between the arylsulfatase A genotype and the clinical phenotype. Two copies of an R allele encoding for an unstable but active arylsulfatase A allow for the mildest course of the disease, namely the adult form of MLD. The mean age at onset is 23 years, with a range of 16–62 years. It is probable that adult MLD is underdiagnosed. The course of the disease is slowly progressive and the mean survival period is at least 12 years, which is longer than in the other forms.

The psychiatric picture may be one of schizophrenia, affective or personality disorder, behavioral abnormalities, manic depressive psychosis, alcoholic dementia, mental deterioration, or dementia. A change in personality and poor job performance often herald the onset of the disease. A frontal lobe syndrome has been described including disinhibition, impulsivity, poor judgment, emotional lability, social inappropriateness, and poor attention span. Complex auditory hallucinations and bizarre delusions may also be described. It is therefore useful to check for homozygous (disease state) and heterozygous (carrier) forms of MLD among populations of psychiatric individuals. The psychiatric

manifestations present in adult MLD may exist in isolation for decades before the onset of neurologic deterioration.

The clinical picture is also reminiscent of multiple sclerosis. The main neurologic symptoms are ataxia and paraparesis. Polyneuropathy is part of the picture in all forms of MLD. In adult MLD, differences in the severity of the neuropathy may exist, some patients having a mild demyelinating neuropathy, others a pronounced one. If the neuropathy is severe, it may become one if not the only presenting symptom of adult MLD. There has been at least one example of adult MLD with polyneuropathy and early life pes cavus deformity before onset of the CNS abnormalities. The existence of white matter lesions, especially in the frontal lobe, will be confirmed on MRI scans. The protein level in the cerebrospinal fluid (CSF) is normal or only slightly elevated. A slowing of the peripheral nerve conduction velocities is observed, with mean values of 24 m/sec and a range of 15–39 m/sec. Storage material may be found by light- and electron microscopy in cutaneous nerve twigs in the skin and in the sural nerve. Increased amounts of sulfatides are excreted in urinary sediments. The assay of arylsulfatase A in leukocytes using the natural substrate cerebroside sulfate is to be recommended rather than the use of the synthetic substrate nitrocatechol sulfate. Attention has to be paid to arylsulfatase A pseudodeficiency caused by homozygosity for the arylsulfatase A pseudodeficiency allele. In that case, enough arylsulfatase A is synthesized to prevent the disease. Therefore one has to demonstrate that there is an accumulation of sulfatides in the organs to confirm the diagnosis of MLD. If the disease is recognized early enough, bone marrow transplantation may be considered depending on the patient's age and deficit, pending progress in gene therapy using adenovirus vectors. Bone marrow transplantation has produced conflicting but sometimes positive results.

Globoid Cell Leukodystrophy

GLD is a galactosylceramide lipidosis caused by a deficiency of the enzyme galactosylceramide β-galactosidase (GALC). The inheritance is autosomal recessive and the gene coding for GALC has been mapped to 14q24.3–q32.1. The enzymatic deficiency produces the accumulation of a related metabolite, galactosylsphingosine or psychosine, which is neurotoxic for the central and peripheral nervous systems. Psychosine provokes the destruction of oligoglial cells and a demyelination in the CNS. The most characteristic feature is the presence of globoid cells in the white matter. Globoid cells are macrophages arising from non-neural mesodermal cells. They contain very characteristic spicular curved inclusions. Peripheral nerves are also affected and spicular inclusions are found in endoneurial macrophages.

Classic GLD affects children during the first months of their lives and includes a first stage with irritability, hyperesthesia, and slowing of nerve conduction velocities, followed by a second period characterized by mental deterioration, opisthotonos, and optic atrophy, ending in a third "burned-out" stage with decerebration and death. A classification of GLD has been devised on the basis of the age at onset of the symptoms: early infantile, late infantile, juvenile, and adolescent or adult type. There is some evidence that both the late infantile and adult types may exist in one family, although there are no strict morphologic or enzymatic clues to prove it. The delayed onset GLD is characterized by an asymmetric tetraparesis, a pseudobulbar palsy, and pallor of the optic disks. Progressive intellectual deterioration including dementia has been described in autopsy-proven cases. A diagnosis of GLD should be considered in individuals with the onset of peripheral weakness, spasticity, ataxia, and dementia with or without seizures.

Alexander's Disease

Classic Alexander's disease, or megalobarencephaly, has been described in infants with enlarged heads and psychomotor retardation. Seizures and spasticity subsequently are noted. Death occurs early. At autopsy, hydrocephalus but also an increase in the brain's weight are present. The most characteristic finding is the presence of homogeneous osmiophilic deposits in astrocytes on hematoxylin-and-eosin–stained slides of the brain. It corresponds to the accumulation of glial filaments, known as Rosenthal fibers. The subpial and perivascular regions are the most severely affected areas of the brain. Immunohistochemistry analysis and EM studies, including immuno-ultrastructural examination, confirm the localization of the Rosenthal fibers in the astrocytes and the presence of very large amounts of tightly packed intermediate filaments merging with aggregates of osmiophilic material. Demyelination is present without signs of myelinoclastic activity. Infantile, juvenile, and adult subgroups have been described with distinctive differences in clinical presentation, prognosis, and morphology. The infantile group is characterized by a progressive enlargement of the head with psychomotor retardation, muscle weakness, pyramidal signs, and convulsions. Rigidity and opisthotonus occur later on. The average age of onset is 6 months, and the average survival after diagnosis is 2 years, 4 months. The juvenile group is characterized by progressive paresis, bulbar signs, and hyperreflexia with more or less intact mental functions. The average age of onset is 9 years, with an average survival of 8 years.

In the adult group, the patients are asymptomatic or have intermittent neurologic dysfunction resembling multiple sclerosis, including ataxia, pyramidal features, or signs of bulbar dysfunction. Neuroimaging may show white matter lesions, but they can hardly be considered specific. In adults, the neuropathologic lesions affect the bulbar pyramids, the cerebellar dentate nuclei, and the subependymal, subpial, and perivascular zones. Rosenthal fibers are often found in the floor of the fourth ventricle. Diagnosis can be achieved with certainty only by brain biopsy in infantile and juvenile cases, and it is doubtful whether a brain biopsy would reveal typical alterations in adult patients unless stereotactic procedures on neuroradiologically defined targets are used. Even then, Rosenthal fibers can be found in a series of conditions, such as multiple sclerosis plaques, pilocytic astrocytomas, cerebral gliomatosis, ependymomas, syringomyelia, or chronic glial reactions. These facts further complicate the problem of differential diagnosis.

Orthochromatic or Sudanophilic Leukodystrophies

Orthochromatic or sudanophilic leukodystrophies represent an ill-defined group of disorders with a poorly understood pathogenesis except for Pelizaeus-Merzbacher disease (PMD), which is caused by mutations in the human proteolipid protein (*PLP*) gene located on chromosome X. The mutations in PMD result in oligodendrocyte death because of the accumulation of PLP in the endoplasmic reticulum. Other mutations cause a total absence of PLP and lead to milder forms of PMD, with prolongation of life into adulthood. The diagnostic criteria are mainly of a neuropathologic nature: a diffuse demyelination or discoloration of the white matter when myelin stains are used and that is not secondary to cortical neuronal losses; a diffuse isomorphic fibrillary gliosis as revealed by Holzer staining or immunohistochemistry analysis using antibodies against glial fibrillary acidic protein; abundant lipofuscin granules in microglia, macrophages, and astrocytes; and minute or large amounts of neutral fats in macroglia, microglia, and perivascular macrophages. PMD is characterized by the presence of islands of relatively preserved myelin. The clinical features are not very specific, with progressive cognitive deterioration and increasing pyramidal signs. Brain imaging shows white matter lesions and a dilatation of the lateral ventricles.

Adult forms of orthochromatic leukodystrophies are very rare. There is an adult form of PMD known as the *Löwenberg-Hill type*, which shares with PMD some morphologic characteristics such as islands of relatively preserved myelin but has a dominant pattern of inheritance instead of the X-linked inheritance of PMD. Similar lesions of the white matter have been occasionally reported in Sjögren-Larsson syndrome, which is characterized by oligophrenia, ichthyosis, and spasticity. Adult sudanophilic leukodystrophy (the classic form of Ferraro or the late-adult type of van Bogaert-Nyssen) is also a very rare disease, some examples being reported as a pigmentary type of orthochromatic leukodystrophy. The onset is in middle age. It can be a sporadic, an autosomal dominant, or a recessive disorder. The clinical presentation is most often one of a frontal lobe-type dementia. Personality changes and bizarre behavior, depression, loss of functional skills, and impairment of memory have been described. Hemiparesis, dysarthria, bilateral pyramidal signs, pseudobulbar features, cerebellar signs, frontal release signs, gait disturbances, ataxia, and sometimes epilepsy may develop. Neuroimaging will show a decrease of volume and density of the white matter, with a resulting dilatation of the lateral ventricles. The diagnosis is difficult to make in the absence of specific tests and results from the exclusion of conditions such as ALD, MLD, GLD, and PMD. Sometimes the autopsy of an affected sibling will give a clue to the diagnosis.

Other Diseases

Cerebrotendinous Xanthomatosis

The hallmarks of cerebrotendinous xanthomatosis (CTX), a rare disease described by van Bogaert and colleagues in 1937, are achilles tendon xanthomas; juvenile cataracts; behavioral problems; epilepsy; psychomotor retardation; dementia; and a series of pyramidal, extrapyramidal, cerebellar, spinal, and peripheral nerve signs. Recurrent attacks of myocardial infarction, angina pectoris, and coronary atherosclerosis are noted in some patients. The symptoms at onset are cataracts (34.8%), achilles tendon xanthomas (33.3%), low intelligence (26.1%), or gait disturbances (5.8%). The clinical symptoms develop insidiously during the second decade of life, but the mean age of the patients is 39.7 ± 9.9 years for men and 38.8 ± 13.4 years for women. Overall, except for tendon xanthomas, most of the clinical manifestations progress with age. In 10–15% of the patients, there will be no xanthomas, and only one-third of the patients will have tendon xanthomas at the onset of the disease.

The enzymatic defect is a block in bile acid synthesis. Mutations in hepatic mitochondrial sterol 27-hydroxylase enzyme underlie CTX. The gene is located on the distal portion of the long arm of chromosome 2. There is abnormal bile synthesis with virtual absence of chenodeoxycholic acid (CDCA) in the bile. The reduced bile acid biosynthesis depresses the activities of other key enzymes, resulting in accumulation of bile acid precursors such as cholestanol and various kinds of bile alcohols and in the enhancement of cholesterol synthesis. The disease results from an increased concentration of cholestanol in plasma and CSF and in the deposition of cholestanol in tendon xanthomas and in different places of the brain, such as the hypothalamus, cerebellum, and mesencephalon. Cholesterol levels are normal or low in plasma, and bile acid precursors are excreted in the bile and urine.

Replacement therapy with CDCA normalizes the biochemical abnormalities, improves the neurologic picture, and halts the clinical deterioration. Coenzyme A reductase inhibitor and low-density lipoprotein apheresis have also been tried in association with CDCA, although the role of low-density lipoprotein apheresis is controversial.

The clinical diagnosis, which is often made very late, is facilitated by the presence of the tendon xanthomas in association with juvenile cataracts and neurologic features. Tendon xanthomas, however, are not pathognomonic and may also be present in familial hyperlipoproteinemia or familial hypercholesterolemia. The high cholestanol concentration in plasma and a normal cholesterol level are typical biochemical findings. Early diagnosis is crucial, because a therapy exists that is more effective if the diagnosis is made early, especially in the presymptomatic stage. Indeed, when the disease is symptomatic, treatment may arrest the progression of the condition, but there is no dramatic effect on clinical manifestations, the xanthomas, or the electrophysiologic findings. Nerve conduction velocities and motor and sensory evoked potentials, which are abnormal in the disease, may be monitored to assess the effect of treatment. MRI scans show brain and cerebellar atrophy; diffuse white matter hypodensities; sometimes more or less symmetric lesions in the basal ganglia, cerebellum, and mesencephalon; and atrophy of the brain stem and corpus callosum. It should be remembered that focal lesions were very prominent in the princeps case. Detection of heterozygotes is only possible by molecular identification of the mutant allele.

Tangier Disease

Tangier disease is a rare autosomal recessive disorder of lipid metabolism characterized by a low serum cholesterol level, a normal or elevated triglyceride level, and nearly absent high-density lipoprotein and apolipoprotein A-I and A-II. The disorder may be discovered in children and adults. Most of the patients have yellowish tonsils, and some may have hepatosplenomegaly, leukopenia, and thrombocytopenia. Myocardial disease and strokes are frequent. Neurologic features include a peripheral neuropathy in two-thirds of the patients and are the presenting symptoms in one-

half of these patients. Mononeuropathy, multiple mononeuropathies, or distal symmetric sensorimotor polyneuropathy or facial diplegia have been described. A syringomyelialike syndrome has also been reported, including wasting of the hand muscles and dissociated sensory loss in the upper trunk. The diagnosis is made thanks to special clinical features such as the enlarged yellowish tonsils, and the assay of high-density lipoprotein and apolipoprotein A-I. A nerve biopsy can document the peripheral nerve involvement but will not show specific features.

Lafora's Disease

The classic age of onset of Lafora's disease is from 6 to 20 years, with a duration of 2–10 years. There are, however, a few reports of progressive myoclonic epilepsy with Lafora bodies characterized by a late onset (17–33 years) and a protracted course (age at death, 42–65 years). Dementia or personality changes are evident from the onset or within the first 10 years of disease and are progressive. The initial symptoms are epileptic seizures, progressive dementia, and later myoclonus. The mode of inheritance is autosomal recessive. The gene for progressive myoclonus epilepsy of the Lafora type maps to chromosome 6q. Characteristic inclusions called *Lafora bodies* are found in neurons present in the CNS but also in the excretory ducts of eccrine or apocrine sweat glands in the skin. Light and EM study of skin biopsy specimens taken at shoulder level or in the axillary region will show inclusions made of a fibrillogranular material in the peripheral duct cells. The skin biopsy specimen might sometimes give negative results. Liver or skeletal muscle biopsies might be considered but could also produce negative findings. We recommend obtaining a skin biopsy specimen first, which, if adequately handled will very likely confirm the diagnosis of Lafora's disease.

Adult Form of Acid Maltase Deficiency

Glycogenosis type II is a recessively inherited lysosomal glycogen storage disease resulting from acid α-glucosidase deficiency. Although the infantile form (Pompe's disease) is rapidly progressive because of the massive lysosomal storage in the skeletal muscles, liver, heart, and nervous system, the juvenile and adult forms manifest as a slowly progressive myopathy with or without respiratory insufficiency. The clinical spectrum ranges from a mild or delayed proximal muscle weakness to a severe weakness and respiratory failure culminating in early death. The symptoms of weakness and dyspnea may progress over several months or may evolve more slowly over many years. The storage of glycogen occurs in skeletal muscle but may vary from muscle to muscle. In general, the level of residual activity of acid maltase correlates with the clinical course. Sometimes a very low enzyme activity can be found in adults with a relatively mild phenotype.

Suggested Reading

Baumann N, Federico A, Suzuki K. Late onset neurometabolic genetic disorders. From clinical to molecular aspects of lysosomal and peroxisomal disorders. Dev Neurosci 1991;13:185.

Berkovic SF, Carpenter S, Andermann F, et al. Kufs' disease: a critical reappraisal. Brain 1988;111:27.

Ceuterick C, Martin J-J. Electron microscopic features of skin in neurometabolic disorders. J Neurol Sci 1992;112:15.

Fressinaud C, Vallat JM, Masson M, et al. Adult-onset metachromatic leukodystrophy presenting as isolated peripheral neuropathy. Neurology 1992;42:1396.

Goebel HH, Lake BD. Symposium: lysosomal and peroxisomal disorders. Brain Pathol 1998;8:73.

Hageman ATM, Gabreels FJM, de Jong JGN, et al. Clinical symptoms of adult metachromatic leukodystrophy and arylsulfatase A pseudodeficiency. Arch Neurol 1995;52:408.

Martin J-J, Guazzi GC. Schilder's diffuse sclerosis. Dev Neurosci 1991;13:267.

Martin J-J. Adult type of neuronal ceroid lipofuscinosis. J Inherit Metab Dis 1993;16:237.

Mitsias P, Levine SR. Cerebrovascular complications of Fabry's disease. Ann Neurol 1996;40:8.

Roels F, Espeel M, Mandel H, et al. Human liver pathology in peroxisomal disorders: a review including novel data. Biochimie 1993;75:281.

Scriver CR Beaudet AL, Sly WS, Valle D. The Metabolic and Molecular Bases of Inherited Disease, 7th edition. McGraw-Hill: New York, 1995.

Van Bogaert L, Scherer HJ, Epstein E. Une Forme Cérébrale de Cholestérinose Généralisée. Paris: Masson, 1937.

Verdru P, Lammens M, Dom R, et al. Globoid cell leukodystrophy: a family with both late-infantile and adult type. Neurology 1991;41:1382.

Chapter 51
Intoxications and Nutritional Deficiencies

Randall R. Long

Chapter Plan

Within most societies, the preponderance of cases of intoxication and nutritional deficiency is encountered within the setting of acute and chronic alcohol (ethanol) overuse. Most people are familiar with the effects of acute alcohol intoxication from firsthand experience on only, it is hoped, a relatively few occasions during early adulthood. For some people, however, alcohol intoxication becomes a recurrent state, and withdrawal syndromes and nutritional deficiencies become relevant issues. It is beyond the scope of this chapter to cover the clinical science of alcohol and other addictions per se, although it emphasizes the diagnosis and management of neurologic syndromes commonly encountered in the setting of chronic alcoholism. Other acute intoxications and deficiency states are also reviewed.

Acute Intoxication

Syndrome of Acute Intoxication

The term *encephalopathy* implies a diffuse disturbance of cerebral function. Acute alcohol intoxication and other intoxications fall within this spectrum. Intoxication may be associated with alterations in both the level of consciousness and the content of consciousness. Intoxicated individuals are typically less responsive than normal, their attention span is often decreased, disorientation is common, and psychotic features may be present (disordered thought and hallucinations). The descriptors "lethargic," "obtunded," "stuporous," and "semi-comatose" are often used, but are imprecise and variably defined. When describing an intoxicated individual, it is preferable to describe specific stimuli and responses, performance, and thought content. Intoxication may also be associated with delirium. Delirious individuals exhibit agitation in addition to confusion, disorientation, and altered thought. Autonomic instability is characteristic of delirium. Intoxicated individuals will sometimes fluctuate between delirium and depressed consciousness. The limit of intoxication is, of course, coma. The clinical phenomenology and management of coma are considered elsewhere (see Chapter 13); acute alcohol and other intoxications should always be considered in the differential diagnosis of coma, just as the differential diagnosis of coma parallels that of encephalopathy.

Acute Ethanol Intoxication

The alteration of consciousness associated with acute alcohol ingestion can be quite variable. Some individuals manifest the features of delirium, whereas in others encephalopathic features are encountered. Variable degrees of dysarthria, clumsiness, and even frank ataxia are common concomitants. Horizontal gaze-evoked nystagmus may be observed. There is only imprecise correlation with blood ethanol levels, however. Although effects are typically more prominent with higher ethanol levels, chronic alcoholics will have few manifestations at a level that would severely compromise an inexperienced drinker.

The management of acute alcohol intoxication is usually passive; alcohol is oxidatively metabolized at a constant rate that increases with body mass. Once intake ceases, the blood level will fall steadily. Respiration and even circulation may be depressed in severe intoxication, however. Respiratory monitoring, control of the airway, and support as needed are crucial during the wait for metabolic clearance. The incoordination that accompanies acute alcohol intoxication may lead to traumatic injury. Occult trauma, particularly closed head injury or cervical spine fracture, should always be considered. Hypothermia may complicate alcohol intoxication. Alcohol induces cutaneous vasodilation and a subjective feeling of warmth, but thereby accentuates convective heat loss. Among chronic alcoholics, occult infection is encountered not infrequently. Ethanol also increases serum osmolality and has a direct diuretic effect. Fluid and electrolyte issues should

always be reviewed. Above all, one must consider the possibility of withdrawal and the complications of nutritional deficiency in chronic alcoholics (see below).

Other Acute Intoxications

Carbon Monoxide

Carbon monoxide poisoning is frequently intentional, the setting suggesting the offending agent. It may also be accidental, however, in association with faulty heating and ventilation systems. Carbon monoxide intoxication presents clinically as an encephalopathy, with cherry red discoloration of the skin and mucous membranes as a key associated feature. An elevated carboxyhemoglobin level confirms the diagnosis.

Methanol

Methanol intoxication is rare, most often encountered typically among disenfranchised alcoholics who turn to methanol as an ethanol substitute. Delirium precedes depression of consciousness in methanol intoxication. Abdominal pain and visual disturbance with optic disc hyperemia commonly occur simultaneously. Kussmaul breathing in association with a striking metabolic acidosis is also characteristic of methanol intoxication. Propylene glycol (an ingredient in many antifreeze preparations) intoxication is less common, but virtually indistinguishable. The goal of specific intervention is to reverse the metabolic acidosis.

Sympathomimetics and Hallucinogens

The major sympathomimetic and hallucinogenic agents seen in intoxication are the amphetamines, cocaine, phencyclidine (PCP), and lysergic acid diethylamide (LSD). Most of these intoxications fall within the spectrum of illicit drug use and addiction, although the amphetamines do have legitimate pharmacologic uses, and inadvertent intoxication may occur in individuals being treated for obesity, hyperactivity, or vestibular disorders. Delirium is the usual presentation, although encephalopathic depression of consciousness and even coma may occur. Frank hallucinations and seizures are common. Cardiac arrhythmias may also occur, particularly with cocaine.

Other Pharmacologic Agents

Benzodiazepines. The benzodiazepines are now among the most commonly prescribed drugs in our society. They are used for conditions ranging from insomnia and anxiety to spasticity and epilepsy. Excess intake, whether accidental, intentional, or iatrogenic, is characterized by drowsiness, clumsiness and incoordination, dysarthria, and end-gaze nystagmus. Respiratory suppression is fortunately a late occurrence. The half-lives of the different benzodiazepines vary greatly and may be quite prolonged in elderly individuals.

Opiates. Naturally occurring and synthetic opiates are major analgesics, but most also induce a euphoria and have a high abuse potential. Acute intoxication may therefore be encountered within patient populations as well as within the setting of drug abuse. The typical manifestations are a depressed sensorium, pupillary constriction, early respiratory suppression, and bradycardia. Naloxone (0.01 mg per kg intravenously) may be administered both diagnostically and therapeutically, reversing most of these manifestations, if only transiently. The dose may be repeated as needed up to a total dose of 10 mg in adults.

Antidepressants. Antidepressant overdose is an all too common occurrence, most individuals presenting with acute intoxication if not coma. These drugs are unfortunately available to the individuals who are at greatest risk of suicide. The initial manifestation of intoxication for all agents in this class (monoamine oxidase [MAO] inhibitors, tricyclics, and selective serotonin reuptake inhibitors) is delirium characterized by restlessness, agitation, and confusion. Many of the tricyclics are potent anticholinergics; pupillary dilatation, dry and red mucous membranes, and hyperthermia are common manifestations. Cardiac arrhythmias and seizures may occur. MAO inhibitors may also be associated with hypertensive crisis secondary to ingestion of foods containing tyramine or other sympathomimetic amines.

Neuroleptics. Neuroleptic intoxication is less common than with antidepressants but may occur in conjunction with and complicate antidepressant overdose. The full spectrum from depressed sensorium to agitated delirium may be encountered. Parkinsonian signs such as rigidity and bradykinesia are expected. Neuroleptic malignant syndrome (NMS) warrants specific mention. Although typically an idiosyncratic rather than a dose-related reaction, NMS may be confused with an intoxication. Affected individuals are typically encephalopathic but also rigid and hyperthermic. Serum creatine kinase levels are quite elevated. Patients may respond to rapid treatment with dantrolene or dopamine agonists such as bromocriptine.

Barbiturates. Barbiturates are prescribed far less frequently than in the past. Intoxication is correspondingly infrequent. It is characterized by depressed sensorium and generalized flaccidity. When coma occurs, brain stem reflexes may be abolished. This may falsely suggest a structural brain stem pathologic state.

An Approach to Management of Acute Intoxication

The clinical management of acute intoxication or any acute alteration of mental state should parallel that of coma. The importance of protecting the airway and supporting respiration and circulation cannot be overemphasized. Once intravenous access is established and appropriate laboratory specimens obtained, glucose, thiamine, and naloxone administration should be considered. If focal central nervous system signs are encountered on examination, structural studies are indicated. Every attempt should be made to contact family or friends for a detailed medical history.

Withdrawal Syndromes

Alcohol Withdrawal

There are actually four fairly distinct alcohol withdrawal syndromes: alcoholic tremulousness ("shakes"), alcoholic hallucinosis ("frights"), alcohol withdrawal seizures ("fits"), and alcohol withdrawal delirium or delirium tremens ("DTs"). Overlap is not uncommon, although the occur-

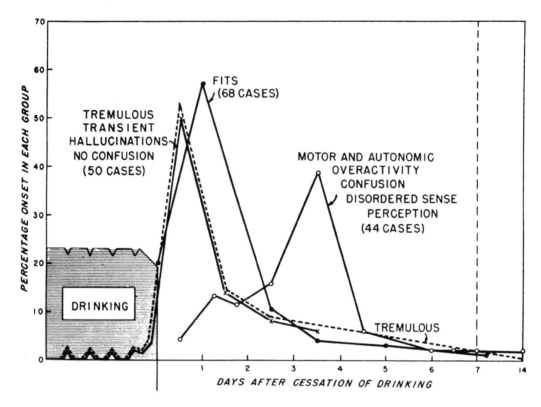

Figure 51-1. Temporal relationship of alcohol withdrawal syndromes to cessation of drinking. (Reprinted with permission from M Victor, RD Adams. The effect of alcohol on the nervous system. Res Publ Assoc Res Nerv Ment Dis 1956;32:526.)

rence of each is relatively fixed in time to the cessation of alcohol intake (Figure 51-1). The occurrence of any of the earlier syndromes indicates a greater risk of the latest, and most serious, delirium tremens.

Tremulousness and Hallucinosis

Withdrawal-associated tremors and hallucinations are most common during the first 36 hours after drinking stops, with a peak incidence at approximately 12 hours. Affected individuals are often anxious and irritable, but their sensorium remains fairly intact. They frequently report nausea. Tachycardia and moderate blood pressure elevation are common. The tremor is a gross accentuation of physiologic action tremor. The hallucinations are typically visual, although somesthetic and even auditory hallucinations may be experienced. The hallucinations of alcohol withdrawal are often rec-

ognized by the affected individual as "unreal." Tremulousness and hallucinosis usually resolve within 24 hours of onset.

Alcohol Withdrawal Seizures

Alcohol withdrawal seizures usually occur between 6 and 48 hours after the last intake of alcohol, with a peak at 24 hours. The seizures are usually brief generalized tonic-clonic seizures. More than one seizure occurs in roughly two-thirds of cases. Once seizures occur, the risk of further seizures subsides after approximately 6 hours. A striking alkalosis and hypomagnesemia are often seen during the interval of withdrawal seizures. The electroencephalogram may show diffuse "postictal" slowing or may appear normal; a photoconvulsive response is commonly seen with photic stimulation. Withdrawal seizures in the absence of seizures at any other time do not warrant ongoing anticonvulsant treatment. Withdrawal seizures are the norm in epileptics who drink, however. Any history of seizures at other times, focal onset, or status epilepticus should suggest more than simple withdrawal seizures.

Delirium Tremens

Delirium tremens, the most threatening and prolonged of the alcohol withdrawal syndromes, tends to appear between 24 hours and 5 days after the last intake of alcohol, the peak incidence falling between 3 and 4 days. Agitated delirium is the norm, consisting of disorientation, altered sensory perception, and frank hallucinations. The delirium is associated with marked autonomic overactivity and instability. Hyperthermia, diaphoresis, tachycardia, and hypertension are common. Withdrawal seizures may occur early in the course of DTs. DTs carries a significant mortality, as high as 15%. Concurrent infection, electrolyte abnormalities, hepatic failure, and cardiovascular crises are usually contributing factors in cases of major morbidity or mortality.

Management of Alcohol Withdrawal

Both prevention and treatment are relevant in managing chronic alcoholics who come to medical attention. If chronic excessive intake is suspected in any patient, preventive measures are in order. Prophylactic use of sedatives, usually benzodiazepines, has been shown to decrease the incidence and severity of all of the alcohol withdrawal syndromes. Lorazepam, diazepam, and chlordiazepoxide are most commonly used. This author prefers lorazepam because of its shorter half-life. A dose of 0.5–2.0 mg lorazepam may be given every 4–6 hours, the dose and interval adjusted to keep the patient calm but easily arousable. If withdrawal signs appear, especially DTs, higher doses are usually needed, invariably via a parenteral route. In the face of DTs, a 1-mg dose of lorazepam should be administered at 5-minute intervals until agitation subsides; doses should then be repeated as often as necessary to maintain a calm state. The benzodiazepines may suppress respiratory drive at high doses; close monitoring of respiratory and cardiovascular status is imperative.

This author also advocates the use of phenytoin for withdrawal seizure prophylaxis. I give a loading dose of 15 mg per kg orally in three divided doses, 4 hours apart. This is followed by a daily maintenance dose of 300–400 mg for 3 days. If the patient presents with withdrawal seizures, intravenous benzodiazepines may be given to break a seizure. Again, longer-term anticonvulsant treatment is not indicated unless there is reason to suspect concurrent epilepsy.

Immediate administration of thiamine is appropriate for all alcoholics whether or not they manifest withdrawal symptoms. Many are thiamine deficient and at risk of developing Wernicke's encephalopathy (see below). A dose of 100 mg should be given intramuscularly each day for 3 days or until normal oral intake is re-established. Surveillance for any comorbidity is also a crucial aspect of management. Again, occult trauma and infection should always be considered. Any patient with delirium and fever should undergo imaging and have a spinal fluid examination; a patient with suspected DTs fits these criteria. Fluid, electrolyte, and acid-base disturbances are the norm in the setting of alcohol withdrawal. Hepatic function and coagulation should always be assessed.

Other Withdrawal States

Barbiturates and Benzodiazepines

If sedative drugs such as the benzodiazepines and barbiturates are consumed at high doses or for long periods of time, abrupt cessation may be associated with a withdrawal syndrome that mimics that of alcohol withdrawal. The higher the dose, the shorter the duration of usage before withdrawal becomes a risk. The shorter the half-life of the drug, the more likely a withdrawal syndrome. Confusion, irritability, and restlessness are common, the onset usually within 1–3 days after cessation of intake. Autonomic hyperactivity may occur. Withdrawal seizures may also be encountered, even in individuals with no history of epilepsy or other central nervous disorder. The management of sedative drug withdrawal parallels that of alcohol withdrawal. An individual at risk should be treated with a similar but longer acting drug. Clonazepam may be used for potential benzodiazepine withdrawal and phenobarbital for barbiturate withdrawal. If active withdrawal occurs and a parenteral drug is needed, diazepam and phenobarbital are readily available. As in alcohol withdrawal, small doses should be repeated frequently until a calm but not obtunded state is reached. Doses are then repeated as necessary to maintain such a state. After several days, the maintenance dose can be gradually tapered. Seizures in the setting of sedative drug withdrawal can also be managed as discussed earlier for alcohol withdrawal seizures.

Opiates

Opiate withdrawal is celebrated in fiction and film—dysphoria, restlessness, myalgias and arthralgias, and even somesthetic hallucinations are common. Gastrointestinal symptoms (nausea, vomiting, and diarrhea) may occur. There may also be autonomic hyperactivity, although usually this is less prominent than in other withdrawal syndromes. It is not a pleasant experience, but opiate withdrawal is associated with far less morbidity and mortality than alcohol or sedative drug withdrawal syndromes. Withdrawal seizures are also uncommon, suggesting underlying epilepsy when they occur. Clonidine (5 mg per kg twice a day for 5–7 days) alleviates many of these manifestations. Alternatively, individuals at risk of opiate withdrawal may be given methadone (10–20 mg twice a day depending on prior intake), and then the methadone can be tapered over 5–7 days.

Nutritional Deficiency in the Setting of Chronic Alcoholism

Wernicke's Encephalopathy

A manifestation of acute thiamine (vitamin B_1) deficiency, Wernicke's encephalopathy is a clinical triad of oculomotor dysfunction, ataxia, and confusion. Although horizontal gaze palsy is the classic eye finding in Wernicke's encephalopathy, almost any combination of oculomotor dysfunction may be encountered. Gaze-evoked nystagmus and sixth nerve palsy are the most common signs. Ataxia affects truncal stability more than limb movements. The encephalopathy may range from mild confusion to coma. Some individuals demonstrate a striking memory deficit (see "Korsakoff's Psychosis"). If untreated, permanent deficits can be expected. Any suggestion of alcoholism or nutritional deficiency

warrants treatment with parenteral thiamine. A dose of 100 mg thiamine should be given intravenously before administration of intravenous fluids containing glucose. Suspected Wernicke's encephalopathy should be treated in the same way, with daily doses continued until symptoms resolve and normal nutritional intake can be ensured.

Korsakoff's Psychosis

Korsakoff's psychosis refers to an amnestic syndrome characterized by both a retrograde and anterograde amnesia. Affected individuals have significant deficits in remote memory and have difficulty learning and retaining new information and experiences. Most individuals have little insight into their deficits. Confabulation may be a striking associated phenomenon but is not always present. There are many causes of Korsakoff's psychosis—that is, any disease process affecting both temporal lobes or their connections—although it is not infrequently seen as a part of Wernicke's encephalopathy and may persist as a long-term sequela.

Other Central Nervous System Deficiency Syndromes in Alcoholics

Cerebellar Degeneration

A syndrome of gradually progressive truncal and lower limb ataxia is sometimes encountered among chronic alcoholics. Other manifestations of chronic alcoholism (cirrhosis, polyneuropathy, and even a history or sequelae of Wernicke's encephalopathy) are frequent in affected individuals. Gait ataxia is the most striking clinical manifestation. Upper limb taxis is usually better preserved, and cerebellar eye signs are typically absent. This reflects atrophic changes and loss of Purkinje cells from the anterior and superior midline cerebellar structures. The condition probably reflects a combination of polynutritional deficiency and a direct toxic effect of alcohol over time.

Other Seldom Seen Central Nervous System Syndromes

Central pontine myelinolysis is a condition of acute to subacute demyelination of central midline structures. Clinical signs include encephalopathy or even coma, long tract signs (usually bilateral), and pontine signs. The most prominent pathologic changes affect myelin pathways in the central pons and midbrain. It is not common but may be encountered among chronic alcoholics or others who are chronically nutritionally deprived. Rapid correction of significant hyponatremia appears to be a major contributing factor. Marchiafava-Bignami disease is a rare degeneration of the corpus callosum reported in chronic alcoholics. There are theories that this condition arises from a combination of nutritional and toxic effects in alcoholics, although systematic epidemiologic and pathologic data are not available. The term "alcoholic dementia" is probably a misnomer, referring to those individuals with a persistent Korsakoff's amnestic syndrome occurring after acute Wernicke's encephalopathy.

Alcoholic Polyneuropathy

Sensorimotor polyneuropathy is common among chronic alcoholics. It probably reflects a polynutritional deficiency, with B-complex deficiencies playing a key role. Distal wasting and weakness, hyporeflexia, and a glove-and-stocking hypesthesia involving all sensory modalities are the cardinal clinical features. Electrodiagnostic and pathologic studies confirm both distal axonal degeneration and demyelination. Chronic thiamine deficiency (beriberi) may be associated with a sensorimotor polyneuropathy indistinguishable from that seen in alcoholics. Some better-nourished alcoholics may present with a "burning foot syndrome," with distal dysesthesias and loss of pain and temperature sensitivity out of proportion to loss of large fiber modalities. There is indirect evidence that this reflects a relative deficiency of pantothenic acid, although a direct toxic effect of ethanol may also contribute.

Other Nutritional Deficiencies with Neurologic Manifestations

Subacute Combined Systems Degeneration/Pernicious Anemia

The classic presentation of pernicious anemia is a macrocytic anemia secondary to malabsorption of vitamin B_{12} (cobalamin) caused by an inherited deficiency of intrinsic factor. If untreated, or in some individuals with only a mild macrocytic picture, the syndrome of subacute combined systems degeneration may be encountered. This syndrome is one of variable components of dementia, visual disturbance, long tract motor and sensory signs, and peripheral polyneuropathy. The syndrome may be seen in classic cases but also in the face of nutritional deficiency secondary to poor dietary intake and other malabsorption syndromes.

The visual disturbance is typically a centrocecal scotoma; optic atrophy may be seen on examination and visual evoked potentials may be delayed. Long tract signs mimic those of cervical cord disease, with various combinations of spinocerebellar and dorsal column signs, spasticity, and extensor plantar responses. Lhermitte's sign may also be elicited. Distal deep tendon reflexes may be depressed because of concurrent peripheral polyneuropathy. The predominant pathologic change at all sites is demyelination. Intensities on T2-weighted images may be seen on magnetic resonance imaging (MRI) scans, and myelin basic protein may be detected on cerebrospinal fluid examination. The differential diagnoses of subacute combined systems degeneration and multiple sclerosis often overlap.

Treatment of vitamin B_{12} deficiency consists of vitamin B_{12} replacement therapy, usually via a parenteral route at the outset and also on an ongoing basis if an absorption deficit is confirmed. A dose of 1,000 µg intramuscularly should be given daily for 2 weeks, weekly for 2 months, and then monthly for life.

Pellagra

Pellagra, nicotinic acid deficiency, is rare outside the developing world and areas of protracted warfare. The syndrome is one of photosensitive dermatitis, diarrhea, anemia, and a mild encephalopathy. Myelopathic and peripheral neuropathic signs are also sometimes encountered.

Pyridoxine Deficiency

Pyridoxine deficiency in adults is usually iatrogenic, secondary to treatment of tuberculosis with isoniazid. There are also reports of pyridoxine deficiency secondary to longer-term treatment with hydralazine, although this is of primarily historical interest. Isolated nutritional deficiency is rare, although pyridoxine deficiency probably contributes to the nutritional polyneuropathy seen in chronic alcoholics. The clinical features of pyridoxine deficiency are a chronic distal symmetric sensorimotor polyneuropathy. Electrodiagnostic and pathologic studies indicate a process of axonal degeneration. Interestingly, pyridoxine excess has also been associated with peripheral nervous system disease, specifically a sensory neuronopathy.

Vitamin E Deficiency

Cases of vitamin E deficiency have been reported in children, usually manifestations of malabsorption or chronic hepatobiliary disease. Various combinations of myelopathy (spasticity with sensory ataxia), peripheral neuropathy, and retinal pigmentary degeneration have been described. Clinical signs improve with replacement therapy.

Suggested Reading

Beck WS. Cobalamin and the nervous system. N Engl J Med 1988;318:1752.

Plum F, Posner J. The Diagnosis of Stupor and Coma. Philadelphia: Davis, 1966.

Victor M. Neurologic Disorders Due to Alcoholism and Malnutrition. In R Joynt, R Griggs (eds), Clinical Neurology. Philadelphia: Lippincott–Raven, 1996.

Chapter 52
Vasculitis and Connective Tissue Diseases

Patricia M. Moore

Chapter Plan

Background

The vasculitides and the connective tissue diseases (CTDs) are immune-mediated disorders
with pleomorphic and occasionally frequent neurologic abnormalities. Early manifestations may
be solely neurologic or, at times, the entire disease is confined to the nervous system. Therefore,
the neurologist should be acquainted with the
clinical and diagnostic features. Much of the nervous system injury in autoimmune diseases arises
through the vasculature. Immune-mediated cerebrovascular disease includes a range of disorders
sharing a central feature of tissue ischemia. Situ-

ated between the immune system and the tissue
parenchyma, the vasculature actively participates
in the physiologic processes of inflammation and
is vulnerable to a variety of pathologic consequences of immune injury. Because reciprocal
interactions between leukocytes and cells in the
vascular wall are critical to numerous normal
functions, distinguishing between a healthy host
response to injury and a pathologic process
requires thoughtful and, often, repeated evaluations. These diseases challenge the researcher and
clinician. This challenge has been met with leaps
in our understanding of cell signals, adhesion
molecules, and cytokines as well the genetic
influences on immune regulation. Unfortunately,
we can only glimpse an era of rational pharmacotherapy. Our standard therapies, the judicious
use of glucocorticoids and immunosuppressants,
although often effective and life prolonging, occasionally produce unacceptable complications or
exacerbate an associated immunodeficiency or
vasculopathy. With continued study and careful
diagnosis, the outlook for improved management
appears promising.

Physiology and Pathophysiology of Immune-Mediated Vascular Processes

Dynamic interactions between endothelial cells,
leukocytes, and platelets contribute to numerous
physiologically important mechanisms. The vascu-

Table 52-1. Processes Implicated in Autoimmune Vascular Diseases

Vasculitis
    Leukocyte-endothelial interactions
    Immune complex deposition
    Autoantibody-mediated changes
    Granulomatosis
    Eosinophilia
Immune-mediated vasculopathies
Microvascular disease

lar endothelium, a highly specialized, metabolically active monolayer of cells, contributes to thromboresistance and vascular tone, directs lymphocyte circulation, and regulates many inflammatory and immune interactions. Endothelial cells communicate with cells of the immune system and tissue parenchyma by expressing a variety of cell surface molecules (e.g., adhesion molecules and homing receptors) and secretion of biologically active substances such as cytokines. The constitutive and inducible expression of these molecules varies with the size of the vessel, the organ, and the genetic makeup of the host. In the development of inflammation, a pivotal step involves leukocyte recruitment and attachment in the presence of blood flow. Leukocyte attachment to the endothelium and infiltration of tissue is mediated by a multiple receptor-ligand system belonging to three families of related proteins: the selectins, the integrins, and the immunoglobulin superfamily. The spatial and temporal appearance of these molecules influences the type and duration of the infiltrate.

Endothelial cells present antigens as well as express molecules that activate, or arm, leukocytes. Reciprocally, T cells can activate endothelial cells primarily through the release of interferon gamma. Vascular smooth muscle and perivascular cells may also signal and initiate inflammation, but the current information about these cells is scantier. This T cell–vessel wall interaction is a physiologic process that is a central part of the body's vigilance against infection; it may also result in vascular disease.

Vasculitis is inflammation of the vessel wall with attendant tissue damage. The clinical features and immunopathogenic mechanisms vary with the underlying disorder (Table 52-1). We can identify three immunopathogenic mechanisms of vasculitis: leukocyte-endothelial interactions, immune complex deposition, and, possibly, autoantibodies. Leukocyte-endothelial interaction, the most clearly defined mechanism of physiologic inflammation, remains the prominent mechanism for vasculitis. Much of our information derives from studies of experimental vascular inflammation, usually infectious, and studies of transplant rejection. In the vasculitides, leukocytes remain in, rather than passing through, the vessel wall. When the leukocytes are directed at antigens within the vessel wall or when they fail to migrate across the vessel wall, tissue damage ensues. However, because all of these events occur over millimeters, they are difficult to detect clinically or serologically. Histologic studies are therefore crucial to analysis of many types of vasculitis. Aspects of vascular inflammation depend in large part on the specific cells involved: neutrophils, lymphocytes, macrophages, eosinophils, and platelets. T-lymphocyte–mediated vascular inflammation may be antigen-specific or antigen-nonspecific. Cytokine-initiated and amplified activation of either lymphocytes or endothelial cells provides a mechanism for cellular attachment in the absence of antigen. One pertinent feature of lymphocytes is their egress from the tissue and re-entry into the circulation. These recirculating lymphocytes impart a pivotal feature of immunologic memory, which enables them to respond more quickly to stimuli and renders them refractory to deletion.

Mononuclear cells, which, when activated, become macrophages, also participate in the development and pathogenesis of vasculitis. These important cells, pivotal in both the processing of antigens and in the progression of inflammation from acute to chronic, are rich sources of cytokines that amplify the recruitment of various cells to the site of injury. Notably, they also possess regulatory functions and contribute cytokines that crucially downregulate the inflammatory responses.

Immune-complex deposition is a second inflammatory process resulting in vasculitis. Immune complexes are a normal, transient phenomenon. They are efficiently cleared from the circulation by several mechanisms. When the body's ability to clear complexes is overwhelmed or the complexes are numerous and persistent, antigen-antibody complexes of certain sizes and valence may deposit in the blood vessels. Deposition of circulating immune complexes or in situ formation (with filtered or planted antigen) of immune complexes both occur. The immune complexes, trapped along the basement membrane, activate complement components. Complement-derived chemotactic factors (C3a, C5a, C567) cause accumulation of the polymorphonuclear neutrophils (PMNs). The PMNs release lysosomal enzymes such as collagenase and elastase that injure the vessel wall. Thrombosis, occlusion, and hemorrhage ensue. Lesions usually heal with prominent scarring. Antigens identified in immune complexes include both heterologous (microbial antigens, sulfonamides) and autoantigens (nuclear antigens and rheumatoid factor). Immune complex–mediated vasculitides, such as hypersensitivity vasculitis (HSV) and, probably, polyarteritis nodosa (PAN), are characterized histologically by mixed neutrophil and mononuclear cell infiltrates with prominent necrosis and evidence of immunoglobulin, complement, and fibrin deposition.

Antibodies alone do not usually cause vascular inflammation. In Kawasaki's disease, anti-endothelial antibodies, not usually pathogenic, are cytotoxic when the high levels of circulating interleukins induce neoantigens on endothelial cells. Another large group of antibodies, antiphospholipid antibodies, bind, at least in vitro, to endothelial cells and theoretically could result in vascular inflammation. Finally, another group of antibodies, antineutrophil cytoplasmic antibodies (ANCAs), associate strongly with a subgroup of vasculitis. ANCAs are typically described by their two histologic patterns, cANCAs and pANCAs, which correlate with the autoantigens proteinase 3 and myeloperoxidase, respectively. cANCAs are at least a marker for Wegener's granulomatosis and microscopic polyarteritis and may participate in the pathogenesis of disease. In vitro, binding of ANCAs to neutrophils or monocytes stimulates a respiratory burst that generates toxic oxygen metabolites and secretes proinflammatory mediators. The neutrophils then degranulate, releasing lytic enzymes that injure the endothelium. ANCAs associated vasculitides are characterized histologically by a neutrophil-rich inflammatory infiltrate.

The common denominator of these immunopathogenic mechanisms is the accrual of cells in the vessel wall with obstruction of the lumen. Tissue ischemia and clinical features may occur acutely, during the active inflammation, or later, when marginally patent, scarred vessels are further compromised by other forms of vascular injury.

Immune-Mediated Degenerative Disease

Not all immune interactions with the vessel wall result in flagrant, histologically demonstrable inflammation. More subtle but equally damaging to the blood vessel wall are the effects of chronic inflammation. The pathophysiologic mechanisms in humans remain undefined. In one animal model, chronic but low levels of circulating immune complexes in a genetically susceptible host result in mural degeneration of medium-sized arteries. In other models of inflammation, serum amyloid A protein and acute phase reactants associated with high-density lipoproteins displace apoprotein A. The diminished capacity to shuttle free fatty acids across the wall results in their deposition in the vessel wall. Concurrent features such as hypertension or corticosteroid therapy may exacerbate this process, resulting in early atherosclerotic disease.

Clinically, the most frequently recognized immune-associated vasculopathies of the nervous system appear in CTDs, particularly systemic lupus erythematosus (SLE). Whether this is related to chronic inflammation, antibodies reactive with the blood vessel wall, or inappropriate activation of adhesion molecules is not known. Histologic evidence of endothelial proliferation, medial hyperplasia of small vessels in the central nervous system (CNS), occurs frequently but inflammation is scanty. The absence of inflammation in the vessel reflects both the chronicity of the circulating immune complexes and immunoglobulins and the relative refractoriness of the CNS vasculature to incite and perpetuate inflammation. Furthermore, studies of the coronary vascular system in autoimmune mice of varying genetic backgrounds provide clues to the mechanism. The consequent histologic features of circulating immune complex deposition depend on the titer and chronicity of the circulating complexes as well as genetic features of the host. Predisposed animals with low levels of immune complexes developed a degenerative process without a cellular infiltrate.

Antiphospholipid antibodies associated or unassociated with clinical SLE have been linked to thrombotic vascular occlusions. This family of antibodies shares reactivity with negatively charged phosphodiester moieties. Potential targets of antiphospholipid antibodies are endothelial cells, prostacyclin, protein C, protein C-S complex, and platelets. Both acute effects on coagulation and chronic effects on the vessel wall are plausible. Whether or not these antibodies are pathogenic remains controversial and a direct pathogenic role of antiphospholipid antibodies in stroke is not established.

Microvascular disease is an important but not easily defined component of autoimmune neurologic disorders. The microvasculature, critically located at the junction of the vascular, coagulation, and immune systems, prominently influences blood flow in response to tissue needs. Thrombotic thrombocytopenic purpura illustrates the clinical and histologic features of a microvascular disorder. It remains likely that there are more primary and secondary microvascular abnormalities than we currently detect clinically. Studies in experimental models of stroke reveal that microvessels mediate many of the postischemia perfusion injuries. Other processes such as hypertension and diabetes contribute to microvascular-initiated tissue ischemia. The immunologic relevance of these interactions exceeds that of autoimmune disease alone as the expression of cell surface molecules on lymphocytes, and endothelial cells in response to trauma and ischemia is the subject of immunomodulatory therapies.

Several events intimately connected with but temporally dispersed from leukocyte recruitment contribute to tissue injury. Increased coagulation and excessive vasomotor reactivity are components of vasculitis. The resting endothelium provides a nonthrombogenic, anticoagulant surface. Additional endothelial antiplatelet and fibrinolytic properties contribute to the maintenance of thromboresistance. During inflammation, the balance changes and the endothelial surface exerts a net procoagulant effect. Interleukin 1 (IL-1) and tumor necrosis factor alpha (TNF-α) activation of the endothelium stimulates the intrinsic and extrinsic coagulation pathways and also reduces its fibrinolytic activity. Furthermore, tissue factor, the principal procoagulant of human brain, is increased during inflammation. Both thrombomodulin and tissue plasminogen activator are decreased. This confluence of procoagulant effects serves a physiologic function. Reduction of blood flow through the inflamed vasculature reduces the cascade that recruits additional cells to the area. Nonetheless, excessive coagulation perpetuates tissue damage from ischemia.

Vascular tone directly affects blood flow. Intrinsic modulation of vascular tone depends in part on elaboration of both vasorelaxants and vasoconstrictors. Endothelins, which are powerful vasoconstrictors, and nitric oxide, which is a potent vasodilator, are part of a balanced system that carefully regulates blood flow in the brain and other organs. Endothelins can provoke a long-lasting vasoconstriction in cerebral vessels of all sizes, including the microcirculation. Potential sources for this vasoconstrictor within the brain are numerous. Nitric oxide, a free radical with high lipid solubility and an extremely short half-life of only a few seconds, is also produced widely within the brain by endothelial cells, astrocytes, and neurons. In inflammation, cytokine- (particularly IL-1) associated release of endothelin induces an overriding vasoconstriction. The functional effect, to reduce flow through the injured vessels, is likely an appropriate acute physiologic response. However, persistent endothelin release also stimulates vascular smooth muscle proliferation. Excessive or persistent vasoconstriction may thus add to ischemic tissue injury.

Other Nonvascular, Immune Mechanisms in Connective Tissue Diseases

The CTDs share a common feature of inflammatory or immune-mediated changes in the joints, muscles, serosal surfaces, and blood vessels. Neurovascular features in the CTD are more likely to result from the immune-mediated degenerative processes or microvascular disease than overt inflammation. Hematologic abnormalities and coagulopathies also contribute to tissue ischemia. However, vascular abnormalities and tissue ischemia are by no means the only pathologic processes in CTD. Other immune effector mechanisms cause neurologic abnormalities; among these are the effects autoantibodies, cytokines, and neuroendocrine molecules have on brain cells.

Autoantibodies to neuronal and non-neuronal targets correlate with clinical features in neuropsychiatric SLE, although there is as yet no definitive evidence for a pathogenic antibody. In other areas of neuroscience, autoantibodies are increasingly recognized for their potential importance in diseases such as paraneoplastic syndromes, Rasmussen's encephalitis, Eaton-Lambert syndrome, myotonic dystrophy, and, possibly, some human peripheral neuropathies.

Cytokines are prominent in the tissue reactions of the CTDs and may contribute to neurologic or psychiatric features of disease. The action of systemic cytokines on the brain is clearly evident in sepsis. Here, IL-1 by its effect on the hypothalamus (inducing corticotropin-releasing hormone and arginine vasopressin) and pituitary (inducing corticotropin) mediates fever, sickness behavior (leading to rest and quiet), and increased production of cortisol from the adrenals. The elevated steroids serve to dampen or limit the underlying inflammation but also directly affect the structure and function of brain cells such as those in the hippocampus. Cytokines, which are produced intracranially in response to systemic stressors or to local processes, also elicit the cascade described above. In addition, they exert autocrine/paracrine effects on cells of the vascular wall, neurons, and glia.

Clinical Presentations of the Vasculitides and Connective Tissue Diseases

Conspicuous among the disorders affecting blood vessels are the vasculitides, which share a central feature of inflammation of the blood vessel wall with attendant tissue damage. Many varieties of vasculitis exist (Table 52-2). Classification of the vasculitides is based on the distribution of clinical features, histopathologic abnormalities, and information about underlying causes or associated diseases. Clinically, preferential involvement of certain organs renders many of the diseases distinctive. Histologic features, including the type and size of vessel, the character of the inflammatory infiltrate, and the presence of necrosis, aneurysm formation, or cicatrization in the vessel wall, contribute information that is useful for diagnosis.

A great variety of clinical symptoms and signs occur in the vasculitides and CTDs, reflecting the

Table 52-2. Classification of the Vasculitides

Idiopathic
    Hypersensitivity vasculitis
    Polyarteritis nodosa
    Churg-Strauss angiitis
    Wegener's granulomatosis
    Henoch-Schönlein purpura
    Temporal arteritis
    Takayasu's arteritis
    Isolated angiitis of the central nervous system
    Behçet's disease
Secondary
    Vasculitis secondary to infection
    Vasculitis secondary to drugs
    Kawasaki's disease
    Vasculitis secondary to malignancy
Associated conditions
    Radiation-associated vasculitis
    Vasculitis associated with connective tissue diseases
    Vasculitis associated with sarcoid
    Vasculitis associated with cryoglobulinemia

numerous mechanisms of tissue injury, the scattered pathologic loci, and the numerous potential complications of therapy. Nonetheless, particular patterns of clinical features or laboratory tests often suggest a specific diagnosis. Examples of this are a triad of headache, visual abnormalities, and jaw claudication in temporal arteritis; hematuria/proteinuria, hypertension, and mononeuropathies multiplex in PAN; and behavioral changes, encephalopathy, arthralgias, and skin lesions in SLE. Firm diagnosis in any of the diseases discussed below requires, in addition to clinical features, histologic data, laboratory studies, and periodic reevaluation.

Idiopathic Vasculitides

PAN, a systemic necrotizing vasculitis, affects medium-sized muscular arteries throughout the body, with the notable exceptions of the spleen and lungs. Systemic symptoms of fever, malaise, and weight loss often herald the disease. More than one-half of patients have either arthralgias or an erythematosus, purpuric, or vasculitic rash. Renal involvement occurs in more than 70% of patients, although an abnormal urinary sediment is more frequent than uremia. Hypertension develops in at least one-half of patients. Histologic characteristics are a segmental, transmural vascular inflammation, with a mixture of lymphomononuclear cells and variable numbers of neutrophils and eosinophils. Fibrinoid necrosis is typical but not diagnostic. Infiltration is followed by intimal proliferation and thrombosis. Strikingly, active necrotizing lesions and proliferative fibrotic healing lesions coexist in close proximity. The lesions have a predilection for vessel bifurcations.

Neurologic abnormalities feature prominently in the morbidity and mortality of the disease. Peripheral neuropathies, often the presenting manifestation of the disease, occur in 50–60% of patients. Classic mononeuritis multiplex and polyneuropathies predominate. A striking ascending sensorimotor quadriparesis occurs resulting from infarction of watershed blood vessels supplying nerves in the mid-arm and mid-thigh. Plexopathies and radiculopathies develop infrequently, and attributable vasculitis only in patients with other known manifestations of disease. Asymptomatic cutaneous neuropathies may be evident on thorough sensory examination. Sural nerve biopsy specimens of carefully selected patients reveal histologic evidence of vascular inflammation in the vasa nervorum with asymmetric involvement between or within fascicles.

CNS abnormalities develop in 40% of patients with PAN, including encephalopathy, focal and multifocal lesions of the brain and spinal cord, subarachnoid hemorrhage, seizures, strokes, and cranial neuropathies. These usually occur later in the course of disease than the peripheral neuropathies. Hypertension sometimes accompanies or follows the encephalopathy, and the additional marginal ischemia may further compromise neurologic function. Visual symptoms are numerous, resulting from inflammation of the choroidal, retinal, or brain parenchymal arteries or the arteries supplying cranial nerves II, III, IV, or VI.

The triad that alerts a physician to a diagnosis of PAN is systemic inflammation, angiographic evidence of enteric vascular diseases, and histologic evidence of vasculitis, often in a peripheral nerve. Diagnosis of PAN may be difficult in the early stages because of the heterogeneity of the disease and the need for invasive tests for accurate diagnosis. Laboratory evidence of systemic inflammation is often associated with the presence of anemia, leukocytosis, thrombocytosis, C reactive proteins, and an elevated sedimentation rate. Anti-nuclear antibodies, present in 20% of patients, are characteristically of low titer and a nonspecific pattern. Although its role in the pathogenesis of PAN is not clear, approximately 20–30% of patients have a hepatitis B antigenemia. ANCAs, particularly to myeloperoxidase, are associated with microscopic polyarteritis, possibly aiding diagnosis. Abnormalities in the urine sediment are common, even if the blood urea nitrogen and creatinine levels are normal. Angiography is an appropriate and rewarding diagnostic tool. Aneurysms, particularly in the hepatic and renal vasculature, occur in 65% of patients. Segmental narrowings of vessels, variations in caliber, and pruning of the vascular tree all occur.

Corticosteroids undoubtedly suppress the inflammation in PAN but most investigators think cyclophosphamide is also necessary to induce a long-term remission. Both oral and intravenous regimens are used. In cases of refractory systemic vasculitis, plasmapheresis, intravenous immunoglobulin, and monoclonal antibody (against a T-cell surface molecule) have been tried.

Churg-Strauss syndrome (CSS), characterized by fever, asthma, eosinophilia, and systemic vasculitis, appears as a vasculitis of small to medium-sized vessels considered clinically distinct from PAN. Pulmonary involvement is typical in CSS and rare in PAN. Similarly, the eosinophilia that is characteristic in CSS is not a feature of PAN. Cutaneous manifestations include palpable purpura, erythema, and subcutaneous nodules.

Histologically, medium and small vessels are affected. The two diagnostically essential lesions are angiitis and extravascular necrotizing granulomas, usually with eosinophilic infiltrates. In any single biopsy specimen, however, the changes may appear very similar to those of PAN.

Neurologic abnormalities, including encephalopathy occurring earlier in the course of the disease than in PAN, probably reflect the smaller size of the affected vessels. The range of reported changes includes memory loss, confusion, seizures, subarachnoid hemorrhage, and chorea as well as visual abnormalities. Peripheral neuropathies occur in 50–75% of patients, usually presenting as mononeuropathy multiplex, but polyneuropathies also occur.

Laboratory features reflect general systemic inflammation. Although the sedimentation rate is elevated and ANA may be present in low titers, no autoantibodies are diagnostic of the disease. ANCAs are not reliably present. Thus, the clinical features again provide important information for diagnosis. Characteristically, the triad of asthma, eosinophilia, and vasculitis in two extrapulmonary organs defines the disease. Many patients with CSS respond satisfactorily to therapy with corticosteroids alone; in severe or refractory disease cyclophosphamide is effective.

HSV, the most frequently encountered of all the vasculitides, is a heterogeneous group of clinical syndromes characterized by inflammation of small vessels, typically venules. Ubiquitous involvement of the skin unifies this group of diseases. Although in many instances the vessel inflammation can be identified as a response to a drug, foreign protein, or microbe, endogenous antigens, such as tumor antigens or serum proteins, can also serve as the sensitizing agent. Clinically, lesions appear as purpura or urticaria. Histologically, the presence of fragmentation and phagocytosis of nuclear debris (leukocytoclasia) is characteristic. Damage to the vessel wall appears to result from deposition of immune complexes with activation of the complement cascade.

Henoch-Schönlein purpura, a predominantly childhood illness, is characterized by vasculitis of the skin as well as the joints, gastrointestinal tract, and kidneys. Evidence of immunoglobulin A (IgA) and C3 in the walls of the arterioles and glomeruli and circulating immune complexes containing IgA support the diagnosis.

Neurologic abnormalities are infrequent. In serum sickness, encephalopathies, seizures, and brachial plexopathies occur although the incidence is unknown. In other HSVs, subarachnoid hemorrhage or seizures are occasionally reported. In most cases of cutaneous venulitis, the nervous system is not affected. To the neurologist and internist, the prominent clinical dilemma in the diagnosis and therapy of HSV is whether the vasculitis will remain restricted to the skin or is the presenting manifestation of systemic vasculitis such as PAN, Churg-Strauss syndrome, or Wegener's granulomatosis. For this reason, evaluation of patients with HSV includes analysis of renal function, immunoglobulins, and autoantibodies that may suggest alternate diseases. Thus, the main goal is to identify any inciting causes, remove the cause, and observe the clinical course. The disease resolves spontaneously in most patients. Evidence of systemic disease (renal, cardiac, gastrointestinal, or neurologic) warrants glucocorticoid or immunosuppressive therapy.

Wegener's granulomatosis is characterized by a necrotizing, granulomatous vasculitis of the upper and lower respiratory tract; glomerulonephritis; and small vessel vasculitis. Patients often present with otitis, epistaxis, rhinorrhea, or sinusitis and may develop a "saddle nose," destruction of the cartilaginous nasal septal support of the bridge of the nose. Systemic symptoms such as fever, malaise, weight loss, and anorexia are almost invariably present. Pulmonary involvement, if not among the presenting symptoms, is almost invariably present on chest films. Renal abnormalities are manifold, varying from mild, abnormal urinary sediment to uremia requiring dialysis.

Neurologic abnormalities, occasionally presenting features of the disease, result from either contiguous extension of the sinus granulomas or a small vessel vasculitis. Cranial neuropathies, reflecting erosion from contiguous granulomas, are prominent and include visual loss, hearing loss, proptosis, ophthalmoplegias, and facial and trigeminal neuropathies. It may be difficult to distinguish an optic neuropathy resulting from granuloma from one secondary to a small vessel vasculitis clinically, but computed tomographic (CT) and magnetic resonance imaging (MRI) scans have greatly aided diagnosis and therapy. The small vessel vasculitis in Wegener's granulomatosis largely affects the peripheral nervous system, resulting in both mononeuropathy multiplex and polyneuropathies, but it may also affect the CNS parenchyma.

Recent data reveal that the histologic features of Wegener's granulomatosis are extremely pleomorphic. Despite early descriptions, neither the extravascular destructive granuloma nor the several types of vasculitis (microvasculitis with prominent infiltration of polymorphonuclear cells, granulomatous vasculitis, and medium vessel vasculitis with fibrinoid necrosis) render the disease specific pathologically. Accurate diagnosis rests with clinical, histologic, and laboratory information. In active disease, the sedimentation rate is invariably elevated, and leukocytosis and thrombocytosis are usually present. The urinary sediment reveals hematuria, sterile pyuria, and red blood cell casts with proteinuria. Autoantibodies, specifically cANCA, appear sufficiently often that they are often considered markers of the disease, although their role in pathogenesis remains uncertain. Chest radiography is useful diagnostically, as is brain MRI.

Cyclophosphamide therapy dramatically reduces the mortality of Wegener's granulomatosis, and a combination of cyclophosphamide and corticosteroid induces remission in a majority of patients. The antimicrobial trimethoprim-sulfamethoxazole appears to be an effective adjunct therapy.

Isolated angiitis of the CNS (IAC) is a recurrent inflammatory disease of the small- and medium-sized blood vessels of the brain and spinal cord. Symptoms and signs are restricted to the nervous system and typically include headaches, encephalopathies, strokes, cranial neuropathies, and myelopathies. Notably, symptoms or laboratory evidence of systemic inflammation are absent. This disease illustrates that in a persistent vascular inflammatory disease the sedimentation rate and levels of ANA, rheumatoid factor, and immune complexes may all be normal (or negative). Neurodiagnostic studies reflect the degree and locations of parenchymal abnormalities. Electroencephalograms and CT scans may appear abnormal but do not specifically suggest or exclude the diagnosis. Similarly, MRI scans often, but not invariably, reveal evidence of parenchymal lesions consistent with ischemic damage. Although MR angiography is potentially useful, much of the disease occurs beyond its current resolution. Studies that yield the most complete information on abnormalities in the cerebral vasculature are angiography and biopsy. Angiography is the gold standard of vasculitis to date, although the results may be normal in up to 10–15% of patients with an exclusively small vessel vasculitis. Features that suggest the diagnosis of vasculitis are recurrent segmental narrowing, abrupt termination of blood vessels, and neovascularization. It is a notable caution that there are no angiographic features that are specific for vasculitis, nor do they distinguish between primary and secondary vasculitides. Biopsy of tissue is important to determine vascular inflammation and to exclude alternate diagnoses such as neoplasia and infection, which are the two prominent causes of similar clinical abnormalities. Clinical situations suggestive of IAC are new onset of headaches, encephalopathy, and multifocal signs. Evidence of recurrent or persistent disease should be confirmed

to distinguish the disease from a self-limited vasculopathy. In our experience, cyclophosphamide combined with low-dose prednisone is the most effective treatment.

Vasculitis restricted to the peripheral nervous system occurs and in some series comprises one-third of all patients with a vasculitic neuropathy. A major difficulty in establishing this as a distinct clinical diagnosis is that vasculitis of the peripheral nerve is often the presenting feature of systemic vasculitis. Because the distribution and histologic features of isolated vasculitis of the peripheral nervous system are identical to that of PAN, it is difficult to determine whether patients, if untreated, would go on to develop systemic disease. Until more information on etiology or pathogenic mechanisms in the peripheral nervous system vasculature is available, careful and repeated studies of these patients, including funduscopic examination; fresh urinalysis for occult blood and protein, creatinine clearances; and evidence of systemic inflammation, are prudent.

Temporal arteritis is a systemic panarteritis that can affect any medium- or large-sized artery, although symptoms below the neck are distinctly unusual. The term *giant cell arteritis* is also used but causes confusion because the term is also applied to Takayasu's arteritis. Temporal arteritis occurs almost invariably in people older than age 50 years; there is a predominance among people of northern European ancestry. A distinctive overlap between temporal arteritis and the systemic inflammatory disease polymyalgia rheumatica exists. Because the two diseases require different dosages of corticosteroids for effective therapy, careful recognition of temporal arteritis remains important. Prominent early symptoms include new onset headache or jaw claudication. Visual abnormalities including visual loss and ophthalmoplegias occur, tragically often, from infarction of branches of the extracranial circulation.

Temporal artery biopsy usually reveals the granulomatous inflammation classically found in the region of the media, but it can extend from the intima to the adventitia. The sensitivity of biopsy varies from 65% to 97%. The fairly nonspecific cellular infiltrate consists of lymphocytes, histiocytes, monocytes, giant cells, and occasional eosinophils. Among the common reasons for negative findings at biopsy are an inadequate specimen and inadequate examination of the specimen obtained. The pathophysiology of temporal arteritis is unclear; the pathologic distribution draws attention to the elastic lamina as an antigenic target. Histologically, the posterior circulation also reveals evidence of vascular inflammation, and this appears to explain the symptoms and signs referable to the posterior fossa. Encephalopathies develop in patients with temporal arteritis but the histologic associations in this older population are not yet clear.

Diagnosis rests with a high index of suspicion of new onset headaches or visual changes in persons older than age 50 years. An elevated sedimentation rate is almost invariable. Elevated values on liver function studies are frequently encountered. Temporal artery angiography has not been as helpful as anticipated, but arteriography in other regions of the body is strongly recommended if symptoms suggest a systemic vasculitis.

Corticosteroids are the mainstay of therapy for symptoms and prevention of serious complications. Prednisone in a single oral dose of 40–60 mg per day usually elicits a prompt clinical response. After the patient is asymptomatic and the sedimentation rate has become normal, prednisone is slowly (over months) tapered to 20 mg per day and the patient monitored for recurrent symptoms. Most authors caution that therapy should be continued for at least 1 year to minimize potentially devastating relapses. After therapy has been tapered, the patient should be followed carefully for at least another year for early recurrence of symptoms.

Takayasu's arteritis is a large vessel arteritis affecting the aortic arch and its branches by a process that is initially inflammatory and later occlusive. Although the disease was first described in young Asian women, it is now recognized worldwide. Takayasu's arteritis is often called the *pulseless disease*, and absence of at least one arterial pulse is identified in 98% of patients. Bruits are often heard. Typically, Takayasu's arteritis is recognized by signs of decreased blood flow to the limbs and viscera. Most of the neurologic abnormalities occur in the later vaso-occlusive stage of the illness. Hypertension exacerbates the vascular disease. Neurologically, strokes, transient ischemic attacks, and syncope are prominent.

Behçet's disease, initially characterized by the triad of relapsing ocular lesions and recurrent oral and genital ulcers, is in fact a systemic disease.

Many organs exhibit a small vessel vasculitis. Thrombophlebitis, arthritis, and erythema nodosum occur frequently. The course is usually frustrating but benign, unless the nervous system is involved. Neurologic involvement increases the morbidity of the disease to a variable degree. Various series report neurologic abnormalities including meningoencephalitis, brain stem abnormalities, and focal CNS changes in 10–50% of patients. The diagnosis is strongly clinical. Various abnormalities on neuroradiographic studies (MRI and CT scans) are nonspecific. Although cerebrospinal fluid analysis frequently reveals inflammation, it has been a reliable monitor of efficacy of therapy. The first line of therapy for Behçet's disease is currently prednisone or chlorambucil. In refractory cases, azathioprine, cyclophosphamide, and cyclosporin B have been used. Both colchicine and dapsone are reportedly successful in alleviating cutaneous lesions.

Secondary Vasculitides

Vasculitis of the nervous systems secondary to an identifiable cause is both frequent and clinically important. The number of patients with a secondary CNS vasculitis far exceeds those with a primary idiopathic vasculitis. A high index of suspicion enables a clinician to institute therapy promptly for a vasculitis secondary to infection, neoplasia, or a toxin.

Infectious agents capable of inducing a prominent vascular inflammation are numerous and include bacteria, fungi, viruses, and protozoa. Mechanisms of infection-mediated inflammation include toxic disruption of the endothelium, immune-mediated cytolysis of infected endothelium, and immune complex– (antibody-infectious organism) mediated inflammation. The prolific inflammation induced by bacteria includes conspicuous accumulation of cells in the vessel wall with associated thrombosis and hemorrhage. This results in the frequent strokes that are part of acute bacterial meningitis and responsible for much of the neurologic sequelae. Other infectious agents causing vasculitis are more indolent and difficult to detect. *Aspergillus, Cryptococcus, Coccidioides immitis, Histoplasma capsulatum,* and *Mucor,* in particular, all infiltrate cerebral vessels. Histologically, inflammation and necrosis of the cerebral blood vessel

Table 52-3. Connective Tissue Diseases

Systemic lupus erythematosus
Sjögren's disease
Polymyositis/dermatomyositis
Rheumatoid arthritis
Progressive systemic sclerosis

wall certainly appear with viruses such as herpes simplex, herpes zoster, cytomegalovirus, and, human immunodeficiency virus. However, viruses such as herpes zoster may also cause vaso-occlusive disease without inflammatory changes.

Toxins are another distinct cause of vasculitis. CNS vasculitis is, however, well reported after a variety of illicit drugs, notably those with a prominent sympathomimetic effect, such as amphetamines. Cocaine and crack cocaine do cause stroke and have occasionally been associated with a vasculitis. Injury or trauma to blood vessels induces a vasocentric inflammatory response.

Neoplasias exert several effects on the blood vessels. Both direct encasement of the vessel by tumor cells and a paraneoplastic inflammation occur. The mechanism of paraneoplastic vasculitis is unknown, but current studies suggest that overexpression of certain cytokines may play a role. Hodgkin's disease is associated with a singular vasculitis that resolves with the treatment of the underlying disease. Other lymphomas, including lymphomatoid granulomatosis and angioendotheliosis, are vasocentric and may present with central or peripheral nervous system abnormalities, illustrating the importance of histologic examination in accurate diagnosis and therapy.

Connective Tissue Diseases

CTDs are a group of multisystem diseases characterized by a central feature of inflammation of joints, muscles, blood vessels, serosal membranes, and skin (Table 52-3). Although vascular inflammation may be a component of these diseases, they are clinically distinct from the vasculitides. The genetic predisposition to these disorders is apparent in the relatives of patients who frequently have in vitro evidence of immunoregulatory abnormalities if not a form of clinical disease. Several of these

diseases spontaneously occur in animals. Neurologic abnormalities, prominent in some disorders, occasionally herald the disease.

SLE is an autoimmune disease characterized by circulating autoantibodies and immune complexes. Features that define SLE are particular patterns of autoantibodies (e.g., those to dsDNA or ribosomal proteins) and evidence of organ system damage, usually through immune complex deposition (e.g., skin, kidneys) or direct autoantibody effects (e.g., anemia, thrombocytopenia). Other nondefining aspects of disease such as fever, arthralgias, and malaise appear to be mediated by cytokines and indicate the presence of systemic inflammation. The epidemiology of SLE is complex, reflecting the multiple genetic, hormonal, and environmental factors that contribute to the manifestation of the disease.

Neuropsychiatric SLE (NP-SLE) refers to the spectrum of neurologic, psychiatric, and behavioral abnormalities occurring in patients with SLE. These clinical disturbances are particularly frustrating because we currently understand little of the pathogenic mechanisms and have few specific tools for diagnosis. Traditionally, identifiable secondary causes of disease such as infections, metabolic abnormalities, and toxins including side effects of medications (which may account for the clinical features of up to one-half of the SLE patients seen in neurologic consultation) are carefully excluded.

Many of the major neurologic abnormalities are readily definable clinically and supported by neurodiagnostic studies. These include the frequently encountered seizures, encephalopathies, strokes, cranial neuropathies, and ataxias as well as the less frequently encountered myelopathy, peripheral neuropathies, and myasthenia gravis. Other features may be more difficult to diagnose, including abnormalities of memory, judgment, and changes in personality. Similarly, psychiatric abnormalities may be clinically obvious, such as major mood disorders with or without coexisting neurologic abnormalities. However, both neurologic and psychiatric abnormalities also appear in more subtle forms. Some investigators attribute these abnormalities to an exacerbation of a preexisting psychiatric disease or exaggeration of an underlying personality trait rather than distinct changes. Furthermore, the complex features of a chronic illness and the strength of social supports do influence behavior.

Seizures, either focal or generalized, occur in many patients with SLE (10–20%) and may be the presenting manifestation of disease in 5%. Typically these are easily controlled with anticonvulsants. Encephalopathies, acute or subacute abnormalities of cognition, attention, or level of arousal sometimes associated with agitated behavior, are frequent but so varied in presentation they often defy classification. Chronic multidomain changes in cognition, sometimes called *dementias*, do occur in SLE, but the contributing factors and incidence remain undefined. Abnormalities in frontal-subcortical circuits may be evident by altered executive functions; disinhibition, distractibility, or apathy may also appear in patients with SLE. There is debate over the appropriate nomenclature for these clinical episodes.

Notably for the clinician, some develop from acute immunologic mechanisms and are treatable; others are the results of chronic injury, and therapy may produce more complications than benefits. Corticosteroids because of their adverse effects on cognition and behavior appear to have more adverse than beneficial effects in CNS disease. Plasmapheresis has been used for short-term improvements. Several series report use of cyclophosphamide for CNS disease. Effective therapies will likely evolve as our understanding of NP-SLE progresses.

Sjögren's syndrome is a chronic autoimmune inflammatory disease characterized by diminished lacrimal and salivary secretion resulting in keratoconjunctivitis sicca and xerostomia. It is usually a relatively benign disease manifested primarily by exocrine gland impairment as a result of destructive mononuclear infiltrates of the lacrimal and salivary glands. In a number of patients, however, visceral involvement occurs and a wide spectrum of extraglandular manifestations may occur as a result of lymphoid infiltration of lung, kidney, skin, thyroid gland, stomach, liver, and muscle. There exists a strong association between Sjögren's syndrome and anti-Ro (SSA) antibodies, although anti-La antibodies also occur. The role of these autoantibodies in disease pathogenesis is uncertain. Diagnosis of Sjögren's syndrome rests on clinical features, lip biopsy demonstrating lymphocyte infiltration, and, usually, presence of circulatory autoantibodies.

Neurologic manifestations occur in up to one-half of patients, according to some reports. Of the various neurologic abnormalities, neuropathies are most frequent and distinctive. Cranial neuropathies, particularly trigeminal neuropathy, quite commonly develop in up to 40% of patients. Although the histologic features are not defined in one series of nerve biopsies, 8 of 11 patients had findings consistent or highly suggestive of vasculitis; other patients had a perivascular inflammatory response. An alternative, distinctive neuropathy in Sjögren's syndrome is not vasculitis but a dorsal root ganglionitis. These patients present with a sensory neuropathy and ataxia usually associated with autonomic insufficiency.

Rheumatoid arthritis consists of progressive erosive inflammation of the joints. Three phases appear: (1) activation of a cellular immune response in the genetically susceptible host; (2) ensuing proliferation of polyclonal B cells results in proliferative synovitis; and (3) cytokine-driven proliferation of synovial cells that invade and destroy articular cartilage. Because the damage to the joints is widespread, secondary injury to the nervous system occurs. Cervical spine abnormalities occur in up to 25% of patients. Potentially devastating is the dissolution of the transverse ligament, allowing forward displacement of the skull and atlas. Physicians must be vigilant in detecting this condition to prevent a high cervical myelopathy in these patients. Peripheral neuropathies develop from compression or ischemia. Compression from swollen tissue and subcutaneous nodules typically results in chronic progressive mononeuropathies. Vascular occlusion, both from vasculitis and obliterative vasculopathy, also causes neuropathies that are usually more acute in onset than the compressive neuropathies. CNS abnormalities are less common and result from subcutaneous nodules or the systemic vasculitis that complicates a small percentage of patients with rheumatoid arthritis.

Progressive systemic sclerosis scleroderma involves the cardinal features of (1) proliferative intimal arterial lesions, (2) obliterative microvascular defects, and (3) atrophy and fibrosis of the involved organs. Largely a cell-mediated (T lymphocytes and mast cells) immune process, some distinctive autoantibodies may be markers of the disease. Neurologic abnormalities are unusual; in one large series they occurred in less than 1% of patients. When clinical neurologic disease does occur, it is usually a consequence of accelerated hypertension, uremia, or pulmonary insufficiency.

Table 52-4. Diagnostic Features and Therapy of Vasculatides

Entity	Organs/Systems Typically Affected	Diagnostic Clues	Treatment
HSV	Skin	History of infection, toxin, skin biopsy	Remove antigen
Polyarteritis nodosa	Kidneys, skin, gut, PNS, eyes, CNS	Evidence of systemic inflammation; angiographic evidence of visceral disease; peripheral neuropathy	Corticosteroids, cyclophosphamide/corticosteroids
Serum sickness	Skin, viscera, PNS	History of infection, immune stimulation	Depends on extent of inflammation
Wegener's granulomatosis	Respiratory tract, kidneys, cranial nerves	History of epistaxis, hemoptysis, abnormal chest x-ray films, abnormal urine sediment, biopsy	Cyclophosphamide/prednisone
Isolated angiitis of the CNS	Brain, cranial nerves, brain stem	Exclude systemic inflammation, angiography, leptomeningeal/cortical biopsy	Cyclophosphamide prednisone
Temporal arteritis	Extracranial vessels, eyes	Sedimentation rate, liver function tests, temporal artery biopsy	Prednisone

HSV = hypersensitivity vasculitis; PNS = peripheral nervous system; CNS = central nervous system.

Rarely, a vasculitis complicates scleroderma and this may involve the CNS.

Usefulness of Diagnostic Testing

Few groups of disorders illustrate the importance of careful selection and prudent interpretation of the numerous available laboratory and radiographic studies as the vasculitides and CTDs (Table 52-4).

A first example is the antinuclear antibody (ANA) test. Positive results on ANA testing do not provide a diagnosis of a specific disease; rather, they reflect a chronic inflammatory process. Its utilization as a screening test should reflect this. In selecting among the other commercially available autoantibody tests, the physician should consider first the differential diagnosis of the patient's clinical features, then select serologic tests that would help narrow the diagnostic field. Because there are no serologic diagnostic studies that confirm or exclude vasculitis, this would avoid the erroneous statement, "I have done a vasculitis screen." ANCAs are a partial exception to this. However, the diagnoses of Wegener's granulomatosis and microscopic polyarteritis still reside in the clinical and histologic features. Serologic abnormalities are far more useful in some of the connective tissue disorders, where a pattern of autoantibodies is often inte-

gral to the diagnosis. An example is anti-dsDNA and anti-Sm autoantibodies that are specific for SLE. Anti-SSA and anti-SSB (Ro and La) continue as useful studies, although clinical features and histologic studies are often still required to distinguish between SLE and Sjögren's disease.

Radiographic studies such as MRI and angiography further illustrate the necessity of thoughtful planning of studies. MRI gives vast information about the parenchyma but little about the blood vessels. MR angiography, which identifies some processes affecting the vascular flow, does not currently have the resolution of angiography. Angiography, which does provide valuable but not infallible information about the vasculature, is expensive and invasive. Yet if a decision about health and potentially life-threatening disease appears necessary, it remains appropriate to choose the study that provides the most useful information. Currently, angiography is a gold standard in the diagnosis of vasculitis.

Finally, when and where to get tissue confirmation deserves attention. Diseases that affect the skin, muscles, or peripheral nervous system are easily accessible to biopsy for tissue analysis. Tissue from organs such as the liver, intestines, and lungs, at slightly higher potential morbidity, is useful and appropriate in numerous diseases. The brain is regarded as inaccessible, although the morbidity of the procedure is low and the tissue often provides the means for diagnosis and the initiation of appropriate therapy. A major reason to obtain brain tissue is to exclude underlying processes that may mimic or present as a CNS vasculitis, such as infections and neoplasia. Excluding these processes before initiating corticosteroid or immunosuppressive therapy is critical. Confirmation of the exact disease process is desirable but not always accomplished, given the patchy nature of the vascular inflammation, particularly in early stages of disease.

Therapy

In current nosology, clinical and pathologic features divide the vasculitides into groups. Perhaps the single most important division to the clinician is that of primary (or idiopathic) and secondary vasculitis. Prompt identification of the secondary vasculitides improves the efficacy of therapy. Both clinical and pathologic features help distinguish among the primary vasculitides. The exact diagnosis may be elusive, however, in the early stages of any of the diseases.

Treatment of vasculitis ranges from the simple measures of removing the cause of the chronic inflammation to corticosteroid/cyclophosphamide immunosuppressive therapy to experimental measures in refractory vasculitis. As information on the mechanisms of vascular inflammation increases, more specific and less toxic therapies can be developed. Physicians treating patients with vasculitis need expertise with the spectrum of vasculitides and autoimmune diseases to appreciate overlap syndromes and the potential evolution of a specific diagnosis over time. Experience in the use of immunosuppressant medications is also important because of the wide range of potential and actual side effects. Side effects occur with any of these agents. Most patients do well on the standard regimens. More difficult are those patients who only partially respond to treatment. The physician must determine whether the clinical effects are from persistent inflammation or other causes. Excluding infection should remain a high priority. Ischemia may result not only from the inflammation but also from chronic changes in the vessel wall accompanied by thrombosis or hemorrhage.

Conclusion

Studies of the vasculitides illustrate recent advances and convergence of information in the biology of inflammation, clinical diagnostic studies, and newer therapies. We anticipate that more focused, less toxic treatments will soon result from our studies of immunopathogenesis today.

Suggested Reading

Boumpas DT, Yamada H, Patronas NJ, Scott D, et al. Pulse cyclophosphamide for severe neuropsychiatric lupus. Q J Med 1991;81:975.

Braquet P, Hosford D, Braquet M, Bourgain R, et al. Role of cytokines and platelet-activating factor in microvascular immune injury. Int Arch Allergy Appl Immunol 1989; 88:88.

Conn DL, Tompkins RB, Nichols WL. Glucocorticoids in the management of vasculitis—a double edge sword? J Rheumatol 1988;15:1181.

Engelhardt A, Lorler H, Neundorfer B. Immunohistochemical findings in vasculitic neuropathies. Acta Neurol Scand 1993;87:318.

Giang DW. Central nervous system vasculitis secondary to infections, toxins, and neoplasms. Semin Neurol 1994; 14:313.

Guillevin L, Le Thi Huong D, Godeau P, Jais P, et al. Clinical findings and prognosis of polyarteritis nodosa and Churg-Strauss angiitis: a study in 165 patients. Br J Rheumatol 1988;27:258.

Hanly JG, Walsh NMG, Sangalang V. Brain pathology in systemic lupus erythematosus. J Rheumatol 1992; 19:732.

Hietaharju A, Yli-Kerttula U, Hakkinen V, Frey H. Nervous system manifestations in Sjogren's syndrome. Acta Neurol Scand 1990;81:144.

Hurst RW, Grossman RI. Neuroradiology of central nervous system vasculitis. Semin Neurol 1994;14:320.

Kissel JT, Riethman JL, Omerza J, Rammohan KW, et al. Peripheral nerve vasculitis: immune characterization of the vascular lesions. Ann Neurol 1989;25:291.

Leung DYM, Geha RS, Newburger JW, Burns JC, et al. Two monokines, interleukin 1 and tumor necrosis factor, render cultured vascular endothelial cells susceptible to lysis by antibodies circulating during Kawasaki syndrome. J Exp Med 1986;164:1958.

Luscher TF, Boulanger CM, Yang Z, Noll G, et al. Interactions between endothelium-derived relaxing and contracting factors in health and cardiovascular disease. Circulation 1993;87:36.

Moore PM. Diagnosis and management of isolated angiitis of the central nervous system. Neurology 1989; 39:167.

Moore PM. Neurological manifestation of vasculitis: update on immunopathogenic mechanisms and clinical features. Ann Neurol 1995;37:S131.

Nishino H, Rubino FA, DeRemee RA, Swanson JW, et al. Neurological involvement in Wegener's granulomatosis: an analysis of 324 consecutive patients at the Mayo Clinic. Ann Neurol 1993;33:4.

O'Duffy JD. Behçet's syndrome. N Engl J Med 1990;322:326.

Osborn L. Leukocyte adhesion to endothelium in inflammation. Cell 1990;62:3.

Sehgal M, Swanson J, DeRemee R, Colby T. Neurologic manifestations of Churg-Strauss syndrome. Mayo Clin Proc 1995;70:337.

Walsh TJ, Hier DB, Caplan LR. Aspergillosis of the central nervous system: clinicopathological analysis of 17 patients. Ann Neurol 1985;18:574.

Watts RA, Carruthers DM, Scott DG. Epidemiology of systemic vasculitis: changing incidence or definition? Semin Arthritis Rheum 1995;25:28.

Index

Note: Page numbers followed by *f* indicate figures; page numbers followed by *t* indicate tables.

Angiopathy, cerebral amyloid, 353t
  intracranial hemorrhage due to, 378, 379f
Angiostrongyliasis, 612
Anomia, color, 328, 328t
Anomic aphasia, 304
Anterograde amnesia, 336, 338
Anterolateral system, 310, 312t
Antibiotic(s), ototoxic, for vertigo, 258t
Antibody(ies)
  antineuronal, in paraneoplastic neurologic syndromes, 643, 644t, 645t
  antineutrophil cytoplasmic, in vasculitis, 819
  antiphospholipid, in vasculitis, 819
  anti–tumor necrosis factor, for neuroimmune diseases, 124t
  CNS, detection of, 182–183, 183t, 185f
Anticholinergic(s), for Parkinson's disease, 427
Anticholinesterase agents, for myasthenia gravis, 553
Anticoagulant(s)
  intracranial hemorrhage due to, 379–381, 380f
  for ischemic stroke, 371
Anticonvulsant(s), for idiopathic trigeminal neuralgia, 231–232
Antidepressant(s)
  in inhibition of neurotransmitter uptake, 140, 142f
  intoxication by, 811
  in vascular dementia prevention, 414
Antiemetic drugs, for migraine, 229
Antiepileptic drugs
  effects on pregnant women, 770–771
  for vertigo, 258t
Antigen(s), exogenous, neuroimmune diseases triggered by, 121, 121t
Antihistaminergic(s), for Parkinson's disease, 425t
Anti-inflammatory drugs, nonsteroidal (NSAIDs), for migraine, 229
Antineuronal antibodies, in paraneoplastic neurologic syndromes, 643, 644t, 645t
Antineutrophil cytoplasmic antibodies (ANCAs), in vasculitis, 819
Antiphospholipid antibodies, in vasculitis, 819
Antiretroviral agents, 630, 630t
Anti–tumor necrosis factor antibodies, for neuroimmune diseases, 124t
Anxiety, 346
Apallic syndrome, defined, 222
Aphasia, 299–308
  amnestic, 304
  anatomy of, 306–307, 307f
  anomic, 304
  atypical, 304–305
  Broca's, 301–302
  clinical evaluation of, 299–301, 301f
  color, 328, 328t
  conduction, 303
  crossed, 306
  defined, 299
  fluent, 302–304
  incidence of, 299
  mixed, 305
  motor, transcortical, 302
  nominal, 304

nonfluent, 301–302
  optic, 326
  sensory, transcortical, 303–304
  subcortical white matter lesions and, 305
  supplementary motor area lesions and, 304
  syndromes of, 301–306
  thalamic lesions and, 304–305
  Wernicke's, 303
Aphemia, 300, 302
Apnea, in brain death, 218
APOE ε4, in Alzheimer's disease, 396
Apomorphine, for Parkinson's disease, 425t, 426, 427
Apoplexy, pituitary, 698, 699f
Appearance, in coma evaluation, 212
Apperceptive agnosia, 324
Apraxia(s), 331–335
  conduction, 331–332
  constructional, 334–335
  defined, 331
  diagnostic, 335
  disorders related to, 335
  dressing, 335
  gait, 272–273, 335
  ideational, 332–333
  ideomotor, 331–333
  kinetic, 331–332
  left hemisphere and, 293–294
  limb, 331–333, 332t
  melokinetic, 331–332
  orofacial, 333–334, 334t
  palpatory, 331
Apraxia of speech, 300
Aqueductal stenosis, hydrocephalus secondary to, 793–794
Arachnoid cyst, 791–793
  differential diagnosis of, 793
  evaluation of, 791f, 792f, 793
  patient presentation with, 791–793
  treatment of, 793
Arbovirus(es)
  causes of, 594t
  characteristics of, 596t–597t
  distribution of, 594t
  encephalitis due to, 592t
Archicerebellum, 39
Arenaviruses, encephalitis due to, 592t
Arousal, alterations in, 206, 206t
Arousal disorders, 737–738
Arrestin, source of, 147
Arterial blood supply to brain, 44–45, 44f
Arterial ischemic stroke, in pregnant women, 760–762, 760f–762f
Arteriosclerosis, 351–352
Arteriovenous fistulas, intradural, 477–479, 478t
Arteriovenous malformations (AVMs)
  intracranial hemorrhage due to, 378–379
  MRI of, 384, 384f
  of spinal cord, 477–478, 478t, 479f
Arteritis
  giant cell, 821t, 824, 828t
    headache due to, 232